10-4-74

OXFORD MEDICAL PUBLICATIONS

DISEASES OF THE
NERVOUS SYSTEM

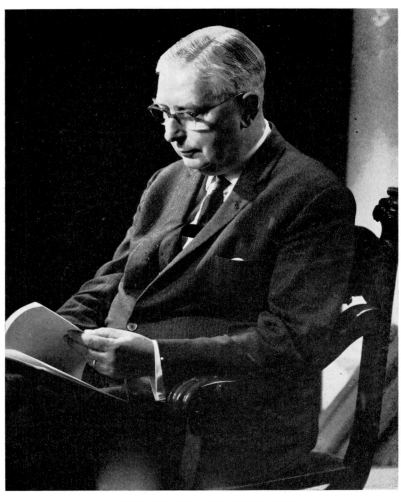

LORD BRAIN OF EYNSHAM
1895–1966

BRAIN'S
DISEASES OF THE
NERVOUS SYSTEM

SEVENTH EDITION

REVISED BY

THE LATE LORD BRAIN

D.M. (OXON.), F.R.C.P. (LONDON), F.R.S.

Formerly Consulting Neurologist to the London Hospital
and Consulting Physician to the
Maida Vale Hospital for Nervous Diseases

AND

JOHN N. WALTON

T.D., M.D. (DURHAM), F.R.C.P. (LONDON)

Professor of Neurology,
University of Newcastle upon Tyne
Neurologist, Regional Neurological Centre,
General Hospital, Newcastle upon Tyne
Physician in Neurology, Royal Victoria Infirmary

LONDON
OXFORD UNIVERSITY PRESS
NEW YORK   TORONTO
1969

Oxford University Press, Ely House, London W. 1

GLASGOW NEW YORK TORONTO MELBOURNE WELLINGTON
CAPE TOWN SALISBURY IBADAN NAIROBI LUSAKA ADDIS ABABA
BOMBAY CALCUTTA MADRAS KARACHI LAHORE DACCA
KUALA LUMPUR SINGAPORE HONG KONG TOKYO

FIRST EDITION 1933
SEVENTH EDITION 1969

PRINTED IN GREAT BRITAIN

CONTENTS

PREFACE TO THE SEVENTH EDITION

BEFORE Lord Brain's untimely death in December 1966 he had revised about one-third of *Diseases of the Nervous System* in preparing for the publication of this Seventh Edition. I am deeply conscious of the honour his executors and publishers have done me by inviting me to complete the preparation of this edition and to assume the authorship of subsequent editions, and am only too well aware of my inadequacy for the task. The previous editions of the book will stand as a permanent monument to Lord Brain's clinical expertise, to his thoughtful approach to neurological medicine and to his outstanding literary skills. This edition will inevitably prove to be something of a hybrid as no two authors can ever hope to agree fully upon the construction and emphasis of such a text and upon the important questions as to what should be included and what should be omitted. I have felt in duty bound to maintain the traditional structure of the volume so carefully conceived by Lord Brain through many editions and have left untouched those sections which he had revised before his death. These include virtually the whole of the original Chapters 1, 2, and 4, the greater part of Chapter 17, some sections in Chapters 3 and 23, and a number of isolated sections of other chapters. But as he had left a note implying that he proposed to include in the new edition an introductory section dealing with general principles I have added such a commentary, based largely upon the opening chapter of my own book *Essentials of Neurology* (Pitman Medical Publishing Company Ltd.) but including also some comments upon the structure, function, and pathology of the neurone and of the glia.

The remaining chapters have been extensively revised, and that on Disorders of Muscle has been completely rewritten, and has been based upon material I have published previously in a review article in *Abstracts of World Medicine* in 1966, and in a chapter entitled 'Some Disorders of Muscle' in the current edition of *Recent Advances in Neurology* (J. & A. Churchill Ltd.), as well as upon the chapter written with Dr. D. Gardner-Medwin in the second edition of *Disorders of Voluntary Muscle* (J. & A. Churchill Ltd.). In the course of my revision some material has been deleted but there have been many extensive additions, particularly in Chapters 3, 6, 10, 11, 13, 18, and 22 in order to bring the book up to date in the light of recent advances in neurological medicine. In each of these chapters many new references to the recent literature have been added.

New illustrations have been included by kind permission of Dr. D. Denny-Brown and the Liverpool University Press, Dr. C. S. Hallpike and the editors and publishers of *Proceedings of the Royal Society of Medicine*, Dr. W. Blackwood and E. & S. Livingstone Ltd., publishers of *Atlas of Neuropathology*, Dr. J. R. Smythies and Blackwell Scientific Publications Ltd., publishers of *The Neurological Foundations of Psychiatry*, and Dr. P. Hudgson and the editors and publishers of *Neurology* (Minneapolis). To all of the authors, editors, and publishers quoted I wish to express my thanks. Dr. G. L. Gryspeerdt and

Dr. G. W. Pearce have also kindly supplied original illustrations and I have provided some of my own for the chapter on 'Disorders of Muscle'; these were prepared in the Department of Photography of the University of Newcastle upon Tyne. I also gladly acknowledge the help and advice upon many topics involved in the preparation of this edition which I have received from innumerable friends and colleagues including Dr. James Bull, Professor E. J. Field, Dr. D. Gardner-Medwin, Professor L. P. Garrod and Professor F. W. O'Grady (for allowing me to see the proofs of their chapter on the antibiotic treatment of meningitis prior to publication), Dr. A. J. McComas, the late Dr. W. V. Macfarlane, and Dr. J. B. Selkon. I am, as always, indebted to my secretary Miss Rosemary Allan for her unfailing help in the preparation of this revised edition and the index, and to Dr. J. C. Gregory and the staff of the Oxford University Press for their patience, understanding, and tolerance during the gestation period. I can but hope that I have done justice to some at least of Lord Brain's aims and intentions for this edition.

JOHN N. WALTON

Newcastle upon Tyne
August 1968

PREFACE TO THE FIRST EDITION

THE last twenty years have witnessed a remarkable development in neurology. Investigation of the effects of war injuries of the spinal cord has greatly increased our knowledge of reflex action in man. The appearance of encephalitis lethargica and the multiplication of forms of acute disseminated encephalitis have added a new field to clinical neurology and brought it into relationship with the new branch of bacteriology which studies the filterable viruses. The discovery of important metabolic centres in the hypothalamus has enhanced the importance of neurology to general medicine. Advances in the technique of neurological surgery have aroused fresh interest in the symptoms and in the pathology of intracranial tumours. Other developments, scarcely less important, have occurred.

Much of this new knowledge is physiological, and in one respect I have departed from the traditional arrangement of a textbook of nervous diseases. Neurology is more dependent than many other branches of medicine upon anatomy and physiology. These subjects, the essential basis of neurological diagnosis, are usually dismissed in a few introductory pages, with the result that much clinical neurology is apt to be both unintelligible and uninteresting to the student. In the first part of this book, as an introduction to the subject, I have discussed—at greater length than usual—the application of anatomy and physiology to the interpretation of the physical signs of nervous disease. Elsewhere will be found sections dealing with anatomy and physiology as introductions to clinical sections. In planning the clinical sections I have used what seemed the most practical, if not always the most logical, arrangement, for there is no entirely satisfactory way of arranging subjects, many of which might be placed in more than one group.

Limitations of space restrict the number of references which it is possible to quote. I have, therefore, chosen only those of special interest and those which form the best introduction to a subject, or are themselves useful sources of references. To the many other writers upon whose work I have freely drawn I express my indebtedness. I am indebted also to a number of my colleagues for the loan of illustrations.

Finally, I welcome this opportunity of expressing my gratitude to my colleagues at the London Hospital for their teaching, encouragement, and help, especially to Dr. Charles Miller, Professor Arthur Ellis, and Dr. George Riddoch, under whom I had the privilege of working on the Medical Unit, and to Mr. Hugh Cairns, Dr. Dorothy Russell, and Dr. S. Phillips Bedson.

W. RUSSELL BRAIN

London
June 1933

1

DISORDERS OF FUNCTION IN THE LIGHT OF ANATOMY AND PHYSIOLOGY

SOME GENERAL CONSIDERATIONS

THOUGH there can be no absolute distinction between diseases of the nervous system and those which affect other organs or systems of the human body, by convention the clinical science of neurology embraces those many disorders which affect the functioning of the central and peripheral nervous systems and the voluntary muscles. In this first chapter it is proposed to review briefly current knowledge of the means by which disorders of nervous function may be brought about by a variety of pathological processes. For the purposes of convenience, this review has been organized on an anatomical and physiological basis so that descriptions of the anatomy and, where necessary, of the physiology of certain structures and pathways in the nervous system will be considered, together with the disorders of function which result when they are diseased. First, however, it is important to recognize that the manifestations of disordered function of the central nervous system may be greatly modified by mental, as by pathological processes, and may also be altered by the influence of the individual's constitution and inherited characteristics. Furthermore, before considering the applied anatomy and physiology of some of the more important pathways in the nervous systems which are commonly affected by disease, it will be necessary to consider the nature of some important units of structure of the nervous system, as well as to classify some of the pathological processes which commonly influence their behaviour.

It must be admitted that there are still many problems in neurology which are not clearly understood. We have, for instance, no definite evidence as to how the brain controls thought processes; while disordered activity of the mind is commonly present and is attributed to dysfunction of the brain even when modern techniques fail to demonstrate any abnormality of structure or any measurable disorder of function in physiological terms, conversely the influence of the mind upon the behaviour of the organs of the body can also be profound. Mental disorders frequently initiate or accentuate symptoms of physical disease, while some organic diseases are regularly accompanied by psychological manifestations. The importance of these mechanisms must be recognized by the physician who deals with sick people, as disease is an abstraction; it is the patient who suffers from the disease who is real and who shows a personal and individual reaction to it. Thus although many physical disorders of the nervous system regularly produce a consistent series of symptoms and physical signs independent of the personality and constitution of the individual, the severity of the resultant symptoms and the rate of recovery or of deterioration, depending upon the pathological process involved, can be influenced by factors which are independent of the physical process present within nervous tissue. While a simple peripheral nerve lesion is likely to produce a consistent clinical syndrome, its effects upon the patient may depend upon the nature of the lesion responsible, in that in industrial injuries, for instance, the patient's disability may be excessive and his recovery unduly delayed, particularly if financial compensation is involved.

In disorders of the nervous system, more perhaps than in any other group of diseases, the physical signs discovered on examination often indicate the anatomical localization of the lesion or lesions responsible for the abnormalities of function which are present, while it is the history of the illness, revealing the detailed evolution of the patient's symptoms, which generally indicates the nature of the pathological process. Thus although the intelligent interpretation of the significance of physical signs demands an adequate knowledge, first, of neuroanatomy for localization of the lesion, and secondly of neurophysiology in order to assess the means by which function has been disordered, it is also necessary that the student should have some understanding of neuropathology in order to be able to analyse the nature of the pathological process which is present. Admittedly there are many neurological disorders, such as migraine and epilepsy, for instance, which give characteristic clinical pictures but in which physical examination may be negative and diagnosis must rest upon analysis of the history alone. Furthermore, as already indicated, the clinical effects of pathological processes are not immutable and the resultant disease can be greatly influenced by the personality and constitution of the individual and by his state of mind. Some patients are born physically and mentally less perfect than others and yet show no obvious defect, but constitutionally they are less capable of resistance to stress, both mental and physical, and are seriously disturbed by environmental influences which would leave others unaffected. Hence the possible effects of fatigue, of ageing processes and of other contributory influences which cannot easily be measured by scientific parameters must be also stressed. In his analysis of the interplay of these many factors, the doctor may be required to bring into play all his reserves of experience and understanding. It is also important to consider at this stage the concept of 'functional' illness or 'functional' disorder. In the strictest anatomical and physiological terms, it would be reasonable to regard as 'functional' those diseases in which there is an important disorder of the function of some organ of the body but which do not depend upon any recognizable pathological change in the organ concerned. By convention, however, the term 'functional disorder' is more often applied in medicine to symptoms and signs which result from a disordered state of mind. Thus headaches due to anxiety or nervous tension are 'functional', and so, too, is hysterical aphonia, while other forms of anxiety or hysterical reaction are commonly included in this category. Functional disorders, therefore, are those conditions in which symptoms and signs result not from any primary physical disease but from conscious or subconscious mental processes; it must be appreciated that these processes may profoundly affect the physical functioning of the body, giving rise to such manifestations as increased cardiac output, tachycardia, perspiration and insomnia. Hence the clinical use of the term 'functional', if not strictly correct in a semantic sense, is hallowed through common usage and can usefully be employed provided the doctor using it understands its meaning and does not regard this as a final diagnosis. It is important also to recognize at this stage that the distinction between organic and functional disease is often one of the most difficult to make in medicine since even when there is clear evidence of a primary physical abnormality, the symptoms may readily be accentuated or distorted by concurrent psychological factors.

Disordered function depends not only upon the localization of pathological change but upon its severity, its extent, and the effects it has upon contiguous nervous tissue and upon interconnected though anatomically remote structures in the nervous system. Thus an acute and extensive lesion may affect a greater area of the brain than its anatomical extent would lead one to expect, for around the edge of the lesion itself the activity of the surrounding nervous tissue is disturbed by oedema, vascular changes, and other ill-defined abnormalities. Furthermore, an acute lesion can produce a state of 'shock' or temporary dissolution of function in related areas of the brain or spinal cord. By contrast, lesions of equal extent which are slow to develop produce far fewer symptoms and physical signs as it is only the structures which are actively invaded or destroyed by the lesion whose function is disturbed; the surrounding tissues have more time to adapt themselves to the presence of the lesion. Adaptation of other forms may also occur, particularly in the cerebral cortex, for here, particularly in children rather than in adults, a function which has been lost through a cortical lesion may be 'adopted', though usually much less efficiently, by another area of the brain. The younger the patient the greater the flexibility of cerebral organization. This type of re-organization is much less likely to occur in the spinal cord for the pathways followed here are more stereotyped and probably less complex. No such adoption of functions can occur in peripheral nerves, but, on the other hand, peripheral nerves are able to regenerate effectively following injury, while effective regeneration does not occur within the spinal cord or brain.

CONSTITUTION AND HEREDITY

It is only too easy to overlook the important influences which may be derived from inherited characteristics. Some neurological disorders are clearly inherited in a strictly Mendelian manner. Diseases such as migraine, Huntington's chorea, peroneal muscular atrophy and facioscapulohumeral muscular dystrophy are generally inherited by an autosomal dominant mechanism, meaning that they result from a dominant gene situated on one of the autosomes and are thus passed on by an affected individual to half his or her children of either sex if penetrance or expressivity of the gene is complete. An autosomal recessive gene, however, can only produce its phenotypic effect if it is paired with a similar gene lying on the other chromosome of the pair. Hence such a disease is only expressed when two unaffected heterozygous carriers marry; usually, therefore, there is no previous history of the disease in the family unless there has been intermarriage between relatives (consanguinity). In such families the likelihood is that the disease will affect 1 in 4 of a series of brothers and sisters;

Friedreich's ataxia, hepatolenticular degeneration (Wilson's disease) and spinal muscular atrophy of infancy are usually inherited in this way. A recessive gene can produce an effect, however, if it is situated on the unpaired portion of the X-chromosome, so that this type of condition occurs in males and is carried by apparently unaffected females. This is the typical pattern of sex-linked recessive (or X-linked) inheritance when the disease may have been found in maternal uncles and now occurs in half the male children of an apparently normal female carrier. Red-green colour blindness, haemophilia and muscular dystrophy of the Duchenne type are inherited in this way. Any inherited disease can, of course, appear anew in a family if a previously normal gene has undergone a process of spontaneous change or mutation. It must also be remembered that apart from those diseases which are clearly inherited by recognizable genetic mechanisms, there are many other disorders of the nervous system in which genetic influences are of importance, though these factors are difficult to define.

Before going on to discuss individual anatomical pathways in the nervous system and the clinical effects of their dysfunction, it will now be important to consider certain units of nervous structure and some of the ways in which they may be affected by pathological processes. This commentary will perforce be superficial and introductory in nature and for fuller information the reader is referred to textbooks on neuroanatomy, neurophysiology and neuropathology.

THE NEURONE

The nerve cell is one of the few types of cell in the human body which cannot be replaced if it is destroyed; it does not undergo division nor is it capable of regeneration after the first few weeks of extra-uterine life. The neurone theory was first proposed by Cajal and his colleagues in 1889–91; this stated that each neurone is a separate cellular entity which consists first of a cell body, secondly of dendrites or short processes which extend for a short distance from the cell, and thirdly of a long (or sometimes short) axon which makes contact by means of nerve endings of various types with the dendrites or cell bodies of other neurones or with muscle or other effector cells. This theory was opposed by many earlier workers who thought that nerve processes merged or became continuous with one another but it has now been shown conclusively that each neuroblast in the embryo forms a single adult nerve cell and that in the mature human and animal synaptic junctions are invariably present when axons and dendrites meet so that neurofibrils never pass from one cell to another. Furthermore, studies of degeneration have shown that neither chromatolysis nor any other form of degeneration in a cell necessarily spreads to involve other neurones. It has also been concluded from tissue culture studies that nerve processes always arise by direct growth from parent cells and not by differentiation from inter-cellular material. Many millions of neurones are present within the central nervous system; they are linked together to form functional conducting pathways and are supported or held together by a framework of specialized but non-conducting cells which constitute the neuroglia.

Neurones vary greatly in size, shape and functional characteristics. Those with long processes are frequently called Golgi Type I, and those with short processes Golgi Type II. The cytoplasm of a neurone contains granules of

Nissl substance which stain with basic dyes such as cresyl violet or toluidine blue, while within its cytoplasm there are minute neurofibrils which extend into its processes and can be demonstrated by special silver stains. Typically the nucleus of a neurone looks pale but it has a single dense central nucleolus [FIG. 1 (a)].

It is now evident that most of the dendrites of a neurone are afferent, while the longer axons are generally efferent. Most dendrites contain small quantities of Nissl substance and have many branches, while axons do not contain Nissl

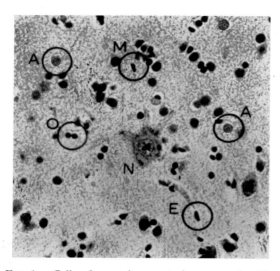

FIG. 1 a. Cells of normal precentral cortex stained by Nissl's method. N = nerve cell; A = astrocyte; O = two oligodendrocytes; M = microglial nucleus; E = capillary endothelial cell nucleus. Thionin, ×350

(FIG. 1 (a–g) is reproduced from Blackwood, W., Dodds, T. C., and Sommerville, J. C. (1964) *Atlas of Neuropathology*, 2nd ed., by kind permission of the authors and E. and S. Livingstone Ltd.)

granules and their main branches come off terminally; the point of origin of the axon from the nerve cell is called the axon hillock [FIG. 1 (b)].

In the central nervous system many large axons, such as those of the pyramidal cells of the cerebral cortex and of the cerebellar Purkinje cells, give off collateral fibres close to their origin, and many large axons of sensory neurones in the posterior root ganglia branch shortly after entering the spinal cord. Close to their termination axons usually divide into a number of fine terminal twigs or telodendria which either enter a peripheral end-organ or else make synaptic contact with the cell bodies or dendrites of other neurones; the resultant ring-like endings are called *boutons terminaux*.

The large axons of the lower motor neurones (α-neurones) which arise from large anterior horn cells in the spinal cord usually divide after entering voluntary muscle (the effector organ) and each main branch then divides further to innervate a group of extrafusal muscle fibres. The lower motor neurone and the groups of muscle fibres which it supplies form a functional unit called the motor unit; the groups of fibres supplied by single large branches constitute so-called sub-units. The intrafusal muscle fibres within the muscle spindles are innervated by axons arising from smaller anterior horn cells (the so-called γ-neurones).

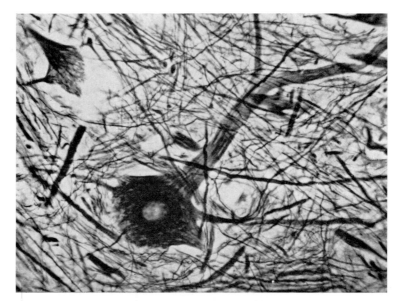

FIG. 1 *b*. Anterior horn cell, spinal cord, showing neurofibrils and the axon. Hortega's silver, $\times 350$

THE MYELIN SHEATH

In the vertebrate central and peripheral nervous systems it appears that all axons with a diameter greater than 1 μ are surrounded by a myelin sheath; this can be seen best in sections stained with osmic acid which demonstrate the myelin but not the axon. The myelin sheath is a complex of lipids and contains cerebroside, sphingomyelin and cholesterol. In the peripheral, but not in the central nervous system, the myelin sheath is enclosed by the processes of Schwann or neurilemmal cells and this sheath is interrupted at regular intervals at the nodes of Ranvier. At this point, though the myelin is interrupted, the Schwann cells nevertheless appear to be continuous. It is the integrity and continuity of the sheath of Schwann around peripheral nerves which allows effective regeneration of axons to occur after injury or degeneration. Whereas in the central nervous system sprouting of damaged axons may also take place when a disease process resolves, these axons cannot be properly directed by a surviving neurilemmal sheath so that such regeneration usually proves to be abortive.

GROUND SUBSTANCE

Apart from the nerve and neuroglial cells and their processes which constitute the grey matter of the central nervous system, it seems that there is also a background substance which probably contains mucopolysaccharides. Though electron microscopy seems to indicate that the cortex is almost wholly made up of the branching processes of neurones and of neuroglial and oligodendroglial cells, there also appears to be a small amount of intercellular fluid (which is increased in cerebral oedema) or ground substance but its function is still unknown.

SYNAPSES OR NEURONAL JUNCTIONS

While peripherally axons may end in effector organs such as muscle, in the central nervous system each small terminal branch or telodendron makes contact with a dendrite (axodendritic contact) or with a cell body (axosomatic contact). In these junctional regions which are called synapses cell membranes are in close contact but do not fuse. As already mentioned, a synaptic contact between a telodendron and a dendrite or a cell body may take the form of a small swelling or ring-like structure (a *bouton terminal*). But a telodendron may make one synaptic contact, in passing, by a *bouton de passage* but then continues to its termination on another part of the same cell or on another cell, so that one axon may have synaptic junctions with many cells. Similarly, a single cell may have many hundreds of surface synaptic contacts derived from many axons. The arrangement and variety of these synapses determine the means by which a nerve cell can be activated, and also, of equal importance in nervous activity, by which it may be inhibited. Physiologically, learning, memory and the acquisition of skills probably depend upon the progressive facilitation of synapses in certain specific pathways in the brain. The method by which transmission of nervous activity occurs across synapses is not yet fully understood. At the synapse most extensively studied, namely the neuromuscular junction, there is convincing evidence that the arrival of a nerve impulse causes a release of acetylcholine, probably from synaptic vesicles in the subneural apparatus, and that this in turn depolarizes the muscle fibre membrane. There is good evidence to suggest that acetylcholine may also be responsible for synaptic transmission within the central nervous system, though this is more difficult to prove.

NEUROGLIA

The supporting cells of the brain and spinal cord are known as the neuroglia. Special silver stains are usually necessary in order to demonstrate fully these glial cells which differ in size and shape and have processes which not only intermingle with the axons and dendrites but which are frequently attached to the wall of blood vessels. Larger stellate neuroglial cells are called astrocytes; they can be divided into protoplasmic and fibrous forms, the fibrous being distinguished from the protoplasmic form chiefly by the presence in the cell body and its processes of fine fibres [FIG. 1 (c)]. The processes of fibrous astrocytes are longer and finer and branch less frequently than do those of the protoplasmic variety, in which the rather thicker and shorter branches which come off at a wider angle give a rather 'mossy' appearance to the cell [FIG. 1 (d)]. Under the light microscope neuroglial fibres seem fine and relatively straight, being seen only with high magnification, but under the electron microscope they are seen to be beaded. Undoubtedly astrocytes have a metabolic function, but their exact role in the metabolism of nervous structure is as yet undetermined. The

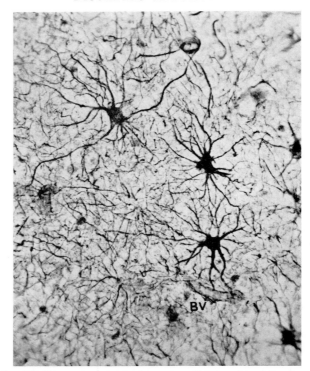

FIG. 1 *c*. Fibrillary astrocytes in the cortex. Cajal's gold sublimate, ×350

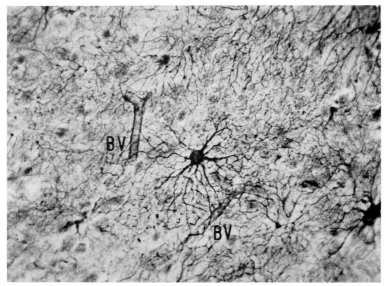

FIG. 1 *d*. Protoplasmic astrocytes in the cortex. Cajal's gold sublimate, ×350

oligodendroglia are smaller neuroglial cells with fewer and shorter processes [FIG. 1 (*a*)]; they may be seen close to axons and around cell bodies but are much more common in the white matter; almost certainly they play an important role in the formation and maintenance of myelin. Microglial cells are much smaller [FIG. 1 (e)] and unlike other glial cells which are of ectodermal origin, they are derived from the mesoderm which is carried into the nervous system by blood vessels. They frequently enlarge and become phagocytic [FIG. 1 (f)] and thus play an important role in removing damaged tissue in the course of pathological processes. The proliferation of neuroglial cells almost always occurs as a reaction to the degeneration of neurones or else as a secondary part of the disease process which causes the neurone to degenerate. The proliferation of astrocytes is called astrocytosis or gliosis, while the proliferation of microglial cells is comparable to the scavenging activity of histiocytes in other organs of the human body.

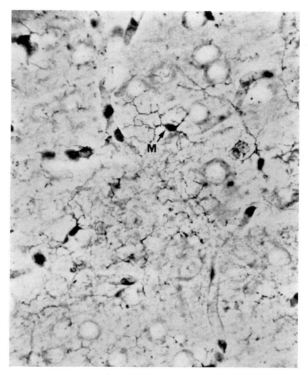

FIG. 1 e. Normal microglia in the cortex of a rabbit (human cells are similar). Hortega's silver, × 450

DEGENERATION AND REGENERATION IN THE NERVOUS SYSTEM

An adult nerve cell, once destroyed, can never be replaced. With increasing age there is undoubtedly a progressive fall-out of certain cortical and spinal neurones. In elderly individuals it is not uncommon to find within the cerebral cortex neurofibrillary tangles or so-called senile argyrophilic plaques which develop in relation to degenerating neurones. Such lesions, if seen in profusion in the cerebral cortex at a relatively early age, are virtually diagnostic of pre-senile dementia and the changes in senile dementia are similar, but it is the age at which they are found and their profusion which is important as they are almost invariably seen to occur in some degree as a result of normal ageing processes in the eighth or ninth decades.

When certain processes of a nerve cell are destroyed, the cell body may survive, but if as a result, say, of peripheral nerve injury, the axon of an anterior horn cell is divided, the Nissl substance in the cell of origin at first aggregates and later disappears (chromatolysis) and the nucleus shifts towards the periphery [FIG. 1 (g)]. These changes are more easily seen in large cells which have abundant Nissl substance; their severity is related to the distance of the axonal

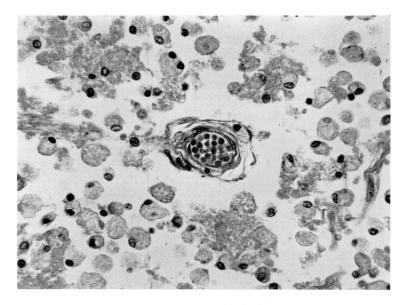

FIG. 1 f. Reactive microglial cells ('compound granular corpuscles' or 'glitter' cells) which are distended with phagocytosed lipid

lesion from the parent cell body and they are more severe when the break is close. It is rare for cells with bodies and processes confined to the central nervous system to survive axonal section and hence these cellular changes may sometimes be used to locate the cells of origin of degenerating axons in a peripheral nerve or in a specific fibre pathway. It is, however, important to recognize that appearances somewhat similar to those of chromatolysis may occasionally be seen in control material and can result from post-mortem autolysis. When degeneration of a cell body proceeds even further, due either to damage to its axon or to a primary degenerative process, it may be surrounded by microglial cells and later disappears leaving only a small glial cluster (neuronophagia).

An axon that has been severed from its cell body undergoes Wallerian degeneration. Within a few days the terminal part of the axis-cylinder begins to swell and subsequently it becomes beaded and then disintegrates. This process of swelling and progressive disintegration then slowly moves proximally (dying back of the neurone). If the axon is myelinated, the myelin sheath begins to break down within a few days and it seems that the neurilemmal cells then proliferate, subsequently appearing to ingest or enfold both the disintegrating axis-cylinder and the myelin within Schwann cell processes. Histiocytes have a phagocytic role and proliferating connective tissue cells also play a part in the degenerative process. Similar axonal changes occur in the central nervous

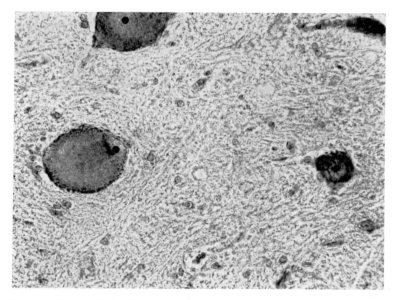

FIG. 1 *g*. Chromatolysis of an anterior horn cell. The cell is swollen and rounded, the Nissl substance is accumulated at the periphery and the nucleus is eccentric.
H & E, ×350

system, except that gliosis results from astrocytic proliferation and the microglia act as phagocytes. The degeneration of myelin secondary to such axonal damage may be identified by certain specific stains which form the basis of the Marchi method which demonstrates degenerating myelinated fibres in such a way that these fibres can be traced in microscopic sections.

In peripheral nerves, soon after an axon has been divided, its tip begins to grow out distally into the surviving neurilemmal sheath which directs its growth. Collateral sprouting often occurs alongside the growing axon, though it is usual for one of these axons to grow distally more rapidly than its collateral sprouts; this distal growth only occurs when the cell body survives and the chromatolytic process is then reversed. Growth occurs at a rate of a millimetre or two a day at first, but after a few weeks it slows down; myelin gradually begins to re-form until eventually the axon re-establishes distal contact. Although profuse axonal sprouting may be seen in the brains or spinal cords of very young animals and infants after injury, it is doubtful as to whether it is ever effective as the axonal sprouts rarely, if ever, make contact with any effector organ.

It must also be recognized that in clinical neurology there are many disease processes which cause demyelination in peripheral nerves or in the central nervous system but which initially leave the axon intact, though incapable of conducting normally. In peripheral nerves such demyelination may begin at or close to the nodes of Ranvier (perinodal demyelination) and may then spread to involve one or many internodal distances. Subsequently if the disease process is reversed, remyelination may occur. In teased specimens of nerve fibres obtained by biopsy or at autopsy in such cases it is often found that the regenerated myelin sheath is thinner than normal and in such areas the internodal distances are often irregular and much shorter than normal. A demyelinating type of neuropathy frequently produces marked slowing of conduction in peripheral nerves, but as the disease process recovers this may eventually return to normal. Demyelination within the central nervous system also affects conduction in the parent axon. The process by means of which remyelination occurs in the central nervous system is unknown, but this process presumably accounts for the remissions which may occur in demyelinating disorders such as multiple sclerosis.

SOME PHYSIOLOGICAL CHARACTERISTICS OF NEURONES

Nerve cells are excitable; this means that they can respond or react to stimuli and these reactions alter the physiological state of the organism. Some cells react specifically; thus stimulation of the lower motor neurone causes muscular contraction while stimulation of neurosecretory neurones causes glandular secretion. In some cells, the change once initiated by the stimulus spreads throughout the cell and its processes and is then independent of the stimulus. This spread or conduction is particularly rapid in muscle and nerve. The conducted response which begins in a nerve cell and spreads along its axon is known as the nerve impulse, while the activity which spreads along a muscle fibre from the neuromuscular junction once depolarization has occurred is called the propagated action potential. These reactions are accompanied by the utilization of oxygen and of glucose, the formation of carbon dioxide and the production of heat and they are also accompanied by certain specific electrical changes.

Nerve and muscle fibres are each normally polarized in such a way that the interior of the fibre is negative to the exterior; the potential difference across the fibre membrane is called the resting membrane potential. This can be measured in a neurone by inserting a micro-electrode into a nerve cell body; in the giant axon of the squid, the axon itself may be impaled. A stimulus adequate to excite the neurone alters the permeability of its membrane to many ions; it develops a high specific permeability to sodium, so that sodium rapidly enters the fibre. In less than a millisecond the polarity of the resting potential is reversed, so that the external surface becomes negative to the interior and the membrane is said to be depolarized. The electrical accompaniment of this change can be recorded as a spike potential and typically the depolarization and this spike potential are propagated along the fibre, forming the so-called nerve action potential. The spread of excitation along a muscle fibre is very similar. As the peak of the action potential moves on, the entry of sodium stops, potassium permeability increases and potassium leaves the fibre so that the original membrane potential is eventually restored. The so-called sodium pump helps slowly to restore the original differences in sodium concentration. A nerve action potential can be measured by means of electrodes inserted into a nerve trunk or, in certain situations, surface electrodes applied to the overlying skin are sufficient. Muscle action potentials can also be recorded with surface electrodes but for diagnostic electromyography needle electrodes are inserted into the muscle. The form of the nerve action potential depends upon recording methods. The conduction velocity in peripheral nerves can be measured either by recording the rate of propagation of the nerve action potential (which is the usual method of measuring conduction in sensory nerves) or by measuring the latencies of the evoked muscle action potential induced by stimulation of a motor nerve at two points a known distance apart. The conduction velocity in a nerve depends upon the fibre diameter. In general, heavily myelinated, thick nerve fibres conduct rapidly and finely myelinated or unmyelinated fibres conduct slowly. In myelinated fibres the nerve impulse passes rapidly from one node of Ranvier to the next. The maximum rate of conduction known is about 100–120 metres per second, but in human peripheral nerves 50–70 metres per second is more usual and the slowest myelinated fibres conduct at about 40 metres per second. Demyelination in peripheral nerves causes marked slowing of conduction. When a nerve impulse has passed, the nerve may show an absolute and a relative refractory period, while small negative and positive after-potentials may be recorded. These after-potentials and accompanying changes in excitability of the nerve are related to the recovery process which follows passage of the impulse. Just as in muscle, miniature end-plate potentials may be recorded close to the neuromuscular junction and are believed to be due to the spontaneous release of amounts of acetylcholine which are insufficient to evoke a propagated action potential, so in a nerve a subthreshold stimulus produces a local excitatory state in a fibre; another subthreshold stimulus may then raise this local excitation to a threshold value and thereby set off a nerve impulse.

It will now be important to consider, as an introduction to the more specific commentaries which follow, some simple principles concerning pathological processes in the nervous system.

SOME PATHOLOGICAL REACTIONS IN THE NERVOUS SYSTEM

Pathological changes in the nervous system can be classified into three broad groups, namely focal lesions, which cause a disturbance in the function of a strictly localized area; diffuse or generalized disorders, whether of metabolic, toxic, vascular or other aetiology, which affect nervous and supporting elements throughout the nervous system; and systemic nervous diseases, in which the pathological process shows a predilection for a particular neuronal structure or group of structures such as, for instance, the anterior horn cells, the cerebellum and its connexions or the pyramidal tracts. Many focal lesions and diffuse disorders affect nervous tissue more or less by accident and many of these are not primarily neurological diseases. Thus cerebral vascular disease, which may produce infarction or haemorrhage, is usually a complication of atherosclerosis or hypertension, while the diffuse pathological changes which occur in the brain in syphilis, for instance, form only one part of the changes resulting from infection of the entire human organism. In the systemic nervous diseases, by contrast, as in motor neurone disease, there is clearly some biochemical or other factor which causes the pathological process to be confined to a particular group of nerve cells or fibre pathways. In this context one must note that the tissues of the nervous system vary considerably in their response to a variety of different noxious influences. Thus ischaemia affects nerve cells more severely than myelin and neuroglia, while plaques of demyelination, as in multiple sclerosis, have a more profound influence upon the nerve fibres of the white matter. There are also considerable differences in the effects of ischaemia, compression and various toxins upon nerve fibres depending upon whether they conduct motor or sensory impulses.

There are a number of methods of classifying pathological processes on an aetiological basis. Thus one can recognize that certain lesions are congenital or due to developmental abnormality. Others may be traumatic, the lesion then being the result of physical or possibly chemical injury. A third large group is that of the inflammatory disorders which in turn may be subdivided according to whether the inflammation is of infective or allergic origin. In either category the infection may be acute, subacute or chronic. Neoplastic disorders are next to be considered and these in turn may be benign or malignant, while malignant processes may involve the nervous system primarily or secondarily as a result of metastasis from a tumour elsewhere. Within a further large group of conditions classified at present as being degenerative because their nature is not yet understood, one must include cerebral vascular disease, but there are also many other conditions of unknown aetiology which must still be so classified. Finally, a variety of metabolic and endocrine disorders may also affect the functioning of the nervous system.

To mention a number of congenital disorders, these are most often apparent as gross disorders of anatomical development and configuration and include such conditions as anencephaly, hydrocephalus and meningomyelocele. Vascular malformations are almost certainly also of congenital origin. Trauma to the nervous system will produce the familiar effects of necrosis, haemorrhage and subsequent scar formation, the scar consisting of proliferated neuroglial cells and fibrils (gliosis) and of mesenchymal fibrous tissue derived from fibroblasts and microglial cells in the supporting tissue of the blood vessels. In the group of acute inflammatory disorders, one must consider the meningitides producing the typical pathological changes of inflammation and exudation of the meninges. It must, however, be noted that meningitis may give rise to superficial degenerative changes in underlying nervous tissue or to ischaemic changes in the nervous parenchyma resulting from an obliterative endarteritis of blood vessels which traverse the subarachnoid space. Pyogenic infection in the brain, as elsewhere, begins with diffuse suppuration, but localization and abscess formation generally follows with the formation of a capsule through gliosis and fibrosis. Most neurotropic viruses, such as those of encephalitis and poliomyelitis, show an affinity for nerve cells and inflammatory changes with perivascular cellular infiltration and degeneration of nerve cells are therefore seen in the grey matter of the brain and/or spinal cord and inclusion bodies may be found within the nucleus or cytoplasm of infected cells. Syphilis, and to a lesser extent tuberculosis, are still two of the most important chronic infections of the central nervous system. The pathological changes they produce will be considered under the appropriate sections later in this volume as they do not differ significantly from the pathological changes produced by these diseases elsewhere, except in so far that in general paresis there are degeneration of nerve cells, gliosis and minimal inflammatory changes in the cerebral cortex, while in tabes dorsalis the most prominent pathological change is gliosis and meningeal fibrosis of the entry zones of the posterior spinal nerve roots with secondary ascending degeneration of the posterior columns of the spinal cord. In allergic or postinfective encephalomyelitis, by contrast to the virus infections, inflammatory changes, consisting largely of perivascular collections of inflammatory cells with loss of myelin, are seen particularly in the white matter of the nervous system. These pathological changes show some resemblance to those observed in the demyelinating disorders of unknown aetiology such as multiple sclerosis and diffuse sclerosis. In these disorders there is patchy loss of myelin of variable extent and severity occurring generally throughout the white matter of the brain and spinal cord. This type of degenerative change in which the axis-cylinders of the nerve fibres are initially preserved is eventually replaced by a glial scar.

So far as neoplastic disorders are concerned, the pathology of these conditions will be considered in greater detail in the sections on intracranial and intraspinal tumours, but it should first be remarked that the commonest benign tumours which compress and distort nervous tissues are the meningioma, which probably arises from cells of the arachnoidal membrane, and the neurofibroma, which grows from the sheath of Schwann of the cranial nerves, spinal roots or peripheral nerves. The commonest of the malignant tumours of the central nervous system is the glioma; these are infiltrating and invasive tumours whose relative malignancy depends upon whether the principal constituent cell of the tumour is a relatively mature astrocyte or one of its more rapidly multiplying primitive precursors. Metastatic malignant neoplasms are also very common in the nervous system.

Vascular disorders are a common cause of pathological change. Bleeding into the subarachnoid space produces an aseptic meningeal inflammation comparable to that of meningitis and sometimes chronic arachnoiditis may result, while chronic bleeding can give rise to a state of haemosiderosis of the meninges. Haemorrhage into the nervous parenchyma gives a central area of total necrosis which is eventually walled off by gliosis and fibrosis. Sometimes a scar results, but more often a cavity is left which is filled with a clear straw-coloured fluid containing bilirubin. An infarct shows an area of central ischaemic necrosis but within 24 hours activated microglial cells invade the necrotic area and soon become distended with the fatty remnants of the necrotic myelin which they have ingested. A minute infarct produced by embolic occlusion of a tiny cortical vessel may consist of nothing more histologically than a small cluster of activated microglial cells, whereas a large one will show an extensive central area of necrosis surrounded by distended phagocytes ('glitter' cells) and proliferating astrocytes. A large area of infarction may eventually be replaced by a contracted glial scar or cavity, while multifocal infarction sometimes leads to the formation of multiple small cavities (status lacunosus).

There remain a large group of degenerative disorders of the central nervous system whose aetiology is at present unknown, but in some of which specific neuropathological changes are seen. In motor neurone disease, for instance, the cells of the motor nuclei of the brain stem and the anterior horn cells of the spinal cord and the corticospinal or pyramidal tracts show a progressive degeneration. In Huntington's chorea there is a selective degeneration of the caudate nucleus and of the nerve cells of the frontal cortex. But in these and in many other disorders which will be considered in the appropriate sections of this volume, though the anatomical distribution of the pathological lesions has been well defined, their nature is little understood. Nor do we know why anoxia should affect particularly the cells of the deepest layer of the cerebral cortex, the Ammon's horn area of the hippocampus, or the Purkinje cells of the cerebellum, nor why hypoglycaemia should also involve the Purkinje cells, or even why deficiency of vitamin B_{12}, as in subacute combined degeneration of the spinal cord, should damage so selectively the posterior columns and pyramidal tracts.

Many metabolic disorders which seriously disturb nervous function produce relatively little pathological change, but in hepatic failure there is astrocytic proliferation, particularly in the basal ganglia but also in the brain stem. The pathological changes in many different forms of polyneuropathy are also non-specific since in some cases the damage is primarily axonal with swelling and fragmentation of axis-cylinders, but in many others it is essentially a demyelinating process.

The purpose of this section has been to comment briefly upon some of the basic pathological reactions which may occur in the diseased nervous system and not to give comprehensive descriptions of the detailed changes which occur in individual disease entities as these will be described in subsequent sections. It will now be convenient to consider in greater detail some of the important neuronal and fibre systems and pathways in the central nervous system and the disorders of function which may be produced by disease in these specific structures.

REFERENCES

BLACKWOOD, W., DODDS, T. C., and SOMMERVILLE, J. C. (1964) *Atlas of Neuropathology*, 2nd ed., Edinburgh.

BLACKWOOD, W., McMENEMEY, W. H., MEYER, A., NORMAN, R. M., and RUSSELL, D. S. (1963) *Greenfield's Neuropathology*, 2nd ed., London.

GARDNER, E. (1968) *Fundamentals of Neurology*, 5th ed., Philadelphia.

GLEES, P. (1961) *Experimental Neurology*, Oxford.

GREENFIELD, J. G., BLACKWOOD, W., McMENEMEY, W. H., MEYER, A., and NORMAN, R. M. (1958) *Neuropathology*, London.

KREIG, W. J. S. (1966) *Functional Neuroanatomy*, 3rd ed., Evanston, Ill.

McKUSICK, W. A. (1964) *Human Genetics*, Englewood Cliffs, N.J.

MATTHEWS, W. B. (1963) *Practical Neurology*, Oxford.

PRATT, R. T. C. (1967) *The Genetics of Neurological Disorders*, London.

WALSH, E. G. (1964) *Physiology of the Nervous System*, 2nd ed., London.

WALTON, J. N. (1966) *Essentials of Neurology*, 2nd ed., London.

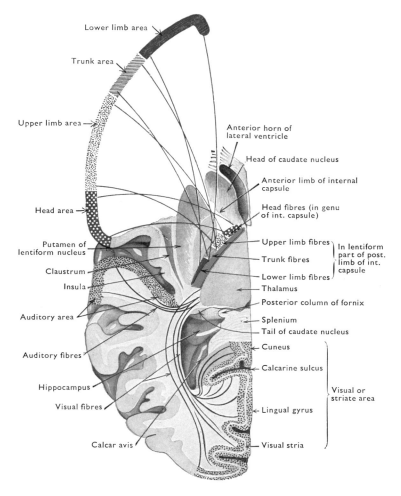

Lower limb area

Trunk area

Upper limb area →

Anterior horn of
lateral ventricle

Head of caudate nucleus

Anterior limb of internal
capsule

Head area →

Head fibres (in genu
of int. capsule)

Putamen of
lentiform nucleus

Upper limb fibres

In lentiform
part of post.
limb of int.
capsule

Trunk fibres

Claustrum

Lower limb fibres

Insula

Thalamus

Posterior column of fornix

Auditory area

Splenium

Tail of caudate nucleus

Auditory fibres

Cuneus

Calcarine sulcus

Hippocampus

Visual or
striate area

Visual fibres

Lingual gyrus

Calcar avis

Visual stria

FIG. 2. Diagram of motor, auditory, and visual areas of left hemisphere
and their relations to the internal capsule

THE CORTICOSPINAL (PYRAMIDAL) TRACT

ANATOMY

THE PRECENTRAL GYRUS

THE corticospinal tracts are the means by which the nervous impulses which excite voluntary movements pass from the cerebral cortex to the lower motor neurones which arise in the brain stem and spinal cord. The corticospinal fibres or upper motor neurones are the axons of cells of the precentral gyrus. It is probable that their cells of origin include not only the Betz cells but also the simple giant cells and the large ordinary pyramidal cells of the fifth layer of the cortex lying anterior to the central sulcus, and extending over Brodmann's areas 4 and 6 (Walshe, 1942).

Since the electrical excitation of different parts of the precentral gyrus evokes movements of different parts of the opposite side of the body, we are justified in speaking of the representation of parts of the body in this part of the brain. The order in which the parts of the body are thus represented is shown in FIGURES 2 and 3.

Individual movements are represented widely and in overlapping areas in the motor cortex, the function of which is the organization of movements in space and time. The cortical centre or focus of a movement is merely the area in which that movement is predominantly represented. Denny-Brown's (1966) observations on stimulation and ablation of area 4 in the monkey and division of the pyramidal tract lead him to the conclusion that 'the pyramidal system is concerned not so much with "discrete" movements of individual muscles, or individual joints as with those spatial adjustments that accurately adapt the movement to the spatial attributes of the stimulus'.

THE INTERNAL CAPSULE

The axons of the corticospinal tract after leaving the grey matter of the cortex pass through the corona radiata and converge upon the internal capsule, a band of white matter lying deep in the substance of the cerebral hemisphere [FIG. 4]. Seen in horizontal section [FIG. 2], it has the head of the caudate nucleus and the optic thalamus on its medial side and the lentiform nucleus on its lateral side. Above, it expands into the corona radiata, and below it is continuous with the cerebral peduncle. The capsule is divided into a shorter, anterior, and a longer, posterior, limb separated by the genu.

The Corticospinal Tract. This occupies the posterior one-third of the anterior limb, the genu, and the anterior two-thirds of the posterior limb. The representation of different parts of the body in the capsule can be seen in FIGURE 2.

The Thalamocortical Tract. This is a sensory tract running from the optic thalamus, a great sensory relay-station, to the cerebral cortex. It is divided into an anterior and a posterior thalamic radiation, the former running in the anterior limb of the capsule to the cortex of the frontal lobe, and the latter in the posterior limb to the postcentral and supramarginal gyri and to the temporal and occipital lobes.

The *optic* and *auditory radiations* are also shown in FIGURE 2.

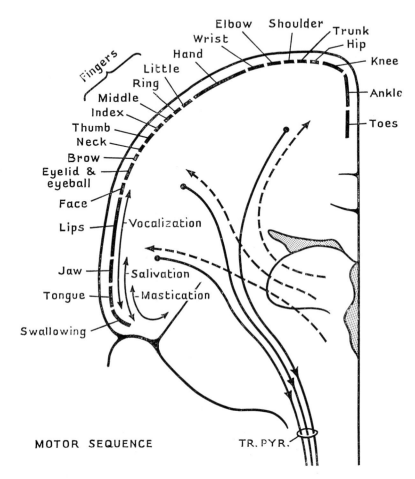

FIG. 3. Corticospinal motor pathway (pyramidal tract). Cross-section through right hemisphere along the plane of the precentral gyrus. The sequence of responses to electrical stimulation of the surface of the cortex (from above down, along the motor strip from toes through arm and face to swallowing) is unvaried from one individual to another

The Frontopontine and the Temporopontine Tracts. These run from the frontal and temporal lobes to lower parts of the nervous system through the anterior and posterior limbs of the capsule respectively.

Fibres of the Corpus Striatum. Fibres linking the optic thalamus and caudate and lentiform nuclei also run in the internal capsule, and the main efferent path of the corpus striatum, the ansa lenticularis, passes in the posterior limb of the capsule from the globus pallidus to the red nucleus, substantia nigra, and subthalamic nucleus.

THE MIDBRAIN

In the midbrain the corticospinal fibres occupy the middle three-fifths of the crus cerebri, the medial fifth being occupied by the frontopontine fibres and

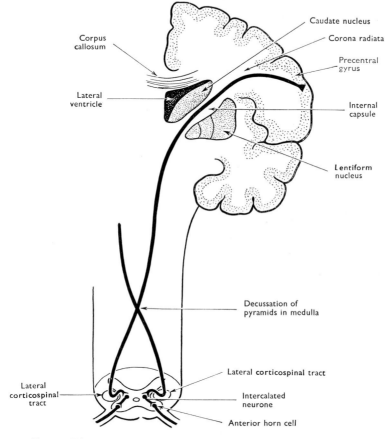

Corpus callosum

Caudate nucleus

Corona radiata

Precentral gyrus

Lateral ventricle

Internal capsule

Lentiform nucleus

Decussation of pyramids in medulla

Lateral corticospinal tract

Lateral corticospinal tract

Intercalated neurone

Anterior horn cell

FIG. 4. Diagram showing course of the crossed corticospinal tracts

the lateral fifth by the temporopontine fibres. The crus cerebri is separated from the tegmen by the substantia nigra, which is thus a posterior relation of the corticospinal tract. Posteromedially to this is the red nucleus, through which pass the bundles of the oculomotor nerve, which emerges from the brain stem on the medial aspect of the crus [FIG. 5].

THE PONS, MEDULLA, AND SPINAL CORD

On entering the pons the corticospinal tract ceases to be compact and becomes broken into scattered bundles by the transverse pontine fibres and the nuclei pontis. At the junction of the pons and the medulla these scattered bundles reunite, and each corticospinal tract constitutes a visible prominence on the anterior aspect of the medulla, the pyramid, which lies between the median fissure and the anterolateral sulcus from the bottom of which emerge the radicles of the hypoglossal nerve.

At the junction of the medulla and the spinal cord the corticospinal tract divides into three parts. (1) The larger medial part decussates with the corresponding fibres of the opposite tract and sinks back to take up a position in the lateral column of the spinal cord, the crossed corticospinal tract. (2) The smaller lateral portion remains in the anterior column of the spinal cord, moving to

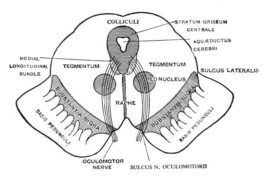

FIG. 5. Diagrammatic view of the cut surface of a transverse section through the superior part of the mesencephalon

a medial position next to the median fissure. Although the medullary decussation is known as the decussation of the pyramids, corticospinal fibres cross the midline at all levels of the brain stem to reach the motor nuclei of the cranial nerves on the opposite side. The fibres of the direct corticospinal tract also gradually cross the midline in the anterior white commissure of the spinal cord, and this tract has usually disappeared in the mid-thoracic region. (3) Uncrossed fibres are also found in the lateral column (Fulton and Sheehan, 1935). The corticospinal fibres ultimately enter the grey matter of the spinal cord. Most of them end, not in relation with the anterior horn cells, but with internuncial fibres in the intermediate zone of the grey matter (Hoff and Hoff, 1934) which enables them to activate inhibitory as well as excitatory fibres; however, some do appear to end directly on anterior horn cells [see FIG. 6, p. 30].

UNILATERAL CORTICOSPINAL LESIONS

HEMIPLEGIA

The commonest cause of hemiplegia is a vascular lesion. We shall therefore consider this as the type of a unilateral corticospinal lesion, pointing out later the distinctive features of lesions in various situations. Let us suppose then that we are investigating a patient two months after such a lesion, when the effects of shock have passed off.

POSITIVE AND NEGATIVE ELEMENTS

We must first consider a conception which we owe to Hughlings Jackson and which is of great importance in the interpretation of nervous symptoms, namely, the distinction between the positive and negative elements in nervous symptomatology. In hemiplegia we find a loss or impairment of certain functions, e.g. voluntary movement. The functions lost, or the negative elements, were clearly dependent upon the integrity of the structures destroyed, i.e. the corticospinal tract. We also observe new phenomena which were not present before the lesion, e.g. muscular hypertonia and an extensor plantar reflex. These, the positive elements, cannot be the direct result of a destructive lesion, but must be manifestations of the activity of other intact parts of the nervous system which have been released or have escaped from control as a result of the damage to the fibres destroyed. If this distinction is borne in mind it will greatly clarify neurological symptomatology.

Negative Signs

Since the corticospinal fibres carry impulses which excite voluntary movements, the negative signs of a corticospinal lesion consist of impairment or loss of such movements.

Ocular Movements. The ocular movements are dealt with in detail in a later chapter [see p. 74]. Immediately after a lesion of the corticospinal fibres in one cerebral hemisphere there is usually weakness of conjugate deviation of the eyes to the side opposite to the lesion. If the patient is unconscious the eyes are deviated to the side of the lesion by the unantagonized action of the ipsilateral lateral rectus and the contralateral medial rectus, which are innervated from the undamaged cerebral hemisphere. These ocular abnormalities usually pass off within a few hours or days of the onset; hence they are not found in the later stages of hemiplegia.

Movements of the Head. Lateral rotation of the head is a movement closely associated physiologically and anatomically with lateral deviation of the eyes. Hence we find that for a short time after a capsular lesion of the corticospinal fibres there is weakness of rotation of the head to the opposite side, and the unconscious patient usually lies with the head, like the eyes, rotated to the side of the lesion by the unantagonized action of the rotating muscles innervated from the normal hemisphere. This abnormal posture is also transitory, disappearing on the recovery of consciousness.

Facial Movements. The facial movements are not all equally weakened by a unilateral corticospinal lesion. Movements of the upper part of the face, such as elevation of the eyebrows and closure of the eyes, are little affected, probably because, like other bilaterally synchronous movements, movements of each side of the upper part of the face are under the control of both cerebral hemispheres. In contrast there is marked weakness of voluntary movements of the lower part of the face, such as retraction of the angle of the mouth in showing the teeth and pursing the lips in whistling. Emotional movements of the lower face, such as smiling and crying, and associated movements, such as involuntary retraction of the angle of the mouth on voluntary closure of the eyes, are little affected because the nervous pathways for these movements do not run with the cortico-spinal fibres.

Movements of the Lower Jaw, Soft Palate, and Tongue. Movements of the lower jaw, soft palate, and tongue are for the most part bilaterally symmetrical and synchronous. We find therefore that they are less affected by a unilateral corticospinal lesion than are movements exclusively under the control of one hemisphere. After such a lesion, however, there is usually slight weakness of the mandibular, palatal, and lingual movements on the opposite side, indicated by deviation of the jaw on opening the mouth and of the tongue on protrusion, to the side opposite to the lesion, while on phonation the palate is less arched on the opposite side and the uvula tends to be drawn to the side of the lesion.

Movements of the Limbs. In the limbs the finer and more skilled movements suffer more than the grosser and less skilled. Hence movements of the fingers and toes are weaker than movements at the proximal joints. After a slight corticospinal lesion clumsiness in carrying out fine movements with the fingers, e.g. buttoning, sewing, or playing the piano, may be more evident than actual weakness. It becomes difficult to move the thumb in isolation from the other digits. This is the basis of *Wartenberg's sign*. If a normal individual is made to flex the terminal phalanges of his fingers against the resistance offered by the observer's fingers similarly flexed, his thumb remains abducted and extended. After a corticospinal lesion, however, the thumb becomes strongly adducted and flexed. After a corticospinal lesion also, movements are not confined to the appropriate parts, but the limbs tend to move as a whole. Finally, probably owing to the distribution of the muscular hypertonia, movements of flexion tend to be stronger than those of extension in the upper limb, while the reverse is the case in the lower limb.

Respiratory Movements. As Hughlings Jackson first demonstrated, during quiet breathing the amplitude of the thoracic expansion tends to be greater on the paralysed than on the normal side, but during vigorous voluntary breathing the opposite occurs.

Gait. The hemiplegic patient in walking circumducts his paralysed leg, swinging it outwards at the hip to obviate the difficulty arising from inability to flex it at the knee. The foot is plantar-flexed, hence the toe tends to drag and the sole of his shoe thus becomes worn at the toe.

Positive Signs

Muscular Hypertonia. Immediately after a vascular lesion the paralysed limbs are usually completely flaccid owing to the occurrence of neural shock. After a variable interval, usually two or three weeks, tone gradually returns to the affected muscles and they ultimately become hypertonic or 'spastic'. This is a state of continuous contraction which manifests itself to the eye in their increased salience, and to the touch in an added tension of the muscles on palpation and in the increased resistance which they offer to passive movements at the joints. The tendon reflexes are exaggerated. Not all muscle groups exhibit hypertonia in equal degree in hemiplegia. In the upper limb the adductors and internal rotators of the shoulder, flexors of the elbow, wrist and fingers, and the pronators of the forearm are usually more spastic than their antagonists. Very rarely the increase of tone is more marked in the extensors of the elbow than in the flexors. In the lower limb the hypertonia predominates in the adductors of the hip, the extensors of the hip and knee, and in the plantar-flexors of the foot and toes. In time contractures tend to develop in the spastic muscles.

It was at one time assumed that hemiplegic spasticity is a release pheno-menon due to corticospinal damage. Tower (1940), however, stated that a pure corticospinal lesion in the monkey causes a flaccid paralysis, and Fulton (1943) believed that a lesion of area 4 leads to flaccid paralysis while ablation of area 6 causes spasticity, amongst other symptoms. The subject has been reviewed by Magoun and Rhines (1947) who regard spasticity as an un-controlled and augmented stretch reflex, produced by loss of descending inhibitory pathways running from area 4s, a suppressor zone between areas 4 and 6, to the bulbar reticular system and thence to the spinal cord, and receiving contributions from the striatum and the cerebellum. These pathways are not corticospinal. Certainly in man upper motor neurone paralysis and spasticity, though usually parallel in severity, sometimes behave as independent variables. Denny-Brown and Botterell (1948) conclude from their ablation studies that spasticity does occur after removal of area 4 alone, but the additional removal of area 6 increases the spasticity in the flexors of the elbow and the extensors of the knee and ankle. Removal of area 6 alone causes a plastic type of rigidity in both flexors and extensors of the upper and lower limb on the affected side.

Denny-Brown's (1966) most recent conclusion is that hemiplegic spasticity is a mixed phenomenon. Its earliest manifestation is a soft, yielding resistance that appears only towards the end of passive stretch and is associated with increased amplitude of tendon reflex. At this stage clonus and its associated repetitive tendon reflex, and the claspknife phenomenon are absent. These together with the hemiplegic posture are 'epiphenomena'. Hemiplegic spasticity resulting from area 4 ablation is a postural automatism resulting from release of subcortical reactions; and its primary basis is direct facilitation of alpha neurones. But a substantial part is due to release of gamma innervation [see p. 30].

Posture. The hemiplegic posture is the outcome of the selective distribution of hypertonia in the limb muscles, the more spastic muscles determining the position of the limb segments. Hence we find the upper limb usually adducted and internally rotated at the shoulder, flexed to a right angle at the elbow, somewhat pronated, and flexed at the wrist and fingers. In the exceptional cases in which hypertonia predominates in the extensors of the upper limb its attitude is one of extension at the elbow, and flexion of the wrist and fingers is less marked. The lower limb is extended, with plantar flexion and often slight inver-sion of the foot. The extensor attitude of the lower limb maintained by hyper-tonia of the extensor muscles may be regarded biologically as the posture of reflex standing, a condition akin to the extensor rigidity of the decerebrate animal.

Reflexes. The tendon reflexes on the paralysed side become exaggerated when shock has passed off, and clonus may be present in the flexors of the fingers, the quadriceps femoris, and the calf muscles. The superficial abdominal and cremasteric reflexes are diminished or lost and the plantar reflex becomes extensor. These reflex changes are more fully described on page 55. Wasting does not occur in the muscles as a result of a lesion of the corticospinal tract.

THE LOCALIZATION OF LESIONS OF THE CORTICOSPINAL TRACT

The following are the distinctive symptoms of lesions of the corticospinal tract at different points in its course.

CORTICAL LESIONS

The chief characteristic of cortical corticospinal lesions arises out of the wide surface distribution of the tract in this region. As a result of this a lesion of moderate size involves only a part of the fibres. In contrast to the conditions obtaining in the internal capsule, where the fibres are so crowded that even a small lesion usually produces a complete hemiplegia, cortical corticospinal lesions usually produce a monoplegia, that is, paralysis of the face or of one limb only, without, or with only slight, implication of parts of the body controlled by adjoining cortical areas.

Jacksonian Convulsions. Since the precentral cortex contains the bodies of the corticospinal cells, a cortical lesion in this region may lead to excitation of the corticospinal fibres, which expresses itself as a convulsion. This is of the well-recognized type described by Hughlings Jackson and hence known as Jacksonian. Such a convulsion begins as a rule with clonic movements, rarely with tonic spasm, of a small part of the opposite side of the body, usually the thumb and index finger, the angle of the mouth, or the great toe, these movements being 'those that have the widest fields of low threshold excitability' (Walshe, 1943).

As the convulsion becomes more severe the initial movement becomes more violent and the movement spreads, in the case of a limb, centripetally, involving the flexor muscles predominantly. A convulsion beginning in a limb then involves the other limb on the same side centrifugally, and the face, and finally may become bilateral, when consciousness is usually lost. Up to a point it is true to say that the spread of the convulsion corresponds to the representation of movements in the motor cortex, but the cortical march must be interpreted in physiological and not in purely anatomical terms (see Walshe, 1943).

SUBCORTICAL LESIONS

In the corona radiata the corticospinal fibres are converging towards the internal capsule and are closer together than in the cortex. Subcortical lesions tend therefore to involve more fibres than cortical lesions of equal size, and it is usual to find that, though the weakness predominates in one limb, the whole of the opposite side of the body is to some extent affected. Adjacent thalamo-cortical sensory fibres may also be involved, causing impairment of postural sensibility and tactile discrimination and localization in the affected limbs. Damage to the optic radiation causes crossed homonymous hemianopia. A lesion in the internal capsule itself is likely to cause motor symptoms on the whole of the opposite side.

LESIONS IN THE MIDBRAIN

Here the proximity of the corticospinal fibres to the third nerve sometimes adds signs of localizing value. Thus we may encounter paralysis of the third nerve with hemiplegia on the opposite side (*Weber's syndrome*). Throughout the brain stem the two corticospinal tracts lie close together. Vascular lesions are often strictly unilateral, but space-occupying lesions, such as tumours, frequently involve both corticospinal tracts. The corticospinal fibres decussate at different levels, those destined for the opposite facial nucleus, for example, crossing at the junction of the midbrain and the pons, while those which are concerned in the movements of the limbs do not cross till they reach the corticospinal decussation in the medulla. A lesion in the midline situated anteriorly at the junction of the midbrain and pons may thus involve only the decussating fibres running to the facial nuclei, and so produce facial diplegia of the supranuclear type. This may be associated with bilateral paralysis of lateral conjugate ocular deviation, the supranuclear fibres for this movement crossing the midline at the same level.

LESIONS IN THE PONS

Owing to the higher level of decussation of the corticofacial fibres a uni-lateral corticospinal lesion in the pons does not cause weakness of the opposite side of the face, but only of the opposite bulbar muscles and limbs. The lesion may, however, also involve the facial nucleus or the intrapontine fibres of the facial nerve on the same side, thus causing one form of 'crossed hemiplegia'. Many forms of this have been described and named after their earliest observers.

Millard-Gubler syndrome consists of paralysis of the lateral rectus, with or without facial paralysis of the lower motor neurone type on one side and supranuclear paralysis of the bulbar muscles and limbs on the opposite side.

Foville's syndrome is similar to Millard-Gubler syndrome, except that paralysis of conjugate ocular deviation to the side of the lesion takes the place of lateral rectus paralysis.

Ipsilateral paralysis of the jaw muscles may be associated with either of these syndromes. When the lesion is situated deeply in the pons, near the midline, involvement of the medial lemniscus causes impairment of postural sensibility on the opposite side of the body. When the lesion is mainly in the lateral region of the pons the lemniscus escapes, but damage to the spinothalamic tract causes crossed analgesia and thermo-anaesthesia, with or without some impairment of sensibility in the trigeminal area on the side of the lesion, owing to involvement of the trigeminal fibres within the pons.

Horner's syndrome, paralysis of the ocular sympathetic, may also result from a lesion in the tegmentum of the pons.

LESIONS IN THE MEDULLA

Many varieties of crossed hemiplegia have been described as a result of unilateral medullary lesions. A lesion near the midline will involve the cortico-spinal fibres to the limbs above their decussation, together with the fibres of the hypoglossal nerve, causing unilateral paralysis of half of the tongue, with crossed hemiplegia of the limbs, to which loss of postural sensibility in the paralysed limbs may be added. When the lateral region of the medulla is affected as well there will also be paralysis of the soft palate and vocal cord, with Horner's syndrome and trigeminal analgesia and thermo-anaesthesia and some cerebellar deficiency, all on the side of the lesion, with loss of appreciation of pain, heat, and cold in the limbs and trunk on the opposite side. Vascular lesions in the midline of the medulla may involve both corticospinal tracts, leading to quadriplegia with unilateral paralysis of the tongue.

SPINAL HEMIPLEGIA

A unilateral lesion of the corticospinal tract in the spinal cord below the medulla and above the fifth cervical segment causes hemiplegia involving the limbs on the affected side but without paralysis of the muscles innervated by the cranial nerves.

DECEREBRATE MAN

Decerebrate rigidity in animals, according to Denny-Brown (1966), is due to overactivity of the gamma efferent fibres to the muscles resulting from release of a structure in the reticular formation of the lower pons from higher control. Its influence is mediated by the medial reticulospinal tract.

A condition which appears to be physiologically homologous with decerebration in the animal may occur in man, either in the form of a convulsion or as a prolonged state of muscular hypertonia without loss of consciousness. The convulsions—'tonic' fits, or 'cerebellar' fits of Hughlings Jackson—are characterized by opisthotonos and rigid extension of all four limbs. The upper limbs are internally rotated at the shoulder, extended at the elbow and hyperpronated, and the fingers are extended at the metacarpophalangeal joints and flexed at the interphalangeal joints. The lower limbs are extended at the hip and knee, and the ankles and toes are plantar flexed. This human decerebrate attitude has been observed to result from lesions at the level of the upper part of the midbrain, such as tumours arising in the midbrain, and pineal tumours and tumours of the cerebellar vermis, which compress the midbrain from without. It may also be produced by diffuse cerebral disturbances, such as anoxia, hydrocephalus and diffuse sclerosis, which grossly damage the functions of both cerebral hemispheres.

REFERENCES

BRAIN, W. R. (1927) On the significance of the flexor posture of the upper limb in hemiplegia, with an account of a quadrupedal extensor reflex, *Brain*, **50**, 113.

CLARK, G. (1948) The mode of representation in the motor cortex, *Brain*, **71**, 320.

DENNY-BROWN, D. (1951) The frontal lobes and their functions, in *Modern Trends in Neurology*, ed. Feiling, A., p. 13, London.

DENNY-BROWN, D. (1966) *The Cerebral Control of Movement*, Liverpool University Press, Liverpool.

DENNY-BROWN, D., and BOTTERELL, E. H. (1948) The motor functions of the agranular frontal cortex, *Res. Publ. Ass. nerv. ment. Dis.*, **27**, 235.

FOERSTER, O. (1931) The cerebral cortex in man, *Lancet*, ii, 309.

FOERSTER, O. (1936) The motor cortex in man in the light of Hughlings Jackson's doctrines, *Brain*, **59**, 135.

FULTON, J. F. (1943) *Physiology of the Nervous System*, 2nd ed., New York.

FULTON, J. F., and SHEEHAN, D. (1935) The uncrossed lateral pyramidal tract in higher primates. *J. Anat. (Lond.)*, **69**, 181.

HOFF, E. C., and HOFF, H. E. (1934) Spinal terminations of the projection fibres from the motor cortex of primates, *Brain*, **57**, 454.

KREIG, W. J. S. (1966) *Functional Neuroanatomy*, 3rd ed., Evanston, Ill.

MAGOUN, H. W., and RHINES, R. (1947) *Spasticity*, Springfield, Ill.

PENFIELD, W., and JASPER, H. (1954) *Epilepsy and the Functional Anatomy of the Human Brain*, p. 60, London.

TOWER, S. S. (1940) Pyramidal lesions in the monkey, *Brain*, **63**, 36.

WALSH, E. G. (1963) *Physiology of the Nervous System*, 2nd ed., London.

WALSHE, F. M. R. (1942) The giant cells of Betz, the motor cortex and the pyramidal tract: a critical review, *Brain*, **65**, 409.

WALSHE, F. M. R. (1943) On the mode of representation of movements in the motor cortex, with special reference to 'convulsions beginning unilaterally' (Jackson), *Brain*, **66**, 104.

WALSHE, F. M. R. (1965) *Further Critical Studies in Neurology*, Edinburgh.

WILSON, S. A. K. (1920) On decerebrate rigidity in man and the occurrence of tonic fits, *Brain*, **43**, 220.

THE LOWER MOTOR NEURONE

The cell bodies of the lower motor neurones (alpha neurones) are situated in the motor nuclei of the brain stem and the anterior horns of the grey matter of the spinal cord. Each motor neurone is influenced by impulses reaching it from many nerve fibres—from the corticospinal tracts by way of interneurones and also from those nerve fibres which act as conductors in the reflex arcs. Between each such nerve terminal and the body of the motor neurone lies a synapse. An excitatory nerve fibre alters the synapse so as to depolarize the cell membrane of the motor neurone; an inhibitory fibre acts by hyperpolarizing it (Eccles, 1957).

The axons of the motor neurones pass into the cranial and spinal nerves, reaching the latter by way of the ventral roots, the motor functions of which were first recognized by Bell in 1811. From the spinal nerves they are distributed to the peripheral nerves, those destined for the limbs passing *en route* through the cervical, lumbar, and sacral plexuses. Each lower motor neurone terminates in relation to a bundle of 150 or more muscle fibres. Injury to the lower motor neurone leads to characteristic symptoms.

SYMPTOMS OF LESIONS OF THE LOWER MOTOR NEURONE

MUSCULAR WEAKNESS AND WASTING

Weakness or complete paralysis occurs in the affected muscles, according to the severity of the lesion. This is an impairment of the function of the muscle itself, and therefore is manifest equally in all movements in which the affected muscle normally plays a part.

MUSCULAR WASTING

Muscular wasting occurs in the affected muscles. This is conspicuous within two or three weeks of an acute lesion, such as acute poliomyelitis or division of a motor nerve, but develops very gradually in chronic disorders such as motor neurone disease.

DISTRIBUTION

The distribution of the weakness and wasting is the outcome of the grouping of the lower motor neurones at the point at which the damage occurs [see p. 31].

HYPOTONIA

Since muscle tone is a state of sustained contraction resulting from impulses reaching the muscles by the lower motor neurones [see p. 30], a lesion of this pathway causes hypotonia, which is manifested in flaccidity and a diminished resistance to stretching of the affected muscles.

REFLEXES

The reflexes in which the affected muscles take part are diminished or lost through interruption of their motor paths. An apparent exception to the rule that hypotonia and loss of reflexes result from lower motor neurone lesions is found when the same patient has also a lesion of the upper motor neurone, as in motor neurone disease. In such cases the hypertonia and increased tendon reflexes produced by the upper motor neurone lesion may more than counter-balance the opposite effects of the lower motor neurone lesion. Such patients may show increased tendon reflexes in the wasted muscles—so-called 'tonic muscular atrophy'.

MUSCULAR FASCICULATION

Fascicular twitching of muscles is seen in its most typical form as a result of chronic degeneration of the anterior horn cells in progressive muscular atrophy. In such cases each twitch involves a group of muscle fibres. It does not occur when these cells are rapidly injured or destroyed as in the acute stage of poliomyelitis; and it is rare when they suffer from compression as in syringo-myelia or spinal tumour. It is occasionally seen in acute inflammatory lesions of the peripheral nerves, for example when the facial nerve is involved in herpes zoster of the geniculate ganglion, and, rarely, in sciatic root compression, but is absent in polyneuritis and the muscular dystrophies. Fascicular twitching of the facial muscles, especially the orbicularis oculi, is common as a transitory occur-rence in normal persons—'live flesh', or myokymia—and is also found in clonic facial spasm, a progressive disorder of unexplained origin. Spasmodic facial contractions are also seen after incomplete recovery from facial paralysis. A few isolated muscular twitchings are often seen in bedridden patients, especially in the calves. Muscular disease may rarely cause fasciculation, e.g. thyrotoxic myopathy and polymyositis.

MUSCULAR CONTRACTURES

Muscular contracture, leading to permanent shortening, may occur in muscles of which the lower motor neurones are damaged, for example in the facial muscles after Bell's paralysis. More often it develops in their antagonists, the action of which is no longer opposed by the paralysed muscles. An example of this is contracture of the calf muscles following paralysis of the anterior tibial group and the peronei in poliomyelitis. Appropriate splinting, passive move-ments, and massage are required to prevent such contractures.

TROPHIC CHANGES

Lesions of the lower motor neurones are often attended by so-called trophic changes. The affected extremity is cold and cyanosed, the finger- and toe-nails are brittle, and the bones are smaller and lighter than normal. These changes are probably due partly to disuse, with loss of the influence of muscular action upon the circulation and the development of the bones, and partly to vasomotor paralysis from destruction of the vasoconstrictor fibres of the sympathetic.

REACTION OF DEGENERATION

Normal muscles respond vigorously to stimulation by the faradic (interrupted) and galvanic (constant) currents. Faradism causes a muscular contraction which persists as long as the current is passing. Galvanism causes a contraction only when the current is made or broken, but not while it is passing. After a lesion of the lower motor neurone a muscle ceases to respond to faradic stimulation of its motor point in from four to seven days. After ten days a normal response to galvanism ceases to be obtainable, but the muscle responds to this form of stimulus by a sluggish, wave-like contraction starting at the point stimulated and requiring a stronger current for its elicitation than the normal muscle. This change is known as 'the reaction of degeneration'. The charting of strength-duration curves has now proved to be more useful than this simple faradic-galvanic test.

ELECTROMYOGRAPHY

Electrical records obtained directly from the muscles by electromyography give much more detailed and accurate information of muscular function than the test for reaction of degeneration, which has been superseded by electromyography in the diagnosis of lesions of the lower motor neurone and muscular disorders. A concentric needle electrode is inserted into a muscle and the electrical potentials amplified and observed on a cathode-ray oscillograph and recorded. The characteristic changes are discussed in the appropriate sections.

MUSCLE TONE

Muscle tone, as Sherrington showed, is reflex in origin. The muscle spindles are the receptors in the muscles which respond to stretch by sending impulses which travel in the largest afferent fibres from the muscles to the spinal cord. The muscle spindles are themselves innervated by the smallest, gamma, efferent fibres in the ventral spinal roots [FIG. 6], and these have been shown to regulate the response of the muscle spindles, acting synergically with external stretch. So by means of the stretch or myotatic reflex and the lengthening and shortening reactions, also described by Sherrington, muscle tone is reflexly maintained and adjusted to the needs of posture and movement. Hence interruption of the reflex arc on its afferent or efferent side leads to hypotonia.

This spinal reflex mechanism is profoundly influenced by higher levels of the nervous system. It is depressed by spinal shock. As the cerebellum is facilitatory to the stretch reflex cerebellar deficiency causes hypotonia. The reticular formation is also facilitatory, as is seen when removal of higher inhibitory control over it causes decerebrate rigidity [see p. 26]. Loss of corticospinal influence

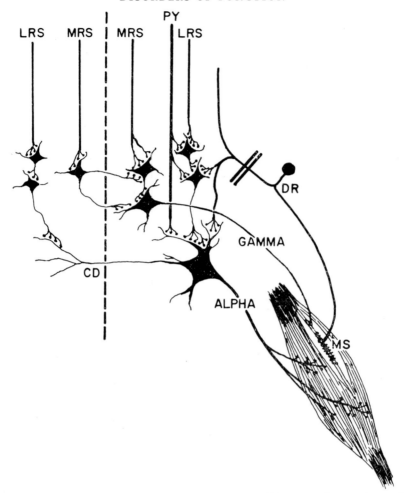

FIG. 6. Diagram to show how the gamma neurone providing motor innervation to the muscle spindle (MS) can, by increasing its sensitivity, facilitate afferent impulses from the annulospinal ending to provide excitation for alpha motor neurones of the same muscle. The medial reticulospinal tracts (MRS) drive the gamma neurone. The lateral reticulospinal tract (LRS) and pyramidal tract (PY) end on the alpha system. The broken line represents the midline. Decussating pathways from the opposite side of spinal cord have access to both types of activation of the alpha motor neurones. Section of the dorsal roots (DR) at the point shown by the bars blocks activation via the gamma neurone. (From Denny-Brown, D. (1966) *The Cerebral Control of Movement*, by kind permission of the author and Liverpool University Press)

also causes spasticity [see p. 23]. The influence of the striatum is complex, but damage to the substantia nigra causes hypertonia (Magoun and Rhines, 1947; Kuffler and Hunt, 1952).

SEGMENTATION IN THE SPINAL CORD

It will be remembered that early in foetal development the body shows a division into a series of segments or metameres. This primitive segmentation to a large extent determines the subsequent plan of the lower motor and first sensory neurones at their emergence from, and entrance into, the spinal cord. Corresponding to each spinal segment is one pair of spinal nerves composed of the ventral and dorsal roots of that segment. The cell bodies of the first sensory neurone, which lie in the dorsal root ganglia, are completely separated in each segment from those of the segments above and below. The cell bodies of the lower motor neurones, however, lie in longitudinal columns in the anterior horns, hence their segmental grouping is less distinct. Nevertheless, the emergence of their axons by a series of separate ventral roots is the basis of a motor segmental arrangement, for we may regard as a segment of the cord from the aspect of motility that group of anterior horn cells of which the axons emerge by one pair of ventral roots and join one pair of spinal nerves.

THE SEGMENTAL REPRESENTATION OF MUSCLES

As we have seen, the cells of the anterior horns lie in longitudinal columns and those which innervate a single muscle commonly extend over more than one segment longitudinally. Further, a number of such longitudinal columns may be recognized cut transversely in a transverse section of the cord. Hence several muscles may be represented in the same segment. It follows that complete destruction of the anterior horn cells in one segment, or of their axons in one ventral root or spinal nerve, causes weakness of all those muscles which are innervated from that segment, but completely paralyses only such as have no nerve supply from adjacent segments.

Through the cervical and lumbosacral plexuses the axons of the lower motor neurones are redistributed and enter into new groupings in the peripheral nerves. Consequently, the fibres from a single spinal segment may reach several peripheral nerves, and conversely, a single peripheral nerve may receive fibres from several spinal segments. Thus we can distinguish between a lesion of a spinal segment, ventral root, or spinal nerve, on the one hand, and a lesion of a peripheral nerve on the other, because the resulting muscular weakness has a distinctive anatomical distribution. For example, the fifth cervical spinal segment innervates the supraspinatus and infraspinatus, deltoid, biceps, brachialis and brachioradialis, muscles which receive their peripheral nerve supply from the suprascapular, axillary, musculocutaneous, and radial nerves respectively. These muscles cannot be paralysed by a lesion involving any single peripheral nerve, nor could a peripheral nerve lesion affect them without affecting others. Such a distribution of muscular weakness indicates a segmental lesion.

On the other hand, if the brachioradialis muscle is paralysed in association with the triceps and the extensors of the wrist and fingers, this grouping points to a lesion of the radial nerve which supplies all these muscles.

MUSCULAR SUPPLY OF PERIPHERAL NERVES

[Modified from Bing, R. (1927).]

A. PLEXUS CERVICALIS (C_1–C_4)

Nn. cervicales	Mm. longus colli	Flexion, extension, and rotation of the neck
	Mm. scaleni	Elevation of ribs (inspiration)
N. phrenicus	Diaphragma	Inspiration

B. Plexus Brachialis (C_5–T_2)

N. thoracic. ant.	M. pect. maj. et min.	Adduction and forward depression of the arm
N. thoracic. long.	M. serrat. ant.	Fixation of the scapula during elevation of the arm
N. dorsalis scap.	M. levator scapul.	Elevation of the scapula
	Mm. rhomboidei	Elevation and drawing inwards of the scapula
N. suprascap.	M. supraspinatus	Elevation and external rotation of the arm
	M. infraspinatus	External rotation of the arm
N. subscapul.	M. latissimus dors. ⎫ M. teres major ⎭	⎰ Internal rotation and dorsal adduction ⎱ of the arm
	M. subscapularis	Internal rotation of the arm
N. axillaris	M. deltoideus	Elevation of the arm to the horizontal
	M. teres minor	External rotation of the arm
N. musculocut.	M. biceps brach.	Flexion and supination of the forearm
	M. coracobrachialis	Flexion and adduction of the forearm
	M. brachialis	Flexion of the forearm
N. medianus	M. pronator teres	Pronation
	M. flexor carpi rad.	Flexion and radial flexion of the hand
	M. palm. long.	Flexion of the hand
	M. flex. digit. superficialis	Flexion of the middle phalanges of the fingers
	M. flex. poll. long.	Flexion of the terminal phalanx of the thumb
	M. flex. digit. (radial portion)	Flexion of the terminal phalanges of the index and middle fingers
	M. abduct. poll. brev.	Abduction of the first metacarpal
	M. flex. poll. brev.	Flexion of the first phalanx of the thumb
	M. opponens poll.	Opposition of the first metacarpal
N. ulnaris	M. flexor carpi uln.	Flexion and ulnar flexion of the hand
	M. flex. digit. prof. (ulnar portion)	Flexion of the terminal phalanges of the ring and little fingers
	M. adductor poll.	Adduction of the first metacarpal
	Mm. hypothenares	Abduction, opposition, and flexion of the little finger
	Mm. lumbricales	Flexion of the first phalanges, extension of the others
	Mm. interossei	The same; in addition, abduction and adduction of the fingers
N. radialis	M. triceps brach.	Extension of the forearm
	M. brachioradialis	Flexion of the forearm
	M. extensor carpi rad.	Extension and radial flexion of the hand
	M. extensor digit.	Extension of the first phalanges of the fingers
	M. extensor digit. minimi	Extension of the first phalanx of the little finger
	M. extensor carpi uln.	Extension and ulnar flexion of the hand
	M. supinator brevis	Supination of the forearm
	M. abduct. poll. longus	Abduction of the first metacarpal
	M. extensor poll. brevis	Extension of the first phalanx of the thumb

	M. extensor poll. longus	Abduction of the first metacarpal and extension of the terminal phalanx of the thumb
	M. extensor indic. prop.	Extension of the first phalanx of the index finger

C. Nn. Thoracales (T$_1$—T$_{12}$)

	Mm. thoracici et abdominales	Elevation of the ribs, expiration, compression of abdominal viscera, &c.

D. Plexus Lumbalis (T$_{12}$—L$_4$)

N. femoralis	M. iliopsoas	Flexion of the hip
	M. sartorius	Internal rotation of the leg
	M. quadriceps	Extension of the leg
N. obturatorius	M. pectineus M. adductor longus M. adductor brevis M. adductor magnus M. gracilis	Adduction of the thigh
	M. obturator extern.	Adduction and external rotation of the thigh

E. Plexus Sacralis (L$_5$—S$_5$)

N. gluteus sup.	M. gluteus med. M. gluteus min.	Abduction and internal rotation of the thigh
	M. tens. fasciae latae	Flexion of the thigh
	M. piriformis	External rotation of the thigh
N. gluteus inf.	M. gluteus max.	Extension of the thigh
N. ischiadicus	M. obturator int. Mm. gemelli M. quadratus fem.	External rotation of the thigh
	M. biceps femoris M. semitendinosus M. semimembranosus	Flexion of the leg
N. peroneus:		
(a) Prof.	M. tibialis ant.	Dorsal flexion and inversion of the foot
	M. extens. digit. long.	Extension of the toes
	M. extens. hall. long.	Extension of the great toe
	M. extens. digit. brev.	Extension of the toes
	M. extens. hall. brev.	Extension of the great toe
(b) Superf.	Mm. peronei	Dorsal flexion and eversion of the foot
N. tibialis	M. gastrocnemius M. soleus	Plantar flexion of the foot
	M. tibialis post.	Plantar flexion and inversion of the foot
	M. flex. digit. long.	Flexion of the terminal phalanges, II–V
	M. flex. halluc. long.	Flexion of the terminal phalanx of the great toe
	M. flex. digit. brev.	Flexion of the middle phalanges, II–V
	M. flex. halluc. brev.	Flexion of the first phalanx of the great toe
	Mm. interossei plant.	Movements of the toes
N. pudendus	Mm. perinei et sphinct.	Closure of sphincters, co-operation in sexual act

SEGMENTAL INNERVATION OF MUSCLES OF UPPER EXTREMITY

[Modified from Bing, R. (1927).]

	CERVICAL SEGMENTS				THORACIC SEGMENTS
	5	**6**	**7**	**8**	**1**
SHOULDER	Supraspinatus				
	Teres minor				
	Deltoid				
	Infraspinatus				
	Subscapularis				
	Teres major				
ARM	Biceps brachii				
	Brachialis				
		Coracobrachialis			
		Triceps brachii			
			Anconeus		
FOREARM	Brachioradialis				
	Supinator				
	Extensores carpi radialis				
	Pronator teres				
	Flexor carpi radialis				
	Flexor pollicis longus				
		Abductor pollicis longus			
		Extensor pollicis brevis			
		Extensor pollicis longus			
		Extensor digitorum communis			
		Extensor indicis			
		Extensor carpi ulnaris			
		Extensor digiti minimi			
			Flexor digitorum superficialis		
			Flexor digitorum profundus		
			Pronator quadratus		
				Flexor carpi ulnaris	
			Palmaris longus		
HAND		Abductor pollicis brevis			
		Flexor pollicis brevis			
		Opponens pollicis			
			Flexor digiti minimi brevis		
			Opponens digiti minimi		
				Adductor pollicis	
				Palmaris brevis	
				Abductor digiti minimi	
				Lumbricales	
				Interossei	

SEGMENTAL INNERVATION OF TRUNK MUSCLES

[Modified from Bing, R. (1927).]

SEGMENTAL INNERVATION OF MUSCLES OF LOWER EXTREMITY

[Modified from Bing, R. (1927).]

	T12	L1	L2	L3	L4	L5	S1	S2
HIP								
Iliopsoas		◼	◼	◼	◼			
Tensor fasciae latae					◼	◼	◼	
Gluteus medius					◼	◼	◼	
Gluteus minimus					◼	◼	◼	
Quadratus femoris					◼	◼	◼	
Gemellus inferior					◼	◼	◼	
Gemellus superior						◼	◼	◼
Gluteus maximus						◼	◼	◼
Obturator internus						◼	◼	◼
Piriformis							◼	◼
THIGH								
Sartorius			◼	◼				
Pectineus			◼	◼				
Adductor longus			◼	◼				
Quadriceps femoris			◼	◼	◼			
Gracilis			◼	◼	◼			
Adductor brevis			◼	◼	◼			
Obturator externus				◼	◼			
Adductor magnus				◼	◼			
Adductor minimus				◼	◼			
Articularis genu				◼	◼			
LEG								
Semitendinosus					◼	◼	◼	◼
Semimembranosus					◼	◼	◼	◼
Biceps femoris						◼	◼	◼
Tibialis anterior					◼	◼		
Extensor hallucis longus					◼	◼	◼	
Popliteus					◼	◼	◼	
Plantaris					◼	◼	◼	
Extensor digitorum longus					◼	◼	◼	
Soleus						◼	◼	◼
Gastrocnemius						◼	◼	◼
Peroneus longus						◼	◼	
Peroneus brevis						◼	◼	
Tibialis posterior						◼	◼	
Flexor digitorum longus						◼	◼	◼
Flexor hallucis longus						◼	◼	◼
FOOT								
Extensor hallucis brevis					◼	◼	◼	
Extensor digitorum brevis					◼	◼	◼	
Flexor digitorum brevis						◼	◼	
Abductor hallucis						◼	◼	
Flexor hallucis brevis						◼	◼	◼
Lumbricales						◼	◼	◼
Abductor hallucis							◼	◼
Abductor digiti minimi							◼	◼
Flexor digiti minimi brevis							◼	◼
Opponens digiti minimi							◼	◼
Quadratus plantae							◼	◼
Interossei							◼	◼

REFERENCES

BING, R. (1927) *Compendium of Regional Diagnosis*, pp. 39–49, London.

DENNY-BROWN, D., and PENNYBACKER, J. B. (1938) Fibrillation and fasciculation in voluntary muscle, *Brain*, **61**, 311.

ECCLES, J. C. (1957) *The Physiology of Nerve Cells*, Baltimore.

KUFFLER, S. W., and HUNT, C. C. (1952) The mammalian small-nerve fibers, a system for efferent nervous regulation of muscle spindle discharge, *Res. Publ. Ass. nerv. ment. Dis.*, **30**, 24.

MAGOUN, H. W., and RHINES, R. (1947) *Spasticity*, Springfield, Ill.

SENSATION

THE EXAMINATION OF SENSATION

The neurologist is concerned with sensibility primarily for the purpose of localizing lesions in the nervous system and determining their nature. His methods of investigation are therefore more 'rough and ready' than those of the experimental psychologist, and have been adopted on account of their practical value for his immediate purpose.

SPONTANEOUS SENSATIONS

The investigation should begin with a careful inquiry whether the patient has experienced any abnormal spontaneous sensations or paraesthesiae. The commonest such sensation is pain, but in addition parts of the body may be described as feeling hot, cold, numb, dead, or heavy, and such abnormal feelings as constriction, itching, tingling, 'pins and needles', and 'electric shocks' may be experienced. When a patient complains of an abnormal sensation it is necessary to ascertain its situation and duration, whether it irradiates and if so in what direction, whether it is excited by movement or by any external stimulus, and whether it is attended by hypersensitiveness of the skin to painful or other stimuli.

'Root-pains' are pains due to a lesion of one or more spinal dorsal roots and are experienced in the segmental areas innervated by the affected roots. They may be excited or intensified by coughing or sneezing or changes of posture.

A patient with a lesion of the posterior columns of the spinal cord in the cervical region may complain of a feeling like an electric shock radiating through the body on flexing or extending the cervical spine.

A strange sensory abnormality is the 'phantom limb'. A patient who has lost a limb by amputation may continue to feel as if the limb were still there, and may even experience pain in the phantom limb. Similarly a patient who has lost postural sensation in a limb or limbs as a result of a lesion of the spinal cord or brain may imagine that he feels his anaesthetic limb and that it occupies a posture different from its real position.

OBJECTIVE SENSORY TESTS

Light Touch. The appreciation of light touch is most conveniently investigated by means of a very small wisp of cotton wool applied to the shaved skin, care being taken that no pressure is exerted upon the skin. The patient with his eyes closed is asked to reply each time he feels a touch.

Pressure Touch. Pressure touch is similarly investigated by pressing with a blunt object such as the unsharpened end of a pencil.

Localization of Touch. The part of the body under investigation is screened from the patient's eyes and after he has been touched he is asked to name the spot or to point to it. For greater accuracy he may indicate it upon a diagram.

Superficial Pain. Superficial pain is investigated by pricking the skin with a pin or needle. It should be noted that this stimulus evokes a tactile sensation of sharpness as well as a feeling of pain. The patient's attention must therefore be directed to the painful element in the feeling. Two sensory effects of pinprick have now been distinguished—an immediate and a slightly delayed sensation of pain, differing somewhat in quality and known as 'first' and 'second' pain. In mapping out cutaneous areas of analgesia or hyperalgesia the point of a pin may be dragged along the skin, the patient being asked to say when the change to normal or exaggerated painful sensibility occurs.

Pressure Pain. Deep pressure, if sufficiently vigorous, normally excites pain. This is most simply tested by compressing a muscle between the fingers and thumb or by squeezing a tendon such as the tendo calcaneus.

Temperature. For testing appreciation of temperature, metal tubes, made of copper or silver, should be used, since glass is a relatively poor conductor of heat. For ordinary purposes one tube should be filled with ice and the other with water at a temperature of 45° C. The tubes are applied to the skin and the patient is asked to describe his sensations. If the water is too hot confusion may arise, since a sensation of pain may be excited.

Perceptual Rivalry. Sometimes loss of cutaneous sensibility may be demonstrable only if corresponding points on both sides of the body are stimulated simultaneously, the stimulus on the abnormal side undergoing extinction [see p. 50].

Postural Sensibility. Postural sensibility, or sense of position, is tested by placing a segment of a limb in a certain position and asking the patient with his eyes closed to describe its posture or imitate it with the opposite limb.

Passive Movement. Power of appreciating passive movement is tested by passively moving a segment of a limb at a joint and finding the angle through which it has to be moved in order that the patient can appreciate the movement. The part to be moved should always be grasped in such a way that the observer's fingers are applied to surfaces parallel to the plane of movement to eliminate the perception of variations in their pressure. Slighter degrees of movement are appreciated at the joints of the fingers and toes than at the more proximal joints of the limbs. Normally a movement of a few degrees is recognized at the interphalangeal and metacarpo- and metatarsophalangeal joints. The patient may also be asked to identify passive movements of the auricle.

Vibration. To test the appreciation of vibration, a tuning-fork C° beating 128 times a second is struck and applied to the part to be investigated. Normally the characteristic tingling sensation is readily felt. Normally also if the patient is asked to say when he ceases to feel the vibration and the fork is then transferred to the opposite limb it again becomes perceptible. When appreciation of vibration is impaired on one side of the body this second response is longer when the fork is transferred from the affected to the normal side than vice versa.

Tactile Discrimination. Tactile discrimination is measured by ascertaining the distance which two compass-points require to be separated in order that the patient may appreciate them as two and not one. Special compasses with blunt points are used, and these are furnished with a scale which indicates the distance the points are separated. The part to be tested is successively touched with two points and with one in a random order, and the number of correct answers and errors noted. The corresponding part on the opposite side, when normal, is used as a control, and to determine the normal threshold, that is, the distance of separation necessary for accurate discrimination. Normally 3–4 mm. of separation is appreciated on the palmar surface of the tips of the thumb and fingers.

Appreciation of Form. Stereognosis, or the appreciation of form in three dimensions, is tested by asking the patient with his eyes closed to recognize common objects placed in his hand. If there is paralysis of the fingers the object must be moved about in the patient's hand by the observer.

THE FIRST SENSORY NEURONE

ANATOMY AND PHYSIOLOGY

The first sensory neurone is the path by which sensory impulses from the periphery reach the central nervous system. The cell bodies of the first sensory neurones are situated in the spinal dorsal root ganglia and in the corresponding sensory ganglia of the cranial nerves. They are bipolar cells, one process being distributed to the periphery and the other entering the spinal cord or brain stem. The peripheral process in some instances enters into relation with sensory end-organs, which are the specific receptors for certain forms of sensibility though there is evidence that some receptors are sensitive to more than one kind of stimulus. The nerve fibres concerned in the appreciation of pain appear to be devoid of end-organs and to terminate as free nerve endings. The receptors for heat and cold are not evenly distributed throughout the skin, but are situated in localized heat and cold spots. Krause's end-bulbs are believed to be the specific endings for cold and Ruffini's corpuscles for heat. Merkel's discs and Meissner's corpuscles are end-organs which are probably concerned in the appreciation of light touch. The hairs are also tactile organs and the hair follicles are richly supplied with nerve endings. Tickle is a form of tactile sensation, and itching is conducted by pain fibres. The Golgi–Mazzoni endings subserve pressure. The Pacinian corpuscles are distributed to the deeper parts of the dermis and to the tendons, periosteum, and the neighbourhood of the joints. These are responsive to mechanical stimuli. In addition muscles and tendons possess specialized sensory end-organs—the muscle and tendon spindles. Each dorsal root fibre breaks up to supply many nerve endings, sometimes hundreds, disposed in three dimensions, i.e. surface area and depth.

Sensibility may be divided into somatic and visceral forms of sensation. Somatic sensibility again may be divided into exteroceptive and proprioceptive forms. Exteroceptive sensibility is concerned with the appreciation of stimuli coming from outside the body and includes cutaneous sensibility and the special senses. Proprioceptive sensibility is the appreciation of the posture and movements of the body itself. Proprioceptive impulses are derived from the labyrinths and the muscles, tendons, and joints. Not all proprioceptive afferent impulses reach consciousness. Many are concerned in reflex activities at the spinal level or influence the cerebellum in its control of movement and posture.

Sensory fibres in the peripheral nerves vary in size and in the rate at which they conduct impulses, which ranges from 100 to 0·5 metres per second. Gasser recognizes three groups of fibres, A, B, and C, in order of diminishing velocity, and distinguishes four subdivisions in A group. Touch and pressure impulses are thought to be carried by A fibres, while pain has a wide range. Two varieties of painful response to a single stimulus have been distinguished—first, pain which is 'bright' or pricking in quality, and second, pain which is burning and is experienced only after a brief delay. These two sensations have been correlated with fibres of different size and rates of conduction (Lewis, 1942) but for a recent discussion of this question see Sinclair (1955). In the skin, pain sensation depends upon a network of interlocking nerve endings so arranged that a given 'sensory spot' is normally supplied from several nerve fibres. Owing to the overlapping distribution of the peripheral nerves themselves it is necessary to distinguish a maximal zone comprising the full distribution of a nerve and an autonomous zone which is the area it exclusively supplies. The difference between them is the intermediate zone.

We can recognize two abnormal forms of painful sensibility. *Hyperalgesia* is present when pain is evoked from skin or deep structures at a lower threshold than normally, and is found when pain endings are exposed owing to injury or surrounded by irritant humoral products. *Protopathic pain*, to use Head's term, is pain of a peculiarly unpleasant and irradiating character usually associated with a raised threshold of stimulation (*hyperpathia*). There is evidence which suggests that protopathic pain, which may be the result of a lesion of a peripheral nerve, the spinothalamic tract, or the thalamus itself, is caused by a reduction in the normal number of conducting pain fibres (Weddell, Sinclair, and Feindel, 1948). *Referred pain*, by which is meant the irradiation of pain, with or without hyperalgesia, into an area of skin when a viscus or muscle is the site of the lesion, is still without a completely satisfactory explanation. Excitation of a common pathway must underlie the phenomenon, but opinions differ as to whether it is in the brain, the spinal cord, or the peripheral nerves (Lewis, 1942; Sinclair, Weddell, and Feindel, 1948).

CUTANEOUS SENSORY SEGMENTATION

Primitive organisms frequently exhibit metameric segmentation of the body, and this arrangement is evident in the human foetus during the early stages of its development. Each somatic segment or metamere is linked to the corresponding segment of the neuraxis by a pair of spinal nerves. In the course of evolution the specialization of the anterior end of the organism to form the head, and the growth of the complicated motor and sensory functions of the limbs have interfered with the primitive metameric segmentation of the nervous system, which in man is now found in its simplest form only in the thoracic region.

Each spinal nerve is formed by a fusion of one ventral and one dorsal spinal root, the ventral root conveying efferent and the dorsal mainly afferent fibres. The sensory character of the dorsal roots was first recognized by Magendie in 1822. After this fusion the spinal nerve divides peripherally into its ventral and dorsal primary divisions, both containing motor and sensory fibres. The dorsal primary division conveys motor fibres to the muscles of the spine and sensory fibres to the overlying cutaneous area. The ventral primary division in its simplest form, for example in the mid-thoracic region, supplies motor fibres to the intercostal muscles and sensory fibres to a narrow zone extending horizontally round the thorax on one side as far as the middle line. At the cervical and lumbosacral enlargements of the cord the arrangement is complicated by the formation of the limb plexuses, in which several of the ventral primary divisions unite and subsequently subdivide to form the peripheral nerves to the limbs. Through the intervention of the plexuses a single spinal nerve may send both motor and sensory contributions to several peripheral nerves, and, conversely, a single peripheral nerve may receive contributions from several spinal nerves. It follows that the sensory loss resulting from interruption of a peripheral nerve differs in its distribution from that produced by interruption of a posterior root or spinal nerve. A segmental or radicular cutaneous area— dermatome—is an area of skin which receives its sensory supply from a single dorsal root and spinal nerve. In the trunk these segmental areas still exhibit a metameric arrangement. In the limbs this has been modified, but as a rule the segmental areas occupy elongated zones in the long axis of the limb [FIG. 7]. Owing to the specialization of the ventral primary divisions of the lower cervical and first thoracic spinal nerves in the innervation of the upper limb, these have lost their cutaneous supply to the trunk anteriorly, and at the level of the second rib the fourth cervical segmental cutaneous area is contiguous with the second thoracic. The lower six thoracic spinal nerves supply the abdominal wall as low as the inguinal ligament. Probably owing to the fact that the dorsal primary divisions of the spinal nerves take no part in the formation of the limb plexuses, all spinal segments appear to be represented in the cutaneous supply of the back.

There is considerable overlapping of contiguous segmental cutaneous areas, hence the division of a single dorsal root does not cause any sensory loss detectable by ordinary clinical methods (Foerster). There is evidence that each root supplies fibres for pain, heat, and cold to a larger area than that to which it supplies fibres for light touch.

In the sensory innervation of the head the trigeminal nerve represents a fusion of the sensory supply of several segments, though the seventh, ninth, and tenth cranial nerves still possess rudimentary sensory branches distributed to the neighbourhood of the auricle. The posterior and inferior boundary of the trigeminal cutaneous area is contiguous with those of the first and second cervical segments respectively.

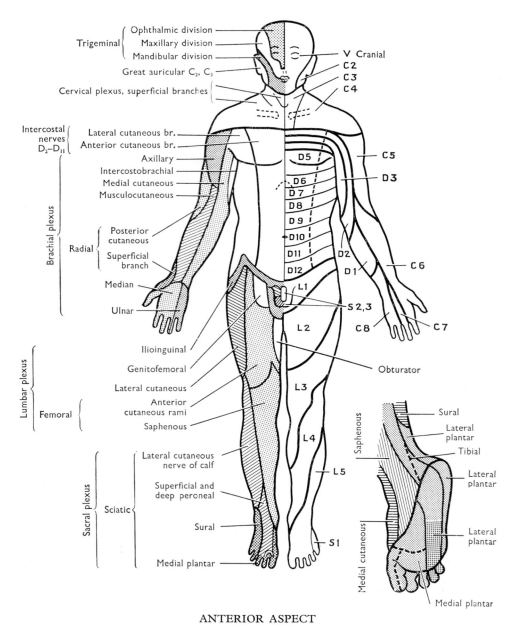

ANTERIOR ASPECT

Fig. 7 *a*. Cutaneous areas of distribution of spinal segments and the peripheral nerves

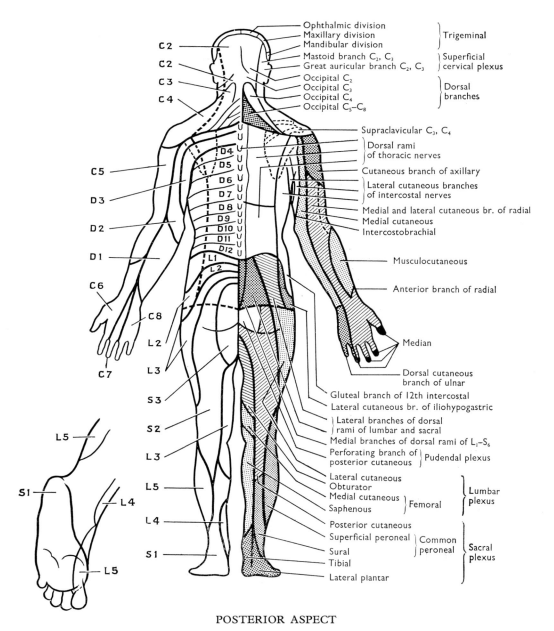

POSTERIOR ASPECT

FIG. 7 *b*. Cutaneous areas of distribution of spinal segments and the peripheral nerves

SENSORY PATHS IN THE SPINAL CORD

As we have seen, all sensory fibres from the limbs and trunk enter the spinal cord by the dorsal roots. After entering the cord these incoming fibres lie on the medial side of the apex of the posterior horn of grey matter, in the outer part of the fasciculus cuneatus, where they divide into ascending and descending branches. The descending branches, which form the comma tract, terminate in the grey matter after passing downwards through a few segments. The ascending fibres pass upwards in the lateral part of the posterior column. They may be divided into three groups in accordance with their respective distributions [FIG. 8].

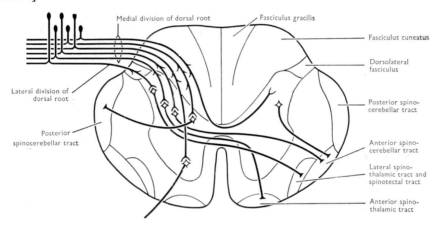

FIG. 8. Spinal cord and dorsal root, showing the divisions of the dorsal root, the collaterals of the dorsal root fibres, and some of the connexions which are established by them

1. Some of these fibres continue to pass upwards in the posterior column of the same side and terminate in the medulla in the nuclei gracilis and cuneatus. In their upward course the fibres of lowest origin pass gradually towards the midline as they are joined on their outer side by fibres from higher roots. Thus the fibres from the sacral roots come to lie nearest the midline, with those from the lumbar roots to their lateral side, and fibres from the cervical roots are the most laterally placed. Those fibres ultimately derived from the lower limb pass upwards in the fasciculus gracilis, while those from the upper limb are found in the fasciculus cuneatus. The fibres of the posterior column convey impulses concerned with the appreciation of posture and passive movements of the joints and of the vibration of a tuning-fork. It is probable that some fibres concerned with the sensation of light touch also pass up in the posterior column as far as the medulla.

The fact that tactile discrimination, i.e. the ability to recognize as two the points of a compass simultaneously applied, and tactile localization may be impaired after lesions of the posterior columns does not mean that these are distinct modalities of sensation mediated by the posterior columns but that they are judgements depending upon the integrity of the pathways subserving light touch.

2. The second group of entering fibres pass up in the posterior column of the same side for a considerable distance, but ultimately enter the posterior horn of grey matter, round the cells in which they terminate. From these cells further fibres take origin and cross the midline in the grey and anterior white commissures to reach the opposite anterior column. There they turn upwards and constitute the anterior spinothalamic tract. These are the remaining fibres concerned in the appreciation of touch.

3. The remaining fibres of the dorsal roots are those which ascend in the posterior column for the shortest distance, usually through only about three segments and never through more than five or six. They also end among the cells of the posterior horn from which fibres of the second relay take origin and, crossing the midline, like those of the previous group, enter the anterolateral column more posteriorly, and turning upwards constitute the lateral spinothalamic tract. These fibres conduct impulses concerned with the appreciation of pain, heat, and cold, those for pain lying dorsal to those for temperature. There is some evidence that there exists a lamination of the fibres of the spinothalamic tracts similar to that of the posterior columns, and that the fibres which convey sensation from the most caudal areas lie nearest to the surface of the cord in each tract and most posteriorly, while those entering at higher levels come to occupy successively deeper and more anterior layers. (For a full discussion see White (1954) and White and Sweet (1955).)

To complete our account of the destinations of the fibres entering the spinal cord by the dorsal roots we must mention two groups of fibres which are not concerned with sensation since they do not conduct impulses to consciousness, namely, those which are relayed upwards in the posterior and anterior spinocerebellar tracts. The end-organs of these fibres are probably mainly, if not exclusively, the proprioceptors of the muscles and tendons, and it is possible that the spinocerebellar tracts are supplied from collaterals of the fibres of the posterior columns. These impulses do not reach consciousness, but provide much of the 'raw material' of proprioceptor information which guides the activities of the cerebellum. Their existence explains why lesions of the dorsal roots and spinal cord may cause ataxia without gross loss of postural sensibility.

BROWN-SÉQUARD SYNDROME

Hemisection of the cord is a rare occurrence, but a lesion mainly involving one half is not uncommon. Destruction of the posterior column causes loss of appreciation of posture and passive movement of the joints, of the vibration of a tuning-fork, and of tactile discrimination below the level of the lesion. Destruction of the lateral spinothalamic tract causes analgesia and thermo-anaesthesia on the opposite side of the body. (Bilateral lesions seriously impair sexual sensibility.) Since fibres entering this tract do not cross the cord for several segments, the upper level of this sensory loss is likely to be a few segments below the level of the lesion. Conversely the fibres entering the cord just below the lesion may be caught before they cross, causing a narrow zone of similar analgesia and thermo-anaesthesia immediately below the lesion on the same side. Owing to the double route of fibres for light touch and tactile localization, partly crossed and partly uncrossed, there is rarely any loss of these forms of sensibility after a unilateral lesion of the cord. Any ataxia which might result from inter-ruption of the spinocerebellar tracts is likely to be masked by that resulting from loss of posterior column sensibility. Hemisection of the cord, of course, interrupts descending as well as ascending tracts, and the clinical picture therefore includes the signs of corticospinal defect below the lesion; and destruction of the anterior horn causes a lower motor neurone lesion with a segmental distribution corre-sponding to the level of the lesion. The signs of this are likely to be conspicuous only when the lesion occurs at the cervical or lumbar enlargements.

SENSORY PATHS IN THE BRAIN STEM

The two principal modifications in the arrangements of the sensory fibres which distinguish the brain stem from the spinal cord are the entrance of the trigeminal nerve and the decussation of the lemniscus. The central connexions of the trigeminal nerve are described elsewhere [see p. 158]. In summary it may be said that fibres concerned in the appreciation of pain, heat, and cold in one trigeminal area, after entering the spinal tract and nucleus of the fifth nerve, cross to the opposite side of the medulla as the trigeminothalamic tract and ascend in close relationship with the medial lemniscus joining the spinothalamic tract in the pons [FIG. 9].

The fibres of the posterior columns of the spinal cord have already been traced to their termination in the nuclei gracilis and cuneatus in the posterior part of the medulla. From these nuclei the second fibres of this sensory path take origin and cross to the opposite side as the internal arcuate fibres or the sensory decussation. After decussating they occupy a position on either side of the mid-line as the medial lemniscus and so pass upwards through the brain stem, to reach the optic thalamus. The medial lemniscus is joined in the pons by fibres from the principal sensory nucleus of the trigeminal nerve which are concerned in the appreciation of light touch, pressure, and postural sensibility over the trigeminal area.

Throughout the brain stem the spinothalamic tract, with which, above the medulla, the trigeminothalamic tract is associated, lies in the tegmentum, external to the medial lemniscus. As a result of this arrangement lesions involving the lateral part of the tegmentum of the brain stem are likely to cause hemi-analgesia and thermo-anaesthesia on the opposite side of the body, leaving postural sensibility and appreciation of passive movement and tactile discrimina-tion intact. When the lesion is situated in the medulla, below the point at which the spinothalamic tract has been joined by the trigeminothalamic tract, analgesia and thermo-anaesthesia involve the opposite side of the body below the face only, while similar sensory loss is likely to occur on the face on the side of the lesion, owing to damage to the spinal tract and nucleus of the trigeminal nerve. Appre-ciation of pain, heat, and cold are frequently affected to a different extent by lesions of the brain stem. Deeply seated lesions may involve the medial lemniscus without the spinothalamic tract, thus producing loss of postural sensibility, of appreciation of passive movement and of tactile discrimination on one or both sides of the body, but leaving appreciation of pain, heat, and cold unimpaired. Massive lesions, such as tumours, are likely to involve all forms of sensibility, though often to a varying extent. In the midbrain the third nerve and red nucleus may be simultaneously involved, leading to *Benedikt's syndrome*—paralysis of the third nerve on one side with hemi-anaesthesia and tremor on the opposite side.

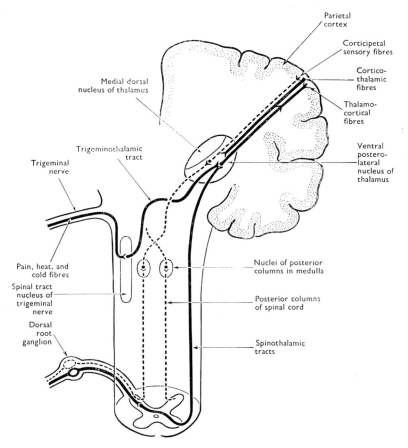

FIG. 9. Diagram showing principal sensory pathways

THE THALAMUS

Walker (1966) has recently reviewed the internal structure and connexions of the thalamus. Fessard and Fessard (1963) suggest that there are two systems of integrative structures at the thalamic level, the associative nuclei on the one hand, thus termed because they project to the association areas of the cortex after receiving afferents from the other nuclei of the thalamus, and on the other hand nuclei of the diffuse projection or non-specific system, comprising the intralaminar nuclei and certain mid-line nuclei. All sensory fibres pass upwards from the brain stem to the optic thalamus, whence many are redistributed in a further relay to the cerebral cortex [see p. 50]. The lateral nuclear mass is divided into a larger ventral and a smaller dorsal part. The ventral part is subdivided into (1) the anterior ventral nucleus with striatal connexions, (2) the lateral ventral, which connects the cerebellum with the motor cortex, and (3) the posterior part again divided into the posteromedial ventral, which receives trigeminothalamic fibres and the posterolateral ventral, which receives the spinothalamic tract and lemniscus. Both of these relay to the post-central gyrus [FIG. 10]. The dorsomedial nucleus is not concerned with direct sensory

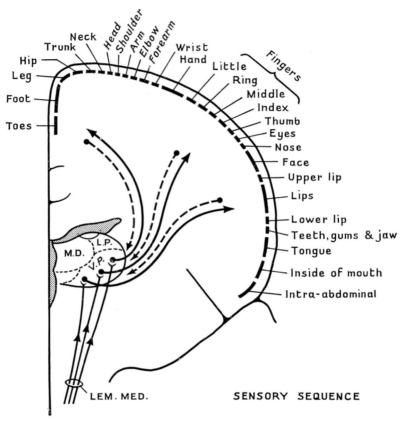

FIG. 10. Somatic sensation. Cross-section of the left hemisphere along the plane of the postcentral gyrus. The afferent pathway for tactile and kinaesthetic sensation is indicated by the unbroken lines coming up, through the medial lemniscus, and the posterolateral ventral nucleus of the thalamus, to the post-central gyrus

awareness, but is probably related to the affective response, especially to pain (see Henson, 1949). It projects to the prefrontal cortex. Since certain forms of sensibility are often unimpaired after lesions of the cerebral cortex, it has been argued that for these the optic thalamus must constitute the end-station: an alternative view is that they are bilaterally represented. These forms of sensation include the qualitative element in the appreciation of pain, heat, and cold, and the affective element, that is the pleasant or unpleasant character, of other forms of stimuli. Nevertheless, electrophysiology has shown that an intimate two-way relationship exists between the thalamus and the cerebral cortex

(Jasper and Ajmone-Marsan, 1952; Jung, Kornhuber, and Fonseca, 1963). Lesions in and near the thalamus are likely to cause loss of various forms of sensibility owing to interruption of the fibres upon which they depend. In addition, peculiarities of sensory response, the interpretation of which has given rise to much discussion, occasionally occur. For the blood supply of the thalamus see page 281.

SENSORY LOSS

A severe and extensive lesion of the thalamus may cause gross impairment of all forms of sensibility on the opposite side of the body, as a result of damage to the ventral nuclei. Less severe lesions may cause less serious sensory disturbance. Appreciation of posture and passive movement usually suffer severely. Appreciation of light touch and its localization are also often impaired. Appreciation of heat and cold may be impaired, both forms of sensibility being affected together, though not always to an equal extent. The threshold for pain may be normal, but is frequently raised, even when painful stimuli cause an exaggerated response.

THALAMIC 'OVER-REACTION' OR 'THALAMIC SYNDROME'

This sensory abnormality which may follow lesions of the thalamus is rare, at least in a fully developed form. It is generally agreed that damage to the lateral nucleus is necessary for it to occur. Pain of central origin may be referred to the opposite side of the body. It may be extremely severe and fail to respond to analgesic drugs, including morphine. Although the threshold to sensory stimuli is usually raised on the affected half of the body, yet such stimuli, when they are effective, excite sensations of a peculiarly unpleasant character. This combination of a raised threshold with over-reaction is known as 'hyperpathia'. The painful stimulation of superficial and deep tissues and of the viscera excites more severe pain on the affected than on the normal side. Extremes of heat and cold similarly excite a feeling of great discomfort on the affected side, and the same is true of such stimuli as scraping, tickling, and a vibrating tuning-fork. Exceptionally, pleasurable stimuli, such as pleasant warmth, have been found to cause increased pleasure on the affected side, and this half of the body has been said to react to emotional states in a manner different from the normal half.

Other symptoms which have been attributed to a lesion of the thalamus include choreo-athetoid movements with slight ataxia and hemiparesis on the opposite side of the body, but it is uncertain whether these symptoms are due to involvement of the thalamus itself or to injury of adjacent regions of the basal ganglia.

Thalamic over-reaction is most often seen after vascular lesions, and is rare with other types of lesion. Its nature has been much discussed and it has been attributed by some workers to irritation of the thalamus, by others to its escape from cortical control. The phenomenon of over-reaction to painful stimuli associated with a raised threshold to such stimuli is not a symptom of thalamic lesions only. It may, in fact, be observed as a result of a lesion involving pain fibres at any point between their endings in the skin and deeper tissues and the thalamus. Thus it occurs during regeneration of a peripheral sensory nerve and as a result of lesions of the spinothalamic tract within the spinal cord and brain stem. It is probably the result of a reduction in the number of pain-conducting fibres, or of defective insulation of those that remain.

SENSATION AT THE SUBCORTICAL LEVEL

A lesion involving the sensory fibres between the thalamus and the cerebral cortex usually causes severe and extensive sensory loss, since the fibres are here more closely crowded together than at the cortex. The appreciation of the qualitative element in pain, heat, and cold is unimpaired if the thalamus is undamaged. Other forms of sensibility are usually severely affected, there being as a rule marked loss of appreciation of posture, passive movement, tactile localization and discrimination, and of the appreciation of size, shape, and form. There may be an impairment of appreciation of temperatures in the middle of the thermal scale. A patient with a subcortical lesion does not exhibit the variability of response and threshold which characterizes patients with cortical lesions.

SENSATION AT THE CORTICAL LEVEL

As Head and his collaborators have shown, the cerebral cortex is concerned chiefly with the spatial and discriminative elements of sensibility, but it is now increasingly recognized that it plays a part in the perception of pain (Henson, 1949). The extent of the cerebral cortex concerned in sensation and the localization therein of different forms of sensory appreciation is somewhat uncertain. There is no doubt that the postcentral gyrus is concerned in the appreciation of the posture and passive movements of the opposite half of the body, parts of which are represented there in a manner similar to their representation for purposes of motility in the precentral gyrus [see FIG. 10]. It is probable that the greater part of the parietal lobe behind the postcentral gyrus is also concerned in sensibility, and Penfield and Rasmussen's (1950) observations on cortical stimulation in the conscious patient have shown that the sensory cortex extends in front of the central sulcus also.

One striking feature of a lesion of the sensory cortex is the extreme variability of the patient's response to sensory stimuli and the difficulty or impossibility of obtaining a threshold. The appreciation of posture and of passive movement is frequently seriously impaired, together with the appreciation of light touch and its accurate localization and the discrimination of the duality of two compass-points. The appreciation of size, shape, form, roughness, and texture often suffers. The qualitative element in pain, heat, and cold is still recognized, but in dealing with thermal stimuli in the middle of the scale the patient may find it difficult to say which of two is the hotter. (For a recent review of sensory anatomy and physiology see Rose and Mountcastle, 1960.)

PERCEPTUAL RIVALRY

This phenomenon, also known as sensory inattention, extinction, or suppression, is characteristic of a lesion of the parietal lobe, when a patient experiences a sensation if a stimulus is applied to the opposite side alone, but fails to experience it when a similar stimulus is simultaneously applied to a spot on the unaffected side of the body, which is the mirror-image of that first stimulated. It has been pointed out by Critchley (1953) and by Denny-Brown, Meyer, and Horenstein (1952) that extinction does not occur if the interval between the two contacts is more than three seconds. (See also Bender (1945) and Henson (1949), who describe a similar suppression of thalamic over-reaction.)

REFERENCES

BENDER, M. B. (1945) Extinction and precipitation of cutaneous sensations, *Arch. Neurol. Psychiat. (Chicago)*, **54**, 1.

BISHOP, G. H. (1946) Neural mechanisms of cutaneous sense, *Physiol. Rev.*, **26**, 77.

CRITCHLEY, M. (1953) *The Parietal Lobes*, London.

DENNY-BROWN, D. (1966) *The Cerebral Control of Movement*, Liverpool University Press, Liverpool.

DENNY-BROWN, D., MEYER, J. S., and HORENSTEIN, S. (1952) The significance of perceptual rivalry resulting from parietal lesion, *Brain*, **75**, 433.

FESSARD, D. A., and FESSARD, A. (1963) in *Progress in Brain Research*, vol. i, ed. Moruzzi, G., Fessard, A., and Jasper, H. H., p. 115, Amsterdam.

FOERSTER, O. (1929) Spezielle Anatomie und Physiologie der peripheren Nerven, LEWANDOWSKY's *Handbuch der Neurologie*, Ergänzungsband, 2, Berlin.

FOERSTER, O. (1933) The dermatomes in man, *Brain*, **56**, 1.

FULTON, J. F. (1943) *The Physiology of the Nervous System*, 2nd ed. Chap. XIV, The thalamus, New York.

HEAD, H. (1920) *Studies in Neurology*, vols. i and ii, London.

HENSON, R. A. (1949) On thalamic dysaesthesiae and their suppression by bilateral stimulation, *Brain*, **72**, 576.

JASPER, H. H., and AJMONE-MARSAN, C. (1952) Thalamocortical integrating mechanisms, *Res. Publ. Ass. nerv. ment. Dis.*, **30**, 493.

JUNG, R., KORNHUBER, H. H., and DA FONSECA, J. S. (1963) in *Progress in Brain Research*, vol. i, ed. Moruzzi, G., Fessard, A., and Jasper, H. H., p. 207, Amsterdam.

LEWIS, T. (1942) *Pain*, New York.

PENFIELD, W., and RASMUSSEN, T. (1950) *The Cerebral Cortex of Man*, New York.

RIDDOCH, G. (1938) The clinical features of central pain, *Lancet*, i, 1093, 1150, 1205.

ROSE, J. E., and MOUNTCASTLE, V. B. (1960) in *Handbook of Physiology*, ed. Field, J., Neurophysiology, vol. i, 387.

SINCLAIR, D. C. (1955) Cutaneous sensation and the doctrine of perceptual rivalry, *Brain*, **78**, 584.

SINCLAIR, D. C., WEDDELL, G., and FEINDEL, W. H. (1948) Referred pain and associated phenomena, *Brain*, **71**, 184.

STOPFORD, J. S. B. (1930) *Sensation and the Sensory Pathway*, London.

WALKER, A. E. (1966) Internal structure and afferent-efferent relations of the thalamus, in *The Thalamus*, ed. Purpura, D. P., and Yahr, M. D., p. 1, New York.

WALSHE, F. M. R. (1942) The anatomy and physiology of cutaneous sensibility: a critical review, *Brain*, **65**, 48.

WEDDELL, G., SINCLAIR, D. C., and FEINDEL, W. H. (1948) An anatomical basis for alterations in quality of pain sensibility, *J. Neurophysiol.*, **2**, 99.

WHITE, J. C. (1954) Conduction of pain in man, *Arch. Neurol. Psychiat. (Chicago)*, **71**, 1.

WHITE, J. C., and SWEET, W. H. (1955) *Pain, its Mechanisms and Neurosurgical Control*, Springfield, Ill.

THE REFLEXES

General Considerations

A reflex is the simplest form of involuntary response to a stimulus. The anatomical basis of a reflex is the reflex arc, which consists of (1) a receptor organ, (2) an afferent path running from the periphery to the brain stem or spinal cord, (3) one or more intercalated neurones in the central nervous system linking the afferent path to (4) the efferent path which leaves the neuraxis by the lower motor neurones to reach (5) the effector organ. The reflex is elicited by a stimulus which may be a touch, a prick, the sudden stretching of a muscle, or some other event which excites an afferent impulse on the reflex arc. The response is a muscular contraction, a modification in muscle tone, glandular secretion, &c., depending upon the nature of the reflex. Important though visceral reflexes are, the neurologist investigating the state of the nervous system is mainly concerned with reflexes which excite responses in the somatic muscula-ture. Reflex action, conceived by Descartes, was first observed by Stephen Hales in a pithed frog about 1730. The concept was elaborated by Robert Whytt in 1755, and later by Marshall Hall in 1833.

A reflex is fundamentally dependent upon the integrity of its reflex arc. Lesions which interrupt this arc at any point cause abolition of the reflex. Loss of a reflex may thus be brought about by interruption of the afferent path by a lesion involving the first sensory neurone in the peripheral nerves, plexuses, spinal nerves, or dorsal roots, by damage to the central paths of the arc in the brain stem or spinal cord, or by lesions of the lower motor neurone at any point between the anterior horn cells and the muscles, or of the muscles them-selves, or by the depression produced by neural shock. The strength of a reflex muscular contraction is influenced by the state of the antagonistic muscles. If these are weak the contraction of the prime movers is enhanced. If the antagon-ists are in tonic contraction, as, for example, in Parkinsonism, the amplitude of the movement normally effected by the prime movers is restricted.

A painful lesion tends to increase the vigour of the reflex activity of neighbour-ing muscles, probably because the incoming stream of painful impulses increases the excitability of the corresponding segments of the spinal cord. Somewhat similarly, one reflex may exert either a reinforcing or an inhibitory effect on another. For example, the flexor withdrawal reflex in the lower limbs in para-plegia tends to inhibit the knee- and ankle-jerks. Higher levels of the nervous system also exert important reinforcing and inhibitory influences upon reflex activities, examples of which will be encountered later.

REFLEXES INVOLVING THE CRANIAL NERVES

The Pupillary Reflexes. These are described on page 89.

The Corneal Reflex. The stimulus which evokes the corneal reflex is a light touch upon the cornea, e.g. with a wisp of cotton wool, and the response is bilateral blinking. The afferent path is through the first division of the fifth cranial nerve; the central path consists of fibres uniting the spinal nucleus of the fifth nerve with both facial nuclei, and the efferent path passes through the facial nerves to both orbiculares oculi muscles. A lesion involving the fifth nerve or its spinal nucleus, since it interrupts the afferent path, causes bilateral loss of blinking in response to stimulation of the cornea on the side of the lesion. A lesion involving the nucleus or fibres of the seventh nerve interrupts the efferent path and hence causes loss of the reflex on the side of the lesion only, and blinking occurs on the opposite side. Loss of the corneal reflex is often an early sign of a lesion of the fifth nerve and may occur before any cutaneous anaesthesia can be detected. Apart from lesions involving the reflex arc, the corneal reflex is lost in states of deep coma.

The Jaw Reflex. In response to a tap upon the chin, depressing the lower jaw, there is a bilateral contraction of the elevators of the jaw. Both afferent and efferent paths pass through the trigeminal nerve. This reflex is a stretch reflex, and, like these, becomes exaggerated as a result of bilateral corticospinal lesions.

The Sucking Reflex. In the infant the contact of an object with the lips evokes the movements of the lips, tongue, and jaw concerned in sucking. This sucking reflex is lost after infancy but may reappear in states of severe cerebral degeneration, for example, the presenile and senile dementias. It may be unilateral, and associated with a grasp reflex on the same side.

The 'Snout' Reflex. A tap on the centre of the closed lips will, in normal infants, provoke a pouting movement of the lips like the formation of a 'snout'. This reflex normally disappears with maturation but may reappear in the presence of bilateral corticospinal tract lesions in or above the upper brain stem and in cerebral degenerative disorders such as those in which the sucking reflex is re-established.

The Palatal Reflex. The palatal ('gag') reflex consists of elevation of the soft palate in response to a touch. The afferent path is by the second division of the fifth nerve; the efferent by the vagus. The palatal reflex is variable in intensity in normal individuals. It is abolished by lesions causing anaesthesia of the palate and by lesions of the vagus nuclei, and in lesions of one vagus nerve the response is unilateral and the uvula is displaced towards the normal side.

The Pharyngeal Reflex. The pharyngeal reflex consists of constriction of the pharynx in response to a touch upon the posterior pharyngeal wall. Its afferent path runs in the glossopharyngeal nerve, its efferent path in the vagus. Like the palatal reflex, it is abolished by lesions causing pharyngeal anaesthesia and by lesions of the vagus nuclei. In cases of unilateral paralysis of the vagus the response is confined to the opposite half of the pharynx.

REFLEXES OF THE LIMBS AND TRUNK
THE TENDON REFLEXES
Physiology

The basis of the tendon reflex is the myotatic reflex which is the reflex contraction of a muscle or part of a muscle in response to stretch. It is monosynaptic, i.e. it is mediated by a reflex arc consisting of two neurones with one synapse between them (Lloyd, 1952).

A so-called 'tendon reflex' is a sharp muscular contraction evoked by suddenly stretching the muscle. The sudden stretch may be brought about by tapping the tendon, or by suddenly displacing the segment of a limb into which the muscle is inserted. The response, a muscular contraction, is most evident in the muscle stretched, but may not be confined to this muscle. A tendon reflex is diminished or abolished by a lesion interrupting either the afferent, central, or efferent paths of the reflex arc or a disorder which makes the muscle incapable of responding to the nervous impulse. Early loss of deep reflexes may be due to desynchronization of impulses reaching the anterior horn cells, i.e. before sensory loss is detectable in cases of polyneuropathy. Higher levels of the nervous system also influence the excitability of the tendon reflexes. This is enhanced by anxiety and by lesions of the corticospinal tracts [see p. 23]. It is diminished by neural shock and by increased intracranial pressure. They may be congenitally absent. The table which follows gives the principal tendon reflexes, their mode of elicitation, and their innervation.

Reflex	Mode of elicitation	Response	Spinal segment	Peripheral nerve
Biceps-jerk	A blow upon the biceps tendon	Flexion of the elbow	Cervical 5–6	Musculo-cutaneous
Triceps-jerk	A blow upon the triceps tendon	Extension of the elbow	Cervical 6–7	Radial
Supinator-jerk or radial reflex	A blow upon the styloid process of the radius	Flexion of the elbow	Cervical 5–6	Radial
Flexor finger-jerk	A blow upon the palmar surface of the semi-flexed fingers	Flexion of the fingers and thumb	Cervical 7–8	Median and ulnar
Knee-jerk	A blow upon the quadriceps tendon	Extension of the knee	Lumbar 2–4	Femoral
Ankle-jerk	A blow upon the tendo calcaneus	Plantar flexion of the ankle	Sacral 1–2	Sciatic

Clonus. Clonus, a rhythmical series of contractions in response to the maintenance of tension in a muscle, is often elicitable when the tendon reflexes are exaggerated after a corticospinal lesion. Clonus of the quadriceps, patellar clonus, is best elicited by a sudden sharp downward displacement of the patella. Ankle clonus is obtained by sharply dorsiflexing the ankle. Clonus of the flexors of the fingers can sometimes be elicited by stretching these muscles by suddenly extending the fingers.

Hoffmann's Reflex. The patient's hand is pronated and the observer grasps the terminal phalanx of the middle finger between his forefinger and thumb. With a sharp flick the phalanx is passively flexed and suddenly released. A positive response consists of a sharp twitch of adduction and flexion of the thumb and flexion of the fingers. This reflex is physiologically identical with the *flexor finger-jerk*, which is elicited by tapping the palmar surface of the slightly flexed fingers. It is an index of muscular hypertonia rather than of a corticospinal lesion as such. It is not always positive in the presence of such a lesion, and may be elicitable in a nervous individual with no organic disease.

In states of muscular hypertonia a reflex response may spread beyond the muscles stretched, as when a tap on the styloid process of the radius elicits a contraction not only of the brachioradialis, but also of the long flexors of the fingers.

CUTANEOUS REFLEXES

The Nociceptive Abdominal Reflexes. These are cutaneous reflexes consisting of a brisk unilateral contraction of a part of the abdominal wall in response to a cutaneous stimulus, such as a touch or a light scratch with a pin. It is convenient to elicit them at three levels on each side—just below the costal margin, at the level of the umbilicus, and at the level of the iliac fossa. Kugelberg and Hagbarth (1958) have shown that the abdominal and erector spinae reflexes are polysynaptic, and are reactions of the trunk to potential injury. They are plurisegmental, and lead to a local withdrawal from the stimulus. They are normally dependent, for a reason which is not fully understood, upon the integrity of the corticospinal tract. Hence a corticospinal lesion is usually associated with diminution or loss of the superficial abdominal reflexes upon the same side. If the corticospinal defect is slight the reflexes may be reduced in vigour but not completely abolished, the reflexes of the lowest segments being most impaired. Superficial abdominal reflexes which have at one time been lost may return later, although the corticospinal lesion persists. The loss of the superficial abdominal reflexes is not always proportional to the severity of the corticospinal lesion. In multiple sclerosis, for example, the reflexes may be lost early, at a stage of the disease when other signs of corticospinal lesions are slight. In congenital diplegia and motor neurone disease, on the other hand, they are usually brisk.

The reflex arcs of the superficial abdominal reflexes are localized in the spinal cord from the seventh to the twelfth dorsal segments. Lesions involving the arcs themselves may produce diminution or loss of the reflexes. The commonest such lesion is damage to the lower motor neurone by poliomyelitis. Little importance can be attached to diminution of the superficial abdominal reflexes in stout people, after repeated pregnancies or abdominal operations, and after middle life.

The Cremasteric Reflex. The cremasteric reflex is a cutaneous reflex closely related to the abdominal reflexes. The appropriate stimulus is a light scratch along the inner aspect of the upper part of the thigh, and the response is a contraction of the cremaster muscle, with elevation of the testicle. This reflex, the arc of which runs through the first lumbar spinal segment, is diminished or abolished by a lesion of the corticospinal tract. It is usually extremely brisk in children, in whom it may sometimes be elicited by a stimulus applied to any part of the lower limb. It is usually diminished or absent on the affected side in a patient with varicocele.

The Gluteal Reflex. The gluteal reflex is physiologically akin to the abdominal reflexes. A scratch on the buttock evokes contraction of the glutei. The spinal segments concerned are lumbar 4 and 5.

The Plantar Reflex. The plantar reflex is one of the most important of all reflexes to the neurologist, because its meaning is unequivocal.

1. *The Flexor Plantar Reflex.* The flexor plantar reflex is normal after the first year of life. The stimulus which evokes it is a scratch upon the sole of the foot, and the response is plantar flexion of the toes usually associated with dorsiflexion of the foot at the ankle, contraction of the tensor fasciae latae muscle, and other variable muscular contractions. It is a spinal segmental reflex mediated by the first sacral segment of the cord and akin to the abdominal reflexes.

2. *The Extensor Plantar Reflex.* Babinski in 1896 first pointed out that in the presence of a corticospinal lesion the normal flexor plantar reflex did not occur, but its place was taken by an upward, extensor movement of the great toe. Riddoch, Walshe, and others showed that the extensor plantar reflex is not an isolated phenomenon, but is part of a general reflex flexion of the whole lower limb, homologous with the flexion reflex of the spinal animal in response to a nocuous or potentially painful stimulus. Recent studies (Brain and Wilkinson, 1959; Landau and Clare, 1959; and Kugelberg, Eklund, and Grimby, 1960) have shown that the distinction between the flexor and extensor plantar reflexes is less clear-cut than was thought. Both are nociceptive reflexes, but 'the unique feature of the pathological extensor response is the recruitment of extensor hallucis longus into contraction with tibialis anterior and extensor digitorum longus' (Kugelberg and Hagbarth, 1958). The afferent focus, i.e. the region of easiest elicitation of this reflex, is the outer border of the sole. The motor focus, or minimal response, is a contraction of the inner hamstring muscles. In its fully developed form the reflex consists of flexion at all joints of the lower limb with dorsiflexion of the great toe and abduction or fanning of the other toes.

Confusion has arisen from the application of the term extensor plantar reflex to a movement which forms part of a flexor reflex of the lower limb. The explanation of this misnomer is that the extensor hallucis longus muscle, though named extensor by the anatomists, is in fact a flexor muscle, since its action is to shorten the limb, and it contracts reflexly in association with other flexor muscles. The term extensor plantar reflex, however, appears to be too firmly established to be altered. 'Positive Babinski reflex' and 'upgoing toe' are alternative terms which are sometimes employed.

Physiological understanding illuminates several points of practical importance in the elicitation of the plantar reflex. The stimulus should always be applied to the outer border of the sole. Since this is the afferent focus of the reflex arc, an extensor response may sometimes be obtained from this region when the inner border of the sole yields a flexor response. The reflex may be more easily obtained after the limb has been passively flexed than when it is lying fully extended. Oppenheim's reflex, dorsiflexion of the great toe, evoked by firm moving pressure on the skin over the tibia, is physiologically the same as Babinski's reflex, differing only in the site of the stimulus. The same is true of

Chaddock's and Gordon's reflexes. The extensor plantar reflex is not an all-or-none reaction: minor degrees of corticospinal tract damage lead to an incomplete flexor response or a failure of the great toe to move up or down.

An extensor plantar reflex is often observed during sleep and deep coma from any cause, for a short time after an epileptic convulsion, and usually in the first year of life, that is, when the corticospinal fibres are either functionally depressed or incompletely developed. In any other circumstances it indicates an organic lesion of the corticospinal tract.

Occasionally in chronic paraplegia a pressure palsy of the peroneal nerve abolishes the extensor plantar reflex.

The Bulbocavernosus Reflex. The bulbocavernosus reflex consists of contraction of the bulbocavernosus muscle, which can be detected by palpation, in response to squeezing the glans penis. The spinal segments concerned are sacral 2, 3, and 4. This reflex is frequently abolished in tabes and in lesions of the cauda equina.

The Anal Reflex. The anal reflex consists of contraction of the external sphincter ani in response to a scratch upon the skin in the perianal region. The spinal segments concerned are sacral 4 and 5.

POSTURAL REFLEXES

'Postural reflexes' is a convenient term to apply to reflexes in which the response consists not of a brief muscular contraction but of a sustained modification in the posture of one or more segments of the body.

Tonic Neck Reflexes. In the decerebrate animal it was found by Magnus and de Kleijn that changes in the position of the head relative to the body caused reflex modifications of the tonus and posture of the limbs. These reflexes, which are excited from the proprioceptors of the cervical spine, are known as *tonic neck reflexes* and may sometimes be observed in hemiplegia.

Associated Reactions. Associated reactions, or associated movements, are automatic modifications of the posture of parts of the body when vigorous voluntary or reflex movement of some other part occurs. They are best observed in the paralysed upper limb in hemiplegia, following a vigorous grasping movement with the sound hand. Other patterns of associated movement occur. Such semi-voluntary activities as yawning, stretching, and coughing often evoke associated movements in the paralysed limbs in hemiplegia, and may arouse in the patient or his friends false hopes of recovery.

FORCED GRASPING AND GROPING

The Grasp Reflex of the Hand. In certain patients the contact of an object with the palmar surface of the fingers, especially the region between the thumb and the index finger, causes reflex flexion of the fingers and thumb so that the hand involuntarily grasps the object. The patient is unable voluntarily to relax his grasp, and efforts to pull the object away only cause it to be more firmly held. The patient may notice that when he is holding an object he is unable to relinquish his hold of it in order to put it down. This phenomenon is known as the *grasp reflex*. In some cases, when the patient's eyes are closed, if the palmar surface of the hand or fingers is lightly touched, the fingers close upon the object and the hand and arm move towards the stimulus and in this way may be drawn in any direction—*forced groping* or the *instinctive grasp reaction*. Even an object presented to vision may be groped for (Massion-Verniory, 1948; Seyffarth and Denny-Brown, 1948).

Forced grasping and groping, which have been considered a regression to the infantile stage of the function of grasping, usually indicate a lesion involving the upper part of the opposite frontal lobe, particularly areas 8s and 24s (Denny-Brown, 1951). This author distinguishes from the true grasp reactions a flexor response to traction which occurs after ablation of the opposite area 4. The commonest causes are neoplasms and vascular lesions. In rare cases the cause has been a tumour in some other part of the brain, but in such instances the functions of the frontal lobe have probably been impaired by increased intra-cranial pressure. A unilateral grasp reflex in a fully conscious patient is of localizing value. When the reflex is bilateral or the patient semi-conscious its value is much less. When the causative lesion produces a progressive hemiplegia the grasp reflex disappears when paralysis becomes complete, which appears to indicate that it utilizes the corticospinal tract as part of its motor path.

The Grasp Reflex of the Foot. An allied grasp reflex may sometimes be observed in the foot, light pressure or a stroking movement applied to the distal half of the sole and plantar surface of the toes evoking tonic flexion and adduction of the toes without other associated movements. Like the fingers, the toes may grasp and hold an object. This reflex is present in the normal infant up to the end of the first year, and in 50 per cent. of children with mongolism. It may occur either with or without the hand-grasp reflex, and is caused by similar lesions.

REFERENCES

ADIE, W. J., and CRITCHLEY, M. (1927) Forced grasping and groping, *Brain*, **50**, 142.
BABINSKI, J. (1922) Réflexes de défense, *Brain*, **45**, 149.
BICKERSTAFF, E. R. (1968) *Neurological Examination in Clinical Practice*, 2nd ed., Oxford.
BRAIN, W. R., and CURRAN, R. D. (1932) The grasp reflex of the foot, *Brain*, **55**, 347.
BRAIN, R., and WILKINSON, M. (1959) Observations on the extensor plantar reflex and its relationship to the functions of the pyramidal tract, *Brain*, **82**, 297.
DENNY-BROWN, D. (1951) in *Modern Trends in Neurology*, ed. Feiling, A., London.
FULTON, J. F. (1938) *Physiology of the Nervous System*, p. 440, New York.
HEAD, H., and RIDDOCH, G. (1917) The automatic bladder, excessive sweating and some other reflex conditions in gross injuries of the spinal cord, *Brain*, **40**, 188.
DE JONG, R. N. (1967) *The Neurologic Examination*, 3rd ed., New York.
KUGELBERG, E., EKLUND, K., and GRIMBY, L. (1960) An electromyographic study of the nociceptive reflexes of the lower limb, *Brain*, **83**, 394.
KUGELBERG, E., and HAGBARTH, K. E. (1958) Spinal mechanism of the abdominal and erector spinae skin reflexes, *Brain*, **81**, 290.
LANDAU, W. M., and CLARE, M. H. (1959) The plantar reflex in man, *Brain*, **82**, 321.
LANGWORTHY, O. R. (1930) The mechanism of the abdominal and cremasteric reflexes, *Arch. Neurol. Psychiat. (Chicago)*, **24**, 1023.
LLOYD, D. P. C. (1952) On reflex actions of muscular origin, *Res. Publ. Ass. nerv. ment. Dis.*, **30**, 48.

MASSION-VERNIORY, L. (1948) Les réflexes de préhension, Supp. ad *Mschr. Psychiat. Neurol.*, Fasc. lxxxviii.

MONRAD-KROHN, G. H. (1918) *Om Abdominalreflexerne*, Christiania.

MONRAD-KROHN, G. H. (1925) Reflexes of different order elicitable from the abdominal region, *Arch. Neurol. Psychiat.* (*Chicago*), **13**, 750.

PAINE, K. S., and OPPÉ, T. E. (1966) *Neurological Examination of Children*, London.

RIDDOCH, G., and BUZZARD, E. F. (1921) Reflex movements and postural reactions in quadriplegia and hemiplegia, with especial reference to those of the upper limb, *Brain*, **44**, 397.

SCHUSTER, P., and PINÉAS, H. (1926) Weitere Beobachtungen über Zwangsgreifen und Nachgreifen und deren Beziehungen zu ähnlichen Bewegungsstörungen, *Dtsch. Z. Nervenheilk.*, **91**, 16.

SEYFFARTH, H., and DENNY-BROWN, D. (1948) The grasp reflex and the instinctive grasp reaction, *Brain*, **71**, 109.

SITTIG, O. (1932) Über die Greifreflexe im Kindesalter, *Med. Klin.*, **28**, 934.

WALSHE, F. M. R. (1914–15) The physiological significance of the reflex phenomena in spastic paralysis of the lower limbs, *Brain*, **37**, 269.

WALSHE, F. M. R. (1919) On the genesis and physiological significance of spasticity and other disorders of motor innervation, with a consideration of the functional relationships of the pyramidal system, *Brain*, **42**, 1.

WALSHE, F. M. R. (1965) *Further Critical Studies in Neurology*, Edinburgh.

WARTENBERG, R. (1945) *The Examination of Reflexes*, Chicago.

THE CEREBELLUM

ANATOMY AND MORPHOLOGY

The cerebellum is situated in the posterior fossa of the skull and is joined to the brain stem by three peduncles, the superior, middle, and inferior. The tentorium cerebelli lies above, and below it is separated from the posterior aspect of the medulla and the dura mater covering the posterior atlanto-occipital membrane by a dilatation of the subarachnoid space, the cerebellomedullary cistern. To the naked eye it is composed of three main divisions, two lateral lobes and a median lobe, the vermis, but this is not a morphological division.

Phylogeny and experimental physiology provide a sounder basis for morphology. According to Larsell (1937) and Fulton and Dow (1937–8) the cerebellum has two primary divisions: (1) the flocculonodular lobe, the most primitive part, with connexions which are entirely vestibular, and (2) the corpus cerebelli, itself divided into (*a*) a palaeocerebellar division, receiving vestibular and spinocerebellar fibres, and composed anteriorly of lingula, lobus centralis, and culmen, and posteriorly of pyramis, uvula, and paraflocculi, and (*b*) a neocerebellar division, constituting the greater part of the corpus cerebelli, with connexions mainly corticopontine. (For recent reviews see Fulton, 1949; Jansen and Brodal, 1954; Kreindler and Steriade, 1958; Brookhart, 1960.)

The cerebellum consists mainly of white matter which is covered with a thin layer of grey matter, the cerebellar cortex, and contains several grey masses, the nuclei. These are divided into lateral nuclei, the nuclei dentatus and emboliformis, and middle and roof nuclei, the nuclei globosus and fastigius.

Microscopically the cortex consists of three principal layers of cells, the molecular layer, which lies most superficially, the granular layer, which is the deepest, and the layer of Purkinje cells, which lies between the two. In the three cortical layers are numerous fibres, impulses from which probably ultimately impinge upon the dendrites of the Purkinje cells. The axons of the latter pass through the white matter of the cerebellar hemispheres and are distributed chiefly to the dentate nuclei.

CEREBELLAR CONNEXIONS

AFFERENT FIBRES

The cerebellum receives numerous afferent fibres which are principally derived from the proprioceptor organs of the body, namely:

Vestibular Fibres. These come from the labyrinth and enter the cerebellum by the inferior peduncles, some being interrupted at the vestibular nuclei. These go mostly to the cortex of the vermis.

Spinal Fibres. These come from the skin and proprioceptors of the muscles and possibly also from the joints and tendons. They reach the cerebellum by the posterior spinocerebellar tract, which ascends in the posterior part of the lateral column of the spinal cord and enters the cerebellum by the inferior peduncle, and by the anterior spinocerebellar tract, which passes up the cord in the antero-lateral column, ascends as high as the midbrain, and turns backwards to the cerebellum through the superior peduncle. The posterior spinocerebellar tract probably receives a contribution from the trigeminal nerve. Fibres from the spinocerebellar tracts end throughout the cerebellar cortex.

Cortical Fibres. Impulses reach the cerebellum from the cerebral cortex by way of the corticospinal tracts with a relay station in the nuclei of the pons, whence fibres pass to the cerebellum by the middle peduncle. They are distributed mainly to the middle lobes.

Olivary Fibres. The olive, which receives spinal and thalamic connexions, is intimately related to the opposite cerebellar hemisphere, to which it sends fibres through the opposite inferior peduncle. Atrophy of one cerebellar hemisphere is usually associated with atrophy of the opposite olive.

Most afferent fibres are distributed to the cerebellar cortex.

EFFERENT FIBRES

Efferent fibres start from the cerebellar nuclei and leave the cerebellum by all three peduncles. The most important outgoing path from the cerebellum passes from the dentate nucleus and from nuclei emboliformis and globosus through the superior peduncle and after decussation is distributed to the opposite red nucleus. From the red nucleus arises the rubrospinal tract, which decussates in the ventral tegmental decussation and passes down through the brain stem to the lateral column of the spinal cord. This is probably the principal route by which the cerebellum influences the lower motor neurone. Each cerebellar hemisphere is thus linked principally with the same side of the body by means of a double decussation in the midbrain. Other fibres from the red nucleus through the ansa lenticularis reach the thalamus and may thus bring the cerebellum into relationship with the basal ganglia and the cerebral cortex.

Other cerebellar efferent fibres reach the reticular formation of the midbrain, the pons, and the medulla by all three peduncles.

THE FUNCTIONS OF THE CEREBELLUM

Our earliest knowledge of the functions of the cerebellum was based upon Rolando's observations of the effects of removal of this organ in 1809. His observations were extended by Flourens in 1824. Luciani, in 1879, summarized the symptoms of cerebellar deficiency as asthenia, atonia, and astasia, that is, weakness and fatigability, diminution of tone, and tremor and a staggering gait. Recent experiments have yielded more precise information concerning cerebellar functions. Rademaker described extensor hypertonia in the limbs after removal of the whole cerebellum and Sherrington found that cerebellar stimulation could inhibit decerebrate rigidity. Denny-Brown, Eccles, and Liddell (1929) by stimulating the cerebellar cortex imposed modifications upon pre-existing spinal reflexes and observed inhibition and excitation of both extensor and flexor muscles, and Miller and Banting (1922) made similar observations in stimulating the cerebellar nuclei. These physiological observations, together with clinical investigation of the effects of cerebellar lesions by Holmes and others, have established the view that the neocerebellum is essentially a reinforcing and co-ordinating organ which plays an important part in graduating and harmonizing muscular contraction, both in voluntary movement and in the maintenance of posture. There is still much to be learned about the details of the physiology of the cerebellum. The subject is fully discussed by Brookhart (1960). Denny-Brown (1966) points out that prolonged depression of the proprioceptive component of all reflexes is the most significant cerebellar defect and that the syndrome of complete cerebellar ablation is the reverse of decerebrate rigidity.

The anterior lobe and the roof nuclei are concerned with the regulation of stretch reflexes and the anti-gravity posture. The flocculonodular lobe is an important equilibratory centre and lesions of this region cause swaying, staggering, and titubation. The neocerebellum regulates voluntary movement.

SYMPTOMS OF CEREBELLAR DEFICIENCY IN MAN

The following are the principal effects of neocerebellar lesions in man:

MUSCULAR HYPOTONIA

Hypotonia is evident in the visible, palpable flaccidity of the muscles, in a diminished resistance to passive movements of the joints, and in the wide excursions occurring at the terminal joints when the limb is vigorously shaken. If the outstretched upper limb receives a sudden tap, it shows a greater displacement than a normal limb. When the lesion is confined to one cerebellar hemisphere the hypotonia is present only on the same side of the body. The hypotonia is probably due to loss of the facilitatory influence of the cerebellum upon the stretch reflex.

DISTURBANCES OF POSTURE

Abnormal Attitudes. With a unilateral cerebellar lesion the shoulder on the affected side is often held at a lower level than the normal shoulder and there may be scoliosis with the concavity towards the side of the lesion. In standing, the weight is thrown on the sound leg and the body is somewhat rotated, with the affected shoulder in advance of the sound one. In severe cases the patient is unable to stand without support and tends to fall towards the side of the lesion. When a lesion involves one cerebellar hemisphere the head is often rotated and flexed, so that the occiput is directed towards the shoulder on the side of the lesion. This rotated posture may be due either to cerebellar deficiency or to a coincident lesion of the vestibular tracts.

Static Tremor. Tremor develops if the patient attempts to maintain a limb in a fixed posture, probably owing to hypotonia of the agonists producing an irregular contraction of the muscles maintaining the attitude.

DISORDERS OF MOVEMENT (ATAXIA)

Several factors combine to produce disturbances of voluntary movement after a lesion of the cerebellum. Muscular contractions are weak and more easily fatigued than normally. Moreover, they are of an irregular, intermittent character, and there is delay both in initiating and in relaxing contractions.

Dysmetria. In dysmetria the range of the movement is inappropriate to its objective. Sometimes the harmonious synthesis of movements at different joints is lost, leading to the phenomenon known as 'decomposition of movement'. When a movement involves the whole arm, instead of its occurring to an appropriate extent at all joints simultaneously, one joint is moved before another.

Tremor. Tremor occurs on voluntary movement, owing partly to faulty fixation and partly to the factors responsible for static tremor. Fine movements, for example movements of the fingers, suffer especially from incoordination due to cerebellar deficiency, and the patient may find it impossible to button his clothes.

Adiadochokinesis. This is the term applied to an inability to carry out alternating movements with rapidity and regularity. For example, the patient is asked alternately to pronate and supinate his forearms or to flex and extend his fingers. After a unilateral cerebellar lesion alternating movements are accomplished slowly and in a jerky, incoordinate fashion on the affected side.

The Rebound Phenomenon. This is a disturbance of movement probably due to muscular hypotonia. If a normal individual is asked to flex his elbow against resistance offered by the observer and his forearm is suddenly released, its excursion in the direction of flexion is quickly arrested by contraction of the triceps. Cerebellar deficiency delays this contraction, with the result that flexion of the elbow is unchecked and the patient may strike himself in the face.

Associated Movements. After a lesion of the cerebellum the normal associated movements which occur on strong voluntary effort may be exaggerated. Vigorous grimaces may accompany speech after a lesion of the cerebellar vermis.

OCULAR DISTURBANCES

In the early stages of a unilateral cerebellar lesion there may be weakness of conjugate ocular deviation to the affected side, but this soon passes off. In cases of severe bilateral lesions, or if the vermis is affected, there may be a temporary impairment of conjugate movement in the vertical plane also.

Skew deviation of the eyes is occasionally observed for a few days after an acute cerebellar lesion. The eye on the affected side is deviated downwards and inwards, while the opposite eye is deviated outwards and upwards. This may be due either to cerebellar deficiency or to interference with the vestibular connexions elsewhere.

Nystagmus is usually present in cerebellar disease. It is most evident when the eyes are deviated horizontally. The slow phase consists of a deviation towards the point of central fixation and the quick phase of a sharp jerk of return to the original position. In the case of unilateral cerebellar lesions the amplitude of the nystagmus is greater and its rate slower when the eyes are deviated towards the side of the lesion than when they are displaced to the opposite side. Nystagmus is usually in the horizontal plane, but there is occasionally a rotatory element also. Nystagmus on vertical deviation is inconspicuous. For a further discussion of nystagmus see page 84.

DISORDERS OF ARTICULATION AND PHONATION

Disturbances of articulation and phonation are more likely to occur when a lesion involves the vermis than when it is confined to one lateral lobe. Articulation is jerky and explosive. The voice is often too loud, and the syllables tend to be separated from each other. At the same time individual syllables are slurred owing to defective formation of consonants. Considerable recovery of speech usually occurs in the case of unilateral lesions.

DISORDERS OF GAIT

The patient with a unilateral lesion tends to stagger towards the affected side and to deviate to this side in walking. This may be well demonstrated by asking him to walk round a chair. When he is turning towards the affected side he tends to fall into the chair, when to the normal side, to move away from the chair in a spiral. The affected lower limb is markedly ataxic.

ABNORMALITIES OF THE REFLEXES

The cutaneous reflexes are unaffected by lesions of the cerebellum. The tendon reflexes, however, often exhibit a characteristic change, which is best seen in the 'pendular' knee-jerk. The knee-jerk is followed by a series of oscillations of the leg, which are normally prevented by the after-shortening of the quadriceps.

BÁRÁNY'S POINTING TEST

The patient, with his eyes closed and one arm outstretched, is asked to move the limb in a given plane and bring his finger back to its original position. Deviation of the limb occurs after a unilateral cerebellar lesion and is most conspicuous when the movement takes place in the vertical plane, the arm deviating outwards on the side of the lesion.

SYMPTOMS OF LESIONS OF THE FLOCCULONODULAR LOBE

Experimental lesions of this region in animals cause swaying, staggering, and titubation, symptoms identical with those of lesions of the vermis in man, especially the medulloblastoma of childhood.

CEREBELLAR VERTIGO

That cerebellar lesions may cause vertigo is not surprising in view of the postural and equilibratory functions of the cerebellum. It is stated that objects seem to move away from the side of the lesion and the sense of rotation of the body is in the same direction with intracerebellar tumours but in the opposite direction with extracerebellar tumours.

LOCALIZATION IN THE CEREBELLUM

Older experiments designed to show localization of function by studying the effects of local ablations were inconclusive. Electroencephalography has made it possible to detect electrical responses in the cerebellum to both peripheral and cerebral stimuli (Dow, 1942; Dow and Anderson, 1942; Adrian, 1943). Adrian found the hind-limb represented in the lobulus simplex on the same side, and the fore-limb behind this in the culmen, while the same areas could be excited from the hind- and fore-limb regions of the cerebral cortex.

ACUTE AND CHRONIC LESIONS

The symptoms of a cerebellar lesion differ markedly in severity according to whether it develops rapidly or slowly. Most of our knowledge of the symptoms of cerebellar deficiency is based upon studies of acute lesions. When the lesion is slowly progressive, such as a tumour, symptoms of cerebellar deficiency are much less severe than when it is acute, and considerable recovery from the effects of an acute lesion can always be expected. These facts seem to imply that other parts of the nervous system can to a considerable extent compensate for loss of cerebellar function.

REFERENCES

ADRIAN, E. D. (1943) Afferent areas in the cerebellum connected with the limbs, *Brain*, **66**, 289.

BAILEY, P. (1944) *The Precentral Motor Cortex*, ed. Bucy, P. C., p. 277, Illinois.

BARD, L. (1925) Du rôle et du mécanisme d'action du cervelet dans la régulation des mouvements, *Rev. neurol. (Paris)*, **32**, 553.

BROOKHART, J. M. (1960) The cerebellum, in *Handbook of Physiology*, ed. Field, J., Sect. 1, Neurophysiology, vol. ii, 1245, Washington, D.C.

CLARKE, R. H. (1926) Experimental stimulation of the cerebellum, *Brain*, **49**, 557.

DENNY-BROWN, D. (1966) *The Cerebral Control of Movement*, Liverpool.

DENNY-BROWN, D., ECCLES, J. C., and LIDDELL, E. G. T. (1929) Observations on electrical stimulation of the cerebellar cortex, *Proc. roy. Soc. Med.*, **104**, 518.

DOW, R. S. (1942) Cerebellar action potentials in response to stimulation of the cerebral cortex in monkeys and cats, *J. Neurophysiol.*, **5**, 121.

DOW, R. S., and ANDERSON, R. (1942) Stimulation of proprioceptors and exteroceptors in the rat, *J. Neurophysiol.*, **5**, 363.

FULTON, J. F. (1949) *Functional Localization in the Frontal Lobes and Cerebellum*, Oxford.

FULTON, J. F., and DOW, R. S. (1937–8) The cerebellum. A summary of functional localization, *Yale J. Biol. Med.*, **10**, 89.

HOLMES, G. (1917) The symptoms of acute cerebellar injuries due to gun-shot injuries, *Brain*, **40**, 461.

HOLMES, G. (1922) Croonian Lectures. The clinical symptoms of cerebellar disease and their interpretation, *Lancet*, i, 1177, 1231; and ii, 59, 111.

HOLMES, G. (1939) The cerebellum of man, *Brain*, **62**, 1.

INGVAR, S. (1923) On cerebellar localization, *Brain*, **46**, 301.

JANSEN, J., and BRODAL, A. (1954) *Aspects of Cerebellar Anatomy*, Oslo.

KREINDLER, A., and STERIADE, M. (1958) *La physiologie et la physiopathologie du cervelet*, Paris.

LARSELL, O. (1937) The cerebellum, *Arch. Neurol. Psychiat. (Chicago)*, **38**, 580.

MILLER, F. R. (1926) The physiology of the cerebellum, *Physiol. Rev.*, **6**, 124.

MILLER, F. R., and BANTING, F. G. (1922) Observations in cerebellar stimulations, *Brain*, **45**, 104.

THE VISUAL FIBRES AND THE VISUAL FIELDS

THE VISUAL FIELDS

Investigation of the extent of the fields of vision and of the degree of visual acuity within them plays an important part in the routine examination of patients suffering from nervous diseases. 'Perimetry' is a term applied to the mapping of the visual fields. This may be carried out in the following ways:

CONFRONTATION PERIMETRY

This method is extremely rough and only gross defects of the visual fields are likely to be detected by it. The observer stands or sits opposite to the patient and about a metre away from him. The patient is instructed to cover one eye with his hand and to fix the gaze of his other eye upon the opposite eye of the observer. The observer then brings a test object, usually his finger, inwards from beyond the periphery of his own visual field, midway between himself and the patient, who is asked to say when he first sees it. This procedure is carried out above, below, and to either side and, if necessary, intermediately, and the observer is able to determine the extent of the patient's visual field relative to his own. Besides ascertaining the outer boundaries of the visual field by the method described, the test object should be made to traverse the field in various directions and the patient should be asked to state if it disappears from view and when it reappears. In this way a *scotoma* or an area of defective vision within the field may be detected.

In young children and uncooperative patients a field defect may sometimes be detected by observing whether the patient notices an object brought in from the periphery in various directions, or whether he blinks in response to a feint with the hand towards the eye—the *menace reflex*.

MECHANICAL PERIMETRY

There are a large number of perimeters in use by which the visual fields can be tested and recorded. The patient is made to gaze at a fixation point and the test object is then moved in the arc of a circle towards the fixation point. The object is at a distance of from 250 to 330 mm. from the eye and is usually between

3 and 10 mm. in diameter. The visual acuity differs in different parts of the visual field. Although a moving object is readily perceived in the peripheral part, central vision for a stationary object is more acute than peripheral vision. Hence the smaller the test object the smaller the visual field in which it is perceptible. The conditions of the test are indicated by the fraction $\dfrac{\text{diameter of object}}{\text{distance}}$. If a 3 mm. test object is used at a distance of 330 mm., this fraction is 3/330. Boundaries of the normal visual field for 3/330 are situated at about 60 degrees up, 60 degrees in, 75 degrees down, and 100 degrees, or a little more, out. The field for colours is smaller than that for white, that for blue and yellow being somewhat larger than that for red and green.

PERIMETRY BY BJERRUM'S SCREEN

A mechanical perimeter is a useful method for determining the boundaries of the visual fields. More refined methods, however, are often necessary for investigating the central portions. Bjerrum's screen enables test objects of 1 and 2 mm. to be used at a distance of 2 metres—1/2000 and 2/2000. In this way very slight defects of visual acuity may be detected and, since they are projected upon a large area, accurately mapped. A depression of visual acuity in the centre of the field may not be demonstrable by tests such as reading types. It is for the detection of such defects that Bjerrum's screen is of special value. The normal field for a 1/2000 test object by this method extends to nearly 26 degrees in all directions. If a defect exists to 1/2000 or 2/2000 objects, larger objects should be used until one is seen in the area of impaired vision.

The term 'hemianopia' indicates a loss of vision in half of the visual field. When this is present in the same half of both fields, for example both right halves, we speak of 'homonymous hemianopia'. When the field defect on one side is a mirror image of that on the other, the hemianopia is said to be bitemporal or binasal, according to the halves affected. A field defect limited to one quadrant is described as 'quadrantic hemianopia' or 'quadrantanopia'. When homonymous field defects are capable of being accurately superimposed one upon another, they are said to be congruous; when their corresponding boundaries differ, they are said to be incongruous.

Closely related disturbances of visual function are—visual inattention or extinction, indicated by a failure to notice movement of an object such as the observer's finger in one half-field, when there is a competing stimulus in the opposite half-field, and visual disorientation, which is inability to localize objects seen, especially to estimate relative distance [see p. 116].

THE PATH OF THE VISUAL FIBRES (FROM THE RETINA TO THE PRIMARY VISUAL CENTRES)

THE OPTIC NERVES

The fibres of the optic nerve are the axons of the ganglion cells of the retina. The macula is the region of most acute vision, and ocular fixation is so regulated as to bring on to the macula the image of any object at which we look. The macular fibres are thus the most important part of the visual afferent system.

In the retina these fibres run from the macula to the temporal side of the optic disc or papilla. Fibres from the upper and lower temporal quadrants of the retina are displaced by the macular fibres to the upper and lower parts of the disc, and fibres from the nasal quadrants occupy the nasal side. The optic nerves pass backwards and inwards through the optic foramina and terminate posteriorly at the optic chiasma.

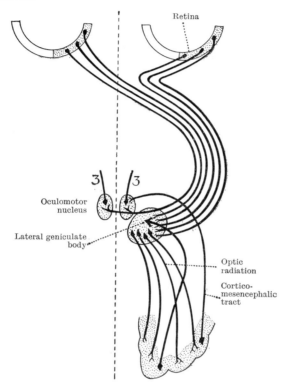

FIG. 11. Diagram of central connexions of the optic nerve and optic tract

THE OPTIC CHIASMA

At the optic chiasma the two optic nerves unite and the decussation of the fibres derived from the nasal halves of the retinae occurs [FIG. 11]. The position of the chiasma is a variable one and assumes importance in relationship to the field defects produced by its compression by tumours in this region. It is usually situated a little behind the tuberculum sellae. It is rarely as far forward as the sulcus chiasmatis and is sometimes much further back behind the dorsum sellae and is then related to the posterior part of the pituitary. The relationship of the chiasma to the sella turcica, pituitary body, and infundibulum is thus variable. The most important of its other relations are, above, the floor of the third ventricle and, laterally, the internal carotid arteries.

The decussating fibres from the nasal half of each retina expand within the chiasma, those from the anterior part of the optic nerve passing inwards and forwards to form a loop, entering the base of the opposite optic nerve before passing backwards to the opposite optic tract, where they are joined by the nasal fibres from the posterior part of the nerve which cross the chiasma more posteriorly. The fibres from the temporal halves of the retinae do not decussate, but are continued backwards on the same side in the optic tract.

THE OPTIC TRACT

Each optic tract is thus composed of fibres from the temporal half of the retina of the same side and from the nasal half of the retina of the opposite side. Within the tract the uncrossed fibres lie dorsolaterally and the crossed fibres ventromesially. Each optic tract sweeps outwards and backwards between the cerebral peduncle and the gyrus parahippocampalis, and finally inwards to terminate in the superior colliculus, the lateral geniculate body, and the pulvinar of the optic thalamus, but experimental evidence throws doubt upon whether the last structure plays any part either in vision or in the optical reflexes. The lateral geniculate body appears to receive the fibres concerned in visual perception, and the superior colliculus those destined to excite reflex activity. Besides the localization in a lateral plane already described, there is in the optic nerves, chiasma, and tracts a considerable degree of localization of the fibres in the vertical plane also, fibres from the lower halves of the retinae lying below, and those from the upper halves above.

VISUAL FIELD DEFECTS DUE TO LESIONS OF THE OPTIC NERVES, CHIASMA, AND TRACTS

We are now in a position to apply the anatomical facts just described to the interpretation of the visual field defects produced by lesions of the optic nerves, chiasma, and tracts.

LESIONS OF THE OPTIC NERVE

A lesion of one optic nerve produces a field defect limited to the same eye, since it lies anterior to the chiasmal decussation. The type of field defect produced varies according to the pathological nature of the lesion and is more fully discussed in a later chapter. In general, inflammatory and compressive lesions of the optic nerve are likely to lead to a central scotoma [FIG. 12] or to a sector defect of irregular shape, but in papilloedema due to increased intracranial pressure the characteristic field defect is an enlargement of the blind spot, together with a peripheral concentric constriction.

LESIONS OF THE CHIASMA

The commonest lesions of the optic chiasma are those due to pressure, either by tumours arising in the pituitary body or above the sella turcica, such as suprasellar cysts and meningiomas. In addition, the chiasma itself may be the site of a gliomatous tumour, or may be compressed by a tumour arising in the third ventricle, by distension of the third ventricle in hydrocephalus, or by an intracranial aneurysm. It may be involved in local chronic arachnoiditis, or in syphilitic meningitis, in demyelinating disorders such as multiple sclerosis and neuromyelitis optica, and, rarely, in vascular lesions and after head injury.

When the point of maximal pressure is in the midline the decussating fibres are first compressed, with the result that at some stage in the development of the growth there is bitemporal hemianopia, for, as we have seen, the decussating fibres are derived from the nasal halves of both retinae, and owing to the refractive effect of the optic lens these parts of the retinae receive images from the temporal halves of the visual fields. When pressure is exerted upon the

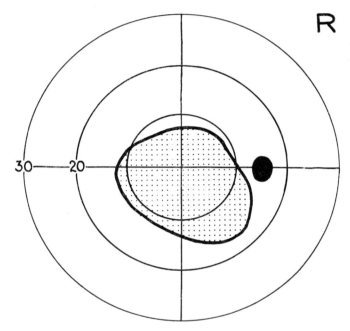

FIG. 12. A central scotoma due to retrobulbar neuritis

chiasma from below, the fibres from the lower nasal quadrants of the retinae are first affected. Hence the field defect begins in the upper temporal quadrants. When the pressure comes from above, the reverse is the case. This rather schematic explanation must now be qualified by the statement that pituitary and suprasellar tumours rarely exert a symmetrical pressure in the midline. Hence the decussating fibres are usually involved on one side before the other. Consequently, in the case of pituitary tumours, the field defect begins as a rule in the upper temporal quadrant on one side as an indentation which may be associated with a paracentral scotoma with which it subsequently fuses. It then spreads to the lower quadrant, while a similar change occurs a little later on the opposite sides [FIGS. 13(a) and (b)]. Further pressure leads to involvement of the nasal field of the eye first affected and at this stage there is blindness of one eye with temporal hemianopia of the other. Finally the remaining nasal field is lost.

Owing to the complicated paths of the fibres in the chiasma and the liability

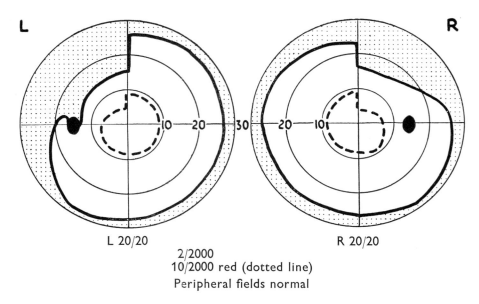

L 20/20   R 20/20

2/2000
10/2000 red (dotted line)
Peripheral fields normal

FIG. 13a. Visual fields of a patient with a chromophobe adenoma of the pituitary, showing early changes in the upper temporal quadrants

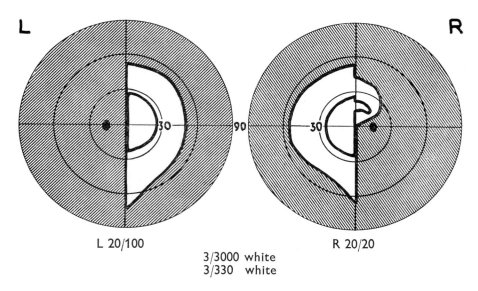

L 20/100   R 20/20

3/3000 white
3/330   white

FIG. 13b. Field changes in a patient with a chromophobe adenoma of the pituitary. The splitting of the macula which occurred in this case is unusual

of pressure to involve also either the optic nerve or tract, many forms of visual field change are encountered.

Rarely compression of the lateral angles of the chiasma may occur, for example, in cases of severe atheroma of the internal carotid arteries. Since the non-decussating fibres are affected, the resulting field defect is binasal hemianopia.

The most characteristic feature of the visual field defects associated with lesions of the chiasma is their asymmetry compared with the more symmetrical character of the defects due to lesions of the optic tracts and radiation.

LESIONS OF THE OPTIC TRACT

Since the optic tracts are composed of fibres from the temporal half of the retina of the same side and the nasal half of the opposite retina, they carry impulses derived from visual images of objects in the opposite half of the visual field. Lesions of one optic tract, therefore, result in a crossed homonymous field defect which usually begins in one quadrant and rarely extends to a complete homonymous hemianopia. The defects in the two visual fields are not as a rule congruous, the visual field defect being usually slightly greater upon the side of the lesion than upon the opposite side. A homonymous field defect occurs in cases of pituitary tumour about half as frequently as bitemporal hemianopia, and the optic tract may also be compressed by other tumours at the base of the brain, including the anterior part of the temporal lobe, and by aneurysm of the internal carotid and posterior communicating arteries; it may also be involved in inflammatory lesions, such as basal syphilitic meningitis.

THE GENICULOCALCARINE PATHWAY

The last stage of the path of the visual fibres to the cortex begins at the lateral geniculate body. From this they enter the posterior limb of the internal capsule, where they lie behind the somatic sensory fibres and internal to the fibres of the auditory radiation. They emerge from the capsule as the optic radiation, or geniculocalcarine pathway, which runs to the area striata of the occipital lobe. This path varies in directness for different fibres. The more dorsal fibres pass directly to the visual cortex, but those situated more ventrally in the optic radiation turn downwards and forwards into the uncinate region of the temporal lobe, and there spread out over the tip of the descending horn of the lateral ventricle before turning back along the inferior aspect of the ventricle to reach the inferior lip of the calcarine sulcus (Falconer and Wilson, 1958; van Buren and Baldwin, 1958). As we have seen, fibres derived from the lower half of the retina remain below those from the upper half throughout the optic chiasma and tracts, and this relationship persists in the geniculocalcarine pathway. Hence the more direct upper fibres of the optic radiation are derived from the upper halves of the retinae and are excited by images from the lower halves of the visual fields, and the reverse is true of the lower fibres, which pass by way of the tip of the temporal lobe. These facts explain the nature of the visual field defects produced by lesions involving the optic radiation in the temporal and parietal lobes respectively. A left temporosphenoidal abscess, for example, tends to damage the lower fibres rather than the upper, and the resulting field defect lies in the upper half

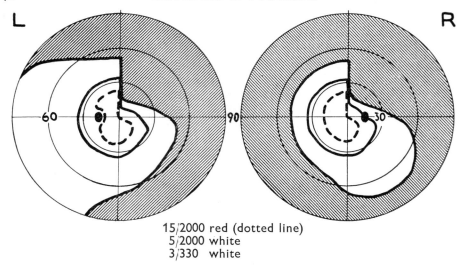

15/2000 red (dotted line)
5/2000 white
3/330 white

FIG. 14. Fields of a patient with a glioma in the left temporo-occipital region

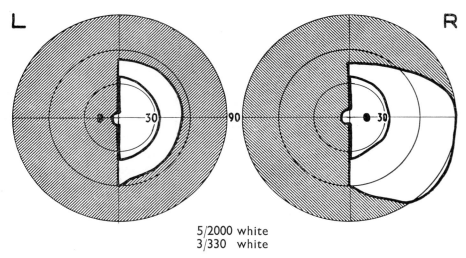

5/2000 white
3/330 white

FIG. 15. Fields of a patient with a metastasis from a breast carcinoma involving the right geniculo-calcarine pathway

of the visual fields. Since a unilateral lesion involves only the fibres concerned in vision in the opposite half-fields, the field defect is a crossed homonymous superior quadrantic one [FIG. 14]. Conversely a lesion involving the optic radiation in the parietal lobe may affect only the upper fibres and produce a crossed inferior quadrantic loss. Complete destruction of one optic radiation produces a crossed homonymous hemianopia. Homonymous field defects due to lesions of the optic radiation are congruous, with escape of a small area around the fixation point—'sparing of the macula' [FIG. 15]. The commonest lesions involving the optic radiation are vascular lesions and tumours. The lower fibres may be involved in abscess of the temporal lobe. The radiations are early affected by degeneration in diffuse sclerosis (Schilder's disease).

THE VISUAL CORTEX

The cortical visual area or 'area striata' is situated above and below the calcarine sulcus and in adjacent portions of the cuneus and lingual gyrus, and sometimes extends slightly on to the lateral surface of the occipital pole. From what has been said previously concerning the representation of the retinae in the optic tracts, it will be realized that the visual cortex on one side receives impulses from the temporal half of the retina on the same side and the nasal half of the opposite retina, that is, those halves of the retinae which are excited by images derived from the opposite halves of the visual fields. Some workers believe that the macula is bilaterally represented at the cortex; others that each half is represented in the opposite visual cortex. The retinae may be regarded as projected upon the visual cortex as follows. The macula occupies a wedge-shaped area of the most posterior part of the visual cortex, extending slightly on to the lateral surface of the occipital lobe, the apex of the wedge being 2 or 3 cm. anterior to the occipital pole. The periphery of the retina is represented in front of the macular area of the cortex, concentric zones of the retina from the macula to the periphery being probably represented from behind forwards in the visual area. The upper quadrants of the retina are represented in the upper part of the visual cortex, above the calcarine sulcus, and the lower quadrants below. From these facts the effects of lesions involving the visual cortex can readily be understood. Lesions of one visual cortex cause crossed homonymous field defects. Lesions involving the upper half, i.e. the area above the calcarine sulcus produce inferior quadrantic field defects, and vice versa. Lesions confined to the occipital pole produce central or paracentral scotomas. Lesions more anteriorly placed tend to produce scotomas involving the periphery of the visual fields, with escape of the central portions, provided the macular fibres of the optic radiation are not injured at the same time. Complete destruction of the visual cortex on one side produces a crossed homonymous hemianopia.

The main arterial supply of the visual cortex is the posterior cerebral artery. Thrombosis of the posterior cerebral artery therefore causes a crossed homonymous hemianopia, with, rarely, escape of the fixation point. Gassel and Williams (1962) suggest that while sparing of the macula may perhaps occur in lesions of the radiation, when it appears to be present in patients with calcarine lesions it is usually an artefact due to inconstancy of gaze during charting of the visual fields; in most calcarine lesions and after hemispherectomy the macular field is split. The commonest lesions of the visual cortex are vascular lesions and tumours. Many cases of gun-shot wound of this part of the brain were observed during the First World War.

REFERENCES

BROUWER, B., and ZEEMAN, W. P. C. (1926) The projection of the retina in the primary optic neuron in monkeys, *Brain*, **49**, 1.
COGAN, D. G., and WILLIAMS, H. W. (1966) *Neurology of the Visual System*, Springfield, Ill.

CUSHING, H. (1921–2) The field defects produced by temporal lobe lesions, *Brain*, **44,** 341.

CUSHING, H., and WALKER, C. B. (1914–15) Distortions of the visual fields in cases of brain tumor (4); chiasmal lesions with especial reference to bitemporal hemianopsia, *Brain*, **37,** 341.

FALCONER, M. A., and WILSON, J. L. (1958) Visual field changes following anterior temporal lobectomy: their significance in relation to 'Meyer's loop' of the optic radiation, *Brain*, **81,** 1.

GASSEL, M. M., and WILLIAMS, D. (1962). Visual function in patients with homonymous hemianopia. Part I, The visual fields, *Brain*, **85,** 175.

HOLMES, G. (1918) Disturbances of vision by cerebral lesions, *Brit. J. Ophthal.*, **2,** 353.

HOLMES, G. (1931) A contribution to the cortical representation of vision, *Brain*, **54,** 470.

HOLMES, G., and LISTER, W. T. (1916) Disturbances of vision from cerebral lesions, with special reference to the cortical representation of the macula, *Brain*, **39,** 34.

HORRAX, G., and PUTNAM, T. J. (1932) Distortion of the visual fields in cases of brain tumour. The field defects and hallucinations produced by tumours of the occipital lobe, *Brain*, **55,** 499.

PUTNAM, T. J. (1926) Studies on the central visual connexions. Part III. The general relationships between the external geniculate body, optic radiation, and visual cortex in man: report of two cases, *Arch. Neurol. Psychiat. (Chicago)*, **16,** 566.

PUTNAM, T. J. (1926) Studies on the central visual system. Part IV. The details of the organization of the geniculo-striate system in man, *Arch. Neurol. Psychiat. (Chicago)*, **16,** 683.

RIDDOCH, G. (1917) Dissociation of visual perceptions due to occipital injuries, with especial reference to appreciation of movement, *Brain*, **40,** 15.

TRAQUAIR, H. M. (1938) *An Introduction to Clinical Perimetry*, 3rd ed., London.

TRAQUAIR, H. M., DOTT, N. M., and RUSSELL, W. R. (1935) Traumatic lesions of the optic chiasma, *Brain*, **58,** 398.

VAN BUREN, J. M., and BALDWIN, M. (1958) The architecture of the optic radiation in the temporal lobe of man, *Brain*, **81,** 15.

THE OCULAR MOVEMENTS

The ocular movements are described as horizontal movement outwards, or abduction; horizontal movement inwards, or adduction; vertical movement upwards, or elevation; vertical movement downwards, or depression. The eye is, of course, capable of diagonal movements at any intermediate angle. The term 'rotation' should be reserved for wheel-like movements around an imaginary pivot passing from before backwards through the centre of the pupil. Such movements of rotation do not normally occur, but are observed only as a result of the unbalanced action of certain muscles. Inward rotation is a movement similar to that of a wheel rolling towards the nose, and outward rotation is the opposite rotatory movement. Normally the movements of the two eyes are harmoniously symmetrical and we then speak of conjugate ocular movements or deviation. Conjugate ocular deviation is described as horizontal or lateral, upward and downward. Conjugate adduction of the two eyes is known as convergence.

THE EXTRINSIC OCULAR MUSCLES

The extrinsic ocular muscles are the four recti, superior and inferior, lateral and medial, and the two obliques, superior and inferior. The action of each of these muscles is shown in the following table and in the diagram [FIG. 16], in which the relative power of the muscles in different directions is indicated by the length of the arrows.

Superior rectus	Medial rectus	Inferior rectus	Inferior oblique	Lateral rectus	Superior oblique
Adductor	Adductor	Adductor	Elevator	..	Depressor
Internal	..	External	External	..	Internal
rotator		rotator	rotator		rotator
Elevator	..	Depressor	Abductor	Abductor	Abductor

It will be seen that only the lateral and medial recti act in a single plane. The other muscles always act in concert with each other in such a way that their conflicting tendencies cancel and a harmonious resultant is produced. Thus when the two obliques aid the lateral rectus in abduction their vertical and

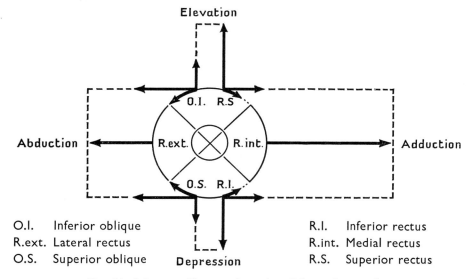

O.I.   Inferior oblique   R.I.   Inferior rectus
R.ext. Lateral rectus   R.int. Medial rectus
O.S.   Superior oblique   R.S.   Superior rectus

FIG. 16. Scheme to illustrate the action of the ocular muscles

rotatory forces cancel each other; and when the superior rectus and inferior oblique contract together in elevating the eye their horizontal and rotatory components also cancel.

But owing to the planes in which the superior and inferior recti and the obliques are placed their actions are influenced by the position of the eye in the orbit. When the eye is rotated outwards 23 degrees the superior rectus is a pure elevator and the inferior rectus a pure depressor. The more it is turned inwards the more they act as internal and external rotators. The converse is true of the obliques. In conjugate deviation there is a harmonious contraction of the appropriate muscles of the two eyes. In lateral conjugate deviation the lateral rectus of one eye and the medial rectus of the other are associated; in conjugate deviation upwards and downwards, the elevators and depressors of the two eyes respectively; and in convergence, the medial recti. Ocular movements must not be regarded as consisting merely of contractions of the prime movers, the muscles actively displacing the eye. There is evidence that graded contraction and relaxation of their antagonists play an important part in orderly movement.

PARALYSIS OF INDIVIDUAL OCULAR MUSCLES

The more important results of paralysis of an ocular muscle are (1) defective ocular movement, (2) squint, (3) erroneous projection of the visual field, and (4) diplopia.

DEFECTIVE OCULAR MOVEMENT

Defective ocular movement is demonstrated by asking the patient to fix his gaze on an object, such as the observer's finger, which is then moved upwards and downwards and to either side, convergence being tested by bringing it towards the patient. The movement is defective in the direction in which the eye is normally moved by the muscle which is paralysed. Slight weakness of a muscle, especially of one of the elevators or depressors, may not lead to any defect of ocular movement evident to the observer.

SQUINT

Squint, or strabismus, is the term applied to a failure of the normal co-ordination of the ocular axes. It is necessary to distinguish paralytic squint from concomitant or spasmodic squint. Paralytic squint may be present when the eyes are at rest, in which case it is due to the unbalanced action of the normal antagonist of the paralysed muscle, for example, the affected eye may be slightly adducted when the lateral rectus is paralysed. More often it is apparent only when the eyes are deviated in the direction in which the eye should be pulled by the paralysed muscle, or if squint is present at rest it is increased by such a movement. Concomitant squint, however, is present at rest and is equal for all positions of the eyes, and, if the fixing eye is covered, the movements of the squinting eye are found to be full. Concomitant squint is not associated with diplopia; paralytic squint, at least in the early stages, usually is.

When the lateral rectus is paralysed the ocular axes converge and the squint is said to be convergent. Paralysis of the medial rectus causes divergent squint. Divergent squint, however, also accompanies myopia, and is often present in an unconscious patient without indicating paralysis of an ocular muscle. The deviation of the axis of the affected eye from parallelism with that of the normal eye is called the 'primary deviation'. If the patient is made to fix an object in a direction requiring the action of the affected muscle and at the same time is prevented from seeing it with his normal eye, the latter is found to deviate too far in the required direction. This is called 'secondary deviation', and is due to the increased effort evoked by his attempt to move the affected eye.

ERRONEOUS PROJECTION OF THE VISUAL FIELD

If we look at a candle straight in front of us and then, turning the eyes but not the head, at a candle placed to one side, in each case the image of the candle falls upon the macula. Let us now consider what happens when the right lateral rectus is paralysed. On conjugate deviation to the right the left eye moves normally and the right eye remains directed forwards. The image of the object regarded falls in the left eye upon the macula, in the right eye upon the nasal half of the retina. The patient is accustomed to regard an object, the image of which falls upon the nasal half of the right retina, as situated to the right of one of which the image falls upon the macula. Consequently he sees two images and projects the false image perceived by his affected eye to the right of the true image perceived by his normal eye. If now his normal eye is covered and he is asked to touch the object, he will direct his finger to the right of its true position. The erroneous projection is always in the normal direction of action of the affected muscle. When it produces sufficient spatial disorientation vertigo results. Hess's screen is an ingenious method of recording the position of the false image.

DIPLOPIA

Erroneous projection of the visual field of the affected eye is responsible for double vision. When both eyes are used, two images are seen, one correctly and one erroneously projected, the true and the false image. Let us apply our previous illustration to the interpretation of diplopia.

In paralysis of the right lateral rectus the right eye is not abducted. If the patient attempts to deviate his eyes horizontally to the right, the image of a small object falls in the left eye upon the macula. In the right eye, which is not displaced, it falls upon the nasal half of the retina, hence it is seen in (or projected into) the temporal field of the right eye. The false image is thus parallel with and to the right of the true image. The further the test object is moved to the right the further into the nasal half of the right retina its image moves, and the further the false image appears to move to the right. From these facts can be deduced two simple rules governing the appearance of diplopia:

1. The separation of the images increases the further the eyes are moved in the normal direction of pull of the paralysed muscle.
2. The false image is displaced in the direction of the plane or planes of action of the paralysed muscle.

It follows from the two rules that when the gaze is so directed that the separation of the images is greatest, the more peripherally situated image is the false one, derived from the affected eye, which can thus be ascertained. The simplest method is to cover one eye with a red, and the other with a green, glass. The patient is then made to look at a light, such as an ophthalmoscope lamp, or a small but well-illuminated piece of white paper. This is moved until the maximal separation of the images is obtained, and they are then distinguishable by their colour. If coloured glass is not available, an intelligent and co-operative patient is usually able to distinguish the images by noticing which disappears when each eye is covered separately.

When the affected eye has been discovered, the paralysed muscle can be determined. It is the muscle which normally displaces the eye in the direction of displacement of the false image. The positions of the false images resulting from paralysis of the various ocular muscles are described below for the right eye. The description will apply to the left eye if right be substituted for left and vice versa. The diplopia is said to be simple, or uncrossed, when the false image lies on the same side of the true image as the affected eye, and crossed when it lies on the opposite side.

POSITION OF FALSE IMAGE IN PARALYSIS OF THE OCULAR MUSCLES OF THE RIGHT EYE

Lateral Rectus. The diplopia is uncrossed and the maximal separation of the images occurs on abduction, when the false image is level with, and parallel with, the true.

Medial Rectus. The diplopia is crossed and the maximal separation of the images occurs on adduction, when the false image is level with, and parallel with, the true.

Superior Rectus. The false image is above and to the left of the true and tilted away from it. Vertical separation of the images is greatest on abduction, the tilting greatest on adduction. The diplopia is crossed.

Inferior Rectus. The false image is below and to the left of the true and tilted towards it. Vertical separation of the images is greatest on abduction, and tilting on adduction. The diplopia is crossed.

Inferior Oblique. The false image is above and to the right of the true and tilted away from it. The diplopia is uncrossed. Vertical separation of the images is greatest on adduction, and tilting on abduction.

Superior Oblique. The false image is below and to the right of the true and tilted towards it. The diplopia is uncrossed. Vertical separation of the images is greatest on adduction, and tilting on abduction. Since the diplopia occurs on looking downwards it is particularly troublesome to the patient when walking downstairs.

A patient suffering from diplopia usually rotates or tilts the head into the position in which the least demand is made upon the paralysed muscle.

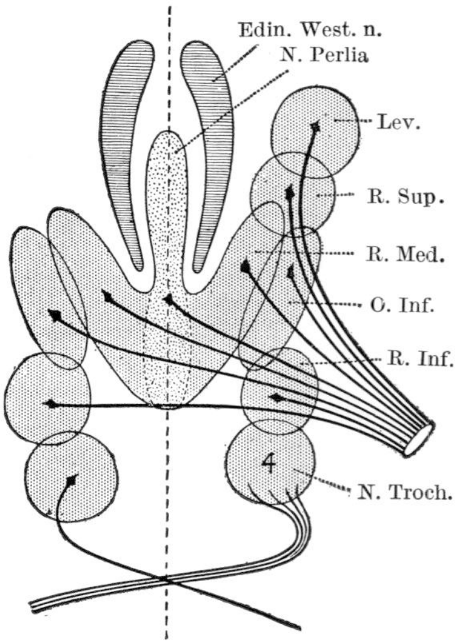

THE NUCLEI OF THE OCULAR MUSCLES

The lower motor neurones which innervate the ocular muscles originate in the nuclei of the third, fourth, and sixth cranial nerves. The first two lie in the midbrain just anterior to the cerebral aqueduct at the level of the superior and inferior colliculi. The nuclei of the sixth nerve lie in the pons beneath the floor of the upper part of the fourth ventricle and partly encircled by the fibres of the seventh nerve.

FIG. 17. Diagram of the oculomotor nucleus

Edin. West. n.
N. Perlia
Lev.
R. Sup.
R. Med.
O. Inf.
R. Inf.
N. Troch.

The precise representation of muscles in the nucleus of the third nerve is still somewhat uncertain, but the diagram [FIG. 17] represents the probable arrangement. The median, unpaired, small-celled nucleus of Perlia is the centre for convergence and accommodation, while the lateral, paired, small-celled nucleus of Edinger-Westphal innervates the constrictor of the pupil. The remainder of the nucleus is the paired, large-celled, lateral nucleus in which the muscles are represented from above downwards as follows: levator palpebrae, superior rectus, inferior oblique, medial rectus, inferior rectus. Decussating fibres unite the lower parts of the nuclei. Immediately below the third nerve nucleus lies that of the fourth nerve which innervates the opposite superior oblique. This nucleus and the adjacent lowest part of the third nerve nucleus innervate the two muscles concerned in depression of the eye, and the two elevating muscles are innervated by mutually adjacent portions of the upper half of the third nerve nucleus.

THE SUPRANUCLEAR AND INTERNUCLEAR PATHS FOR OCULAR MOVEMENT

CONJUGATE LATERAL DEVIATION

Movements of the eyes can be evoked from two areas of the cerebral cortex by electrical stimulation. One supranuclear path of the motor fibres concerned in conjugate lateral deviation begins in the posterior part of the middle frontal gyrus, anterior to the precentral gyrus. Electrical stimulation of this area produces deviation of the eyes to the opposite side. From the middle frontal gyrus the supranuclear path runs through the corona radiata to the internal capsule, where it is situated near the genu, and then to the cerebral peduncle. In the midbrain the fibres decussate and pass downwards into the upper part of the pons. Just above the sixth nucleus the path divides, some fibres running into that nucleus, while others cross the midline, turn upwards in the posterior longitudinal bundle, and terminate in that part of the third nerve nucleus which innervates the opposite medial rectus. Thus excitation of the supranuclear fibres causes a contraction of the opposite lateral rectus and the ipsilateral medial rectus, and so produces conjugate ocular deviation to the opposite side.

The other cortical area for eye movements is in or near the visual cortex in the occipital lobe. From here fibres have been traced through the pulvinar to the midbrain.

CONJUGATE VERTICAL DEVIATION

Less is known about the supranuclear paths for conjugate vertical than about those for conjugate lateral deviation. Probably they also originate in the middle frontal gyrus, but on electrical excitation of this region the more powerful lateral movement of the eyes overpowers the vertical movements. The fibres probably run through the internal capsule and decussate in the upper part of the midbrain. Those concerned in conjugate elevation appear to cross at a higher level than those concerned in conjugate depression. After decussating they terminate in the appropriate regions of the third nerve nucleus and in the fourth nerve nucleus.

CONJUGATE CONVERGENCE

The supranuclear paths for conjugate convergence are also incompletely known. Since convergence is normally the response to the perception or imagination of a visual image, the path of excitation probably runs through the visual cortex, and then, possibly passing through the middle frontal gyrus, by a descending route with the corticospinal fibres to the midbrain, to terminate after decussation in the nuclei of the medial recti.

REFLEX OCULAR FIXATION

In voluntary ocular deviation, the patient turns the eyes spontaneously or in response to a command. In addition, conjugate ocular deviation may be excited by various stimuli.

Retinal Stimulation. The retinal stimulus may be either (*a*) macular, or (*b*) peripheral.

(*a*) The patient's head is kept motionless and he is told to fix his gaze upon an object which is then moved in various directions. Appropriate conjugate ocular deviation occurs to keep the image of the object upon the macula.

(*b*) It is an everyday experience that a moving object in the periphery of the visual field excites deviation of the head and eyes so directed that its image is brought upon the macula.

Auditory Stimulation. In response to a sound the eyes are deviated in the direction from which the sound appears to come.

Labyrinthine Stimulation. Caloric, rotatory, and electrical excitation of the labyrinth evokes conjugate ocular deviation.

Passive Movement of the Head. The patient is made to fix an object with his gaze and the head is then rotated, flexed, or extended at the neck. Afferent impulses from the cervical spine excite appropriate ocular deviation to keep the image of the object on the macula, whatever the position of the head. For example, if the head is passively rotated to the left, the eyes become deviated to the right.

The regions concerned in ocular fixation are the visual cortex and the descending path to the midbrain via the pulvinar and the posterior longitudinal bundle.

THE MEDIAL LONGITUDINAL FASCICULUS

The medial longitudinal fasciculus is an important path linking the oculomotor nuclei. It connects the lateral rectus with the opposite medial rectus in conjugate lateral deviation, and it carries impulses concerned in the reflex ocular movements described in the last section. It links together the cochlear and the vestibular parts of the eighth nerve with the oculomotor nuclei and the muscles which rotate the head.

SUPRANUCLEAR AND INTERNUCLEAR LESIONS

Dissociation of Voluntary Ocular Movement and Reflex Fixation.
Bilateral lesions of the frontal centres or their descending paths interfere with voluntary movement of the eyes, which, however, can still follow a slowly moving

object, or fix an object while the head is moved. In such cases reflex fixation is overactive and the eyes tend to remain fixed on an object until the gaze is obscured. The converse condition, a lesion interfering with reflex fixation, makes it impossible for the subject to fix, and hence to see clearly, a moving object or an object when he himself is moving (Holmes, 1938).

CONJUGATE LATERAL MOVEMENT

We may encounter either spasm, paralysis, or dissociation of conjugate lateral movement of the eyes.

Spasm of conjugate lateral movement may occur as an element in a focal epileptic attack, of which it may be the first symptom, when the exciting lesion is situated in the middle frontal gyrus, the eyes being deviated to the opposite side. It may occur in convulsions excited by an occipital lesion, in which case there is usually a visual aura. It is commonly observed also in the generalized convulsions of epilepsy. Spasmodic lateral deviation occasionally occurs in Parkinsonism due to encephalitis lethargica, though in this condition vertical deviation is more frequent. It may be excited reflexly by a lesion of the labyrinth, the eyes in this case being usually deviated towards the side of the lesion. In paralysis of conjugate lateral movement in an unconscious patient the eyes are often deviated to the non-paralysed side by the unbalanced action of the normal hemisphere.

Paralysis of conjugate lateral movement to one side may occur as a result of a lesion of the supranuclear fibres at any point in their course, but the effects of a unilateral lesion above the pons are always transitory. When the lesion is situated above the decussation of these fibres in the lower midbrain, lateral movement to the opposite side is paralysed. When the lesion is below the decussation, i.e. in the pons just above the sixth nucleus, the paralysis is to the same side as the lesion. A lesion involving the decussation leads to bilateral paralysis, and this may also occur as a result of one extending to both sides of the pons. It must be remembered that the supranuclear fibres are concerned with voluntary movement of the eyes, and the true test of their conductivity is to tell the patient to look to one or the other side. To ask him to follow a moving finger with his gaze is to introduce a reflex element into the response. It is common to find in a patient, unconscious from a haemorrhage into the internal capsule, evidence of a paralysis of conjugate ocular deviation which apparently quickly disappears when he recovers consciousness. Such patients, however, often show slowness or weakness in deviating the eyes to the opposite side on command, though they are able to follow with their eyes a moving object.

A pontine lesion usually abolishes reflex conjugate lateral deviation as well as the voluntary movement—a point in favour of the existence in this region of a 'centre', from which starts a final common path shared by both voluntary and reflex movements.

In paralysis of conjugate lateral deviation the affected medial rectus contracts normally on convergence, unless the supranuclear path for convergence, which is separate from that for lateral deviation, should also be involved. This is an example of the rule that supranuclear lesions cause paralysis of movements and not of muscles.

Dissociation of conjugate lateral movement occurs when either the lateral or the medial rectus contracts more strongly than its conjugate fellow, and the normal harmony of the two eyes is disturbed. Most commonly the lateral rectus contracts normally, but the opposite medial rectus is weak or paralysed for conjugate lateral movement but contracts normally on convergence. The lesion, usually due to multiple sclerosis, has been thought to involve the ascending fibres of the medial longitudinal fasciculus linking the two muscles together, while the supranuclear path for convergence which terminates at a higher level escapes (ophthalmoplegia internuclearis anterior of Lhermitte). A lesion involving the nucleus of the medial rectus muscle in the third nerve nucleus, or the fibres running to this muscle in the third nerve, of course paralyses the muscle both for conjugate lateral movement and for convergence. A lesion of the sixth nerve or its nucleus causes paralysis of the lateral rectus, but the opposite medial rectus contracts normally on conjugate lateral deviation and on convergence.

Causes of Conjugate Lateral Paralysis

The commonest cause of conjugate lateral paralysis is tumour involving the pontine centre. It may also be produced by encephalitis, though less often than vertical paralysis, and by multiple sclerosis, in which disease dissociation of lateral movement is common, the medial rectus contracting less strongly than the lateral. Vascular lesions account for most of the remaining cases.

CONJUGATE VERTICAL MOVEMENTS

Spasm of conjugate vertical movement upwards may occur in an epileptic fit or in an attack of petit mal. It is also the commonest form of oculogyral spasm found in encephalitic Parkinsonism, though downward and lateral spasm occasionally occur. Upward deviation of the eyes also occurs normally during sleep, and on voluntary closure of the eyelids and blinking.

Paralysis of conjugate vertical movement seems not to occur as a result of lesions above the midbrain. At the level of the superior colliculus there exist supranuclear mechanisms for the conjugate vertical movements and for convergence, since any of these movements may be abolished separately and without evidence of a nuclear lesion. Moreover, as in the case of conjugate lateral deviation, voluntary vertical deviation may be lost while the movement can still be excited reflexly, for example by flexing or extending the head when the patient's gaze is fixed upon a motionless object. Such a loss of voluntary, with retention of reflex, movement indicates a lesion of the supranuclear path, while the final common path from the hypothetical midbrain 'centre' remains intact. The centre for vertical movement upwards is situated at a higher level in the midbrain than that for downward movement, since a tumour arising in the third ventricle and impinging upon the midbrain from above impairs the former before the latter. Upward deviation is much more frequently lost than downward deviation, and, as Collier has pointed out, its loss is sometimes associated with retraction of the upper lids. In some cases the defect is congenital. It may result from encephalitis, neoplasm of the third ventricle, midbrain or pineal body, and vascular and other lesions of the upper midbrain.

PARALYSIS OF CONVERGENCE

Paralysis of convergence is rarely observed as a result of lesions of the cerebral hemispheres, probably because its supranuclear paths are bilateral. It is common, however, in extrapyramidal syndromes associated with rigidity, especially in Parkinsonism due to encephalitis lethargica. It is also met with as a result of lesions involving the convergence centre in the midbrain and may occur after head injury. In such cases there may be an isolated loss of convergence and accommodation. More often loss of convergence is associated with loss of vertical conjugate movement, and sometimes with loss of the reaction of the pupils to light. Loss of convergence is occasionally, and spasm of convergence usually hysterical. Loss of convergence may cause diplopia.

NUCLEAR OPHTHALMOPLEGIA

By nuclear ophthalmoplegia is meant a paralysis of ocular muscles due to a lesion involving the nuclei of the oculomotor nerves. When the extrinsic ocular muscles are involved, the term external ophthalmoplegia is used: paralysis of the pupillary and ciliary muscles is known as internal ophthalmoplegia. When both are affected together we speak of total ophthalmoplegia. Internal ophthalmoplegia is dealt with in a later section. We are here concerned only with external ophthalmoplegia, including ptosis.

Nuclear ophthalmoplegia must be distinguished from supranuclear lesions and from lesions of the oculomotor nerve trunks. As we have seen, supranuclear lesions cause disturbances of conjugate ocular movement. Consequently the ocular axes remain parallel and diplopia is not produced. Nuclear lesions may be unilateral, but are more often bilateral. When bilateral they are not symmetrical, and loss of parallelism of the ocular axes and diplopia occur. The varied degree of paralysis of the muscles of both eyes, with or without internal ophthalmoplegia, rarely simulates a lesion of the third nerve trunks, in which as a rule the muscles innervated by the nerve are all affected to an equal extent. Nuclear ophthalmoplegia confined to the fourth nerve has probably never been verified. Since the sixth nerve supplies only one muscle, an isolated lesion of the sixth nerve nucleus can only be distinguished from a lesion of the nerve trunk by the presence of associated symptoms of a lesion of the pons.

The following are the principal causes of nuclear ophthalmoplegia:

1. *Massive lesions involving the brain stem*, especially tumours of the third ventricle, midbrain, pineal body and pons, and vascular lesions.

2. *Avitaminosis.* The condition described by Wernicke as acute superior haemorrhagic polio-encephalitis is now ascribed to avitaminosis.

3. *Infections.* In this group fall syphilis, encephalitis lethargica, and disseminated encephalomyelitis. Syphilitic nuclear ophthalmoplegia may be vascular in origin, but a degenerative type sometimes occurs in tabes and in general paresis.

4. *Progressive ophthalmoplegia* is the term which has been applied to a group of ophthalmoplegias of unknown origin, and, possibly, mixed aetiology, characterized by the insidious onset and slowly progressive course of ptosis and external ophthalmoplegia. The disorder may start at any age and is sometimes

familial. Myopathy of the external ocular muscles accounts for most cases. Lead poisoning is a rare cause.

5. *Syringobulbia* rarely produces ophthalmoplegia.

6. *Head injury* is a rare cause of nuclear ophthalmoplegia, which may result from contusion of the brain stem.

7. *Congenital defects* of ocular movement occur. These may be hereditary and associated with other hereditary abnormalities.

NYSTAGMUS

Nystagmus is a disturbance of ocular posture characterized by a more or less rhythmical oscillation of the eyes. This movement may be of the same rate in both directions, or quicker in one direction than in the other. In the latter case the movements are distinguished as the quick and the slow phases. The quick phase is taken to indicate the direction of the nystagmus, so that if the slow phase is to the left and the quick to the right, the patient is said to exhibit nystagmus to the right. Nystagmus may occur when the eyes are in the position of rest, or only on deviation in certain directions or on convergence, or only when the head is in a certain position—positional nystagmus. The movement may be confined to one plane, horizontal or vertical, or occur in more than one plane—rotary nystagmus. Nystagmus may be associated with a rapid rotary tremor of the head, or with jerky vertical movements of the eyelids. The acquired forms may cause an apparent movement of objects seen by the patient. Nystagmus can be recorded by electronystagmography.

The nature of nystagmus can be best appreciated by recalling the statement made in a previous section [on p. 80] that the posture of the eyes is influenced reflexly by a number of factors of which the most important are impulses derived from the retinae, the labyrinths, and the cervical spine. Nystagmus is a disturbance of ocular posture which may be due to (1) defective or abnormal retinal impulses, (2) abnormal labyrinthine impulses, (3) lesions of the cervical spinal cord, (4) lesions involving the central paths concerned in ocular posture, and (5) weakness of the ocular muscles. (6) It may also be a congenital abnormality of unknown aetiology, and (7) it is rarely hysterical.

NYSTAGMUS OF RETINAL ORIGIN

1. *Amblyopia* coming on in early life may cause nystagmus if some vision is retained, and especially if macular vision is impaired. The visual impairment renders ocular fixation defective, and a pendular nystagmus results.

2. *Miners' nystagmus* has been attributed to the relative inefficiency of macular vision in a dim light as a result of the absence of rods in the macula. On this hypothesis the defectiveness of macular vision causes defective fixation. It is also believed that neurosis plays a part in maintaining, if not in originating, the disturbance.

3. *Optokinetic nystagmus.* Optokinetic nystagmus is the term applied to the nystagmus evoked by a succession of moving objects passing before the eyes. A familiar example is the nystagmus which occurs in an individual looking out of the window of a moving train. The slow phase is in the direction in which the landscape appears to move and the quick phase is in the direction in which the

train moves. To test for optokinetic nystagmus a Bárány drum is used. This is a revolving, striped cylinder, the speed and direction of which can be altered easily. Horizontal and vertical nystagmus in each direction is produced by revolving the drum at the same speed. The amplitude and regularity of the nystagmus in each direction is noted.

Optokinetic nystagmus is a brain stem reflex, quite distinct from that for vestibular nystagmus and independent of the vestibular nuclei (Dix, Hallpike, and Harrison, 1949). The cortical centre for optokinetic nystagmus is in the supramarginal and angular gyri (Carmichael, Dix, and Hallpike, 1956). Optokinetic nystagmus to the opposite side is suppressed in lesions of this area. Brain stem lesions involving the medial longitudinal fasciculus on one side are associated with changes in optokinetic nystagmus. Thus these changes are sometimes found in multiple sclerosis and intramedullary tumour.

LABYRINTHINE NYSTAGMUS

The clinical aspects of labyrinthine nystagmus are considered on page 177. Appropriate stimulation of the horizontal semicircular canals evokes horizontal nystagmus, and of the vertical canals, rotary nystagmus. Acute lesions of the internal ear, whether primary or secondary to disease of the middle ear, cause nystagmus, usually rotary, and with the quick phase as a rule towards the opposite side. The amplitude of the oscillation is increased when the eyes are deviated in the direction of the quick phase and diminished on fixation in the direction of the slow phase. Chronic labyrinthine lesions often lead to fine rotary nystagmus on lateral fixation to one or both sides, especially to the side of the lesion.

NYSTAGMUS DUE TO SPINAL CORD LESIONS

Nystagmus is very rarely seen after a lesion of the cervical region of the spinal cord, and has then been attributed to a defect of afferent impulses from the cervical spine. Many authorities have questioned whether an isolated lesion of the spinal cord alone can cause this sign.

NYSTAGMUS DUE TO CENTRAL LESIONS

Nystagmus is a common symptom of lesions of the brain stem and cerebellum. With cerebellar lesions nystagmus may occur on fixation in any direction, the slow phase being towards the position of rest, and the quick phase towards the periphery. With a unilateral cerebellar lesion it is present in both eyes and is most marked on conjugate deviation to the side of the lesion. It may occur as a result of lesions involving the cerebellar connexions within the brain stem, the vestibular nucleus, and the posterior longitudinal bundle. Multiple sclerosis is the commonest cause. Nystagmus of central origin also occurs in cases of Friedreich's ataxia and other hereditary ataxias, encephalitis, syringomyelia, tumours, and vascular lesions of the brain stem and cerebellum. It is rare in syphilis.

Positional nystagmus [see p. 178] has been used to distinguish central from labyrinthine lesions. A change in the direction of the nystagmus produced by a change in the position of the head favours a central lesion. A positional nystagmus which does not change with changes in the position of the head but may appear only in certain positions or be influenced in intensity by head-posture may be either central or peripheral in origin (Nylén, 1939; Lindsay, 1945).

NYSTAGMUS DUE TO WEAKNESS OF THE OCULAR MUSCLES

A peripheral cause of nystagmus, in weakness of the ocular muscles required to maintain a posture of conjugate deviation, seems the best explanation of its occurrence in such conditions as polyneuritis, especially alcoholic polyneuritis, myasthenia gravis, botulism, and various forms of poisoning.

CONGENITAL AND FAMILIAL NYSTAGMUS

Nystagmus may be present from birth, and in several members of the same family, sometimes in successive generations. Congenital nystagmus is usually a fine pendular oscillation present at rest and increased on deviation in all directions, but more than one variety occurs. There may be an associated oscillation of the head. There is usually no subjective movement of objects. Its cause is unknown, but it may be associated with other ocular defects involving poor vision such as albinism, astigmatism, or amblyopia. It may be inherited as a Mendelian dominant or as a sex-linked recessive, and males are affected three times as often as females.

HYSTERICAL 'NYSTAGMUS'

Hysterical movement of the eyes superficially resembling nystagmus disappear when ocular fixation is unconscious and reappear on testing the eye movements. They may be associated with spasm of convergence.

REFERENCES

ANDRÉ-THOMAS (1924) La paralysie horizontale du regard; les voies oculomotrices; le faisceau longitudinal postérieur; à propos d'une observation clinique suivie d'autopsie, *Rev. Oto-neuro-ophtal.*, **2**, 241.

BENDER, M. B. (1964) *The Oculomotor System*, New York.

CARMICHAEL, E. A., DIX, M. R., and HALLPIKE, C. S.(1956) Pathology, symptomatology, and diagnosis of organic affections of the eighth nerve system, *Brit. med. Bull.*, **12**, 146.

COGAN, D. G. (1956) *Neurology of the Ocular Muscles*, 2nd ed. Springfield, Ill.

COGAN, D. G., and WILLIAMS, H. W. (1966) *Neurology of the Visual System*, Springfield, Ill.

DIX, M. R., HALLPIKE, C. S., and HARRISON, W. S. (1949) Some observations on the otological effects of streptomycin intoxication, *Brain*, **72**, 241.

FAVILL, J. (1928) The twenty-six normally possible forms of rotationally induced nystagmus, *Arch. Neurol. Psychiat. (Chicago)*, **19**, 318.

HÖGYES, A. (1931) Du mécanisme nerveux des mouvements associés des yeux, *Rev. Oto-neuro-ophtal.*, **9**, 477.

HOLMES, G. (1938) The cerebral integration of the ocular movements, *Brit. med. J.*, **2**, 107.

LINDSAY, J. R. (1945) The significance of positional nystagmus in otoneurological diagnosis, *Laryngoscope (St. Louis)*, **55**, 527.

LYLE, T. K., and JACKSON, S. (1949) *Practical Orthoptics in the Treatment of Squint*, 3rd ed., London.

MONCREIFF, W. F. (1931) Ophthalmoplegia internuclearis and other supranuclear paralyses of the eye movements, *Arch. Neurol. Psychiat. (Chicago)*, **25**, 148.

MYERS, I. L. (1925) Nystagmus: neuro-otologic studies concerning its seat of origin, *Amer. J. med. Sci.*, **169**, 742.

NYLÉN, C. O. (1939) The otoneurological diagnosis of tumours of the brain, *Acta oto-laryng. (Stockh.)*, Suppl. 33.

RADEMAKER, G. G. J., and TER BRAAK, J. W. G. (1948). On the central mechanism of some optic reactions, *Brain*, **71**, 48.

SMITH, J. LAWTON (1963) *Optokinetic Nystagmus*, Springfield, Ill.

SPILLER, W. G. (1924) Ophthalmoplegia internuclearis anterior: a case with necropsy, *Brain*, **47**, 345.

VAN GEHUCHTEN, P. (1930) Un cas de paralysie latérale du regard par lésion protubér-antielle, *Rev. Oto-neuro-ophtal.*, **8**, 701.

THE PUPILS AND THE EYELIDS

THE INNERVATION OF THE PUPILS

The size of the pupil is under the control of two mutually antagonistic muscles: the circular muscle of the iris, the sphincter pupillae, which causes contraction and is innervated by the third nerve, and the radial fibres of the iris which cause dilatation and receive their nerve supply from the cervical sympathetic.

THE IRIDODILATOR FIBRES

Little is known about the innervation of the pupil above the midbrain. The experimental work of Karplus and Kreidl, however, points to a path for pupillary dilatation from the frontal cortex to the hypothalamus and thence into the cerebral peduncle. Such a corticofugal path appears necessary to explain the occurrence of pupillary dilatation in states of emotion. The iridodilator fibres continue downwards in the tegmentum of the pons, medulla, and the cervical cord to the lateral horn of the grey matter of the eighth cervical and first and second thoracic segments. From the cells of these lateral horns the preganglionic fibres take origin, and leave the cord by the corresponding ventral roots. From the spinal nerves they pass by the white rami communicantes of the sympathetic to the cervical sympathetic nerve trunk to end in the superior cervical ganglion. The postganglionic fibres start from this ganglion and join the internal carotid plexus with which they enter the skull, and from which some pass to the ophthalmic division of the trigeminal nerve and reach the pupil by the nasociliary and long ciliary nerves, while others go from the carotid plexus through the ciliary ganglion without interruption, and into the short ciliary nerves.

THE IRIDOCONSTRICTOR AND CILIARY FIBRES

The iridoconstrictor fibres probably originate in the nuclei of Edinger-Westphal [see FIG. 17, p. 78]. Entering the third nerve, they terminate in the ciliary ganglion, from which postganglionic fibres arise which pass by the short ciliary nerves to the circular muscle of the iris. It is possible that this is true only of the fibres concerned in the reaction to light and that those involved in the reaction on accommodation by-pass the ciliary ganglion (see below). The ciliary fibres follow the same route except that they probably arise in the median nucleus of

Perlia and terminate in the ciliary muscle, contraction of which allows the lens to become more convex and so accommodates the eye for near vision.

PARALYSIS OF THE SPHINCTER PUPILLAE

The constrictor muscle of the iris may be paralysed as a result of a lesion involving the iridoconstrictor fibres at any point between the nucleus of Edinger-Westphal and the eye. The pupil is widely dilated owing to the unantagonized action of the iridodilator muscle, and the reaction to both light and accommodation is lost. Paralysis of the sphincter pupillae occurring without paralysis of the extra-ocular muscles is usually due to a lesion either of the nucleus of Edinger-Westphal or of the ciliary ganglion.

PARALYSIS OF THE DILATOR PUPILLAE: OCULAR-SYMPA-THETIC PARALYSIS

Paralysis of pupillary dilatation is due to a lesion of the iridodilator fibres of the sympathetic. The pupil is constricted—myosis—by the unopposed iridoconstrictor muscle, and fails to exhibit the normal dilatation when the eye is shaded, in states of pain and emotional excitement, and reflexly when the skin of the same side of the neck is scratched with a pin—the ciliospinal reflex. The iridodilator fibres throughout their course are close to the other fibres of the ocular sympathetic, viz. those which produce tonic elevation of the upper lid and tonic protrusion of the eyeball by means of the unstriped muscle of the orbit. Paralysis of the dilator of the iris is therefore usually associated with paralysis of these muscles also, manifested in slight ptosis and enophthalmos (Horner's syndrome).

The myosis of the Argyll Robertson pupil has been attributed to a lesion of the iridodilator fibres in the midbrain. Myosis may also occur with lesions of the pons, as in the pin-point pupils of pontine haemorrhage, and of the lateral part of the medulla, as in thrombosis of the posterior inferior cerebellar artery. In the spinal cord the lateral horns of the upper dorsal region may be involved in a variety of lesions. The sympathetic white rami may be destroyed by trauma, as in the Klumpke type of birth palsy of the brachial plexus; and the cervical sympathetic may be damaged in the neck by trauma or pressure, especially from enlarged cervical lymph nodes.

Within the cranium the postganglionic fibres may be damaged by the pressure of a tumour or aneurysm behind the orbit.

Apart from lesions of the sympathetic, the pupils are usually small in the elderly and in patients suffering from hypertension.

PARALYSIS OF ACCOMMODATION

Paralysis of accommodation may be produced by lesions involving the median nucleus of Perlia, the third nerve, or the ciliary ganglion. As an isolated ocular phenomenon it is found in diphtheria, in which condition the lesion is according to some authorities nuclear, according to others neuritic, and according to yet others in the ciliary muscle.

INEQUALITY OF THE PUPILS

Inequality of the pupils may occur when one is either pathologically small or pathologically large, or when one is of moderate size but fails to react to light; in which case the normal one will be the larger when it is dilated and the smaller when it is constricted. These various abnormalities can be interpreted in the light of the facts set out above. Irregularity of the pupils is frequently present in syphilis, and sometimes in encephalitis lethargica. In such cases it is probably due to lesions at or near the nucleus and must be distinguished from the irregularity produced by local lesions of the iris, especially iritis.

ACTION OF DRUGS ON THE PUPIL AND CILIARY MUSCLE

Certain drugs influence the pupil and accommodation when applied to the eye. Pilocarpine and physostigmine (eserine) cause constriction of the pupil and spasm of accommodation by stimulating the nerve endings of the third nerve in the pupil and ciliary muscle. Atropine causes dilatation of the pupil and paralysis of accommodation by paralysing the same nerve endings. I have seen several patients with iridoplegia produced by belladonna accidentally introduced into the eye by the fingers after using belladonna liniment. Cocaine causes dilatation of the pupil by stimulating the nerve endings of the sympathetic fibres. The action of morphine in causing iridoconstriction is central, not peripheral.

THE PUPILLARY REACTIONS
THE LIGHT REFLEX

If one eye is exposed to light, a constriction of both pupils normally occurs. The response of the pupil of the eye upon which the light falls is called the direct reaction, that of the opposite pupil the consensual reaction. In eliciting the light reflex the patient should be asked to look at a distant object in order to eliminate the contraction of the pupil on accommodation, and the eye not being tested should be covered in order to eliminate the consensual reaction. The afferent impulses from the retina follow the path of the visual afferent fibres as far as the optic tracts, with a similar decussation of those from the nasal halves of the retina at the optic chiasma. It is unknown whether the reflex fibres are identical with those concerned in vision, or whether, as some have supposed, two separate sets of fibres exist for these functions. Fibres in the optic nerve vary in size and, correspondingly, in speed of conduction, and it has been shown in the cat that retinal impulses to the lateral geniculate body are conveyed by coarse fast-conducting fibres, while those passing to the midbrain centres are fine and slowly conducting (Clark, 1944). On leaving the optic tracts the reflex fibres separate from the visual and according to Magoun *et al.* (1936) in the monkey they pass through the brachium of the superior colliculus, but do not enter it, turning rostrally and medially into the pretectal region and then descending to the oculomotor nuclei. The decussating fibres cross, some in the posterior commissure and some ventral to the aqueduct near the nuclei. It is clear that both optic tracts must be connected with both oculomotor nuclei since a beam of light falling upon either half of either retina evokes a contraction of both pupils. The efferent path of the reflex runs from the nuclei of Edinger-Westphal by the iridoconstrictor fibres already described.

THE REACTION ON ACCOMMODATION

When the gaze is directed from a distant to a near object, contraction of the medial recti brings about a convergence of the ocular axes and, in association with this, accommodation occurs by contraction of the ciliary muscle, and the pupil contracts. In these circumstances contraction of the pupil is in the nature of an associated movement, which is probably the outcome of impulses originating in the visual cortex and descending either directly or by way of the second frontal gyrus to the midbrain, there to terminate in the nuclei of Edinger-Westphal. In eliciting this reaction the patient is asked to look at a distant object and then at the examiner's finger, which is gradually brought to within two inches of the eyes.

The pupillary reaction on accommodation will be impaired parallel with the reaction to light by any lesion involving all the iridoconstrictor fibres. Its selective impairment, with preservation of the light reflex, indicates a midbrain lesion. Impairment or loss of the pupillary reaction on accommodation may be associated with weakness of convergence, as, commonly, in encephalitic Parkinsonism, but the reaction on accommodation may be preserved though convergence is paralysed, or conversely. A rare disturbance of this reflex is the myotonic pupillary reaction of Saenger, in which pupillary constriction on accommodation, though it is slow in developing, is long sustained and may last for half a minute or more. This abnormality is most frequently encountered in the condition of tonic pupil with absent tendon reflexes described below.

REFLEX IRIDOPLEGIA AND THE ARGYLL ROBERTSON PUPIL

The term 'reflex iridoplegia' indicates a failure of the pupil to react to light. The term 'Argyll Robertson pupil' should be reserved for a special form of reflex iridoplegia in which, as described by Argyll Robertson, the pupil 'is small . . . constant in size, and unaltered by light or shade; it contracts promptly and fully on convergence and dilates again promptly when the effort to converge is relaxed; it dilates slowly and imperfectly to mydriatics' (Adie). Most of the features had been described many years before Argyll Robertson by Romberg. Very rarely the Argyll Robertson pupil reacts paradoxically to light by a slight dilatation.

Loss of the pupillary light reflex depends upon a lesion at some point on the reflex path, and the preservation of the reaction on accommodation implies that the lesion does not involve the fibres concerned in this reaction. Reflex iridoplegia may occur as a result of lesions in the following situations.

Lesions of the Optic Nerve. Accommodation, convergence, and the associated iridoconstriction can occur in the absence of vision, for example, if an individual who has become blind tries to look at the end of his nose. Consequently a lesion of the optic nerve severe enough to impair the conduction of the afferent impulses concerned in the light reflex can cause loss of that reflex with retention of the reaction on accommodation.

Lesions of the Optic Tract. Destruction of one optic tract causes loss of the light reflex when the temporal half of the ipsilateral retina and the nasal half of the contralateral retina are illuminated, though the reflex remains elicitable from the other half of each retina. Homonymous hemianopia due to a lesion of the optic tract can sometimes thus be distinguished from a similar hemianopia due to a lesion of the optic radiation which does not interrupt the light reflex. (Wernicke's hemianopic reaction.)

Central Lesions. There is abundant evidence that reflex iridoplegia may be produced by lesions of the upper part of the midbrain. It has been observed in cases of tumour involving this region, as a result of vascular lesions, in encephalitis lethargica, as a rare manifestation of multiple sclerosis and syringomyelia, and as a result of a traumatic lesion of the upper midbrain. Syphilis is, of course, far the commonest cause of the Argyll Robertson pupil as above defined, which is usually present in general paresis and tabes and frequently in meningovascular syphilis. The site of the lesion responsible for this sign in syphilis of the nervous system is disputed. One hypothesis would place it in the upper half of the midbrain, near the cerebral aqueduct, where it may be supposed to interrupt the fibres approaching the iridoconstrictor nucleus.

Lesions of the Motor Path. An alternative and more acceptable view is that the lesion lies in the ciliary ganglion, the fibres concerned in the reaction on accommodation reaching the ciliary body without passing through the ganglion and so escaping damage (Nathan and Turner, 1942). It is stated that lesions of the third nerve may abolish the reaction of the pupil to light without that on accommodation. Such a dissociation can unquestionably occur as a result of lesions in or behind the eye, and it has been described in a number of cases of trauma involving the eye, and I have seen it as a sequel of herpes zoster ophthalmicus. The explanation is probably the same as in the syphilitic Argyll Robertson pupil.

Reflex iridoplegia is occasionally seen in alcoholic polyneuritis, chronic hypertrophic polyneuritis, and diabetes, but the site of the lesion in these conditions is unknown.

Myosis is not necessarily associated with loss of the pupillary light reflex. The Argyll Robertson pupil of tabes, however, is much contracted, and its constriction is probably due to associated involvement of the fibres of the ocular sympathetic, which also explains the loss of reflex dilatation in response to painful stimuli, and the ptosis, so characteristic in tabes. An almost constant feature of the Argyll Robertson pupil in tabes is a patchy depigmentation of the iris and there is usually loss of the ciliospinal reflex.

REFERENCES

CLARK, W. E. LE G. (1944) Discussion on the visual pathways, *Proc. roy. Soc. Med.,* **37,** 392.

COGAN, D. G., and WILLIAMS, H. W. (1966) *Neurology of the Visual System,* Springfield, Ill.

HARRIS, W. (1935) The fibres of the pupillary reflex and the Argyll Robertson pupil, *Arch. Neurol. Psychiat. (Chicago),* **39,** 1195.

MAGOUN, H. W., ATLAS, D., HARE, W. K., and RANSON, S. W. (1936) The afferent path of the pupillary light reflex in the monkey, *Brain,* **59,** 234.

MERRITT, H. H., and MOORE, M. (1933) The Argyll Robertson pupil: an anatomic-physiologic explanation of the phenomenon, with a survey of its occurrence in neurosyphilis, *Arch. Neurol. Psychiat.* (*Chicago*), **30,** 357.

NATHAN, P. W., and TURNER, J. W. A. (1942) The efferent pathway for pupillary contraction, *Brain*, **65,** 343.

PARSONS, J. H. (1904–6) The innervation of the pupil, *Roy. Lond. ophthal. Hosp. Rep.*, **16,** 20.

PATON, L., and MANN, I. C. (1925) The development of the third nerve nucleus and its bearing on the Argyll Robertson pupil, *Trans. ophthal. Soc. U.K.*, **45,** 610.

WILSON, S. A. K. (1928) Argyll Robertson pupil, *Modern Problems in Neurology*, p. 332, London.

TONIC PUPILS AND ABSENT TENDON REFLEXES

Definition. A syndrome of unknown aetiology and pathology characterized in its fully developed form by abnormalities in the reactions of one or both pupils to light and accommodation and absence of the tendon reflexes. The features of the tonic pupil were first described by Ware in 1813. They were rediscovered in 1902 by Strasburger and Saenger independently. An example of the complete syndrome was shown by Markus in 1905. Our present knowledge is based chiefly upon clinical observations of Moore (1924, 1931), Holmes (1931), and Adie (1931 *a*, 1931 *b*, and 1932).

Synonym. The Holmes–Adie syndrome.

AETIOLOGY AND PATHOLOGY

The disorder occurs almost exclusively in females and the age of onset is usually during the third decade. Beyond this nothing is known as to its aetiology. Adie thought the lesion responsible for the pupillary abnormalities must be in the vegetative portion of the oculomotor nucleus. Russell's (1956) work suggests that the lesion is in the efferent parasympathetic pathway to the eye, probably postganglionic. Harriman and Garland (1968) have reported a case of tonic pupil which came to autopsy. The pupil affected was the right one and the right ciliary ganglion, in contrast to the left, showed degeneration of neurones, most of which were replaced by clumps of capsular cells. There was also a loss of large axons though many fine axons still traversed the ganglion.

SYMPTOMS

The onset is usually sudden, the patient or her friends noticing that one pupil has become larger than the other. Sometimes the first complaint is of mistiness of vision in one eye. The pupillary abnormality is unilateral in about 80 per cent. of cases. The affected pupil is moderately dilated and is therefore usually larger than its fellow. When tested by ordinary methods the reaction of the affected pupil to light, both direct and consensual, is either completely or almost completely absent. Sometimes, however, a sluggish reaction to light can be elicited after the patient has remained in a dark room for about half an hour. The characteristic feature, however, is the response of the pupil to accommodation. Whereas a hasty examination may suggest that the pupil does not react at all on accommodation, nevertheless, if the patient be made to gaze fixedly at a near object, the pupil, sometimes after slight delay, contracts very slowly through a range which is often greater than normal, so that the affected pupil actually becomes smaller than the normal one. When accommodation is relaxed, dilatation of the pupil begins either at once or after a slight delay and proceeds even more slowly than contraction. This is the tonic pupillary reaction.

The tonic pupillary reaction, however, is not always present, but may be replaced by sluggishness or even absence of the reaction on accommodation. The pupil may thus be fixed to light and on accommodation. Russell (1956) distinguishes a 'paralytic' type of pupil attributed to parasympathetic paralysis and a 'tonic' type, due to supersensitization of the sphincter pupillae to acetylcholine liberated by intact parasympathetic fibres. The paralytic phase may thus be succeeded by the tonic phase. Accommodation may also be tonic, so that, after the gaze has been fixed on a near object, some seconds may elapse before this becomes clear. Russell (1958) explains the tonic ciliary muscle in the same way as the tonic pupil.

Some abnormality in the tendon reflexes is usually present, the ankle-jerks, knee-jerks, and arm-jerks being diminished or lost in this order of frequency. Occasionally the tonic pupil occurs with normal reflexes or, less frequently, normal pupils with absent tendon reflexes. Usually no other abnormality is found in the nervous system or elsewhere.

DIAGNOSIS

It is important to distinguish the tonic pupil from the Argyll Robertson pupil, but this is not difficult if it is borne in mind that the Argyll Robertson pupil is smaller than normal, does not react to light, and reacts promptly and fully on convergence, and dilates incompletely to mydriatics, differing in all these respects from the typical tonic pupil.

PROGNOSIS

The syndrome is permanent but has no ill effect beyond the inconvenience attaching to tonic accommodation. Patients have been observed in whom the condition of the pupil has remained unchanged for thirty or forty years. Occasionally it spontaneously changes its size and, rarely, the other eye becomes affected some time after the first.

TREATMENT

No treatment is of any value, but eserine drops may be used if the dilated pupil leads to discomfort.

REFERENCES

ADIE, W. J. (1931 a) Pseudo-Argyll Robertson pupils with absent tendon reflexes, *Brit. med. J.*, **1**, 928.

ADIE, W. J. (1931 b) Argyll Robertson pupils true and false, *Brit. med. J.*, **2**, 136.

ADIE, W. J. (1932) Tonic pupils and absent tendon reflexes. A benign disorder *sui generis*; its complete and incomplete forms, *Brain*, **55**, 98.

ALAJOUANINE, T., and MORAX, P. V. (1938) La pupille tonique et ses rapports avec la syndrome d'Adie, *Ann. Oculist. (Paris)*, **175**, 205, 277.

HARRIMAN, D. G. F., and GARLAND, H. G. (1968) The pathology of Adie's syndrome, *Brain*, **91**, 401.

HOLMES, G. (1931) Partial iridoplegia associated with symptoms of other disease of the nervous system, *Trans. ophthal. Soc. U.K.*, **41**, 209.

MOORE, R. F. (1924) Discussion on the pupil from the ophthalmological point of view, *Trans. ophthal. Soc. U.K.*, **44**, 38.

MOORE, R. F. (1931) The non-luetic Argyll Robertson pupil, *Trans. ophthal. Soc. U.K.*, **51**, 203.

RUSSELL, G. F. M. (1956) The pupillary changes in the Holmes–Adie syndrome, *J. Neurol. Neurosurg. Psychiat.*, **19**, 289.

RUSSELL, G. F. M. (1958) Accommodation in the Holmes–Adie syndrome, *J. Neurol. Neurosurg. Psychiat.*, **21**, 290.

THE INNERVATION OF THE EYELIDS

Two muscles act as elevators of the upper eyelid, the levator palpebrae superioris, which is innervated by the third nerve, and Müller's palpebral muscle, part of the smooth muscle of the orbit, which receives its nerve supply from the cervical sympathetic. Closure of the lids is brought about by the orbicularis oculi, the motor nerve of which is the facial.

RETRACTION OF THE UPPER LID

Retraction of the upper lid is attributable to a relative or absolute shortening of the elevating muscles, perhaps especially of the smooth muscle. When present it is exaggerated when the patient voluntarily elevates his eyes, and it is responsible for the lag of the upper lid in following the downward movement of the eye, which is known as von Graefe's sign. Lid retraction is most frequently encountered in exophthalmic goitre, but, as Collier has pointed out, it may be produced by a lesion in the upper part of the midbrain, especially one involving the posterior commissure. It may follow a vascular lesion in this situation and it is also sometimes met with in tabes, multiple sclerosis, encephalitis lethargica (especially the Parkinsonian form), tumour of the midbrain, myasthenia gravis, and as a congenital abnormality.

Retraction of the upper lid may be unilateral or bilateral and may occur with or without exophthalmos. When it is due to a lesion in the upper part of the midbrain it may be associated with weakness of conjugate elevation of the eyes or with reflex iridoplegia.

PTOSIS OF THE UPPER LID

Ptosis of the upper lid may be the result of paralysis of either the levator palpebrae superioris or of the orbital smooth muscle. In the latter case the drooping of the lid is comparatively slight. Complete paralysis of the levator, however, causes closure of the eye. It is necessary to distinguish between ptosis due to a lesion of the sympathetic and that due to paresis of the levator. This may be done by observing the reaction of the lid when the patient voluntarily elevates the eyes. Normally, elevation of the upper lid occurs as an associated movement with elevation of the eyes. In ptosis of sympathetic origin the amplitude of this associated movement is normal. In ptosis due to paresis of the levator it is diminished. Over-action of the frontal belly of the occipitofrontalis muscle is commonly present in a patient with ptosis. This muscle normally contracts in association with the levator palpebrae, and when the latter muscle is paralysed the increased effort made by the patient to elevate the lid involves an increased contraction of the frontalis muscle, physiologically comparable to secondary deviation of a conjugate ocular muscle in paralytic strabismus. Paralysis of the levator may be due to a lesion involving the nucleus of the third nerve or the third nerve trunk or its superior division within the orbit or to disorder of function at the myoneural junction in myasthenia gravis. It may be congenital. A lesion of the ocular sympathetic responsible for ptosis may occur within the brain stem, spinal cord, and eighth cervical and first and second thoracic ventral roots and spinal nerves, and the cervical sympathetic trunk. It is usually associated with other signs of ocular sympathetic paralysis, namely myosis and enophthalmos.

EXOPHTHALMOS AND ENOPHTHALMOS

The smooth muscle of the orbit is normally in a state of sufficient tonic contraction to produce some protrusion of the eyeball. Paralysis of this muscle causes slight enophthalmos: it is unlikely that exophthalmos is ever due to its over-activity. The commoner causes of exophthalmos are: (1) exophthalmic goitre; and (2) the closely related exophthalmic ophthalmoplegia; (3) pseudotumour of the orbit; (4) primary tumours within the orbit, especially of the optic nerve and its sheath; (5) diseases of the nasal air sinuses, empyema, mucocele, and carcinoma; (6) retro-orbital intracranial tumours, especially meningiomas and aneurysms. Less common causes are carotid-cavernous sinus aneurysm, craniostenosis, xanthomatosis, Wegener's granulomatosis, chloroma, and metastatic tumour from the suprarenal (Hutchison type) (see van Buren, Poppen, and Horrax (1957)).

REFERENCES

BRAIN, W. R. (1955) Exophthalmic ophthalmoplegia, *Trans. ophthal. Soc. U.K.*, **55,** 351.

BUREN, J. VAN, POPPEN, J. L., and HORRAX, G. (1957) Unilateral exophthalmos, *Brain*, **80,** 139.

COLLIER, J. (1927) Nuclear ophthalmoplegia with especial reference to retraction of the lids and to lesions of the posterior commissure, *Brain*, **50,** 488.

POCHIN, E. E. (1939) Ocular effects of sympathetic stimulation in man, *Clin. Sci.*, **4,** 79.

POCHIN, E. E. (1939) The mechanism of lid retraction in Graves' disease, *Clin. Sci.*, **4,** 91.

SPEECH AND ITS DISORDERS

THE NATURE OF SPEECH

PSYCHOLOGICAL CONSIDERATIONS

Speech is an extremely complex activity. In order to understand its nature it is necessary to trace its development in the individual from infancy. Infant speech goes through a number of phases including babbling which is the spontaneous production of sounds, and echolalia, which is the imitation of sounds made by others. The foundation of speech is thus sensorimotor—the sounds produced by others causing the child to produce sounds which it hears itself and which are linked with proprioceptor impulses from its own muscles of articulation. The next stage is the long one of learning the meanings of words, which involves associating the sounds of the words with objects which are perceived in abstraction from their environment, and later increasing abstraction is involved in naming qualities, actions, and relationships. The meaning of words is also influenced by their arrangements in sentences, i.e. by their grammatical and syntactical modifications.

When the child learns to read it does so by associating visual signs, i.e. letters and words, with the sounds which it has already learned. Through reading aloud, written words become linked with heard words, and with the kinaesthetic sensations of speech. In writing, movements of the hand are employed to reproduce visual signs similar to those which form the basis of reading. Since in writing one reads as one writes there exists a close link between the perception of the visual signs which constitute letters and words, and the kinaesthetic sensations derived from the fingers.

Words therefore are symbols. A spoken word is to the hearer an auditory symbol of an object, action, or relationship; a written word in the first instance acquires its symbolic significance through its association with heard speech, that is, symbolic sounds. Words as symbols possess meanings, but these meanings are of an elementary nature. In fully developed speech individual words possess significance only in relationship with other words. The unit of meaning is then a sentence or even a series of sentences. Speech, therefore, is the communication of meanings by means of symbols, which usually take the form of spoken or written words. Meaning may, however, be communicated by gesture, and gesture meanings have been especially elaborated in the manual speech of the deaf and dumb. In reading Braille print the blind utilize tactile instead of visual sensations. Mathematics and music also involve the use of written symbols.

Hughlings Jackson first pointed out that speech is not always used for the communication of meanings—propositional speech, as he called it—but may also constitute the expression of feeling, in which case it may have no propositional value.

How far is thought dependent upon speech? It has been maintained that we think in words and that normal speech functions are therefore necessary for thought. The process of logical thought is probably subject to large individual variations depending upon whether the thinker chiefly utilizes visual or auditory images. It appears to be true, however, that internal verbal formulation is not necessary, at least for the simpler forms of logical thought. It is probably required for more abstract thinking, and is necessary for the communication of the products of thought to others.

PHYSIOLOGICAL AND ANATOMICAL CONSIDERATIONS

At the psychological level the meaning of a written or a spoken word is the outcome of the association of the given visual and auditory sensations with other forms of sensation in the past. A meaning is thus based upon a constellation of associations built up by experience. At the physiological and anatomical levels the basis of such meanings is presumably a linkage of neurones. Visual impulses reach the cerebral cortex in the region of the calcarine sulcus of the occipital lobes; auditory impulses in the posterior part of the superior temporal gyrus. Kinaesthetic impulses from the muscles of articulation and from the upper limb terminate in the lower half of the postcentral gyrus. It is to be expected therefore that the anatomical linkages of neurones upon which verbal meanings depend will join together these regions of the cerebral cortex, and these are found in the tracts of white matter known as association fibres, which underlie the grey matter of the cerebral cortex.

For reasons which are little understood, about 90 per cent. of persons are right-handed, and in these the left cerebral hemisphere plays the predominant role in speech and is known as the dominant or major hemisphere: it is the site of the speech functions in a proportion of left-handed people also. In the remainder of the left-handers the right hemisphere is the dominant one for speech, or speech functions may be bilaterally represented. The important associational paths just described are therefore situated in the left hemisphere in right-handed persons, but sensory impulses concerned in the reception of speech also reach the auditory and visual regions of the right cerebral cortex, which are linked to the left hemisphere by paths passing through the corpus callosum.

Their importance has recently been demonstrated by Gazzaniga, Bogen, and Sperry (1965), who found that, after division of the corpus callosum and the other commissural connexions in man, speech could deal only with perceptual information reaching the left cerebral hemisphere. The right cerebral hemisphere still had capacities of its own but was isolated from verbal expression. (See also Geschwind, 1965.)

The posterior half of the left cerebral hemisphere is thus the site of those neuronal linkages which underlie the elaboration of meanings in response to auditory and visual stimuli, i.e. the comprehension of heard and written speech. Since articulated speech is the expression of meanings it must be the outcome of the activity of a part of the brain which at least overlaps that concerned in the reception of speech, for the anatomical basis of meanings is common to both. Articulation involves movements of the jaw, lips, tongue, palate, larynx, and the respiratory muscles, which are represented in the lowest part of the precentral gyrus. If meanings are to gain articulate expression the posterior half of the left hemisphere must be linked to the lowest part of the precentral gyrus. An important part in this association is played by the external capsule, which is a band of white matter running from the tip of the temporal lobe beneath the cortex of the insula to the lower part of the precentral gyrus and the posterior part of the middle and inferior frontal gyri. Speech requires co-ordinated bilateral movements of the muscles of articulation, and this co-ordination is effected by fibres passing from the lower part of the left frontal lobe to the corresponding region of the right hemisphere by the corpus callosum. From the lower part of the precentral gyri the motor fibres concerned in articulation pass downwards in the corticospinal tracts and after decussation end in the trigeminal and facial nuclei, the nuclei ambigui and the hypoglossal nuclei in the pons and medulla, whence the lower motor neurones run in the corresponding cranial nerves to the lips, soft palate, tongue, and larynx. Corticospinal fibres similarly innervate the diaphragm and intercostal muscles. As in the case of other motor activities, the cerebellum and striatum exercise a regulating influence upon articulation.

DYSARTHRIA

We are now in a position to draw a distinction between speech and articulation. Speech is the term employed for the whole process by which meanings are comprehended and expressed in words. Articulation is the motor function whereby words, having been formulated, are converted into sounds. Dysarthria is a disorder of articulation. It therefore does not involve any disturbance in the proper construction and use of words. In the dysarthric patient symbolic verbal formulation is normal: only the mechanism of verbal sound production is faulty. When this is so severely affected that the patient is totally unable to articulate, he is said to be anarthric.

The following are the principal causes of dysarthria:

UPPER MOTOR NEURONE LESIONS

The articulatory muscles on each side appear to be innervated by both cerebral hemispheres. Hence a unilateral corticospinal lesion, for example in the internal capsule, may cause temporary but not permanent dysarthria. Dysarthria is produced, however, by bilateral corticospinal lesions, due, for example, to congenital diplegia, vascular lesions of both internal capsules, degeneration of both corticospinal tracts, as in motor neurone disease, and lesions such as tumours involving both corticospinal tracts together in the midbrain. With such lesions the articulatory muscles are weak and spastic and the tongue appears smaller and firmer than normal. The jaw-jerk and the palatal and pharyngeal reflexes are exaggerated. Speech is slurred, production of consonants, especially labials and dentals, being severely affected. Spastic dysarthria is usually associated with dysphagia and often with impairment of voluntary control over emotional expression, a syndrome which has received the unsatisfactory name of 'pseudo-bulbar palsy'.

LESIONS OF THE CORPUS STRIATUM

With lesions of the corpus striatum articulation is impaired, partly at least, as a result of muscular rigidity. Thus in hepatolenticular degeneration and in Parkinsonism articulation is slow and slurred owing to immobility of the lips and tongue and the pitch of the voice is monotonous. In severe cases speech may be unintelligible.

DISORDERS OF CO-ORDINATION

The co-ordination of articulation suffers severely when the vermis of the cerebellum is damaged and also when lesions involve the cerebellar connexions in the brain stem. Speech in such cases is often explosive and associated with violent grimaces. Syllables may be slurred or unduly separated—scanning or syllabic speech. Ataxic dysarthria of this character is seen after acute lesions of the cerebellar vermis and in multiple sclerosis and the hereditary ataxias. Ataxic speech also occurs in chorea and athetosis, and in these disorders irregular respiration contributes to the dysarthria.

LOWER MOTOR NEURONE LESIONS

Lower motor neurone lesions cause wasting and weakness of the muscles of articulation. In the early stages the pronunciation of labials suffers most. Later, progressive weakness of the tongue impairs the production of dentals and gutturals, and weakness of the soft palate gives the voice a nasal quality. To this may be added impairment of phonation, and finally speech becomes completely impossible. Progressive bulbar palsy is the commonest example of this. It may also occur in syringobulbia and the bulbar form of poliomyelitis, and with tumours of the medulla.

Combinations of these varieties of dysarthria are common, for example, in multiple sclerosis the articulatory muscles may be both spastic and ataxic and in motor neurone disease a combination of upper and lower motor neurone lesions may be present.

MYOPATHIES

Disease of the muscles, such as occurs in myasthenia gravis and muscular dystrophy involving facial muscles, leads to dysarthria similar to that resulting from lesions of the lower motor neurones. In myasthenia fatigability may cause increasing slurring of speech if the patient is asked to count. In the myotonias tonic muscular contraction may add a spastic character to the speech.

TREATMENT

Little can be done when dysarthria is due to a progressive disorder, but in children suffering from congenital dysarthria or dysarthria due to diplegia, athetosis, and chorea much can be accomplished. Speech training must consist of (1) vocal gymnastics, (2) breathing exercises, and (3) the practice of muscular relaxation, and should be combined with general remedial physical exercises.

PALILALIA

Palilalia is a rare disorder of speech, the nature of which is obscure. As its name implies (from the Greek *palin*, again; *lalein*, to chatter), it is characterized by repetition of a phrase which the patient reiterates with increasing rapidity. Palilalia most frequently occurs as a symptom of the Parkinsonian syndrome following encephalitis lethargica, and in pseudobulbar palsy due to vascular lesions. In one of my patients it occurred as a temporary phenomenon as a result of compression of the medulla. It is difficult to understand why a lesion involving the lower motor mechanisms of speech should cause a disorder of the formation of phrases.

MUTISM

Mutism is the term applied to a complete loss of speech in a conscious patient. It occurs in akinetic mutism in which there is an abnormal state of consciousness [see p. 970] but also in a variety of cerebral lesions with full preservation of consciousness, e.g. after severe head injury, after certain cerebrovascular lesions, in advanced Parkinsonism, after bilateral thalamotomy, and after anoxic states due to many causes, e.g. carbon monoxide poisoning. It also occurs in the psychoses, for example in cyclothymia, as a result of extreme depression or mental retardation, and in schizophrenia. It is also met with in hysteria. In the psychoses the severity of the mental disorder is always apparent and the mute patient is usually unable to write. In hysterical mutism other hysterical symptoms such as convulsions, rigidity, and anaesthesia are usually present.

The treatment of hysterical mutism involves the general treatment of the hysterical state. The treatment of the symptom consists of re-education in speech, the patient being shown how to place his lips and tongue, then induced to phonate and so convinced that he is able to speak. It is sometimes possible to restore speech by giving a small dose of an intravenous anaesthetic.

APHONIA

In aphonia phonation is lost but articulation is preserved; hence the patient talks in a whisper. Aphonia may be the result of organic disease causing bilateral paralysis of the adductors of the vocal cords [see p. 193] or of disease of the larynx, for example, laryngitis. It is most commonly a symptom of hysteria, in which case the patient, though unable to phonate when speaking, can do so when coughing.

The treatment of hysterical aphonia involves the general treatment of the hysterical state [see p. 1004] and re-education in phonation. By making the patient modulate his cough he may be brought to phonate vowels at different pitches and may then be induced to combine these with the consonants which he is able to whisper.

APHASIA

Whereas dysarthria is a disorder of the motor mechanism of articulation, aphasia is a disturbance of the higher and much more complex functions, described on pages 95–6, by which meanings are comprehended and expressed. It is thus a disorder of the use of symbols in speech. Since aphasia strictly interpreted means absence of speech, the term dysphasia, meaning disorder of speech, is sometimes employed. The present state of opinion on disturbances of speech has been well characterized by Head as 'chaos'. The terminology employed in the description of aphasia is still to a large extent in bondage to old-fashioned views concerning the psychological nature of speech and outworn conceptions of cerebral localization. Confusion springs from a failure to distinguish between psychological, physiological and anatomical accounts of speech and its disorders, and to recognize the complexity of the relations between them.

The Development of Thought about Aphasia

It is impossible to understand the terminology of aphasia without some knowledge of its historical development, which is described in more detail by Head (1920, 1926) and Weisenburg and McBride (1935).

The first attempt to localize functions in different parts of the brain was made by Gall (1758–1828), who distinguished six varieties of memory, including name-memory, verbal, and grammatical memory, all of which he localized in the frontal lobes. Dax in 1836 first drew attention to the special importance of the left cerebral hemisphere for speech. Broca (1824–80) in 1861 reported two cases which led him to take the view that the faculty of articulation was located in the inferior frontal gyrus (Broca's area). Damage to this area caused what he called 'aphemia'—a term altered by Trousseau to 'aphasia'. Broca distinguished two forms of speech disturbance—aphemia and verbal amnesia, the former being a defect of verbal expression and the latter a loss of memory for both spoken and written words.

Hughlings Jackson's (1835–1911) first paper on disorder of speech was published in 1864. It is difficult to summarize his views, which he elaborated in a long series of communications. His great contribution was the introduction of a dynamic conception of speech and aphasia. Like Broca he recognized two main groups of aphasic patients. In one group speech is lost or gravely damaged; in the other the patient has numerous words but uses them wrongly. He pointed out that the higher and more voluntary aspects of speech tend to suffer more than the lower and automatic, and he distinguished what he called 'propositional' speech from emotional speech. Aphasia is essentially an inability to 'propositionize' in speech, and the same fundamental difficulty underlies spoken speech, reading, and writing. Internal speech is affected like external speech and the thinking of the aphasic patient is therefore hampered also, but in most cases of aphasia mental images are unimpaired.

Hughlings Jackson's work was little appreciated at the time and the main line of development of thought about aphasia was in the direction of increasing localization of function. Bastian (1837–1915) in 1869 maintained that we think in words and that words are revived in the cerebral hemispheres as remembered sounds. He localized auditory and visual word centres as well as other centres linked by association paths. He was thus the most notable of the 'diagram-makers' as Head calls them. He prepared the way for the conceptions of word-deafness and word-blindness—terms introduced by Kussmaul—caused by lesions of these centres. Wernicke (1848–1905) in 1874 localized the centre for auditory images in the left superior temporal gyrus and described three varieties of aphasia— sensory, due to destruction of this centre, motor, due to a lesion of Broca's area, and a third due to interference with conduction between these two centres. When both centres were destroyed there was total aphasia.

In 1906 Pierre Marie (1853–1940) reopened the question of aphasia by maintaining that lesions of Broca's area had nothing to do with speech disorders. He contended that there was only one form of aphasia—the sensory aphasia of Wernicke, which was not a special loss of word memories but a defect of general intelligence, and of special intelligence of language. He considered the motor speech disturbance to be an anarthria caused by a lesion of 'the lenticular zone'. Henschen and Kleist are among the modern workers who may be classed as localizationists.

Henry Head (1861–1940) returned to and developed the dynamic concepts of Jackson. He expressly avoided the question of localization, and developed a functional approach, seeking to discover by a specially devised series of tests how the function of speech broke down in aphasia, which he regarded as a disorder of 'symbolic formulation and expression'. In Head's (1926) view, 'disorders of language of this kind cannot be classified as isolated affections of speaking, reading, and writing, for these acts are more or less disturbed whatever the primary nature of the defect. Nor can they be attributed directly to destruction of auditory or visual images or to any other analogous processes, which belong to a relatively low order in the psychical hierarchy. Each clinical variety represents some partial affection of symbolic formulation and expression; the form it assumes depends upon the particular modes of behaviour which are disturbed or remain intact.' Head recognized four such forms of disturbance, which he termed verbal, nominal, syntactical, and semantic.

Some other points of view remain to be mentioned. Liepmann at one time regarded expressive aphasia as a form of apraxia, and word-deafness and word-blindness as forms of agnosia. Though he later abandoned this view it was subsequently adopted by Kinnier Wilson. Goldstein (1948) and others explain the various symptoms of aphasia in terms of the Gestalt theory as manifestations of a single functional disorder, loss of the ability to grasp the essential nature of a process, impairment of abstract attitude, &c.

Recent workers have applied to aphasic utterances phonetic analysis (Alajouanine and Mozziconacci, 1948; Alajouanine, 1956; and Bay, 1957), psychological testing (Bay, 1960), and the Gestalt theory (Conrad, 1954). For a review of the whole subject see Brain (1965).

The Nature and Classification of Aphasia

Aphasia is a disorder of function and must therefore be interpreted in functional terms. The older conceptions of aphasia were mostly inadequate because they treated of speech and its breakdown in terms of consciousness, i.e. of words and their auditory, visual, and kinaesthetic images. The neurophysiology of speech, however, embraces complex functions to which there is often no counterpart in consciousness, and which need new concepts for their interpretation (Goldstein, 1948; Alajouanine and Mozziconacci, 1948; Brain, 1961). A word is something more to the nervous system than any one of the innumerable ways in which it can be pronounced or written: its basis is a neurophysiological disposition, which I have called a word-schema, and through which any specific instance of a word is able to evoke its appropriate meaning. Speech involves auditory phoneme-schemas, central word-schemas, sentence-schemas, meaning-schemas, and motor phoneme-schemas, and aphasia results from a breakdown of their receptive or expressive functions, or of both. It rarely happens, however, that a localized cerebral lesion disturbs only one physiological function, and the same psychological disorder may be the result of more than one kind of physiological disturbance. Hence the inadequacy of psychological classifications of aphasia and the failure of attempts to correlate anatomical lesions with clear-cut disorders of function. We have to fall back upon an empirical classification of aphasia. Experience shows that on the whole a lesion in one part of the brain disturbs speech in certain ways and a lesion in another situation in different ways. Hence there exists an anatomical classification of aphasia which roughly corresponds to a functional one. The functions disordered by such focal lesions, however, are rarely so simple or 'psychological' that they can be adequately described as 'expressive', 'receptive', &c. Yet to introduce new terms at this stage would be confusing, and is unnecessary for practical purposes. I have therefore retained the older functional terminology for the most part, adding the corresponding anatomical and other synonyms in brackets. As there is no functional term for the combination of word-blindness and agraphia produced by a lesion of the angular gyrus I have used 'visual asymbolia' for this. Goldstein's conception of 'central aphasia' is a valuable one. This is a disorder of inner speech resulting from the disorganization of word- and sentence-schemas and so affecting speech in all its receptive and expressive aspects.

It is an old observation that aphasia in polyglots tends to impair the mother tongue less, and for a shorter time than, foreign languages. This is not always so, however.

SYMPTOMATOLOGY

Pure Word-Deafness and Word-Blindness

Since the two sensory channels concerned in the reception of heard and written language reach the temporal and occipital cortex respectively, and between these lie association paths and nodal points, the area of cortex devoted to the understanding of speech is much larger than that occupied with its expression. Consequently lesions, especially small vascular or traumatic lesions, can damage the comprehension of speech selectively. Within the area lying between the superior temporal gyrus in front and the area striata behind, the more posteriorly a lesion is situated the more will it affect the comprehension of written speech, while the more anteriorly it is placed the more will the understanding of spoken speech suffer. This is the justification for the conception of word-deafness (auditory aphasia) and word-blindness (visual aphasia). It has been contended that pure forms of these do not occur. Certainly they are very rare. On the one hand they merge into the more general disorders of auditory and visual agnosia, on the other hand, they are often associated with other forms of speech disturbance.

In *pure* or *subcortical word-deafness* the patient distinguishes words from other sounds but does not understand them, so that his own language sounds to him like a foreign tongue. Sometimes he recognizes the meaning of an individual word, but not of a whole sentence. Owing to this defect he cannot repeat words or write to dictation, but there is no other change in speaking, reading, or spontaneous writing. A case of this kind was reported by Hemphill and Stengel (1940). The lesion is thought to be in the subcortical white matter beneath the posterior part of the left superior temporal gyrus. In *pure* or *subcortical word-blindness*, or visual aphasia, the patient cannot recognize words, letters, or colours, but can visualize colours. He cannot copy but can write spontaneously. The lesion is in the lingual gyrus and involvement of the optic radiation causes an associated right homonymous hemianopia. Pure word-blindness is very rare and in most cases other symptoms are present, especially agraphia [see p. 105] Inability to read is termed *alexia*.

Visual Asymbolia

Visual asymbolia or *cortical word-blindness* describes the combination of visual aphasia with agraphia produced by a lesion of the left angular gyrus.

Central Aphasia (Syntactical Aphasia)

In central aphasia, the difficulty in understanding spoken speech is associated with gross disorder of thought and expression. Spoken speech is fluent, in marked contrast to the speech of the patient with expressive aphasia, but it is disordered by verbal and grammatical confusions—paragrammatism—difficulty in evoking words as names for objects, actions, and qualities, and the utterance of non-existent or incorrect words—paraphasia (the syntactical aphasia of Head). The comprehension of spoken speech is impaired, but reading is less affected, and the patient can usually understand what he reads silently, though if he reads aloud he may be confused by the inaccuracies in his verbal expression of what he sees. Writing is usually less affected than articulate speech. Defective comprehension of spoken speech prevents the patient from noticing his own errors in speaking, and in severe cases he pours forth a stream of unintelligible jargon (jargon aphasia). The lesion responsible for central aphasia is situated in the left temporoparietal region.

Mixed forms of aphasia are common, since the lesion responsible for the aphasia is often large. Thus Wernicke's *sensory aphasia*, also called *receptive aphasia* and *cortical word-deafness*, due to a cortical lesion in the posterior one-third of the left superior temporal gyrus is a mixture, as Goldstein points out, of pure word-deafness with central aphasia and some degree of nominal aphasia.

Total aphasia results from massive destruction of the frontotemporal region of the left hemisphere.

Nominal Aphasia (Amnestic Aphasia)

Difficulty in finding names occurs sufficiently often in relative isolation to have been distinguished as amnestic or nominal aphasia. The inability to appreciate the symbolic significance of names is most evident when the patient is asked to name an object which is held before him. In severe cases he is quite unable to do so; in milder cases he succeeds with familiar, but fails with less familiar, objects. Characteristically he rejects a wrong name suggested by the examiner. He usually insists that he knows what the object is, but cannot name it, and frequently attempts to convey his recognition by some periphrasis. For example, a patient suffering from nominal aphasia, when shown a pair of spectacles, pointed to his ears and said, 'That's what you put on. Shows more strongly for yourself. If you cannot see enough, so you put it on.'

The structure of words is not impaired. Writing exhibits the same nominal defect as articulated speech. There is much difficulty in comprehending spoken and written language owing to failure to recognize the meaning of words.

When nominal aphasia is the result of a focal cerebral lesion this usually lies between the angular gyrus and the posterior part of the superior temporal gyrus on the left side.

Expressive Aphasia (Cortical Motor Aphasia, Verbal Aphasia, Broca's Aphasia)

In this form of aphasia the expressive aspect of speech suffers severely. In severe cases the patient may be completely speechless or able to say only 'yes' or 'no', and even these words may be inappropriately used, and cannot be repeated to order. He may be limited to the same phrase constantly repeated—a recurring utterance. Emotional speech suffers less than 'propositional', and an otherwise almost speechless individual may be able to swear or utter other emotional ejaculations. With improvement the power of expression gradually returns, but speech is slow, interrupted by pauses, and words are badly pronounced. When the patient cannot think of the right word himself he will recognize it when it is offered to him. Polysyllables tend to be slurred. The significance of words as names is unimpaired, however, and grammar is unaffected. In reading aloud, speech suffers in the same way as in spontaneous utterance. In writing also the patient exhibits errors in verbal formulation. Written words tend to be incomplete, and spelling is defective. Superficially the comprehension of both heard and written speech may appear to be normal. Nevertheless, there is often difficulty in grasping complex meanings, probably because the power of internal verbal formulation is faulty.

There is general agreement that expressive aphasia is usually produced by lesions situated in the posterior part of the inferior frontal gyrus (Broca's area) and the lower part of the precentral gyrus but the lesion may be elsewhere, especially on either side of the central sulcus (Conrad, 1954).

Pure Word-Dumbness (Subcortical Motor Aphasia)

In this form of speech disturbance there is a gross impairment of articulation or even complete loss of spoken speech, but inner speech is intact, comprehension is unimpaired, and writing is normal. In its pure form it is rare; more often inner speech and writing are relatively well preserved in comparison with uttered speech. The lesion has been thought to lie in the white matter deep in Broca's area. Another view regards this as a functional variant of Broca's aphasia resulting from an identical lesion, and Conrad's work quoted above shows that the causal lesions of the two may be co-extensive.

The Transcortical Aphasias and Echolalia

The characteristic feature of the transcortical aphasias is the preservation or relative preservation of the power of repetition, though either spontaneous speech or comprehension is more severely affected—transcortical motor and sensory aphasia respectively. Lichtheim's explanation of the disorder as the result of a lesion of transcortical pathways is doubtful. *Echolalia* means an automatic and compulsive repetition of words in the absence of understanding of their meaning: it differs from the transcortical aphasias in the absence of an intention to repeat.

Agraphia, Acalculia, and Amusia

Agraphia is the term first used by Ogle to describe the loss of the ability to express meanings in written language. To establish the presence of agraphia, which is not infrequently associated with paralysis of the right arm, it must be shown that the patient cannot write with the left hand. Writing is a complex function closely related to the comprehension of written speech, and a patient who suffers from visual asymbolia is unable to write correctly. Pure agraphia is a disorder independent of word-blindness. Several varieties have been described (Kleist, 1922; Herrmann and Pötzl, 1926). An idiokinetic agraphia results from a lesion of the left angular gyrus in a right-handed person. Copying is more successful than spontaneous writing and writing from dictation. Agraphia may also be produced by a lesion in the posterior part of the middle frontal gyrus, which interferes with nervous impulses reaching the area of the precentral gyrus concerned in movements of the hand. Such a lesion no doubt was responsible for the association of agraphia with aphasia in the case of Dr. Samuel Johnson, who, writing to Mrs. Thrale two days after his 'stroke', said: 'In penning this note, I had some difficulty; my hand, I knew not how or why, made wrong letters.' There is also an apraxic agraphia.

Acalculia is the term applied to a defect in the use of mathematical symbols which is usually present in aphasia of the expressive type and may also occur after a left parietal lesion as part of Gerstmann's syndrome [see p. 116].

Amusia, the term applied to a defect of musical expression or appreciation when due to a cerebral lesion, like aphasia may be either expressive or receptive. It is rarer than aphasia and may sometimes follow a right-sided lesion in a right-handed person.

Examination of a Patient with Aphasia

Examination of a patient with aphasia requires care and patience and should be carried out in a systematic manner. The following scheme of investigation fulfils all ordinary clinical requirements.

(1) Is the patient right- or left-handed, and, if the latter, did he write with the right hand? (2) What was the state of education as regards reading, writing, and foreign tongues? (3) Does he understand the nature and uses of objects, and can he understand pantomime and gesture, or express his wants thereby? (4) Is he deaf? If so, to what extent and on one or both sides? (5) Can he recognize ordinary sounds and noises? (6) Can he comprehend language spoken? If so, does he at once attempt to answer a question? (7) Is spontaneous speech good? If not, to what extent and in what manner is it impaired? Does he make use of wrong words, recurring utterances, or jargon? (8) Can he repeat words uttered in his hearing? (9) Is the sight good or bad; is there hemianopia, or papilloedema? (10) Does he recognize written or printed speech and obey a written command? If not, does he recognize words, letters, or numerals? (11) Can he write spontaneously? What mistakes occur in writing? Is there paragraphia? Can he read his own writing some time after he has written it? (12) Can he copy written words, or from print into printing? Can he write numerals or perform simple mathematical calculations? (13) Can he read aloud? (14) Can he name at sight words, letters, numerals, and common objects? (15) Can he write from dictation? (16) Can he match an object with its name, spoken or written, when a series of objects and names are simultaneously presented? (17) Any other tests, emotional, rhythmical, or musical, which may raise the physiological level of the speech centres. (18) Any other means of proving in what way he can receive and express ideas.

THE CAUSES OF APHASIA

Apart from developmental disturbances of speech described below, aphasia is rare in childhood and increases in frequency with increasing age. It is most frequently met with after middle life, since the commonest cause is a vascular lesion, especially ischaemic. Cerebral haemorrhage causes aphasia less often than thrombosis, because haemorrhage occurs deep in the white matter of the hemisphere more often than in the cortex or subcortical regions. Transitory attacks of aphasia may occur as a result of temporary disturbances of cerebral circulation in patients suffering from hypertension or cerebral atheroma, and transitory aphasia occurring in migraine can probably be similarly explained. Cerebral embolism may cause aphasia, but is uncommon compared with other cerebral vascular lesions. The varieties of aphasia due to obstruction of the different cerebral arteries are described elsewhere [see pp. 293–6].

Intracranial tumour is the commonest cause of aphasia during the first half of adult life, when cerebral vascular lesions are rare. Abscess of the left temporal lobe may also cause aphasia, and so may traumatic lesions involving the 'speech areas'. Apart from abscess, infective lesions of the brain rarely cause aphasia, though it occurs occasionally in encephalitis, and acute cerebral lesions causing hemiplegia and attributed to encephalitis or vascular occlusion are almost the only cause of aphasia in childhood. Neurosyphilis may cause aphasia, either by leading to cerebral thrombosis or to general paresis. In the latter, transitory aphasia may occur as a symptom of a congestive attack, and a profound disintegration of speech may develop as a result of the widespread deterioration of cortical function in the later stages, comparable to that which occurs in degenerative cortical disorders, such as Alzheimer's disease and Pick's disease.

PROGNOSIS

The prognosis of aphasia depends largely upon its cause. When it develops as a result of a vascular lesion, neural shock is responsible for part of the immediate disturbance of function. Consequently a considerable improvement may be anticipated as this passes off. The prognosis appears to be better when aphasia is due to haemorrhage than when an important artery has been obstructed by thrombosis or embolism, and the outlook is better also when the aphasia is of the expressive, than when it is of the receptive, type and in the left-handed than in the right-handed. The prognosis is good when aphasia is due to an extracerebral tumour, such as a meningioma, which has compressed but not invaded the brain. In the case of an intracerebral tumour, even if the tumour can be removed, the operation is likely to be followed by an exacerbation of the speech disturbance and little ultimate improvement can be expected. Recovery often occurs from aphasia due to acute infections of the brain, and any lesion of the dominant hemisphere during the first four years of life.

TREATMENT

The treatment of aphasia requires unlimited patience and is likely to be more successful when the disturbance of speech affects the expressive than when it involves the receptive function. In the latter type of aphasia not only has the patient difficulty in understanding what is required of him, but he also fails to understand his own attempts at speech. The aphasic patient requires to be taught on lines similar to those used in teaching a backward child. The various vowel and consonant sounds must be taught separately, the patient being directed to watch the movements of his teacher's lips and tongue. He is then taught to pronounce the names of common objects when he sees them. The names have then to be associated with pictures and finally with simple written words. The scheme of instruction must be adapted to meet the requirements of each individual case and to utilize to the best effect those elements of speech which are least seriously impaired. Details are described by Weisenburg and McBride (1935), Goldstein (1942, 1948), and Alajouanine and Mozziconacci (1948).

REFERENCES

ALAJOUANINE, T. (1956) Verbal realization in aphasia, *Brain*, **79**, 1.

ALAJOUANINE, T., and MOZZICONACCI, P. (1948) *L'Aphasie et la désintégration fonctionnelle du langage*, Paris.

BAY, E. (1957) Die corticale Dysarthrie und ihre Beziehungen zur sog. motorischen Aphasie, *Dtsch. Z. Nervenheilk.*, **176**, 553.

BAY, E. (1960) Zur Methodik der Aphasie-Untersuchung, *Nervenarzt*, **31**, 145.

BRAIN, W. R. (1945) Speech and handedness, *Lancet*, ii, 837.

BRAIN, LORD (1965) *Speech Disorders*, 2nd ed., London.

CONRAD, K. (1954) Some problems of aphasia, *Brain*, **77**, 491.

COLLIER, J. S. (1929) Aphasia and other defects of speech, in *A Textbook of the Practice of Medicine*, ed. Price, F. W., 3rd ed. p. 1460, London.

CRITCHLEY, M. (1927–8) On palilalia, *J. Neurol. Psychopath.*, **8**, 23.

EWING, A. W. G. (1930) *Aphasia in Children*, London.

GAZZANIGA, M. S., BOGEN, J. E., and SPERRY, R. W. (1965) Observations on visual perception after disconnexion of the cerebral hemispheres in man, *Brain*, **88**, 221.

GESCHWIND, N. (1965) Disconnexion syndromes in animals and man, *Brain*, **88**, 237 585.

GOLDSTEIN, K. (1942) *After-effects of Brain Injuries in War*, London.

GOLDSTEIN, K. (1948) *Language and Language Disturbances*, New York.

HEAD, H. (1920) Aphasia: an historical review, *Brain*, **43**, 390.

HEAD, H. (1926) *Aphasia and Kindred Disorders of Speech* (2 vols.), Cambridge.

HEMPHILL, R. E., and STENGEL, E. (1940) A study on pure word-deafness, *J. Neurol. Psychiat.*, **3**, 251.

HENSCHEN, S. E. (1925) Clinical and anatomical contributions on brain pathology. Abstracts and comments by W. F. Schaller, 5th Part. Aphasia, amusia, and acalculia *Arch. Neurol. Psychiat. (Chicago)*, **13**, 226.

HENSCHEN, S. E. (1926) On the function of the right hemisphere of the brain in relation to the left in speech, music and calculation, *Brain*, **49**, 110.

HENSCHEN, S. E. (1927) Aphasiesysteme, *Mschr. Psychiat. Neurol.*, **65**, 87.

HERRMANN, G., and PÖTZL, O. (1926) Über die Agraphie, *Abhandlung aus der Neurol. Psychiat., Psychol. und ihr Grenzgetret*, Berlin.

JACKSON, J. H. (1932) *Selected Writings*, vol. ii, London.

KLEIST, K. (1922) *Handbuch der ärztlichen Erfahrungen im Weltkriege*, iv, 491, Leipzig.

NIELSEN, J. M. (1946) *Agnosia, Apraxia, Aphasia. Their Value in Cerebral Localization*, 2nd ed., New York.

WEISENBURG, T. H., and MCBRIDE, K. E. (1935) *Aphasia*, New York.

WILSON, S. A. K. (1926) *Aphasia*, London.

DEVELOPMENTAL SPEECH DISORDERS

Developmental speech disorders are of considerable importance, since, unless a correct diagnosis is made, the sufferer may be wrongly regarded as mentally defective, and valuable opportunities of treatment may be missed.

Developmental expressive aphasia (Orton) is rare, developmental aphasia being usually of the receptive type. Two varieties of this, congenital word-deafness and developmental dyslexia, are distinguished, but combined forms occur.

DEVELOPMENTAL RECEPTIVE APHASIA

Congenital word-deafness, or congenital auditory imperception, as it has recently been called, is a rare inborn defect of speech. It is frequently familial and may appear in different members of successive generations of a family. Males are affected more frequently than females in the proportion of 5 to 1. The essential disturbance of function appears to be an inability to appreciate the significance of sounds, although hearing is normal. It may be supposed that there is a lack of the anatomical mechanism whereby sounds become associated with other sensory impressions and with kinaesthetic sensations produced by speech and so acquire meanings. Since the disorder is more profound than merely a lack of appreciation of the significance of words, the term 'congenital auditory imperception' has been proposed for it by Worster-Drought and Allen (1928–9). There is no evidence as to the pathological nature of the disorder, but it appears likely to be due to an inability to discriminate sounds in spite of normal hearing.

The defect is present from birth but is not as a rule noticed until the age at which a normal child begins to understand speech and to learn to speak. It is then found that the patient takes no notice when spoken to and does not learn to repeat words. Hearing, however, is normal and the child responds to noises. Spoken language is not understood provided the patient has not learned to lip-read. The appreciation of musical sounds may or may not be defective. Worster-Drought and Allen have pointed out that associated with the word-deafness there may be a defect in appreciating the meaning of written and printed symbols. This is not surprising in view of the large part which hearing plays in learning to read in normal individuals. Speech suffers seriously as a result of auditory imperception. For a number of years the child may not speak at all. Sooner or later, however, most patients acquire a vocabulary of their own, which is comprehensible only to those who have been closely associated with them. The words spoken bear little resemblance to normal words, though they possess meaning for the speaker. This defective form of speech has been called 'idioglossia' and 'lalling'. A well-known example of idioglossia is the pronunciation of the Lord's Prayer by one of Colman's patients, which was as follows: 'Oue tabde ne nah e nedde, anne de di na; i tede ta, i du de di on eeth a te e edde. Te ut te da oue dade de, e didde ap tetedde, a ne adin to tetedde adase us, ne notte totate, mime, utte enu, to i aitevene, pore e dande, to edde a edde. Ame.'

Although sufferers from congenital word-deafness are frequently found in institutions for the mentally subnormal, they do not necessarily suffer from any defect in mental capacity but are severely handicapped by the inadequacy of the primary channel through which we learn the meaning of things around us. It is not surprising therefore that the victims of this disorder tend to develop abnormal psychological reactions to their surroundings, especially when they are treated as lazy or mentally subnormal.

The diagnosis is from general mental subnormality, and from high-tone deafness which can be excluded by audiometry.

The education of the congenitally word-deaf requires much care, and an intelligent appreciation of the nature of their disorder. As in the case of the deaf, they must be educated principally through the sense of sight and should be taught lip-reading, while their sense of touch may also be used to educate them in correct articulation. It is important that attempts should also be made to educate the sense of hearing. The nature of the disability must be taken into account in planning an occupation.

DEVELOPMENTAL DYSLEXIA

Developmental dyslexia seems the best term to apply to a mixed group of individuals who possess in common a defect in learning to read. This condition has been called congenital word-blindness, but a defect which can rightly be so described is the cause in only a small proportion of cases.

Developmental dyslexia is much commoner than congenital word-deafness, and Thomas has estimated that it is present in 1 in every 2,000 London school-children. Like congenital word-deafness it is not uncommonly familial and may occur in more than one generation of the same family. In some cases it may be due to a congenital lack of the ability to appreciate the significance of visual symbols. In many patients, however, visual symbolization appears to be normal, and the defect appears to consist in an inability to differentiate the spoken word into its sounds and to break up a written word into its sounds and letters (Schilder, 1944). Consequently the printed word is wrongly pronounced, and conversely a dictated word is wrongly spelled. The writing of dyslexic children is very abnormal. The subject has been reviewed by Money (1962) and Critchley (1964).

Developmental dyslexia usually becomes apparent owing to the child's backwardness in learning to read. This may be wrongly attributed to a general defect of intelligence or to laziness. Yet by intelligence tests these children are frequently normal and their power of visual imagery is unimpaired. Such children are apt to develop psychoneurotic reactions to their environment owing to lack of understanding of their disability.

MIRROR-WRITING

This is the term applied to script which runs from right to left, the letters being reversed and forming mirror-images of normal script. Normal individuals can frequently carry out mirror-writing with the left hand, either when writing with the left hand alone or with both hands simultaneously. Since this capacity is present without previous training we must assume that the education of the right hand in normal writing involves the unconscious education of the left hand to perform the same movements in the opposite direction. Such mirror-writing with the left hand may become evident in right-handed individuals who have developed right hemiplegia, and I have known it follow an injury of the occipital region of the brain.

The situation is more complicated than this, however, in patients suffering from developmental dyslexia who exhibit mirror-writing, for in such individuals mirror-writing appears to be secondary to mirror-reading, as shown by Orton. These children tend to read words from right to left and pronounce them accordingly. For example, 'not' is pronounced 'ton', and if asked to copy words they frequently do so in the reversed order, with or without reversal of single letters. The frequent association of left-handedness with mirror-reading and writing suggests that these disorders may be secondary to a lesion of the left hemisphere which is normally dominant and to a substituted dominance of the right hemisphere. Many normal children pass through a temporary phase of mirror-writing, at least of certain letters, when first learning to write.

TREATMENT

Treatment must be based upon an understanding of the nature of the child's disability. Attention must be paid to educating the child in the association of syllables with the articulatory movements employed in their pronunciation. The phonetic method of teaching spelling, in which the child learns letters by their sounds and not by their names, should be employed. Special care must be taken in teaching the child to read from left to right. The teacher should point to the letters in this order and the child should be encouraged to do the same with the forefinger of the right hand. (For details see Schonell, 1948, and Schiffman, 1962.)

Stress should be laid upon reading for amusement, and in dictation the child should not depend solely upon ear, but should sit by a normal child and be allowed to see what he has written. Educational authorities throughout the child's career should be informed of his disability in order that allowances may be made, especially in examinations.

STUTTERING

Definition. A dysrythmia of speech leading to a disturbance of articulation characterized by abrupt interruptions of the flow of speech, or the repetition of sounds or syllables.

AETIOLOGY

The association of stuttering with left-handedness indicates that in many cases it possesses an anatomico-physiological basis which is confirmed by its rare occurrence in association with expressive aphasia. Orton states that stuttering children fall into four groups: (1) those in whom an enforced shift from the left to the right hand has been carried out by parents or nurse; (2) those who have been slow in selecting a master-hand and show considerable inter-grading; (3) those who fulfil neither of these conditions and have a strong family history of stuttering; and (4) those with no shift of handedness and no family history of stuttering. In this group, however, other types of speech defect or left-handedness can usually be found in the family. Moreover, stuttering usually begins either at the age of two or three when the child is beginning to talk and to develop a master-hand or between the ages of six and eight in a child that has hitherto spoken fluently, i.e. at the age at which reading and writing are being acquired. It is thus clear that the localization of the speech 'centres' in the right cerebral hemisphere tends to cause stuttering, especially if the dominance of the right hemisphere is impaired by an attempt to make the right the master-hand.

The role of neurosis stressed for example by Johnson (1959) is difficult to assess since stuttering in itself is likely to evoke shyness and neurotic reactions. Orton maintains that child stutterers who are investigated before the overlay of neurosis has developed show no more psychological abnormalities than other children. Boys suffer four times as often as girls and several surveys report an incidence of 1 per cent. of stutterers among British schoolchildren.

SYMPTOMS

The flow of speech may be broken by pauses, during which it is entirely arrested, or by the repetition of sounds or syllables. The pause may be filled with grunts or hisses, and stuttering is frequently associated with facial contractions or tics involving the limbs or even the whole body. The spastic element is usually called *tonus* and the repetitive *clonus*. Various stages in the development of stutter have been described. It is generally agreed that the first consists of reiteration of syllables. Stein (1942) describes six phases in the second stage. Dentals (t, d), labials (p, b), and gutturals $(k$ and hard $g)$ are the consonants which are usually the most troublesome to the stutterer, especially when they occur at the beginning of a word. Stutterers often go out of their way to avoid certain words by reconstructing sentences and may employ tricks to enable them to achieve correct pronunciation, for example, spelling a word before pronouncing it. They can usually sing, and may be able to recite without hesitancy.

PROGNOSIS

Mild stuttering tends to disappear spontaneously. In severe cases considerable improvement and often complete cure can be achieved by thorough treatment.

TREATMENT

When stuttering occurs in a left-handed child who has been made to use the right hand, a return to left-handedness often produces great improvement. Re-education of speech by a trained teacher is essential. Abnormalities in the upper respiratory passages, if present, should first receive appropriate treatment. The role of muscular spasm in the production of stuttering must be explained to the patient, who should be taught to practise relaxation of the muscles concerned in speech. Relaxation should be followed by breathing exercises and by vocal gymnastics, exercises being prescribed in which the lips, tongue, jaw, and palate are moved without the production of sounds. Later the patient begins to practise words, and articulation may at first be facilitated by various devices such as singing, or speaking through a megaphone or in time with a metronome. The use of syllabic speech under the supervision of a trained speech therapist has proved to be remarkably successful in some cases.

In children psychological difficulties at home and at school should be inquired for, and in adults psychological treatment may be required to straighten a warped personality. At all ages suggestion born of the faith and enthusiasm of the teacher is an essential element in treatment. (See Travis, 1959; Morley, 1957; and Andrews and Harris, 1964.)

REFERENCES

ANDREWS, G., and HARRIS, M. (1964) *The Syndrome of Stuttering*, London.

BRAIN, W. R. (1945) Speech and handedness, *Lancet*, ii, 837.

CRITCHLEY, M. (1964) *Developmental Dyslexia*, London.

FILDES, L. G. (1921) A psychological inquiry into the nature of the condition known as congenital word-blindness, *Brain*, **44**, 286.

JOHNSON, W. (1959) in *Handbook of Speech Pathology*, ed. Travis, L. E., p. 897, London.

MONEY, J. (1962) *Reading Disability. Progress and Research Needs in Dyslexia*, Baltimore.

MORLEY, M. E. (1957) *The Development and Disorders of Speech in Children*, London.

ORTON, S. T. (1925) 'Word-blindness' in school children, *Arch. Neurol. Psychiat. (Chicago)*, **14**, 581.

ORTON, S. T. (1937) *Reading, Writing and Speech Problems in Children*, London.

RONNE, H. (1936) Congenital word-blindness in school children, *Trans. ophthal. Soc. U.K.*, **56**, 311.

SCHIFFMAN, G. (1962) in *Reading Disability. Progress and Research Needs in Dyslexia*, ed. Money, J., p. 45, Baltimore.

SCHILDER, P. (1944) Congenital alexia and its relation to optic perception, *J. genet. Psychol.*, **65**, 67.

SCHONELL, F. J. (1948) *Backwardness in the Basic Subjects*, 4th ed., Edinburgh.

STEIN, L. (1942) *Speech and Voice*, London.

THOMAS, C. J. (1905) Congenital 'word-blindness' and its treatment, *Ophthalmoscope*, **3**, 380.

TRAVIS, L. E. (1959) *Handbook of Speech Pathology*, London.

WEST, R. W., KENNEDY, L., and CARR, A. (1937) *The Rehabilitation of Speech*, New York.

WORSTER-DROUGHT, C., and ALLEN, I. M. (1928–9) Congenital auditory imperception, *J. Neurol. Psychopath.*, **60**, 193 and 289.

APRAXIA AND AGNOSIA

APRAXIA

Apraxia may be defined as an inability to carry out a purposive movement, the nature of which the patient understands, in the absence of severe motor paralysis, sensory loss, and ataxia. For example, a patient who is asked to protrude his tongue is unable to do so on request, though he may carry out inappropriate movements such as opening his mouth. A moment later he spontaneously protrudes his tongue to lick his lips. Apraxia may involve any movement normally voluntarily initiated—movements of the eyes, face, muscles of articulation, chewing and swallowing, manipulation of objects, gestures with the upper limb, walking, or sitting down.

Normal purposive movements depend upon the integrity not only of the corticobulbar and corticospinal tracts, but also of association tracts whereby these efferent paths are excited. The idea of the movement, whether formulated spontaneously or in response to an external command, thus passes into action. Apraxia is the result of interruption of the pathways thus acting as ideomotor links. In right-handed individuals purposive motor activity appears thus to be controlled by the posterior part of the left hemisphere, especially by the supramarginal gyrus. Thence fibres pass forwards in the left hemisphere to the precentral gyrus and cross to the same gyrus on the right side, through the corpus callosum. Lesions in the left parietal lobe are therefore likely to produce bilateral apraxia. Lesions between this region and the left precentral gyrus may lead to apraxia of the limbs on the right side, and lesions involving the anterior part of the corpus callosum or of the subcortical white matter on the right side may cause left-sided apraxia. The commonest form of apraxia is that involving the lips and tongue, which is frequently encountered in association with right hemiplegia due to a lesion of the left hemisphere. Apraxia for dressing is usually the result of a lesion of the right parietal lobe.

Apraxia has been analysed by Liepmann (1905 *b*) into limb-kinetic apraxia, due to loss of kinetic memories of part of the body, ideokinetic apraxia, due to a dissociation between ideational and kinaesthetic processes, and ideational apraxia, in which the general conception of the movement is imperfect, its component parts being correctly carried out but wrongly combined.

Apraxia is usually associated with an impairment of the power to imitate movements. The disturbance of function which underlies apraxia is essentially the same as that responsible for motor aphasia, which may justly be regarded as an apraxia of the purposive movements concerned in speech. The nature of apraxia has recently been discussed by Geschwind (1965).

A special form of apraxia has been named by Kleist (1922) constructional or optical apraxia. There is no apraxia of single movements but the spatial disposition of the action is disordered. The patient, for example, cannot copy a simple arrangement of matches, but recognizes his mistakes.

Apraxia is most frequently seen as a result of localized lesions of the brain, especially vascular lesions and tumours. It may also be a symptom of diffuse cerebral inflammatory or degenerative states, such as general paresis and the presenile cerebral degenerations.

AGNOSIA

The arrival of nerve impulses at the cortical areas concerned in vision, hearing, and cutaneous and postural sensibility excites crude sensations which have not yet attained the perceptual level involved in the recognition of objects. This is brought about by the association of the sensations excited through one sensory channel with memories of sensations derived from other sensory channels during previous experiences of the object, which include our actions in regard to it. The perception of an object seen or felt is thus a constellation of sensory images and memories directed towards action, and the recognition of an object as having been seen before, and of its use, depends upon the capacity of the primary visual or tactile sensations which it evokes to excite the right motor schemas. When, by reason of disease of the brain, this secondary process fails to occur, the patient fails to recognize the object. This defect is known as agnosia or mind-blindness. Its nature has recently been discussed by Geschwind (1965).

Visual agnosia is present when the patient, in whom the paths from the retina to the occipital cortex are intact and the latter is undamaged, nevertheless fails to recognize common objects which he clearly sees. This condition may result from lesions in the left parieto-occipital region in right-handed persons. Prosopagnosia is a restricted form of visual agnosia in which the patient is unable to recognize faces. Auditory agnosia implies the failure to recognize sounds in a patient who is nevertheless not deaf. An individual suffering from this disability in a severe form will fail to appreciate not only the nature of words but also musical tunes. This results from a lesion of the left temporal lobe in right-handed persons. Tactile agnosia is one form of the disorders comprised under the more general term astereognosis. The patient, though not suffering from gross sensory defect in the fingers or hand, is nevertheless unable to recognize an object placed in the hand. This may be produced by a lesion of the parietal lobe situated posteriorly to the post-central gyrus at the level of the hand area. Agnosia usually only affects the recognition of objects through one sensory channel. Thus a patient suffering from visual agnosia, who cannot recognize a key when he sees it, can usually recognize it when it is placed in his hand. Conversely, a patient who cannot recognize objects placed in his hand recognizes them readily when he sees them.

REFERENCES

BRAIN, W. R. (1941) Visual object-agnosia, with special reference to the Gestalt theory, *Brain*, **64**, 43.

BRAIN, LORD (1965) *Speech Disorders*, 2nd ed., London.

GESCHWIND, N. (1965) Disconnexion syndromes in animals and man, *Brain*, **88**, 237, 585.

KLEIST, K. (1922) Die psychomotorischen Störungen und ihr Verhältnis zu den Motilitätsstörungen bei Erkrankungen der Stammganglien, *Mschr. Psychiat. Neurol.*, **52**, 253.

LIEPMANN, H. (1905 *a*) Der weitere Krankheitsverlauf bei dem einseitig Apraktischen und der Gehirnbefund auf Grund von Serienschnitten, *Mschr. Psychiat. Neurol.*, **17**, 289.

LIEPMANN, H. (1905 *b*) *Über Störungen des Handelns bei Gehirnkranken*, Berlin.

LIEPMANN, H. (1908) *Drei Aufsätze aus dem Apraxiegebiet*, Berlin.

NATHAN, P. W. (1947) Facial apraxia and apraxic dysarthria, *Brain*, **70**, 449.

NIELSEN, J. M. (1937) Unilateral cerebral dominance as related to mind-blindness, *Arch. Neurol. Psychiat.* (*Chicago*), **38**, 108.

NIELSEN, J. M. (1938) Gerstmann syndrome: finger agnosia, agraphia, confusion of right and left and acalculia, *Arch. Neurol. Psychiat.* (*Chicago*), **39**, 536.

NIELSEN, J. M. (1946) *Agnosia, Apraxia, Aphasia. Their Value in Cerebral Localization*, 2nd ed., New York.

NIELSEN, J. M., and FITZGIBBON, J. P. (1936) Agnosia, apraxia, aphasia: their value in cerebral localisation, *Bull. Los Angeles neurol. Soc.*, **7**, 210.

SITTIG, O. (1931) *Über Apraxie: eine klinische Studie*, Berlin.

WILSON, S. A. K., and WALSHE, F. M. R. (1914–15) The phenomenon of 'tonic innervation' and its relation to motor apraxia, *Brain*, **37**, 199.

DISORDERS OF THE BODY-IMAGE

We are aware of the existence of our bodies, their position in space, and the relation of their parts to one another because we receive sense-data through numerous sensory channels, which include vision, cutaneous sensibility, and proprioceptor impulses from the muscles and joints and from the labyrinths. The paths carrying the somatic impulses pass by way of the ventral nucleus of the optic thalamus to the supramarginal gyrus which is thus concerned with awareness of the opposite half of the body. This presentation of the body to consciousness is known as the body-image or body-schema.

Symptoms of disorder of the body-image may be positive or negative. The chief positive symptom is the phantom—an illusion of the persistence of a part of the body which has been lost by amputation, e.g. a phantom limb, or an illusory awareness of part of the body from which sensation has been lost owing to interruption of afferent pathways. Phantom limbs after amputation may be painless or painful (Riddoch, 1941). The painless phantom soon becomes less obtrusive, and gradually shortens, to disappear into the stump. A painful phantom is usually associated with abnormalities of the stump, especially large and tender end-bulbs and interstitial neuritis of the divided nerves. Painful phantoms may persist indefinitely and cause much distress. A phantom limb may be abolished by a lesion of the area of the opposite parietal cortex concerned with representation of the body-image.

Lesions of this part of the brain are responsible for some of the most bizarre psychophysiological disturbances. Thus the patient may be unaware of the opposite half of his body—*autotopagnosia*. Often he also neglects objects in the same half of extrapersonal space and in drawing a clock face he will insert the figures in one half of the circle only, ignoring the other. When shown his arm he may deny that it belongs to him. If he is hemiplegic he may deny this also. These symptoms in right-handed persons are observed only after lesions of the right parietal lobe and therefore refer to the left side of the body. The disorder of awareness of the body image which occurs after left parietal (angular gyrus) lesions in right-handed persons is finger agnosia (Gerstmann, 1924, 1940), characterized by an inability to recognize and select individual fingers when looking at both hands. This may apply to both the patient's and the observer's fingers and is usually associated with agraphia, acalculia, and a failure to discriminate between right and left (Gerstmann's syndrome). Constructional apraxia is also observed in many such cases. The rejection of evidence of bodily disease, e.g. hemiplegia, blindness, is known as *anosognosia* (Anton's syndrome).

REFERENCES

GERSTMANN, J. (1924) Fingeragnosie. Eine umschriebene Störung der Orientierung am eigenen Körper, *Wien. klin. Wschr.*, **37**, 1010.

GERSTMANN, J. (1940) Syndrome of finger agnosia, disorientation for right and left, agraphia and acalculia, *Arch. Neurol. Psychiat. (Chicago)*, **44**, 398.

HEAD, H., and HOLMES, G. (1920) *Studies in Neurology*, ii, p. 605.

LHERMITTE, J. (1939) *L'Image de notre corps*, Paris.

NIELSEN, J. M. (1938) Disturbances of the body scheme: their physiologic mechanism, *Bull. Los Angeles neurol. Soc.*, **3**, 127.

RANEY, A. A., and NIELSEN, J. M. (1942) Denial of blindness (Anton's syndrome), *Bull. Los Angeles neurol. Soc.*, **7**, 150.

REDLICH, F. C., and DORSEY, J. F. (1945) Denial of blindness by patients with cerebral disease, *Arch. Neurol. Psychiat. (Chicago)*, **53**, 407.

RIDDOCH, G. (1941) Phantom limbs and body shape, *Brain*, **64**, 197.

SCHILDER, P. (1935) *The Image and Appearance of the Human Body*, London.

VISUAL DISORIENTATION

Visual disorientation is a loose term covering a variety of disorders of an agnostic kind usually following a parieto-occipital lesion (Brain, 1941). It includes (*a*) defective visual localization of objects in the opposite half-fields, (*b*) agnosia for the left half of space—usually the result of a right parieto-occipital lesion, (*c*) loss of topographical memory, (*d*) loss of orientation secondary to visual agnosia for objects, (*e*) mixed and undefined forms occurring, for example, in mental confusion. In the more severe forms of visual disorientation the patient cannot find his way about.

REFERENCE

BRAIN, W. R. (1941) Visual disorientation with special reference to lesions of the right cerebral hemisphere, *Brain*, **64**, 244.

THE SIGNS OF LOCAL LESIONS OF THE BRAIN

It is customary in textbooks on nervous diseases to describe in a separate section the signs of local lesions of the brain. Since these are dealt with in connexion with anatomy and physiology, tumours, and vascular lesions, to avoid reduplication they will not be repeated, but for the convenience of the reader references are here given to the parts of the book in which are described the signs of local lesions in various situations.

The Prefrontal Lobe:
Tumours of the frontal lobe, pp. 240–1.
Syndromes of the cerebral arteries—anterior cerebral artery, p. 295.
Spasticity, p. 24. The grasp reflex, p. 57. Mental functions, p. 963.

The Precentral Gyrus:
The corticospinal tract, p. 17.
Tumours of the precentral gyrus, pp. 241–2.
Syndromes of the cerebral arteries—the middle cerebral artery, p. 296.

The Temporal Lobe:
Tumours of the temporal lobe, p. 243.
The geniculocalcarine pathway, p. 71.

The Parietal Lobe:
Tumours of the parietal lobe, p. 244.
Sensation at the cortical level, p. 50.
The geniculocalcarine pathway, p. 71.

The Occipital Lobe:
Tumours of the occipital lobe, p. 245.
The visual cortex, p. 73.
Syndromes of the cerebral arteries—the posterior cerebral artery, p. 297.

The Corpus Callosum:
Tumours of the corpus callosum, p. 245.

The Basal Ganglia:
The corpus striatum, p. 513.
Sensation—the thalamus, p. 49.

THE CEREBROSPINAL FLUID

ANATOMY AND PHYSIOLOGY

FORMATION, CIRCULATION, AND ABSORPTION

Clinical and experimental observation has established that the cerebrospinal fluid is mainly formed by the choroid plexuses of the cerebral ventricles. That formed by the plexuses of the lateral ventricles passes through the interventricular foramina into the third ventricle. Thence the fluid flows through the cerebral aqueduct into the fourth ventricle, which it leaves by the median and two lateral foramina of the fourth ventricle to reach the subarachnoid space. The subarachnoid space, which lies between the arachnoid membrane externally and the pia mater internally, constitutes a vessel which carries the fluid from the cerebral ventricles to its points of absorption. The inner surface of the arachnoid and the outer surface of the pia mater are covered with flattened mesothelial cells and these also cover the numerous trabeculae, which bridge the subarachnoid space, and the nerves and blood vessels which pass across it. The subarachnoid space is deepest at the base of the brain and between the inferior surface of the cerebellum and the medulla. In these regions its expansions constitute the various cisterns, the largest of which is the cerebellomedullary cistern beneath the cerebellum.

The subarachnoid space extends superficially over the whole surface of the brain and spinal cord. It is also prolonged into the substance of the nervous system by means of extensions which are known as the perivascular spaces. Every blood vessel entering or leaving the nervous system must pass across the subarachnoid space. In so doing it carries with it into the nervous system a sleeve of arachnoid immediately surrounding the vessel and a sleeve of pia mater more externally. Between the two lies the extension of the subarachnoid space, which is known as the perivascular space and which subdivides on each division of the vessel to terminate where the pia mater and arachnoid become continuous. It is probable that products of metabolism and cell-containing inflammatory exudates pass from the perivascular spaces to mingle with the cerebrospinal fluid in the subarachnoid space, and it is the perivascular spaces which are seen to form cuffs round the vessels packed with inflammatory cells in microscopic sections taken from the nervous system in infective conditions such as syphilis, encephalitis, and poliomyelitis.

The cerebrospinal fluid of the subarachnoid space probably receives a contribution from the perivascular spaces, and possibly also from the lymphatics of the cranial and other peripheral nerves. After bathing the surface of the spinal cord and the base of the brain it passes upwards over the convexity of the hemispheres, to be absorbed into the intracranial venous sinuses. The bulk of the evidence shows that absorption takes place through the microscopic arachnoid villi, which are minute projections of the subarachnoid space into the lumen of the sinuses, and the recent work of Welch and Friedman (1960) shows that these operate as valves, opening in response to a rise of pressure of the cerebrospinal fluid.

CHEMICAL COMPOSITION OF THE CEREBROSPINAL FLUID

The following table, based upon the investigations of Fremont-Smith and Cohen, shows the principal differences in chemical composition between the cerebrospinal fluid and the blood plasma. It used to be thought that the cerebrospinal fluid was a dialysate of plasma, but Davson (1967) reviews the evidence that secretory activity is required to explain its chemical composition. Sweet *et al.* (1954) consider that it is both a secretion and an ultrafiltrate. Recent work (see Davson, 1967) has also defined comparative concentrations of amino acids in plasma and cerebrospinal fluid, and information upon the enzyme activity (LDH, GOT, CPK) in the fluid in health and disease is now being accumulated.

VOLUME AND RATE OF FORMATION

The volume of the cerebrospinal fluid in adults is normally about 130 ml. Its rate of formation can only be estimated by artificial methods, the accuracy

Comparison of Blood Plasma and Cerebrospinal Fluid

	Blood Plasma	Cerebrospinal Fluid
Group 1. (Substances normally present in greater quantity in the plasma than in the fluid.)	Protein, 6–7/100 ml.	Ventricular, 5–15 mg./100 ml. Cisternal, 15–25 mg./100 ml. Lumbar, 15–45 mg./100 ml.
	Inorganic phosphorus, 2–4 mg./100 ml.	1·25–2 mg./100 ml.
	Uric acid, 2–4 mg./100 ml.	Trace.
	Cholesterol, 150 mg./100 ml.	Trace.
	Calcium, 10 mg./100 ml.	5–6 mg /100 ml.
	Sulphates, 4 mg./100 ml.	1 mg./100 ml.
	Glucose, 100 mg./100 ml.	50–80 mg./100 ml.
Group 2. (Substances normally present in greater quantity in the fluid than in the plasma.)	Chlorine (as NaCl), 560–620 mg./100 ml.	725–750/mg. 100 ml.
Group 3. (Substances approximately equally distributed between plasma and fluid.)	Sodium, potassium, CO_2, urea, lactic acid, sulphonamides.	
Group 4. (Substances which do not pass from the plasma to the fluid except in minute traces.)	Fibrinogen, iodides, salicylates, nitrates, lipoids, bile pigments, organic arsenic, most ferments, many enzymes, immune bodies, penicillin, streptomycin.	

of which is doubtful. It is probable that the total volume is completely replaced several times a day.

FUNCTIONS OF CEREBROSPINAL FLUID

Many functions have been attributed to the cerebrospinal fluid though most of them are somewhat speculative. There is no doubt, however, about its importance mechanically in protecting the nervous system from jars and shocks. Probably also it acts as a regulator of the intracranial pressure and as a support to the venous sinuses in postures in which the intracranial venous pressure is raised. It is likely that it plays a part in the nutrition and metabolism of the nervous system, though this aspect of its functions is little understood.

METHODS OF OBTAINING CEREBROSPINAL FLUID

To obtain cerebrospinal fluid for examination it is necessary to puncture either the cerebral ventricles or the subarachnoid space, which may be reached most easily either in the cerebellomedullary cistern or in the lumbar cul-de-sac, where it extends beyond the lower end of the spinal cord.

LUMBAR PUNCTURE

Lumbar puncture is the simplest method of obtaining access to the subarachnoid space and is so frequently used that every practitioner of medicine should be capable of carrying it out. The spinal cord terminates at the lower border of the first lumbar vertebra in the adult, and at a slightly lower level in the child. The arachnoid is continued downwards below the termination of the spinal cord as far as the second sacral vertebra, and forms a lumbar cul-de-sac of the subarachnoid space normally containing cerebrospinal fluid and crossed by the roots of the cauda equina. A needle can be introduced into this space without risk of injury to the spinal cord.

Indications and Contra-indications

Lumbar puncture is carried out for the following purposes: (1) to obtain cerebrospinal fluid for cytological, chemical, and other investigations and to estimate its pressure; (2) in the relief of intracranial pressure and the removal of toxic, inflammatory, or other irritative substances in the cerebrospinal fluid, in the various forms of encephalitis and meningitis, intracranial haemorrhage, external hydrocephalus, uraemia, eclampsia, &c.; (3) to introduce into the subarachnoid space therapeutic substances or local anaesthetics; (4) to introduce into the subarachnoid space air for radiographic purposes—encephalography and myelography—or for treatment; (5) to introduce opaque media for radiography.

There are several important contra-indications to lumbar puncture. In the presence of increased intracranial pressure, especially when there is reason to suspect a tumour in the posterior fossa of the skull, sudden withdrawal of fluid from the spinal canal may cause herniation of the medulla into the foramen magnum—the 'cerebellar pressure cone'—with fatal results. When a space-occupying lesion is present or suspected in one cerebral hemisphere a herniation of the medial part of the temporal lobe may occur through the tentorial hiatus and the resultant compression and distortion of the upper brain stem may be equally disastrous. Thus the investigation is better avoided if intracranial tumour, abscess or haematoma are likely to be present and should be performed in such cases only if essential information can be obtained in no other way, and if immediate neurosurgical aid is at hand. In such cases ventricle puncture is the only really safe method of obtaining cerebrospinal fluid. The presence of infection in the lumbar region is a contra-indication to lumbar puncture, owing to the risk of infecting the spinal canal. Marked spinal deformity in the dorsal or lumbar regions may render lumbar puncture difficult or impossible.

Preparation for Lumbar Puncture

There are a number of patterns of lumbar puncture needle. Their gauge ranges from 17 to 19; a good length is 8 cm. Harris's needles for trigeminal injection made by Messrs. Weiss are excellent. The Dattner needle consists of a fine inner needle, 25, within an outer one, 20, the use of which is described below. A needle of large diameter may be required in cases of meningitis when thick pus, containing flakes of fibrin, is to be withdrawn.

Method of Puncture

Lumbar puncture may be performed with the patient either sitting or lying on one side. As many patients cannot sit up, it is best to accustom oneself to performing the operation with the patient lying on his left side. In either position the most important point is to secure the greatest possible degree of flexion of the lumbar spine. If the patient is conscious and co-operative he should be asked to bend his legs until his knees approach his chin and then to clasp his hands beneath his knees, or an assistant can aid flexion of the spine by applying pressure with one hand behind the neck and the other beneath the knees. When the patient is in position the next step is to find the landmarks. A line joining the highest points of the iliac crests, which may be marked with a swab dipped in iodine or other suitable antiseptic, usually passes between the third and fourth lumbar spinous processes, and the puncture can be performed either at this point or between the fourth and fifth spines. The skin is now cleaned with alcohol and ether and painted with iodine. A local anaesthetic is not essential, but renders the proceeding more comfortable for the patient. The skin should be anaesthetized with 1 per cent. procaine solution. A general anaesthetic is necessary only in the case of delirious or excitable patients who cannot be maintained in position, or when there exists a spasmodic extension of the spine which cannot otherwise be overcome, as may happen in meningitis.

The needle, with the stylet in position, is now introduced midway between the spinous processes in the selected interspace and either in the midline, or, as some prefer, half an inch to one side. The cutting edges of the bevelled point should be directed upwards and downwards and not transversely, since the fibres of the ligamenta flava and of the dura run longitudinally and are less likely to be divided in the former case. After its point has entered the skin the needle is passed forwards and slightly upwards in the sagittal plane. If it has been introduced to one side of the midline slight inward deviation is also necessary. It is of assistance in keeping in the right direction if one glances at the whole length of the patient's spine. At an average depth of about 4·5 cm. the point of the needle encounters the increased resistance of the ligamentum flavum, and after penetrating a further $\frac{1}{2}$ cm. it should enter the subarachnoid space. The stylet is now withdrawn and laid upon a sterile towel and if the puncture has been successful cerebrospinal fluid drips from the butt of the needle. After the pressure has been measured as described on page 125 the fluid is collected in two sterile test-tubes consecutively, about 3 ml. being allowed to run into each. Five ml. is sufficient for diagnostic purposes, and no more should be withdrawn except for purposes of treatment. The needle is then withdrawn. The patient sometimes complains of pain in one leg when the needle enters the subarachnoid space. This is due to the point having come into contact with one of the roots of the cauda equina, which, however, is not likely to be damaged. Care should be taken not to introduce the needle too far lest an intervertebral disk should be injured.

The Dattner needle is designed to avoid headache after lumbar puncture by making the hole as small as possible. When the ligamentum flavum is reached, the inner needle is advanced for the actual puncture and the fluid withdrawn by means of a syringe.

A Dry Tap

In almost all cases the failure to obtain fluid means that the puncture has been incorrectly carried out. The point of the needle may not have entered the subarachnoid space either because it has been introduced too obliquely in the longitudinal plane or because it has deviated to one side or because, on account of scoliosis or arthritis, the interspace is difficult to find. It may not have penetrated far enough, or it may have gone too far, the point having come into contact with the posterior wall of the body of the vertebra where puncture of a vein is the commonest cause of blood in the fluid. The stylet should be passed into the needle again to remove any possible obstruction and the depth of the point varied. If no fluid comes, the needle should be withdrawn and reinserted either in the same interspace or in the one above or below. A genuine dry tap, when the point of the needle is actually in the subarachnoid space, may occur when the spinal subarachnoid space is blocked at a higher level and hence the pressure of the fluid in the lumbar sac is low, or when the lumbar sac itself is filled by a neoplasm or by a congenital abnormality, as in spina bifida.

Sequels of Lumbar Puncture

The only common sequel of lumbar puncture is headache, which comes on after a few hours, is throbbing in character, and may be associated with nausea, vomiting, giddiness, and pain in the neck and back. In severe cases it is literally prostrating, being much intensified by sitting up, and lasting for days or even exceptionally for weeks. It is most likely to occur when a normal fluid is withdrawn and is very rare in syphilitic patients. It is due to lowered intracranial tension produced by a continued leakage of cerebrospinal fluid through the puncture wound in the theca. When the Dattner needle was used, headaches occurred in only 3 per cent. of patients punctured as out-patients and allowed to go home (Erskine and Johnson, 1938). With an ordinary needle certain precautions will do much to prevent the development of 'lumbar puncture headache'. The needle used should be small in calibre, and introduced with the cutting edges in the sagittal plane. The minimal amount of fluid should be withdrawn; in any case not more than 10 ml., unless the object of the puncture is to reduce the intracranial pressure. The patient, who should be kept in bed for up to four hours after the puncture, should be without a pillow for several hours and the foot of the bed may be raised. Some workers feel that if the patient lies prone rather than supine a positive rather than a negative pressure in the extradural space is produced and discourages leakage of fluid. If in spite of these precautions headache develops, treatment is directed to raising the intracranial pressure by promoting the formation of cerebrospinal fluid. This is best accomplished by drinking fluid in large quantities.

Lumbar puncture occasionally causes an intensification of symptoms of the disease from which the patient is suffering. Root pains, if present, may be intensified, and this is especially liable to occur in the presence of a lesion compressing the spinal cord, any of the symptoms of which may be exacerbated by the alterations of pressure induced by the withdrawal of fluid. In multiple sclerosis relapses have sometimes been attributed to lumbar puncture, and in this disease the procedure has sometimes appeared to precipitate a terminal acute encephalomyelitis. These events, however, are too rare to operate as contra-indications. The risks attendant upon lumbar puncture when the intracranial pressure is greatly increased, especially when there is a tumour in the posterior fossa, have already been described. Meningitis following lumbar puncture is fortunately rare and is due to a failure to preserve asepsis during the operation.

VENTRICLE PUNCTURE

The following are the principal indications for ventricle puncture: (1) the relief of increased intracranial pressure before operation for intracranial tumour; (2) the injection of air into the ventricles for ventriculography for the diagnosis of hydrocephalus or intracranial tumour; (3) the injection of an antibiotic; (4) for comparison of the pressure or chemical composition of the fluid in the two lateral ventricles or of the ventricular and spinal fluids; (5) in rare cases to obtain fluid for examination when there is a contra-indication to both cistern and lumbar puncture. The first and second are the purposes for which ventricle puncture is most frequently carried out.

CISTERN PUNCTURE

The cerebellomedullary cistern which is penetrated in cistern puncture, is a dilatation of the subarachnoid space lying between the inferior surface of the cerebellum above, the posterior surface of the medulla in front, and the dura mater covering the posterior atlanto-occipital membrane below and behind.

Indications and Contra-indications for Cistern Puncture

The principal indications for cistern puncture are: (1) to obtain cerebrospinal fluid for examination when lumbar puncture is for some reason impossible, for example, on account of deformity of the spine; (2) for comparison of the composition or pressure of the cisternal and lumbar fluids; (3) for the injection of opaque media in the radiographic investigation of blockage of the spinal subarachnoid space and particularly when lumbar myelography is impossible, or when the upper as well as the lower limits of a spinal lesion producing block must be defined; (4) for the introduction of therapeutic substances, such as an antibiotic; (5) to introduce air for encephalography. Cistern puncture should never be carried out when there is reason to suspect a tumour or abscess in the posterior fossa, when there is a marked rise of intracranial pressure, or when the cerebellomedullary cistern is likely to be obliterated by inflammatory adhesions, or to be the site of a congenital abnormality.

Method of Cistern Puncture

The patient is prepared by shaving the scalp up to a horizontal line at the level of the external occipital protuberance. The skin is then cleaned with alcohol and ether and painted with iodine or other suitable antiseptic. The patient should be seated and his head is held by an assistant with both hands and well flexed. The operator places the tip of the forefinger of his left hand upon the spinous process of the second cervical vertebra, which is the highest palpable spinous process. A spot half an inch above this point is anaesthetized with ethyl chloride or with a 1 per cent. solution of procaine. A lumbar puncture needle with the stylet in position is then inserted at this point and passed forwards in a plane which passes through the point of introduction, the middle of the external acoustic meatus, and the nasion. At a depth of about 3 cm. the point of the needle will encounter the posterior atlanto-occipital membrane, which offers considerable resistance. On gently introducing it a further $\frac{1}{2}$ cm. it should penetrate the cerebellomedullary cistern, and on withdrawal of the stylet cerebrospinal fluid usually drips from the needle. Often, however, although the point of the needle is in the cistern, there is no flow of fluid. This may be promoted by exerting gentle suction with a syringe inserted into the butt of the needle. The medulla lies at a depth of about 3 cm. in front of the posterior atlanto-occipital membrane. With care, therefore, there is no risk that the point of the needle will enter the medulla. It should not, however, be introduced more than 6 cm. from the surface of the skin. If the operator is unaccustomed to cistern puncture it is often rendered easier by directing the point of the needle slightly above the plane described, so that it comes into contact with the occipital bone. It is then slightly depressed to pass through the membrane. After withdrawal of the needle the point of puncture can be closed with collodion. Headache may follow cistern puncture. Its prophylaxis and treatment are the same as those described below for lumbar puncture.

ROUTINE EXAMINATION OF THE CEREBROSPINAL FLUID PRESSURE

Method of Determination. The pressure of the cerebrospinal fluid is best determined by means of a simple manometer. A graduated glass tube is attached to the lumbar puncture needle and the observer reads the height to which the fluid ascends in the tube. The instrument designed by Greenfield consists of a lumbar puncture needle with a two-way stopcock which permits fluid to be withdrawn without removing the manometer. A glass tube 30 cm. long is attached to the needle by a small piece of rubber tubing. To estimate pressures of more than 300 mm. it is necessary to connect a second length of tubing. For routine purposes the pressure is determined with the patient lying on the left side, and it is important to see that the head is supported at the same level as the lumbar spine. Lumbar puncture having been performed in the usual way, the tap is turned so that the fluid rises in the manometer. At this point the patient should be allowed to straighten his spine and should be directed to relax his muscles and breathe quietly and regularly, as muscular tension and holding the breath raise the pressure. Pressure is measured in millimetres of cerebrospinal fluid and normally shows oscillations corresponding to respiration and finer variations synchronous with the arterial pulse. The normal pressure of the cerebrospinal fluid in adults in the horizontal position is 60–150 mm. of fluid. According to Levinson it is lower in children, in whom it is normally from 45 to 90 mm. of fluid. In adults in the sitting posture the normal pressure is from 200 to 250 mm. of fluid, which, it should be noted, is usually less than the height of the vertex above the needle. Hence in the sitting posture the pressure in the ventricles and cerebellomedullary cistern may be negative.

Pathological Variations of Pressure. An abnormally high cerebrospinal fluid pressure is found in cases of intracranial tumour and haemorrhage, hypertensive encephalopathy, benign intracranial hypertension, and hypervitaminosis A, hydrocephalus, intracranial sinus thrombosis, meningism, and the various forms of meningitis and encephalitis, including the more acute forms of syphilitic meningitis and general paresis. The pressure may also be raised in uraemia and in some cases of emphysema. In intracranial tumour the pressure may be as high as 500–1,000 mm. of fluid.

A subnormal pressure is sometimes a sequel of head injury and may be found in cases of subdural haematoma. It is also encountered in conditions in which the lumbar subarachnoid space is cut off from communication with the cerebral subarachnoid space. This is most commonly met with in cases of spinal sub-arachnoid block due to spinal tumour or localized spinal meningitis. It may also occur when a block exists at the region of the foramen magnum as a result of a tumour in this situation or of meningeal adhesions following meningitis. The cerebrospinal fluid pressure may also be abnormally low if a second lumbar punc-ture is performed within a few days after a previous one.

Queckenstedt's Test. Normally if one compresses the jugular veins of a patient during lumbar puncture there is an immediate and rapid rise in the pres-sure of the cerebrospinal fluid which quickly reaches 300 mm. of fluid and almost as rapidly falls to normal when the veins are no longer compressed. The effect of compressing the veins is to cause a temporary congestion of the intracranial venous sinuses and hence to raise the intracranial pressure. The communica-tion of this raised pressure to the manometer attached to the lumbar puncture needle depends upon the patency of the subarachnoid space between the cranial cavity and the lumbar sac. In cases of obstruction of the subarachnoid space in the region of the foramen magnum or within the spinal canal the rise of pressure normally produced by jugular compression is either absent or slight in extent and slow in appearing, according to whether the block is complete or in-complete. In such cases also the normal variations in pressure due to respiration and the arterial pulse are also diminished or absent, but compression of the abdomen may cause an exaggerated rise of pressure.

Compression of either jugular vein separately may yield valuable evidence of thrombosis of the transverse sinus, for if the sinus is obstructed there will usually be no rise of pressure in the fluid when the jugular vein on the affected side is compressed.

NAKED-EYE APPEARANCE

Turbidity. The normal cerebrospinal fluid is clear and colourless and resembles water. Turbidity, when present, is usually due to an excess of polymorphonu-clear cells. In acute meningitis these are often present in such numbers that a deposit of pus forms at the bottom of the tube and the supernatant fluid may be yellow. It is very rare for an excess of lymphocytes to cause turbidity, but this may occasionally be due to micro-organisms.

Fibrin Clot. The development of a clot of fibrin in a specimen of fluid implies the presence of fibrinogen and of fibrin ferment. Such a clot may occur either in a fluid of which the protein content is only slightly raised or in the highly albuminous fluids characteristic of spinal subarachnoid block, and sometimes occurring in polyneuritis. In the former case the clot forms a faint 'cobweb' which takes from twelve to twenty-four hours to appear. It is most frequently seen in tuberculous meningitis, but also occurs occasionally in other forms of meningitis and has been described in syphilitic meningitis and in poliomyelitis. The clot which forms in highly albuminous fluids may solidify the whole specimen. In such cases clotting may be precipitated by the addition of fibrin ferment in the shape of a drop of fresh blood.

Blood. Blood may be present in the cerebrospinal fluid, either as an accidental result of injury to an intrathecal vein by the lumbar puncture needle, or as the product of pre-existing haemorrhage into the subarachnoid space. This distinction is obviously of great importance. When a vein is injured at lumbar puncture the specimen of fluid collected in the first tube is often blood-stained, but the second usually shows no visible blood, whereas after subarachnoid haemorrhage both specimens are uniformly blood-stained. Further, in the former case if the red cells are given time to settle, the supernatant fluid is seen to be colourless, whereas within a few hours of subarachnoid haemorrhage the supernatant fluid shows a yellow coloration. In practice there is seldom any difficulty in distinguishing the accidental contamination of the specimen with blood from subarachnoid haemorrhage. *Subarachnoid haemorrhage* is usually due to head injury, or to the rupture of an intracranial aneurysm or angioma into the subarachnoid space, or to the bursting of an intracerebral haemorrhage either into the ventricular system or into the subarachnoid space. In rare cases an intense 'haemorrhagic' form of encephalitis may lead to the presence of small amounts of blood in the cerebrospinal fluid. After subarachnoid haemorrhage the yellow coloration of the fluid appears in a few hours and reaches its greatest intensity at the end of about a week. It has usually disappeared in two to four weeks. The red cells generally disappear from the fluid in three to seven days. The presence of blood in contact with the leptomeninges excites a cellular reaction, and the fluid therefore usually contains a moderate excess of cells. As a rule these are all mononuclear, but polymorphonuclear cells may be found if the haemorrhage has invaded the brain substance.

Xanthochromia. Xanthochromia, or yellow coloration of the cerebrospinal fluid, is found, as just described, after subarachnoid haemorrhage and also when pus is present in considerable amount in the fluid. Xanthochromic fluid is also often found after an intracerebral haemorrhage, or cerebral infarction, in some cases of intracranial tumour, especially when the tumour is near the ventricular system, and sometimes in the case of tumours of the eighth nerve. It is also characteristic of obstruction of the spinal subarachnoid space and may also be seen in fluid from above a tumour of the cauda equina and sometimes in polyneuritis. A slight yellow coloration of the fluid may be present in cases of jaundice of long standing.

CYTOLOGICAL AND CHEMICAL ABNORMALITIES

Since this is a textbook of clinical neurology, methods of carrying out cell counts and chemical investigations on the cerebrospinal fluid will not be described in more detail than is necessary for a discussion of their interpretation. Those who wish to acquaint themselves with the technique of these examinations are referred to the textbooks on the cerebrospinal fluid (see references).

Cells

The normal cerebrospinal fluid contains a small number of cells. These are lymphocytes or large mononuclear cells and should not exceed three per cubic millimetre. In pathological states a greater variety of cells may be present and these may occur in very large numbers. Those most frequently encountered are lymphocytes, large mononuclear cells and polymorphonuclear cells. Less frequently eosinophils, plasma cells, macrophages, and compound granular corpuscles and fibroblasts are found. Tumour cells are rare but when present are of great diagnostic importance. Yeasts, actinomycotic granules, echinococci, and cysticerci have been observed in cases of infection of the nervous system with these organisms.

Significance of Cell Content. Certain generalizations may be made with regard to the presence and numbers of different types of cell in the fluid. The majority of cells are probably derived from the meninges, though some may take origin within the nerve tissue and pass into the subarachnoid space from the perivascular spaces. In general a pleocytosis, or excess of cells in the spinal fluid, indicates meningeal irritation, though this does not necessarily imply the presence of meningeal infection. Whether the cellular increase is polymorphonuclear depends partly upon the acuteness of the pathological process and partly upon the nature of the infecting organism. A predominantly polymorphonuclear count is usually found in acute infections and in acute exacerbations of chronic infections, while a mononuclear count is characteristic of chronic infections. But while pyogenic organisms excite a mainly polymorphonuclear leucocytosis except in their most chronic stages, a mononuclear pleocytosis is characteristic of infection with neurotropic viruses, though polymorphonuclear cells are sometimes present when the infection is most acute. We thus encounter predominantly polymorphonuclear, predominantly mononuclear, and mixed cell counts.

A predominantly polymorphonuclear pleocytosis is found in meningitis due to pyogenic organisms, including the meningococcus, staphylococcus, streptococcus, pneumococcus, *Escherichia coli, Bacillus typhosus, Listeria monocytogenes*, and *Haemophilus influenzae*. In these conditions the polymorphonuclear cells are usually present in very large numbers. A very acute syphilitic meningitis may also excite a polymorphonuclear reaction in which the cells may number several thousands per cubic millimetre. Mononuclear pleocytosis rarely exceeds 200 cells per mm.[3] and more commonly lies between 10 and 50 cells per mm.[3] Counts of up to 1,000 per mm.[3], however, may occur in various forms of virus meningitis. It is characteristic of syphilis of the nervous system, encephalitis lethargica, multiple sclerosis, poliomyelitis (after the first few days of the infection), herpes zoster, acute lymphocytic choriomeningitis, and some cases of tuberculous meningitis. It may also be present in mumps, and has been described in infectious mononucleosis, whooping cough, malaria, trypanosomiasis, relapsing fever, and leptospirosis canicola or icterohaemorrhagica. Cerebral tumour may cause a slight mononuclear pleocytosis, especially when the tumour is in contact with the meninges. So also may cerebral abscess, intracranial sinus thrombosis, and subarachnoid haemorrhage. The mixed type of pleocytosis, in which polymorphonuclear and mononuclear cells are present in approximately equal numbers, is found in cerebral abscess, in which case the number of cells is often small, and in cases of infection of the bones of the skull in the neighbourhood of the meninges. A mixed cell count is also present in many cases of tuberculous meningitis, in poliomyelitis during the first few days, and in the more acute forms of syphilitic meningitis.

Protein

The total protein content of the normal cerebrospinal fluid is from 0·015 to 0·045 g. per 100 ml. This consists of albumin and globulin in a ratio of 8 to 1 (Hewitt). Increase of the protein of the fluid is extremely common. A moderate increase, usually to below 0·2 g. per 100 ml. is found in inflammatory diseases of the nervous tissue and meninges, such as the various forms of meningitis, encephalitis, poliomyelitis, multiple sclerosis, and syphilis of the nervous system. Intracranial tumour and cerebral haemorrhage and infarction may also cause a moderate rise of protein content. A marked rise is less common.

Froin originally described the syndrome which is known by his name and in which a high protein content of fluid is associated with xanthochromia, massive coagulation, and pleocytosis. Froin's cases were examples of obstruction of the spinal subarachnoid space, due to localized spinal meningitis, which was responsible for the pleocytosis. The essential part of the syndrome is now known to be the great excess of protein, and Greenfield and Carmichael (1925) proposed that the term Froin's syndrome should be applied only to fluids which contain 0·5 g. per 100 ml. of protein or more, and which are not frankly purulent. Thus defined it occurs, according to these authors, in three classes of disease: (1) chronic, especially syphilitic, meningitis, and more rarely acute and subacute meningitis; (2) obstruction of the spinal subarachnoid space, due to tumour of the cord or its envelopes, spinal caries, and epidural abscess, whether tuberculous or staphylococcal; (3) acute or subacute polyneuritis. It may also occur in fluid withdrawn above the level of a tumour of the cauda equina. The characteristic changes in the spinal fluid which occur in obstruction of the spinal subarachnoid space are attributable to several anatomical factors. Spinal block cuts off the fluid below the obstruction from the normal course of circulation and absorption. Compression of the spinal veins by a tumour or similar lesion causes chronic venous congestion of the cord below the level of the obstruction, since the venous drainage of the cord is from below upwards in the longitudinal veins which have few anastomoses. The spinal arteries on the other hand, although they run longitudinally, anastomose freely with the radicular arteries, which enter the spinal canal through the intervertebral foramina. Further, blood plasma may pass into the spinal fluid from the blood vessels of a tumour, or as inflammatory exudate when the obstructive lesion is a meningitis.

The Albumin-Globulin Ratio

Several reactions designed to demonstrate an excess of globulin in the cerebrospinal fluid are in common use. In the *Nonne-Apelt reaction* ammonium sulphate is the reagent employed. A positive reaction ranges from a slight opalescence to actual precipitation of the globulin. In *Noguchi's reaction* the globulin if present in excess is precipitated by butyric acid. In *Pandy's reaction* a solution of carbolic acid is used and positive reactions range from opalescence to milky turbidity. Similar positive reactions are obtained in *Weichbrodt's reaction* with a solution of mercuric chloride. These reactions are not quantitative. Pandy's reaction is the most sensitive, and may yield a weakly positive result with normal fluids.

In normal fluids the greater part of the globulin present is pseudoglobulin. In pathological fluids an increase of globulin is usually associated with an increase in albumin, and the increase of the former is often proportionately greater than that of the latter. Euglobulin shows a much greater increase than pseudoglobulin, especially in general paresis. Electrophoresis is now being used to study the globulins of the cerebrospinal fluid (Deneker and Swahn, 1961). Many different globulin fractions have now been identified using techniques of disc electrophoresis and immunoelectrophoresis. Normally the fluid contains, when compared with serum, a high proportion of β-globulin and a relatively low proportion of γ-globulin. In normal fluid the γ-globulin does not usually exceed 20 per cent. of the total protein and is generally substantially less. Proportions in excess of 25 per cent. are found in more than 50 per cent. of cases of multiple sclerosis and similar increases have been observed in active neurosyphilis and subacute encephalitis. Thus estimation of the γ-globulin in the fluid is being increasingly used for diagnostic purposes (see Davson, 1967; and Link, 1967).

Phospholipids

The total phospholipid content of the fluid may be increased in a number of neurological diseases but a relative rise in the content of cephalin is seen in patients with demyelinating processes (Zilkha and McArdle, 1963).

Glucose

The normal glucose content of the cerebrospinal fluid is somewhat lower than that of the blood and lies between 50 and 85 mg. per 100 ml. Diminution of the glucose content of the fluid is found in meningitis. It is probable that glucose in the fluid is consumed by the infecting organisms. In pyogenic meningitis, indeed, sugar is usually absent from the fluid. A moderate decrease in glucose content to 10–50 mg. per 100 ml. is characteristic of tuberculous meningitis, certain other chronic meningitides (e.g. torulosis) and carcinomatosis of the meninges. A rise in the glucose content of the fluid is found in diabetes parallel to that obtaining in the blood.

Chlorides

The chlorides are the only chemical constituent of the cerebrospinal fluid which is maintained at a higher concentration than in the blood. The normal chloride content of the fluid is 720 to 750 mg. per 100 ml. estimated as sodium chloride. In purulent meningitis this figure is reduced to an average of from 650 to 680 mg. per 100 ml. The reduction is much greater in tuberculous meningitis, in which condition Fremont-Smith and his collaborators obtained an average reading of 610 mg. per 100 ml. and a minimum of 520 mg. In the early stages of tuberculous meningitis the reduction is less marked. The chloride content of the fluid was in the past regarded as of diagnostic value in distinguishing tuberculous meningitis both from conditions such as poliomyelitis in which the chloride content of the fluid is normal and also from other conditions of meningeal inflammation in which the fall is less marked. However, it is now recognized that the fall of chloride content in the fluid is usually due to frequent vomiting and that when the chloride content of the blood plasma varies from normal a corresponding change occurs in the chlorides of the fluid. Similarly we find the chloride content of the fluid to be above normal in many cases of nephritis, especially in the stage of uraemia, and below normal in meningism.

COLLOIDAL REACTIONS

Lange's Colloidal Gold Reaction. Lange's colloidal gold reaction is often of great diagnostic value, although its theoretical basis is incompletely understood and it has been largely superseded in most laboratories by estimation of the various globulin fractions (particularly γ-globulin) in the fluid. It is based upon the observation that the cerebrospinal fluid in certain pathological states possesses the property of precipitating a preparation of colloidal gold and that the degree of precipitation varies according to the concentration of cerebrospinal fluid used.

In carrying out the test ten, or sometimes six, test-tubes are employed, each of which contains the same amount of the colloidal gold solution. Cerebrospinal fluid is then added so that in the first tube it is present in a concentration of 1 in 10 and in each subsequent tube this concentration is progressively reduced by one-half. The result is a series of ten tubes each containing the same amount of colloidal gold solution, but containing concentrations of cerebrospinal fluid ranging from 1 in 10 to 1 in 5,120. The unchanged colloidal gold solution is cherry-red in colour, and this colour changes in proportion to the degree of precipitation, through purple and blue to complete decolorization of the supernatant fluid with a bluish precipitate. These changes are numerically expressed, 0 signifying no change and the figures 1 to 5 denoting progressive degrees of alteration. In reading the result of the test the tube containing the highest concentration of cerebrospinal fluid is placed on the left and the concentration diminishes in the series from the left to the right.

The following types of colloidal curve may be encountered:

1. Normal fluids cause no precipitation, except possibly to the slightest extent in the middle of the curve, and are thus reported as 0000000000 or 0000110000.

2. The 'paretic' curve. In this type of curve complete precipitation occurs in the first four or five tubes and none in the last two or three. A typical series would be 5555321000. The 'paretic' curve is so called from its constancy in general paresis. It may be present in meningovascular syphilis and in tabes. It is also found in some 50 per cent. of cases of multiple sclerosis and sometimes following subarachnoid haemorrhage.

3. The luetic or tabetic curve. This is represented by the figures 1233210000 and is the type of curve usually encountered in tabes and sometimes in meningovascular syphilis.

4. The meningitic curve shows a plateau further to the right than the preceding and is represented by the figures 0012344310. This type of curve is that usually found in syphilitic and bacterial meningitis.

The principal value of the colloidal gold curve lies in its assistance in differentiating general paresis from other types of neurosyphilis and in the support which it sometimes yields for a diagnosis of multiple sclerosis. A paretic curve is always found in untreated cases of general paresis, and though it is sometimes present in other forms of neurosyphilis it is much more readily altered by treatment in the latter than in the former. In a suspected case of multiple sclerosis the presence of a paretic curve in the cerebrospinal fluid in association with a negative Wassermann reaction is to be taken as confirmatory evidence of the diagnosis.

The explanation of the varying degree of precipitation of the colloidal gold solution by different dilutions of the cerebrospinal fluid in pathological states depends upon the relative concentration of albumin and globulins in the fluid.

SEROLOGICAL REACTIONS

The Wassermann and V.D.R.L. reactions in the cerebrospinal fluid are discussed in the section on syphilis.

BACTERIOLOGICAL EXAMINATION

In cases of infection of the nervous system and the meninges with pyogenic organisms and with the tubercle bacillus a bacteriological examination of the cerebrospinal fluid may be necessary, especially to determine the causal organism in meningitis.

When dealing with a fluid which is frankly purulent it is sufficient to make a film with a platinum loop and to stain it in the usual way. When there is no visible pus, and in suspected cases of tuberculous meningitis, it is advisable to centrifuge the fluid before examining it. Cultures should also be made, both for the further identification of an organism which is seen in the film and also because when the film yields a negative result an organism can sometimes be isolated by culturing. Animal inoculation is sometimes called for.

REFERENCES

COHEN, H. (1927) Chemical studies bearing on the formation of cerebrospinal fluid, *Brain*, **50**, 601.

DAVSON, H. (1958) Some aspects of the relationship between the cerebrospinal fluid and the central nervous system, in *Ciba Foundation Symposium on the Cerebrospinal Fluid*, p. 189, London.

DAVSON, H. (1967) *The Physiology of the Cerebrospinal Fluid*, London.

DENEKER, S. J., and SWAHN, B. (1961) *Clinical Value of Protein Analysis in Cerebrospinal Fluid*, London.

ERSKINE, D., and JOHNSON, A. G. (1938) Lumbar puncture in out-patients, *Lancet*, ii, 371.

GREENFIELD, J. G., and CARMICHAEL, E. A. (1925) *The Cerebrospinal Fluid in Clinical Diagnosis*, London.

LINK, H. (1967) Immunoglobulin G and low molecular weight proteins in human cerebrospinal fluid, *Acta neurol. scand.*, **43**, Suppl. 28.

MERRITT, H. H., and FREMONT-SMITH, F. (1937) *The Cerebrospinal Fluid*, Philadelphia.

MILLEN, J. W., and WOOLLAM, D. H. M. (1962) *The Anatomy of the Cerebrospinal Fluid*, London.

SWEET, W. H., BROWNELL G. L., SCHOLL, J. A., BOWSHER, D. R., BENDA, P., and STICKLEY, E. E. (1954) The formation, flow and absorption of cerebrospinal fluid, newer concepts based on studies with isotopes, *Res. Publ. Ass. nerv. ment. Dis.*, **34**, 101.

VON STORCH, T. J. C., CARMICHAEL, E. A., and BANKS, T. E. (1937) Factors producing lumbar cerebrospinal fluid pressure in man in the erect posture, *Arch. Neurol. Psychiat. (Chicago)*, **38**, 1158.

WEED, L. H. (1935) Certain anatomical and physiological aspects of the meninges and cerebrospinal fluid, *Brain*, **58**, 383.

WELCH, K., and FRIEDMAN, V. (1960) The cerebrospinal fluid valves, *Brain*, **83**, 454.

WOLSTENHOLME, G. E. W., and O'CONNOR, C. M. (1958) *Ciba Foundation Symposium on the Cerebrospinal Fluid Production, Circulation and Absorption*, London.

ZILKHA, K. J., and MCARDLE, B. (1963) The phospholipid composition of cerebrospinal fluid in diseases associated with demyelination, *Quart. J. Med.*, **32**, 79.

HISTORY AND EXAMINATION

THE HISTORY OF THE ILLNESS

GENERAL CONSIDERATIONS

In the diagnosis of nervous diseases the history of the patient's illness is often of greater importance than the discovery of his abnormal physical signs. The group of physical signs may be common to several disorders, and only an accurate knowledge of their mode of development may enable the correct diagnosis to be made. The history obtained from the patient should always be supplemented, if possible, by an account of his illness given by a relative or by some one who knows him well. This is essential when the patient suffers from mental impairment and also when his complaint includes attacks in which he loses consciousness, but it is always desirable, since a relative or friend will often remember an important point which the patient himself has forgotten to mention.

First note the patient's name and address, age, and exact details of his occupation. The last named is often of importance as a source of exposure to injury or to toxic substances. Ascertain if he is right-handed.

It is well to begin by asking the patient of what he complains and when he was last in normal health, in this way fixing, at least provisionally, the date of onset of his symptoms. After this he should be allowed to relate the story of his illness as far as possible without interruption, questions being put to him afterwards to expand his statements and to elicit additional information. In the case of all symptoms it is important to ascertain not only the date but also the mode of onset, whether sudden, rapid, or gradual, whether the symptom since its first appearance has fluctuated in intensity and whether the patient's condition is improving, stationary, or deteriorating at the time of examination.

HISTORY OF PRESENT ILLNESS

Inquiry should always be made with regard to the following symptoms, whether or not the patient mentions them spontaneously:

Mental State. The patient's mental history should be ascertained, not only as far as possible from himself, but also from relatives or friends, on the lines laid down below for the examination of his mental condition. If mental abnormality is suspected it is necessary to ascertain the patient's normal level of intelligence and temperament.

Sleep. Has he suffered from disturbances of sleep, either from paroxysmal or persistent sleepiness or from insomnia?

Speech. Has he had difficulty in speaking? If so, of what nature? Has he been able to understand what is said to him and to read? Has his writing been affected? [see p. 106].

Attacks of Loss of Consciousness. Has he suffered from attacks of loss or impairment of consciousness? If so, for further inquiries see pages 257 and 922.

Headache. Has he suffered from headache? If so, further inquiries should be made as described on page 266.

Special Senses. Has he had hallucinations of smell or taste or noticed an impairment of these senses? Has he had visual hallucinations? If so, what has been their character and distribution in the visual fields? Has there been any visual impairment: if so, of one or both eyes and of what nature? Has it been transitory or progressive? Has he had double vision? If so, has this been transitory or progressive and has he noticed this symptom when looking in any special direction? Is his hearing impaired? If so, is this unilateral or bilateral and is the deafness associated with tinnitus? Does he suffer from giddiness? If so, he should describe precisely its nature and state whether it is associated with a sense of rotation of himself or of his surroundings, and with deafness, tinnitus, or vomiting.

Movement and Sensibility. Does he complain of muscular weakness, of loss of control over the limbs or of involuntary movements, and if so, what is the distribution of these symptoms? Has his gait been abnormal, and if so, how? Has he tended to fall, and if so, in what direction? Has he had any spontaneous sensory disturbances, especially pain, numbness, or tingling? If so, further inquiries should be made, as described on page 37.

The Sphincters and Reproductive Functions. Has there been any disturbance of sphincter control? Has he experienced difficulty in holding or passing urine or faeces? Has he had polyuria? In the case of a man, is his sexual power normal for his age? In the case of a woman, has there been any abnormality in menstruation, especially amenorrhoea?

Nutrition. Is the weight stationary, diminishing, or increasing?

HISTORY OF PREVIOUS ILLNESSES

Inquiry as to previous illnesses should always include, in the case of a male patient, a specific inquiry as to venereal disease. A history of aural discharge or of tuberculosis may be important in relation to intracranial abscess or tuberculous meningitis. A history of convulsions or of meningitis in childhood or of encephalitis lethargica may be significant in relation to a later illness. A history of 'influenza' should be amplified by details of the illness thus described. Inquiry should always be made for a history of accidental injury, especially to the head and spine. A difficult birth may be significant in relation to epilepsy.

SOCIAL HISTORY

This should include inquiry as to the patient's educational and occupational career, adjustments to family life, military service career, residence abroad, and personal habits in respect of recreation, tobacco, and alcohol. If alcoholic excess is admitted, its amount and duration should be ascertained.

FAMILY HISTORY

The family history is often of great importance, since many diseases of the nervous system are hereditary. The patient should always be asked whether cases of nervous or mental disease have occurred among his relatives and if so the precise nature of the illness should, if possible, be ascertained. Consanguinity in the parents should be inquired for. If the patient is married, inquiry should be made as to the state of health of the spouse. Death of husband or wife from general paralysis or aneurysm may afford an important clue to a syphilitic disorder in a patient. For the same reason the number of children and the occurrence of miscarriages and stillbirths should be ascertained.

EXAMINATION OF THE PATIENT

STATE OF CONSCIOUSNESS

Is the patient conscious or unconscious [see p. 970]? If unconscious, how far does he respond to stimuli, such as pinching the skin? Can he be roused, and if so, when he is roused is his mental condition normal or abnormal? How far can he think with normal clarity and speed, and perceive, respond to, and remember current stimuli? Can he swallow? The following psychological investigations are, of course, applicable only to conscious patients.

INTELLECTUAL FUNCTIONS

Is the patient orientated in space and time? Does he recognize his surroundings and does he know the date? Is his memory normal, and, if impaired, is it better for remote than for recent events? Does he fill gaps in his memory by confabulating, that is, by relating imaginary events? Retentiveness may be tested by asking the patient to retain and repeat a series of digits—normally seven can be repeated—or retain a name, address, and the name of a flower for five minutes.

What is his level of intelligence? Is he in touch with current events? Can he grasp the meaning of a passage which he reads from a newspaper, or of a picture depicting an incident?

Does he suffer from delusions or hallucinations? A delusion is an erroneous belief which cannot be corrected by an appeal to reason and is not shared by others of the patient's education and station. An hallucination is a sensory impression occurring in the absence of a corresponding external stimulus. A patient may conceal both delusions and hallucinations. The latter may sometimes be suspected on account of his behaviour. For example, a patient who is subject to visual hallucinations may behave as though manipulating invisible objects, while one who is experiencing auditory hallucinations, for example voices, may adopt a listening attitude.

EMOTIONAL STATE

Is the patient's emotional state normal? Is he excited or depressed? If excited, is his condition one of elation, that is, excitement associated with a sense of well-being, or of fear and anxiety? Apart from excitement, does he experience an abnormal sense of well-being—euphoria? Is he anxious and, if so, to what does he attribute his anxiety? Is he irritable? Is he emotionally indifferent and apathetic? Does he take normal care of his dress and appearance, or is he indifferent and dirty?

SPEECH AND ARTICULATION

Are speech and articulation normal? If there is reason to suspect that the patient is suffering from aphasia, the appropriate tests must be carried out [see p. 106].

THE CRANIAL NERVES

Test the sense of smell for each nostril separately [see p. 141].

Test the visual acuity and visual fields [see pp. 65–6].

Examine the ocular fundi [see p. 143].

Are the pupils equal, central, and regular? Are they abnormally dilated or contracted? Test the reactions to light, both direct and consensual, of each eye separately, and the reaction on accommodation.

Test the ocular movements, upwards and downwards and to either side, and ocular convergence. Is squint, diplopia, or nystagmus present? Note the size of the palpebral fissures. Does the patient exhibit ptosis or retraction of the upper lids? Is exophthalmos present?

Is there wasting of the temporal muscles and masseters? Test the jaw movements and the jaw-jerk.

Examine sensibility to light touch, pin-prick, heat and cold over the trigeminal area, and test the corneal reflexes.

Is the facial expression normal? Is there wasting of the facial muscles? Is the face the site of involuntary movements? Test the following voluntary movements —closure of the eyes, elevation of the eyebrows, frowning, retraction of the lips, pursing the lips, whistling. Test emotional facial movements—smiling. In some cases of facial paralysis it is necessary to test the sense of taste [see p. 190].

Test the hearing, both air-conduction and bone-conduction. If hearing is defective, apply both Weber's and Rinne's tests [see p. 173]. In certain cases it may be necessary to test the vestibular reactions [see p. 177].

Is the soft palate elevated normally on phonation? Test the palatal and pharyngeal reflexes.

Examine the movements of the vocal cords, if necessary.

Test the movements of the sternomastoids and trapezii.

Examine the tongue. Is it wasted? Is fasciculation present? Is it tremulous? Is it protruded normally?

Note the presence or absence of head retraction and test for cervical rigidity.

THE LIMBS AND TRUNK

The following is a convenient routine for the examination of the limbs and trunk. Examine the upper limbs while the patient is lying down; then ask him to sit up, or, if he is unable to do so, to turn on to one side, and examine the scapular muscles and the back; then ask him to lie down again and examine the front of the thorax and the abdomen, and finally the lower limbs. Sensibility as well as motor functions should first be examined in this order, but in many cases, especially when there is reason to suspect a lesion of the spinal cord, it may be convenient to review the sensibility of the body as a whole.

Muscular Power and Co-ordination. In examining the limbs note first their *posture* and the presence or absence of *muscular wasting* and *fasciculation*. Next note the presence or absence of *involuntary movements*, of which the following are those most commonly encountered. A tic is a co-ordinated, repetitive movement involving as a rule a number of muscles in their normal synergic relationships. Choreic movements are quasi-purposive, jerky, irregular, and non-repetitive, and are characterized by dissociation of normal muscular synergy. Athetosis consists of slow, writhing movements, which are most marked in the peripheral segments of the limbs. Tremor is a rhythmical movement at a joint, brought about by alternating contractions of antagonistic groups of muscles. Myoclonus is a shock-like muscular contraction affecting part or the whole of the muscle independently of its antagonists. If involuntary movements are present, note their relationship to rest, posture, and voluntary movement.

Next examine *muscle tone* by passive movement at the various joints and note the presence or absence of *muscular contractures*. Next test voluntary power by asking the patient to carry out against resistance the movements possible at the various joints, comparing successively the same movement on the two sides of the body. If it is desired to record the degree of power present in a muscle the following scale may be used: no contraction, 0; flicker or trace of contraction, 1; active movement, with gravity eliminated, 2; active movement against gravity, 3; active movement against gravity and resistance, 4; normal power, 5.

Muscular co-ordination is tested in the upper limbs by asking the patient to touch the tip of his nose with the tip of his forefinger, first with the eyes open and then with the eyes closed. He should also be asked to carry out alternating movements of flexion and extension of the fingers, or pronation and supination of the forearms simultaneously on both sides. When the patient is in bed, co-ordination of the lower limbs may be tested by asking him to place one heel on the opposite knee, or to raise the leg from the bed and touch the observer's finger with his toe.

Movements of the abdominal wall are tested by asking the patient to raise his head from the bed against resistance and noting by palpation the degree of contraction of the abdominal muscles and also whether displacement of the umbilicus occurs.

Sensibility. As a routine, the patient's appreciation of light touch, pin-prick, heat and cold, posture, passive movement, and vibration should be tested, attention being paid not only to defective sensibility but also to the presence of tenderness of the superficial and deep structures. In some cases additional tests may be needed [see p. 38]. Since the spinal segmental areas run longitudinally along the long axis of the upper limbs, sensibility on the ulnar border should be compared with that on the radial border, either by applying successive stimuli transversely to the limb, or by dragging the stimulus, for example a pin, along the skin. On the trunk the segmental areas are distributed almost horizontally. Changes of sensibility are therefore best detected by moving the stimulus from below upwards or vice versa. In the lower limbs the sacral segmental areas, which are represented on the sole and the posterior aspect of the limb, should always be tested.

The Reflexes. The following reflexes should be examined as a routine: in the upper limbs, the supinator-, biceps- and triceps-jerks; on the trunk, the abdominal reflexes; in the lower limbs, the knee- and ankle-jerks and the plantar reflexes; at the same time tests for patellar and ankle clonus should be carried out.

The Sphincters. Note the state of the sphincters and examine the abdomen for evidence of distension of the bladder.

Trophic Disturbances. Note the state of the patient's nutrition, especially the presence of wasting or excessive obesity and the condition of the external genitalia. Note the distribution of hair on the body, anomalies of sweating, and the presence or absence of cutaneous pigmentation and trophic lesions of the skin, nails, and joints.

Examine the *scalp* and *skull* [see p. 231] and also the *spine*, noting the presence of deformity, rigidity, and tenderness in the latter and auscultating for a bruit.

A complete general physical examination should be made. Examination of the peripheral blood vessels, especially the carotids, is important. Inequality of carotid pulsation should be noted, and auscultation for a bruit should be carried out over each carotid, mastoid process, and eye. If a bruit is present, can it be abolished by carotid compression?

GAIT

If the patient is well enough to leave his bed, observe whether he is able to stand without support with the feet together, and whether the steadiness of his stance is affected when he closes his eyes. Ask him to walk, if necessary with support, and note the presence of spasticity or ataxia of the lower limbs in walking. Slight disturbances of stance and gait may be detected by asking the patient to stand first on one foot and then on the other, first with the eyes open and then with the eyes closed; and to walk along a line, placing one heel in front of the toes of the other foot.

ELECTROENCEPHALOGRAPHY

The observation of Berger (1929) that it was possible to record changes of electrical potential occurring in the human brain has already led to important advances in knowledge. The changes of electrical potential recorded are usually of the order of from 5 to 50 millivolts, and have a duration of from 1 second down to 20 milliseconds. The recording of such small electrical changes has been

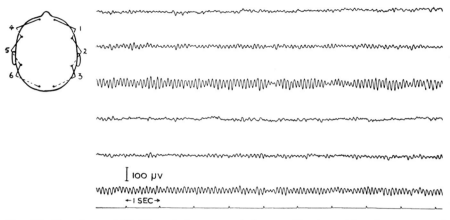

FIG. 18. Female, aged 23. Normal electroencephalogram. Dominant 10 cycles per second alpha activity in the posterocentral regions

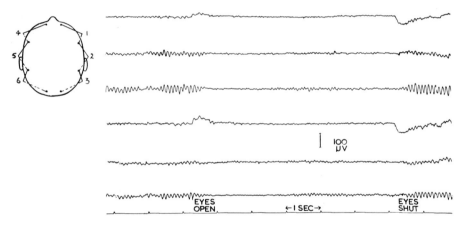

FIG. 19. Female, aged 23. Normal electroencephalogram. Almost complete blocking of the dominant alpha rhythm to eye opening

rendered possible by the development of thermionic valve amplification. For ordinary purposes electrodes are applied to the unshaved scalp.

The first electrical rhythm, described by Berger as the alpha rhythm, and later referred to by Adrian and others as the Berger rhythm, consists of an almost sinusoidal discharge with a frequency of about 10 per second and with a potential varying irregularly from zero to about 100 microvolts in some subjects [FIGS. 18 and 19]. The area of the alpha discharge is usually limited to the parieto-occipital region of both hemispheres, but it may be seen elsewhere. It has been demonstrated by Berger and by Adrian that the alpha rhythm is inhibited by visual activity and it is also decreased or abolished when the eyes are shut, by intellectual concentration, such as that required for mental arithmetic, and also by a startling external stimulus, such as a noise or sensation. It is, therefore, suggested that the alpha rhythm is an indication of physiological rest in that area of the occipital cortex concerned with the integration of visual stimuli. Other rhythms have been described. Electroencephalography may reveal localized or diffuse brain damage, or abnormal discharges, which are described in the appropriate sections (see also Hill and Driver, 1962).

REFERENCES

ADRIAN, E. D., and MATTHEWS, B. H. C. (1934) The Berger rhythm: potential changes from the occipital lobes in man, *Brain*, **57**, 355.

ADRIAN, E. D., and YAMAGIWA, K. (1935) The origin of the Berger rhythm, *Brain*, **58**, 323.

BERGER, H. (1929) Über das Elektrenkephalogramm des Menschen, *Arch. Psychiat. Nervenkr.*, **87**, 527.

HILL, D., and DRIVER, M. V. (1962) in *Recent Advances in Neurology and Neuropsychiatry*, 7th ed., ed. Brain, Lord, p. 169, London.

HILL, D., and PARR, G. (1963) *Electro-encephalography*, 2nd ed., London.

KILOH, L. G., and OSSELTON, J. W. (1967) *Clinical Electroencephalography*, 2nd ed., London.

WALTER, W. G. (1938) The technique and application of electro-encephalography, *J. Neurol. Neurosurg. Psychiat.*, N.S. **1**, 359.

WALTER, W. G., and DOVEY, V. J. (1944) Electro-encephalography in cases of sub-cortical tumour, *J. Neurol. Neurosurg. Psychiat.*, N.S. **7**, 57.

2

THE CRANIAL NERVES

THE FIRST OR OLFACTORY NERVE

THE OLFACTORY FIBRES

THE olfactory portion of the nasal mucous membrane contains bipolar sensory cells which constitute the olfactory neurones of the first order. Their central processes, which are unmyelinated, form small bundles, the filaments of the olfactory nerve, which pass through the cribriform plates of the ethmoid bone and enter the olfactory bulb. From the olfactory bulb further fibres reach the brain through the olfactory tract (for details see Le Gros Clark, 1947). As this approaches the cerebral hemisphere it divides into a median and a lateral root on either side of the anterior perforated space. The lateral root is the more important in man and carries fibres to the olfactory area of the cerebral cortex, which consists of the peri-amygdaloid and pre-piriform areas of the so-called piriform lobe and, in spite of long tradition, does not include the hippocampus (Brodal, 1947). The anterior commissure unites the olfactory cortical regions of the two hemispheres and probably also carries fibres from each olfactory tract to the opposite hemisphere.

DISTURBANCES OF THE SENSE OF SMELL

By the sense of smell we perceive not only scents but also flavours, the sense of taste being concerned only with the recognition of the four primary tastes—sweet, bitter, salt, and acid. It is a commonplace observation that a cold in the head, which abolishes the sense of smell, abolishes also flavours but not the primary tastes.

In testing the sense of smell small bottles containing coffee, oil of peppermint, oil of cloves, camphorated oil, and other scents are applied in turn to each nostril, and the patient is asked if he recognizes them. It must be remembered that many normal individuals with an acute sense of smell find difficulty in naming scents.

Anosmia, or loss of the olfactory sense, is occasionally congenital, and sometimes hereditary. It may occur either temporarily or permanently as a result of infections of the nose. The sense of smell is lost when the olfactory tract is interrupted. Complete or partial loss may occur on one or both sides as a result of head injury either with or without fracture of the base of the skull in the anterior fossa. Sumner (1964) found an incidence of 7·5 per cent., the liability increasing with increasing severity of the head injury. The olfactory tract may be compressed by tumours, especially by meningiomas growing from the olfactory groove, or less frequently by tumours of the frontal lobe or in the region of the optic chiasma, or by the distended cerebral hemispheres in obstructive hydrocephalus. It may be involved in meningitis, both purulent and syphilitic and, like the optic nerves, degenerate in tabes. It is doubtful whether complete anosmia is produced by lesions of the olfactory cortex on one side, probably because fibres from each olfactory tract reach both cerebral hemispheres. A lesion of one uncus, however, may cause a reduction in olfactory acuity in the nostril of the same side. Irritative lesions in the neighbourhood of the uncus are liable to cause olfactory hallucinations, which are usually associated with disturbance of consciousness and involuntary convulsive movements of the lips, jaw, tongue, and pharynx—uncinate fits [see p. 243].

Parosmia may occur especially after head injury. Strong scents then smell abnormal, usually unpleasant, and a persistent unpleasant olfactory hallucination may be experienced. A similar symptom sometimes occurs in depressive illness.

The treatment of anosmia is that of the causative lesion. Sumner found that in all but severe injuries about 50 per cent. recover, but with a post-traumatic amnesia of over 24 hours when traumatic anosmia occurs it is permanent in 90 per cent. of cases.

REFERENCES

BRODAL, A. (1947) The hippocampus and the sense of smell, *Brain*, **70,** 179.
CLARK, W. E. LE G. (1947) *Anatomical Pattern as the Essential Basis of Sensory Discrimination*, Oxford.
DANA, C. L. (1889) The olfactory nerve, *N.Y. med. J.*, **50**, 253.
ELSBERG, C. A. (1937) The newer aspects of olfactory physiology and their diagnostic applications, *Arch. Neurol. Psychiat.* (*Chicago*), **37,** 223.
ELSBERG, C. A., and STEWART, J. (1938) Quantitative olfactory tests: value in localization and diagnosis of tumors of the brain with analysis of results in three hundred patients. *Arch. Neurol. Psychiat.* (*Chicago*), **40,** 471.
LEIGH, A. D. (1943) Defects of smell after head injury, *Lancet*, i, 38.
SUMNER, D. (1964) Post-traumatic anosmia, *Brain*, **87,** 107.

THE SECOND OR OPTIC NERVE

The course of the optic nerve and the situation of the retinal fibres within it are described on page 66.

THE VISUAL ACUITY

Distant vision may be estimated by testing the patient's power of reading Snellen's type at a distance of 6 metres. The visual acuity is expressed as a fraction, the distance of the eye from the type, i.e. 6 metres, being divided by the distance at which the patient should be capable of reading the smallest type he can read. Normal visual acuity is thus 6/6ths. If at 6 metres the patient can only read type which he should be capable of reading at 60 metres, the visual acuity is said to be 6/60ths. Near vision is tested by Jaeger's types. For more accurate investigation of the visual acuity perimetry is necessary.

THE VISUAL FIELDS

Methods of investigating the visual fields are described on pages 65–6.

Ophthalmoscopy

Examination of the fundus oculi is of such importance in the investigation of cases of nervous disease that it should form part of the routine examination of every patient. Except when the pupil is greatly contracted, it is usually possible to examine the optic disc; but to make a complete examination of the macular region and of the periphery of the retina, the pupil should previously be dilated with homatropine. The normal optic disc is circular and rosy pink in colour, though slightly paler than the surrounding retina. It possesses a well-defined edge and a depression—the physiological cup—from which the arteries and veins emerge. The normal appearance of the disc and its vessels can be learned only from experience. The following are the most important abnormalities. The disc may be pinker than normal, from hyperaemia, or abnormally pale from optic atrophy. Its edge may be indistinct. The physiological cup may be filled or the disc may be actually swollen above the level of the surrounding retina, the swelling being measured in dioptres. The veins of the disc may be congested, the arteries may be thickened and tortuous, or both arteries and veins may be abnormally fine and narrow. Pulsation of the arteries is abnormal, but pulsation of the veins is sometimes seen in normal individuals. Finally, the disc and surrounding area of the retina may be the site of exudate or haemorrhages.

The macular region is situated about two disc-breadths horizontally outwards from the outer edge of the disc. It is somewhat darker than the rest of the fundus and is almost devoid of blood vessels. The principal abnormalities to be found in the macula are an extension of oedema from the optic disc—the macular 'fan'—and a stippled, star-shaped, or haemorrhagic exudate in cases of hypertensive retinopathy. A cherry-red spot is seen at the macula in cases of obstruction of the central artery of the retina and in the infantile form of cerebromacular degeneration, and pigmentation is seen in the late infantile and juvenile forms of this disease. Since the macula is the most sensitive part of the retina and is concerned in central vision, macular lesions cause great impairment of visual acuity.

Finally the whole of the periphery of the retina should be inspected. The condition of the arteries and the veins should be noted. Retinal arteriosclerosis first manifests itself in displacement of the veins at the point where they are crossed by the arteries, with congestion of the portion distal to the crossing. Greater degrees of arterial thickening lead to tortuosity and irregularity of the arteries, with an increased light refraction from their surface—silver-wire arteries. In retinal arteriosclerosis and hypertensive retinopathy haemorrhages and exudate may be seen in the peripheral parts of the retina. Black pigmentation is characteristic of the various forms of choroidoretinitis. A retinal angioblastoma may sometimes be seen in cases of Lindau's disease and a phakoma in tuberous sclerosis, and in cases of general miliary tuberculosis and tuberculous meningitis tubercles may be seen in the retina as roundish, yellow bodies about half the size of the disc.

LESIONS OF THE OPTIC NERVE

PAPILLOEDEMA (CHOKED DISC)

By papilloedema is meant simply an oedema of the optic papilla or disc, without reference to its underlying cause. Like oedema in other parts of the body, papilloedema may be due to different pathological states, of which the following are the most important:

1. Increased intracranial pressure.
2. Inflammatory conditions of the optic nerve, optic neuritis, and retrobulbar neuritis.
3. Oedema associated with disease of the retinal arteries and retinal exudation, as in malignant hypertension and giant-cell arteritis.
4. Venous obstruction, due to neoplasms and gumma of the orbit, thrombosis of the central vein of the retina, some cases of cavernous sinus thrombosis, traumatic arteriovenous aneurysm of the internal carotid artery and the cavernous sinus, intrathoracic venous obstruction, as by neoplasms, aneurysm of the aorta.
5. In conditions associated with a massive increase in the protein content of the cerebrospinal fluid (e.g. some cases of the Guillain-Barré syndrome).
6. Changes in the composition of the blood, as in severe anaemia, erythraemia, and severe emphysema.
7. Obscure causes. Disseminated lupus erythematosus, carcinomatous neuropathy, the reticuloses, and infective endocarditis.

For the study of nervous diseases the papilloedema due to increased intracranial pressure and that associated with optic and retrobulbar neuritis are the forms of greatest importance.

Papilloedema due to Increased Intracranial Pressure

The optic nerve, which developmentally and histologically is part of the brain, is surrounded like the brain by the three meninges. Immediately covering the nerve is the pia mater and superficially to that the arachnoid, both of which are prolonged forwards to fuse with the sclerotic. Outside both is the dura mater, which is continuous anteriorly with the periosteum of the orbit. The optic nerve, therefore, is surrounded by a subarachnoid space which is continuous with the cerebral subarachnoid space. A rise in the pressure in the cerebrospinal subarachnoid space is freely conducted to the optic subarachnoid space, where it has a double effect, causing compression of the central vein of the retina where it crosses the space, and impeding lymphatic drainage from the retina and optic nerve (Paton and Holmes, 1910). The result of this combined venous and lymphatic obstruction is congestion and oedema of the optic disc and retina.

This question has recently been discussed by Behrman (1966), who has also drawn attention to the production of papilloedema by general brain swelling conducted to the optic nerves. The following are the principal causes of increased intracranial pressure leading to papilloedema:

Intracranial Tumour. Not all intracranial tumours cause papilloedema. The presence or absence of this symptom and its severity when present may, therefore, be an aid to the localization of a tumour. Generally speaking, the occurrence of papilloedema depends upon whether the tumour is so placed as to cause a rise in the tension of the cerebrospinal fluid, and also upon its rate of growth. It is almost constantly present in the case of tumours occupying the temporal lobe, the cerebellum, and the fourth ventricle, but is absent in about half the cases of subcortical and pontine tumours. It is frequently late in developing when the tumour is in the prefrontal region or arises near the vertex. Cerebellar tumours give rise to papilloedema of the greatest severity. The more rapidly a tumour grows the more likely is it to cause papilloedema. I have known papilloedema absent in patients with a very large but slowly growing angio-blastomatous cyst of the cerebellum. Inequality of the degree of oedema in the two eyes is not uncommon, but if the difference is not great it is of no localizing value. A tumour arising near one optic foramen tends to prevent the development of papilloedema in that eye by cutting off the optic sheath from communication with the cerebral subarachnoid space. In such cases primary optic atrophy may develop on the side of the tumour and may be associated with papilloedema on the opposite side (syndrome of Gowers, Paton, and Foster Kennedy).

Cerebral Abscess. Papilloedema is inconstant in cerebral abscess and may be late in developing.

Hydrocephalus. Hydrocephalus from any cause may lead to papilloedema, but in some cases the pressure of the distended floor of the third ventricle upon the optic chiasma and nerves causes primary optic atrophy.

Meningitis. Meningitis causes papilloedema less frequently than might be expected in view of the rise in pressure of the cerebrospinal fluid, which occurs in this condition, possibly because meningeal adhesions tend to wall off the optic sheaths. Papilloedema is often absent in tuberculous meningitis and is most frequent in meningitis of long duration. In any form of meningitis the infecting organism may penetrate the optic nerve, causing optic neuritis.

Intracranial Sinus Thrombosis. This leads to an increase in the pressure of the cerebrospinal fluid by diminishing its paths of absorption into the intracranial venous system.

Subarachnoid Haemorrhage. Haemorrhage into the subarachnoid space may cause papilloedema, the blood being driven into, and distending, the subarach-noid space of the optic sheaths. The commonest cause of this condition is leakage from an intracranial aneurysm.

Some Unusual Causes. Rarely emphysema leads to papilloedema by raising the pressure of the cerebrospinal fluid, so may hypervitaminosis A, and tetany due to hypoparathyroidism. The cause of benign intracranial hypertension is unknown.

Ophthalmoscopic Appearances of Papilloedema

In the earliest stage of papilloedema the retinal veins appear congested and the optic disc is pinker than normal. The disc edge appears blurred at its upper and lower margins, and this blurring extends to the nasal side before the temporal. An increase in the oedema causes filling of the physiological cup, and later the nerve head becomes elevated above the general retinal level, sometimes by as much as 8 or even 10 dioptres. The oedema in severe cases spreads into the retina causing a macular 'fan'. Distension of the retinal veins is extreme, and haemorrhages may be found on the retina and on the disc itself. If the intra-cranial pressure does not subside, the condition progresses to optic atrophy. The swelling of the disc diminishes, and it becomes paler. The arteries become constricted and the perivascular lymph spaces thickened. Finally, in a typical case, the disc is pale and flat, the physiological cup remaining filled, and the edges of the disc being less distinct than formerly. The arteries are constricted, but the veins often remain congested for a considerable time—secondary optic atrophy.

The Visual Fields in Papilloedema

In the earlier stages of papilloedema the only change in the visual fields may be enlargement of the blind spots. Later concentric constriction of the fields sets in, with a diminution in the visual acuity of the remainder, terminating ultimately in blindness. It should be noted that papilloedema may be associated with other changes in the visual fields due to lesions involving other parts of the visual fibres.

OPTIC NEURITIS AND RETROBULBAR NEURITIS

The term 'optic neuritis' used to be employed for all conditions associated with oedema of the optic disc, so that 'optic neuritis' was described as a symptom of intracranial tumour. Since neuritis implies inflammation this was a misnomer, and the name is now confined to infective or toxi-infective conditions of the optic nerve. The distinction between optic neuritis and retrobulbar neuritis is based upon an ophthalmoscopic rather than a pathological difference, and is apt to be misleading. If a neuritis of the optic nerve is sufficiently anterior to cause oedema of the disc it is described as optic neuritis or papillitis; if it is more posteriorly situated so that the direct effects of the inflammation are not visible ophthalmoscopically it is called retrobulbar neuritis. This accident of localization is in many cases of no pathological import.

Causes of Optic and Retrobulbar Neuritis

The causes of optic and retrobulbar neuritis are few.

Multiple Sclerosis. This must be placed first in frequency, and most cases are undoubtedly due to this disease. The optic nerve lesion, which is usually but not always unilateral, may be the first symptom and precede other manifestations by many years. In other cases other signs may have preceded it and may be found on routine examination of the nervous system, for example, nystagmus, intention tremor, diminution or absence of the abdominal reflexes, and extensor plantar responses. Examination of the cerebrospinal fluid may show abnormalities suggestive of multiple sclerosis, especially an abnormal γ-globulin or colloidal gold curve. The changes in the optic nerve are the same as those of multiple sclerosis elsewhere in the nervous system, namely, demyelination of the nerve fibres, with inflammatory exudation and, later, gliosis. Vision is hardly ever permanently lost as a result of this disease.

Disseminated Myelitis with Optic Neuritis (Devic's Disease or Neuro-myelitis Optica). This is a rare disease, closely allied to multiple sclerosis, both clinically and pathologically. Bilateral optic or retrobulbar neuritis is associated with transverse myelitis. Acute bilateral retrobulbar neuritis occurring without other lesions of the nervous system is probably a closely related disorder, but it sometimes occurs also in diffuse sclerosis and in multiple sclerosis.

Syphilis. A syphilitic lesion of the optic nerve, with the characteristic endarteritis, is a rare cause of retrobulbar neuritis. Diagnosis with the aid of serological tests is usually easy.

Zoster. Optic neuritis, going on to atrophy, with complete loss of vision, has been described in ophthalmic herpes zoster.

Orbital Infections. The optic nerve may be involved in inflammation spreading directly from the orbit, where it may be secondary to infection of the nasal air sinuses or dental abscess.

Meningitis and Encephalitis. As we have seen, infection may spread into the nerve from the meninges in any form of meningitis, and optic neuritis sometimes occurs in acute disseminated encephalomyelitis and in Schilder's disease.

Vitamin Deficiency. Bilateral retrobulbar neuritis followed by optic atrophy has been attributed to vitamin B deficiency (Moore, 1937; Spillane and Scott, 1945). Retrobulbar neuritis in pernicious anaemia has been attributed to a combination of vitamin B_{12} deficiency and tobacco amblyopia (Freeman and Heaton, 1961).

Toxic Causes. No hard-and-fast line can be drawn between retrobulbar neuritis and toxic optic atrophy [see p. 149].

Clinical Features of Optic and Retrobulbar Neuritis

Acute inflammation of the optic nerve leads to pain in and behind the eye on ocular movement and on pressure. If the inflammation extends to the optic disc it causes papillitis, with the appearances of papilloedema, though the swelling of the disc is usually slight, and haemorrhages are uncommon. When the inflammation is confined to the retrobulbar portion of the nerve the disc appears normal until signs of atrophy appear. This occurs in most cases, and is indicated by pallor of the disc, involving, in mild cases the temporal fibres, in severe cases the whole disc. Even after papillitis the physiological cup is usually restored and the disc edge and vessels appear normal.

In inflammation of the optic nerve the macular fibres suffer most, either because the central part of the nerve is most involved or because, being the most highly evolved part of the visual afferent system, they are the most susceptible to damage. In consequence the characteristic visual field defect is a central scotoma, the loss for red and green objects being greater than that for white. In most cases improvement occurs in a few weeks, but the functional manifestation of the residual atrophy is often a central scotoma, much smaller than that of the acute phase. Helpful points of distinction between optic neuritis with papillitis, and papilloedema due to increased intracranial pressure, are that in the former the swelling of the disc is slight in comparison with the loss of vision, in the latter the reverse is usually the case; and in optic neuritis the usual field defect is a central scotoma, in papilloedema a peripheral concentric constriction.

OPTIC ATROPHY

'Primary' and 'Secondary' Optic Atrophy

As the foregoing sections of this chapter show, optic atrophy may follow a variety of pathological states, and other causes have yet to be mentioned. When the pathological causes of optic atrophy were less understood a confusing distinction was drawn between 'primary' and 'secondary' optic atrophy. This is purely an ophthalmoscopic distinction, 'secondary' optic atrophy being the term used when atrophy follows some observable change in the optic disc which influences the appearance of the atrophied nerve, and 'primary' atrophy when no such cause is ophthalmoscopically obvious. We now recognize that even the 'primary' atrophies are secondary to some pathological state such as pressure upon or poisoning of the optic nerve. The term 'consecutive' optic atrophy is sometimes used when the atrophy is consecutive upon retinal lesions.

Causes of Optic Atrophy

Familial Disorders. In these obscure diseases the optic atrophy is probably due to a primary degeneration which affects various parts of the nervous system including the retinae and optic nerves.

1. *Cerebromacular Degeneration.* This infantile form, amaurotic family idiocy or Tay-Sachs disease [see p. 568], is characterized by a lipoid degeneration of the ganglion cells of the retina, atrophy of which at the macula is responsible for the cherry-red spot.

In the late infantile and juvenile forms (Batten-Mayou type) the cherry-red spot is absent, but the macula may be pigmented. Macular degeneration may occur also at puberty or early in adult life as an inherited disorder (Behr).

2. *The Hereditary Ataxias* [see p. 586]. In this group of closely related disorders there is degeneration of various parts of the nervous system, especially of the cerebellum and its tracts. Any form of hereditary ataxia may be associated with optic atrophy.

3. *Retinitis Pigmentosa.* This is an hereditary disease which is inherited in some sibships as a Mendelian dominant, less often as a recessive. It is often associated with nerve deafness and with a family history of epilepsy. There is a characteristic spidery black pigmentation of the periphery of the retina, and the optic disc exhibits a yellowish waxy pallor and much reduction in the calibre of the vessels. The victims of this disease suffer from night-blindness and progressive concentric constriction of the visual fields.

Retinitis pigmentosa is also a feature of the Laurence–Moon–Biedl syndrome.

4. *Leber's Hereditary Optic Atrophy.* This is a rare hereditary disease which affects young males (Francois, 1961). There is a sudden onset of bilateral visual impairment, usually between the ages of 15 and 30. The fields of vision show central scotomas. Papillitis may be present in the acute stage: later the discs are atrophic. Improvement occurs in less than one-third of those attacked, and complete recovery is rare. The optic nerve lesions are now known to be part of a more general disorder.

5. *Congenital Optic Atrophy.* This may be hereditary (Thompson and Cashell, 1934–5) or an element in congenital diplegia.

Consecutive Optic Atrophy. In this group the cause of the optic atrophy is obvious on retinoscopy. It includes the various forms of retinitis and choroidoretinitis and vascular lesions of the retina, especially obstruction of the central artery.

Secondary Optic Atrophy following Papilloedema. Optic atrophy following papilloedema has been described in a previous section of this chapter [see p. 146].

Optic Atrophy following Acute Optic and Retrobulbar Neuritis. The causes of this are discussed on page 146.

Syphilitic Optic Atrophy. Syphilis used to be the cause in 40 per cent. of all cases of primary optic atrophy, but this is no longer true in Great Britain. Optic atrophy occurs in 10 to 15 per cent. of cases of tabes and 50 per cent. of cases of congenital tabes and congenital general paresis, but is rare in acquired general paresis unless tabes is present also. Both eyes are affected, but not always equally at first. The lesion begins in the marginal fibres of the optic nerve, distal to the chiasma. Some workers think that the primary change is an inflammation of the pial sheath of the optic nerves and that the myelin sheaths suffer before the axis cylinders (Stargadt, Behr). Others believe, however, that there is some primary degeneration of the nerve fibres. Optochiasmatic arachnoiditis is not the cause (Bruetsch, 1948).

Paton distinguishes two types: a parenchymatous degeneration with slow onset, losses in the peripheral fields and maintenance of good central visual acuity for a long period, and an interstitial lesion with fairly rapid loss of central vision and little involvement of the peripheral fields for white. The disc is grey or white, often with a bluish tint. The physiological cup is preserved; the stippling of the lamina cribrosa is visible. The disc edge and vessels are normal.

Secondary optic atrophy occurs in syphilis after papilloedema, when, as occasionally happens, this is caused by the meningovascular form of the infection.

For the prognosis and treatment of syphilitic optic atrophy see pages 426, 431.

Toxic Optic Atrophy. The optic nerve fibres are susceptible to a number of poisons, though their mode and site of action are little understood. Among these are tobacco, lead, arsenic (especially tryparsamide), methyl mercuric iodide, toxic substances associated with methyl alcohol, carbon bisulphide, thallium, certain insecticides [see p. 810], quinine, and aspidium filix mas. It is uncertain whether tobacco, methyl alcohol, and carbon bisulphide cause degeneration of the retinal ganglion cells or act on the nerve fibres. Tobacco appears to act through its content of cyanide which may produce conditioned vitamin B_{12} deficiency. The optic atrophy which rarely results from isoniazid administration is probably due to vitamin B_6 deficiency while the retinopathy resulting from sensitivity to chloroquine may be accompanied by pallor of the optic discs. Quinine and aspidium filix mas are said to produce spasm of the retinal arteries and hence retinal atrophy. Any severe anaemia, especially that following severe internal haemorrhage, may cause optic atrophy, probably by causing the death of the ganglion cells. So, too, may diabetes. Chronic alcoholism is sometimes a cause,

Pressure. Pressure is a common and important cause. In the eye itself it is produced by glaucoma. It may occur in the optic canal, if this is narrowed by bony overgrowth, as in Paget's osteitis, or if a tumour arises from the optic nerve or its sheath, or even as the result of a thickened ophthalmic artery. Behind the foramen the commonest cause of pressure is a tumour, either of the hypophysis, or of the craniopharyngeal pouch, or a meningioma arising above the sella turcica or in the olfactory groove, or a glioma of the optic chiasma, of the frontal lobe, or of the tip of the temporal lobe. Pressure may also arise from localized arachnoiditis of the optic chiasma, the distended floor of the third ventricle in obstructive hydrocephalus, from an intracranial aneurysm, or from arteriosclerotic internal carotid arteries. In the diagnosis of pressure upon the optic nerve the radiography of the optic canals is often of value.

Trauma. Primary optic atrophy may occur after head injury, usually in only one eye. The lesion is the immediate result of the blow, and since there is often no radiographic evidence of fracture it is probably caused by rupture of vessels. The eye may be completely blind, or there may be a localized visual field defect, usually temporal.

Visual Fields in Optic Atrophy

No generalization can be made about the visual fields in optic atrophy, since they depend entirely upon the cause. After papilloedema there are usually enlargement of the blind spot and peripheral concentric constriction. Retrobulbar neuritis and the toxic amblyopias are usually associated with central scotomas, but in poisoning with quinine and aspidium filix mas the peripheral part of the fields suffers more than the central. In tobacco amblyopia the scotoma is centrocaecal. Pressure lesions may produce central scotoma or other partial field defects. It must be remembered, too, that optic atrophy following both papilloedema and pressure upon the optic nerve may indirectly be due to an intracranial lesion which involves the visual fibres more posteriorly also, and itself causes visual field defects.

Prognosis of Optic Nerve Lesions

The prognosis of lesions of the optic nerve depends chiefly upon the extent to which the cause can be removed. When papilloedema is due to increased intracranial pressure, relief of this is usually followed by marked improvement in vision, provided optic atrophy has not already developed. Similarly, great improvement in vision often follows quite rapidly the removal of direct pressure upon the optic nerve. A considerable degree of recovery can usually be expected in optic neuritis and retrobulbar neuritis due to multiple sclerosis, and also in sporadic cases of acute bilateral optic and retrobulbar neuritis, though occasionally vision is permanently lost in this condition. The outlook is less satisfactory in optic atrophy of toxic origin, though some improvement may occur if exposure to the toxin can be terminated; recovery from tobacco amblyopia is usually satisfactory. Tabetic optic atrophy, when severe enough to cause visual impairment, often progresses in spite of all treatment.

Treatment of Optic Nerve Lesions

The treatment of lesions of the optic nerve is primarily that of the causal disorder. Corticosteroids have proved to be of value for acute optic and retrobulbar neuritis in some cases.

REFERENCES

ADIE, W. J. (1932) The aetiology and symptomatology of disseminated sclerosis, *Brit. med. J.*, **2**, 997.

BEHRMAN, S. (1966) Pathology of papilloedema, *Brain*, **89**, 1.

BELL, J. (1931) Hereditary optic atrophy (Leber's disease), *Treasury of Human Inheritance*, vol. ii, part iv, Cambridge.

BRUETSCH, W. L. (1948) Surgical treatment of syphilitic primary atrophy of the optic nerves (syphilitic optochiasmatic arachnoiditis), *Arch. Ophthal. (Chicago)*, **38**, 735.

DUPUY-DUTEMPS, L. (1930) Stase papillaire. Critique des théories par oedème propagé ou par rétention lymphatique, *Ann. Oculist. (Paris)*, **167**, 134.

FERGUSON, F. R., and CRITCHLEY, M. (1928–9) Leber's optic atrophy and its relationship with the heredo-familial ataxias, *J. Neurol. Psychopath.*, **9**, 120.

FRANCOIS, J. (1961) *Heredity in Ophthalmology*, p. 500, St. Louis.

FREEMAN, A. G., and HEATON, J. M. (1961) The aetiology of retrobulbar neuritis in Addisonian pernicious anaemia. *Lancet*, i, 908.

GREENFIELD, J. G., and EPSTEIN, S. H. (1937) A case of syphilitic optic atrophy with hemianopic field defect in less affected eye, *Trans. ophthal. Soc. U.K.*, **57**, 127.

MOORE, D. F. (1937) Nutritional retrobulbar neuritis, followed by partial optic atrophy, *Lancet*, i, 1225.

MOORE, J. E. (1932) The syphilitic optic atrophies, *Medicine (Baltimore)*, **11**, 263.

PATON, L. (1909) A clinical study of optic neuritis in its relationship to intracranial tumours, *Brain*, **32**, 65.

PATON, L. (1930–1) Classification of the optic atrophies, *Proc. roy. Soc. Med.*, **24**, 25.

PATON, L., and HOLMES, G. (1910–11) The pathology of papilloedema: a histological study of sixty eyes, *Brain*, **33**, 389.

SPILLANE, J. D., and SCOTT, G. I. (1945) Obscure neuropathy in the Middle East, *Lancet*, ii, 261.

THOMPSON, A. H., and CASHELL, G. T. W. (1934–5) A pedigree of congenital optic atrophy embracing sixteen affected cases in six generations, *Proc. roy. Soc. Med.*, **28**, 1415.

TRAQUAIR, H. M. (1938) *An Introduction to Clinical Perimetry*, 3rd ed., London.

THE THIRD, FOURTH, AND SIXTH NERVES

THIRD-NERVE PARALYSIS

After leaving the nucleus [see p. 78] the fibres of the third nerve sweep outwards and forwards through the medial longitudinal fasciculus, the red nucleus, and the medial margin of the substantia nigra to emerge from the brain stem along the bottom of the sulcus oculomotorius on the medial aspect of the crus cerebri [FIG. 5, p. 20]. The nerve passes forwards between the posterior cerebral and superior cerebellar arteries, close to the posterior communicating artery, and pierces the dura mater beside the posterior clinoid process in a small triangular space between the free and attached borders of the tentorium cerebelli. It then passes through the lateral wall of the cavernous sinus, where it lies close to the fourth, sixth, and first division of the fifth nerves, and enters the orbit through the superior orbital fissure between the two heads of the lateral rectus muscle. Here it divides into two branches, the upper supplying the levator palpebrae and the superior rectus, and the lower the medial and inferior recti and the inferior oblique, the nerve to which supplies the short root to the ciliary ganglion.

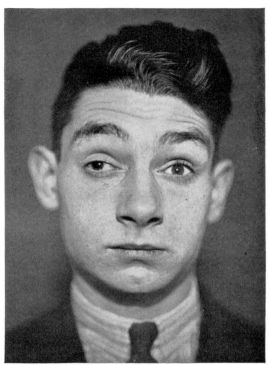

FIG. 20. Recovering third-nerve palsy on right side in a case of ophthalmoplegic migraine. (Note the ptosis, dilated pupil, and abduction of the eye due to un-opposed action of the lateral rectus, and the over-action of the frontal belly of the occipitofrontalis muscle.)

Paralysis of the third nerve causes ptosis, complete internal ophthalmoplegia, and paralysis of the superior, medial, and inferior recti, and inferior oblique. The pupil is widely dilated owing to paralysis of the sphincter pupillae and the unantagonized action of the dilator, and fails to react. Accommodation is paralysed. The unantagonized lateral rectus causes outward deviation of the eye, and the only possible ocular movements are abduction, carried out by the lateral rectus, and a movement of depression, internal rotation, and abduction by the superior oblique. Paralysis of the levator palpebrae superioris causes ptosis of the upper lid, and the resulting closure of the eye masks the diplopia, which becomes evident to the patient when the lid is passively raised [FIG. 20].

Although lesions of the third nerve usually cause both external and internal ophthalmoplegia, it may happen that in a partial lesion the iridoconstrictor fibres escape, or that in recovery from a complete lesion the intrinsic fibres may recover before the extrinsic. When both the third nerve and the ocular sympathetic are injured, as may happen with a lesion just behind the orbit, the pupil is not dilated.

FOURTH-NERVE PARALYSIS

The fibres of the fourth nerve after leaving the nucleus turn backwards through the peri-aqueductal grey matter on the medial aspect of the mesencephalic root of the trigeminal nerve, and then downwards and medially to decussate in the anterior medullary velum, whence the nerve emerges just behind the colliculi. It then passes round the cerebral peduncle, lying between the peduncle and the temporal lobe, and pierces the free border of the tentorium cerebelli lateral to the third nerve to enter the lateral wall of the cavernous sinus. It enters the orbit through the superior orbital fissure above the ocular muscles and terminates in the superior oblique. A lesion of the fourth nerve causes paralysis of this muscle with weakness of movement of the eye downwards and outwards. For the character of the resulting diplopia, see page 78. When the lesion involves the nucleus or the fibres of the nerve within the midbrain before their decussation in the anterior medullary velum, the paralysis of the superior oblique is on the opposite side to the lesion. When the nerve is damaged in its extracerebral course the paralysis is ipsilateral.

SIXTH-NERVE PARALYSIS

The fibres of the sixth nerve, after leaving the nucleus just below the floor of the fourth ventricle, pass forwards through the pons to emerge at its inferior border above the lateral side of the pyramid of the medulla. It has a long extracerebral course along the base of the brain before it pierces the dura mater of the posterior fossa, just below the dorsum sellae. Like the third and fourth nerves, it lies in the lateral wall of the cavernous sinus, whence it passes through the superior orbital fissure to terminate in the lateral rectus muscle. A lesion of the sixth nerve causes paralysis of this muscle with loss of abduction of the eye, which is deviated inwards by the unantagonized medial rectus [FIG. 21]. For the character of the resulting diplopia, see page 78.

CAUSES OF PARALYSIS OF THE THIRD, FOURTH, AND SIXTH NERVES

The third, fourth, and sixth nerves may be damaged singly or together, and on one or both sides.

Within the brain stem their nuclei or intracerebral fibres may be damaged by trauma, neoplasms, vascular lesions, encephalitis, or multiple sclerosis, and in the case of the sixth nerve, syringobulbia. Congenital aplasia of the nuclei may cause bilateral ptosis, absence of elevation of the eyes, or lateral rectus paralysis with or without facial paralysis (Moebius syndrome).

Intracranial tumour may cause direct compression of the nerves at any point in their course, but, in addition,

Increased intracranial pressure due to intracranial tumour or abscess remote from the nerves, or to hydrocephalus, may indirectly impair their conductivity. The sixth nerve most often suffers in this way, and sixth-nerve paralysis may occur with a tumour in any situation. Supratentorial tumours probably cause this by displacing the brain stem downwards and so stretching the nerve. The third nerve may also suffer, especially with tumours of the temporal lobe. In such cases the third nerve is compressed as it tracks across the free edge of the tentorium cerebelli and a partial or complete third-nerve palsy is an important warning sign of herniation of the temporal lobe through the tentorial hiatus;

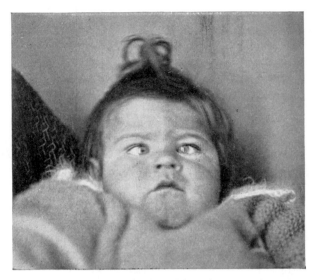

FIG. 21. Congenital bilateral lateral rectus palsies

a fixed dilated pupil may be an important early sign of this phenomenon. The fourth nerve escapes.

Neoplastic infiltration of the meninges may compress the nerves in their passage across the base of the skull and through the dura mater. Such meningeal metastases may be derived from a primary glioma in the brain, which is rare, or by extension of a primary growth of the nasopharynx, or by metastasis from a tumour elsewhere, e.g. in the lung, breast, stomach, or prostate.

Intracranial aneurysm, especially when arising near the circle of Willis, may directly compress one or more of the oculomotor nerves, especially the third nerve, or they may be subjected to pressure by extravasated blood or clot after rupture of the aneurysmal sac. Compression may arise from a vessel which is congenitally abnormal in position (Sunderland, 1948).

Ophthalmoplegic migraine is the term applied to cases of recurrent ocular palsy, the onset of which is associated with severe headache, and which tend to recover in the course of days or weeks, only to relapse subsequently, finally becoming permanent. The third, fourth, or sixth nerve may be involved. The relationship of this condition to true migraine is doubtful [see p. 274].

Syphilis is a cause of ocular palsies through implication of the nerves in syphilitic meningitis and is a common cause of a painless third-nerve palsy.

In *meningitis*, either pyogenic or tuberculous, both infection and compression of the nerves may occur. Extension of infection from the middle ear to the inferior petrosal sinus is responsible for sixth-nerve paralysis, with or without trigeminal neuritis, occasionally associated with mastoiditis—Gradenigo's syndrome. The basal meninges and cranial nerves may be more extensively involved in a spread of infection from osteitis of the bones of the base of the skull.

In *encephalitis* and *multiple sclerosis* the inflammatory process may occasionally involve the oculomotor nerves, and the sixth nerve may suffer in poliomyelitis, which may be the cause of some cases of lateral rectus palsy of sudden but unexplained onset in children.

Polyneuritis. The cranial nerves, including those supplying the ocular muscles, may be the site of polyneuritis, either with or without polyneuritis involving the limbs, *polyneuritis cranialis*. The sixth nerve is occasionally paralysed in diphtheria.

'*Rheumatic*' *neuritis* is a term which has been applied to certain ocular palsies of unexplained pathology which seem akin to Bell's palsy of the facial muscles. The paralysis, which usually involves the lateral rectus, often recovers completely.

Vascular lesions of the oculomotor nerves are not uncommon in elderly patients, especially those with high blood pressure. Either the third, fourth, or sixth may be involved. The lesion may be either haemorrhage or infarction, and complete recovery of function in two or three months is the rule.

Diabetic ocular palsies are probably of the same nature.

Within the *cavernous sinus* the oculomotor nerves may be paralysed as a result of thrombophlebitis of the sinus, or of the pressure or rupture of an aneurysm of the internal carotid artery.

Paralysis of one of the oculomotor nerves, usually the sixth, occasionally follows the administration of a *spinal anaesthetic*. Its precise cause is unknown. Recovery occurs in a few weeks.

Ophthalmoplegia has been attributed to *orbital periostitis* especially in the superior orbital fissure, but in some cases so described in the past the cause has probably been a retro-orbital aneurysm or a *parasellar meningioma*. An intra-orbital cause of ophthalmoplegia is the invasion of the orbit by *carcinoma arising in a nasal sinus*. The onset is gradual and steadily progressive, there is much pain, and proptosis usually develops. A similar clinical picture may result from a non-malignant *mucocele* of the *ethmoid* sinus, but this is usually painless.

Finally *head injury* may damage the third, fourth, or sixth nerve.

TREATMENT OF LESIONS OF THE OCULOMOTOR NERVES

Treatment is primarily that of the causal condition. When diplopia is present the patient should wear a shade or a frosted glass in front of one eye for the relief of discomfort and vertigo. Orthoptic exercises are helpful and it is sometimes possible to diminish diplopia by the use of a prism. During the acute stage of periostitis of the superior orbital fissure analgesics will be required and recent evidence suggests that corticosteroid drugs are indicated.

REFERENCES

CAIRNS, H. (1938) Peripheral ocular palsies from the neuro-surgical point of view, *Trans. ophthal. Soc. U.K.*, **58**, 464.

CHAVASSE, F. B. (1938) The ocular palsies. Some clinical sequels of ocular palsy, *Trans. ophthal. Soc. U.K.*, **58**, 483.

COGAN, D. G. (1956) *Neurology of the Ocular Muscles*, 2nd ed., Springfield, Ill.

LYLE, T. K., and JACKSON, S. (1949) *Practical Orthoptics in the Treatment of Squint*, 3rd ed., London.

SUNDERLAND, S. (1948) Neurovascular relations and anomalies at the base of the brain, *J. Neurol. Neurosurg. Psychiat.*, **11**, 243.

THE FIFTH OR TRIGEMINAL NERVE

PERIPHERAL DISTRIBUTION

The fifth nerve contains both motor and sensory fibres. It is the principal sensory cranial nerve and represents a fusion of the sensory nerves of a number of metameric segments. It arises from the inferior surface of the pons on its lateral aspect by two roots, a large sensory root and a small motor root. The two roots pass forwards in the posterior fossa and, piercing the dura mater beneath the attachment of the tentorium to the tip of the petrous part of the temporal bone, enter a cavity in the dura mater overlying the apex of the petrous bone. Here the sensory root expands to form the trigeminal ganglion, which contains the ganglion cells of the sensory fibres and is homologous with the dorsal root ganglia of the spinal nerves. The ganglion gives rise to three large nerve trunks, which constitute the three divisions of the trigeminal nerve, namely the ophthalmic or first division, the maxillary or second, and the mandibular or third [FIG. 22]. The motor root of the nerve passes forwards beneath the ganglion and becomes fused with the third division.

THE OPHTHALMIC NERVE

The ophthalmic nerve, after lying in the lateral wall of the cavernous sinus together with the third, fourth, and sixth nerves, enters the orbit through the superior orbital fissure. It supplies the skin of the face and scalp, as follows: a narrow zone adjacent to the midline throughout the length of the nose; the upper eyelid and the scalp from the base of the nose and the eyelid as far back as the lambdoidal suture in the midline and for about 3 inches laterally to this. The first division also supplies sensory fibres to the eye, including the conjunctiva and the cornea, to the iris, and to the mucous membrane of the frontal sinuses and the upper part of the nose. It is uncertain whether secretory fibres to the lacrimal gland are derived from the fifth nerve or from the geniculate ganglion of the facial nerve, reaching the gland by the greater petrosal, the pterygopalatine ganglion, the second division of the trigeminal and the anastomosis between the temporomalar and the lacrimal nerves.

THE MAXILLARY NERVE

The maxillary nerve after leaving the trigeminal ganglion passes through the foramen rotundum into the pterygopalatine fossa. It enters the orbit as the infra-orbital nerve through the inferior orbital fissure, and then passing through the infra-orbital canal reaches the face through the infra-orbital foramen. It supplies the skin of the upper lip as far as the midline and the skin of the cheek between the area on the nose supplied by the ophthalmic nerve and a line passing upwards and slightly outwards from the angle of the mouth, crossing the zygoma about midway between the outer canthus of the eye and the ear, and continuing

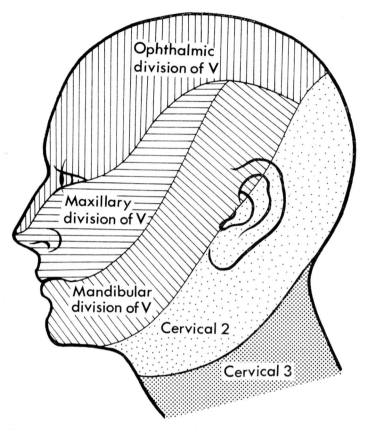

FIG. 22. Cutaneous distribution of the three divisions of the trigeminal nerve and the second cervical spinal segment

upwards to join the lateral boundary of the area of supply of the first division on the scalp, about the middle of the temporal ridge. The maxillary division also supplies the mucous membrane of the maxillary sinus and of the lower part of the nose, together with the mucous membrane of the upper lip, the hard palate, and the soft palate, except its posterior aspect, together with the teeth of the upper jaw.

THE MANDIBULAR NERVE

The mandibular nerve is formed by a fusion of the third division of the trigeminal ganglion with the motor root. These two roots pass out of the skull by the foramen ovale and unite to form a single trunk in the infratemporal fossa.

The mandibular nerve supplies the skin of the lower lip and chin, together with a zone of the cheek about an inch wide laterally to the lateral boundary of the cutaneous supply of the maxillary nerve and bounded below by the border of the area supplied by the cervical plexus. Above this its distribution expands to include the tympanic membrane, and the external acoustic meatus and the skin of the temple, where its distribution is bounded anteriorly by the lateral border of the second division, above by the lateral border of the first division, and behind by a line drawn upwards from the external acoustic meatus to the vertex in the region of the lambdoidal suture. Anatomical and embryological evidence indicates supply of the tragus and upper part of the pinna by the auriculotemporal branch of the mandibular division. Clinical evidence suggests that there may be some variation in the precise distribution of this nerve and the possibility of overlap cannot be excluded. In addition to this cutaneous area the mandibular nerve supplies the mucous membrane of the cheek, lower jaw, floor of the mouth, and anterior two-thirds of the tongue, and the teeth of the lower jaw. From the chorda tympani taste fibres pass to the anterior two-thirds of the tongue by the lingual nerve, which is a branch of the mandibular nerve. Meningeal branches from the trigeminal nerve supply the dura mater of the greater part of the skull above the tentorium and of the tentorium itself.

The cervical plexus supplies a zone of the cheek about one inch wide overlying the angle of the jaw.

THE MOTOR ROOT

The motor root of the trigeminal nerve innervates the following muscles: the temporal, the masseter, the medial and lateral pterygoids, the anterior belly of the digastric and the mylohyoid muscle, the tensor tympani and the tensor veli palatini.

CENTRAL CONNEXIONS

The motor nucleus of the trigeminal nerve lies in the lateral part of the tegmental portion of the pons. The mesencephalic root is probably also motor. Incoming sensory fibres of the trigeminal divide, some passing into the principal sensory nucleus, which is situated in the substantia gelatinosa in the lateral part of the tegmentum of the pons, while others turn downwards to form the spinal tract which descends on the lateral side of the substantia gelatinosa. As the spinal tract passes downwards its fibres gradually terminate in the substantia gelatinosa which constitutes its terminal nucleus, the nucleus of the spinal tract. Both the spinal tract and its nucleus end in the upper part of the spinal cord about the level of the second spinal nerve. The sensory fibres entering the principal sensory nucleus are concerned with tactile and postural sensibility. From this nucleus relay fibres cross the midline and form the trigeminothalamic tract or trigeminal lemniscus at the inner end of the medial lemniscus. The descending fibres of the spinal tract are concerned with the appreciation of pain and thermal sensibility. Fibres from the ophthalmic division end in the lowest part of the spinal nucleus, fibres from the mandibular division in the highest part and those from the maxillary division intermediately. Relay fibres from this nucleus cross the midline and pass upwards in close relationship with the medial lemniscus to join the spinothalamic tract in the pons [see p. 46].

LESIONS OF THE TRIGEMINAL NERVE

PERIPHERAL LESIONS

The nerve may be involved between the pons and the trigeminal ganglion in inflammatory lesions such as syphilitic meningitis, or it may be compressed by a tumour or an aneurysm. This part of the nerve commonly undergoes degeneration in tabes. In the trigeminal ganglion it may be compressed by a tumour of the ganglion itself or of the hypophysis, or by a meningioma arising in its neighbourhood, or damaged by fracture of the base of the skull involving the middle fossa. With the sixth nerve it may be involved in inflammation spreading from the petrous bone in mastoiditis to the inferior petrosal sinus—Gradenigo's syndrome. Inflammation of the ganglion occurs in trigeminal herpes zoster. The peripheral branches of the nerve distal to the ganglion may be injured as a result of fracture of the bones of the face. Lesions of the nerve often cause pain, which is referred to the cutaneous area of its distribution, and may be associated with cutaneous anaesthesia and analgesia. When the nerve is involved between the pons and the ganglion, all three divisions are likely to be affected, but lesions involving the ganglion itself may lead to symptoms which are confined to one division, most frequently the first. Lesions of the motor root cause weakness and wasting of the muscles of mastication on the affected side. Wasting of the temporal muscle and of the masseter leads to hollowing above and below the zygoma, and, when the patient is made to clench his teeth, palpation reveals that contraction of these muscles is less vigorous than on the normal side. When the mouth is opened, the jaw deviates to the paralysed side as a result of the unantagonized action of the lateral pterygoid on the opposite side.

CENTRAL LESIONS

The central connexions of the trigeminal nerve may be involved in lesions, especially tumours, syringobulbia and vascular lesions, affecting the pons, medulla, and uppermost cervical segments of the spinal cord. The motor nucleus may be affected by a lesion in the lateral part of the tegmentum of the pons, in which case weakness of the muscles of mastication is usually associated with paresis of the lateral rectus and facial paresis on the affected side. Owing to the divergence of the sensory fibres of the trigeminal nerve within the brain stem, dissociation of sensibility over the face commonly results from central lesions. A lesion of the pons which involves the principal sensory nucleus will cause anaesthesia to light touch over the trigeminal distribution, with preservation of appreciation of pain, heat, and cold. On the other hand, lesions involving the medulla and the upper cervical segments of the spinal cord, by injuring the spinal tract and its nucleus, will cause analgesia and thermo-anaesthesia, with preservation of sensibility to light touch and sometimes severe and persistent spontaneous pain referred to the trigeminal area. This latter dissociation is characteristic of syringobulbia and of thrombosis of the posterior inferior cerebellar artery. Since the first division of the nerve is represented lowest and the third division highest in the nucleus of the spinal tract a lesion of the lowest part of the medulla will cause analgesia limited to the first and second divisions only. Syringobulbia, however, leads to a characteristic progressive advance of the border of the analgesia, which begins posteriorly and gradually converges upon the tip of the nose and the upper lip, these being usually the last places to lose painful sensibility.

A lesion of the pons may also cause analgesia and thermo-anaesthesia on the opposite side of the face through damage to the crossed trigeminothalamic tract.

NEUROPATHIC KERATITIS

Neuropathic keratitis is a degenerative lesion of the cornea which may follow a lesion of the fifth nerve in any part of its course, including the pons, provided corneal analgesia results. Neuropathic keratitis is most frequently seen as a sequel of alcoholic injection of the trigeminal ganglion for trigeminal neuralgia. It may also occur as a result of vascular lesions or of tumours involving the pons and medulla and of compression of the fifth nerve in its peripheral course by a tumour, or of extension of inflammation to it in syphilitic or pyogenic meningitis. In some cases it occurs in association with corneal analgesia for which no cause can be found. At the onset the whole corneal surface becomes faintly stippled and hazy and the cornea begins to lose its surface epithelium. Secondary infections may follow, resulting in more severe changes.

TRIGEMINAL NEURALGIA

Synonym. Tic douloureux.

Definition. A disorder characterized by paroxysmal brief attacks of severe pain within the distribution of one or more divisions of the trigeminal nerve usually without evidence of organic disease of the nerve.

AETIOLOGY AND PATHOLOGY

The cause of trigeminal neuralgia is obscure. Histological examination of the trigeminal ganglion has revealed no changes which can be held responsible. Kugelberg and Lindblom (1959) have brought forward evidence that 'the mechanism responsible for the paroxysmal pain is situated centrally, probably in the brain stem in structures related to the spinal V nucleus'. Females are affected more frequently than males in the proportion of three to two. Heredity plays a part in causation in some cases. In 2 per cent. of Harris's cases one of the patient's parents had been a sufferer.

Rarely trigeminal neuralgia is a symptom of organic nervous disease. Unilateral or bilateral trigeminal neuralgia associated with spastic paraplegia is a distinctive syndrome, which in some cases has been proved to be due to multiple sclerosis, and characteristic attacks rarely occur as a result of compression of the nerve by a tumour or in association with peroneal muscular atrophy, neurofibromatosis, facial hemiatrophy, facial myoclonus, or Paget's osteitis.

Trigeminal neuralgia may begin at any age, but it is rare before middle life and in most cases the onset occurs at about the age of 50, but may be as late as 70 or even later. Sometimes emotion, exposure to cold, or a blow on the face appears to precipitate the first attack.

SYMPTOMS

The characteristic feature of trigeminal neuralgia is the occurrence of brief, severe paroxysms of pain, which are usually for a long time confined to the distribution of one division of the nerve. The second and third divisions are the site of the pain with approximately equal frequency. The first division is rarely affected and then usually only after the second division has been involved. Whether the pain first involves the second or third division, it usually in the course of time spreads to the other of the two lower divisions. In a small proportion of cases it is bilateral, though rarely from the onset.

In an attack the pain is usually most intense in, and may be confined to, part of the region supplied by the affected division. Thus it may be most marked in the cheek, the upper jaw, the lower jaw, or the tongue. It tends to spread, however, through the rest of the divisional area. It is usually described as burning or stabbing. One of the most striking features of the attacks is that they tend to be precipitated by chill, by touching the face, as in washing, by talking, mastication, and swallowing. Many patients describe 'trigger zones', touching which will invariably excite an attack. The attacks are always brief and do not last longer than one or two minutes. The pain is very severe and during the attack the patient may be in agony. The pain often reflexly evokes spasm of the muscles of the face on the affected side, hence the term 'tic douloureux'. Flushing of the skin, lacrimation, and salivation may also occur.

In trigeminal neuralgia there is no reduction of sensibility over the distribution of the nerve. So-called trophic changes in the skin have been described, but it is probable that these are the result of the patient rubbing the face during the attack or of remedies which have been applied in his attempts to relieve the pain. The attacks may interfere with the taking of food, and the recurrence of severe pain over a long period tends to cause loss of weight and depression. Fortunately the attacks usually cease at night, though they sometimes awaken the patient from sleep. Long periods of freedom from pain, lasting weeks or months, are the rule in the early stages.

DIAGNOSIS

There is usually little difficulty in diagnosis if attention is paid to the cardinal symptoms, especially the paroxysmal character of the attacks with freedom from pain in the intervals, the factors which precipitate them, and the absence of signs of an organic lesion of the nerve. In the rare cases in which this syndrome is associated with organic disease, for example, multiple sclerosis or tumour of the eighth nerve, other signs of these disorders are usually present. It is important to distinguish trigeminal neuralgia from the pain due to a gross lesion of the nerve, especially compression by a tumour. In such cases the pain is more persistent and is usually associated with impairment of sensibility in the distribution of the nerve, and weakness of the muscles supplied by the nerve is often present. Trigeminal pain may follow lesions of the central connexions of the nerve within the brain stem, for example, thrombosis of the posterior inferior cerebellar artery. In such cases, however, other signs of a brain stem lesion are present. Post-herpetic pain of trigeminal distribution is distinguished by the history of the zoster eruption, which leaves characteristic residual cutaneous scars, by the persistence of the pain, and by the impairment of sensibility. Tabes dorsalis is an occasional cause of paroxysmal attacks of pain within the trigeminal area. The characteristic signs of tabes, however, render the diagnosis of the cause of the pain easy. Neuritis of branches of the trigeminal nerve, especially of the supra-orbital and of the auriculotemporal, causes pain within the distribution of the branch affected. In cases of neuritis there is a history of a recent acute onset; the attacks of pain tend to last for hours, with paroxysmal exacerbations; the affected nerve is tender on pressure; and there is often hyperalgesia, or more rarely relative analgesia, over the cutaneous area supplied by the nerve.

Referred pain is extremely common within the trigeminal distribution, and possible causes of this must always be excluded. Frontal sinusitis and infection of the maxillary sinus tend to cause pain which is referred to the areas of the first and second divisions respectively. In such cases there may be oedema of the tissues overlying the infected air sinus and in addition to tenderness of the supra-orbital and infra-orbital nerves the bone also is tender. Radiography of the sinuses, and examination of the nose may be necessary to establish the diagnosis. Diseases of the eye may cause severe referred pain, especially glaucoma, in which the pain is referred to the temple. Examination of the eye immediately reveals the cause of the trouble. The teeth are a common source of referred pain. In addition to dental caries, which is easily detected, pain may be due to a peri-apical abscess or to an unerupted tooth. In case of doubt, radiograms of the teeth should be taken. Pain may also be referred to the face from lesions of the heart and lungs.

Psychogenic pain in the face may lead to diagnostic difficulties. It fails to conform to the characters either of trigeminal neuralgia or of any form of pain due to an organic disease, signs of which are absent, nor does it respond to analgesic drugs, often not even to morphine. Other psychogenic symptoms may be present, and the patient's mental state usually affords a clue to the nature of the pain.

Migrainous neuralgia causes severe paroxysmal pain within the trigeminal distribution [p. 278], but is distinguished from trigeminal neuralgia by its periodicity, the absence of precipitating factors, and the much longer duration of each paroxysm.

PROGNOSIS

Spontaneous recovery from trigeminal neuralgia is extremely rare. The interval between the bouts of pain may be long, remissions lasting months or even years. As a rule, however, once the disorder is established attacks follow each other fairly frequently and the intervals between them tend to become shorter. Finally there may be many attacks during the day. Trigeminal neuralgia caused by multiple sclerosis may cease spontaneously, however.

TREATMENT

The first step in treatment is to eliminate as far as possible all sources of infection within the area of the trigeminal nerve. It must be confessed, however, that this usually fails to influence the course of the disorder and the wholesale extraction of sound teeth is quite unjustifiable. Medicinal treatment is often effective in controlling the pain and rendering life tolerable in the milder cases. It should, therefore, always be tried. The most effective drug is carbamazepine (*Tegretol*) in doses of 200 mg. three or four times daily depending upon tolerance

(Blom, 1962). Phenytoin sodium is sometimes helpful. Morphine should not be prescribed regularly in view of the risk of habit formation. An old remedy is the following:

Potassium bromide	. .	600 mg.
Tincture of gelsemium .	.	0·6 ml.
Phenazone	. . .	450 mg.
Water to 10 ml., thrice daily.		

If the pain cannot be controlled by medicinal measures, it will become necessary to interrupt conductivity in the fifth nerve. This may be done by alcoholic injections of the nerve at various points or by surgical division of the nerve. Alcoholic injection is the simpler procedure and has the advantage that if surgical treatment is necessary later the patient already has experience of the resulting numbness. It is the method to be preferred, therefore, in most cases, unless the patient is going abroad and must have relief which is certain to be permanent. For the methods of injection the reader is referred to the papers by Harris (1926, 1937, 1938) and Penman (1949, 1950). The disadvantages of alcoholic injection are first, that for the inexperienced operator it may be difficult to spare the cornea and secondly, that recurrence of pain in 1–3 years is not infrequent. Hence some physicians prefer to advise surgical treatment at the outset in younger patients not responding to carbamazepine and reserve alcoholic injections for use in the elderly.

The surgical operation now usually employed for the relief of trigeminal neuralgia is extradural division of the sensory root, behind the trigeminal ganglion. The motor root can be spared and relief from pain is permanent. It has been suggested that when the first division is not involved an attempt should be made to save these fibres in order to avoid the risk of neuropathic keratitis. This attempt, however, may lead to sparing some fibres of the second division, or pain may develop later in the first division. Other treatments are Sjöqvist's (1937) operation of tractotomy, division of the spinal tract of the trigeminal nerve in the medulla, and Taarnhøj's operation of decompression of the sensory root (Woolsey, 1955). In some cases in which the pain is limited to the distribution of a single trigeminal branch (supra-orbital, infra-orbital, inferior dental nerves) alcoholic injection of the branch or surgical division of the nerve in its peripheral course may relieve symptoms completely but this relief is usually temporary.

TRIGEMINAL NEUROPATHY

This term has been used by Spillane and Wells (1959) to describe a disorder characterized by 'persistent sensory disturbance of the face, usually numbness in the territory of one or more divisions of the trigeminus'. Pain may occur, and in one case there was trophic ulceration of the nose. Hughes (1958) has found at operation on similar cases evidence of a chronic inflammatory process causing atrophy of the sensory root.

REFERENCES

BLOM, S. (1962) Trigeminal neuralgia; its treatment with a new anticonvulsant drug (G32883), *Lancet*, ii, 839.

CAMPBELL, F. G., GRAHAM, T. G., and ZILKHA, K. J. (1966) Clinical trial of carbamaze-pine (Tegretol) in trigeminal neuralgia, *J. Neurol. Neurosurg. Psychiat.*, **29**, 265.

DANDY, W. E. (1929) An operation for the cure of tic douloureux, *Arch. Surg. (Chicago)*, **18**, 687.

FRAZIER, C. H. (1925) Subtotal resection of sensory root for relief of major trigeminal neuralgia, *Arch. Neurol. Psychiat. (Chicago)*, **13**, 378.

FRAZIER, C. H. (1926) Division of sensory root on both sides, *J. Amer. med. Ass.*, **87**, 1730.

GOLDSTEIN, N. P., GIBILISCO, J. A., and RUSHTON, J. G. (1963) Trigeminal neuropathy and neuritis, *J. Amer. med. Ass.*, **184**, 458.

HARRIS, W. (1926) *Neuritis and Neuralgia*, London.

HARRIS, W. (1937) *The Facial Neuralgias*, London.

HARRIS, W. (1938) Alcohol injection in inoperable malignant growths of the jaws and tongue, *Brit. med. J.*, **2**, 831.

HUGHES, B. (1958) Chronic benign trigeminal paresis, *Proc. roy. Soc. Med.*, **51**, 529.

JEFFERSON, G. (1931) Surgical treatment of trigeminal neuralgia, *Brit. med. J.*, **2**, 309.

JEFFERSON, G. (1931) Observations on trigeminal neuralgia, *Brit. med. J.*, **2**, 879.

KUGELBERG, E., and LINDBLOM, U. (1959) The mechanism of the pain in trigeminal neuralgia, *J. Neurol. Neurosurg. Psychiat.*, **22**, 36.

PATON, L. (1926) The trigeminal and its ocular lesions, *Brit. J. Ophthal.*, **10**, 305.

PENMAN, J. (1949) A simple radiological aid to Gasserian injection, *Lancet*, ii, 268.

PENMAN, J. (1950) The differential diagnosis and treatment of tic douloureux, *Post-grad. med. J.*, **26**, 627.

PENMAN, J., and SMITH, M. C. (1950) Degeneration of the primary and secondary sen-sory nerves after trigeminal injection, *J. Neurol. Neurosurg. Psychiat.*, **13**, 36.

SJÖQVIST, O. (1937) Eine neue Operationsmethode bei Trigeminusneuralgie: Durch-schneidung des Tractus spinalis trigemini, *Zbl. Neurochir.*, i–ii, 274.

SMYTH, G. E. (1939) The systematization and central connections of the spinal tract and nucleus of the trigeminal nerve, *Brain*, **62**, 41.

SPILLANE, J. D., and WELLS, C. E. C. (1959) Isolated trigeminal neuropathy, *Brain*, **82**, 391.

WOOLSEY, R. D. (1955) Trigeminal neuralgia: treatment by decompression of the posterior root, *J. Amer. med. Ass.*, **159**, 1733.

THE SEVENTH OR FACIAL NERVE

ORIGIN, COURSE, AND DISTRIBUTION

The seventh cranial nerve contains motor fibres only, though it is associated in part of its course with a small number of sensory fibres going to the external acoustic meatus, with fibres which excite salivary secretion, and with others which convey taste impulses from the anterior two-thirds of the tongue. These secretory and gustatory fibres travel in the nervus intermedius. The motor nucleus is situated in the ventral part of the tegmentum of the pons. The fibres which take origin from this nucleus pass backwards in the pons almost as far as the floor of the fourth ventricle, where they form a loop around the nucleus of the sixth nerve before turning forwards to emerge from the lateral aspect of the lower border of the pons, on the medial side of the eighth nerve, from which the seventh is separated by the nervus intermedius [FIG. 23]. The three nerves then pass together from the pons to the internal acoustic meatus. Within the petrous portion of the temporal bone the facial nerve occupies the aqueductus Fallopii or facial canal. After passing outwards it turns sharply back-wards on the medial side of the middle ear and then downwards behind it to emerge from the skull at the stylomastoid foramen. At the backward turn of the

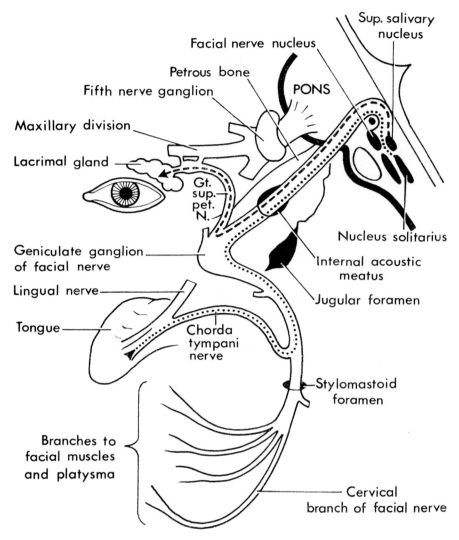

Sup. salivary nucleus

Facial nerve nucleus

Petrous bone

Fifth nerve ganglion

PONS

Maxillary division

Lacrimal gland

Gt. sup. pet. N.

Nucleus solitarius

Geniculate ganglion of facial nerve

Internal acoustic meatus

Lingual nerve

Jugular foramen

Tongue

Chorda tympani nerve

Stylomastoid foramen

Branches to facial muscles and platysma

Cervical branch of facial nerve

FIG. 23. The facial nerve

Lesions involving the facial nerve trunk above the geniculate ganglion will cause loss of lacrimation (greater petrosal nerve), and loss of taste in the anterior two-thirds of the tongue (chorda tympani nerve), as well as paralysis of both upper and lower facial muscles.

Lesions between the geniculate ganglion and the point where the chorda tympani nerve leaves the facial nerve (6 mm. above the stylomastoid foramen), will cause loss of taste sensation in the anterior two-thirds of the tongue, as well as paralysis of the facial muscles, but lacrimation will still be present.

Lesions below the point where the chorda tympani nerve leaves the facial nerve will cause paralysis of the facial muscles, but both taste and lacrimation will be present

(Redrawn from an original drawing by Mr. Charles Keogh.)

nerve it expands to form the geniculate ganglion which receives the nervus inter-medius and which contains the ganglion cells of the taste fibres of the chorda tympani. It sends branches to the pterygopalatine and otic ganglia, carrying fibres for the secretion of saliva. Within the facial canal the facial nerve gives off a nerve to the stapedius muscle, and the chorda tympani nerve which carries gustatory fibres to the anterior two-thirds of the tongue. The chorda tympani after crossing the tympanic cavity emerges from the skull by the anterior canali-culus for the chorda tympani and unites with the lingual nerve, a branch of the mandibular nerve, beneath the lateral pterygoid muscle. The facial nerve after emerging from the stylomastoid foramen gives branches to the stylohyoid muscle, to the posterior belly of the digastric and the occipital belly of the occipito-frontalis, and then turns forwards to divide within the parotid gland into a number of branches which innervate the muscles of expression, including the buccinator and the platysma.

FACIAL PARALYSIS

Facial paralysis may be due to:

1. A supranuclear lesion involving the corticospinal fibres concerned in voluntary facial movement.
2. A supranuclear lesion involving the fibres concerned in emotional move-ment of the face—mimic paralysis.
3. Nuclear and infranuclear lesions involving the lower motor neurones.
4. Primary degeneration or disorder of function of the facial muscles.

1. *Facial paralysis due to a supranuclear corticospinal lesion* is distinguished by the fact that movements of the lower part of the face are affected more severely than those of the upper part, and that although voluntary retraction of the angle of the mouth is weak, emotional and associated movements of the face are little, if at all, affected. Reaction of degeneration does not occur in the facial muscles.

2. The occasional occurrence of *weakness or abolition of emotional movements of the face* with retention of voluntary movements and the escape of the former after corticospinal lesions indicates that the nervous impulses concerned in emotional movement of the face employ a different supranuclear path from the corticospinal tract. This path appears to originate in the frontal lobe, anterior to the precentral gyrus, and most cases of mimic facial palsy are due to lesions of the anterior part of the frontal lobe. This dissociated form of facial weakness has also been described as a result of lesions in the neighbourhood of the thalamus.

3. *Lesions involving the lower motor neurones* supplying the facial muscles, since they destroy the final common path, affect to an equal extent all forms of facial movement, and as a rule the upper and lower facial muscles are equally weakened. The symptoms of facial paralysis due to lower motor neurone lesions are described in detail in the section dealing with Bell's paralysis. The facial lower motor neurones may be involved by a lesion:

(*a*) within the pons;
(*b*) within the posterior fossa, between the pons and the internal acoustic meatus;

(c) within the temporal bone;
(d) after emergence from the skull;
(e) they may be the site of neuritis throughout their length.

(a) *Pontine lesions.* Massive lesions involving the facial nucleus or the fibres of the facial nerve inevitably affect neighbouring structures as well. Facial paralysis due to such lesions is, therefore, usually associated with paralysis of the lateral rectus, or of conjugate ocular deviation to the same side, and often with paralysis of the ipsilateral jaw muscles. There may also be sensory loss due to involvement of the spinal tract and nucleus of the trigeminal nerve and of the spinothalamic tract, or a corticospinal lesion of the upper and lower limbs on the opposite side. Acute and chronic degenerative lesions of the facial nuclei are likely to involve other bulbar motor nuclei. Pontine lesions causing facial paralysis include tumours, syringobulbia, vascular lesions, poliomyelitis, Landry's paralysis, multiple sclerosis, and motor neurone disease. Bilateral facial paralysis occasionally occurs as a congenital abnormality, probably due to a failure of development of the facial nuclei, and is then usually associated with congenital ocular palsies.

(b) *Within the posterior fossa* the proximity of the facial nerve to the nervus intermedius and the eighth nerve is responsible for the fact that these nerves usually suffer together. Lesions in this situation, therefore, usually cause deafness and loss of taste in the anterior two-thirds of the tongue, in association with facial paralysis. The commonest of such lesions are acoustic neuroma and other tumours in the region of the cerebellopontine angle.

(c) *Within the temporal bone* the facial nerve may be involved in fractures of the skull, and is exposed to infections of the middle ear and mastoid, and facial paralysis may be the direct result of spread of infection from the middle ear to the facial canal, or may follow surgical operations on the ear, in which case the nerve may be merely contused or actually divided or exposed to invasion by the infecting organism. Slow progressive facial palsy may be caused by an epidermoid within the temporal bone, and is then associated with deafness (Jefferson and Smalley, 1938). Herpes zoster infecting the geniculate ganglion usually causes facial paralysis through secondary involvement of the motor fibres of the nerve (syndrome of Ramsay Hunt). Facial paralysis caused by a lesion within the middle ear is usually associated with loss of taste in the anterior two-thirds of the tongue, as a result of interruption of the fibres of the chorda tympani within the facial nerve, or in its passage through the middle ear. Inflammation of the facial nerve within the stylomastoid foramen is the cause of facial paralysis occurring spontaneously or following exposure to cold and known as Bell's palsy.

(d) *After leaving the skull* the fibres of the facial nerve may be involved in inflammation from suppurating glands behind the angle of the jaw or in compression by tumours of the parotid gland. They are exposed to traumatic lesions in the face, including compression by forceps during delivery.

(e) *Neuritis of the facial nerve* may occur in tetanus, polyneuritis cranialis, acute leukaemia and sarcoidosis.

4. *Primary degeneration or disorder of function of the facial muscles* is seen in myasthenia gravis, in which the retractors of the angle of the mouth suffer

earlier and more severely than the elevators and depressors of the lips, in the
facioscapulohumeral type of muscular dystrophy, and in dystrophia myotonica.
Facial muscle weakness rarely occurs in polymyositis and involvement of the
orbicularis oculi is usual in cases of ocular myopathy.

BELL'S PALSY (FACIAL PARALYSIS)

Definition. Facial paralysis of acute onset due to non-suppurative inflammation
of the facial nerve within the stylomastoid foramen.

AETIOLOGY AND PATHOLOGY

The most plausible explanation of Bell's paralysis (named after Sir Charles
Bell, 1774–1842) is that it is due to an acute inflammation involving the nerve
within the stylomastoid foramen. It is uncertain whether the lesion is primarily
in the nerve, interstitial neuritis, or in the bone, a periostitis. In either case
oedema must lead to compression of the nerve fibres, with resulting paralysis.
At first the nerve is swollen, later it is reduced to a fibrous cord (Morris, 1938,
1939).

Bell's paralysis may occur at any age from infancy to old age. It appears to
be most common in young adults, and males are affected more frequently
than females.

In some cases no predisposing cause can be found, but not uncommonly there
is a history of exposure to chill, for example, riding in a vehicle or sleeping next
to an open window. In other cases the paralysis follows an acute infection of the
nasopharynx, and in a small proportion of cases it has been shown to be due
to the virus of herpes zoster.

SYMPTOMS

Bell's palsy is almost always unilateral, very rarely bilateral. The onset is
sudden and frequently the patient awakens in the morning to find the face
paralysed. He or his friends observe that his mouth is drawn to one side. There
is frequently pain at the onset within the ear, in the mastoid region, or around
the angle of the jaw.

There is paralysis of the muscles of expression [FIG. 24]. The upper and lower
facial muscles are usually equally affected and the muscles are paralysed to an
equal extent for voluntary, emotional, and associated movements. The eyebrow
droops, and the wrinkles of the brow are smoothed out. Frowning and raising the
eyebrow are impossible. Owing to paralysis of the orbicularis oculi the palpebral
fissure is wider on the affected than on the normal side and closure of the eye
is impossible. Eversion of the lower lid, and lack of approximation of the punc-
tum to the conjunctiva impair the absorption of tears, which tend to overflow
the lower lid. The nasolabial furrow is smoothed out, and the mouth is drawn
over to the sound side. The patient is unable to retract the angle of the mouth,
and to purse the lips, as in whistling. Owing to paralysis of the buccinator the
cheek is puffed out in respiration, and food tends to accumulate between
the teeth and the cheek. The displacement of the mouth causes deviation of the

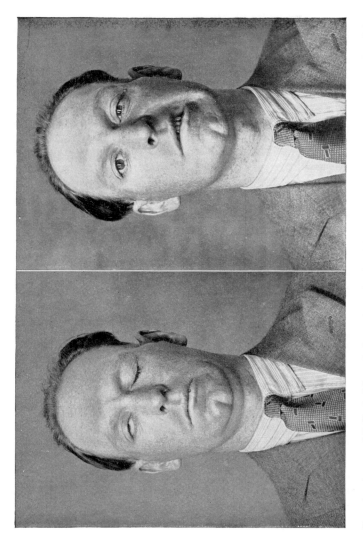

Fig. 24. A case of Bell's facial paralysis on the right side. (Note weakness of the orbicularis oculi and of the retractors of the angle of the mouth.)

tongue to the sound side when it is protruded, and may thus cause paralysis of the tongue to be suspected in error.

When the inflammation spreads up from the stylomastoid foramen to involve the facial nerve above the point at which the chorda tympani leaves it, there is loss of taste on the anterior two-thirds of the tongue, and when the branch to the stapedius is also involved the patient may complain of hyperacusis, an intensification of loud noises.

DIAGNOSIS

Bell's palsy of the facial nerve is distinguished from facial paralysis due to a lesion of the pons by the presence in the latter case of symptoms of involvement of other pontine nuclei, especially the fifth and sixth, and sometimes of the long tracts. Lesions in the posterior fossa usually involve the eighth nerve as well. A history of aural discharge and examination of the tympanic membrane makes it easy to recognize facial paralysis secondary to otitis media. Unilateral facial palsy is sometimes an early symptom of multiple sclerosis, especially in young adults, and is occasionally due to syphilis. A recurrent form associated with headache has been termed 'facioplegic migraine'.

PROGNOSIS

In many cases of Bell's palsy complete recovery occurs, though this may take months. In Taverner's (1955) series about half the patients made a complete recovery. If at the end of three weeks from the onset there is some return of voluntary power in the face or some response to faradic stimulation of the facial muscles, recovery is likely to be rapid and will probably be complete in a few weeks. Electromyography is a useful guide to prognosis. In those cases in which recovery is never complete, contracture usually develops in the paralysed muscles, and this does much to improve the appearance of the face at rest, although the paralysis is evident when the patient smiles. When marked contracture develops, the nasolabial furrow may become actually deeper on the paralysed side than on the normal side and the affected eyebrow may be drawn downwards. Clonic facial spasm is an occasional sequel of incomplete recovery, but usually is not very severe. The syndrome of 'crocodile tears'—unilateral lacrimation on eating—occurs in a small proportion of cases. It is due to regenerating facial nerve fibres running from the geniculate ganglion through the greater petrosal nerve and the pterygopalatine ganglion to the lacrimal gland. Recurrent facial palsy is rare. I have known it occur first on one side and a year later on the other, while very occasionally it may develop simultaneously on the two sides.

TREATMENT

When the patient is seen during the acute stage, treatment should be directed to relieving the inflammation. Robison and Moss (1954) advocate the use of cortisone but Taverner et al. (1966) have found, in a controlled trial, that ACTH is more effective if given early enough. It is sound treatment to try to prevent stretching of the paralysed muscles, which occurs when the mouth is drawn over to the sound side. The usual wire splint is unphysiological. It is better to apply two strips of adhesive strapping or transparent tape ('Sellotape' or 'Scotch Tape') above and below the mouth to counteract the pull of the muscles on the normal side (Pickerill and Pickerill, 1945).

As soon as the acute stage is past and pain has disappeared, galvanic current may be used to stimulate the facial muscles. The negative electrode is held beneath the mastoid and the positive electrode is used to stroke the face, a current of about 3 milliamperes being all that is necessary. This treatment has been recommended for some years but doubt is now being cast upon its value and many workers believe that it may even predispose to contracture; they prefer to give no electrical treatment at all. As soon as voluntary power shows some sign of return the patient should be encouraged to practise closing the eye and retracting the angle of the mouth in front of the looking-glass.

If in six to eight weeks there is no recovery or if reaction of degeneration has set in, surgical treatment may be considered, viz. Ballance and Duel's operation of decompression of the facial canal, and incision of the nerve sheath (Morris, 1938, 1939). However, it now seems likely that this operation is only likely to be effective if carried out within a few days of the onset of paralysis at a time when there is no certain method of knowing which cases (the minority) are unlikely to show rapid recovery. An autograft may be used in late cases when the nerve is fibrotic. Plastic surgery may be helpful in irrecoverable cases.

CLONIC FACIAL SPASM (HEMIFACIAL SPASM)

Definition. A disorder which chiefly affects middle-aged or elderly women. There are frequent shock-like contractions of the facial muscles, usually limited to one side. Its cause is unknown.

AETIOLOGY AND PATHOLOGY

The causation of clonic facial spasm is a matter of hypothesis. It is probably the result of an irritative lesion at some point in the course of the nerve and has been ascribed to a lesion of the geniculate ganglion. Others suggest that it is due to a compressive lesion of the nerve (usually fibrosis of unknown aetiology) within its canal. Similar spasms certainly occur for a brief period in some cases of herpes zoster of the geniculate ganglion.

SYMPTOMS

Clonic facial spasm is much more common in women than in men and is rare before middle life. It usually begins in the orbicularis oculi as a fine intermittent twitching resembling that which occurs in normal individuals in states of debility and fatigue and which is known as 'live flesh'. The spread of the spasm is extremely slow, but gradually the muscles of the lower part of the face are involved, especially the retractors of the angle of the mouth. Finally strong spasms involve all the facial muscles on one side almost continuously. At this stage there is always slight weakness and wasting of the facial musculature. Taste may be lost over the anterior two-thirds of the tongue. Bilateral clonic facial spasm is less common: in such cases one side is usually affected after the other. The involuntary closure of both eyes in such cases causes much inconvenience. Clonic facial spasm may be associated with trigeminal neuralgia on the same or the opposite side.

DIAGNOSIS

Clonic facial spasm must be distinguished from other involuntary movements involving the face. The commonest of these is habit spasm, a brief compulsive movement usually seen in children and young adults. When the face is the site of habit spasm the movements are bilateral. Blepharospasm, prolonged spasm of the orbicularis oculi, is usually seen in elderly women, and in this case also the movements are bilateral and there is no clonic twitching of the lower facial muscles. However, it may sometimes be associated with choreic movements of the lips in cases of senile chorea while intermittent blepharospasm is a common 'hysterical' phenomenon and may sometimes be severe and disabling in patients of either sex suffering from severe depression or anxiety. The involuntary movements of chorea and athetosis are also bilateral, and are usually associated with similar movements in the limbs.

PROGNOSIS

In the absence of treatment clonic facial spasm is a slowly progressive disorder and spontaneous recovery does not occur. It may terminate after many years in complete facial paralysis on the affected side, and the twitching then ceases.

TREATMENT

Drugs are of no lasting value although the condition is accentuated by tension and embarrassment so that chlordiazepoxide (*Librium*) in doses of 5–10 mg. three times a day, or diazepam (*Valium*) 2–5 mg. three times a day, are sometimes helpful. Relief can be sometimes obtained by means of a temporary interruption of conduction in the facial nerve by alcoholic injection. The method of injection of the nerve trunk in the region of the stylomastoid foramen is described by Harris (1926). A selective paresis can be produced by the simple procedure of injecting with alcohol the appropriate branches of the nerve as they lie behind the mandible.

Alcoholic injection of the branches of the facial nerve gives relief from the involuntary movements for a period of from six to twelve months, but also produces a greater or less degree of facial paralysis and the movements are liable to recur as the muscles recover their power. Harris and Wright (1932) recommended faciohypoglossal anastomosis, but the results of the operation are unsatisfactory and many patients are better left without any form of definitive treatment as the movements have no more than a minor nuisance value in the majority. Decompression of the nerve in the facial canal is more logical and is sometimes successful.

REFERENCES

ADSON, A. W. (1925) Surgical treatment of facial paralysis, *Arch. Otolaryng. (Chicago)*, **2**, 217.
HARRIS, W. (1926) *Neuritis and Neuralgia*, p. 371, London.
HARRIS, W., and WRIGHT, A. D. (1932) Treatment of clonic facial spasm, *Lancet*, i, 657.

JEFFERSON, G., and SMALLEY, A. A. (1938) Progressive facial palsy produced by intra-temporal epidermoids, *J. Laryng.*, **53**, 417.

MORRIS, W. M. (1938) Surgical treatment of Bell's palsy, *Lancet*, i, 429.

MORRIS, W. M. (1939) Surgical treatment of facial paralysis, *Lancet*, ii, 558.

PICKERILL, H. S., and PICKERILL, C. M. (1945) Early treatment of Bell's palsy, *Brit. med. J.*, **2**, 457.

ROBISON, W. P., and MOSS, B. F. (1954) Treatment of Bell's palsy with cortisone, *J. Amer. med. Ass.*, **154**, 142.

TAVERNER, D. (1955) Bell's palsy. A clinical and electromyographic study, *Brain*, **78**, 209.

TAVERNER, D., FEARNLEY, M. E., KEMBLE, F., MILES, D. W., and PEIRIS, O. A. (1966) Prevention of denervation in Bell's palsy, *Brit. med. J.*, **1**, 391.

THE EIGHTH OR VESTIBULOCOCHLEAR NERVE

The eighth nerve contains two groups of fibres, those which supply the cochlea and are concerned in hearing, and those which supply the semicircular canals, the utricle and the saccule, and are concerned in postural and equilibratory functions. These two parts of the eighth nerve are described as the cochlear and the vestibular nerves. They run together in the eighth nerve from the internal acoustic meatus to its entry into the brain stem in the lateral aspect of the lower border of the pons, but they differ in their peripheral distribution and their central connexions. The eighth nerve in its passage across the posterior fossa lies on the lateral side of the seventh nerve, from which it is separated by the nervus intermedius.

THE COCHLEAR FIBRES

The ganglion cells of the cochlear nerve are situated in the spiral ganglion of the cochlea. These are bipolar cells of which the peripheral processes terminate in relationship with the cells of the spiral organ. Their central processes pass through the eighth nerve into the pons, where they terminate in the cochlear nucleus. Relay neurones originate in the cochlear nucleus and cross to the opposite side by two alternative paths. Fibres from the more dorsal portion of the nucleus cross just beneath the floor of the fourth ventricle, where they form the striae acousticae; those from the ventral portion enter the olive of the same side, whence arise further neurones which cross in the ventral region of the pons and are known as the fibres of the trapezium. Both dorsal and ventral fibres meet in the lateral lemniscus in which they pass upwards through the brain stem to the inferior colliculus and the medial geniculate body, whence further fibres are distributed to the cortical auditory centre in the transverse temporal gyrus and adjacent portion of the superior temporal gyrus.

TESTS OF AUDITORY FUNCTION

Interruption of the cochlear fibres causes impairment of hearing—nerve deafness. Since loss of hearing is also a symptom of lesions involving the auditory conducting mechanism in the middle ear, it is necessary to distinguish nerve deafness from middle-ear deafness. For this purpose the following tests are employed.

Weber's Test. A vibrating tuning-fork (C = 256) is applied to the forehead or vertex in the midline and the patient is asked whether the sound is heard in the midline or is localized in one ear. In normal individuals the sound appears to be in the midline. In middle-ear deafness it is usually localized in the affected ear, in nerve deafness in the normal ear. This is due to the fact that in nerve deafness bone-conduction of sound is reduced as well as air-conduction, whereas in middle-ear deafness air-conduction is reduced but bone-conduction is relatively enhanced.

Rinne's Test. This is based upon the same fact. A vibrating tuning-fork is applied to the patient's mastoid process, the ear being closed by the observer's finger. The patient is asked to say when he ceases to hear the sound, and the fork is then held at the acoustic meatus. In middle-ear deafness the sound cannot be heard by air-conduction after bone-conduction has ceased to transmit it. In nerve deafness, as in normal individuals, the reverse is the case.

A further distinction between nerve deafness and middle-ear deafness is that in the former loss of hearing is most marked for high-pitched tones; in the latter for low-pitched tones.

Loudness Recruitment. This test is applied to patients who are deaf in one ear. A sound of the same frequency but differing intensities is presented to either ear alternately, and the patient is asked to say when the sound heard with the deaf ear sounds as loud as that heard with the normal one. In conductive deafness the ratio between the intensities required to produce equal loudness in the two ears remains the same for all intensities. In nerve deafness, as the intensity rises, the difference between the two ears diminishes and may disappear. This is known as loudness recruitment. It is characteristic of a lesion of the sensory end-organs in the cochlea, and is usually absent in cases of lesion of the vestibulocochlear nerve (Dix, 1956; Hallpike, 1965).

Other tests of auditory function are the speech test, specially valuable in the detection of lesions of the vestibulocochlear nerve (Johnson and House, 1964), Békèsy audiometry (Jerger, 1960), the tone decay test (Rosenberg, 1958; Green, 1963), and the SISI (short increment sensitivity index) (Jerger, Shedd, and Harford, 1959).

LESIONS RESPONSIBLE FOR NERVE DEAFNESS

Nerve deafness may result from involvement of the terminals of the cochlear part of the eighth nerve in lesions of the internal ear. Such lesions include trauma, chronic otitis interna, which sometimes follows low-grade infections of the middle ear, and acute labyrinthitis, which may be either primary or secondary to acute purulent otitis media, meningococcal meningitis, or mumps. The internal ear may also be involved in congenital syphilis, in congenital deaf-mutism, one form of which is associated with adenoma of the thyroid, in otosclerosis and in atheroma. It is uncertain whether streptomycin causes deafness by damaging the vestibulocochlear nerve or the acoustic centres in the pons. The vestibulocochlear nerve may be damaged within the petrous bone by fractures of the skull or by an intratemporal epidermoid, in both of which cases deafness may be associated with facial palsy, and is sometimes compressed by bony hyperplasia of the internal acoustic meatus in osteitis deformans. In its passage across the posterior fossa the eighth nerve may be the site of a tumour, an acoustic neuroma, or may be involved in an inflammatory lesion, e.g. due to meningovascular syphilis. Rare causes are avitaminosis and polyneuritis cranialis, the deafness in both being bilateral. Deafness is a rare symptom of lesions within the central nervous system, though I have known unilateral deafness to be caused by a vascular lesion of the pons, and by multiple sclerosis, and total bilateral deafness and loss of vestibular function to be associated in the other signs of brain-stem damage in a case of head injury. Compression of the midbrain in the region of the inferior colliculi by tumours of the midbrain or pineal body may cause impairment of hearing. Deafness does not occur as a result of lesions of the temporal lobe unless the lesion is bilateral. Central deafness in childhood may be due to birth injury, anoxia following labour or kernicterus.

TINNITUS

Tinnitus is a sensation of noise caused by abnormal excitation of the acoustic apparatus or of its afferent paths or cortical areas. Tinnitus may be continuous or intermittent, unilateral or bilateral. The noise heard may be high- or low-pitched and is variously described as hissing, whistling, or, in severe cases, as resembling the noise made by a steam-engine or by machinery. It may possess a rhythm corresponding to that of the pulse. Apart from associated deafness, tinnitus when severe may interfere with hearing, and is most evident to the patient at night, when objective noises are diminished. Persistent tinnitus sometimes leads to much distress and depression in elderly people, while there is evidence to suggest that sometimes it is a manifestation of endogenous depression in such cases and it may be relieved by appropriate treatment of the depression. Tinnitus is frequently associated with deafness and sometimes with vertigo.

The causes of tinnitus are various. Wax in the external acoustic meatus, catarrh of the Eustachian tube, and acute otitis media probably act by causing obstruction of the conducting apparatus of the ear. The tinnitus produced by forcible contraction of the orbicularis oculi is attributed to an associated spasm of the stapedius. In a large group of cases tinnitus is due to a disturbance of the circulation of the internal ear, and this is probably the cause of that produced by drugs, for example, quinine, salicylates, and amyl nitrite, by acute labyrinthitis, generalized arteriosclerosis, severe anaemia, aortic incompetence, and otosclerosis. Tinnitus precedes the deafness sometimes caused by streptomycin [see p. 174]. Abnormal sounds arising within the cranium may be conducted to the ear and so cause tinnitus. Thus a rhythmical bruit is sometimes heard by the patient in cases of rupture of the internal carotid into the cavernous sinus, congenital intracranial aneurysm, and arterial angioma. Irritation of the acoustic afferent paths may lead to tinnitus when the eighth nerve is the site of a tumour or is involved in inflammation due, for example, to syphilitic meningitis. Tinnitus is rarely the result of a lesion of the central nervous system, but may occur in association with deafness after vascular or other lesions of the lateral part of the tegmentum of the pons. Noises heard as a result of irritative lesions of the auditory cortex in the temporal lobe are usually more complex than those caused by irritation of the acoustic apparatus and its lower pathways. In this group fall auditory hallucinations comprising the aura of an epileptic fit and those which sometimes occur as symptoms of a neoplasm or other lesion involving the temporal lobe. But Frazier and Rowe (1932) say that tinnitus occurred in 25 per cent. of their fifty-one verified cases of temporal lobe tumour.

The treatment of tinnitus is disappointing. Local lesions of the ear should receive appropriate treatment. Sedatives such as phenobarbitone usually have some palliative action and in appropriate cases in which no organic cause for the complaint can be demonstrated, and in which depression is severe, anti-depressive drugs are sometimes dramatically successful. In severe cases, in which the tinnitus is intolerable, it may be justifiable to destroy the cochlea or divide the eighth nerve, but the patient must be informed that complete deafness in the ear thus treated will result and that tinnitus may persist in spite of the operation.

THE VESTIBULAR FIBRES AND THE FUNCTIONS OF THE LABYRINTH

The membranous labyrinth is concerned with hearing and balance. The end-organs for balance are the semicircular canals, utricle and saccule. This membranous structure is a closed system surrounded by perilymph, lying within the bony labyrinth of the temporal bone. It is filled with endolymph, which has a high potassium and low sodium content closely resembling intracellular fluid (Citron, Exley, and Hallpike, 1956). On the wall of the canal of the cochlea is a gland-like structure, the stria vascularis, which is thought to be concerned with the production of endolymph. Perilymph has a composition similar to extracellular fluid and it communicates with the subarachnoid space through the saccus endolymphaticus.

The parts of the labyrinth concerned with balance are the semicircular canals, utricle and saccule. The semicircular canals, three in number, are arranged approximately in the three planes of space at right angles to one another, and are so placed that, when the head is inclined 30 degrees forwards from the erect position, the lateral canal is horizontal. The anterior canal lies in a plane midway between the frontal and sagittal planes with the outermost portion anteriorly and runs inwards and backwards. The posterior canal lies in a vertical plane at right angles to the anterior canal with its outermost part posteriorly and runs inwards and forwards. Each canal exhibits a dilatation, the ampulla, which contains epithelium, and the crista, bearing hair cells, which are the vestibular receptors. Somewhat similar receptors, the maculae, exist in the utricle and saccule, but in these the hair cells are in contact with small crystals, the otoliths. The semicircular canals are excited by movements, especially angular acceleration. The precise way in which this stimulates the hair cells is still unsettled, but the best working hypothesis is that they respond to movements of the endolymph. The utricle conveys information concerning the position of the head in space. The position of the otoliths with reference to the hair cells varies under the influence of gravity. The saccule may be concerned with vibration.

The vestibular nerve arises from cells in the vestibular ganglion and is joined in the internal meatus by the cochlear nerve which arises from cells in the spiral ganglion of the cochlea. These two nerves form the eighth cranial nerve. On reaching the cranial cavity this nerve crosses the cerebellopontine angle and enters the pons. The vestibular division passes medial to the cochlear division which soon becomes separated from it by the inferior cerebellar peduncle. The vestibular fibres terminate in a group of nuclei in the brain stem.

Recent research and clinical observation have led to the concept that each vestibular system is divided into two functional parts, the canal and tonus elements. The right and left canal or phasic elements, from the semicircular canals, go to nuclei in the brain stem and from there to the eye muscles. This is the pathway taken when nystagmus is evoked during the caloric test. The right and left tonus elements, from the utricles, are believed to have their own brain-stem nuclei and cortical centres in the posterior parts of the temporal lobes. Each tonus system is functionally opposed and balanced by the other. The brain-stem nuclei of the canal, and the tonus elements, are interconnected. A knowledge of this hypothesis is necessary for the interpretation of the caloric test for vestibular function.

EXAMINATION FOR VESTIBULAR DYSFUNCTION

Examination for vestibular dysfunction must include observations for spontaneous manifestations—nystagmus, disorders of gait and of muscular control—as well as induced manifestations. Investigation of cochlear function should accompany this examination.

Spontaneous Vestibular Nystagmus

Spontaneous nystagmus consists of a slow and a rapid component. It is described by the direction of the rapid component. It may be first, second, or third degree.

First-degree nystagmus to the left is seen only on looking to the left.

Second-degree nystagmus to the left is present on looking straight ahead and is increased on looking to the left.

Third-degree nystagmus to the left is present on looking straight ahead, is increased to the left, and is present, though decreased, on looking to the right.

Observation for spontaneous nystagmus should always be made with the patient's head in the erect position. The lateral gaze must not be extended beyond the limits of binocular vision.

In dysfunction of the semicircular canals or their peripheral neurones, the nystagmus is always accompanied by vertigo and is limited in duration because central compensation occurs. If nystagmus persists for more than a few weeks it is usually due to change in the central vestibular pathway. With central lesions the subjective symptoms are frequently less severe.

Induced Manifestations of Vestibular Dysfunction

Induced manifestations are shown by various clinical tests for vestibular function. The caloric test, tests for positional and optokinetic nystagmus are necessary for diagnosis. Electronystagmography makes it possible to record details of the nystagmus.

Caloric Test. The caloric test of Fitzgerald and Hallpike is a means of demon strating dysfunction of the canal and tonus elements of the vestibular system. The results remain remarkably constant regardless of repetition.

A moderate but effective thermal stimulus is applied to each labyrinth separately. The stimulus used is water at 7° C. below and 7° C. above body temperature. This produces equal and opposite horizontal nystagmus lasting approximately two minutes in the normal individual.

During the test the patient lies on a couch with his head raised 30 degrees from the horizontal. In this position the lateral semicircular canals are vertical, the position of maximal thermal sensitivity. The patient is asked to look at a suitable spot so that a fixed gaze is maintained. Water at 30° C. is run into one ear continuously for 40 seconds, not less than 250 ml. being used. In the normal subject second-degree nystagmus away from the stimulated labyrinth occurs. The time is recorded in seconds from the beginning of irrigation to the point when second-degree nystagmus can no longer be seen with a good light at a distance of 10 inches. Irrigation at 30° C. is repeated in the other ear. Water at 44° C. is then used in each ear in turn, when the induced nystagmus is towards the irrigated side. Accuracy of temperature and duration of irrigation are essential in this test. Experience in observation of the end point and in interpretation of the caloric patterns is necessary for reaching a correct diagnosis.

The caloric test is of great value in the diagnosis of organic lesions at all levels of the vestibular system. It may show suppression of activity on one side, canal paresis, or a directional preponderance of nystagmus, which means that nystagmus in one direction, from whichever canal it is obtained, is stronger than in the other direction, according to whether the canal or tonus elements of the vestibular system are affected. Combined responses showing directional preponderance and canal paresis frequently occur [FIGS. 25–9].

In cerebral lesions involving the posterior part of the temporal lobe, the cortical centre for the tonus pathway, marked directional preponderance of caloric nystagmus towards the side of the lesion is found (Carmichael, Dix, and Hallpike, 1956).

In brain-stem lesions directional preponderance away from the lesion is found more frequently than canal paresis, which occurs when the lesion is at or above the level of the entry of the eighth nerve. Combined responses sometimes occur (Carmichael, Dix, and Hallpike, 1965).

In peripheral lesions the commonest abnormality found is canal paresis, due to a lesion of the lateral semicircular canal or its peripheral neurones. Canal paresis is found in a high proportion of patients with Ménière's disease, vestibular neuronitis and acoustic neuroma. Combined lesions indicating a change in the utricle or its peripheral neurones as well as the lateral canal occur in 21 per cent. of cases of Ménière's disease (Hallpike, 1950). Directional preponderance of caloric nystagmus alone is found less commonly in peripheral disease.

Positional Tests. In recent years it has been shown (Dix and Hallpike, 1952) that nystagmus on sudden movement of the head in certain directions, is produced by changes in the otolith organ of the utricle. The cause of this change is thought to be either an alteration in the blood supply or low-grade infection. This syndrome is now known as benign paroxysmal positional nystagmus.

Tests for otolith function cannot be confined to one ear, but there is a useful and easily performed test to elicit positional nystagmus. The patient is seated on a couch. His head is held and he is briskly laid back so that his head becomes 30 degrees below the horizontal and rotated 30 to 40 degrees towards the observer [Fig. 30]. In the normal subject no nystagmus or vertigo occur. In benign paroxysmal positional nystagmus, after a short, characteristic latent period, severe vertigo and rotary nystagmus towards the lowermost ear (the

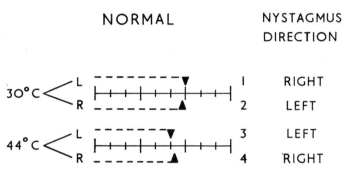

Fig. 25. Caloric responses: normal. (From Fitzgerald, G., and Hallpike, C. S. (1942) *Brain*, **65**, 115. By kind permission of the Authors and Editor.)

affected one) occur and last for several seconds. If the critical position is maintained, the nystagmus and vertigo gradually stop. On returning to a sitting position a similar, though usually less severe, episode occurs. If the test is then repeated the phenomenon may not be observed, as adaptation occurs rapidly.

Positional nystagmus is sometimes seen in posterior fossa lesions. These patients have less subjective vertigo and the nystagmus, which is more prolonged, does not show adaptation and often changes direction when the position of the head is altered.

REFERENCES

CARMICHAEL, E. A., DIX, M. R., and HALLPIKE, C. S. (1956) Pathology, symptomatology and diagnosis of organic affections of the eighth nerve system, *Brit. med. Bull.*, **12**, 146.

CARMICHAEL, E. A., DIX, M. R., and HALLPIKE, C. S. (1965) Observations upon the neurological mechanism of directional preponderance of caloric nystagmus resulting from vascular lesions of the brain-stem, *Brain*, **88**, 51.

CITRON, L., EXLEY, D., and HALLPIKE, C. S. (1956) Formation, circulation and properties of the labyrinthine fluids, *Brit. med. Bull.*, **12**, 101.

DIX, M. R. (1956) Loudness recruitment, *Brit. med. Bull.*, **12**, 119.

DIX, M. R., and HALLPIKE, C. S. (1952) The pathology, symptomatology and diagnosis of certain disorders of the vestibular system, *Proc. roy. Soc. Med.*, **45**, 341.

DIX, M. R., HALLPIKE, C. S., and HARRISON, M. S. (1949) Some observations upon the otological effects of streptomycin intoxication, *Brain*, **72**, 241.

FRAZIER, C. S., and ROWE, S. N. (1932) Certain observations upon the localization in 51 verified tumours of the temporal lobe, *Res. Publ. Ass. nerv. ment. Dis.*, **13**, 251.

GREEN, D. S. (1963) Modified tone decay test (MTDT) as screening procedure for eighth nerve lesions, *Speech Hearing Dis.*, **28**, 31.

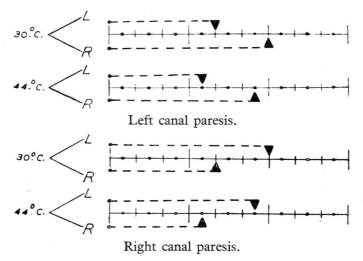

Left canal paresis.

Right canal paresis.

FIG. 26. Caloric responses: canal paresis. (From Fitzgerald, G., and Hallpike, C. S. (1942) *Brain*, **65**, 115. By kind permission of the Authors and Editor.)

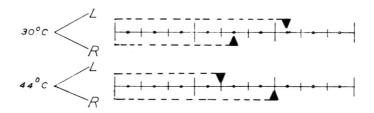

DIRECTIONAL PREPONDERANCE TO RIGHT.

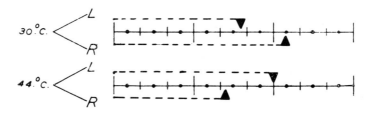

DIRECTIONAL PREPONDERANCE TO LEFT.

FIG. 27. Caloric responses: directional preponderance. (From Fitzgerald, G., and Hallpike, C. S. (1942) *Brain*, **65**, 115. By kind permission of the Authors and Editor.)

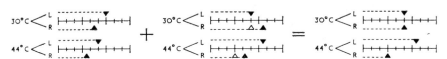

FIG. 28. Caloric responses: from a case of Ménière's disease of the right labyrinth. Combination of right canal paresis (1) and directional preponderance to the left (2). (From Hallpike, C. S. (1965) *Proc. roy. Soc. Med.*, **58**, 185. By kind permission of the Author and Editor.)

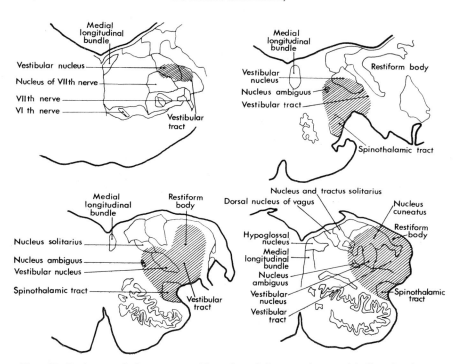

FIG. 29. Brain-stem lesion; a case of lateral medullary syndrome with directional preponderance of the caloric responses to the left. (From Carmichael, E. A., Dix, M. R., and Hallpike, C. S. (1965) *Brain*, **88**, 51. By kind permission of the Authors and Editor.)

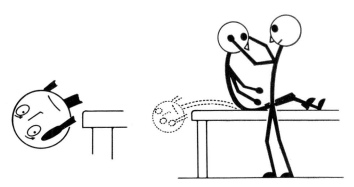

FIG. 30. The method of eliciting positional nystagmus. (From Hallpike, C. S. (1955) *Postgrad. med. J.*, **31**, 330. By kind permission of the Author and Editor.)

HALLPIKE, C. S. (1950) in Discussion on the medical treatment of Ménière's disease, *Proc. roy. Soc. Med.*, **43**, 288.

HALLPIKE, C. S. (1955) Ménière's disease, *Postgrad. med. J.*, **31**, 330.

HALLPIKE, C. S. (1965) Clinical otoneurology and its contributions to theory and practice, *Proc. roy. Soc. Med.*, **58**, 185.

HALLPIKE, C. S. (1967) Some types of ocular nystagmus and their neurological mechanisms, *Proc. roy. Soc. Med.*, **60**, 1043.

HOUSE, W. F. (1965) Subarachnoid shunt for drainage of hydrops, *Laryngoscope (St. Louis)*, **75**, 1547.

JERGER, J. F. (1960) Békèsy audiometry in analysis of auditory disorders, *J. Speech Res.*, **3**, 275.

JERGER, J. F., SHEDD, J. L., and HARFORD, E. (1959) On the detection of extremely small changes in sound intensity, *Arch. Otolaryng.*, **69**, 200.

JOHNSON, E. W., and HOUSE, W. F. (1964) Auditory findings in 53 cases of acoustic neuromas, *Arch. Otolaryng.*, **80**, 667.

ROSENBERG, P. E. (1958) Clinical Measurement of Tone Decay: read before the American Speech and Hearing Association Convention, 1958.

VERTIGO

THE NATURE OF VERTIGO

Vertigo may be defined as the consciousness of disordered orientation of the body in space. The derivation of the term implies a sense of rotation of the patient or of his surroundings, but this, though frequently present, is not the only form of vertigo as just defined. There are three ways in which the spatial orientation of the body may be felt to be disordered.

1. The external world may appear to move, often in a rotatory fashion, but other forms of movement, such as oscillation, may be experienced.

2. The body itself may be felt to be moving, either in rotation or as a sensation of falling, or the movement may be referred to within the body, e.g. within the head.

3. The postures and movements of the limbs, especially the lower limbs, are felt to be ill-adjusted and unsteady.

The motor accompaniments of vertigo consist of forced movements of the body, such as falling, and disordered orientation of parts of the body, manifested in the eyes as nystagmus and sometimes diplopia, and in the limbs as pass-pointing, while visceral disturbances, such as pallor, sweating, alterations in the pulse rate and blood pressure, nausea, vomiting, and diarrhoea may be present. Temporary amaurosis and even loss of consciousness may occur in severe attacks.

Since vertigo is due to a disturbance of spatial orientation, a brief review of the organization of this function is desirable. The maintenance of an appropriate position of the body in space depends in man upon several groups of afferent impulses, of which the following are the most important.

1. From the retinae are derived visual impulses which, in contributing to our perception of visual space, are intimately concerned in spatial orientation.

2. The labyrinth is a highly specialized spatial proprioceptor. The otoliths are mainly concerned in the orientation of the organism with reference to gravity, while the semicircular canals respond to movement and to angular momentum.

3. The proprioceptors of the joints and muscles of the neck are of importance

in relating labyrinthine impulses, which convey information solely concerning the position of the head, to the attitude of the rest of the body.

4. The proprioceptors of the lower limbs and trunk are concerned with the position of the body in relation to the acts of sitting, standing, and walking.

The afferent impulses derived from these various sense organs are mutually related by central mechanisms, of which the cerebellum, the vestibular nuclei, the medial longitudinal fasciculus, and the red nuclei are probably the most important, and which constitute reflex paths by which the position of the body is normally appropriately orientated. From these lower centres impulses reach the cerebral cortex mainly in the temporal and parietal lobes and so influence voluntary movement. Vertigo may result from the disordered function either of the sensory end-organs or of the afferent paths or of the central mechanisms concerned.

THE CAUSES OF VERTIGO

It is clear from the anatomical and physiological considerations outlined above that vertigo may be the result of a disturbance of function at many different levels. We may therefore recognize (1) psychogenic vertigo, (2) vertigo due to cortical disturbances, (3) vertigo of ocular origin, (4) vertigo of cerebellar origin, (5) vertigo due to brain-stem lesions, (6) vertigo due to lesions of the eighth nerve, and (7) aural vertigo. In diffuse conditions, such as head injury and circulatory disease, it may be difficult to say what is the site of origin of the symptoms.

Psychogenic Vertigo

'Giddiness' is a common symptom among sufferers from anxiety neurosis. There is no sensation of rotation but the symptom consists of a feeling of instability associated with a sense of anxiety and the symptoms of over-activity of the sympathetic nervous system. Vertigo may also occur as a conversion symptom in hysteria.

Vertigo due to Cortical Disturbances

The aura of an epileptic attack may be a feeling of giddiness, as is not uncommon in minor epilepsy of temporal lobe origin. Vertigo may also occur in basilar artery migraine and in association with localized cerebral lesions. It may be caused by an intracranial tumour in any situation.

Vertigo of Ocular Origin

Vertigo may occur in normal individuals in consequence of unusual visual perceptions. Giddiness at heights and on looking from the platform at a swiftly moving train are examples of this. Paralysis of one or more external ocular muscles is often associated with vertigo. This is due to the spatial disorientation which is produced by false projection of the visual fields [see p. 77].

Vertigo of Cerebellar Origin

Vertigo may be slight or absent in spite of a massive lesion of the cerebellum, especially if this is limited to the lateral lobe. A cerebellar lesion is most likely to cause vertigo when it involves the flocculonodular lobe which is closely linked anatomically with the vestibular system. Thus severe vertigo may occur at the onset of thrombosis of the posterior inferior cerebellar artery and it is an invariable symptom in primary intracerebellar haemorrhage.

Vertigo due to Brain-Stem Lesions

Vascular or neoplastic lesions of the brain stem may cause vertigo if they involve the vestibular connexions. A plaque of multiple sclerosis in the pons may cause severe vertigo with conspicuous nystagmus, vomiting, and prostration: so too may syringobulbia. There is evidence that streptomycin may damage the vestibular nuclei and the Purkinje cells and nuclei of the cerebellum, and this is probably the cause of the vertigo and ataxia which may follow the administration of this antibiotic (see Winston *et al.*, 1948; Burns and Westlake, 1949). Transitory ischaemia of the brain stem is the probable cause of the vertigo evoked by head movement in patients with atheroma of the vertebral arteries especially in the presence of cervical spondylosis.

Vestibular Neuronitis and Epidemic Vertigo

Dix and Hallpike (1952) have applied the term vestibular neuronitis to a disorder causing paroxysmal vertigo or a sense of loss of balance while walking and unassociated with deafness or tinnitus. Tests of cochlear function showed no abnormality: the caloric vestibular responses, however, were abnormal, often grossly so, on one or both sides. The onset was often associated with an infective illness and the prognosis was good.

Epidemic vertigo produces a very similar clinical picture occurring in epidemics sometimes with symptoms of gastro-intestinal or respiratory infection. There is evidence that it may be due to a mild encephalitis affecting the brain stem (Leishman, 1955; Pedersen, 1959).

Vertigo due to Lesions of the Eighth Nerve

Since the eighth nerve carries the vestibular fibres, lesions of this nerve may cause giddiness associated with deafness and tinnitus. The commonest such lesion is an acoustic neuroma, but the nerve may also be compressed by abnormal vessels or involved in inflammation in meningitis or meningovascular syphilis.

Aural Vertigo

The agencies which may cause vertigo by disturbing the functions of the labyrinth are numerous. They include (1) wax in the external acoustic meatus, (2) blockage of the Eustachian tube and sudden changes in atmospheric pressure, (3) acute and chronic suppurative otitis media, (4) otosclerosis, (5) drugs, especially quinine and salicylate, (6) impairment of blood supply due to atheroma with or without high blood pressure, vasomotor instability, severe anaemia and increased intracranial pressure, (7) head injury, (8) herpes zoster of the geniculate ganglion, (9) acute non-suppurative labyrinthitis, (10) recurrent aural vertigo (Ménière's syndrome), (11) motion-sickness, (12) benign positional vertigo.

Benign Positional Vertigo

Benign positional vertigo usually comes on acutely between the ages of 30 and 60. It is attributed to irritation of the otolith apparatus, and may be associated with middle-ear disease or labyrinthine trauma. Giddiness occurs on head movement and may be evoked by the test described on page 179. The prognosis on the whole is good.

MÉNIÈRE'S DISEASE

Definition. The characteristic feature is the recurrence of attacks of severe giddiness leading to vomiting and prostration, and usually associated with tinnitus and increasing deafness. The disorder runs a protracted course with a tendency to disappearance of the vertigo as the deafness increases. All these characteristics were described by Ménière (1860–1).

AETIOLOGY AND PATHOLOGY

Men suffer from Ménière's syndrome more often than women in a proportion of about 3 to 2. It is a disorder of middle age, especially late middle age, the average age of onset being 49, and more than one-third of all patients are first affected after the age of 60. Little is certainly known about the aetiology. Focal sepsis in the teeth, tonsils, and nasal sinuses is certainly important in some cases. The affinity between recurrent aural vertigo and migraine was first pointed out by Ménière himself. Allergy may possibly be a common basis in some cases (Atkinson, 1941, 1943).

Pathological investigations by Hallpike and Cairns (1938) demonstrated a gross dilatation of the endolymph system of the internal ear, the cause of which is unknown.

SYMPTOMS

The usual history is that the patient has suffered from slowly progressive deafness and tinnitus in one or both ears for months or even years, and then suddenly has an attack of giddiness. In some cases the giddiness develops so rapidly that the patient may fall; more often it takes a few minutes to become severe. In a severe attack the patient is literally prostrated, and there is an intense sensation of rotation of the surroundings, less often of the patient himself. Vomiting soon develops with severe nausea, and lasts as long as the patient remains giddy. Rarely there is also diarrhoea. The pulse may be rapid or slow, and the blood pressure raised or lowered, and there may be profuse sweating. Double vision may occur, and in very severe cases consciousness may be lost. Deafness and tinnitus are sometimes intensified during the attack. The vertigo may last from half an hour to many hours, and then gradually subsides. On attempting to stand and walk the patient is unsteady and staggers.

During the attack the patient usually lies on the sound side and exhibits a rotary nystagmus which is most evident on looking towards the affected ear. In the intervals between the attacks giddiness is liable to be brought on by sudden movements of the head and there is often a fine rotary nystagmus on extreme lateral fixation to either side. There may be some persistent unsteadiness, indicated by an inability to stand steadily with the eyes closed or to walk heel-and-toe. Deafness may be unilateral or bilateral. Both air- and bone-conduction are usually impaired and there is a selective loss of the higher tones. Loudness recruitment is always present.

The common response to the caloric test is a canal paresis in the ear with the worse hearing. Directional preponderance is less frequent. Less often still both are present.

DIAGNOSIS

Aural vertigo may sometimes be confused with minor epilepsy, but when giddiness is a symptom of the latter condition the attacks last only a few seconds, consciousness is always impaired or lost, and the giddiness disappears as rapidly as it develops. In Ménière's disease tinnitus and some impairment of hearing are almost always present, and a lesion which involves both the cochlear and the vestibular functions must be situated either in the internal ear or in the eighth nerve. A lesion in the latter situation almost always interferes with the functions of the facial nerve, and often of the fifth nerve on the same side as well as of the cerebellum. When vertigo is due to lesions of the brain stem or cerebellum hearing is usually unimpaired and other symptoms of lesions in these situations are usually present.

PROGNOSIS

The attacks tend to recur at irregular intervals and with varying severity. Usually the intervals of freedom last only a few weeks; in rare cases the patient is free from attacks for years. There is a tendency for the attacks to diminish in severity spontaneously, and finally to cease *pari passu* with an increase of the deafness. Exceptionally, in the absence of radical treatment, the attacks continue for many years.

TREATMENT

During an attack the patient must rest lying perfectly still. An intramuscular injection of 50 mg. of chlorpromazine will relieve the discomfort in severe cases. Phenobarbitone, prochlorperazine and various antihistamines are used as vestibular sedatives. Some advocate vasodilators, and histamine itself. A careful search for focal sepsis in the teeth, tonsils, or nasal sinuses should be carried out and any infection found appropriately treated. A salt-free diet combined with a restriction of fluid intake may be helpful. The patient should be warned about the risk of a sudden attack. If, after six months, there is no response to medical measures, and especially if the vertigo incapacitates him from following his occupation, surgical treatment should be considered. Section of the vestibular nerve abolishes the vertigo while preserving the hearing and the tinnitus. Ultrasonic irradiation destroys vestibular function. Some reduction of hearing occurs in one-third of cases. Endolymphatic subarachnoid shunt is a method of correcting the causal endolymphatic hydrops with good results (House, 1962). Removal of the utricle is a simple method of destroying vestibular function, suitable when hearing is already seriously impaired since it also causes deafness.

REFERENCES

ATKINSON, M. (1941) Observations on the aetiology and treatment of Ménière's syndrome, *J. Amer. med. Ass.*, **116**, 1753.

ATKINSON, M. (1943) Ménière and migraine. Observations on a common causal relationship, *Ann. intern. Med.*, **18**, 797.

BRAIN, W. R. (1938) Vertigo. Its neurological, otological, circulatory, and surgical aspects, *Brit. med. J.*, **2**, 605.

BURNS, P. A., and WESTLAKE, R. E. (1949) in *Streptomycin*, ed. Waksman, S. A., p. 524, Baltimore.

CAIRNS, H., and BRAIN, W. R. (1933) Aural vertigo. Treatment by division of eighth nerve, *Lancet*, i, 946.

CAWTHORNE, T. E., FITZGERALD, G., and HALLPIKE, C. S. (1942) Studies in human vestibular function: III. Observations on the clinical features of 'Ménière's' disease: with especial reference to the results of the caloric tests, *Brain*, **65**, 161.

DANDY, W. E. (1933) Treatment of Ménière's disease by section of only the vestibular portion of the acoustic nerve, *Bull. Johns Hopk. Hosp.*, **53**, 52.

DANDY, W. E. (1934) Ménière's disease, *Arch. Otolaryng. (Chicago)*, **20**, 1.

DANDY, W. E. (1937) Pathologic changes in Ménière's disease, *J. Amer. med. Ass.*, **108**, 931.

DIX, M. R., and HALLPIKE, C. S. (1952) The pathology, symptomatology and diagnosis of certain disorders of the vestibular system, *Proc. roy. Soc. Med.*, **45**, 341.

FITZGERALD, G., and HALLPIKE, C. S. (1942) Studies in human vestibular function: II. Observations on the directional preponderance ('Nystagmusbereitschaft') of caloric nystagmus resulting from cerebral lesions, *Brain*, **65**, 115.

FRAZIER, C. S., and ROWE, S. N. (1934) Certain observations upon the localization in 51 verified tumours of the temporal lobe. In *A.R.N.M.D.* Localization of function in the cerebral cortex, p. 251, Baltimore.

HALLPIKE, C. S. (1965) Clinical otoneurology and its contributions to theory and practice, *Proc. roy. Soc. Med.*, **58**, 185.

HALLPIKE, C. S., and CAIRNS, H. (1937–8) Observations on the pathology of Ménière's syndrome, *Proc. roy. Soc. Med.*, **31**, 1317, also (1938) *J. Laryng.*, **53**, 625.

HOUSE, W. F. (1962) Subarachnoid shunt for drainage of endolymphatic hydrops, a preliminary report, *Laryngoscope*, **72**, 713.

LEISHMAN, A. W. D. (1955) 'Epidemic vertigo' with oculomotor complication, *Lancet*, i, 228.

PEDERSEN, E. (1959) Epidemic vertigo, *Brain*, **82**, 566.

WINSTON, J., LEWEY, F. H., PARENTEAU, A., MARDEN, P. A., and CRAMER, F. B. (1948) An experimental study of the toxic effects of streptomycin on the vestibular apparatus of the cat, *Ann. Otol. (St. Louis)*, **57**, 738.

WRIGHT, A. J. (1938) Aural vertigo, *J. Laryng.*, **53**, 97.

WRIGHT, A. J. (1938) Labyrinthine giddiness: its nature and treatment, *Brit. med. J.*, **1**, 668.

THE NINTH OR GLOSSOPHARYNGEAL NERVE

The glossopharyngeal nerve contains both sensory and motor fibres. The ganglion cells of the former are situated in the inferior ganglion of the nerve. Their central processes mostly pass into the tractus solitarius and terminate in the nucleus of this tract. A few also enter the dorsal nucleus of the vagus. The motor fibres originate partly in the inferior salivary nucleus and partly in the nucleus ambiguus. The glossopharyngeal nerve arises by a series of radicles from the posterior lateral sulcus of the medulla between the fibres of origin of the vagus and accessory nerves [FIG. 31]. After crossing the posterior fossa

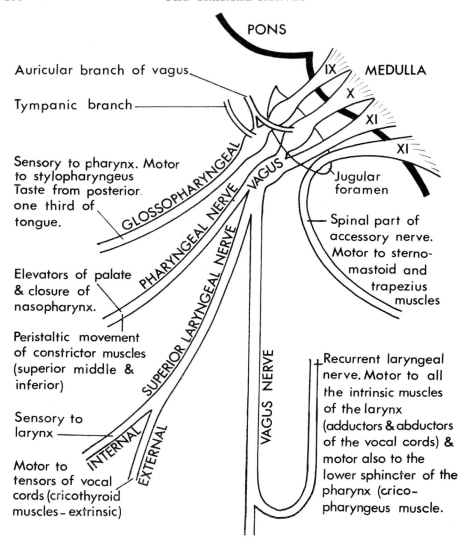

FIG. 31. The motor and sensory nerves supplying the pharynx and larynx, explaining the various patterns of paralysis commonly met with. (Redrawn from an original drawing by Mr. Charles Keogh.)

of the skull it emerges through the anterior compartment of the jugular foramen. In the neck it arches downwards and forwards between the internal carotid artery and the internal jugular vein, and then between the internal and external carotid arteries to the side of the pharynx. Within the skull it gives off the tympanic nerve which enters the tympanic cavity, to which it supplies sensation, and joins the tympanic plexus, from which the lesser petrosal nerve carries to the otic ganglion fibres which excite salivary secretion. In the neck the glossopharyngeal nerve gives a branch to the stylopharyngeus muscle, its sole motor supply, and branches to the mucous membrane of the pharynx. The terminal branches of the nerve supply the tonsil, the lower border and posterior surface of the soft palate, and the posterior third of the tongue. The glossopharyngeal nerve is thus the motor nerve of the stylopharyngeus and carries fibres concerned in the secretion of saliva, especially by the parotid gland. It supplies common sensibility to the posterior third of the tongue, the tonsils, and the pharynx, and taste-fibres to the same region.

Isolated lesions of the glossopharyngeal nerve are almost unknown. It is most frequently damaged in association with the vagus and accessory nerves at the jugular foramen (see below).

GLOSSOPHARYNGEAL NEURALGIA

The glossopharyngeal nerve is occasionally subject to paroxysmal neuralgia, which in its general characteristics resembles the much commoner paroxysmal trigeminal neuralgia. We owe the recognition of this syndrome to Harris. As in trigeminal neuralgia, the pain occurs in brief attacks, which may be of great severity. It usually begins in the side of the throat and radiates down the side of the neck in front of the ear and to the back of the lower jaw. Exceptionally, the pain may begin deep in the ear. Attacks tend to be precipitated by swallowing or by protruding the tongue, and the ear may be extremely sensitive to touch.

Glossopharyngeal neuralgia is distinguished from trigeminal neuralgia by the situation of the pain and the precipitation of the attacks by swallowing. Pain of a similar distribution may occur as a result of new growths involving the tonsil and pharynx, and this cause must therefore be excluded. In glossopharyngeal neuralgia there is often a long history of pain.

Carbamazepine (*Tegretol*) in doses of 200 mg. three or four times daily may completely control the pain. If it fails, treatment consists in interruption of the afferent fibres of the nerve. Harris has successfully injected the nerve with alcohol after its emergence from the skull, but this is a difficult procedure, and does not reach the fibres of the tympanic nerve which leave the glossopharyngeal within the skull. To obtain permanent relief it is better to carry out surgical avulsion of the nerve, which may be performed in the neck when the pain is predominantly pharyngeal, but should be carried out intracranially in the posterior fossa when the deep part of the ear also is the site of pain (Jefferson, 1931). Chawla and Falconer (1967) give reasons for suggesting that the condition is more aptly named glossopharyngeal and vagal neuralgia as the areas of supply of the auricular and pharyngeal branches of the vagus nerve are also involved. They recommend intracranial section of the glossopharyngeal nerve and of the upper two rootlets of the vagus as the operation of choice.

REFERENCES

ADSON, A. W. (1924) The surgical treatment of glossopharyngeal neuralgia, *Arch. Neurol. Psychiat.* (*Chicago*), **12**, 487.

CHAWLA, J. C., and FALCONER, M. A. (1967) Glossopharyngeal and vagal neuralgia, *Brit. med. J.*, **3**, 529.

DANA, C. L. (1926) The story of the glossopharyngeal nerve and four centuries of research concerning the cranial nerves of man, *Arch. Neurol. Psychiat.* (*Chicago*), **15**, 675.

DANDY, W. E. (1927) Glossopharyngeal neuralgia (tic douloureux), *Arch. Surg.* (*Chicago*), **15**, 198.

FAY, T. (1927–8) Observations and results from intracranial section of the glossopharyngeus and vagus nerves in man, *J. Neurol. Psychopath.*, **8**, 110.

HARRIS, W. (1926) *Neuritis and Neuralgia*, London.

JEFFERSON, G. (1931) Glossopharyngeal neuralgia, *Lancet*, ii, 397.

STOOKEY, B. (1928) Glossopharyngeal neuralgia, *Arch. Neurol. Psychiat.* (*Chicago*), **20**, 702.

THE SENSE OF TASTE

There are only four tastes: sweet, salt, bitter, and acid. All other flavours are olfactory sensations.

The sense of taste is tested by means of weak solutions of sugar, common salt, quinine, and acetic acid or vinegar. The patient must keep his tongue protruded and must reply to questions by nodding or shaking his head. It is convenient to have the names of the four tastes written on cards, to which he can point. The protruded tongue is dried and a drop of the testing solution applied to the lateral border on one side. The patient is then asked to indicate what he tastes. The anterior two-thirds and the posterior one-third of the tongue must be tested separately. The tongue is dried between successive tests.

THE TASTE FIBRES

PERIPHERAL PATH

The peripheral path of the taste fibres is still a matter of controversy. Their usual route is probably as follows. The fibres carrying taste impulses from the anterior two-thirds of the tongue pass at first through the lingual nerve to the chorda tympani, through which they reach the facial nerve, and the geniculate ganglion which contains their ganglion cells. From the geniculate ganglion they pass to the pons by the nervus intermedius. In certain cases alcoholic injection of the trigeminal ganglion and third division of the trigeminal nerve at the foramen ovale has been followed by loss of taste on the anterior two-thirds of the tongue, though this loss is often only temporary. It is possible that the loss of taste in such circumstances is not due to an interruption of the taste fibres but to secondary trophic effects on the tongue of the lesion of the mandibular nerve. On the other hand, it has been suggested that the taste fibres, after reaching the geniculate ganglion by the route already described, pass by the lesser petrosal nerve to the otic ganglion, and ultimately reach the pons through the third division of the fifth nerve.

Taste fibres from the posterior one-third of the tongue, from the pharynx, and from the lower border of the soft palate are carried by the glossopharyngeal nerve.

CENTRAL CONNEXIONS

The taste fibres after entering the pons pass into the tractus solitarius, the upper part of which, sometimes called the gustatory nucleus of the trigeminal, may receive taste fibres from the trigeminal nerve, while the middle part receives fibres from the nervus intermedius, and the lower part fibres from the glossopharyngeal. The fibres of the tractus solitarius terminate in a column of grey matter known as the nucleus of this tract, from which relay-neurones arise, which cross the midline and turn upwards in the tegmentum of the pons and medulla to form the gustatory lemniscus, which lies near the midline to the outer side of the medial longitudinal fasciculus. The gustatory lemniscus ascends to the thalamus, from which taste fibres are further relayed to the cortical centre for taste at the foot of the postcentral gyrus.

LOSS OF TASTE

Loss of taste—ageusia—on the anterior two-thirds of the tongue may occur as a result of lesions of the chorda tympani or of the geniculate ganglion and in some cases of the mandibular nerve. There is no clear evidence as to whether or not it results from lesions of the nervus intermedius. Lesions of the glossopharyngeal nerve cause loss of taste on the posterior one-third of the tongue. Lesions of the tractus solitarius and its nucleus cause unilateral ageusia, and lesions near the midline of the pons may cause bilateral loss of taste from destruction of both gustatory lemnisci (Harris).

Little is known with regard to loss of taste resulting from cerebral lesions, though taste is occasionally lost, together with the sense of smell, as a result of head injury. Sumner (1967) has recently described 10 cases of post-traumatic ageusia, 9 of which also had anosmia and has postulated the existence of a cerebral centre for both taste and smell which may be damaged by head injury. Rarely ageusia follows bilateral thalamotomy for Parkinsonism.

Hallucinations of taste may occur in association with those of smell as a result of an irritative lesion involving the neighbourhood of the uncus. Lesions in this region may also cause parageusia, a perversion of taste in which many substances possess the same unpleasant flavour.

REFERENCES

HARRIS, W. (1926) *Neuritis and Neuralgia*, London.
SCHWARTZ, H. G., and WEDDELL, G. (1938) Observations in the pathways transmitting the sensation of taste, *Brain*, **61**, 99.
SUMNER, D. (1967) Post-traumatic ageusia, *Brain*, **90**, 187.

THE TENTH OR VAGUS NERVE

CENTRAL CONNEXIONS

The vagus nerve contains both sensory and motor fibres. The ganglion cells of the former are situated in the superior ganglion and in the inferior ganglion of the nerve. The cells of the superior ganglion are concerned in the supply of common sensibility to part of the external ear and terminate in relation with the spinal tract of the trigeminal nerve and its nucleus. The cells of the inferior ganglion are concerned in the carriage of afferent impulses from the pharynx, larynx, trachea, oesophagus, and thoracic and abdominal viscera. Their central processes terminate in relation with the tractus solitarius, and the dorsal nucleus of the vagus. The motor fibres of the vagus are derived from two nuclei in the medulla. The dorsal nucleus of the vagus is situated near the midline, a little beneath the floor of the fourth ventricle. It sends fibres to the para-sympathetic ganglia of the vagal plexuses for the innervation of the thoracic and abdominal viscera. The nucleus ambiguus is an elongated column of grey matter situated deep in the medulla between the dorsal accessory olive and the spinal nucleus of the trigeminal nerve. Its fibres are distributed through the glossopharyngeal, vagus, and accessory nerves to the striated muscles of the palate, pharynx, and larynx.

PERIPHERAL DISTRIBUTION

THE VAGUS TRUNK

The vagus leaves the medulla by a series of radicles at the anterior margin of the inferior cerebellar peduncle and in series with the roots of the glossopharyn-geal nerve above and the accessory below [FIG. 31]. The roots form a single trunk, which leaves the skull through the jugular foramen, in which it occupies the same compartment as the accessory nerve. Within the neck it occupies the carotid sheath, lying behind the carotid arteries and the internal jugular vein. It enters the thorax behind the large veins, on the right side crossing over the subclavian artery, on the left side occupying the interval between the left common carotid and subclavian arteries. In the thorax the relations of the two nerves differ. The right nerve passes downwards beside the brachiocephalic trunk and the trachea and behind the right brachiocephalic vein and superior vena cava to the posterior surface of the root of the lung. The left nerve passes downwards between the left common carotid and subclavian arteries and behind the left brachiocephalic vein and the phrenic nerve. It passes over the aortic arch to the posterior surface of the root of the left lung. In the posterior mediastinum both nerves contribute to the pulmonary and oesophageal plexuses, and at the oesophageal opening of the diaphragm they enter the abdomen, the left nerve in front of the oesophagus and the right behind it, and terminate by supplying the stomach and other abdominal organs.

Branches. The superior ganglion of the vagus gives off a meningeal branch, which supplies the dura mater of the posterior fossa, and an auricular branch which supplies common sensibility to the back of the auricle and external acoustic meatus. The inferior ganglion supplies a pharyngeal branch which combines with the pharyngeal branches of the glossopharyngeal and superior cervical ganglion of the sympathetic to form the pharyngeal plexus, to which it contributes motor fibres destined for the muscles of the pharynx and soft palate, except the stylopharyngeus and the tensor veli palatini. The superior laryngeal nerve is derived from the inferior ganglion, and divides into internal and external branches. The internal laryngeal branch is the principal sensory nerve of the larynx. The external laryngeal branch, after supplying fibres to the inferior constrictor of the pharynx, innervates the cricothyroid muscle.

Within the neck the vagus gives off cardiac branches, and the recurrent laryngeal nerves, which pursue a different course on the two sides. The right recurrent laryngeal nerve arises at the root of the neck, where the vagus crosses the subclavian artery, around which it passes upwards and immediately behind the subclavian, the common carotid, and the thyroid gland. The left recurrent laryngeal nerve leaves the vagus as it crosses the aortic arch, and after passing beneath the arch turns upwards in the superior mediastinum, between the trachea and the oesophagus to the neck, where its course is the same as that of the right nerve. The terminal branches of the recurrent laryngeal nerves innervate all the muscles of the larynx (with the exception of the cricothyroid muscles, and possibly some fibres of the transverse arytenoid muscles), and also supply the cricopharyngeus muscles which form the lower sphincter of the pharynx.

SYMPTOMS OF LESIONS OF THE VAGUS
THE PHARYNX AND LARYNX

The function and neurology of the pharynx and larynx are so closely linked together that it is best to consider them together.

A common form of paralysis involves the soft palate, the three constrictors of the pharynx, the larynx, and the lower sphincter of the pharynx, often on one side only. The difficulties that a patient experiences in the way of postnasal catarrh, snoring, coughing and clearing the voice, and swallowing, will not be understood unless this is realized.

The pharynx functions as a muscular peristaltic tube in the second (involuntary) stage of deglutition. In the anterior wall of the pharynx are (a) the opening into the mouth and the back of the tongue, and (b) the opening into the larynx, and the thyroid and cricoid cartilages. Above is the nasopharyngeal sphincter, separating the pharynx from the nasal passages, and below is the cricopharyngeal sphincter, separating the pharynx from the oesophagus. During respiration the nasopharyngeal sphincter and the larynx remain open and the cricopharyngeal sphincter is closed. In the act of swallowing the nasopharyngeal sphincter and the larynx are closed, and the cricopharyngeal sphincter opens.

PARALYSIS OF THE PALATE

The motor fibres to the soft palate originate in the upper part of the nucleus ambiguus and leave the vagus trunk at the inferior ganglion, just below the jugular foramen, in the pharyngeal nerve. Lesions of the vagus above the ganglion, or lesions involving the pharyngeal nerves, cause paralysis of the palate. It must be remembered that the tensors of the palate are supplied by the fifth nerve, and are unaffected by lesions of the vagus.

Unilateral palatal paralysis causes few apparent symptoms, because of the efficient compensation by the paired unparalysed muscles of the opposite side. Nevertheless the slight changes may be of importance to the patient: postnasal catarrh due to inefficient drainage of the nasopharynx, snoring, slight changes in phonation in singers, and ultimately slight changes in hearing because of inefficient function of the Eustachian tube on the same side.

Unilateral paralysis is detected on examination of the throat by the fact that when the patient phonates, for example in saying 'ah', elevation of the palate fails to occur on the affected side, and the uvula is drawn over to the normal side.

Bilateral palatal paralysis causes regurgitation of food into the nose on swallowing, because the nasopharyngeal sphincter fails to close off the nasal passages. The voice takes on a nasal resonance for the same reason, and there is an alteration in the pronunciation of consonants for the correct utterance of which the nasal passages should be occluded. This is most evident in the pronunciation of *b* and *g*, *rub* becoming *rum*, and *egg*, *eng*. There is a tendency to mouth-breathing and snoring at night, and there is difficulty in draining mucus from the nasal passages into the pharynx. There is no elevation of the paralysed palate, and the palatal reflex is lost.

The commonest causes of palatal paralysis are poliomyelitis affecting the nuclei in the medulla, diphtheria affecting the nerve endings, and brain-stem infarction. 'Nystagmus' of the soft palate, a rhythmical myoclonus, forms part of a syndrome associated with lesions of the olivodentate system [see p. 955].

PARALYSIS OF THE PHARYNX

The motor fibres to the three paired constrictors of the pharynx, which are the muscles mainly responsible for propelling food into the oesophagus, originate in the middle part of the nucleus ambiguus and leave the vagus trunk at the inferior ganglion. Lesions above the ganglion cause pharyngeal paralysis. The palatal muscles (superior sphincter of the pharynx), the laryngeal muscles (sphincter of the larynx), and the cricopharyngeal muscles (lower sphincter of the pharynx), are often involved in the same lesion. The pharyngeal wall droops on the affected side, and the pharyngeal reflex is present only on the unaffected side.

There is a tendency to collect frothy mucus above the opening of the oeso-phagus indicating delay in emptying the pharynx into the oesophagus. This mucus overflows into the larynx causing troublesome efforts to clear the voice, and difficulty with swallowing. Compensation by the constrictor muscles on the unaffected side is often efficient, but the patient will find it easier to sleep on the affected side to prevent irritation to the larynx from mucus, and there is always difficulty in clearing the throat, and swallowing has to be deliberate.

Bilateral pharyngeal paralysis causes marked dysphagia and bilateral loss of the pharyngeal reflex. Soft pulpy foods are sometimes more readily swallowed than the usual solids and liquids.

PARALYSIS OF THE LARYNX

The motor fibres to the larynx originate in the lowest part of the nucleus ambiguus and some at least probably leave the medulla by the accessory fibres of the accessory nerve, subsequently joining the vagus in the jugular foramen. The fibres destined for the cricothyroid muscle, which acts as a tensor of the vocal cords, leave the vagus by the superior laryngeal nerve and reach the muscle through its external branch. Fibres which innervate the abductors and adductors of the vocal cords leave the vagus by the recurrent laryngeal nerves.

Abduction of the vocal cords occurs during inspiration, and the cords are adducted in phonation and coughing. Reflex adduction occurs in response to irritation of the larynx.

Supranuclear Lesions

Little is known regarding the occurrence of paralysis of the larynx as a result of supranuclear lesions. Hemiplegia does not impair the movement of the vocal cords. Bilateral lesions involving the laryngeal centre in the cortex at the base of the precentral gyrus may do so. In such cases respiratory and reflex laryngeal movements are unaffected.

Nuclear and Infranuclear Lesions

The old terms adductor and abductor paralysis are misleading. The position of the vocal cords in varying forms of paralysis depends upon the site of the lesion, and the extent to which different peripheral nerves are involved, and whether wasting of paralysed muscles has taken place. The ability of the larynx to overcome the handicap of varying forms of paralysis is a remarkable example of compensation by unparalysed muscle groups.

The following varieties of laryngeal paralysis may occur:

Unilateral Paralysis. (1) If the lesion affects the recurrent laryngeal nerve on one side only, there will be paralysis of all the muscles of the larynx with the exception of the tensors of the cords (cricothyroids) which are supplied by the external branch of the superior laryngeal nerve. The lower sphincter of the pharynx (cricopharyngeus) will also be paralysed on the same side. The appearance of the larynx when viewed through a laryngeal mirror shortly after the lesion [FIG. 32] shows a paralysed vocal cord lying near the midline, with the unparalysed cord coming across to meet it when the patient tries to say E. There will be pooling of frothy mucus round the opening of the oesophagus on the same side, showing delay in emptying the pharynx into the oesophagus. As compensation becomes established, this tendency to collect mucus may disappear. At first there is slight weakness of the voice and slight difficulty with swallowing fluids, but compensation by the unparalysed paired muscles is so efficient that the voice may appear normal, although it may tend to tire. For this reason unilateral paralysis of the larynx often remains undiagnosed. Slight movement can be seen on the affected side, because the tensors of the paralysed cord are still functioning, and the paralysed arytenoid will come to lie just in front of the arytenoid on the unparalysed side. This is a useful diagnostic aid. The presence of some motor fibres running in the internal branch of the superior laryngeal nerve to the transversus arytenoideus has been suggested, and this could account for some of the slight movements seen in the affected cord.

(2) If the lesion involves the superior laryngeal nerve as well as the recurrent laryngeal nerve (that is between the nucleus ambiguus and the inferior ganglion of the vagus) total paralysis of one half of the larynx will be present. Paralysis of the pharynx and palate on the same side will almost always be present, because the pharyngeal branch of the vagus is involved in the lesion. The vocal cord on the affected side will lie at rest slightly to one side of the midline, and the arytenoid cartilage on the same side will appear to lie in front of its fellow on the opposite side, and will often bend slightly inwards over the vocal process. There will be frothy mucus round the opening of the oesophagus. Cinematograph X-rays of patients swallowing opaque meals show that there is a tendency for the majority of the food to pass down one piriform recess into the oesophagus. The cricopharyngeus is seen to close firmly, shutting off the pharynx from the oesophagus, and oesophageal peristalsis continues to propel

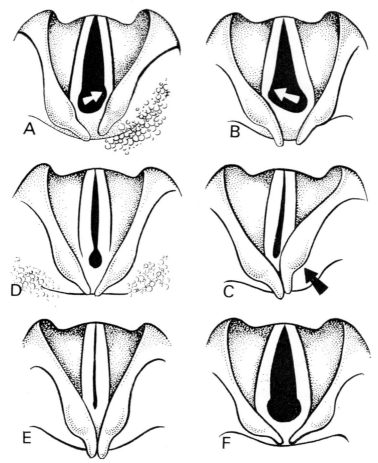

FIG. 32. Paralysis of the Larynx
(as seen through a laryngeal mirror)

(A) Paralysis of the left recurrent laryngeal nerve. (Neurofibroma)
    The paralysed arytenoid always lies slightly in front of the non-paralysed right arytenoid. Froth tends to collect round the opening of the oesophagus, owing to paralysis of the left cricopharyngeus muscle (lower sphincter of the pharynx, supplied by the same recurrent laryngeal nerve). On adduction the non-paralysed right vocal cord moves across to meet the paralysed left cord.

(B) Paralysis of the right recurrent laryngeal nerve. (Thyroidectomy)
    There is no collected froth at the opening of the oesophagus because compensation is so good by the intact left paired cricopharyngeus muscle that it has been able to overcome the delay due to the paralysis of the right cricopharyngeus muscle.

(c) The same case showing closure of the larynx on adduction.
    The left non-paralysed cord now moves up to the paralysed cord, and the non-paralysed arytenoid now lies in front of the paralysed arytenoid.

(D) Paralysis of both vocal cords at the same time. (Thyroidectomy)
    The cords are held in adduction because their muscles are all paralysed except for the chief tensors of the cords, the cricothyroid muscles (supplied by the external branch of the superior laryngeal nerve).

(E) Normal closure of the vocal cords as seen in a laryngeal mirror.

(F) Normal abduction of the vocal cords as seen in a laryngeal mirror.

(Redrawn from an original drawing by Mr. Charles Keogh.)

the food down the oesophagus. If the cricopharyngeus muscle is paralysed partly, or wholly, there is inefficient closure of this sphincter of the cricopharyngeus, and some food regurgitates back into the pharynx. This accounts for the presence of frothy mucus in the lower pharynx in paralysis of the recurrent laryngeal nerves.

Bilateral Paralysis. This may be produced by bilateral lesions at any point between the nucleus ambiguus and the recurrent laryngeal nerves, but if the paralysis is really complete the lesions must be above the inferior ganglion of the vagus on both sides.

1. If the bilateral lesions are below the inferior ganglion, the motor fibres in the superior laryngeal nerve will escape, and the main tensors of both cords will then be intact and unopposed, because all the other muscles are paralysed. As described above, some motor fibres may run in the internal branch of the superior laryngeal nerve to the transversus arytenoideus. The cords are held close together, not more than 2 mm. apart. Some apparent adduction can take place because the tensors are active, but abduction is impossible. There is pooling of mucus at the opening of the oesophagus indicating delay in emptying the pharynx into the oesophagus, because the lower sphincter of the pharynx (cricopharyngeus) is paralysed. The voice is weak but remarkably clear; there is dyspnoea on exertion, and inspiratory stridor on deep inspiration [FIG. 33]. Patients differ very greatly in their disabilities, some being unable to under-

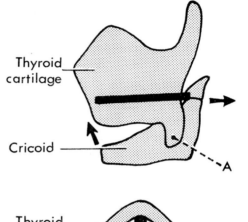

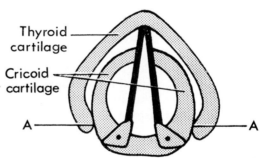

FIG. 33. Diagram of the mechanism of the larynx to explain why there is severe respiratory stridor when both recurrent laryngeal nerves are paralysed. The unopposed contraction of the non-paralysed cricothyroid muscles tilt the posterior border of the cricoid cartilage backwards, tensing the vocal cords and drawing them together.
A–A shows the axis of tilt.

take ordinary duties without stridor and breathlessness and distress, whilst others manage very well except for breathlessness on exertion, and distress during upper respiratory infections.

2. If bilateral paralysis of the larynx is complete, the lesions must involve both superior laryngeal nerves and both recurrent laryngeal nerves. The lesions are usually above the inferior ganglion of the vagus on both sides, or involve all four of the above peripheral nerves. Paralysis of the palate and pharynx often accompanies complete bilateral paralysis of the larynx. The cords are immobile and lie just to the side of the midline in the so-called cadaveric position.

The voice is weak but clear. The airway is adequate for most normal duties. There is difficulty in clearing the cords of mucus, coughing is not efficient, and swallowing is difficult partly because there is overflow into the paralysed larynx, and partly because there is paralysis of the cricopharyngeus and the pharynx cannot empty itself properly.

Speech in Laryngeal Paralysis

It must be remembered that patients can develop quite astonishingly good voices after complete removal of the larynx for carcinoma with permanent tracheostomy. With practice, air is sucked into the open oesophagus on deep inspiration, and expelled through folds in the pharynx. It is not surprising therefore that patients retain remarkably clear voices in all forms of paralysis of the vocal cords, even though the voice may be weak and hoarse.

Recovery in Paralysis of the Recurrent Laryngeal Nerves

Paralysis of the recurrent laryngeal nerves most commonly follows thyroid operations or results from poliomyelitis or from involvement of the left nerve in the mediastinum by lymph node metastases from bronchial carcinoma. Occasionally paralysis of one nerve may take place without any apparent cause, even after exhaustive and skilled examination. It is probable that forms of paralysis of this nerve resemble Bell's palsy in the facial nerve. Recovery can take place after paralysis of the recurrent laryngeal nerves. Axons may be ruptured during thyroid operations without loss of gross continuity of the epineurium of a recurrent laryngeal nerve. This is shown when recovery takes place after paralysis. Degrees of paralysis may depend on the number of axons damaged in a single recurrent nerve. After prolonged paralysis of the larynx, wasting of the laryngeal muscles may occur with some subluxation of the crico-arytenoid joints. Indrawing of the arytenoid eminences and folds may then occur on forced inspiration.

Visceral Functions of the Vagus

Little is known concerning the effects of high lesions of the vagus upon its visceral functions. In animals section of both vagi is usually fatal. In man tachycardia may follow bilateral lesions of the vagus, for example, in the case of subtentorial tumours, and in various forms of polyneuritis.

LESIONS INVOLVING THE VAGUS
Nuclear Lesions

Lesions of the nucleus ambiguus may occur in posterior inferior cerebellar thrombosis, syringobulbia, medullary tumour, motor neurone disease, encephalitis, poliomyelitis, rabies, Landry's paralysis, and diphtheritic and other forms of polyneuritis.

Nuclear lesions usually cause an associated paralysis of the soft palate, pharynx, and larynx, though when the upper part of the nucleus only is affected the larynx escapes (palatopharyngeal paralysis: syndrome of Avellis).

Bilateral paralysis of the larynx may be due to a nuclear lesion, of which the commonest cause is tabes. It may also occur as a symptom of lead poisoning and of vitamin B deficiency.

Lesions in the Posterior Fossa

Lesions which involve the vagus between its emergence from the medulla and its exit from the skull in the jugular foramen almost invariably affect neighbouring cranial nerves, especially the ninth, eleventh, and twelfth. Such lesions include tumours, and syphilis, and the extension of infection from the middle ear to the bone or dura mater of the posterior fossa. The commonest combinations of associated cranial nerve lesions in this region are glossopharyngeal, vagus, and accessory (the syndrome of the jugular foramen, and of Vernet); vagus and accessory (the syndrome of Schmidt); vagus, accessory, and hypoglossal (the syndrome of Hughlings Jackson).

Lesions of the Trunk

Lesions of the trunk of the vagus above the origin of the superior laryngeal nerve cause unilateral anaesthesia of the larynx, with total paralysis of the ipsilateral vocal cord.

Lesions of the Recurrent Laryngeal Nerve

Lesions of the recurrent laryngeal nerve do not affect the sensibility of the larynx. They may cause total paralysis of the larynx or paralysis of abduction. The left recurrent laryngeal nerve, owing to its longer course, is more exposed to damage than the right. Within the thorax it may be compressed by aneurysm of the aorta, and rarely by the enlarged left atrium in mitral stenosis, or by neoplasm of the mediastinum or enlargement of mediastinal glands due to neoplastic metastases, lymphosarcoma, or Hodgkin's disease. Within the neck both recurrent laryngeal nerves are exposed to surgical trauma, to the pressure of enlarged deep cervical glands, whether malignant or inflammatory, and of an enlarged thyroid, and may be involved in carcinoma of the oesophagus.

The Superior Laryngeal Nerve

Lesions of this nerve are of no importance, but the nerve may require to be injected with alcohol for the relief of pain, due to tuberculosis or neoplasia of the larynx, at the point where the internal laryngeal branch pierces the thyrohyoid membrane.

REFERENCES

FAY, T. (1927) Observations and results from intracranial section of the glossopharyngeus and vagus nerves in man, *J. Neurol. Psychopath.*, **8**, 110.

FERRACOL, EUZIÈRE, and PAGES (1930) Les paralysies laryngées, *Rev. Oto-neuro-ophtal.*, **8**, 241.

SCHUGT, H. P. (1926) Tuberculosis of the larynx. Treatment by surgical intervention in the superior and inferior laryngeal (recurrent) nerve, *Arch. Otolaryng. (Chicago)*, **4**, 479.

THE ELEVENTH OR ACCESSORY NERVE

ORIGIN AND DISTRIBUTION

The accessory is a purely motor nerve, which arises partly from the medulla and partly from the spinal cord. The cranial portion, or internal branch, is derived from cells of origin which are situated in the lower part of the nucleus ambiguus of the medulla. The spinal portion, or external branch, is derived from cells situated in the lateral part of the anterior horn of grey matter of the spinal cord, from the first cervical down to the fifth cervical segment. The cranial fibres emerge from the lateral aspect of the medulla below the roots of the vagus nerve. The spinal fibres emerge from the lateral aspect of the spinal cord between the ventral and dorsal roots. The spinal rootlets unite to form a trunk, which ascends in the spinal subdural space, posterior to the ligamentum denticulatum, to the foramen magnum, where it joins the cranial portion to form a single trunk, which leaves the skull through the jugular foramen in the same compartment as the vagus. In the jugular foramen the cranial fibres join the vagus, and their subsequent course to the pharynx and larynx has already been described. The spinal portion, or external branch, enters the neck between the internal carotid artery and the internal jugular vein. Passing downwards and laterally across the latter it descends beneath the sternomastoid muscle, which it supplies as it pierces it on its deep aspect. After crossing the posterior triangle, the nerve ends by entering the trapezius on its deep surface. In its course it communicates with branches of the second, third, and fourth cervical nerves.

LESIONS OF THE ACCESSORY NERVE

NUCLEAR LESIONS

Lesions of the nucleus ambiguus, the nucleus of origin of the cranial fibres, have been described in the section dealing with the vagus nerve. The cells of origin of the spinal fibres in the anterior horns of the grey matter of the upper five cervical segments may undergo degeneration in poliomyelitis and motor neurone disease, or may be compressed in syringomyelia or by tumours involving the spinal cord in the cervical region.

LESIONS OF THE NERVE TRUNK

Within the posterior fossa the nerve trunk may be damaged by the pressure of tumours, by syphilis, and by the spread of infection from the middle ear, usually suffering in association with neighbouring cranial nerves, especially the ninth, tenth, and twelfth, as described in the section on the vagus nerve. After emerging from the skull the nerve trunk may be compressed or involved in inflammation by the upper deep cervical glands, or may be severed in operations in this region. When the lesion is deep to the sternomastoid, both sternomastoid and trapezius are paralysed; when it is in the posterior triangle of the neck the sternomastoid escapes.

LESIONS OF THE SPINAL BRANCH

UNILATERAL LESIONS

Paralysis of one sternomastoid causes no abnormality in the position of the head at rest. The muscle is wasted and is less salient than its fellow on the normal side. There is weakness of rotation of the head to the opposite side, and when the patient flexes the neck the chin is slightly turned to the paralysed side by the unopposed action of the normal opposite muscle. A lesion of the accessory nerve causes paralysis of only the upper fibres of the trapezius. This part of the muscle is wasted and the normal curve formed on the back of the neck by the lateral border of the trapezius becomes flattened. The shoulder is lowered on the affected side, and the scapula becomes rotated downwards, and outwards, the lower angle being nearer the midline than the upper. There is also slight winging of the scapula, which disappears when the serratus anterior is brought into action. There is weakness of elevation and retraction of the shoulder, and the patient is unable to raise the arm above the head after it has been abducted by the deltoid. It can still be raised above the head in front of the body, however, a movement in which the serratus anterior takes part.

BILATERAL LESIONS

Bilateral paralysis of the sternomastoids causes weakness of flexion of the neck, and the head tends to fall backwards when the patient is erect. Weakness of the sternomastoids is conspicuous in dystrophia myotonica. Paralysis of both trapezii causes weakness of extension of the neck, and the head tends to fall forwards. This is most frequently seen in motor neurone disease, polymyositis and myasthenia gravis.

REFERENCES

SHERREN, J. (1906) *Injuries of Nerves and Their Treatment*, London.
STRAUSS, W. L., and HOWELL, A. B. (1936) The spinal accessory nerve and its musculature, *Quart. Rev. Biol.*, **11**, 387.

THE TWELFTH OR HYPOGLOSSAL NERVE

ORIGIN AND DISTRIBUTION

The hypoglossal nerve is the motor nerve of the tongue. Its fibres originate in the hypoglossal nucleus of the medulla, which represents an upward continuation of the anterior horn of grey matter of the spinal cord. It is an elongated column of grey matter, which in its upper part is subjacent to the floor of the fourth ventricle, near the midline, and below is situated on the anterolateral aspect of the central canal. The nerve fibres after leaving the nucleus pass forwards through the medulla to emerge from its ventral aspect between the olive and the pyramid. After a short course across the posterior fossa the rootlets of the nerve unite in the hypoglossal canal through which it leaves the skull. In the neck the nerve passes downwards and forwards towards the hyoid bone, and then turns medially towards the tongue, passing forwards and downwards over the two carotid arteries, lying beneath the digastric and stylohyoid muscles. It then passes between the mylohyoid and hypoglossus muscles to reach the tongue.

The chief branch of the hypoglossal nerve, its descending branch, passes downwards in the anterior triangle to join the descending cervical nerve and form the ansa hypoglossi, from which branches are distributed to the majority of the infrahyoid muscles. A further branch of the hypoglossal nerve supplies the thyrohyoid muscle but the fibres which leave the nerve by both the descending and the thyrohyoid branch are derived from a communication from the first and second cervical nerves.

LESIONS OF THE HYPOGLOSSAL NERVE

A unilateral lesion of the hypoglossal nerve causes weakness and wasting of the corresponding half of the tongue. The wasting of the tongue muscles throws

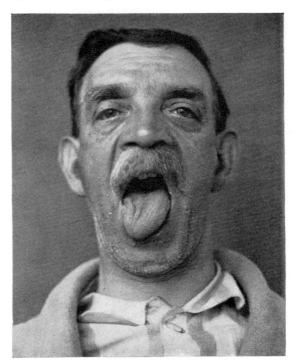

FIG. 34. Paralysis and wasting of the right side of the tongue, due to a lesion of the right hypoglossal nerve. (Note the deviation of the tongue to the paralysed side on protrusion.)

the epithelium on the affected side into folds, and owing to the relative thickening of the epithelium fur tends to accumulate on the paralysed half of the tongue. The median raphe becomes concave towards the paralysed side, to which the tip is deviated. The tongue deviates to the paralysed side on protrusion [FIG. 34]. Unilateral paralysis of the tongue does not impair articulation.

Bilateral lower motor neurone lesions of the tongue cause marked wasting of both sides, associated, when the lesion is due to a progressive degeneration of the cells of the nuclei, with fasciculation. In severe cases of bilateral paralysis the tongue lies on the floor of the mouth and protrusion is impossible. Dysarthria and some degree of dysphagia are present. In dysarthria due to bilateral palsy of the tongue alone the patient finds it difficult to pronounce t and d, and the anteriorly produced lingual vowels, $\breve{e}$, $\bar{a}$, $\breve{i}$, and $\bar{e}$. But bilateral paralysis of the tongue is not usually an isolated phenomenon, and in such cases dysphagia and dysarthria are therefore due in part to paralysis of other muscles.

Unilateral lower motor neurone lesions of the tongue may occur as a result of lesions involving the hypoglossal nucleus or the fibres of the nerve in their course through the medulla, for example, acute poliomyelitis, syringobulbia, and thrombosis of median branches of the vertebral artery. In the last case one or both corticospinal tracts are usually also involved. Between the medulla and the hypoglossal canal the nerve roots may be compressed by a tumour or by an aneurysm of the vertebral artery, or may be involved in syphilitic meningitis, or by extension of infection from the middle ear to the basilar part of the occipital bone or to the dura mater overlying it. In such cases the glossopharyngeal, vagus, and accessory nerves are likely to suffer in association with the hypoglossal (syndrome of Hughlings Jackson). Unilateral or, less often, bilateral atrophy and fasciculation of the tongue may also be due to congenital anomalies in the neighbourhood of the foramen magnum (the Arnold–Chiari malformation, basilar impression of the skull).

Unilateral hypoglossal paralysis has been ascribed to a periostitis of the hypoglossal canal analogous to the lesion of the stylomastoid foramen responsible for Bell's facial paralysis. It is a rare sequel of head injury. In the neck the nerve may be injured in operations in this region, accidentally or intentionally, as in the operation of hypoglossofacial anastomosis. Hemiatrophy of the tongue may occur as part of the syndrome of facial hemiatrophy.

The commonest cause of a bilateral lower motor neurone lesion of the tongue is involvement of the medullary nuclei in motor neurone disease—progressive bulbar palsy. In such cases fasciculation is conspicuous as long as active degeneration is occurring. It may also be caused by subluxation of the odontoid process or may follow retropharyngeal infection.

There should be no difficulty in distinguishing upper from lower motor neurone lesions involving the tongue. Bilateral upper motor neurone paralysis occurs as a result of lesions involving both corticospinal tracts above the medulla and forms part of the syndrome known as pseudobulbar palsy. The commonest causes are double hemiplegia of vascular origin, multiple sclerosis, motor neurone disease, and tumours of the brain stem. The tongue is somewhat smaller than normal owing to spastic contraction of the muscles, but true wasting does not occur. Neighbouring muscles are also the site of spastic paralysis and the jaw-jerk is exaggerated.

REFERENCE

GOLDENBERG, N. A., and SANDLER, J. G. (1931) Isolated paralysis of the hypoglossal nerve, *Rev. Oto-neuro-ophtal.*, **9,** 429.

3

HYDROCEPHALUS AND INTRACRANIAL TUMOUR

HYDROCEPHALUS

Definition. An increase in the volume of the cerebrospinal fluid within the skull.

AETIOLOGY

It is important at the outset to distinguish (1) increase in the volume of cerebrospinal fluid without increase in its pressure, and (2) increase in the volume with increase in the pressure.

1. *Increase in the volume of the cerebrospinal fluid without increase of pressure* is generally of no clinical importance. In such cases the excess of fluid is compensatory to atrophy of the brain, and this condition is observed in cases of congenital cerebral hypoplasia and of acquired cerebral atrophy due to diffuse sclerosis, general paresis, and senile or presenile degenerative changes, after severe head injury, and in some epileptics. There is an excess of fluid occupying the subarachnoid space over the shrunken gyri, and there is also usually some distension of the cerebral ventricles, which, however, is not due to increased intraventricular pressure but is a passive result of atrophy of the white matter of the hemispheres.

2. *Increased volume of the cerebrospinal fluid with increased pressure* is due to a disturbance of the formation, circulation, or absorption of the fluid. In some cases one, in others more than one, of these factors operate.

As we have seen in a previous section, the cerebrospinal fluid is formed by the choroid plexuses of the cerebral ventricles, flows through the ventricular system, reaches the subarachnoid space by the medial and lateral apertures of the fourth ventricle, bathes the surface of the brain and spinal cord, and is resorbed into the blood stream by the arachnoid villi of the intracranial venous sinuses.

Increased Formation

We know little about causes of increase in the rate of formation of the cerebrospinal fluid. Bedford's work renders it unlikely that hydrocephalus can be caused by obstruction of the great cerebral vein. Increased formation of fluid occurs, however, when the osmotic tension of the blood is lowered as in meningism, and may be caused by a papilloma of the choroid plexus.

There is evidence that both lack and excess of vitamin A may lead to increased pressure of cerebrospinal fluid, possibly by increasing its production (Millen and Woollam, 1958).

Obstructed Circulation

Obstruction to the circulation of the cerebrospinal fluid may occur at any point of its course. Within the ventricles the commonest cause is a neoplasm which may compress one or both interventricular foramina or fill the third ventricle. The cerebral aqueduct may be obstructed by a tumour arising in the third ventricle, in the midbrain, or in the pineal body, or may be congenitally narrowed or even absent. Owing to the small calibre of the cerebral aqueduct, slight swelling of its ependymal lining may lead to its obstruction, and cases have been reported in which hydrocephalus has been due to gliosis caused by ependymitis in this region. Aqueduct stenosis is one of the commonest causes of infantile hydrocephalus and may even give rise to symptoms of increased intracranial pressure for the first time in adult life (McHugh, 1964). The cause is unknown but the recent demonstration by Johnson et al. (1967) that aqueduct stenosis and hydrocephalus can be induced in suckling hamsters by the inoculation of mumps virus may be relevant.

Subtentorial tumours may obstruct the fourth ventricle. The foramina of the fourth ventricle may be blocked by a congenital septum (the Dandy–Walker syndrome) or by adhesions following meningitis or by displacement of the medulla into the foramen magnum by the pressure of a tumour. Within the subarachnoid space obstruction may again be due to tumour, to adhesions following trauma, inflammation, or haemorrhage, or to congenital abnormalities such as basilar impression or the Arnold–Chiari malformation.

The last-named is a tongue of cerebellar tissue with an elongated medulla oblongata which protrudes into the spinal canal [FIG. 35]. The essential feature is that the cerebellar tonsils on either side of the medulla extend downwards into the cervical spinal canal. Russell and Donald (1935) suggest that the malformation prevents the cerebrospinal fluid from flowing upwards into the cerebral subarachnoid space and so interferes with its absorption. This abnormality is sometimes associated with meningomyelocele and lumbosacral spina bifida, or with simple meningocele but it is now recognized that it may occur as an isolated anomaly. To remove the sac in such cases of spina bifida may precipitate hydrocephalus if this is not present already, because, it is suggested, the sac is capable of absorbing some cerebrospinal fluid. MacFarlane and Maloney (1957) have observed congenital narrowing of the cerebral aqueduct sufficient to cause hydrocephalus in half of 20 cases of Arnold–Chiari malformation. Gardner (1965) has suggested that a Chiari malformation or, less often, the Dandy–Walker syndrome may result in dilatation of the central canal of the spinal cord early in life (hydromyelia) and that this, in turn, is the commonest mechanism by means of which syringomyelia is produced. The observations of Appleby et al. (1968) give some support to this view.

Impaired Absorption

Absorption of fluid from the arachnoid villi may be impaired by a rise in the intracranial venous pressure, due to compression of venous sinuses by an intracranial tumour, or impediment to the venous drainage from the head by raised intrathoracic pressure in cases of pulmonary neoplasm or aneurysm of the aorta. Thrombosis of the superior sagittal sinus by extension of inflammation from the transverse sinus seems the probable cause of the condition described as 'otitic hydrocephalus' in which symptoms of hydrocephalus complicate otitis media or mastoiditis (Symonds, 1931, 1937) but Foley (1955) states that in such cases the

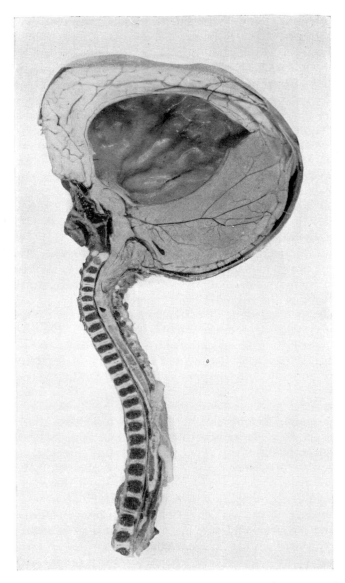

FIG. 35 Sagittal section of the nervous system in a case of
hydrocephalus due to the Arnold–Chiari malformation. Note
the abnormal cerebellum and the spina bifida. (By courtesy of the
Photographic Department of the Hospital for Sick Children
Great Ormond Street, London.)

ventricles are not enlarged and the condition therefore should not be called hydrocephalus. [See also p. 211.] Obliteration of the arachnoid villi by inflammatory material may occur in meningitis.

We can thus distinguish the following varieties of hydrocephalus:

1. Increased volume of cerebrospinal fluid with normal pressure—*compensatory hydrocephalus.*

2. Increased volume of cerebrospinal fluid with increased pressure—*hypertensive hydrocephalus.*

Hypertensive hydrocephalus can be further subdivided into:

(*a*) *Obstructive hydrocephalus,* in which there is an obstruction to the circulation of the cerebrospinal fluid, either within the ventricles or at the outlet from the fourth ventricle, which prevents free communication between the ventricles and the subarachnoid space, and

(*b*) *Communicating hydrocephalus,* in which free communication between the ventricles and the subarachnoid space exists and hydrocephalus is due either to disturbance in the formation and absorption of cerebrospinal fluid, or to an obstruction to its circulation in the subarachnoid space itself. Hakim and Adams (1965) have recently distinguished a form of communicating hydrocephalus of unknown aetiology, usually occurring in late life, which they have called *low-pressure hydrocephalus* since although the cerebral ventricles are dilated the pressure within them is either normal or only slightly raised (see below).

The terms internal and external hydrocephalus are incompletely descriptive, since the ventricles are usually dilated in all forms of hydrocephalus, both compensatory and hypertensive, and an increased volume of fluid in some parts of the subarachnoid space is common to both compensatory and hypertensive communicating hydrocephalus.

Laurence (1959) in 100 consecutive post-mortem examinations found that malformation alone was the cause in only 14 per cent. of cases, but in association with infection or trauma it accounted for 46 per cent. Inflammatory reaction due to infection or haemorrhage without malformation accounted for another 50 per cent., the remaining 4 per cent. being due to tumours. Thus malformation was present in 46 per cent. and inflammation in 82 per cent. Cohen (1965) reviewing the radiological findings in Macnab's (1962) series of 200 found that 18 per cent. were due to aqueduct block, 42 per cent. to cistern block, and 40 per cent. were associated with an Arnold–Chiari malformation [FIG. 35].

In the past, a distinction has been made between 'congenital' and 'acquired' hydrocephalus. What has just been said, however, shows that this distinction is an artificial one. A congenital abnormality alone is the most likely cause of hydrocephalus developing before birth but as the work of Laurence shows, both congenital and acquired factors frequently contribute to hydrocephalus in infancy. Nor do congenital factors cease to operate in later life since hydrocephalus developing in adult life may be the late result of a congenital abnormality of the aqueduct or an Arnold–Chiari malformation.

The commoner causes of hydrocephalus developing in the absence of congenital abnormalities are adhesions of the leptomeninges following meningitis, especially meningococcal meningitis, and arachnoiditis of obscure origin, thrombosis of the intracranial venous sinuses, and intracranial tumour. Syphilitic meningitis or arachnoiditis following subarachnoid bleeding are rare causes. Obstruction within the third or fourth ventricle or in the subarachnoid space, is occasionally due to parasitic cysts.

PATHOLOGY

As we have seen, the causes of hydrocephalus are pathologically various, and they need not be described in detail. Distension of the cerebral ventricles is the most conspicuous feature. When obstruction occurs in the cerebral aqueduct only the lateral and third ventricles are distended. When the obstruction is more caudally situated the cerebral aqueduct and the fourth ventricle may also be enlarged. Ventricular distension causes thinning of the cerebral hemispheres, which in severe cases may be extreme and is associated with some atrophy of the cortical ganglion cells. The ependyma of the ventricles is normal, except in inflammatory cases, when a localized or more or less diffuse ependymitis may be present. Meningeal adhesions indicate a previous meningitis. Distension of the ventricles leads to pressure upon the bones of the skull, which become thin, especially where they overlie the cerebral gyri. Separation of the sutures occurs when hydrocephalus develops in early life, but is not as a rule seen after the age of 18. Compression of the base of the skull causes erosion of the clinoid processes and excavation of the sella turcica. The olfactory tracts and optic nerves are usually atrophic.

SYMPTOMS

Infantile Hydrocephalus

Enlargement of the head is the most conspicuous symptom in infantile hydrocephalus [FIG. 36]. It may occur before birth, but is usually noticed during the first few months of life owing to the large head, prominent scalp veins, and turning down of the eyes ('rising sun sign'). In most cases it is slowly progressive and the head may attain a huge size, with a circumference of 30 inches or even more. The cranial sutures are widely separated and the anterior fontanelle is much enlarged. There is marked congestion of the veins of the scalp. In extreme cases the head may be translucent and may yield a fluid thrill on percussion and an audible murmur on auscultation. Enlargement of the head occurs in all its diameters. The frontal region bulges forwards, and downward pressure upon the orbital plates causes the eyes to be protruded forwards and downwards. As the head becomes too heavy for the child to lift it, gravity, acting upon it in the supine position, in time causes it to become relatively larger in the coronal than in the sagittal plane.

Owing to the expansibility of the skull in infancy, the familiar symptoms of increased intracranial pressure are slight or absent. Hydrocephalic children seem little troubled by headache and rarely vomit. Convulsions are common. Bilateral anosmia may occur. Optic atrophy due to pressure upon the nerves is usually present, but in some cases there is papilloedema, and this may be superimposed upon optic atrophy. Papilloedema does not occur when the subarachnoid space is blocked. Visual acuity may be progressively reduced until in severe cases the child may become blind. Paralysis of other cranial nerves may occur, and squint is not uncommon. Nystagmus may be present. In the limbs there are usually some weakness and incoordination, which are generally more marked in the lower than in the upper limbs. Spasticity with exaggeration of tendon reflexes is common in the lower limbs, though sometimes the tendon reflexes are lost. The plantar reflexes are usually extensor. There is little or no disturbance of sensibility. The mental state varies in different cases. In severe cases there is usually mental deficiency, but in milder cases this may be slight or absent. It has been shown that intelligence may be unimpaired even when the ventricular

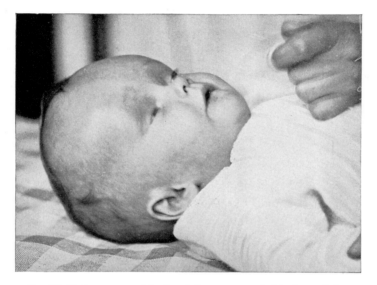

FIG. 36. Enlargement of the head due to congenital hydrocephalus

dilatation is such that only one centimetre thickness of cerebral substance remains between the ventricles and the inner table of the skull. In milder cases there may be obesity due to compression of the hypothalamus and hypophysis. In more severe cases there is usually wasting. Cerebrospinal rhinorrhoea is a rare complication.

Hydrocephalus after Infancy

The clinical picture of hydrocephalus after infancy varies somewhat with its cause. In obstructive hydrocephalus symptoms of increased intracranial pressure are conspicuous. Headache and vomiting are the earliest symptoms and are followed after a short interval by the development of papilloedema. The headache is at first paroxysmal, but later becomes constant, and there are sometimes intense exacerbations characterized by severe headache radiating down the neck and associated with head retraction and even with opisthotonos, vomiting, and impairment of consciousness. Giddiness is a common symptom. Some mental deterioration usually occurs after a time, especially in later life, and hallucinations, delusions, and disturbances of emotional mood may occur. Convulsions are less common than in the infantile variety, and enlargement of the head is less conspicuous on account of the greater age of the patient, and does not occur after the age of 18. Before that age there is often slight separation of the cranial sutures, yielding a 'cracked-pot sound' on percussion and associated with venous congestion of the scalp. Cranial nerve palsies may occur, especially paralysis of the sixth and seventh nerves, and often fluctuate in severity from day to day. Slight exophthalmos is not uncommon. Gross weakness of the limbs is absent, though clumsiness and slight incoordination are common.

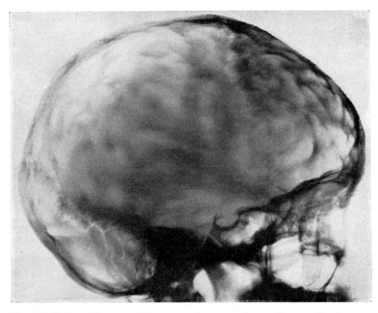

FIG. 37. A rise of intracranial pressure has caused great increase in the convolutional markings. There is separation of the sutures especially well illustrated in the region of the coronal suture and the junction of the basisphenoid. There is general thinning of the skull. A child suffering from a stricture of the cerebral aqueduct. (Radiogram by Dr. Jupe.)

The tendon reflexes may be exaggerated or diminished. The plantar reflexes are frequently extensor. There is as a rule no sensory loss. Symptoms of hypopituitarism, obesity, and genital atrophy, are common in children and adolescents.

The pressure of cerebrospinal fluid is generally increased in communicating hydrocephalus, but is often normal or may even be diminished in obstructive hydrocephalus. In the syndrome of 'low-pressure hydrocephalus' (Hakim and Adams, 1965) fluctuating confusion, ataxia, and progressive dementia are the most prominent features; characteristically such patients often deteriorate strikingly following air encephalography which demonstrates marked dilatation of all the ventricles but no air diffuses over the cortex. Most such cases arise in middle or late life and striking improvement may follow a shunt operation (see below). The fluid is usually normal in composition. Radiograms of the skull [FIG. 37] may show enlargement of the calvarium, with thinning, and exaggeration of the convolutional markings. Separation of the sutures may be present in children. The clinoid processes are often eroded and the sella turcica is deepened and expanded anteroposteriorly. Ventriculograms show enormous dilatation of the ventricular system [FIGS. 38 and 39] and the concavity of the anterior cerebral arteries is increased in the angiograms. Ventriculography with *Myodil* may be needed to show the site of an obstruction. Isotope ventriculography may also be useful in the diagnosis of obstructive and communicating hydrocephalus (Spoerri and Rösler, 1966; and Bannister, Gilford, and Kocen, 1967).

DIAGNOSIS

The diagnosis of infantile hydrocephalus is not usually difficult. Owing to the enlargement of the head it may be confused with rickets, but in rickets the enlargement of the head is due to localized thickening of the bone and other characteristic bony abnormalities are present elsewhere. The rare condition megalencephaly can be distinguished only by ventriculography.

After infancy hydrocephalus is frequently present as a complication of conditions causing increased intracranial pressure. The recognition of the existence of hydrocephalus is usually a simple matter. The discovery of its cause calls for the appropriate investigations.

When the cause of hydrocephalus is a tumour focal signs of the tumour may be lacking, and in hydrocephalus of long standing confusion may arise from the presence of signs produced by the hydrocephalus itself. Spina bifida should suggest the presence of the Arnold–Chiari malformation.

Benign Intracranial Hypertension

This term is used by Foley (1955) to describe a persistent rise of pressure of the cerebrospinal fluid in the absence of a space-occupying lesion and with ventricles of normal size, which makes the term hydrocephalus unsuitable. This syndrome, also called 'toxic hydrocephalus', occurs in two groups of patients. One consists predominantly of women, with a peak incidence in the fourth decade. The patient is often obese, and there is an association with pregnancy and miscarriage: in a smaller group, affecting the sexes equally, there is a previous history of infection or mild head injury. In so-called 'otitic hydrocephalus', which appears to be due to transverse or sagittal sinus thrombosis secondary to otitis, again the pressure of the fluid is raised without ventricular enlargement. Papilloedema is constant, headache and vomiting are common though often not severe and diplopia may occur. Visual failure is commoner than in the non-otitic groups, and central scotomas may occur. The disorder usually lasts months, sometimes more than a year, but is benign apart from the risk of visual failure.

PROGNOSIS

In most cases untreated infantile hydrocephalus proves fatal during the first few years of life, but Macnab (1966) quotes figures showing that the average hydrocephalic alive at 3 months has a 26 per cent. chance of reaching adult life without surgery, and if he survives to between 1 and 2 years he has a 50 per cent. chance. Some who survive suffer from mental subnormality, epilepsy or blindness. In the past many children with the Arnold–Chiari malformation and

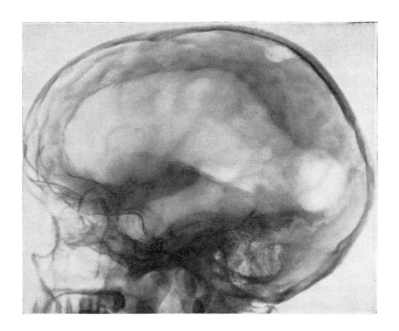

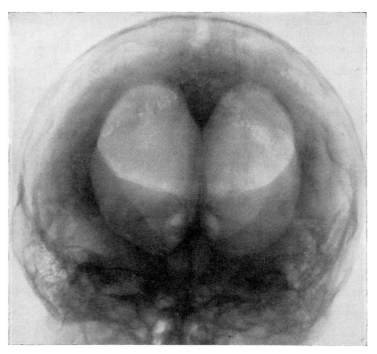

FIGS. 38 and 39. Hydrocephalus: ventriculograms showing enormous dilatation of the ventricular system, the lateral and third ventricles being clearly seen. The anterior end of the third ventricle has encroached on the hypophysial fossa so that the dorsum sellae is eroded and the whole fossa deepened. (Radiograms by Dr. Jupe.)

myelomeningocele died either from infection of the sac or coning of the mal-formation in the foramen magnum. The introduction of the Spitz–Holter valve has reduced the mortality of hydrocephalus with myelomeningocele to 30 per cent. at the end of 2 years and that of uncomplicated hydrocephalus to 20 per cent. The prognosis of hydrocephalus after infancy depends upon its cause and how far this is amenable to treatment.

TREATMENT

Infantile Hydrocephalus

In spite of many and varied attempts to deal surgically with infantile obstruc-tive hydrocephalus the results of treatment have hitherto been disappointing. Treatment has been directed to permitting the escape of fluid from the distended ventricles. Probably it has failed because the channels of absorption are defective. Openings have been made in the corpus callosum and in the floor of the third ventricle. Dandy has excised the choroid plexuses of the lateral ventricles. Attempts have been made to drain the cerebrospinal fluid into the ureter and the peritoneal cavity. The latter, and drainage from a ventricle into the jugular vein by a Spitz–Holter or Pudenz valve, are the most effective methods. The Arnold–Chiari abnormality may be successfully treated by suboccipital decompression. The Spitz–Holter and Pudenz–Heyer valves, made of silastic, were introduced into Great Britain in 1958. These valves have made possible the atrioventricular drainage of hydrocephalus via the jugular vein. This revolutionized the treatment of myelomeningocele associated with hydro-cephalus, for with adequate drainage of the hydrocephalus an infant with myelomeningocele could have the neural tissue replaced in the spinal canal, the spinal defect covered with fascial flaps and the area covered with healthy skin within 12 months of birth. A complication of the use of the valve is bacterial infection.

Hydrocephalus after Infancy

The appropriate treatment of hydrocephalus after infancy depends upon its cause. When it is due to an intracranial tumour this must receive appropriate surgical treatment. In congenital and acquired narrowing of the cerebral aque-duct one lateral ventricle may be drained by catheter into the cerebellomedullary cistern (Torkildsen's operation of ventriculocisternostomy). Obliteration of the apertures of the fourth ventricle has been successfully treated by the construc-tion of a new aperture. Benign intracranial hypertension and otitic hydrocephalus should be treated by corticosteroid drugs and/or repeated lumbar puncture, and diuretics may also be tried. Failing vision may necessitate cranial decompression. Treatment has recently been reviewed fully by Scarff (1963).

REFERENCES

APPLEBY, A., FOSTER, J. B., HAWKINSON, J., and HUDGSON, P. (1968) The diagnosis and management of the Chiari anomalies in adult life, *Brain*, **91**, 131.
BANNISTER, R., GILFORD, E., and KOCEN, R. (1967) Isotope encephalography in the diagnosis of dementia due to communicating hydrocephalus, *Lancet*, ii, 1014.

COHEN, S. J. (1965) *see* MACNAB, G. H. (1966).

CUSHING, H. (1926) *Studies in Intracranial Physiology and Surgery*, London.

DANDY, W. E. (1918) Extirpation of the choroid plexus of the lateral ventricles in communicating hydrocephalus, *Ann. Surg.*, **68**, 569.

DANDY, W. E. (1919) Experimental hydrocephalus, *Ann. Surg.*, **70**, 129.

DANDY, W. E. (1921) The cause of so-called idiopathic hydrocephalus, *Bull. Johns Hopk. Hosp.*, **32**, 67.

FOLEY, J. (1955) Benign forms of intracranial hypertension in 'toxic' and 'otitic' hydrocephalus, *Brain*, **78**, 1.

GARDNER, W. J. (1965) Hydrodynamic mechanism in syringomyelia: its relationship to myelocele, *J. Neurol. Psychiat.*, **28**, 247.

GLOBUS, J. H. (1928) Communicating hydrocephalus (so-called idiopathic hydrocephalus), *Amer. J. Dis. Child.*, **36**, 680.

GLOBUS, J. H., and STRAUSS, I. (1928) Subacute diffuse ependymitis, *Arch. Neurol. Psychiat.* (*Chicago*), **19**, 623.

HAKIM, S., and ADAMS, R. D. (1965) The special clinical problem of symptomatic hydrocephalus with normal cerebrospinal fluid pressure, *J. neurol. Sci.*, **2**, 307.

HASSIN, G. B. (1930) Hydrocephalus, *Arch. Neurol. Psychiat.* (*Chicago*), **24**, 1164.

JOHNSON, R. T., JOHNSON, K. P., and EDMONDS, C. J. (1967) Virus-induced hydrocephalus: development of aqueductal stenosis in hamsters after mumps infection, *Science*, **157**, 1066.

LAURENCE, K. M. (1959) The pathology of hydrocephalus, *Ann. roy. Coll. Surg. Engl.* **24**, 388.

MACFARLANE, A., and MALONEY, A. F. J. (1957) The appearance of the aqueduct and its relationship to hydrocephalus in the Arnold–Chiari malformation, *Brain* **80**, 479.

McHUGH, P. R. (1964) Occult hydrocephalus, *Quart. J. Med.*, **33**, 297.

MACNAB, G. H. (1962) *see* MACNAB, G. H. (1966).

MACNAB, G. H. (1966) The development of the knowledge and treatment of hydrocephalus, in *Hydrocephalus and Spina Bifida*, National Spastics Society, p. 1, London.

MILLEN, J. W., and WOOLLAM, D. H. M. (1958) Vitamins and the cerebrospinal fluid, *Ciba Foundation Symposium on the Cerebrospinal Fluid*, p. 168, London.

RUSSELL, D. S. (1949) Observations on the pathology of hydrocephalus, *Spec. Rep. Ser. med. Res. Coun.* (*Lond.*), No. 265.

RUSSELL, D. S. (1954) Hydrocephalus, *Res. Publ. Ass. nerv. ment. Dis.*, **34**, 160.

RUSSELL, D. S. and DONALD, C. (1935) The mechanism of internal hydrocephalus in spina bifida, *Brain*, **58**, 203.

SCARFF, J. E. (1963) Treatment of hydrocephalus; an historical and critical review of methods and results, *J. Neurol. Psychiat.*, **26**, 1.

SHELDON, W. D., PARKER, H. L., and KERNOHAN, J. W. (1930) Occlusion of the aqueduct of Sylvius, *Arch. Neurol. Psychiat.* (*Chicago*), **23**, 1183.

SPOERRI, O., and RÖSLER, H. (1966) Isotope ventriculography with I^{131} and I^{125} in the evaluation of hydrocephalus, in *Hydrocephalus and Spina Bifida*, National Spastics Society, p. 88, London.

SYMONDS, C. P. (1931) Otitic hydrocephalus, *Brain*, **54**, 55.

SYMONDS, C. P. (1937) Hydrocephalic and focal cerebral symptoms in relation to thrombophlebitis of the dural sinuses and cerebral veins, *Brain*, **60**, 531.

TORKILDSEN, A. (1947) *Ventriculocisternostomy*, Oslo.

INTRACRANIAL TUMOUR

Definition. The term 'intracranial tumour' is conveniently applied to localized intracranial lesions, whether of neoplastic or of chronic inflammatory origin, which by occupying space within the skull tend to cause a rise in intracranial pressure.

AETIOLOGY

Over 1 per cent. of all deaths are due to intracranial tumours, which form about 10 per cent. of all malignant neoplasms in man. Apart from those of inflammatory origin, the aetiology of intracranial tumours is little understood. In a minority of cases congenital abnormality appears to play an important part in causation, especially in the angiomatous malformations and the angioblastomas, the ganglioneuromas, the cholesteatomas, and tumours of the craniopharyngeal pouch. The causation of the gliomas is as obscure as that of neoplasms in general. It is uncertain whether the primitive character of the cells of which some gliomas are composed should be regarded as an indication that they are derived from embryonic cell rests, or should be considered as a cellular regression. There is no evidence that trauma is a predisposing factor, except, rarely, in the case of meningiomas which have been known to arise beneath the site of a previous head injury.

An intracranial tumour may occur at any age, though, as will be seen later, certain types of glioma tend to exhibit a characteristic age incidence. The frequent occurrence of some forms of glioma in childhood is responsible for the fact that the age incidence of intracranial tumours differs from that of most other malignant neoplasms, which are rare before middle life. Tuberculomas appear to be relatively more common in childhood than in adult life. Intracranial tumour affects the sexes with equal frequency.

PATHOLOGY

The pathology of intracranial neoplasms has made great advances during the present century, chiefly owing to the researches of Cajal, Hortega, and Cushing and his pupils, and has assumed considerable clinical importance. It has been learned that the different types of tumour, even the different varieties of glioma, often exhibit a characteristic age incidence and rate of growth and a predilection for certain situations in the brain. Hence it is becoming possible for the clinician with increasing frequency to diagnose not only the presence and situation of an intracranial tumour, but also its precise pathological nature, and to form an accurate estimate of its prospects of removal, of the peculiar difficulties likely to be encountered in the task, and of its probable malignancy. Histological examination during and after removal of the growth, especially in the case of the gliomas, throws further light on the last point and yields information as to the prospects of a recurrence and the likelihood that the tumour will respond favourably to irradiation therapy.

The following figures indicating the relative frequency of the various kinds of intracranial tumour are based upon the findings of Cushing and upon the data obtained from the National Hospital, Queen Square, by Walshe (1931). The percentages are about the same in the two groups with the exception of those referring to hypophysial adenoma.

Glioma	about 41·0	per cent.
Meningioma	,, 13·0	,,
Acoustic neuroma	,, 10·0	,,
Hypophysial duct tumour	,, 7·0	,,

Sarcoma . . .	about	$7 \cdot 0^1$	per cent.
Secondary carcinoma .	,,	$5 \cdot 0$	,,
Hypophysial adenoma .	,,	$4 \cdot 6^1$	,,
,, ,, .	,,	$19 \cdot 2^2$	,,
Tuberculoma ⎫ Granuloma ⎬ . .	,,	$2 \cdot 5$	,,
Blood vessel tumour .	,,	$1 \cdot 7$	,,
Choroid plexus tumour less than		$1 \cdot 0$	,,
Cholesteatoma . . ,,	,,	$1 \cdot 0$	,,

[1] National Hospital figures.   [2] Cushing's figures.

Few other reported series have contained such a high proportion of sarcomas, which are now accepted as being rare, and most recent series have contained a much higher percentage of metastatic tumours than that given in the above table (Russell and Rubinstein, 1959). There is now general agreement that gliomas constitute 40–45 per cent. of all intracranial neoplasms, metastases about 15 per cent., meningiomas about 10 per cent., and acoustic neuromas and pituitary tumours about 5 per cent. each.

Gliomas

The gliomas are tumours derived from the cells which constitute the supporting tissue of the nervous system, but unlike connective-tissue tumours elsewhere they are of epiblastic origin. The precise classification of the gliomas is still unsettled. Bailey and Cushing (1926) proposed a classification based upon the development of the glial cell, but this was criticized by Scherer (1940 *a* and *b*). He pointed out that too much stress had been laid upon specific staining methods, and that immature or anaplastic glioma cells cannot be identified with certainty. Systematic examination of complete tumours reveals different types of cell in a single tumour. Moreover, tumours which are histologically identical may behave quite differently, e.g. the cerebral and cerebellar astrocytomas and the more and less rapidly growing oligodendrogliomas. Sometimes a glioma seems to arise diffusely, as in so-called 'gliomatosis cerebri', or from multiple centres at the same time. Kernohan *et al.* (1949) recognize only five main groups of primary brain tumours, distinguishing within the group grades of malignancy.

With the exception of the ependymoma the gliomas are all infiltrative tumours. This explains the great difficulty of complete surgical removal and the liability to recurrence after operation. Moreover, the fact that the glioma may leave nervous tissue which it infiltrates intact explains why a tumour may be much more extensive than would be supposed from the symptoms and physical signs. For clinical purposes the following are the most important of the gliomas. Those most frequently encountered are the astrocytomas, about 36 per cent., glioblastomas, about 34 per cent., and medulloblastomas, about 11 per cent., of Bailey and Cushing's series of gliomas.

Medulloblastoma. These are rapidly growing tumours which are most frequently encountered in the cerebellum in children, where they arise in the region of the roof of the fourth ventricle, but they are also encountered rarely in adults. They are composed of masses of rounded undifferentiated cells [FIG. 40] and show a marked tendency to become disseminated through the subarachnoid space both of the brain and of the spinal cord. This subarachnoid metastasis is not peculiar to the medulloblastoma but apparently may occur much less often in the case of any of the gliomas. The medulloblastoma is one of the more malignant gliomas, and the average duration of illness is six months before and six months after operation though, especially in adults, survival for several years is not uncommon. Radiation appears to be of considerable value in retarding the growth of this tumour.

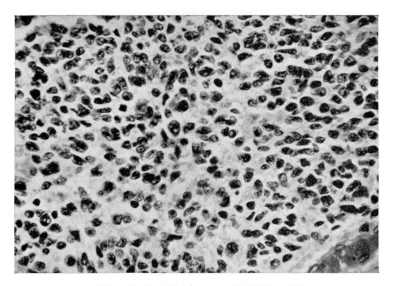

FIG. 40. Medulloblastoma. H. & E. ×350

Glioblastoma (Spongioblastoma) Multiforme. This is an extremely malignant glioma arising in middle life and almost invariably found in the cerebral hemispheres. It tends to infiltrate the brain extensively and often attains an enormous size. It is a reddish, highly vascular tumour, and often exhibits haemorrhages and areas of necrosis [FIG. 41]. Microscopically it consists of relatively undifferentiated round or oval cells, together with spongioblastic and astroblastic forms. No form of treatment prolongs life for more than a few months, and the average survival period for those treated surgically is twelve months.

Astrocytoma. Five types of astrocytoma are recognized by Russell and Rubinstein (1959). They are white, infiltrating growths which may occur at any age, and in either the cerebral or the cerebellar hemispheres. They grow slowly, and are relatively benign, and the average survival period after the first symptom is 67 months in the case of the former and 89 months in the case of the latter. The cerebellar astrocytoma of childhood is a particularly benign tumour. Microscopically [FIG. 42] they exhibit abundant astrocytes and, in the case of the fibrillary astrocytomas, a dense fibril network, and the tumour cells exhibit attachments to the blood vessels characteristic of the astrocyte. Astrocytomas

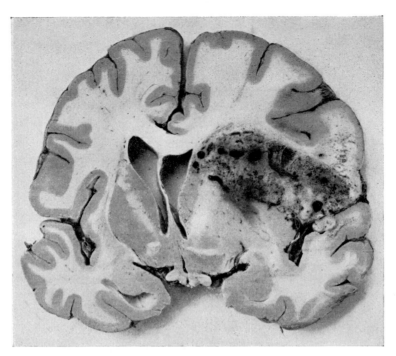

FIG. 41. Glioblastoma multiforme. Note haemorrhagic areas and displacement of ventricular system

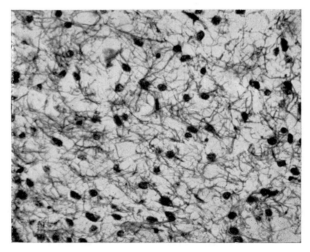

FIG. 42. Astrocytoma

are particularly liable to undergo cystic transformation. Gliomatous cysts, therefore, have on the whole a favourable prognosis, though cystic change is fairly
common in the glioblastomas.

Less common gliomas are:

Oligodendroglioma. This is a rare, slowly growing, usually relatively benign
tumour occurring in the cerebral hemispheres in young adults. The cells of
which it is composed exhibit features which are held to relate them to oligodendroglia. An oligodendroglioma may undergo malignant anaplasia.

Ependymoma. This is a firm, whitish tumour, sometimes papilliferous, arising
from the ependyma, frequently in the roof of the fourth ventricle and sometimes
from the walls of the other ventricles or from the central canal of the spinal cord.
Histologically it shows a characteristic 'rosette' formation.

Ganglioglioma. This rare tumour is composed of ganglion cells surrounded
by glioma tissue composed of astrocytes and astroblasts. The *astroblastoma* is
commonly found in the white matter of the cerebral hemispheres. The *polar
spongioblastoma* is a tumour of childhood and early adult life, relatively slowly
growing, and found, according to Bailey, especially in the optic nerves, chiasma
and tract, and the midbrain.

Neuroblastomas and Ganglioneuromas. Though not glial in origin, these
may conveniently be mentioned here. Both are rare tumours, the former consisting of neuroblasts and the latter of ganglion cells and in some instances of
nerve fibres, which are usually unmyelinated.

Meningioma

These tumours were at one time thought to arise from the dura mater and
hence were known as dural endotheliomas. It is now believed, however, that,
although they are attached to the dura, many arise from the arachnoid cells which
penetrate the dura to form the arachnoid villi, projecting into the dural venous
sinuses. They are composed of specialized connective-tissue cells resembling the
cells which constitute the arachnoid villus. These cells are present in columns
or whorls [FIG. 43], and the tumour sometimes contains fibroglia together with
collagen fibres and small calcified concretions known as psammoma bodies. They
have therefore been termed 'meningeal fibroblastoma' and 'arachnoid fibroblastoma'. The term 'meningioma', however, though less completely descriptive,
is more convenient.

Commonly the meningioma is a single, large, more or less irregularly lobulated
growth, but less frequently it may form a flat plaque spreading over the inner
surface of the dura. A distinctive feature of the meningiomas is their relationship
to the bones of the skull. Though hyperostosis may occur as a reaction in the overlying bone without its having been invaded, these tumours tend to invade bone
in about 20 per cent. of cases, absorption of bone and new bone formation occurring simultaneously. In this process the outer table of the skull may be absorbed
and rebuilt so as to constitute a bony boss [FIG. 53, p. 241]. Microscopically,
meningioma cells fill the Haversian canals and spaces. New bone is laid down
in spicules perpendicularly to the surface of the skull, the osteogenetic cells being

derived from the outer layers of the dura or from the bone itself. In rare cases a meningioma may perforate the skull and infiltrate the extracranial tissues. The meningioma, which is of mesodermal origin, does not usually invade the brain but compresses it, and the resulting disturbance of cerebral function is as a rule much less marked in proportion to the size of the tumour than is the case with the gliomas. A malignant invasive form (sarcomatous change) is described.

Since the meningiomas arise from the cells of the arachnoid villi they are commonly found along the course of the intracranial venous sinuses, and their sites of greatest predilection are the superior sagittal sinus—parasagittal

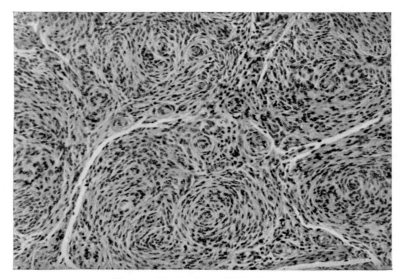

FIG. 43. Meningioma. H. & E. × 133

meningiomas; the sphenoparietal sinus and the middle meningeal vessels—meningiomas of the convexities; the olfactory groove of the ethmoid; and the circle of sinuses around the sella turcica—suprasellar meningiomas. Meningiomas are uncommon below the tentorium but may arise from the tentorium itself or at the torcula. Occasionally they are found within the lateral ventricles. All meningiomas are commoner in women than in men. Multiple meningiomas may occur in association with multiple neurofibromas [see p. 581].

Acoustic Neuroma

Acoustic neuromas are usually unilateral. Rarely they are bilateral and are then usually, though not always, manifestations of generalized neurofibromatosis and may be associated with multiple meningiomas [see p. 581]. Familial examples of bilateral acoustic neuroma have been reported. Penfield believes that the solitary acoustic neuroma can be differentiated histologically from that associated with generalized neurofibromatosis. A solitary tumour consists of elongated cells like spindle fibroblasts with much collagen and reticulum, and exhibits marked palisading and parallelism of nuclei. Some workers believe that these tumours arise from the perineurial or endoneurial connective tissue and that the fibroblast is their type cell. They have therefore been termed 'perineurial fibroblastomas'. Russell and Rubinstein (1959), deriving them from the Schwann cells, call them schwannomas. Though the eighth cranial nerve is their commonest site, similar tumours may be found upon other cranial nerves, especially the optic and the trigeminal, upon spinal nerve roots, usually the dorsal, and upon peripheral nerves. The neurofibroma of von Recklinghausen is thought by Penfield to differ from the tumour just described in that nerve fibres are found within it. For clinical purposes the term 'acoustic neuroma' may conveniently be used to include both types of tumour, if indeed they are histologically distinct.

Blood Vessel Tumours

The blood vessel tumours of the brain have been subjected to detailed study only comparatively recently and any classification is necessarily to some extent provisional. The following forms are encountered:

1. The angiomatous malformations, including the cirsoid aneurysms.
2. The cavernous haemangiomas.
3. The haemangioblastomas.
4. The Sturge–Weber syndrome.

The first two groups are collectively known as blood vessel hamartomas.

1. *The Angiomatous Malformations.* These are probably to be regarded as congenital abnormalities of vascular development rather than as true neoplasms. They may be divided into (*a*) telangiectases, (*b*) arteriovenous malformations.

(*a*) *Telangiectases*, or capillary angiomas, consist of groups of greatly dilated capillaries. They may be associated with Osler's hereditary telangiectasia and are usually accidental post-mortem findings, though rupture has been known to cause death through haemorrhage.

(*b*) *Arteriovenous Malformations.* These consist of a mass of enlarged and tortuous cortical vessels, supplied by one or more large arteries usually derived from the blood supply of one, but sometimes of both, hemispheres, and sometimes fed also from below the tentorium, and drained by one or more large veins. These malformations are most frequently encountered in the field of the middle cerebral artery, but may involve the brain stem (Logue and Monckton, 1954).

Angiography has revealed that the angiomatous malformations are commoner than used to be thought. Verified angiomas accounted in one series for 6·5 per cent. of 200 cases of cerebral vascular disease. Increased vascularity of the scalp, with large and pulsating arteries, and hypertrophy of one or both carotids may be present, and even secondary cardiac hypertrophy may occur. A bruit is commonly heard over one or both carotid arteries in the neck and on the scalp overlying the angioma.

2. *The Cavernous Haemangiomas.* The cavernous haemangiomas appear to be congenital abnormalities rather than true neoplasms. They usually occur above the tentorium. They form a lobulated mass consisting of small and large spaces containing blood.

3. *The Haemangioblastomas.* The haemangioblastomas are tumours which, according to Cushing and Bailey (1928), are composed of angioblasts, the primitive

cells which normally form the foetal blood vessels. They usually consist of vascular channels and spaces with sparse intercapillary tissue containing swollen fat-laden endothelial cells. They exhibit a marked tendency to form cysts in the surrounding nerve tissue, the cyst containing xanthochromic fluid which is probably an exudate from the vessels of the tumour. The cyst may be large and the tumour a small nodule in its wall, which must be excised if the cyst is not to refill. The haemangioblastomas are almost invariably subtentorial tumours, though two examples have been observed above the tentorium. They are usually single, but there may be multiple growths in the cerebellum or in addition to a cerebellar tumour a tumour in the medulla or spinal cord. An important feature of the haemangioblastomas is their association with abnormalities in other parts of the body. The most important of these, because the most easily observed, is a haemangioblastoma of the retina (von Hippel's disease). This is a small tumour usually situated in the periphery of the retina and supplied by an enlarged artery and vein. Secondary proliferative changes in, and rarely even detachment of, the retina may render it difficult to recognize. Other abnormalities which may coexist are haemangioblastoma of the spinal cord, cysts of the pancreas and kidneys, hypernephromas of the kidneys or the suprarenal glands. The coincidence of these abnormalities is known as Lindau's disease and is familial in about 20 per cent. of cases. Polycythaemia may occur.

4. *The Sturge–Weber Syndrome.* In the fully developed form of this disorder an extensive capillary-venous malformation affects one hemisphere, particularly in the parieto-occipital region and is associated with a characteristic 'wavy' pattern of subcortical calcification which outlines the gyri and is visible radiologically after the third to fifth year of life. There is a 'port-wine' stain on the face on the affected side, often with an associated buphthalmos (ox eye), while most patients have a contralateral hemiparesis and epilepsy.

Craniopharyngioma

These tumours are also described as tumours of the craniopharyngeal, or Rathke's, pouch, adamantinomas, and hypophysial epidermoids. In order to understand their origin it is necessary briefly to review the development of the hypophysis in the embryo.

The hypophysis develops as a result of fusion of an evagination of the ectoderm of the stomodaeum with a process which extends downwards from the floor of the forebrain. The former loses its opening into the mouth cavity and becomes a closed sac from which are derived the anterior lobe and the pars intermedia of the hypophysis. The process from the forebrain forms the posterior lobe and the infundibulum. The remnants of the craniopharyngeal pouch remain, and, owing to rotation of the developing gland, come to lie anterior to the infundibulum and at the upper angle of the anterior lobe. They may also be found within the sella turcica itself.

Tumours arising from these embryonic relics show characteristics resulting from their origin in the stomodaeum. They contain cells resembling those of the buccal epithelium of the embryo, including the ameloblasts of the embryonic enamel organ. These tumours are very liable to undergo cystic degeneration and calcification and may even develop bone. They usually arise above the sellar diaphragm, and extend upwards into the third ventricle and hypothalamic region, but occasionally are seen within the sella itself.

Tumours of the Hypophysis

The cells of the anterior lobe of the hypophysis are the alpha, eosinophil, or acidophil cells, which secrete the growth hormone, the luteinizing hormone and prolactin; the beta or basophil cells, which secrete the follicle-stimulating hormone, corticotrophin and thyrotrophin, and the poorly staining chromophobe cells. It is now thought that the small chromophobe cell may be a stem cell, the large chromophobe being an actively secreting cell (see Hubble, 1961).

The common hypophysial tumours are adenomas. The commonest of these is the chromophobe adenoma, composed of cells which sometimes show alveolar formation and resemble the chromophobe cells of the normal gland. The endocrine disturbances associated with chromophobe tumour are those of 'hypo-pituitarism'. The chromophil adenoma is composed of cells resembling the acidophil cells of the normal gland. It sometimes undergoes cystic degeneration. This tumour gives rise to symptoms of hyperpituitarism—gigantism if it develops before puberty and acromegaly in adults. The basophil adenoma is usually microscopic in size and only rarely gives rise to pressure symptoms.

The hypophysial adenomas arise within the sella turcica, which they expand, and later may pass through the sellar diaphragm and attain a considerable size, compressing the structures at the base of the brain.

Adenocarcinoma of the hypophysis is a rare, rapidly growing tumour which gives rise to metastases.

The occurrence within the sella turcica of metastases from extracranial tumours is rare and has been most frequently recorded in cases of carcinoma of the breast.

Osteoma and Osteochondroma

Ivory osteomas may develop in the frontal or ethmoidal sinuses and may occasionally be large enough to compress the frontal lobe. Osteochondroma of the base of the skull rarely gives neurological manifestations but has been known to produce subarachnoid haemorrhage.

Cholesteatoma

The cholesteatoma, or cerebrospinal epidermoid, is a rare tumour of adult life which affects males more frequently than females. It is regarded as a foetal epithelial inclusion and is most frequently found in the subarachnoid cisterns at the base of the brain. Those arising below the tentorium, a common site, may be situated either in the cerebellopontine angle or in the midline on the ventral aspect of the cerebellum, or within the fourth ventricle or in the temporal bone. The naked-eye appearance of the tumour in the fresh state is highly characteristic. It is pearly white, smooth, and glistening, firm but brittle. Microscopically a cholesteatoma is composed of several layers, of which the most characteristic—the stratum granulosum—consisting of several rows of large, finely granular cells, probably corresponds to the dermis.

Pinealoma

Tumours of the pineal gland are rare. The commonest form contains two types of cell, a large cell with a clear cytoplasm and smaller cells resembling small lymphocytes. Russell (1944) considers that these are atypical teratomas. In addition to the two types of cell just described, epithelial cells and keratin may be present. True pinealomas are very rare.

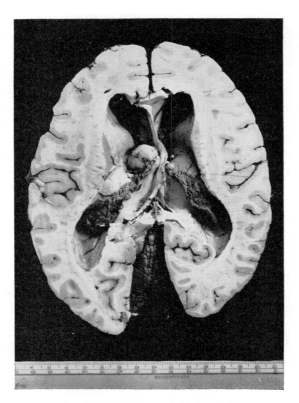

FIG. 44. Colloid cyst of third ventricle

Colloid Cysts of the Third Ventricle

These are rounded cystic tumours measuring from 1 to 3 cm. in diameter and arising from the paraphysis, ependyma or choroid plexus [FIG. 44]. They are lined with ciliated epithelium and contain thick glairy fluid or gelatinous material. Owing to their position they readily cause hydrocephalus. Papilloma of the choroid plexus may also occur.

Rare forms of intracranial tumour are chordomas; osteomas, arising from the inner table of the skull; primary sarcomas, especially chondromyxosarcomas; and intracranial dermoids.

Chordomas are tumours derived from remnants of the notochord. Within the skull they are found in the region of the clivus.

Papilloma of the Choroid Plexus

Up to half of these benign vascular tumours occur in the fourth ventricle, about one-third in the lateral ventricles (usually left) and one-sixth in the third ventricle. Recurrent or chronic subarachnoid bleeding and communicating hydrocephalus may result.

Glomus Tumours

These tumours arise from the glomus jugulare and may invade the middle ear or the posterior fossa giving rise to unilateral deafness and multiple palsies of lower cranial nerves; erosion of the base of the skull is often visible radiologically (Henson, Crawford, and Cavanagh, 1953). Glomus intravagale tumours also occur but, like the histologically-similar carotid body tumours, are usually extracranial. Though they are similar pathologically to chromaffinomas in other sites these neoplasms rarely, if ever, secrete noradrenaline.

Metastatic Tumours

About 15–20 per cent. of cerebral neoplasms are secondary to a primary growth elsewhere, usually in the lung, breast, stomach, prostate, kidney, or thyroid. The lung appears to be the commonest source of metastatic cerebral tumour and not infrequently the symptoms of the cerebral growth are more conspicuous than those of the primary. Secondary cerebral carcinomas are usually multiple and rapidly growing. Hence the history of symptoms is usually short. They are pinkish, rounded tumours, well defined from the oedematous and softened surrounding brain tissue. Metastases within the fourth ventricle may give in middle or late life the same triad of symptoms (morning headache, morning vomiting and postural vertigo) as is seen in younger patients with ependymomas in the same site. An important variety of secondary carcinoma within the skull is constituted by a group of cases in which the tumour cells infiltrate the dura at the base of the skull and spread into the leptomeninges and the bones of the base. This condition is sometimes described as carcinomatosis of the meninges and may rarely lead to subdural haematoma. More often many of the cranial nerves are compressed or infiltrated and multiple cranial nerve palsies are accompanied by neck stiffness, headache and confusion. The hypophysis may be invaded and the tuber cinereum compressed, leading to metabolic and endocrine disorders. In such cases metastatic deposits may be present in the uppermost cervical lymph nodes. Secondary sarcoma of the brain is much rarer than secondary carcinoma. Melanotic sarcoma may metastasize with great rapidity to the brain and meninges and can produce subarachnoid haemorrhage.

Tumours of Infective Origin

Tuberculoma. Tuberculoma of the brain appears to be much less frequent in Britain than a generation ago, when it was regarded as one of the commonest of intracranial tumours. It is still one of the commonest intracranial tumours on the Indian sub-continent. Cerebral tuberculomas are more frequently subtentorial than supratentorial and vary in size from small nodules up to large masses which may occupy more than one lobe of the brain. They are usually at some point subjacent to the pia mater. There is a yellow caseous centre surrounded by a pinkish-grey outer zone. Microscopically, cerebral tuberculomas show the features characteristic of tuberculous lesions elsewhere. The caseous centre is surrounded by a zone containing giant cells and epithelioid cells and vessels showing endarteritis. Outside this area infiltration with compound granular corpuscles and fibrosis are conspicuous.

Gumma. Gumma of the brain is extremely rare. It is generally connected with the meninges, probably arising initially as a circumscribed patch of gummatous meningitis. Its pathology is described in the section on cerebral syphilis.

Parasitic Cysts. Intracranial hydatid cysts are rare even in countries in which hydatid infection is common, the brain being infected in only 5 per cent. of cases. They may be single or multiple. They sometimes occur outside the dura, and in one patient, whom I saw, an extradural collection of hydatids eroded the frontal bone, and some cysts were extruded through the scalp. More often the cysts, which frequently attain the size of a hen's egg, occupy the substance of the cerebral hemispheres or lie within the ventricles. Cysticercus cellulosae and coenurus cerebralis cysts may cause symptoms of increased intracranial pressure. Either may occur in the ventricles or cause an adhesive arachnoiditis in the posterior fossa. Cysticercus cellulosae may also behave as a space-occupying lesion in the cerebral hemisphere (Kuper *et al.*,1958) [see also p. 399]. Rarely infection of the brain with the ova of *Schistosoma japonicum* may cause tumour-like masses.

PATHOLOGICAL PHYSIOLOGY

The functions of the brain depend upon the maintenance of the circulation of the blood and of the cerebrospinal fluid at their appropriate pressures. The brain is unique among the viscera in being confined within a rigid box, the cranium. It follows that the total volume of the intracranial contents, the brain and its coverings, the blood vessels and the blood, and the cerebrospinal fluid is constant, and that an increase in the volume of any one of them can only occur at the expense of the others. The intracranial contents, however, do not respond passively to changes in their volume or pressure, but react in complicated ways, so that any such alteration has far-reaching consequences. Four factors which influence the intracranial pressure require consideration—the mass of the brain, the circulatory system, the cerebrospinal fluid, and the rigidity of the skull.

The Mass of the Brain

An intracranial tumour usually increases the mass of the brain, though in the case of certain slowly growing infiltrating tumours the increase in mass may be very slight, with the result that symptoms of increased intracranial pressure are slight or absent. The direct local effects of the increased mass of the brain produced by a tumour play a comparatively small part in raising intracranial pressure. Owing to the partial division of the cranial cavity into compartments by the falx and the tentorium, the local rise of pressure is to a considerable extent limited to the cranial compartment in which the tumour arises though it may cause local herniations, e.g. of the cingulate gyrus of the frontal lobe beneath the falx cerebri—subfalcial herniation, of the medial temporal lobe into the opening in the tentorium—tentorial herniation, or of the cerebellar tonsils into the foramen magnum—the cerebellar pressure cone.

The Cerebral Circulation

The vascular channels first compressed are naturally those in which the blood pressure is lowest, namely, the veins and venous sinuses. Compression of veins in the neighbourhood of a tumour causes oedema of surrounding nervous tissue and so adds to the local rise of pressure. It also causes a diversion of the venous blood stream into other channels, and this leads indirectly to a general rise in intracranial venous pressure. This tends to increase the formation and impede the absorption of cerebrospinal fluid.

The Cerebrospinal Fluid

Besides causing increase in the pressure of cerebrospinal fluid through the disturbance of the cerebral circulation just described, a tumour may lead to hydrocephalus by obstructing the circulation of the fluid, as described in the section on hydrocephalus.

The Rigidity of the Skull

In the adult after union of the cranial sutures the skull is rigid and unyielding, and by preserving the volume of the intracranial contents constant is responsible for the far-reaching effects of a disturbance of the intracranial pressure. In the child the non-union of the sutures provides a partial safety-valve, and allows of some expansion. Hence a marked rise of intracranial pressure in childhood leads to separation of the sutures, and the skull yields a 'cracked-pot sound' on percussion. Some relief of the pressure results and other signs of raised intracranial pressure are often slighter in childhood than in later life.

MODE OF ONSET

The mode of onset of symptoms depends upon the nature and site of the tumour. It is slowest in the case of astrocytomas, oligodendrogliomas, meningiomas, acoustic neuromas and hypophysial adenomas which may be present for years before the patient consults a doctor, and most rapid in glioblastoma multiforme and secondary carcinoma. The commonest modes of onset are (1) progressive focal symptoms, e.g. focal epilepsy, monoplegia, hemiplegia, aphasia, cerebellar deficiency, associated with symptoms of increased intracranial pressure; (2) symptoms of increased intracranial pressure alone; (3) progressive focal symptoms alone, e.g. visual failure, unilateral deafness, dementia; (4) generalized epileptic attacks preceding other symptoms by many years; both slowly-growing gliomas and meningiomas may cause epilepsy for as long as 20 years, before causing other symptoms; (5) an apoplectiform onset with loss of consciousness, and perhaps hemiplegia.

SYMPTOMS OF INCREASED INTRACRANIAL PRESSURE

The symptoms of an intracranial tumour are conveniently divided into symptoms attributable to increased intracranial pressure, and focal symptoms which are due to the local effects of the growth. It might be expected that focal symptoms would arise before a tumour was large enough to disturb the intracranial pressure. More frequently, however, the reverse is the case, and the general symptoms often indicate the presence of a tumour which it is by no means easy to localize by physical examination alone. Headache, papilloedema, and vomiting may be described as the classical triad of symptoms of increased intracranial pressure, but they are not found with equal frequency. In one series headache was present in 88 per cent., papilloedema in 75 per cent., and vomiting in 65 per cent. of cases of cerebral tumour. All three were found together in only 60 per cent. It is clearly unnecessary that all, or indeed any, of these symptoms should be present in order to diagnose an intracranial tumour.

Headache. The headache of intracranial tumour is probably mainly due to abnormal states of tension in the cerebral blood vessels (Northfield, 1938) though compression or distortion of the dura also plays a part. It is paroxysmal, at least in the earlier stages. It is often described as a throbbing or a 'bursting' pain. It occurs chiefly during the night and in the early morning. Often the patient awakens with a headache which lasts from a few minutes to a few hours and then passes off, to recur the next day. With the gradual enlargement of the growth the headaches tend to become more prolonged and may ultimately be continuous. They always tend to be intensified by any activities which raise the intracranial pressure, such as exertion, excitement, coughing, sneezing, vomiting, stooping, and straining at stool. They may be influenced by posture, being worse when the patient is lying down, or lying upon one side, and may be relieved by adopting a sitting attitude.

Owing to the early occurrence of a diffuse rise of intracranial pressure in many cases of cerebral tumour, headache is of little localizing significance. The pain due to the local pressure of the growth may be predominantly unilateral, on the side of the tumour, and is occasionally associated with tenderness of the skull on percussion over a limited area overlying it. In the case of subtentorial tumours the headache in the early stages may be mainly suboccipital, with a tendency to radiate down the back of the neck. In such cases flexion of the neck may increase the pain and this sign may be a warning of a cerebellar pressure cone. As the intracranial pressure rises, the headache tends to be diffuse, and hydrocephalus may lead to paroxysms of severe diffuse pain radiating down the neck and sometimes associated with head retraction. Pressure upon the trigeminal nerve leads to unilateral pain, most commonly following the distribution of the first division and associated with hyperalgesia or analgesia over the same area.

Papilloedema. The pathogenesis and appearances of papilloedema are described on pages 143–6. Its incidence varies according to the situation of the tumour. It is almost constant in tumours of the cerebellum, fourth ventricle, and temporal lobes, but is absent in half the cases of pontine and subcortical tumours. It is usually late in developing in the case of prefrontal tumours, and is often more severe with extracerebral than with intracerebral growths. Cerebellar tumours cause papilloedema of the greatest severity. A slight difference in the degree of swelling of the two optic discs is not uncommon, but is of little value as an indication of the situation of the tumour. A tumour arising sufficiently near the optic canal to cut off the subarachnoid space of the optic nerve from communication with the cerebral subarachnoid space causes primary optic atrophy on the affected side and occasionally contralateral papilloedema results from the general effect of the tumour (Foster Kennedy syndrome, often due to an olfactory groove meningioma).

The changes in the visual fields due to papilloedema consist of enlargement of the blind spot with concentric constriction at the periphery of the field. Visual acuity deteriorates, and, if the condition progresses, optic atrophy and complete blindness are likely to result. Patients with papilloedema are liable to brief transitory attacks of blindness which are probably due to a temporary increase in the obstruction to the venous drainage of the retina.

Vomiting. Vomiting, when due to intracranial tumour, usually occurs during the night or in the early morning when the headache is especially severe. Though sometimes, especially in children, it is preceded by little nausea, there is no ground for the belief that vomiting of cerebral origin is always of this precipitate character.

Epileptiform Convulsions. Generalized epileptiform convulsions may be a symptom of increased intracranial pressure, e.g. in hydrocephalus, but it is often impossible to decide whether the convulsions are due to the increased pressure, or are local effects of the cerebral tumour responsible for it. They occur in some 30 per cent. of cases (Nattrass, 1949; Hoefer *et al.*, 1947) and are the first symptoms in 68 per cent. of cases of astrocytoma, 60 per cent. of cases of meningioma, and 51 per cent. of cases of glioblastoma (Hoefer *et al.*).

Vertigo. Vertigo, when a symptom of increased intracranial pressure, is not often a subjective sense of rotation, but more frequently a feeling of unsteadiness, with a tendency to fall on stooping.

Disturbances of Pulse Rate and Blood Pressure. An acute or subacute rise of intracranial pressure, such as that due to intracranial haemorrhage or meningitis, often causes slowing of the pulse rate, usually to between 50 and 60 beats a minute. If the pressure continues to increase the pulse becomes extremely rapid. In either case it may be irregular. A gradual increase in the intracranial pressure, such as that due to an intracranial tumour, does not usually cause bradycardia, but moderate tachycardia is not uncommonly found in cases of subtentorial tumour.

A rapid rise of intracranial pressure usually causes a rise of blood pressure. Thus in intracranial haemorrhage a progressive rise of blood pressure probably indicates that the bleeding is continuing. Chronic rise of intracranial pressure does not have this effect, and in patients with intracranial tumour, especially when the lesion is below the tentorium, the blood pressure is often subnormal.

Respiratory Rate. A gradual rise of intracranial pressure does not at first affect the respiratory rate. A rise of sufficient rapidity and severity to produce loss of consciousness usually leads at first to slow and deep respirations. Later the respiratory rate may become irregular, e.g. of the Cheyne-Stokes type, in which periods of apnoea alternate with a series of respirations which wax and wane in amplitude. In the terminal stage of a fatal increase of intracranial pressure the respirations are rapid and shallow.

'Hypopituitarism.' Any state of increased intracranial pressure associated with internal hydrocephalus may lead to symptoms of 'hypopituitarism', namely, adiposity and genital atrophy in some cases, loss of body hair and hypoadrenalism with hypothyroidism in others. This is due to downward pressure of the floor of the distended third ventricle, which may erode the clinoid processes and diaphragma sellae and compress the hypophysis. These symptoms commonly arise in children and are most frequently seen in cases of cerebellar tumour. It is not easy to say whether they should be ascribed to compression of the hypothalamus or of the hypophysis itself. Possibly both are in part responsible.

Radiography of the skull in such cases shows erosion of the clinoid processes and slight general enlargement of the sella turcica. This group of symptoms, if misinterpreted, may lead to the erroneous diagnosis of a hypophysial or suprasellar tumour.

Somnolence. Persistent somnolence is seen when hydrocephalus is pronounced and with tumours near the hypothalamus. Narcolepsy is uncommon.

Glycosuria. Glycosuria is occasionally encountered, sometimes with hyperglycaemia, more often with a normal blood-sugar and a lowered renal threshold.

Mental Symptoms. The most varied mental symptoms may be associated with increased intracranial pressure. If the pressure rises sufficiently high all mental activity is suspended in coma, and the more rapid the rise the more likely is this to occur. An acute or subacute rise of pressure insufficient to produce coma usually leads to mental confusion with disorientation in space and time. Chronic rise of intracranial pressure may lead to progressive dementia, with a failure of intellectual capacity, emotional apathy, carelessness with regard to the person, and incontinence of urine and faeces. Or the mental state may rather be one of confusion, with disorientation and hallucinations. Less frequently, marked disturbances of emotional mood are conspicuous, and the patient suffers from outbreaks of excitement in which he may be violent, or from depression in which he may be suicidal. In the mildest cases some impairment of memory and of power to concentrate, with irritability, may be the only mental symptoms.

In cases of intracranial tumour mental symptoms are most likely to occur when the tumour is situated in the frontal lobe or corpus callosum or leads to a considerable degree of aphasia; but they may be produced by a tumour in any situation which causes a rise of intracranial pressure. Thus any of the mental disturbances described may be produced by a tumour of the cerebellum. Mental symptoms as a result of increased intracranial pressure are more likely to occur in the middle-aged and elderly than in younger patients.

False Localizing Signs

Collier first drew attention to the importance of symptoms, especially cranial nerve palsies, produced by intracranial tumours in other ways than by direct compression. Since these, unless properly interpreted, may lead to mistakes in localization, he termed them 'false localizing signs'. A sixth-nerve palsy on one or both sides, and, less frequently, a third-nerve palsy, may be thus produced and have been variously attributed to stretching of the nerves, to their compression by arteries, and to other modes of interference with their function resulting from displacement of the cranial contents, e.g. tentorial herniation compressing one third nerve at the edge of the tentorium. Other false localizing signs include bilateral extensor plantar responses or bilateral grasp reflexes resulting from interference with the function of the cerebral hemispheres by distension of the ventricles in hydrocephalus; 'hypopituitarism' resulting from hydrocephalus, as already described; an extensor plantar response occurring on the same side as a tumour of one cerebral hemisphere produced by compression of the opposite cerebral peduncle against the tentorium; cerebellar symptoms resulting from tumours of the frontal lobe, and midbrain symptoms, especially fixed dilated pupils, produced by a tumour of the cerebellar vermis.

EXAMINATION OF THE HEAD

Examination of the head may yield important information in cases of intracranial tumour and should never be neglected. There may be visible enlargement when hydrocephalus develops before the union of the cranial sutures. In such cases separation of the sutures may yield a 'cracked-pot sound' on percussion. Local tenderness of the skull may be present in the region overlying the tumour. A bony boss may overlie a meningioma [FIG. 53, p. 241]. Venous congestion of the scalp is a not uncommon result of increased intracranial pressure and is most evident in children. When there is a marked rise of intracranial pressure with separation of the sutures, extreme venous congestion of the scalp occasionally occurs. Dilatation and tortuosity of the arteries of the scalp are sometimes associated with a vascular intracranial tumour, especially a meningioma or an angioma. Such arterial congestion is usually confined to the side of the tumour and is often most evident in the superficial temporal artery. An audible bruit should be sought by auscultation. It is most frequently present over an arterial angioma, much less frequently over a highly vascularized meningioma, very rarely in the presence of an aneurysm. However, cranial bruits are not infrequently heard in normal children while bruits heard in the neck in adults and resulting from stenosis of major vessels (carotid, vertebral, subclavian) may rarely be transmitted along temporal vessels so that auscultation of the neck is also essential. A bruit over the orbit is usually present, along with pulsating exophthalmos in cases of carotico-cavernous fistula.

Facial naevus may be associated with venous angioma, retinal haemangioblastoma with haemangioblastoma of the cerebellum, and cutaneous pigmentation with neurofibromatosis.

Attention should be paid to the presence or absence of exophthalmos.

Accessory Methods of Investigation

Radiography. In every suspected case of intracranial tumour lateral, antero-posterior, and postero-anterior views should be taken, and other positions, including basal views and Towne's view, are usually included in routine skull surveys (Cairns and Jupe, 1939; Bull, 1951). Radiographic examination of the skull may reveal abnormalities in the bones, calcification in the tumour, or displacement of the pineal body. In selected cases further radiograms may be taken after the injection of air into the cerebral ventricles, pneumoventriculography, or into the spinal subarachnoid space, pneumoencephalography. A common abnormality observed in the bones of the skull is a general erosion or 'convolutional thinning' [FIG. 37, p. 210]. The radiograms show many rounded areas of rarefaction, sometimes described as 'finger-printing' or a 'beaten silver' appearance. The rarefied areas are thought to be produced by the pressure of the summits of the gyri. Convolutional thinning may be an indication of a considerable generalized rise of intracranial pressure but this change must be interpreted with care as a somewhat similar appearance is normal in children and may persist up to the twenty-fifth year or even later in some normal individuals. Separation of the sutures may be seen when a rise of intracranial pressure occurs before the age at which these unite. It is most commonly seen in childhood. Erosion of the posterior clinoid processes and erosion or decalcification of the dorsum sellae is a safer guide to the presence of raised intracranial pressure (see below) but decalcification in this area is also a common result of normal ageing processes. Local erosion of bone is most frequently seen in the region of the skull superficial to a meningioma. Around the eroded area new bone formation occurs, often taking the form of spicules, perpendicular to the vault, and surrounding this there is frequently a network of deepened vascular channels in the bone. The petrous portion of the temporal bone may be eroded by an acoustic neuroma which may lead to unilateral enlargement of the internal acoustic meatus. Bony changes in the region of the sella turcica are produced not only by tumours of the hypophysis itself and those arising in its neighbourhood, but also by a general increase in the intracranial pressure. Hypophysial tumours cause a uniform expansion of the sella turcica with thinning of its walls. The ballooned sella projects downwards and forwards into the sphenoidal sinuses, and the upward pressure of the growth may erode the clinoid processes. Tumours arising outside the sella, but immediately above it, cause erosion of the clinoid processes and flattening of the sella, which is not, however, uniformly enlarged unless invaded by the tumour [Fig. 45]; while the downward pressure of the floor of the distended third ventricle in internal hydrocephalus results in a very similar radiographic appearance.

Calcification is most frequently observed in cysts of the craniopharyngeal pouch, in which it is visible as a radiographic opacity in 75 per cent. of cases. These tumours may exhibit on the X-ray film merely a few opaque flecks, or a mass the size of a hen's egg.

Calcification may occur also in the angiomas, which may sometimes present a characteristic convoluted appearance due to the deposit of calcium in the walls of the vessels composing the tumour but more often the pattern is non-specific. Meningiomas also sometimes show calcified areas, and these may be encountered, though less frequently, in gliomas [FIG. 46], teratomas, tumours of the choroid plexuses, and tuberculomas. Chronic intracerebral haematomas, and, very rarely, subdural haematomas may also calcify. A typical form of calcification is also seen in the very rare lipoma of the corpus callosum while bilateral calcification in the basal ganglia may be familial or can occur in pseudohypoparathyroidism.

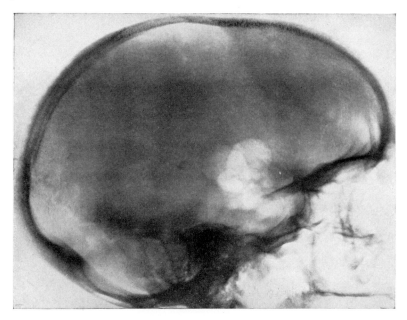

FIG. 45. Cystic hypophysial epidermoid tumour filled with air after eroding the sella turcica, and rupture into the sphenoidal sinus

The pineal body is normally sufficiently calcified to be visible radiographically in 60 per cent. of adults and is to be seen in the midline above and behind the sella turcica. It may be displaced to the opposite side by a neoplasm of one cerebral hemisphere. Calcification may also be seen in the normal choroid plexuses, in the petroclinoid ligaments, tuberculum sellae and falx cerebri, and even in the dura mater of the vault of the skull.

Ventriculography. When the introduction of air, through a needle inserted into one lateral ventricle through a burr hole, is completed, radiograms of the skull are taken, comprising right and left lateral [FIG. 51], antero-posterior [FIG. 47], and postero-anterior views and others as may be necessary. In some cases ventriculography with an opaque substance (*Myodil* or *Pantopaque*) may be helpful.

Intracranial tumours may cause symmetrical or asymmetrical changes in the size, shape, and position of the ventricles. Symmetrical dilatation of the lateral ventricles [FIGS. 38 and 39] indicates internal hydrocephalus, which may be due to a tumour of the third ventricle, midbrain, or pineal body, or a subtentorial

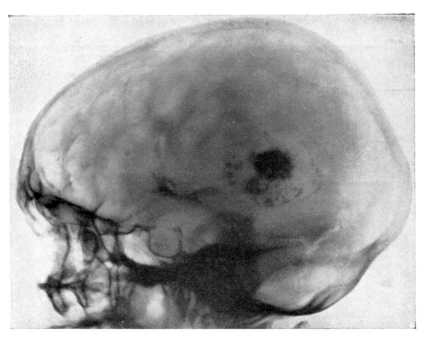

FIG. 46. Extensive calcification in an oligodendroglioma situated in the left temporo-parietal region. The convolutional markings due to increased intracranial pressure and the enlargement of the pituitary fossa are well seen. (Radiogram by Dr. Jupe.)

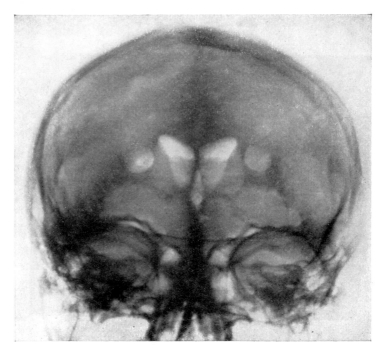

FIG. 47. Normal ventriculogram. Antero-posterior position. The anterior horns are seen with the bodies of the lateral ventricles showing through them. The third ventricle is seen lying below and between the lateral ventricles. (Radiogram by Dr. Jupe.)

growth. Tumours of one cerebral hemisphere usually cause a filling defect of the ipsilateral ventricle, varying from obliteration of part of the ventricle to collapse of the whole, with displacement of the ventricular system to the opposite side and some dilatation of the opposite ventricle [FIGS. 48–50]. The third ventricle may be obliterated by a tumour arising within it or invading it from the interpeduncular space. Ventriculography is not without risk, and may lead to an acute rise of the intracranial pressure. It is advisable that it should only be performed when the patient is so situated that cerebral exploration can be performed without delay if it should become necessary.

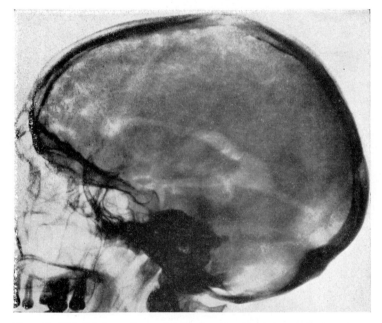

FIG. 48. The left lateral ventricle is depressed and encroached on by a left parietal tumour (glioblastoma). (Radiogram by Dr. Jupe.)

Pneumoencephalography. The injection of air into the lumbar subarachnoid space or cerebellomedullary cistern is a much simpler procedure than its introduction directly into the ventricles, and by this means air may be induced to enter not only the cerebral ventricles but also the cerebral subarachnoid space. Radiography after the lumbar injection of air is known as air encephalography. It is more liable to cause headache than ventriculography, and it is usually contra-indicated when the intracranial pressure is high and in most cases when a subtentorial tumour is suspected, on account of the risk of herniation of the medulla into the foramen magnum. It may also be dangerous in the presence of a supratentorial tumour because of the risk of tentorial herniation. In some centres air encephalography is regularly performed using only small amounts of air without removal of cerebrospinal fluid even in the presence of papilloedema ('fractional air encephalography'). This method has the advantage that filling of the fourth ventricle and basal cisterns may be rapidly demonstrated during the passage of

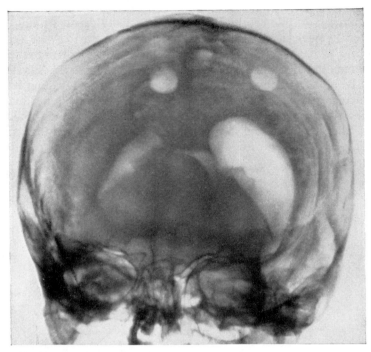

FIG. 49. Large basal ganglia tumour rising from the floor of the right ventricle and partly filling its lumen. The whole ventricular system is displaced away from the side of the lesion. (Radiogram by Dr. Jupe.)

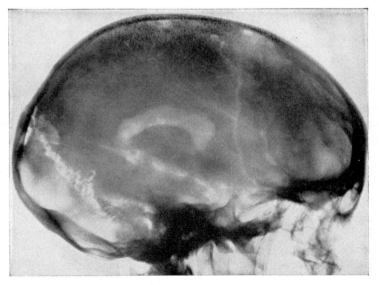

FIG. 50. Frontal glioma causing a filling defect and slight depression of the anterior horn. (Radiogram by Dr. Jupe.)

the bubble of air but it can only be performed if skilled neurosurgical aid is immediately at hand and hence, because of its potential hazards, ventriculography is generally preferred whenever there is any suspicion of raised intracranial pressure. The method is indicated instead of ventriculography in suspected cases of atrophy of the cerebral hemispheres and in other conditions when it is desired to demonstrate the presence of abnormalities in the cerebral subarachnoid space.

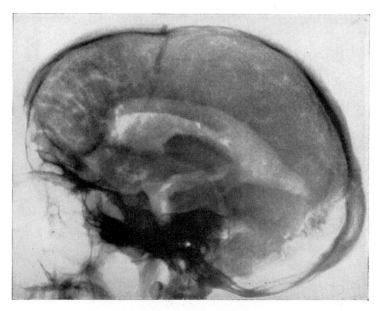

FIG. 51. Normal encephalogram showing the lateral, third, and fourth ventricles. (Radiogram by Dr. Jupe.)

The patient should be given a preliminary injection of pethidine, 100 mg., while a general anaesthetic is to be preferred in children or in uncooperative adults. Lumbar puncture is performed in the usual way with the patient seated in an upright position. Ten ml. of spinal fluid are withdrawn and replaced by the injection of air. A further quantity of fluid is then withdrawn and more air is injected. During the injection the head is held with the neck slightly flexed when it is desired to fill the ventricles and extended when it is desired to fill the subarachnoid space. Usually 30 ml. of air is enough to give all the information needed. Radiograms are taken and interpreted as after ventriculography [FIG. 51].

Initial radiographs are usually taken as the air enters the fourth ventricle and basal cisterns, and various positions of the head are utilized to demonstrate other parts of the ventricular system.

Neither ventriculography nor encephalography is devoid of risk, and fatalities have been reported. They are only to be recommended, therefore, when neither clinical investigation nor simple radiography has rendered possible the localization of a suspected intracranial tumour and when angiography has not yielded, or is thought unlikely to yield, the necessary information. As already mentioned, ventriculography is possible when encephalography is contra-indicated. When either is applicable, encephalography is usually to be preferred as it does not involve shaving the skull and a surgical operation.

Cerebral Angiography. Moniz devised a method of investigating radiographically the distribution of the cerebral arterial supply, radiograms being taken immediately after the injection into the common carotid artery of *Thorotrast,* a solution opaque to X-rays. This has now been replaced by iodine

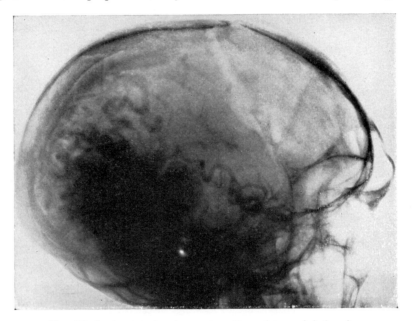

FIG. 52. Angiogram showing angioma in parieto-occipital region

compounds. The percutaneous technique has taken the place of the open operation and various alternative routes are now employed. It may thus be possible to demonstrate abnormal vascularity in an aneurysm, angioma [FIG. 52], vascular glioma, or meningioma, or the displacement of cerebral arteries by an avascular tumour. The procedure is less disturbing to the patient than ventriculography and encephalography, and may yield more information about the site, size, and nature of a supratentorial tumour than air injection does. Vertebral artery angiography may yield information about a subtentorial tumour especially by visualizing displacements of the basilar artery. Arch aortography carried out by insertion of a catheter into a limb artery, the catheter then being advanced into the aortic arch, is particularly applicable in the investigation of occlusive or stenotic vascular disease in major vessels in the neck, but certain tumours in the neck (e.g. carotid body tumours) may be visualized by this method or by carotid angiography.

Electroencephalography. Electroencephalography may yield localizing evidence of a cortical tumour in the shape of a focus of large delta waves corresponding to the site of the growth (Walter, 1936–7). A tumour involving the basal ganglia may yield a 6 per second theta rhythm (Walter and Dovey, 1944). Many other features of localizing value have been described (Kiloh and Osselton, 1966) and occasionally give a clue to the nature of the lesion (Fischer-Williams *et al.*, 1962).

Isotope Encephalography. Isotope encephalography ('brain-scanning') depends upon the excessive uptake by a tumour or other brain lesion of a radioactive substance which can be detected radiographically. Bull and Marryat (1965) record their experience with 100 cases, using ^{203}Hg chlormerodrin. A positive finding is highly significant. A negative one does not exclude a tumour. The procedure is especially valuable in the detection of multiple metastases. Isotope ventriculography, in which similar scans are performed after the injection of radio-iodinated serum albumin by lumbar puncture is particularly useful in the investigation of communicating hydrocephalus.

Sonoencephalography. Sonoencephalography is the use of ultrasound to provide information about the intracranial contents. A-Scope SEG, its simplest form, is useful for the detection of the displacement of the midline structures, e.g. by a space-occupying lesion. B-Scope and B-Scan SEG are refinements of the technique (Grossman, 1966).

The Cerebrospinal Fluid. Lumbar puncture should be avoided as a rule in suspected cases of intracranial tumour, especially when there is a marked rise of intracranial pressure, and when there is reason to suspect that the tumour is in the posterior fossa. The rapid withdrawal of cerebrospinal fluid from the lumbar subarachnoid space may cause the medulla and cerebellar tonsils to be driven downwards into the foramen magnum, forming the so-called 'cerebellar pressure cone', with possibly fatal results. Herniation of the medial temporal lobe through the tentorial hiatus (tentorial herniation) may also be fatal in cases of supratentorial tumour. When the possibility of an intracranial tumour seems remote and lumbar puncture is indicated for diagnostic purposes the pressure of the cerebrospinal fluid should be determined by manometry, as if it is raised above normal this may suggest that a tumour could after all be present. Usually the rise of pressure of the cerebrospinal fluid is proportional to the severity of the signs of increased intracranial pressure. The protein of the cerebrospinal fluid may be normal but not uncommonly is above normal, though it is not usually higher than 0·1 per cent. In some cases, however, it may be considerably above this figure, and highly albuminous xanthochromic fluids are occasionally observed. A great increase in the protein content of the fluid seems most likely to occur when the tumour is in the neighbourhood of the ventricular system. It is not uncommon in tumours of the corpus callosum, but has also been observed in cases of acoustic neuroma. The cell content of the fluid is usually normal, but a mononuclear pleocytosis may be found when the tumour is closely related to the meninges, especially in metastatic carcinoma of the brain and often in the presence of parasitic cysts. Exceptionally, tumour cells exhibiting active mitosis are found in the fluid. The glucose and chloride contents of the fluid are usually normal and there is no characteristic change in the colloidal gold curve or γ-globulin.

Other Investigations. Other investigations include those necessary to exclude an extracerebral primary tumour, especially radiography of the lungs, which should be carried out in every case.

FOCAL SYMPTOMS

Frontal Lobe

Prefrontal Tumours. By prefrontal tumours are meant tumours confined to that part of the frontal lobe lying anterior to the precentral gyrus. Headache as a rule occurs early, but papilloedema and vomiting usually develop late and may be absent. As we have seen, mental symptoms may occur with a tumour in any situation, even below the tentorium. There is evidence, however, that they are more likely to occur when the tumour is in the corpus callosum or frontal lobe than when it is elsewhere. Moreover, in the absence of other localizing signs the development of mental symptoms before signs of increased intracranial pressure favours a frontal localization. The mental disturbance is a progressive dementia, of which the characteristic feature is a defective grasp of situations as a whole, a failure of the synthetic function of thought. In more severe cases the patient's intellectual capacity suffers more seriously. He becomes stupid, fails to appreciate the gravity of his illness, is careless of his dress and appearance, and develops incontinence of urine and faeces without exhibiting any sense of impropriety. Such patients are sometimes jocular and facetious and repeatedly make simple jokes or puns (Witzelsucht). Irritability of temper and depression are not uncommon.

Generalized convulsions occur in up to 50 per cent. of cases. When the tumour is situated near the base the patient may experience an aura associated with speech. He may feel as if he wishes to speak but cannot do so, and may actually stammer before losing consciousness. There may be a sensation of something gripping the throat. When the tumour is situated towards the superior aspect of the lobe the motor element in the convulsion is likely to consist of turning of the head and eyes to the opposite side with complex clonic and tonic movements of the contralateral limbs.

Catatonia is a symptom which occurs more frequently with frontal lobe tumours than with tumours elsewhere. The patient tends to become immobilized for some time in one attitude; or may maintain indefinitely an attitude into which his limbs have been manipulated by the observer—waxy flexibility.

Expressive aphasia may occur when the tumour involves the posterior part of the inferior frontal gyrus.

The grasp reflex is an important sign, when present, as it is probably pathognomonic of a frontal lobe lesion. It is most frequently observed in the opposite hand, but may be found only in the foot when the tumour is situated in the superior part of the lobe.

A rare sign of a lesion of the frontal lobe which must not be confused with the grasp reflex is tonic innervation or perseveration, which consists of a persistence of muscular contraction voluntarily initiated, due to a failure of relaxation. Tonic perseveration is usually most evident after flexion of the fingers, but may occur after movements of other parts of the body on the side opposite to the lesion. Muscular relaxation is slow and may not be complete for several seconds.

Pressure upon neighbouring corticospinal fibres may lead to weakness upon the opposite side of the body, usually most marked in the face and tongue, and tremor may be present in the limbs either of the same or of the opposite side.

Pressure upon the olfactory nerve, lying upon the floor of the anterior fossa, may lead to anosmia on the side of the lesion. This is most likely to occur in

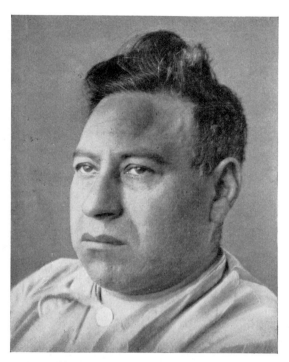

FIG. 53. Erosion of bone and new bone formation leading
to a bony boss overlying a left frontal meningioma

the case of meningiomas arising from the olfactory groove. Such tumours extending backwards may compress the optic nerve, causing primary optic atrophy on the side of the lesion, while the rise of intracranial pressure causes papilloedema on the opposite side (the Foster Kennedy syndrome). Cerebellar symptoms may occur and constitute a false localizing sign.

Precentral Tumours. Precentral tumours are perhaps the easiest to localize on account of the early development of symptoms of excitation and destruction of the corticospinal fibres.

Corticospinal excitation finds expression in a focal convulsion, of which several forms are encountered. In the typical Jacksonian fit [FIG. 54] the convulsion begins with clonic movements, rarely with tonic spasm, in a limited area of the opposite side of the body, e.g. the thumb, and slowly spreads, involving other parts in the order in which they are represented in the precentral gyrus [see p. 18]. When the whole of one side of the body is convulsed the opposite side may become involved, and at this stage consciousness is usually lost. Partial Jacksonian attacks may occur, in which the convulsion is limited to a small part of one side of the body, without loss of consciousness. Such a convulsion may be continuous—'epilepsia partialis continua'. Jacksonian attacks may occur at long intervals, or with great frequency, even up to several hundreds a day—serial Jacksonian epilepsy. When consciousness is not regained between successive attacks the condition is described as Jacksonian status epilepticus.

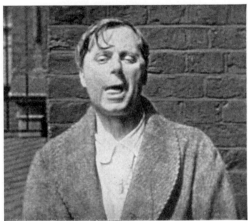

FIG. 54. Jacksonian convulsion beginning in the left side of the face, due to a tumour in the lower part of the right precentral gyrus

Motor weakness is the result of the destruction of the corticospinal fibres by the tumour, and exhibits a regional distribution corresponding to the representation of parts of the body in the precentral gyrus. Owing to the large surface extent of the corticospinal cells on the cortex, even a large cortical tumour is likely to cause weakness of only a part of the opposite side of the body, that is, a monoplegia. With inferiorly placed tumours there is weakness, often accompanied by apraxia, of the face and tongue on the opposite side, and weakness of movements of the thumb, which is represented in the adjacent area. If the tumour is at a higher level the thumb may escape, though the fingers and arm are affected, while a tumour involving principally the medial aspect of the hemisphere is likely to cause a monoplegia involving only the foot or the whole lower limb. The usual reflex changes associated with a corticospinal lesion are found, and such reflex abnormalities may be limited to the paretic part.

A tumour of the falx in the region of the paracentral lobule (a parasagittal meningioma) is likely to produce weakness of both lower limbs, beginning in the feet, one being usually affected more than the other. Retention of urine may occur owing to compression of the cortical centres for the detrusor of the bladder. There may be an impairment of postural sensibility in the toes when the sensory area of the paracentral lobule is involved.

Jacksonian convulsions are usually associated with permanent weakness of the part of the body which is the focus of the fit, but after each convulsion there is often a temporary extension of this weakness to other parts (Todd's paralysis). Sensory loss is absent, unless the tumour extends to the postcentral gyrus.

Temporal Lobe

The focal symptoms of temporal lobe tumours are often slight, especially when the tumour is on the right side. When the lesion is anteriorly situated and involves the uncus there is often a very characteristic group of symptoms. This is the cortical centre for taste and smell, and the closely associated motor functions of licking, mastication, and swallowing are also represented in this region. Tumours of the uncus may cause so-called uncinate fits which are characterized by (1) an olfactory or gustatory aura, (2) certain motor concomitants, and (3) an abnormal state of consciousness.

1. The aura consists of an hallucination of taste or smell which is usually unpleasant but occasionally pleasant. It may be described as resembling paint, gas, acetylene, 'something burning', or even, as one patient put it, the monkey house at the Zoo. There may be abnormal sensations referred to the epigastrium.

2. Involuntary licking, smacking the lips, or tasting movements frequently accompany the olfactory or gustatory aura and form the motor component of the uncinate fit.

3. The patient presents a dazed or dreamy appearance and usually stops what he is doing, but does not fall. He may have no recollection of the attack afterwards or he may describe peculiar disturbances of memory, for example, the *déjà vu* phenomenon, a feeling that everything that is happening has happened before, or experience a recurrent dream, or he may in a very short time relive in detail a large part of his past life. He may experience illusions relating to the external world or his own body. Objects may appear larger or smaller or more distant than normally, or unreal. There may be visual or auditory hallucinations. A sense of depersonalization or unreality (*jamais vu*) may occur. Emotional disturbances include fear and depression.

Destruction in the region of the uncus leads to an impairment of taste and smell on the side of the lesion, though this does not as a rule proceed to complete loss. Generalized convulsions may also occur when a tumour involves the temporal lobe.

Visual field defects may be produced by tumours of the temporal lobe. They are absent in at least half of all cases, but when present are of great localizing value. The lower fibres of the optic radiation are likely to be caught in their path around the tip of the inferior horn of the ventricle. The characteristic defect is therefore a crossed upper quadrantic hemianopia, the loss being usually more extensive in the ipsilateral field. Although the cortical centre for hearing is situated in the posterior part of the temporal lobe, temporal tumours do not cause complete deafness in either ear, though a unilateral lesion in this situation may lead to some bilateral impairment of hearing. Temporal tumours may cause tinnitus or auditory hallucinations, in which the patient may imagine that the words which he seems to hear are addressed to him by a person who happens to be in the room. Left-sided temporal lobe tumours cause aphasia in about 50 per cent. of cases. This may merely take the form of a defect in naming objects. In more severe cases central aphasia, with or without word-deafness, is present [see p. 103]. The patient is unable to understand spoken words and this disability may extend to written words also. When speech is even more severely disordered the patient speaks jargon, his speech consisting often of a voluble outpouring of meaningless phrases and words of his own construction. Apraxia sometimes occurs.

Neighbourhood symptoms include weakness of conjugate deviation of the eyes to the opposite side, signs of a corticospinal lesion on the opposite side, especially weakness of the face, and tremor either on the same or on the opposite side of the body. Myosis and slight ptosis due to compression of the ocular sympathetic may be seen in the early stages and may give place to mydriasis and other signs of third-nerve palsy. Diminution of the corneal reflex on the affected side may be the only evidence of compression of the trigeminal nerve.

Parietal Lobe

The parietal lobe is the principal sensory area of the cerebral cortex. Sensory disturbances therefore constitute a prominent part of the symptoms of tumours of this region. The postcentral gyrus is the part of the parietal lobe most concerned with sensation. Parts of the body are here represented for purposes of sensation in a manner similar to their motor representation in the precentral gyrus. From below upwards we encounter in the following order the larynx and pharynx, the tongue, the buccal cavity, the face, neck, thumb, index, second, third, and fourth fingers, the hand, forearm, upper arm, shoulder, chest, abdomen, thigh, and leg. The foci of the foot and toes are situated at the superior border of the hemisphere, and on the medial aspect, in the paracentral lobule, lie the foci of the bladder, rectum, and genital organs [see p. 18].

Irritation of the postcentral gyrus causes sensory Jacksonian fits which consist usually of paraesthesiae, such as tingling or 'electric shocks', rarely of pain, and which begin in that part of the opposite side of the body corresponding to the focus of excitation. The paraesthesiae then spread to other parts in the order of their representation in the gyrus. Such sensory fits may occur alone, or may be followed by a similar spreading motor discharge due to the extension of the excitation to the precentral gyrus, in which case the clonic convulsion often lags behind the advance of the paraesthesiae.

A destructive lesion of the postcentral gyrus leads to sensory loss, the extent of which corresponds in distribution to the extent of the cortical lesion. The sensory loss is of the cortical type, that is, it involves the spatial and discriminative aspects of sensation, especially postural sensibility and tactile discrimination, while the crude appreciation of pain, heat, and cold is left intact. As a result of sensory loss the patient may be unable to recognize objects placed in his affected hand—'astereognosis'.

Postcentral lesions lead also to hypotonia and wasting of the affected parts and to both static and kinetic ataxia. When the patient is at rest there is often a conspicuous restlessness of the affected upper limb, sometimes amounting to 'pseudo-athetosis', and he may gesticulate exaggeratedly with the affected hand. There is likely to be considerable ataxia in the finger–nose test—'sensory ataxia'.

Parietal tumours reaching deep into the white matter may lead to 'thalamic over-reaction', an exaggerated response to unpleasant stimuli on the opposite side of the body, though this is usually present to only a slight extent. Involvement of the fibres of the optic radiation causes a crossed homonymous defect of the visual fields; and since the upper fibres are the more likely to be caught, the field defect may be confined to the lower quadrant.

The posterior part of the parietal lobe constitutes a 'watershed' between the three great cortical sensory areas, the optic, acoustic, and somatic. A left-sided lesion of this area may therefore be expected to cause considerable disturbance of speech on its receptive side. Lesions of the left angular gyrus usually cause alexia and agraphia with which may be associated finger-agnosia and acalculia. Lesions of the same area on the right side cause disturbances of awareness of the opposite side of the body and half of space [see pp. 115 and 116]. Lesions of the left supramarginal gyrus may cause ideational apraxia.

Occipital Lobe

Tumours of the occipital lobe are comparatively rare. Headache is an early symptom, and other signs of increased intracranial pressure are usually conspicuous. Epileptiform convulsions occur in a considerable proportion of cases —50 per cent. in one series. They may be preceded by a visual aura, such as flashes of light moving from one side towards the middle line, but this is not constant. Such attacks may begin with turning of the eyes to the opposite side. The characteristic focal sign of an occipital tumour is a visual field defect. This may consist of a crossed homonymous hemianopia extending up to the fixation point, or of a crossed homonymous quadrantic defect, or of a crescentic loss in the periphery of the opposite half-fields. Hemianopia may have been discovered by the patient owing to his collisions with people or objects on his blind side.

Lesions in the left lateral occipital region cause visual object-agnosia and agnosia for colours. Extension of the tumour to the region of the angular gyrus on the left side leads to the symptoms described in the preceding section. Neighbourhood symptoms may be present. The commonest of these are auditory hallucinations with word-deafness when the posterior part of the temporal lobe is involved; impairment of taste and smell; sensory impairment of cortical type, and slight motor weakness, both on the opposite side; and nystagmus, hypotonia, and inco-ordination on the same side, the result of pressure transmitted to the cerebellum.

Corpus Callosum

Tumours of the corpus callosum are more common than is generally realized. Bull (1967) has recently pointed out that one quarter of all hemisphere astrocytomas show macroscopic or microscopic evidence of invasion of the corpus callosum. Sometimes they yield a distinctive clinical picture but more often the clinical presentation is non-specific. Mental symptoms are prominent and are often the first symptoms to be noticed. It is said that mental changes are more frequently observed in cases of tumour of the corpus callosum than when the tumour is situated in any other part of the brain, including the frontal lobe. Apathy, drowsiness, and defect of memory are the commonest mental disturbances, but any of the mental symptoms already described as occurring in cases of cerebral tumour may be present. The defect of memory may be so severe that a patient who has suffered from an intense headache may in a few minutes have forgotten it completely. General convulsions are common. Indeed, a combination of progressive dementia with major (or focal) attacks of epilepsy must always raise the possibility of a tumour in this position. The situation of the tumour in the midline extending laterally into the central white matter on both sides leads early to damage to the corticospinal tracts. This is usually asymmetrical in the early stages, and it is then common to find hemiplegia on one side, while the other exhibits the reflex changes resulting from a corticospinal lesion, with little loss of power. Later, double hemiplegia may be found. Anteriorly placed tumours extending into the frontal lobes may cause a grasp reflex on one or both sides. Apraxia is present in a small proportion of cases. It may occur on the left side only, owing to interruption of fibres linking the left supramarginal gyrus with the right corticospinal tract. Tremor and choreiform movements sometimes occur and are probably due to involvement of the corpus striatum. Signs of increased intracranial pressure are often late in developing. The protein content of the cerebrospinal fluid is likely to be high.

Centrum Semiovale and Basal Ganglia

The centrum semiovale consists mainly of corticospinal fibres converging on the internal capsule, and sensory fibres diverging from the latter to the various cortical sensory areas. Tumours in this region may cause little disturbance of the intracranial pressure, but they usually cause motor or sensory symptoms early. Owing to the concentration of fibres near the internal capsule the whole of the opposite side of the body is likely to be affected. Anteriorly placed tumours cause a progressive spastic hemiplegia. When the tumour is situated more posteriorly the presenting symptoms are sensory, and all forms of sensibility are usually impaired on the opposite side, and sensory ataxia is present. Hemianopia may be added if the optic radiation is involved. Somnolence is not uncommon when the tumour invades the region of the thalamus; and signs of pressure upon the upper part of the midbrain may be found, especially weakness of conjugate deviation upwards and inequality of the pupils. The invasion of the third ventricle by the tumour is rapidly followed by the development of signs of increased intracranial pressure if these have not been present before (see McKissock and Paine, 1958).

Third Ventricle

The third ventricle may be the primary site of a tumour, e.g. a colloid cyst, or it may be invaded by a tumour arising below, in the interpeduncular space, above, in the falx or corpus callosum, or laterally, in the basal ganglia. Such extraventricular tumours usually yield ample evidence of their presence before they invade the ventricle. Tumours arising in the ventricle, however, are often difficult to localize. Hydrocephalus may be acute, subacute, intermittent, or chronic. Severe paroxysmal headaches are common, and may be influenced by changes in the position of the head. Headache and papilloedema may be the only symptoms. Progressive dementia may occur, or coma may suddenly develop. Impairment of memory, including a Korsakow-like syndrome, may occur.

Somnolence, polyuria, hyperglycaemia and glycosuria, obesity, sexual regression, and irregular pyrexia may be produced by downward pressure by a tumour upon the tuber cinereum and pituitary body. Lateral extension of the growth in the region of the internal capsule causes signs of corticospinal defect on one or both sides.

Midbrain

Tumours arising in the midbrain usually cause internal hydrocephalus early owing to obstruction of the cerebral aqueduct. Headache, papilloedema, and vomiting are therefore conspicuous. Owing to the concentration in this region of the nuclei of the third and fourth cranial nerves and the supranuclear paths converging upon them, ocular abnormalities are prominent. Lesions of the upper part of the midbrain usually cause a paresis of conjugate ocular deviation upwards, and retraction of the upper lids may be associated with this. Lesions of the lower half cause paresis of conjugate ocular deviation downwards with which ptosis and paresis of convergence may be combined. Conjugate lateral movement of the eyes usually escapes, at least in the early stages, though a lesion just above the pons may involve the supranuclear fibres for lateral movement at their decussation and so cause a bilateral paralysis of lateral conjugate gaze.

The pupils are often unequal and tend to be dilated. The reactions both to light and on convergence-accommodation may be lost, or the latter may be preserved when the former is lost. Asymmetrical nuclear ophthalmoplegia may occur.

The corticospinal tracts are usually involved on both sides, though one is often more severely affected than the other. The characteristic reflex changes of corticospinal lesions are present. Weakness and spasticity, slight in the early stages, progress until in some cases a condition of virtual decerebrate rigidity supervenes. 'Tonic' fits characterized by opisthotonos with extension of all four limbs and loss of consciousness may occur. Tremor is common, and nystagmus and ataxia result from injury to the cerebellar connexions. Choreiform movements are occasionally observed.

Sensory changes are due to damage to the long ascending sensory paths. Extensive areas of analgesia and defects of postural sensibility may be encountered. Compression of the lateral lemniscus may lead to unilateral or bilateral deafness.

Pineal Body

The symptoms of tumours of the pineal body consist of (1) signs of increased intracranial pressure, (2) signs of pressure upon neighbouring parts of the brain, and (3) in exceptional cases disturbances of growth and development. Since the pineal body is situated between the splenium of the corpus callosum above and the superior colliculi below, its enlargement speedily causes internal hydrocephalus, owing to obstruction to the drainage of the third ventricle, and symptoms of compression of the upper part of the midbrain. Signs of increased intracranial pressure therefore occur early, and are associated with the signs of a midbrain lesion as described in the previous section, namely, defect of conjugate ocular deviation upwards, less often downwards and laterally; paresis of convergence; retraction or ptosis of the upper lids; inequality of the pupils, which are usually dilated; reflex iridoplegia; bilateral signs of corticospinal lesion; nystagmus and ataxia; tremor and sensory loss, including deafness.

The disturbances of growth are found only when the tumour develops in young boys, and not always then, occurring in only about 14 per cent. of all cases. They consist of mental precocity, abnormal growth of the skeleton, and premature development of the genitalia and secondary sexual characteristics, a syndrome which has received the name 'macrogenitosomia praecox'. The cause of these symptoms is unknown. There is some recent evidence to suggest that tumours in this area may rarely secrete aldosterone, or perhaps stimulate the output of aldosterone from the adrenals, giving the manifestations of aldosteronism.

The internal hydrocephalus caused by a pineal tumour may lead to 'hypopituitarism', and obesity may thus complicate the clinical picture.

The Region of the Optic Chiasma

The small region at the base of the brain lying between the optic chiasma and the cerebral peduncles is the site of tumours arising in four situations, namely, (1) tumours of the hypophysis, (2) craniopharyngiomas, (3) suprasellar meningiomas, and (4) gliomas of the optic chiasma. Since these tumours are distinguished by differences in the general and focal symptoms to which they give rise it is convenient to consider them separately.

Tumours of the Hypophysis. As already described, three pathological types of hypophysial tumour commonly occur, namely, (a) chromophil, (b) chromophobe, thus described in terms of the reaction of their cells to eosin staining, and (c) basophil adenomas. The symptoms of these tumours may be divided into (1) endocrine disturbances which vary according to the pathological nature of the tumour, (2) pressure symptoms, and (3) alterations in radiographic appearance, which, though varying in severity, are common to the first two tumours in virtue of their situation within the sella turcica.

1. *Endocrine Disturbances.* (a) *Chromophil Adenoma.* In this tumour the eosinophil cells characteristic of the anterior lobe of the normal hypophysis predominate, though chromophobe cells may also be present. The endocrine symptoms are commonly regarded as due to an overproduction of the growth hormone of the gland, that is to say, as pathological hyperpituitarism. When the tumour arises before growth has ceased, gigantism occurs; when, as more frequently happens, the tumour begins during adult life, acromegaly is the result [FIG. 55]. This is characterized by slow changes in the skin and subcutaneous tissues, bones, viscera, general metabolism, and sexual activity. The skin and subcutaneous tissues, especially of the fingers, lips, ears, and tongue, exhibit a fibrous hyperplasia, and paraesthesiae may occur in the fingers. Overgrowth of the bones is most evident in the skull, face, mandible, and at the periphery of the extremities. The calvarium is thickened and the bony ridges and points of attachment of muscles are increased in size. The zygomatic bones enlarge, and

as a result of overgrowth of the mandible the lower jaw becomes prognathous, and separation of the teeth occurs. The hands become broad and spade-like and hyperostoses may develop on the terminal phalanges ('tufting'). Similar changes occur in the feet, and the patient frequently notices that he requires a larger size in gloves and boots. Compression of the median nerves in the carpal tunnels may occur. Kyphosis in the upper dorsal spine is common and hypertrophy

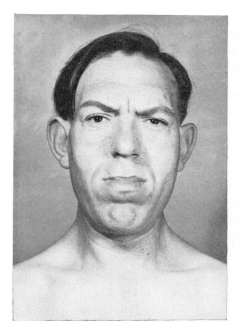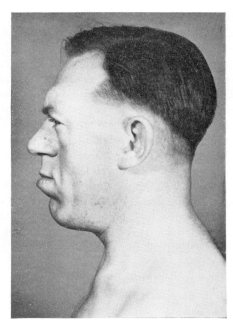

FIG. 55. Acromegaly

of many of the viscera has been described. Sugar metabolism is often disturbed, leading to hyperglycaemia and glycosuria, which frequently responds less to insulin than is the case in diabetes mellitus. Thyrotoxicosis may occur, and hypertrichosis may be present. Impairment of sexual function occurs in both gigantism and acromegaly, impotence in the male and relative or complete amenorrhoea in the female being the rule. Enlargement of the breasts, and lactation persisting for months, and occurring even in nulliparous women, have been described in association with hypophysial tumours, presumably due to an overproduction of prolactin.

(b) *Chromophobe Adenoma.* These tumours occur almost exclusively in adult life and according to Cushing are three times as common as the chromophil tumour which is associated with acromegaly. Since both their endocrine and their pressure symptoms are apt to be less obtrusive, the diagnosis is much more likely to be missed. The endocrine symptoms of the chromophobe tumour are usually ascribed to its destructive effect upon hypophysial function, that is, they are regarded as due to hypopituitarism. The first symptom is usually a depression of sexual function, which in women takes the form of scanty menstruation,

progressing to complete amenorrhoea, and in men to impotence. Women sometimes give a history of a late onset as well as an early cessation of menstruation.
The skin becomes soft and pliable and there is often a loss of hair over the
limbs and trunks (particularly in the axillae and pubic regions), and over the
face in men. Moderate obesity often develops, associated with a lowered metabolic rate and increased sugar tolerance. The biochemical changes of hypothyroidism, hypo-adrenalism, and hypogonadism will be found. These symptoms
may be present for many years before pressure symptoms occur. Rarely a
chromophobe adenoma is associated with Cushing's syndrome.

(c) *Basophil Adenoma*. The basophil adenoma rarely attains a sufficient size
to cause pressure symptoms. It has been found in association with a syndrome
(Cushing's syndrome) characterized by remarkable metabolic disorders, but
Crooke (1935) has found that a hyaline change in the basophil cells of the
anterior lobe of the hypophysis is the only feature common to patients exhibiting
the syndrome hitherto attributed to the basophil adenoma, whether this is
associated with basophil adenoma of the hypophysis, hyperplasia or neoplasm of
the suprarenal cortex, tumour of the thymus, or bronchial carcinoma. Recently,
however, true basophil adenomas have been discovered in patients who had
previously undergone adrenalectomy for Cushing's syndrome. The individuals
affected are usually young women, and their symptoms, to which Cushing drew
attention, include painful, plethoric adiposity, associated with cutaneous striae
and purpuric patches, hirsuties, amenorrhoea, hyperglycaemia, hypertension,
polycythaemia, and osteoporosis.

2. *Pressure Symptoms*. Pressure symptoms may be entirely absent particularly
in the case of the basophil adenoma and less often with the chromophil (acidophil)
adenoma which may for some time produce only endocrine effects. Headache
is usually an early symptom of hypophysial tumour, and is more marked as
a rule when the tumour is of the chromophil, than when it is of the chromophobe,
type. In the early stages it is due to expansion of the sella and is usually described
as a 'bursting' headache with a bitemporal distribution. If later the tumour
extends beyond the diaphragma sellae the headache is due to general increase
of intracranial pressure. Vomiting is usually absent, except in the later stages.
Since the optic chiasma lies above the diaphragma sellae, visual field defects
are an important and early symptom of hypophysial tumours. Usually the
tumour as it enlarges upwards first compresses the decussating fibres of the
chiasma, hence bitemporal hemianopia is the field defect most frequently
encountered [see p. 53]. This is as a rule asymmetrical, the defect beginning in
the periphery of the upper temporal quadrant on one side, whence it extends
towards the fixation point and downwards into the lower temporal quadrant.
A similar change occurs either simultaneously or subsequently on the opposite
side. In other cases the defect may begin as a scotoma on the temporal side of
the fixation point. As the tumour grows, the nasal field of the eye first affected
is encroached upon so that the patient often passes through a stage of complete
blindness in one eye with a temporal hemianopia on the opposite side. Later,
if the pressure is not relieved, the second eye also becomes blind. Less frequently one or other optic tract is compressed before the chiasma with the production of a homonymous hemianopia. Rarely the visual paths escape damage.

Compression of the optic chiasma causes primary optic atrophy, which is often more advanced in one eye than in the other. As the pressure at the same time obliterates the subarachnoid sheath of the optic nerves, papilloedema rarely occurs. In the later stages of the development of the growth ocular palsies may be produced by compression of the third or sixth cranial nerves, and trigeminal pain, usually referred to the first division of the nerve and sometimes associated with analgesia.

Cerebral symptoms do not occur until the tumour has expanded beyond the sella, when compression of the cerebral peduncles or invasion of one hemisphere from below may lead to unilateral or bilateral signs of corticospinal defect; uncinate fits may result from compression of the uncus, and pressure upon the frontal lobe may lead to marked mental deterioration, with or without abnormal emotional reactions.

3. *Radiographic Appearances*. Adenoma of the hypophysis, except the basophil variety, causes a uniform expansion of the sella, with thinning of its walls [see p. 232].

Craniopharyngioma. The pathology of these tumours has already been described. Since they depend upon abnormalities of development, symptoms often appear at an early age, and in more than one-third of the cases the patient comes for treatment before the age of 15. Less frequently, however, they cause no symptoms until middle life or even old age. These tumours usually arise above the sellar diaphragm, but exceptionally they develop within the sella itself.

1. *Endocrine Disturbances*. Since they are situated between the floor of the third ventricle and the hypophysis and develop at an early age, they may produce a large variety of disturbances of growth and metabolism, which may be due to their compression either of the hypophysis or of the tuber cinereum, or of both of these structures. In Cushing's words, 'the patient may show extreme degrees of adiposity or emaciation, of polyuria or the reverse, of dwarfism, of sexual infantilism or of premature physical senility'. In the later stages the patient may be drowsy, and urticaria and hyperpyrexia have not uncommonly followed operative interference with the growth. When the tumour first produces symptoms later in life endocrine disturbances may, by contrast, be few, though diabetes insipidus may occur.

2. *Pressure Symptoms*. Symptoms of increased intracranial pressure are much more conspicuous than in the case of hypophysial tumours. When the tumour arises in childhood the skull may be enlarged and the sutures separated. Headache and vomiting may be severe, and papilloedema is rather commoner than optic atrophy. The tumour may compress the optic nerves, chiasma, or tracts leading to corresponding field defects. The optic chiasma is compressed from above, hence the resulting bitemporal hemianopia usually begins in the lower quadrants. The frontal lobes, temporal lobes, and cerebral peduncles may also be compressed.

3. *Radiographic Appearances*. These consist of (i) general signs of increased intracranial pressure, such as convolutional thinning, (ii) erosion of the clinoid processes and flattening of the sella turcica, the result of downward pressure by the tumour, (iii) radiographic evidence of calcification within the tumour, which is present in about 75 per cent. of cases and varies from faint, opaque flecks to

a mass the size of a hen's egg, lying above the sella turcica. Occasionally there are also areas of calcification within the sella.

Suprasellar Meningioma. Suprasellar meningiomas are tumours of adult life arising from the meninges which cover the circle of venous sinuses around the diaphragma sellae. Headache is not as a rule severe and endocrine symptoms are usually absent. The principal symptoms are visual and are due to compression of the optic nerve, chiasma, or tract, according to the position of the tumour. Primary optic atrophy is the rule and the visual field defects may consist either of hemianopia or a central or temporal paracentral scotoma. One eye is usually affected before the other and to a greater extent. Pressure of the tumour upon the base of the brain may lead to uncinate attacks, general convulsions, and hemiparesis. Radiograms may show no abnormality, or the optic canal or clinoid processes may be eroded and the sella flattened, and there may be opacities due to calcification within the growth.

Glioma of the Optic Chiasma. This is a rare tumour which usually occurs in childhood, and may be associated with generalized neurofibromatosis. Owing to the situation of the tumour visual deterioration usually draws attention to its presence before a marked rise of intracranial pressure occurs. Primary optic atrophy is the rule and the visual field defects are often bizarre, and may not conform to the more familiar bitemporal or homonymous hemianopia. Exophthalmos may occur. Endocrine disturbances are absent. Radiograms usually show enlargement of one optic foramen and less often enlargement of the sella turcica forwards beneath the anterior clinoid processes.

Cerebellum

The cerebellum is a common site of tumour, especially in childhood. Medulloblastomas are usually found in the cerebellum during the first decade of life. They arise in the midline in the region of the roof of the fourth ventricle. Astrocytomas, though they may occur either in the cerebrum or in the cerebellum, are also most frequently encountered in the latter during childhood or early adult life, and are often cystic. Haemangioblastomas are almost exclusively cerebellar tumours, and are also usually cystic.

Cerebellar tumours arise in the midline but many then extend into one or other hemisphere. The symptoms differ considerably according to whether the tumour is median or lateral.

Midline Cerebellar Tumours. In this group the history is usually short and the patient, generally a child, is likely to be brought for examination within a few weeks of the onset. Symptoms of increased intracranial pressure occur early, and often become severe. Headache, vomiting, and papilloedema are conspicuous, and in children hydrocephalus often leads to enlargement of the skull, with separation of the sutures. Symptoms of cerebellar deficiency are usually most marked on standing and walking (truncal ataxia), and there may be little or no ataxia of the limbs on examination. Giddiness is common, and there is usually unsteadiness on standing, especially with the eyes closed. The patient usually tends to fall backwards, sometimes forwards. The gait tends to be broad-based and unsteady, especially on turning. Nystagmus is often absent, but there is usually muscular hypotonia which may be unequal in degree upon the two sides of the body. Compression of the midbrain may lead to 'tonic fits', characterized by extension of all four limbs and opisthotonos, with loss of consciousness, and the pupils are occasionally dilated and exhibit sluggish reactions, a misleading sign which may suggest a tumour of the third ventricle or pineal body. The remaining cranial nerves are often little affected, though weakness of one or both lateral recti and slight facial weakness may be encountered. There is as a rule little weakness of the limbs, though an extensor plantar response on one or both sides may be found. The tendon reflexes may be sluggish, probably as a result of raised intracranial pressure. Sensory loss is exceptional.

Tumours of the Cerebellar Hemisphere. As in the case of midline cerebellar tumours signs of increased intracranial pressure usually occur early, but a cystic haemangioblastoma may attain a large size without causing conspicuous symptoms. In addition to suboccipital headache early symptoms include clumsiness of the ipsilateral hand, a tendency to stagger to the side of the lesion, and giddiness on turning the head.

Nystagmus is usually marked and is most evident on conjugate lateral ocular deviation to the side of the lesion. The quick phase is directed towards the periphery and the slow phase towards the centre. Nystagmus is usually confined to the plane in which the eyes are deviated, but may occasionally be rotary. Other signs of a deficiency of cerebellar function are most marked in, and often confined to, the limbs on the side of the lesion. Hypotonia is usually conspicuous. The outstretched upper limb on the affected side tends to sway if unsupported. Ataxia is present on the affected side, being most evident in the upper limb on carrying out fine movements, for example in the finger–nose test, and in the lower limb in walking. The gait is unsteady. The patient tends to walk with a wide base and deviate to the affected side, and is liable to fall to the affected side when standing up with the feet together and the eyes closed. Rapid alternating movements are carried out with the affected limb in an irregular, jerky manner or may even be impossible. The shoulder on the affected side is sometimes held lower than the normal shoulder, and there may be scoliosis with the concavity towards the side of the lesion.

There is occasionally an abnormal attitude of the head, which is flexed to one side and rotated so that the occiput is directed towards the shoulder, towards which the head is flexed. This rotated, or, as it is sometimes called, 'cerebellar', posture of the head may occur in the absence of a lesion of the cerebellum, and is due to an interruption of afferent impulses derived from the otolith organs of the internal ear. In the early stages of a lateral cerebellar tumour the head is usually flexed and rotated to the side of the lesion. Later, when the tumour is sufficiently large to exert pressure upon the brain stem, the head is rotated to the opposite side. Speech is usually little affected in cerebellar tumours, whether of the midline or lateral lobes. [For other symptoms of cerebellar deficiency see p. 61.]

The symptoms of cerebellar deficiency associated with a tumour of the cerebellum often appear to be disproportionately slight with reference to the size of the tumour. It is known that after ablation of the cerebellum a considerable recovery of function may occur, and it is probable that the slow growth of the tumour permits a gradual compensation for cerebellar deficiency by other parts of the nervous system.

Neighbourhood symptoms are usually more conspicuous in the case of lateral cerebellar tumours than when the tumour is in the midline. Forward pressure by the tumour may cause a disturbance of function of any of the cranial nerves from the fifth to the twelfth on the same side, the fifth, sixth, and seventh being most frequently affected. Pressure upon the ipsilateral half of the pons and medulla not infrequently leads to slight signs of corticospinal defect on the opposite side of the body and occasionally to sensory loss, especially impairment of postural sensibility, though this is rarely marked. Sometimes ipsilateral signs of corticospinal tract dysfunction arise due to pressure of the contralateral crus cerebri against the free edge of the tentorium.

Eighth Nerve

Tumours of the eighth nerve (acoustic neuromas) may be either unilateral or bilateral. In the latter case they are usually manifestations of general neurofibromatosis. They rarely give rise to symptoms before the third decade of life and most commonly during the fifth decade. They are tumours of slow growth, and focal symptoms commonly exist for years before those of increased intracranial pressure develop. Owing to the situation of the tumour upon the eighth nerve the first symptoms are due to a disturbance of the functions of this nerve, and this feature is so constant that if a tumour situated in the cerebellopontine angle manifests itself through some other inaugural symptom it is unlikely to be an acoustic neuroma. Tinnitus is usually the first symptom, followed by progressive deafness, through sometimes labyrinthine symptoms, for example giddiness, precede disturbances of hearing. It is not uncommon to find that a patient, when he first comes under observation, is completely deaf in the affected ear. Headache at first is usually occipital, but sometimes frontal, and tends to radiate from back to front through the mastoid region. In the late stages it becomes general and there may be attacks of severe occipital pain radiating down the spine and associated with retraction of the head and neck, respiratory embarrassment, and, sometimes, loss of consciousness. Papilloedema and vomiting are comparatively late in developing. The patient may complain of paraesthesiae referred to the face on one or both sides, and attacks of facial spasm may occur. Diplopia is not uncommon. Dysphagia is a late symptom.

On examination there are signs of impaired conductivity in the affected eighth nerve. Hearing is much reduced and may be completely lost. Tests of vestibular function usually show loss of sensitivity—a canal paresis. This usually occurs alone but sometimes in combination with a directional preponderance to the unaffected side (Carmichael, Dix, and Hallpike, 1956). The head is sometimes rotated so that the occiput is directed towards the shoulder of the affected side.

Other signs result from pressure by the tumour upon neighbouring cranial nerves. There is usually some facial weakness on the affected side, though this may be slight. Sensory loss may occur in the trigeminal distribution, but reduction or loss of the corneal reflex may be the only sign of involvement of the fifth nerve. Weakness of the lateral rectus may be present as a result of compression of the sixth nerve. The remaining cranial nerves are usually unaffected. Disturbance of function of the fifth, sixth, seventh, and eighth cranial nerves may occur on the opposite side as well as on the side of the tumour. Compression of the ipsilateral cerebellar hemisphere causes symptoms of cerebellar deficiency on the side of the tumour. Signs of compression of the brain stem are not as a rule conspicuous, but crossed hemiparesis and hemianaesthesia may occur as a result of compression of the long descending and ascending tracts, and weakness of conjugate ocular deviation to the side of the tumour, as a result of compression of the pons.

Atypical symptoms, occurring when the tumour arises more medially than usual, include acute or chronic hydrocephalus, causing rapid visual failure and slow mental deterioration, respectively, also paroxysmal disorders of consciousness, including epilepsy (Shephard and Wadia, 1956). Radiographic examination may show erosion of the petrous portion of the temporal bone or of the internal acoustic meatus by the tumour.

Pons and Medulla

The commonest tumour of the brain stem is the pontine astrocytoma of childhood. Owing to the close association in the pons and medulla of important cranial nerve nuclei as well as of the descending and ascending fibre tracts, tumours in this region soon give rise to localizing signs and symptoms. Possibly for this reason signs of increased intracranial pressure are often slight when the patient first comes under observation. Vomiting is often absent, and papilloedema appears in under 50 per cent. of cases. Headache, which in the early stages is mainly occipital, and vertigo are common, and both may be intensified by rotation of the head. Diplopia is usually the first focal symptom, a point of distinction from cerebellar medulloblastoma. At first the signs may point to a lesion confined to one-half of the brain stem but they soon become bilateral. Weakness of the lateral rectus on one or both sides usually develops early, and may be followed by paresis of conjugate ocular deviation, or the latter may occur alone. Crossed paralysis is usually seen at an early stage, the distribution of the paresis on the two sides of the body depending upon the level of the tumour. Most frequently there is weakness of the jaw and facial muscles on one side and of the soft palate, tongue, and limbs on the other. Later bilateral paralysis of the bulbar muscles and limbs usually develops. Sensory loss in the region of the trigeminal distribution with reduction of the corneal reflex is usually present on one or both sides, and impairment of hearing may occur. Sensory loss on the limbs and trunk is variable. Analgesia and thermo-anaesthesia may occur without loss of postural sensibility or vice versa, or all forms of sensibility may be affected. Sensory changes may be predominantly unilateral or bilateral. Nystagmus and some degree of ataxia of the limbs are common, even though the cerebellum is not itself invaded. A rotated posture of the head is not uncommon, the head being flexed and rotated towards the side less affected by the tumour. Paralysis of the ocular sympathetic on one or both sides is frequent, and the visceral functions of the medulla may be disordered, leading to tachy-cardia or cardiac irregularity, alterations in the respiratory rate and rhythm, hiccup, and glycosuria. The course of the illness due to these tumours is some-times protracted, lasting for several years, as many of them are very slow-growing (the condition which used to be called 'benign hypertrophy of the pons' is now known to be due to a slow-growing astrocytoma).

Fourth Ventricle

Tumours arising in the fourth ventricle itself are usually ependymomas originating in the ependymal cells, though the fourth ventricle may be invaded by tumours arising in the vermis of the cerebellum or in the pons. The charac-teristic triad of symptoms are headache, morning vomiting and vertigo, with nystagmus increased or elicited by change in position of the head. In young patients ependymoma is the commonest cause but over the age of 50 the same syndrome may result from metastases in the fourth ventricle (usually from bronchial carcinoma). Headache is an early symptom and is liable to paroxysmal exacerbations, the pain radiating to the neck and even to the shoulders and arms. Vomiting and papilloedema and other evidences of hydrocephalus usually develop rapidly. But headache and papilloedema may be absent: one patient had no symptoms except vomiting, for which he had had a laparotomy, and an ataxic gait. There is often stiffness of the cervical muscles and disorders of equilibrium are prominent. The patient often tends to fall backwards, and the gait may be ataxic. Symptoms of cerebellar deficiency in the limbs may be slight or absent. 'Tonic fits' may occur. Disturbance of function of the cranial nerves is often slight, though there may be paresis of one or both lateral recti, and trismus may occur. The tumour may lead to disturbances of the visceral centres of the medulla, causing attacks of tachycardia, dyspnoea and irregular respiration, hiccup, sweating, and vasomotor disturbances, polyuria, and glyco-suria. Sudden death may occur.

In some cases the tumour grows out from the fourth ventricle and surrounds and compresses the spinal cord at the level of the foramen magnum, producing analgesia and thermo-anaesthesia of the face and upper limbs, with signs of corticospinal involvement, and leading to a clinical picture closely resembling syringobulbia. In such cases Queckenstedt's test may reveal a blockage of the subarachnoid space.

Basal Meninges

Neoplastic infiltration of the basal meninges leads to a fairly distinctive clinical picture. This condition may be due to metastases from extracranial neoplasms, or to extension to within the cranial cavity of a primary carcinoma of a nasal sinus or other nasopharyngeal growth. It leads to progressive cranial nerve palsies, which are usually bilateral but often asymmetrical. Papilloedema may be present or absent. Invasion of the hypophysis and tuber cinereum may cause polyuria, drowsiness, and other symptoms of hypothalamic disturbance. In some cases cervical rigidity and pyrexia are present, the clinical picture then resembling that of tuberculous meningitis (carcinomatosis of the meninges). Neoplastic infiltration of the basal meninges may also be associated with focal symptoms due to metastases within the brain, and metastases should be looked for in the cervical lymph nodes.

DIAGNOSIS

Other conditions may be confused with intracranial tumour, either because they give rise to increased intracranial pressure or because they lead to a progressive cerebral lesion, or for both of these reasons. The following are the conditions most likely to be mistaken for a growth.

Intracranial Abscess

In most cases intracranial abscess is readily distinguished from tumour, since its development is usually acute or subacute and a primary focus of infection is almost always to be found either in the ears, sinuses, lungs or elsewhere. Rarely, however, a chronic abscess may arise, its source of infection being latent or having disappeared. In such cases the diagnosis from tumour may be impossible and the nature of the lesion may be unsuspected until operation. A sudden or apoplectiform onset, the occurrence of a leucocytosis in the blood and of a slight pleocytosis in the cerebrospinal fluid, and the presence of slight pyrexia are points in favour of an abscess, but none of these is constantly present. The EEG is more often severely abnormal in the case of brain abscess than in intracranial tumour.

Arachnoiditis

The terms 'arachnoiditis', and 'meningitis circumscripta serosa', have been applied to a condition the pathogenesis of which is obscure, but which in some cases at least is probably inflammatory in origin, and which recently has been observed to follow acute lymphocytic choriomeningitis. Localized cystic collections of cerebrospinal fluid in the subarachnoid space may be indistinguishable from intracranial tumour before operation. Not uncommonly they occur in the cerebellopontine angle and at the base of the brain, where the optic chiasma may be involved. Pre-operative diagnosis from tumour may be impossible.

Benign Intracranial Hypertension

The raised pressure of the cerebrospinal fluid in this condition due to venous sinus occlusion or cerebral oedema of cause unknown causes papilloedema, headache, and vomiting, but there are no progressive focal signs, the electro-encephalogram may be normal (Foley, 1955) and the ventricles will be neither enlarged nor displaced; in fact they are usually small. The same is true of 'otitic hydrocephalus'.

Cerebral Arterial Disease

Cerebral softening due to vascular occlusion usually causes symptoms apparently referable to a single lesion, though there is sometimes evidence that the lesions are multiple. The onset of symptoms with a slight 'stroke' is valuable evidence of their vascular origin, and confirmation is found in evidence of arteriosclerosis elsewhere. However, in some cases of cerebral infarction, particularly due to carotid occlusion, the evolution of symptoms is slow and diagnosis from tumour is difficult or impossible without contrast radiology. In malignant hypertension severe headache and papilloedema may coexist with a focal cerebral lesion, but the blood pressure is high. In some cases the diagnosis remains in doubt until ventriculography demonstrates the absence of a space-occupying lesion, but it must be remembered that in later life an intracranial tumour may coexist with arteriosclerosis and raised blood pressure.

Neurosyphilis

The meningovascular form of neurosyphilis may be mistaken for tumour on account of the presence of headache and papilloedema associated with an intracranial lesion, while the mental deterioration and convulsions of general paresis may suggest a tumour of the frontal lobe or corpus callosum. In both forms of neurosyphilis, however, reflex iridoplegia is likely to be present, and the Wassermann reaction and other characteristic changes in the cerebrospinal fluid reveal the true nature of the disorder. Gumma of the brain is extremely rare, and the coexistence of symptoms of an intracranial tumour with a positive Wassermann reaction must not be regarded as necessarily or even probably indicating that the patient is suffering from cerebral gumma. Syphilis and cerebral tumour sometimes occur in the same individual.

Epilepsy

Since epileptiform convulsions are a common symptom of intracranial tumour, the differential diagnosis of tumour from other causes of epilepsy frequently arises. Constitutional epilepsy usually begins before the age of 25, though even in later life no cause may be found for the fits even after prolonged observation of the patient. Convulsions beginning after this age should always suggest the possibility of tumour, though in late middle life and old age cerebral arteriosclerosis is probably the commonest cause. In epilepsy headache is absent, except immediately after the fits, and signs of a focal lesion of the nervous system are usually absent, and if present are non-progressive. A focal onset of the fits is of little diagnostic value, since it is not peculiar to intracranial tumour. Full investigations should always be carried out in doubtful cases.

Migraine

Headache, vomiting, visual hallucinations, and visual field defects are common both to migraine and to tumours in the neighbourhood of the visual cortex of the occipital lobe, especially angioma. As a rule the field defects of migraine are transitory, lasting only for from one-half to one hour, but occasionally an exceptionally severe attack is followed by a permanent scotoma or hemianopia. Usually migraine begins at puberty, and there is often a family history of the disorder. Signs of increased intracranial pressure are absent and there is no evidence of a progressive intracranial lesion. Visual field defect associated with an occipital tumour is persistent. A bruit is sometimes to be heard over an angioma, and X-rays may show calcification or abnormal vascular markings in the skull. Angiography usually settles the question.

Retrobulbar Neuritis

Acute bilateral retrobulbar neuritis may simulate intracranial tumour, because it causes disc swelling with impairment of vision. It is distinguished, however, by the acute onset and by the fact that the visual loss is disproportionately great compared with the papilloedema, which is usually slight. Moreover, the field defect is central, whereas in papilloedema due to increased intracranial pressure, if present at all it is peripheral. Headache is absent in retrobulbar neuritis, but pain in the eyes may be considerable, and they are usually tender on pressure.

Diffuse Sclerosis

Diffuse sclerosis may simulate tumour when papilloedema is present. However, the onset in early life, usually with visual failure of subcortical origin, and the bilateral distribution of the symptoms should enable the two conditions to be distinguished.

Chronic Subdural Haematoma

Since this is a slowly progressive space-occupying lesion it may be indistinguishable from tumour in the absence of a history of trauma. Electro-encephalography may be helpful, and angiography usually settles the diagnosis.

DIAGNOSIS OF THE NATURE OF THE TUMOUR

Medulloblastoma

This is a rapidly growing, malignant tumour, most frequently found in the neighbourhood of the roof of the fourth ventricle in childhood. It should be suspected in children who present the symptoms of a midline cerebellar tumour with a history of a few months' duration.

Glioblastoma Multiforme

This is a malignant and rapidly growing tumour arising in middle life and usually found in the cerebral hemispheres. It should be suspected in middle-aged persons presenting the symptoms of a tumour of one cerebral hemisphere with a history of a few months' duration.

Astrocytoma

The astrocytoma is a slowly growing tumour which may arise either in the cerebral or cerebellar hemispheres. In most cases in which the history of an intracranial tumour in either of these situations extends over several years, the growth is an astrocytoma or an oligodendroglioma but the latter is more liable to show calcification on plain X-rays than the former. Owing to its situation, the cerebellar astrocytoma is likely to bring the patient under observation sooner than one situated in the cerebral hemisphere.

Meningioma

Meningiomas are almost exclusively supratentorial tumours and exhibit certain sites of election which have already been described. They are rare before middle life. There may be a very long history, e.g. of epilepsy for many years.

Owing to their extracerebral origin they compress but do not invade the brain. The focal symptoms to which they give rise are less severe in relation to the size of the tumour than is the case with the gliomas. Meningiomas, therefore, frequently cause a marked increase in intracranial pressure, with comparatively slight signs of a focal lesion. Their proximity to the skull leads to erosion of bone in 20 per cent. of cases, and this is often demonstrable on radiographic examination, which may also show calcification within the tumour. The meningiomas are usually associated with increased vascularity, which may be extracranial as well as intracranial, the latter being visible radiographically. Radiographs may also show enlargement of the foramen spinosum in the base of the skull and of the middle meningeal channels in the vault.

Angioma

Since angiomas originate in a congenital abnormality two-thirds cause symptoms below the age of 30. Epilepsy, intracerebral or subarachnoid haemorrhage and hemiparesis are the commonest presenting symptoms. The diagnosis is confirmed by angiography (Mackenzie, 1953).

Haemangioblastoma

These tumours are almost exclusively cerebellar and are sometimes associated with haemangioblastoma of the retina and spinal cord, and with cysts of the pancreas and kidneys, and hypernephromas of the kidneys or suprarenal glands. Only the first of these associated abnormalities, however, is likely to be discoverable clinically.

Tumours in the neighbourhood of the Hypophysis

The diagnosis of the pathological nature of these tumours is described in the section dealing with their symptomatology.

Acoustic Neuroma

The clinical picture of this tumour, which commonly arises in middle-aged persons, is highly distinctive, since the first symptoms are those of destruction of the eighth nerve on one side.

Metastatic Tumours

Metastatic tumours should be suspected in middle-aged or elderly individuals who present the history of a rapidly developing intracranial growth. In all such cases a thorough clinical and radiographic search for a primary neoplasm should be made. A history of marked loss of weight is suggestive. Not infrequently an intracranial metastasis gives rise to symptoms before the primary lesion, especially when this is in the lung, and sometimes the primary lesion is not discovered until autopsy.

Tuberculoma

Tuberculoma may occur at any age, but is most frequent in childhood and early adult life. It is now rare in Europe and the U.S.A. but is still common in India (Dastur and Desai, 1965). It begins as a circumscribed patch of tuberculous leptomeningitis and is therefore cortical or subcortical in the cerebral or cerebellar hemispheres and first involves the superficial regions when it is situated in the brain stem. Remissions and relapses in the development of symptoms are somewhat characteristic, and increase in intracranial pressure is often disproportionately slight. A pleocytosis may be found in the cerebrospinal fluid. The presence of a tuberculous lesion elsewhere will afford some confirmatory evidence, but this is so common that it may coexist with a glioma.

Gumma

Gumma is a very rare tumour of the brain. Both glioma and syphilitic infection are comparatively common and both may occur in the same individual. The association of a positive Wassermann reaction with the symptoms of an intracranial growth should not be interpreted as meaning that the latter is necessarily or even probably a gumma. Intracranial gumma usually responds little to antisyphilitic treatment. It cannot safely be diagnosed before operation.

Parasitic Cysts

The possibility that the symptoms of an intracranial tumour may be due to parasitic cysts should always be considered in a patient who has been exposed to the infestation. The presence of such cysts elsewhere in the body affords strong confirmatory evidence, and the cerebrospinal fluid often shows a mononuclear pleocytosis. The blood may exhibit an eosinophilia. Complement fixation and flocculation tests, and Casoni's intradermal sensitization test may be of diagnostic value in suspected cases of hydatid infection.

PROGNOSIS

The prognosis of intracranial tumour is influenced by the nature of the growth and its accessibility to the surgeon. In the absence of surgical interference almost all intracranial tumours increase in size, their rate of growth depending upon their nature. The resulting increase of intracranial pressure and destruction of brain tissue ultimately prove fatal. When papilloedema is severe, death may be preceded by blindness. The more malignant gliomas, such as the medulloblastomas and the glioblastomas, grow rapidly and usually prove fatal within a year. The slowly growing astrocytomas may cause symptoms for many years before leading to a marked increase in intracranial pressure. (See Penman and Smith, 1954.)

Sudden death in cases of intracranial tumour is rare, but is an eventuality which should always be borne in mind. It may occur in the absence of marked papilloedema, though there is usually a history of headaches of increasing severity. The patient may without warning become first drowsy and then comatose and die within a few hours of losing consciousness; these events are usually due to tentorial or cerebellar herniation with consequent brain-stem compression or haemorrhage. A dilating pupil or occipital pain and neck stiffness are useful alerting signs indicating a need for measures to be undertaken rapidly to reduce the intracranial pressure.

The recent improvement in neurosurgical techniques has greatly increased the range of cerebral surgery, and in the best hands the immediate mortality of operations for the removal of intracranial tumour is under 10 per cent. Extra-cerebral tumours can frequently be removed without damage to the underlying brain, and in such cases complete recovery may occur. Removal of an intra-cerebral tumour, on the other hand, necessitates considerable cerebral trauma. The risk of residual symptoms is proportionately increased. Mental deterioration and aphasia are likely to follow the removal of a large intracerebral tumour of the left hemisphere. Tumours in the interpeduncular region are relatively inaccessible to surgery, and tumours which infiltrate the brain stem cannot be removed. The more malignant the tumour, the greater the likelihood of its recurrence after its attempted removal. Recurrence of the more rapidly growing gliomas is the rule, and even meningiomas may recur.

The prognosis is naturally bad in the case of metastatic tumours on account of the primary growth and the frequency of metastases elsewhere.

Tuberculomas may become quiescent. Chemotherapy has rendered their surgical removal much safer.

TREATMENT

The ideal treatment of an intracranial tumour is its surgical removal, though for the reasons given in the previous section this is not always practicable. However, an attempt should be made to remove all accessible meningiomas. Most neurosurgeons now feel that any attempt to remove gliomas (except in the cerebellum) is unwise though partial removal may prolong life by producing internal decompression. If biopsy confirms the diagnosis of a benign astrocytoma the prognosis of these tumours is better without radical surgery. Subtemporal decompression, once widely practised, has now been largely discarded as brain hernias almost invariably result. An attempt should always be made to remove cerebellar tumours, whether in the midline or hemispheres, and the same is true of most ependymomas of the fourth ventricle. Exploration and drainage of the cyst in cases of craniopharyngioma is often indicated and many pituitary tumours can be successfully removed. Except in the elderly with focal signs but little evidence of raised pressure all acoustic neuromas demand surgery though surgeons differ as to whether total or intracapsular removal is preferable; much depends upon the size of the growth and the circumstances of the individual case.

Intracranial gumma responds little, if at all, to antisyphilitic treatment and the indications for surgical interference are the same as in the case of intra-cranial neoplasms.

It is doubtful if the mere presence of an intracranial tuberculoma justifies operation unless there is evidence of increased intracranial pressure. The systemic chemotherapy of tuberculosis may be first given a trial.

The scope of radiotherapy in the treatment of intracranial tumour is as yet undefined. Irradiation is indicated in most cases of hypophysial adenoma and of medulloblastoma of the cerebellum, for which it should be used in association with surgical treatment. It is generally contra-indicated in cases of slowly- or rapidly-growing glioma except for those in the pons which may be benefited. Some glomus tumours are radiosensitive and metastases in the cerebral hemi-spheres or posterior fossa respond dramatically though temporarily, depending upon the site of the primary growth. Much work is now in progress upon the effects of antimitotic agents (e.g. cyclophosphamide, vincristine sulphate) which seem to be particularly beneficial in cases of medulloblastoma.

Dehydration is of value for the temporary reduction of increased intracranial pressure and also as a palliative measure in inoperable cases. Dehydration is especially useful in emergencies, for example to restore to consciousness a semi-comatose patient, in order that a complete clinical examination may be carried out; to combat rapidly developing cerebral oedema and to lower the intracranial pressure in a patient awaiting operation. A simple method of lowering the intracranial pressure used in the past was rectal magnesium sulphate but this is now outmoded.

To obtain a more rapid reduction of the intracranial pressure it is necessary to inject a hypertonic solution intravenously and sucrose and mannitol have both been used: Javid (1958) advised urea for this purpose. The usual dose is 1 G. per kilogramme of body weight. It is given intravenously as a 30 per cent. solution in 10 per cent. invert sugar, at a rate of 60 drops per minute. It can also be given by the mouth. Poor renal function and active intracranial bleeding are contra-indications and it seems that though rapid reduction in pressure occurs there may be 'rebound' oedema subsequently. Now most workers prefer steroid drugs in large dosage; dexamethasone, 5 mg. three times daily initially, is often remarkably successful and may be continued in diminishing dosage for as long as may be required.

REFERENCES

ALEXANDER, G. L., and NORMAN, R. M. (1960) *The Sturge-Weber Syndrome*, Bristol.

ALLEN, I. M. (1930) A clinical study of tumours involving the occipital lobe, *Brain*, **53,** 194.

BAILEY, P. (1932) Histologic diagnosis of tumors of the brain, *Arch. Neurol. Psychiat. (Chicago)*, **27,** 1290.

BAILEY, P. (1948) *Intracranial Tumors*, 2nd ed., Springfield, Ill.

BAILEY, P., and BUCY, P. C. (1931) The origin and nature of meningeal tumors, *Amer. J. Cancer*, **15,** 15.

BAILEY, P., and CUSHING, H. (1925) Medulloblastoma cerebelli, a common type of mid-cerebellar glioma of childhood, *Arch. Neurol. Psychiat. (Chicago)*, **14,** 192.

BAILEY, P., and CUSHING, H. (1926) *A Classification of the Tumours of the Glioma Group*, London.

BECKMANN, J. W., and KUBIE, L. S. (1929) A clinical study of twenty-one cases of tumour of the hypophyseal stalk, *Brain*, **52,** 127.

DU BOULAY, G. H. (1965) *Principles of X-ray Diagnosis of the Skull*, London.

BRADY, J. I., and RODRIGUEZ, F. (1961) Cerebellar hemangioblastoma and polycythemia, *Amer. J. med. Sci.*, **242,** 579.

BULL, J. W. D. (1951) Diagnostic neuroradiology, in *Modern Trends in Neurology*, 1st Series, ed. FEILING, A., London.

BULL, J. W. D. (1967) The corpus callosum, *Clin. Radiol.*, **18,** 2.

BULL, J. W. D., and MARRYAT, J. (1965) Isotope encephalography: experience with 100 cases, *Brit. med. J.*, **1,** 473.

CAIRNS, H. (1935–6) The ultimate results of operations for intracranial tumors, *Yale J. Biol. Med.*, **8,** 421.

CAIRNS, H., and JUPE, M. H. (1939) The central nervous system, in *A Textbook of X-ray Diagnosis by British Authors*, iii, pp. 3–198, London.

CAIRNS, H., and RUSSELL, D. S. (1931) Intracranial and spinal metastases in gliomas of the brain, *Brain*, **54,** 377.

CARMICHAEL, E. A., DIX, M. R., and HALLPIKE, C. S. (1956) Pathology, symptomatology and diagnosis of organic affections of the eighth nerve system, *Brit. med. Bull.*, **12**, 146.

COURVILLE, C. B. (1967) Intracranial tumors. Notes upon a series of three thousand verified cases with some current observations obtaining to their mortality, *Bull. Los Angeles neurol. Soc.*, **32**, Suppl. No. 2.

CRITCHLEY, M., and FERGUSON, F. R. (1928) The cerebrospinal epidermoids (cholesteatomata), *Brain*, **51**, 334.

CRITCHLEY, M., and IRONSIDE, R. N. (1926) The pituitary adamantinomata, *Brain*, **49**, 437.

CROOKE, A. C. (1935) A change in the basophil cells of the pituitary gland common to conditions which exhibit the syndrome attributed to basophil adenoma, *J. Path. Bact.*, **41**, 339.

CUSHING, H. (1912) *The Pituitary Body and its Disorders*, Philadelphia.

CUSHING, H. (1917) *Tumors of the Nervus Acusticus and the Syndrome of the Cerebello-Pontile Angle*, Philadelphia.

CUSHING, H. (1921) Further concerning the acoustic neuromas, *Laryngoscope (St. Louis)*, **31**, 209.

CUSHING, H. (1927) Acromegaly from a surgical standpoint, *Brit. med. J.*, **2**, 1 and 48.

CUSHING, H. (1930) The chiasmal syndrome of primary optic atrophy and bitemporal defects in adults with a normal sella turcica, *Arch. Ophthal. (Chicago)*, **2**, 505 and 707.

CUSHING, H. (1932 *a*) The basophil adenomas of the pituitary body and their clinical manifestations (pituitary basophilism), *Bull. Johns Hopk. Hosp.*, **1**, 137.

CUSHING, H. (1932 *b*) *Intracranial Tumours. Notes upon a Series of Two Thousand Verified Cases with Surgical-mortality Percentages Pertaining Thereto*, Springfield, Ill.

CUSHING, H., and BAILEY, P. (1928) *Tumors Arising from the Blood-vessels of the Brain*, Springfield, Ill.

CUSHING, H., and EISENHARDT, L. (1938) *Meningiomas, their Classification, Regional Behaviour, Life History, and Surgical End Results*, Springfield, Ill.

DANDY, W. E. (1928) Arteriovenous aneurysm of the brain and venous abnormalities and angiomas of the brain, *Arch. Surg. (Chicago)*, **17**, 190 and 715.

DANDY, W. E. (1933) *Benign Tumors in the Third Ventricle of the Brain*, London.

DASTUR, H. M., and DESAI, A. D. (1965) A comparative study of brain tuberculomas and gliomas based upon 107 case records of each, *Brain*, **88**, 375.

DAVIDOFF, L. M., and DYKE, C. G. (1937) *The Normal Encephalogram*, London.

DOTT, N. M., and BAILEY, P. (1925–6) A consideration of the hypophyseal adenomata, *Brit. J. Surg.*, **13**, 314.

EDWARDS, C. H., and PATERSON, J. H. (1951) A review of the symptoms and signs of acoustic neurofibromata, *Brain*, **74**, 144.

FIELDS, W. S., and SHANKLY, P. C. (1962) *The Biology and Treatment of Intracranial Tumors*, Springfield, Ill.

FISCHER-WILLIAMS, M., LAST, S. L., LYBERI, G., and NORTHFIELD, D. W. C. (1962) Clinico-EEG study of 128 gliomas and 50 intracranial metastatic tumours, *Brain*, **85**, 1.

FOERSTER, O., GAGEL, O., and MAHONEY, W. (1939) Die encephalen Tumoren des verlängerten Markes, der Brücke und des Mittelhirns, *Arch. Psychiat. Nervenkr.*, **110**, 1.

FOLEY, J. (1955) Benign forms of intracranial hypertension, *Brain*, **78**, 1.

FORD, R., and AMBROSE, J. (1963) Echoencephalography. The measurement of the position of midline structures in the skull with high-frequency pulsed ultrasound, *Brain*, **86**, 189.

GARDNER, W. J., and FRAZIER, C. H. (1930) Bilateral acoustic neurofibromas, *Arch. Neurol. Psychiat. (Chicago)*, **23**, 266.

GLASER, M. A. (1929) Tumours of the pineal, corpora quadrigemina and third ventricle, the inter-relationship of their syndromes and their surgical treatment, *Brain*, **52**, 226.

GLOBUS, J. H., and SILBERT, S. (1931) Pinealomas, *Arch. Neurol. Psychiat (Chicago)*, **25,** 937.

GROSSMAN, C. C. (1966) *The Use of Ultrasound in Brain Disorders*, Springfield, Ill.

HENSON, R. A., CRAWFORD, J. V., and CAVANAGH, J. B. (1953) Tumours of the glomus jugulare, *J. Neurol. Neurosurg. Psychiat.*, N.S. **16,** 127.

HOEFER, P. B., SCHLESINGER, E. B., and PENNES, H. H. (1947) Epilepsy, *Res. Publ. Ass. nerv. ment. Dis.*, **26,** 50.

HORRAX, G. (1924) Generalized cisternal arachnoiditis simulating cerebellar tumor, *Arch. Surg. (Chicago)*, **9,** 95.

HORRAX, G. (1939) Meningiomas of the brain, *Arch. Neurol. Psychiat. (Chicago)*, **41,** 140.

HORRAX, G., and BAILEY, P. (1925) Tumors of the pineal body, *Arch. Neurol. Psychiat. (Chicago)*, **13,** 423.

HOUDART, R., and LE BESNERAIS, Y. (1963) *Les Anévrismes artérioveineux des hémisphères cérébraux*, Paris.

HUBBLE, D. (1961) The endocrine orchestra, *Brit. med. J.*, **1,** 523.

IRONSIDE, R., and GUTTMACHER, M. (1929) The corpus callosum and its tumours, *Brain*, **52,** 442.

JAVID, M. (1958) Urea—new use of an old agent, *Surg. Clin. N. Amer.*, **38,** 907.

KELLY, R. (1951) Colloid cysts of the third ventricle, *Brain*, **74,** 23.

KERNOHAN, J. W., MABON, R. F., SVIEN, H. J., and ADSON, A. W. (1949) A simplified classification of the gliomas, *Proc. Mayo Clin.*, **24,** 71.

KILOH, L. G., and OSSELTON, J. W. (1966) *Clinical Electroencephalography*, 2nd ed., London.

KOLODNY, A. (1928) The symptomatology of tumours of the temporal lobe, *Brain*, **51,** 385.

KOLODNY, A. (1929) Symptomatology of tumor of the frontal lobe, *Arch. Neurol. Psychiat. (Chicago)*, **21,** 1107.

KRAYENBUHL, H., and YASARGIL, M. G. (1965) *Die zerebrale Angiographie*, Stuttgart.

KUPER, S., MENDELOW, H., and PROCTOR, N. S. F. (1958) Internal hydrocephalus caused by parasitic cysts, *Brain*, **81,** 235.

LINDAU, A. (1921) Studien über Kleinhirncysten. Bau, Pathogenese und Beziehungen zur Angiomatosis Retinae, *Acta path. microbiol. scand.*, Supp. i. 1.

LOGUE, V., and MONCKTON, G. (1954) Posterior fossa angiomas, *Brain*, **77,** 252.

LYSHOLM, E. (1935–7) *Das Ventrikulogram* (Parts 1–3), Stockholm: also *Acta radiol. (Stockh.)*, Supps. 24–26.

MACKENZIE, I. (1953) The clinical presentation of the cerebral angiomas, *Brain*, **76,** 184.

McKISSOCK, W., and PAINE, K. W. E. (1958) Primary tumours of the thalamus, *Brain*, **81,** 41.

MICHAUX, L., and FELD, M. (1963) *Les Phakomatoses cérébrales*, Paris.

MONIZ, E. (1931) *Diagnostic des tumeurs cérébrales et épreuve de l'encéphalographie artérielle*, Paris.

MULLAN, S. (1962) Mortality of the surgical treatment of brain tumors, *J. Amer. med. Ass.*, **182,** 601.

NATTRASS, F. J. (1949) Clinical and social problems of epilepsy, *Brit. med. J.*, **1,** 1.

NORTHFIELD, D. W. C. (1938) Some observations on headache, *Brain*, **61,** 133.

PARKER, H. L. (1927) Involvement of central nervous system, secondary to primary carcinoma of lung, *Arch. Neurol. Psychiat. (Chicago)*, **17,** 198.

PENDERGRASS, E. P., SCHAEFFER, J. P., and HODES, J. P. (1956) *The Head and Neck in Roentgen Diagnosis*, 2nd ed., Oxford.

PENFIELD, W. (1927) The encapsulated tumors of the nervous system, *Surg. Gynec. Obstet.*, **45,** 178.

PENFIELD, W. (1931) A paper on classification of brain tumours and its practical application, *Brit. med. J.*, **1,** 337.

PENFIELD, W. (1932) Tumors of the sheaths of the nervous system, *Arch. Neurol. Psychiat. (Chicago)*, **27,** 1298.

PENMAN, J., and SMITH, M. C. (1954) Intracranial gliomata, *Spec. Rep. Ser. med. Res. Coun. (Lond.)*, No. 284.

RAIMONDI, A. J. (1966) Ultrastructure of brain tumours, in *Progress in Neurological Surgery*, ed. KRAYENBUHL, H., MASPES, P. E., and SWEET, W. H., Basle.

ROBERTSON, E. G. (1967) *Pneumoencephalography*, 2nd ed., Springfield, Ill.

ROUSSY, G., and OBERLING, C. (1931) *Les Tumeurs des centres nerveux et des nerfs périohériques*, Paris.

ROUSSY, G., and OBERLING, C. (1932) Histologic classification of tumors of the central nervous system, *Arch. Neurol. Psychiat. (Chicago)*, **27**, 1281.

RUSSELL, D. S. (1944) The pinealoma: its relationship to teratoma, *J. Path. Bact.*, **56**, 145.

RUSSELL, D. S., and CAIRNS, H. (1930) Spinal metastases in a case of cerebral glioma of the type known as astrocytoma fibrillare, *J. Path. Bact.*, **33**, 383.

RUSSELL, D. S., and RUBINSTEIN, L. J. (1959) *Pathology of Tumours of the Nervous System*, London.

SCHERER, H. J. (1940 a) The pathology of cerebral gliomas, *J. Neurol. Psychiat.*, N.S. **3**, 147.

SCHERER, H. J. (1940 b) The forms of growth in gliomas and their practical significance, *Brain*, **63**, 1.

SHEPHARD, R. H., and WADIA, N. H. (1956) Some observations on atypical features in acoustic neuroma, *Brain*, **79**, 282.

SPENCER, R. (1965) Scintiscanning in space-occupying lesions of the skull, *Brit. J. Radiol.*, **38**, 1.

TAVERAS, J. M., and WOOD, E. H. (1964) *Diagnostic Neuroradiology*, Baltimore.

VORIS, H. C., and ADSON, A. W. (1935) Tumors of the corpus callosum, *Arch. Neurol. Psychiat. (Chicago)*, **34**, 965.

WAGENEN VAN, W. P. (1927) Tuberculoma of the brain, *Arch. Neurol. Psychiat. (Chicago)*, **17**, 57.

WALSHE, F. M. R. (1931) Intracranial tumours; a critical review, *Quart. J. Med.*, **24**, 587.

WALTER, W. G. (1936–7) The electroencephalogram in cases of cerebral tumour, *Proc. roy. Soc. Med.*, **30**, 579.

WALTER, W. G., and DOVEY, V. J. (1944) Electroencephalography in cases of subcortical tumour, *J. Neurol. Psychiat.*, N.S. **7**, 57.

WORSTER-DROUGHT, C., DICKSON, W. E. C., and McMENEMY, W. H. (1937) Multiple meningeal and perineural tumours with analogous changes in the glia and ependyma (Neurofibroblastomatosis), *Brain*, **60**, 85.

ZÜLCH, K. J. (1965) *Brain Tumors: Their Biology and Pathology*, New York.

HEADACHE

THE INVESTIGATION OF A CASE OF HEADACHE

Headache is one of the commonest symptoms. Though it is frequently a trivial disorder, it is also at times a symptom of the gravest significance. Every patient suffering from headache requires, therefore, careful consideration and sometimes thorough investigation. In taking the history, attention must be paid to the following points. How long has the patient suffered from headache? Is it increasing in severity? Is it constant or paroxysmal, and if paroxysmal what is the duration of the paroxysms, and do they occur at any special time of day? Are they precipitated by any circumstance or activity, and how, if at all, can they be relieved? What is the character of the headache, and what is its situation? Is it associated with tenderness of the scalp or skull, with visual disturbances, vomiting, or vertigo? Has there been an injury of the head? Are there symptoms of nasal obstruction or of a discharge, either from the nostrils or into the pharynx? Is there a history of syphilis?

The investigation of a case of headache involves a complete examination of all the systems of the body, special attention being paid to the ocular fundi, the nose and nasal air sinuses, the blood pressure, and the urine. Radiography of the skull, including the nasal sinuses, and examination of the cerebrospinal fluid and blood Wassermann reaction may be required in appropriate cases.

THE MODE OF PRODUCTION OF HEADACHE

All the tissues covering the cranium are sensitive to pain, especially the arteries but also the muscles and pericranium. The skull bone itself is insensitive. Within the cranium the venous sinuses and their tributaries, the dura mater and the cerebral arteries, the fifth, ninth, and tenth cranial nerves are the chief pain-sensitive structures.

The main factors in the causation of headache are (1) inflammation of or about the pain-sensitive structures of the head, (2) referred pain, (3) meningeal irritation, (4) traction on or dilatation of the above-mentioned vessels, (5) direct pressure by tumours upon sensory nerves in the head, and (6) psychological causes when the pain is often due to a state of tension in the muscles of the scalp and neck. The following is a convenient pathological classification.

THE CAUSES OF HEADACHE

Disease of the Bones of the Cranium

Osteitis of the cranial bones is an occasional cause of headache. Syphilitic osteitis and osteitis deformans of Paget should especially be borne in mind. Headache due to osteitis is of a burning, boring character and is associated with tenderness of the skull, which often feels warmer than normal. Local or general thickening of the cranium is often present, and the characteristic changes in the bones are demonstrable by radiography. Craniostenosis, which may cause headache owing to premature synostosis of the sutures, is readily recognized by the abnormal shape of the skull.

Neuritis and Neuralgia

Pain in the head may be due to neuritis or neuralgia of the sensory nerves of the scalp. The supraorbital, auriculotemporal, posterior auricular, and great occipital nerves may be the site of such processes. The pain in such cases is usually paroxysmal and radiates along the course of the nerve, which is tender on pressure. Cutaneous hyperalgesia corresponding to the sensory distribution of the nerve affected is usually present. Tic douloureux is a form of trigeminal neuralgia which may involve the scalp when it attacks the first division of the nerve. This, however, is less frequently involved than the second and third divisions. Herpes zoster of the trigeminal ganglion is sometimes a cause of severe and persistent neuralgic pain. After the acute stage the scars of the eruption remain visible, and there is usually cutaneous anaesthesia. Pain in the distribution of the trigeminal nerve may be due to pressure upon it in its intracranial course by intracranial neoplasm or aneurysm, or to its involvement in meningovascular syphilis or tabes. Moreover, its central fibres may be involved in a lesion within the medulla. Thrombosis of the posterior inferior cerebellar artery, and syringobulbia, may in this way cause neuralgic pain over the face and scalp.

Referred Pain

Lesions of many viscera are attended by pain referred to the superficial tissues remote from the viscus involved, but innervated by the same segment of the nervous system. In this way visceral disease in many situations may be attended by pain in the head and localized hyperalgesia of the face or scalp. These symptoms may be produced by eye-strain, iritis, glaucoma, lesions of the middle ear, nasal sinuses, teeth including unerupted teeth, pharynx, and tongue, and also by disease of the intrathoracic and intra-abdominal viscera [see p. 40]. The explanation of this reference of pain to the head from remote organs is that the trigeminal is the somatic sensory nerve corresponding to the vagus, by which so many viscera are innervated. Nasal obstruction, apart from infection of the nasal sinuses, is a common cause of persistent frontal headache. Occipital headache is often present in cases of cervical spondylosis.

Meningeal Irritation

Meningeal irritation is responsible for some of the most severe headaches. It may be due to the various forms of meningitis, including syphilitic meningitis, or to the presence of non-infective irritant products such as extravasated blood in contact with the meninges. The pain is constant, severe, and throbbing or 'bursting', and is usually associated with hyperalgesia of the scalp, and in the case of acute meningitis with other signs of meningeal irritation, such as cervical rigidity and Kernig's sign.

Headaches of Vascular Origin

Paroxysmal throbbing or 'bursting' headaches may occur in patients with malignant hypertension, when the headache is not directly related to the height of the blood pressure but to the degree of stretch evoked at the time in the cranial arteries (Wolff and Wolf, 1948). Intracranial aneurysm is rarely large enough to cause increased intracranial pressure before rupture. It may cause pain in the head, however, by compression of the trigeminal nerve. After rupture, subarachnoid haemorrhage leads to headache by causing both increased intracranial pressure and meningeal irritation.

Changes in the calibre and permeability of the cranial vessels are probably responsible for the headaches which accompany or follow numerous toxic states such as severe infections, alcoholic over-indulgence, general anaesthetics, uraemia, and diffuse cerebral inflammations—the various forms of encephalitis. In the 'hangover' headache dehydration and reduced intracranial pressure probably play a part. Sudden prostrating headache simulating that of subarachnoid haemorrhage has been described in patients who have eaten cheese or broad beans while taking mono-amine oxidase inhibitor drugs, mainly tranylcypromine, for the treatment of depression.

Migraine is probably also a vasomotor disorder, and on this hypothesis the headache is due to vascular dilatation following a preliminary constriction. The characteristics of migrainous headache are described on page 273.

The headache experimentally induced by histamine has been studied by Pickering (1933). Some workers believe that histamine headache occurs clinically (Horton, 1941) or that histamine plays a part in the production of migraine [see p. 271].

Headache may also be caused by temporal or cranial arteritis [see p. 328].

Intracranial Space-occupying Lesions

The mode of production of headache by intracranial neoplasm and abscess and its characteristics are considered elsewhere [see p. 228].

Trauma

In the more severe degrees of head injury headache is apt to be masked by impaired consciousness. It is a prominent symptom following concussion or cerebral contusion, and in this so-called post-concussional syndrome it may be paroxysmal, tends to be precipitated by noise, excitement, exertion, and stooping, and is often associated with irritability, nervousness, and giddiness.

Lowered Intracranial Pressure

This may cause headache, as, for example, after lumbar puncture. Such headache is throbbing and may be literally prostrating, since it is intensified by sitting or standing and relieved by lying flat or with the feet raised above the level of the head. The pain may radiate from the head to the neck or dorsal spine.

Cough Headache

This is a very distinctive, brief, but often severe 'bursting' kind of pain experienced after coughing, usually by a middle-aged man, who may clasp his head when he coughs in an attempt to relieve it. Its cause is obscure, but rarely it is a symptom of an intracranial tumour. In most cases, however, it is benign and disappears spontaneously.

Psychogenic Headache

Numerous abnormal cranial sensations are described by neurotic and psychotic patients. The commonest is a sense of pressure at the vertex, frequently encountered in anxiety states. One source of anxiety-headache is persistent contraction of the frontal belly of the occipitofrontalis muscle. Such tension headaches are typically dull and aching in character; they may be continuous but more often come on towards the end of the day, although in depressed patients the headache may be present on waking. Persistent 'neuralgic' pains associated with hyperaesthesia of the scalp and failing to respond to all analgesics may be encountered in hysteria as may bizarre headaches described in a florid manner ('like a nail being driven into the skull or an engine lifting off the top of the head'). Patients suffering from depressive states sometimes describe 'terrible pains in the head' of which they can give no more precise description [see also Chapter 23].

TREATMENT

Apart from palliative treatment with analgesics, which can safely be used in most cases, the treatment of headache is that of the causal disorder.

REFERENCES

DRAKE, F. R. (1956) Tension headache; a review, *Amer. J. med. Soc.*, **232**, 105.

HORTON, B. J. (1941) Histamine cephalalgia, *J. Amer. med. Ass.*, **116**, 377.

KUNKLE, E. C., and WOLFF, H. G. (1951) Headache, in *Modern Trends in Neurology*, 1st Series, ed. FEILING, A., London.

NORTHFIELD, D. W. C. (1938) Some observations on headache, *Brain*, **61**, 133.

PICKERING, G. W. (1933) Observations on the mechanism of the headache produced by histamine, *Clin. Sci.*, **1**, 77.

PICKERING, G. W. (1939) Experimental observations on headache, *Brit. med. J.*, **1**, 907.

SCHUMACHER, G. A., and WOLFF, H. G. (1941) Experimental studies in headache, *Arch. Neurol. Psychiat* (*Chicago*), **45**, 199.

WOLFF, H. G. (1963) *Headache and Other Head Pain*, 2nd ed., New York.

WOLFF, H. G., and WOLF, S. (1948) *Pain*, p. 37, Springfield, Ill.

MIGRAINE

Synonyms. Hemicrania; bilious attack; sick headache.

Definition. A paroxysmal disorder characterized in its fully developed form by visual hallucinations, scotomas, and other disturbances of cerebral function, associated with unilateral headache and vomiting.

AETIOLOGY AND PATHOLOGY

Migraine has been known to medical science for nearly 2,000 years. In the first century of the Christian era Aretaeus of Cappadocia described it as heterocrania, and the term hemicrania, from which the word migraine was derived was introduced by Galen (A.D. 131–201). Among modern studies Liveing's (1873) is a classic.

The aetiology of migraine is complex and difficult. It is not a fatal disease and pathological investigations are therefore scanty. Moreover, since it appears to be primarily a disorder of function little information is likely to be gained from morbid anatomy.

The Intracranial Disturbance of Function

It has long been held that the most plausible hypothetical explanation of migraine is that it is due to arterial spasm, followed by dilatation, occurring within the distribution of the common carotid artery. This view has now been confirmed. During the scotomatous phase of an attack focal electroencephalographic changes have been observed in the opposite cerebral cortex, consistent with cortical ischaemia (Engel, Ferris, and Romano, 1945), and during this phase it has also been observed that amyl nitrite will temporarily abolish the scotoma (Schumacher and Wolff, 1941). It appears, therefore, that arterial spasm is responsible for the subjective visual disturbances and other cortical symptoms at the onset of the attack, while subsequent vasodilatation causes the headache and is manifest in flushing of the face, congestion of the superficial temporal artery and of the conjunctiva, and nasal mucosa on the side of the headache. Schumacher and Wolff have shown that the headache in migraine is due to dilatation mainly of the extracerebral arteries of the dura and scalp, branches of the external carotid, whereas histamine headache comes from dilatation of the large cerebral arteries. The specific effect of ergotamine tartrate on the headache is attributed to its increasing the tone of the branches of the external carotid artery. It is clear that the intracranial disturbance may be precipitated by more than one factor, and it is probable that in susceptible individuals more than one sort of stimulus may cause an attack, though in different patients different causal factors predominate.

Ocular Factors

Refractive errors and defective ocular muscle balance are often blamed for migraine, though probably usually with little justification. Attacks may certainly be precipitated, however, by unusual visual stimuli, especially looking at a bright light.

Allergy

The importance of allergy has been stressed by Balyeat (1933). Sufferers from migraine may often be shown to be sensitive to one or more food protein or other allergens, including pollen and tobacco, and may suffer from other disorders of an allergic nature.

Dietetic Factors

While allergy may explain the precipitation of attacks by protein to which the patient is sensitive, other dietary factors may play a part. Thus the excessive consumption of animal fat or of alcohol may be followed by an attack; so, too, may missing a meal.

Psychological Factors

Sufferers from migraine, though often mentally well balanced, and among the most intelligent and industrious members of the community, are not uncommonly of an introverted or obsessional temperament, and attacks of migraine may be precipitated by mental fatigue or anxiety, or by other forms of stress. Many women suffering frequent attacks at about the time of the menopause are found to be depressed and treatment of the depression is then beneficial.

Endocrine Factors

On the whole there is little evidence that endocrine abnormality is important. The occurrence of 'menstrual migraine' has been quoted in favour of an ovarian disturbance. Water-retention occurs in some cases (Goldzieher, 1941). Sicuteri, Testi, and Anselmi (1961) showed that the urinary excretion of 5-hydroxyindol-acetic acid may be increased in severe attacks suggesting an intermittent release of 5-hydroxytryptamine (serotonin) into the circulation (Curzon, Theaker, and Phillips, 1966).

Heredity

Hereditary predisposition is all-important. Migraine is often an hereditary disorder and is inherited as a Mendelian dominant. Here again appears a link with allergy, since asthma, hay fever, and other allergic disorders are common among the relatives of the migrainous.

Association with Epilepsy

Much stress has been laid by some writers on the alleged association of migraine with epilepsy. Both are common disorders and it is doubtful if their association in the same individual or in the same family occurs more frequently than can be explained by chance. Occasionally, however, a severe attack of migraine may terminate in an epileptic attack but loss of consciousness at the height of an attack is more often syncopal.

Age and Sex

The age of onset is usually at or shortly after puberty, much less frequently in middle life or later, though an onset at about the menopause is not very uncommon in women. Migraine is rare before puberty, but cyclical vomiting and travel-sickness are common in childhood in those who subsequently develop migraine. Women are slightly more subject to migraine than men and usually suffer more severely.

SYMPTOMS

The Onset

Prodromal symptoms may be present or absent. The commonest of these are drowsiness and lassitude, hunger, and constipation or slight looseness of the bowels. Sometimes the subject feels exceptionally well before an attack. The onset may occur during the day, which is usually the case in migraine with a sensory aura. When headache is not preceded by such manifestations, the patient often awakens with it in the morning from a particularly heavy sleep.

Symptoms of Cortical Origin

Sensory symptoms, though not constant, are highly characteristic. Visual disturbances are the commonest. These usually have a homonymous distribution, involving the corresponding halves of both visual fields. They usually consist of a gradually developing hemianopia, which may be preceded by positive symptoms such as flashes of light. The hemianopia may begin in the periphery of the field and spread towards the centre, or vice versa. A common mode of onset is the appearance of a bright spot near the centre. This gradually expands towards the periphery, the advancing edge exhibiting scintillating figures which may be coloured and angular—*teichopsia*, or *fortification spectra*. The spreading scintillation leaves behind it an area of blindness, so that when it reaches the periphery of the half-fields the patient is left with homonymous hemianopia. The spread of these visual symptoms occupies from fifteen to twenty minutes, and the hemianopia then gradually fades away in the order of its development, the whole disturbance lasting about half an hour, though objects in the affected fields may appear less bright than normally for several hours. Many varieties of migrainous visual disturbance occur. The symptoms may have a homonymous quadrantic distribution. Very rarely peripheral vision is lost in the whole of both fields, leaving only a 'telescopic' central field of vision. Exceptionally also the hemianopia is bilateral and leads to temporary complete blindness. In certain cases permanent visual field defects (hemianopia or a quadrantic defect) may persist after a severe attack.

Paraesthesiae and numbness of parts of the body occur next in frequency to visual disturbances. These symptoms possess a cortical distribution, involving the periphery of the limbs and the circumoral region. The upper limb is most often affected, a tingling sensation beginning in the periphery and gradually spreading up the limb, taking fifteen or twenty minutes to do so. The lips, face, and tongue may be subsequently affected on one or both sides, or may be involved without the upper limb. The lower limb is rarely the site of paraesthesiae. Paraesthesiae usually develop shortly after the onset of the visual disturbances, but may occur without the latter as the first symptom. Less frequently they do not develop until after the headache has been present for several hours.

Gustatory and auditory hallucinations have occasionally been reported, but are rare.

Weakness of a limb, usually the upper, or of half of the body may develop and usually follows the paraesthesiae and in very occasional cases recurrent attacks are each accompanied by transient hemiparesis ('hemiplegic migraine').

Aphasia, usually of the expressive, less often of the receptive, type, may occur. In right-handed people it may be associated with visual disturbances in the right half-fields, and paraesthesiae on the right side of the body. There may be temporary disorientation in space.

Transitory diplopia may be complained of during an attack. Giddiness is not uncommon, and there may be slight mental confusion. Loss of consciousness or even an epileptiform attack rarely occurs.

When the symptoms of the aura suggest ischaemia in the distribution of the hind-brain circulation the condition has been called 'basilar artery migraine' (Bickerstaff, 1961).

It is often assumed that in patients who show a permanent visual field defect, aphasia, ophthalmoplegia (see below) or motor weakness persisting after an attack of migraine it is likely that an intracranial vascular anomaly (e.g. aneurysm or angioma) will be present but a recent investigation of cases of 'complicated migraine' (Pearce and Foster, 1965) has shown that investigations designed to demonstrate such lesions are usually negative.

Headache

Headache is the most characteristic symptom of migraine and the one from which it derives its name. It may be the only manifestation of the disorder, or may follow the sensory symptoms just described. It usually occurs as a boring pain in a localized area on one side, often in the temple, and gradually spreads till the whole of the affected side of the head is involved. Headache occurs on the side opposite to that to which the sensory symptoms are referred. Sometimes it extends to the whole head. It gradually increases in intensity and acquires a throbbing character, being intensified by stooping and by all forms of exertion. In milder cases it lasts for several hours but passes away if the patient can sleep, or after a night's rest. In more severe cases it persists for days.

Nausea is usually present during the stage of headache, and vomiting may or may not occur. In milder cases it seems to relieve the headache.

Vasomotor changes are often conspicuous. The face is often pale and the extremities are cold, until improvement begins, but congestion of the face, conjunctiva, and nasal mucous membrane may occur, and is often confined to the side of the headache. There may be subconjunctival haemorrhage or even bruising around the eyes. The superficial temporal artery on the affected side is congested and exhibits vigorous pulsation.

There is often polyuria following the attack.

Electroencephalography

Dow and Whitty (1947) found a persistently abnormal EEG between the attacks in 30 of 51 patients examined.

VARIETIES OF MIGRAINE

The commonest form of migraine is characterized by headache alone, or by headache and vomiting without other symptoms. Somewhat less frequently visual or sensory disturbances precede the headache. Less often still the visual or sensory symptoms, motor weakness, or aphasia are not followed by headache. Exceptionally vomiting may occur alone or in association with abdominal pain.

Ophthalmoplegic Migraine

This term has been applied to recurrent attacks of headache associated with paralysis of one or more oculomotor nerves, which persists for days or weeks after the attack and tends to become permanent. Although transitory diplopia is occasionally associated with true migraine the diagnosis of migraine should be received with great suspicion when it is used to cover ocular palsies lasting more than an hour or two. Probably many cases hitherto described as ophthalmoplegic migraine have been examples of intracranial aneurysm, intracranial angioma, or some other slowly progressive organic lesion.

However, in a review of the ophthalmological complications of migraine Pearce (1967) has found that ophthalmoplegia, either isolated or recurrent, occurring in attacks of migraine, may remain unexplained despite full investigation.

Facioplegic Migraine

Recurrent facial palsy associated with migraine is very rare. It is probably to be explained by ischaemia of the nerve trunk or compression of it by a dilated artery as is ophthalmoplegic migraine.

Retinal Migraine

Retinal vascular lesions in migraine are fortunately rare. I have seen thrombosis of the central artery of the retina, and of single branches, and have known recurrent attacks of retinal ischaemia to lead to bilateral optic atrophy with an irregular peripheral constriction of the visual fields. Retinal and vitreous haemorrhages may also occur.

COURSE AND PROGNOSIS

The frequency of attacks of migraine varies considerably in different patients. Often the disorder seems to possess a rhythm which is little influenced by outside factors. The attacks may occur once a week, once a fortnight, or once a month, with great regularity. Attacks in which headache occurs alone are usually more frequent than those in which it is preceded by sensory symptoms. The latter usually recur at intervals of several months. Occasionally a patient has repeated frequent attacks, a condition which may be called status hemicranialis, by analogy with status epilepticus. Headache preceded by visual symptoms may occur more than once a day for a period of days. Apart from treatment, attacks tend to grow less frequent and less severe as the patient grows older and usually cease in late middle life. It is not uncommon for the character of the attack to change. For example, visual symptoms may cease to appear or occur without headache.

Migraine does not shorten life, but in severe cases in women a state of chronic exhaustion may occur. In a small number of cases permanent hemianopia or other visual field defects have followed an exceptionally severe attack. In such cases teichopsia may persist for weeks. Very rarely permanent aphasia and hemiplegia have been said to occur, but this should suggest an organic lesion rather than migraine.

DIAGNOSIS

It is important to distinguish migraine from similar symptoms resulting from organic disease of the brain. The early onset is an important point of distinction, since migraine usually begins at puberty whereas most organic conditions with which it may be confused are encountered in adult life. A tumour of the occipital lobe, especially an angioma, may lead to attacks of visual hallucinations associated with headache and vomiting. In these cases, however, careful perimetry usually shows a visual field defect, which persists between the attacks, and increases. Moreover, signs of increased intracranial pressure are likely to develop, and there may be evidence of pressure exerted by the tumour upon the neighbouring parts of the brain, and in a case of an arterial angioma a cranial bruit. Also I have seen migraine simulated by an aneurysm of the internal carotid artery compressing the optic nerve.

Migraine is occasionally confused with epilepsy, since visual hallucinations may constitute the prodromal symptoms of both. In migraine, however, the progress of the attack is slow, in epilepsy it is rapid; and the retention of consciousness in the former should put the diagnosis beyond doubt.

When transitory attacks of paraesthesiae, weakness, and aphasia occur in migraine without headache, the diagnosis may be difficult. Such disturbances may simulate cerebral ischaemia due to vascular lesions. In migraine, however, there is usually a history of previous attacks of headache, dating from an early age. The transitory ischaemic attacks of cerebral vascular disease occur chiefly in late middle age and old age, and attacks of paraesthesiae in multiple sclerosis, which usually last for several days or weeks, thus differ from those of migraine, which usually last only half an hour or at the most a few hours. When headache occurs alone, it must be distinguished from pain in the head due to other causes: see pages 266–70.

TREATMENT

The sufferer from migraine should endeavour to regulate his life so as to avoid both mental and physical fatigue as far as possible. Refractive errors, if present, should be corrected. Diet is important, but individual idiosyncrasies are marked. Some patients benefit from a diet in which animal fats are restricted; and other articles of diet likely to precipitate attacks include eggs, chocolate, and raw fruit, especially apples and oranges. When protein sensitivity is shown to exist, specific desensitization may be tried. Meals should be taken regularly, and glucose may with advantage be added to the diet. In contrast there are some patients who improve on a ketogenic diet.

Drug treatment can be divided into two categories, namely treatment of the attack and prophylaxis. While some attacks may be controlled by aspirin, paracetamol or compound codeine tablets, the single most useful remedy is ergotamine tartrate which may be taken by mouth, sublingually, by suppository, by inhalation of a fine powder or by intramuscular injection (0·5 mg.). Useful commercial preparations in which ergotamine is combined with antihistamine or anti-emetic preparations include *Migril, Cafergot Q, Cafergot* suppositories, *Orgraine* and *Medihaler ergotamine*. Often trial and error is necessary to find the most appropriate remedy for each individual patient. All such remedies must however be given early and preferably when the aura begins, if the attack is to be aborted. Vomiting is sometimes a troublesome side-effect. Some intelligent patients can be taught to inject themselves if oral medication fails.

In prophylaxis, antihistamine drugs such as prochlorperazine (*Stemetil*), 5 mg. three times daily, are helpful in mild cases as are compound tablets containing ergotamine, atropine and a barbiturate sedative (e.g. *Bellergal,* one tablet three times daily) while *Gowers' Mixture* still has its advocates and is occasionally very successful:

Sodium bromide	.	.	.	600 mg.
Trinitrin solution	.	.	.	0·03–0·06 ml.
Tincture of nux vomica		.	.	0·3 ml.
Tincture of gelsemium .		.	.	0·6 ml.
Nitric acid or hydrobromic acid, dilute				0·3 ml.
Chloroform water	.	.	.	to 10 ml.

To be taken thrice daily

The most effective prophylactic remedy yet introduced is dimethysergide (Curran and Lance, 1964) which is given in a dosage of 1–3 mg. three times daily. There is, however, a risk that retroperitoneal fibrosis may result from prolonged ingestion of this drug which should not therefore be given in a dose of more than 3 mg. daily for more than three months at a time. Other prophylactic remedies can be continued over much longer periods. In anxious and tense patients at any age, tranquillizing remedies such as trifluoperazine, 1 mg. three times daily, or chlordiazepoxide, 5–10 mg. three times daily, may be helpful while in the many women in the paramenopausal age group in whom frequent attacks of migraine and depression coexist a similar tranquillizer along with phenelzine, 15 mg. three times daily, or amitriptyline, 25–50 mg. three times daily, may be dramatically successful in reducing the frequency and severity of attacks.

REFERENCES

ADIE, W. J. (1930) Permanent hemianopia in migraine and subarachnoid haemorrhage, *Lancet*, ii, 237.

ALLAN, W. (1927) The neuropathic taint in migraine, *Arch. Neurol. Psychiat. (Chicago)*, **18**, 587.

ALLAN, W. (1928) The inheritance of migraine, *Arch. intern. Med.*, **42, 590.**

BALYEAT, R. M. (1933) *Migraine, Diagnosis and Treatment*, Philadelphia.

BICKERSTAFF, E. R. (1961) Basilar artery migraine, *Lancet*, i, 15.

BICKERSTAFF, E. R. (1961) Impairment of consciousness in migraine, *Lancet*, ii, 1057.

BRADSHAW, P., and PARSONS, M. (1965) Hemiplegic migraine, *Quart. J. Med.*, **34**, 65.

CURRAN, D. A., and LANCE, J. W. (1964) Clinical trial of methysergide and other preparations in the management of migraine, *J. Neurol. Neurosurg. Psychiat.*, **27,** 463.

CURSCHMANN, H. (1931) Zur Frage der allergischen Migräne, *Nervenarzt*, **4,** 71.

CURZON, G., THEAKER, P., and PHILLIPS, B. (1966) Excretion of 5-hydroxyindolyl acetic acid (5 HIAA) in migraine, *J. Neurol. Psychiat.*, **29, 85.**

DALESSIO, D. J. (1962) On migraine headache, serotonin and serotonin antagonism, *J. Amer. med. Ass.*, **181, 318.**

DOW, D. J., and WHITTY, C. W. M. (1947) Electroencephalographic changes in migraine, *Lancet*, ii, 52.

ENGEL, G. L., FERRIS, E. B., JR., and ROMANO, J. (1945) Focal encephalographic changes during scotomas of migraine, *Amer. J. med. Sci.*, **209,** 650.

FRIEDMAN, A. P. (1963) The pathogenesis of migraine headache, *Bull. Los Angeles neurol. Soc.*, **28,** 191.

FRIEDMAN, A. P., and ELKIND, A. H. (1963) Methysergide in treatment of vascular headaches of migraine type, *J. Amer. med. Ass.*, **184,** 125.

GOLDZIEHER, M. A. (1941) Endocrine aspects of headaches, *J. Lab. clin. Med.*, **27,** 150.

LIVEING, E. (1873) *On Megrim, Sick-Headache, and Some Allied Disorders*, London.

O'SULLIVAN, M. E. (1936) Termination of one thousand attacks of migraine with ergotamine tartrate, *J. Amer. med. Ass.*, **107,** 1208.

PEARCE, J. (1968) The ophthalmological complications of migraine, *J. neurol. Sci.*, 6 73.

PEARCE, J. M. S., and FOSTER, J. B. (1965) An investigation of complicated migraine, *Neurology (Minneap.)*, **15,** 333.

RILEY, H. A. (1932) Migraine, *Bull. neurol. Inst. N.Y.*, **2, 429.**

RILEY, H. A., BRICKNER, R. M., and SOLTS, S. E. (1934–6) Unusual types of migraine, *Bull. neurol. Inst. N.Y.*, **4,** 403.

SCHUMACHER, G. A., and WOLFF, H. G. (1941) Experimental studies in headache, *Arch. Neurol. Psychiat. (Chicago)*, **45,** 199.

SICUTERI, F., TESTI, A., and ANSELMI, B. (1961) Biochemical investigations in headache; increase in the hydroxyindolacetic acid excretion during migraine attacks, *Int. Arch. Allergy*, **19,** 55.

VON STORCH, T. J. C. (1937) The migraine syndrome, *New Engl. J. Med.*, **117,** 247.

VON STORCH, T. J. C. (1938) Complications following the use of ergotamine tartrate, *J. Amer. med. Ass.*, **111, 293.**

WOLFF, H. G. (1963) *Headache and Other Head Pain*, 2nd ed., New York.

MIGRAINOUS NEURALGIA

This term was applied by Harris (1926) to a highly distinctive type of headache involving chiefly the eye and frontal region on one side and characterized by its periodicity. Attacks may occur once or several times in twenty-four hours and last from one to several hours. A bout tends to last for several weeks after which the patient is free from symptoms for months or even one or two years when the headache recurs in the same way. Lacrimation and nasal congestion on the affected side are apt to occur in the attacks. There are no abnormal physical signs. The condition must be distinguished from intracranial tumour, and local causes of headache in the eye or nasal sinuses.

It now seems certain that the condition which has been variously referred to as 'histamine headache' (Horton, 1941) or 'cluster headache' (Wolff, 1963) is the same condition as periodic migrainous neuralgia and this syndrome also embraces the syndromes of ciliary neuralgia, vidian neuralgia, and spheno-palatine neuralgia described by the earlier neurologists. Harris (1940) recommended alcohol injection of the Gasserian ganglion but Symonds (1956) showed that ergotamine tartrate, 0·5 mg., given by subcutaneous injection once, twice, or even three times daily completely relieved the attacks. The injections are given for as long as may be necessary until the bout is over; this can only be determined by reducing or withdrawing treatment to see whether the attacks recur. Fortunately ergotism seems to be very rare in such cases. Balla and Walton (1964) found that in many cases ergotamine by mouth (*Migril*) was equally effective if given regularly or, if this failed, dimethysergide, 1–2 mg. three times daily. Probably oral medication should be tried first before going on to treatment with injections.

REFERENCES

BALLA, J. I., and WALTON, J. N. (1964) Periodic migrainous neuralgia. *Brit. med. J.*, i, 219.

HARRIS, W. (1926) *Neuritis and Neuralgia*, London.

HARRIS, W. (1940) Alcohol injection of the Gasserian ganglion for migrainous neuralgia, *Lancet*, ii, 481.

HORTON, B. T. (1941) Histamine cephalagia, *J. Amer. med. Ass.*, **116**, 377.

SYMONDS, C. (1956) A particular variety of headache, *Brain*, **79**, 217.

WOLFF, H. G. (1963) *Headache and Other Head Pain*, 2nd ed., New York.

4

DISORDERS OF THE CEREBRAL CIRCULATION

THE CEREBRAL ARTERIAL CIRCULATION

THE intracranial blood supply is derived from the two internal carotid arteries and the two vertebral arteries which unite anteriorly to form the basilar artery. The circulus arteriosus cerebri (circle of Willis) which is situated at the base of the brain is formed by anastomoses between the internal carotid arteries, the basilar artery, and their branches, as follows.

The basilar artery divides into the two posterior cerebrals, which are joined to the two internal carotids by the posterior communicating arteries. The internal carotids give off the two anterior cerebral arteries, which are united by the single anterior communicating artery, which thus completes the circle.

The principal intracranial arteries and their areas of distribution [see PLATES 1 and 2] are:

ARTERIES OF THE CEREBRAL HEMISPHERES

The Internal Carotid Artery

The internal carotid artery after entering the cranium gives off small branches to the wall of the cavernous sinus, and to the third, fourth, fifth, and sixth cranial nerves, including the trigeminal ganglion, the hypophysis, and the dura mater of the middle fossa. The next branch is the *ophthalmic artery*, from which the central artery of the retina is derived. The internal carotid next gives off the *posterior communicating artery*, which unites it with the posterior cerebral artery. The posterior communicating artery supplies the optic chiasma, hypophysis, tuber cinereum, and hypothalamic region, the lower part of the anterior third of the posterior limb of the internal capsule, part of the lateral nucleus of the thalamus, the anterior third of the crus cerebri, and part of the midbrain, including the subthalamic nucleus and Forel's field. The *anterior choroidal artery* passes backwards and outwards from the internal carotid to enter the anterior extremity of the descending horn of the lateral ventricle, where it supplies the choroid plexus. It is distributed also to the optic tract, to the uncus, to the posterior two-thirds of the posterior limb of the internal capsule, and the origin of the optic radiation, to part of the lentiform nucleus, and sometimes to the anterior third of the crus cerebri, which is usually supplied by the posterior communicating; sometimes it also supplies the posterior two-thirds of the crus cerebri which is more often supplied by the posterior cerebral.

The Anterior Cerebral Artery

The anterior cerebral artery passes forwards and medially from the internal carotid, turns round the genu of the corpus callosum, above which it runs backwards to terminate posteriorly, usually one inch anterior to the parieto-occipital sulcus. It gives off the following principal branches: (1) Basal branches, of which the most important has been called the recurrent branch (Heubner's artery). This branch enters the anterior perforated substance and supplies the anterior part of the caudate nucleus, the anterior one-third of the putamen, and the inferior half of the anterior limb of the internal capsule. (2) The anterior communicating artery, which is a short branch uniting the two anterior cerebrals and which gives off no branches. (3) Branches to the frontal and parietal lobes. These supply the medial aspect of the hemisphere and the upper part of its lateral aspect for from three-quarters to one inch from the median edge throughout the length of the artery and a corresponding area of the white matter of the frontal and parietal lobes, including the olfactory tract and lobe. The most important cortical branch of the anterior cerebral supplies the paracentral lobule, which contains the leg area of the motor cortex. Other branches of the anterior cerebral pass downwards to supply the genu, rostrum, and body of the corpus callosum.

The Middle Cerebral Artery

The middle cerebral artery passes laterally from the internal carotid in the stem of the lateral sulcus to the surface of the insula, where it divides into its terminal cortical branches. When crossing the base of the brain it gives off its striate branches. These branches supply part of the lentiform nucleus, the upper part of both anterior and posterior limbs of the internal capsule, and the horizontal part of the caudate nucleus behind the head. The cortical distribution of the middle cerebral artery is coterminous with that of the anterior cerebral as far back as the middle of the superior parietal lobule. It then extends to the edge of the median surface or is bounded by the territory of the posterior cerebral artery, passing downwards between the intraparietal sulcus and the occipital lobe to reach the middle of the inferior temporal or the lower border of the middle temporal gyrus. In about half of all cases the area of the middle cerebral artery extends to the occipital pole, or half an inch anterior to it. It also supplies the tapetum of the corpus callosum and the white matter of the centrum semiovale corresponding to its cortical distribution. The cortical branches of the middle cerebral artery are the orbital, the frontal, which supply the inferior and middle frontal gyri, and are distributed to the precentral gyrus and the posterior part of the middle frontal gyrus; the parietal, which supply the postcentral gyrus and the adjacent superior parietal lobule; continuing in the direction of the main stem of the artery these also supply the inferior parietal lobule, part of the lateral surface of the occipital lobe, and the posterior part of the temporal lobe; finally there are temporal branches, which supply the superior and middle temporal gyri.

The Posterior Cerebral Artery

The two posterior cerebral arteries are the terminal branches of the basilar. They run backwards and upwards around the cerebral peduncles and beneath the splenium of the corpus callosum to the calcarine sulcus of the occipital lobe. Close to its origin the posterior cerebral artery gives off basal branches which

PLATE 1

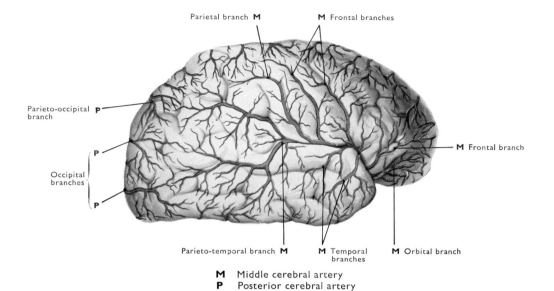

Parietal branch **M**   **M** Frontal branches

Parieto-occipital **P** branch

P

Occipital branches

P

M Frontal branch

Parieto-temporal branch **M**   **M** Temporal branches   **M** Orbital branch

M   Middle cerebral artery
P   Posterior cerebral artery

Distribution of cerebral arteries on the supero-lateral surface
of the right cerebral hemisphere

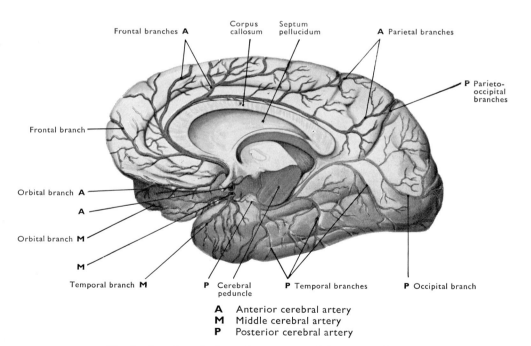

Frontal branches **A**   Corpus callosum   Septum pellucidum   **A** Parietal branches

P Parieto-occipital branches

Frontal branch

Orbital branch **A**

A

Orbital branch **M**

M

Temporal branch **M**   **P** Cerebral peduncle   **P** Temporal branches   **P** Occipital branch

A   Anterior cerebral artery
M   Middle cerebral artery
P   Posterior cerebral artery

Distribution of cerebral arteries on the medial and tentorial surfaces
of the right cerebal hemisphere

PLATE 2

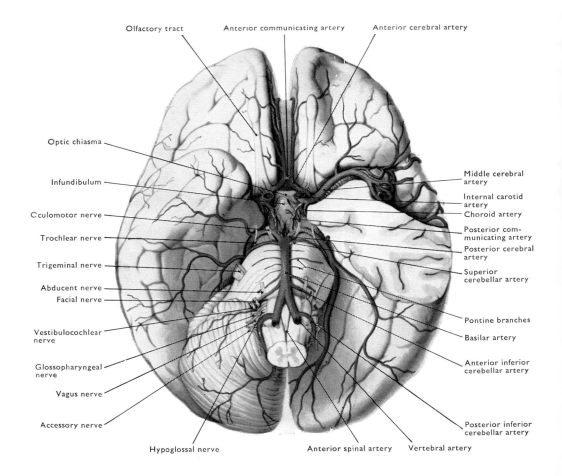

Olfactory tract

Anterior communicating artery

Anterior cerebral artery

Optic chiasma

Infundibulum

Cculomotor nerve

Trochlear nerve

Trigeminal nerve

Abducent nerve

Facial nerve

Vestibulocochlear nerve

Glossopharyngeal nerve

Vagus nerve

Accessory nerve

Middle cerebral artery

Internal carotid artery

Choroid artery

Posterior communicating artery

Posterior cerebral artery

Superior cerebellar artery

Pontine branches

Basilar artery

Anterior inferior cerebellar artery

Posterior inferior cerebellar artery

Hypoglossal nerve

Anterior spinal artery

Vertebral artery

Arteries of the base of the brain

supply the posterior part of the thalamus, including the pulvinar, the posterior two-thirds of the crus cerebri, and the red nucleus. Other branches pass around the brain stem to supply the colliculi and the geniculate bodies. The *posterior choroidal arteries*, of which there are usually two, supply some branches to the thalamus, the brain stem, and the third ventricle, and terminate in the choroid plexus of the third and lateral ventricles. There are four *cortical branches* of the posterior cerebral: the anterior temporal and the posterior temporal, which supply especially the uncus; the calcarine branch, which passes along the calcarine sulcus and is distributed to the visual area of the cerebral cortex, and the parieto-occipital branch, which passes along the corresponding sulcus. The cortical area supplied by the posterior cerebral includes the medial surface of the temporal lobe, and of the occipital lobe as far forwards as the internal parieto-occipital sulcus, or to a point one inch anterior to this. The most anterior part of the temporal lobe, however, is supplied by the middle cerebral, and the anterior end of the uncus by the anterior choroidal artery. The cortical area of the posterior cerebral extends on to the outer surface for a distance of from three-quarters to one inch, being here bounded by the posterior limits of the anterior and middle cerebral arteries. Above, it usually extends anteriorly as far as the external parieto-occipital sulcus or in some cases to half-way along the superior parietal lobule; below, it supplies the medial aspect of the temporal lobe to within an inch of the tip.

Blood Supply of Internal Capsule, Basal Ganglia, and Optic Radiation

The superior half of the anterior limb of the *internal capsule* is supplied by the middle cerebral artery, the inferior half by the anterior cerebral; the posterior limb is supplied as follows: the superior half by the middle cerebral, the anterior one-third of the inferior half by the posterior communicating, the posterior two-thirds by the anterior choroidal. The *thalamus* is supplied by vessels derived from the posterior cerebral, the posterior communicating, the anterior and posterior choroidal arteries, and the middle cerebral. The posterior half of the lateral nucleus is supplied by the middle and posterior cerebral arteries, the anterior half by the middle cerebral and posterior communicating arteries. The posterior half of the lateral nucleus is supplied by the lenticulo-optic, retromamillary, and thalamo-geniculate (the artery of the thalamic syndrome), the anterior half by the lenticulo-optic and thalamo-tuberal vessels. The oral one-third of the *caudate nucleus* and *putamen* is supplied by perforating branches of the anterior cerebral, the rest by the striate branches of the middle cerebral. The greater part of the *globus pallidus* is supplied by the anterior choroidal. The *optic radiation* at its origin is supplied by the anterior choroidal artery: of the rest, the superior three-quarters is supplied by the middle cerebral and the inferior one-quarter by the posterior cerebral, unless the middle cerebral does not reach so far back, when the posterior cerebral supplies the whole.

ARTERIES OF THE BRAIN STEM

The arteries of the brain stem are mostly derived from the *basilar* and the two *vertebral arteries*, though the upper part of the midbrain receives in addition contributions from the posterior communicating artery, the anterior choroidal artery, and the posterior cerebral and its branches. The vertebral arteries enter a canal in the cervical spine at the level of the sixth cervical vertebra and then pass upwards to emerge at the level of the atlas and form a considerable loop before entering the foramen magnum. They fuse at the level of the junction between the pons and the medulla to form the *basilar artery*, which terminates at the upper border of the pons by dividing into the two posterior cerebrals. The arteries of the brain stem show considerable variations of distribution, but conform on the whole to the following general scheme:

Paramedian arteries enter the brain stem near the midline anteriorly and supply a narrow zone extending from before backwards close to the midline. Short circumferential arteries supply an area, often wedge-shaped, on the lateral aspect, and long circumferential arteries are distributed to the posterior part and to the cerebellum.

The superior cerebellar artery is the highest branch derived from the basilar before its bifurcation. It passes outwards and backwards around the brain stem, giving small branches to the cerebral peduncle and the colliculi, and terminates by dividing to supply the upper surface of the vermis and of the lateral lobe of the cerebellum.

The anterior inferior cerebellar artery arises from the middle of the basilar and passes backwards to supply part of the pons, including the lateral tegmental region and the anterior part of the lower surface of the lateral lobes of the cerebellum. The *internal auditory artery* leaves the anterior inferior cerebellar artery, or less often the basilar or the vertebral, to accompany the cochlear part of the eighth nerve and enters the internal acoustic meatus to supply the internal ear.

Throughout its length the basilar gives off small vessels to the anterior part of the pons.

Its lowest lateral branch supplies a wedge-shaped area of the lateral aspect of the upper part of the medulla corresponding to the area supplied by the posterior inferior cerebellar artery in the lower part of the medulla.

The posterior inferior cerebellar artery is the largest branch of the vertebral. Its site of origin is variable, but it usually arises from this artery a little distance below the lower border of the pons. It then passes outwards and backwards around the medulla, giving branches which supply a wedge-shaped area of the lateral aspect of the medulla, the base of which is on the surface, and the apex postero-internally, and the lower part of the inferior cerebellar peduncle. It also supplies the choroid plexus of the fourth ventricle. The main trunk divides into two terminal branches which supply the inferior vermis and the lower surface of the cerebellar hemisphere.

The vertebral artery, besides supplying the lateral aspect of the medulla through the posterior inferior cerebellar, gives off branches to the paramedian region, a narrow zone adjacent to the middle line, including the pyramids of the medulla and extending backwards as far as the floor of the fourth ventricle. This paramedian area at the lowest medullary level is supplied by the *anterior spinal artery,* which arises by the fusion of a branch from each vertebral artery.

PHYSIOLOGY OF THE CEREBRAL CIRCULATION

The experiments of McDonald and Potter (1951) show that the internal carotid and vertebral arteries share the blood supply to their own half of the brain in such a way that there is normally no interchange of blood between them. Their respective streams meet in the posterior communicating artery at a 'dead point' at which the pressure of the two is equal, and do not mix there. If, however, both internal carotid or both vertebral arteries are occluded, blood passes backwards or forwards from the pair which are still patent. Similarly, if one internal carotid or one vertebral artery is occluded, blood crosses the middle line so that the area which would otherwise be deprived of blood is supplied by the contralateral fellow. The circulus arteriosus cerebri thus provides an important anastomotic circulation. Another exists in the distal anastomoses between the three major cerebral arteries at the periphery of their cortical fields of supply (Van der Eecken, 1959). Once within the brain no artery appears ever to join another. Thus whereas cortical arteries have profuse meningeal anastomoses at the 'water-shed' regions, perforating vessels appear to be true 'end-arteries'. Normally, the two streams from the vertebral arteries remain each on its own side of the basilar unmixed, like the Blue and White Nile for some miles below their union at Khartoum.

Schmidt (1950) states that the cerebral circulation normally tends to follow passively upon changes in the arterial pressure to a greater extent than that of most other organs. There is no evidence that the cerebral blood flow is affected by cervicothoracic ganglion block. The cerebral vessels are dilated by products of metabolism, especially CO_2, and constricted by increased O_2, and diminished CO_2. Schmidt concludes that CO_2 is the dominant influence in regulating the tone of the cerebral vessels, and that these are relatively insusceptible to the ordinary vasoconstrictor and vasodilator drugs. In recent years much new information concerning cerebral blood flow in health and disease has been derived from investigations using the Kety–Schmidt nitrous oxide method and more recently with the aid of various techniques using radioactive substances which can be utilized to measure general or regional blood flow. Fazekas et al. (1955) showed that cerebral blood flow diminished from a mean value of 57·5 ml./100 g. of brain per minute in the 18- to 47-year age group, to 47·5 ml./100 g. of brain per minute in individuals over 57 years of age. Findings in patients with hypertension and cerebral vascular disease have been reviewed by McHenry (1966).

The Blood-brain Barrier

It is an old observation that many substances injected into the blood stream do not enter the brain: the dye trypan blue has been extensively used for these tests. The existence of a blood-brain barrier between the blood vessels and the nerve cells has been postulated to explain this, but its nature is still obscure. It has been shown that brain damage, whether produced by experimental injuries or disease, impairs the blood-brain barrier (see Hess, 1955; Millen and Hess, 1958; Meyer, 1958). Taylor, Smith, and Hunter (1954) have used increased permeability of the meninges to bromide in meningitis as a test. Lassen and Ingvar (1963) have injected Kr.85 or Xenon 133 dissolved in saline into the internal carotid artery and have followed the clearance of the isotope from different regions of the brain by collimated external scintillation detectors. This technique not only gives some indication of regional blood flow but some conclusions concerning the blood-brain barrier may be inferred.

REFERENCES

ALEXANDER, L. (1942) The vascular supply of the strio-pallidum, *Res. Publ. Ass. nerv. ment. Dis.*, **21**, 77.

ATKINSON, W. J. (1949) The anterior inferior cerebellar artery, *J. Neurol. Neurosurg. Psychiat.*, **21**, 137.

BEEVOR, C. E. (1907) The cerebral arterial supply, *Brain*, **30**, 403.

BRAIN, W. R. (1957) Order and disorder of the cerebral circulation, *Lancet*, ii, 857.

CRITCHLEY, M. (1930) The anterior cerebral artery and its syndromes, *Brain*, **53**, 120.

FAY, T. (1925) The cerebral vasculature, *J. Amer. med. Ass.*, **84**, 1727.

FAZEKAS, J. F., KLEN, J., and FINNERTY, F. A. (1955) Influence of age and vascular disease on cerebral hemodynamics and metabolism, *Amer. J. Med.*, **18**, 477.

FOIX, C. (1925) Irrigation de la couche optique, *C.R. Soc. Biol. (Paris)*, **92**, 55.

FOIX, C., and HILLEMAND, P. (1925) Les artères de l'axe encéphalique jusqu'au diencéphale inclusivement, *Rev. Neurol. (Paris)*, **32**, 705.

HESS, A. (1955) Blood-brain barrier and ground substance of central nervous system, *Arch. Neurol. Psychiat. (Chicago)*, **74**, 149.

LASSEN, N. A., and INGVAR, D. H. (1963) Regional cerebral blood flow measurement in man: a review, *Arch. Neurol. (Chic.)*, **9**, 615.

McDONALD, D. A., and POTTER, J. M. (1951) The distribution of blood to the brain, *J. Physiol. (Lond.)*, **114**, 356.

McHENRY, L. C., JR. (1966) Cerebral blood flow studies in cerebrovascular disease, *Arch. intern. Med.*, **117**, 546.

MEYER, A. (1958) in *Neuropathology*, by Greenfield, J. G., Blackwood, W., McMenemey, W. H., Meyer, A., and Norman, R. M., p. 230, London.

MILLEN, J. W., and HESS, A. (1958) The blood-brain barrier: an experimental study with vital dyes, *Brain*, **81**, 248.

SCHMIDT, C. F. (1950) *The Cerebral Circulation in Health and Disease*, Springfield, Ill.

SHELLSHEAR, J. L. (1927) A contribution to our knowledge of the arterial supply of the cerebral cortex in man, *Brain*, **50**, 236.

STOPFORD, J. S. B. (1915–16 and 1916–17) The arteries of the pons and medulla oblongata, *J. Anat. Physiol.*, **50**, 131; and **51**, 250.

TAYLOR, L. M., SMITH, H. V., and HUNTER, G. (1954) The blood-c.s.f. barrier to bromide in diagnosis of tuberculous meningitis, *Lancet*, i, 700.

VAN DER EECKEN, H. M. (1959) *The Anastomoses between the Leptomeningeal Arteries of the Brain*, Springfield, Ill.

CEREBRAL ISCHAEMIA

Cerebral ischaemia, or impairment of the blood supply to the brain, may be produced in a number of different ways. (1) Since, as we have seen, the cerebral blood flow is directly related to the blood pressure, a sudden fall of blood pressure from any cause may produce symptoms of cerebral ischaemia. The cause of this is discussed below. (2) The defective blood supply may be the result of disease of the cerebral arteries themselves due, for example, to atheroma or endarteritis. (3) A cerebral vessel may be obstructed by a substance carried into it from elsewhere by the circulation—cerebral embolism.

COMPLETE CIRCULATORY ARREST

The brain is highly vulnerable to any interruption of its circulation. This most commonly occurs on the operating table in a patient under an anaesthetic. Here the situation is complex since the metabolism of the brain is already abnormal by reason of the anaesthetic, and the patient has sometimes been anoxic before the cardiac arrest occurs. How long it takes for irreversible brain damage to occur in such circumstances is uncertain; it is probably at the most two minutes at normal body temperature, but may be very much longer in hypothermia. Meyer (1958) reports a case in which severe brain damage followed respiratory and cardiac arrest in only one minute. Patients who survive may live for many months in a state of decerebration, or decortication, or, if they are conscious, with severe dementia. Anoxia is less dangerous than complete circulatory arrest because in the latter the general nutrition of the nerve cells, and the removal of waste products, are also interfered with.

SYNCOPE

Definition. Syncope is a brief and transitory loss of consciousness, due to impairment of the cerebral circulation, and usually occurring in the absence of organic disease of the brain. If the fall in the cerebral circulation is sufficiently prolonged convulsions occur. Hence an isolated convulsion may sometimes be precipitated by circumstances which more usually cause syncope, but in pathogenesis, and electroencephalographically, syncope and epilepsy are quite distinct.

AETIOLOGY

The essential feature of syncope is a temporary fall in the cerebral circulation below the level necessary for the maintenance of consciousness. Apart from narrowing of the cerebral arteries, syncope is always the result of low cardiac output, which may be produced in a number of ways, some of them complex.

Postural Hypotension

This is a convenient term for the pathogenesis of fainting in a variety of circumstances which have this in common. Venous return to the heart is impaired because the blood accumulates in the veins in rapidly growing adolescents in hot rooms or in church, in young soldiers immobilized on parade, especially in hot weather, in patients getting up after long confinement to bed, in elderly men after emptying the bladder in the night (micturition syncope, *Lancet*, 1962), in those too rapidly assuming the erect posture after sympathectomy, hypotensive drugs, spinal anaesthesia and high spinal cord injuries, and in certain diseases, e.g. tabes, polyneuritis, and porphyria. In all these conditions the reflex postural regulation of the blood pressure is inadequate. The reasons are often complex. The pressor reflexes may be interrupted on their afferent side in tabes and polyneuritis, or centrally depressed by alcohol or other drugs, including phenothiazines and amine-oxidase inhibitors. The condition may be familial (Johnson, Lee, Oppenheimer, and Spalding, 1966). Brigden, Howarth, and Sharpey-Schafer (1950) discuss the physiology of fainting induced by change of posture. In chronic orthostatic hypotension, a rare disorder believed to be due to an abnormality of the autonomic nervous system, the blood pressure falls as soon as the patient assumes the upright posture but there is no compensatory vasoconstriction of peripheral vessels so that pallor, sweating, and tachycardia do not occur and there is abrupt loss of consciousness. The senses are regained as soon as the patient lies down; after frequent attacks confusion, dysarthria, and other neurological signs may develop (Shy and Drager, 1960; Hohl, Frame, and Schatz, 1965).

Cough Syncope

Cough syncope or 'laryngeal epilepsy' is syncope or epilepsy produced by prolonged coughing, usually in middle-aged men. The changes in intrathoracic pressure produced by coughing interfere with the venous return of blood to the heart, and there is often atheromatous narrowing of the cerebral arteries as well. Another 'mechanical' mode of producing syncope by interfering with venous return is by stretching with the arms extended and raised and the spine hyperextended—'stretch syncope'—which may occur in young people.

Psychological Causes

The occurrence of syncope as an immediate effect of sudden psychological shock is well known. Rook (1947) attributed nearly half the faints occurring in airmen during the last war to emotional causes. Here again there is a fall of blood pressure due to complex factors. Reflexly induced pooling in the peripheral circulation may be the most important, but McHenry, Fazekas, and Sullivan (1961) draw attention to the fact that hyperventilation, a common accompaniment of anxiety, may lead to cerebral ischaemia by lowering the CO_2 content of the blood. Tachycardia, also due to anxiety, may lower the cardiac output. Fainting may be a conditioned reaction to particular circumstances.

Physical Shock

A wide diversity of physical stimuli are capable of causing syncope, and in some cases it may be artificial to distinguish the physical from the psychological factor. Severe pain may cause loss of consciousness, but many stimuli which cause little or no pain may be equally effective, such as venepuncture, cisternal and lumbar puncture, and pleural puncture ('pleural epilepsy').

Anaemia of Sudden Onset

Anaemia due to severe haemorrhage may cause syncope, though an equally severe anaemia of gradual onset does not.

Polycythaemia Vera

In cases of polycythaemia vera the increased viscosity of the blood may predispose to cerebral infarction but many patients also experience episodes of cerebral or brain-stem ischaemia similar to those of carotid or vertebro-basilar insufficiency (see below) (Silverstein, Gilbert, and Wasserman, 1962).

Cardiac Disorder

Syncope may be caused by the impairment of the cerebral circulation resulting from low cardiac output caused by disorder of the rate and rhythm of the heart in heart-block, auricular flutter, and paroxysmal tachycardia. Syncope and epilepsy in heart-block—Stokes–Adams syndrome—are the best known of these disturbances. The loss of consciousness is most likely to occur during the cardiac asystole which may develop in the transition between partial heart-block and complete block, and the attacks may cease when the block is complete, but do not always do so. Many attacks may occur in a day. They usually occur when the patient is at rest and not during physical effort. Typically loss of consciousness and pallor occur during asystole and flushing with a few myoclonic jerks of the extremities occur when the pulse returns and consciousness is quickly restored. These attacks rarely occur in patients with bundle-branch block. In addition low cardiac output may be due to massive pulmonary embolism, mechanical obstruction of the mitral valve, and severe aortic stenosis.

Carotid Sinus Syncope

The important part played in the regulation of the circulation by the carotid sinus, the slight dilatation of the carotid in the region of the bifurcation, was first pointed out by Hering, though previously the vagus had been held responsible for the effects now known to originate in the sinus. A rise of pressure within the sinus causes a reflex fall in blood pressure with slowing of the heart rate, while a fall of pressure within the sinus has the opposite effect. These reflex changes are mediated by the nerve to the carotid sinus, a branch of the glossopharyngeal nerve, and the medullary vasomotor centres. Disease in the neighbourhood of the sinus, or even hypersensitivity of the reflex mechanism may cause syncopal attacks which can be reproduced by digital pressure in this region. Precipitation of the attacks by spontaneous movements of the head is mentioned by Turner and Learmonth (1948).

Ferris, Capps, and Weiss (1935) have described three types of carotid sinus syncope: (1) 'vagal' attacks in which unconsciousness is due to cerebral anoxaemia resulting from reflex cardiac asystole; (2) attacks of a depressor type in which loss of consciousness is due to cerebral anoxaemia caused by a fall in blood pressure; and (3) a cerebral type of attack in which unconsciousness occurs without any significant change in heart rate or blood pressure and without change in the cerebral blood flow, but the occurrence of this is doubtful. Hutchinson and Stock (1960), reporting sixteen cases, all male, classified the symptoms as (1) vertigo, (2) syncopal attacks—sometimes with convulsions, (3) 'focal' attacks of cerebral symptoms, and (4) mental changes. Attacks might be brought on by turning the head. In none of their cases did symptoms occur without circulatory change. (See also Reese, Green, and Elliott, 1962.)

The causes of carotid sinus attacks include lesions in the neighbourhood of the sinus, such as scarring from tuberculous adenitis, atheroma of the artery, and rarely carotid body tumour. Among more general causes are the menopause and dietary deficiency associated with chronic alcoholism.

Cerebral Atheroma

Temporary cerebral ischaemia resulting from atheroma of the cerebral arteries is an unusual cause of syncope and is unlikely to occur unless the cerebral circulation as a whole is gravely impaired, or the ischaemia particularly involves the central reticular formation. Faintness may then be brought on particularly by turning the head or extending the neck, through impairment of the blood supply through one or other internal carotid or vertebral artery or both, independently of the carotid sinus reflex. Fainting attacks due to brain-stem ischaemia are particularly liable to occur when occlusion of the left subclavian artery close to its origin results in retrograde flow of blood down the homolateral vertebral artery in order to supply the upper limb (the 'subclavian steal syndrome').

SYMPTOMS

The onset of an attack of syncope may be sudden, but it often takes a quarter of a minute to develop. There may be prodromal symptoms such as coldness or tingling in the extremities, sweating, or loss of vision. The patient becomes cold and limp, and at the onset of loss of consciousness sinks to the ground, though the premonitory symptoms often enable him to sit or lie down first. Respiration is usually sighing, the pulse is generally slow, and its tension low. The pupils may be dilated and react sluggishly to light, and the corneal reflexes are likely to be lost and the tendon reflexes diminished. Muscular twitching and urinary incontinence may occur, or, if the cerebral ischaemia is sufficiently prolonged, a general convulsion.

Electroencephalography

In syncope due to impairment of the cerebral blood flow slow waves of high voltage develop in the EEG concurrently with the loss of consciousness (Hill and Driver, 1962) and this is followed by complete flattening of the EEG record while clonic or tonic convulsions occur (Gastaut and Fischer-Williams, 1957).

DIAGNOSIS

When syncope leads only to loss of consciousness it must be distinguished from epilepsy. Syncope, being secondary to a circulatory change, is usually more gradual in its onset and its cessation than an attack of petit mal. Convulsive movements do not occur as a rule, and the patient is limp rather than rigid, as in epilepsy. Syncopal convulsions, however, need to be distinguished from epilepsy. In many cases the cause of the syncopal attacks is obvious. Syncope of carotid sinus origin can be reproduced by pressure on the sinus, which, however, is no longer effective after procaine has been injected into this region. In the stage of partial heart-block the diagnosis may be impossible without an electrocardiogram: in complete block the heart rate is usually from 26 to 30. The EEG dysrhythmia characteristic of epilepsy is absent: if syncope can be induced, e.g. by ocular compression, the EEG changes are those described above.

PROGNOSIS

A syncopal attack in itself is rarely fatal and leaves no sequelae. However, prolonged and diffuse cerebral ischaemia which may, for example, occur during anaesthesia, particularly in the elderly, may lead to permanent anoxic brain damage. The prognosis is that of the causal condition.

TREATMENT

Little treatment is required for the ordinary attack of syncope, which is self-limiting. The patient should be placed in a horizontal posture. Smelling salts and brandy (if he can swallow) act reflexly as cardio-accelerators. Any causal condition will require treatment. Syncope of carotid sinus origin is best treated with anticholinergic or sympathomimetic drugs of which the former, such as atropine, 0·5 mg. two or three times daily or propantheline bromide, 15 mg. three times a day, are usually the most successful. In intractable cases it may be justifiable to denervate the sinus.

REFERENCES

BRIGDEN, W., HOWARTH, S., and SHARPEY-SCHAFER, E. P. (1950) Postural changes in the peripheral blood-flow of normal subjects with observations on vaso-vagal fainting reactions as a result of tilting, the lordotic posture, pregnancy and spinal anaesthesia, *Clin. Sci.*, **60, 79.**

FERRIS, E. B. (1937) The relation of the carotid sinus to the autonomic nervous system and the neuroses, *Arch. Neurol. Psychiat. (Chicago),* **37, 365.**

FERRIS, E. B., Jr., CAPPS, R. B., and WEISS, S. (1935) Carotid sinus syncope and its bearing on the mechanism of the unconscious state and convulsions: a study of thirty-two additional cases, *Medicine (Baltimore),* **14, 377.**

GASTAUT, H., and FISCHER-WILLIAMS, M. (1957) Electroencephalographic study of syncope, *Lancet,* ii, 1018.

HILL, D., and DRIVER, M. V. (1962) in *Recent Advances in Neurology and Neuropsychiatry,* 7th ed., ed. Lord Brain, p. 219, London.

HOHL, R. D., FRAME, B., and SCHATZ, I. J. (1965) The Shy-Drager variant of idiopathic orthostatic hypotension, *Amer. J. Med.,* **39, 134.**

HUTCHINSON, E. C., and STOCK, J. P. P. (1960) The carotid-sinus syndrome, *Lancet,* ii, 445.

JOHNSON, R. H., LEE, G. DE J., OPPENHEIMER, W. R., and SPALDING, J. M. K. (1966) Autonomic failure due to intermedio-lateral column degeneration, *Quart. J. Med.,* **35, 276.**

KERSHMAN, J. (1949) Syncope and seizures, *J. Neurol. Neurosurg. Psychiat,* **12, 25.**

LANCET (1962) Fainting on micturition, Leader, *Lancet,* ii, 286.

MCHENRY, L. C., Jr., FAZEKAS, J. F., and SULLIVAN, J. F. (1961) Cerebral haemodynamics of syncope, *Amer. J. med. Sci.,* **241, 173.**

MEYER, A. (1958) in *Neuropathology,* by Greenfield, J. G., Blackwood, W., McMenemey, W. H., Meyer, A., and Norman, R. M., p. 241, London.

REESE, C. L., GREEN, J. B., and ELLIOTT, F. A. (1962) The cerebral form of carotid sinus syncope, *Neurology (Minneap.),* **12, 492.**

ROOK, A. F. (1947) Fainting and flying, *Quart. J. Med.,* **40, 181.**

SHARPEY-SCHAFER, E. P. (1953) The mechanism of syncope after coughing, *Brit. med. J.,* **2, 860.**

SHY, G. M., and DRAGER, G. A. (1960) A neurological syndrome associated with orthostatic hypotension, *Arch. Neurol. (Chic.),* **2, 511.**

SILVERSTEIN, A., GILBERT, H., and WASSERMAN, L. R. (1962) Hemiplegic complications of polycythaemia, *Ann. intern. Med.,* **57, 909.**

TURNER, R., and LEARMONTH, J. R. (1948) Carotid-sinus syndrome, *Lancet,* ii, 644.

WEISS, S., and BAKER, J. P. (1933). The carotid sinus reflex in health and disease. Its role in the causation of fainting and convulsions, *Medicine (Baltimore),* **12, 297.**

ATHEROMA OF THE ARTERIES SUPPLYING THE BRAIN

AETIOLOGY AND PATHOLOGY

The term 'cerebral arteriosclerosis' is usually limited to degenerative changes in the arteries of the brain. Strictly interpreted, however, as arterial thickening it occurs also in inflammatory conditions. The following are the most important causes of arteriosclerosis: (1) *Primary degeneration of the intima*. This takes the form of atheroma. There is degeneration of the intima with the production of fat debris and some reactionary fibrosis. Calcification may occur in the degenerated area. There is usually some medial degeneration. The causes of primary atheroma are still the subject of debate. It occurs principally in late middle age and old age, yet some very old individuals may show little. Metabolic diseases, such as diabetes and myxoedema are usually associated with widespread atheroma. (2) *Degeneration secondary to high blood pressure*. High blood pressure is associated with hypertrophy of the media of the arteries and the hypertrophied media undergoes degeneration. Atheroma occurs partly as a result of medial degeneration and partly as the effect of the raised blood pressure itself. (3) *Endarteritis* causes thickening, especially of the intima. The main cause is syphilis. It is therefore more fully described in the section on syphilis of the nervous system. It may follow tuberculous meningitis. (4) *Thrombo-angiitis obliterans* is an inflammatory disease affecting all the coats of the blood vessels and leading to thrombosis and fibrous occlusion of the lumen. The disease is generalized throughout the blood vessels, but cerebral symptoms, though they occasionally occur, are rare. (5) *Polyarteritis nodosa* and *giant cell arteritis* are also rare causes. This section will be concerned only with atheroma.

Progressive occlusion of the arteries supplying the brain tends to impair the cerebral circulation. As already mentioned, impairment of the cerebral circulation from this cause may be the result of atheroma affecting the extracranial course of these arteries, i.e. the common carotids, internal carotids and vertebrals, as well as of involvement of these vessels or their branches within the skull. Progressive occlusion of these blood vessels impairs the circulation in the regions they supply. The effects of this depend upon the size and situation of the vessel, and the rate of onset of the occlusion particularly in relation to the collateral circulation. Actual obstruction of an artery by atheroma, with or without subsequent thrombosis, causes softening of the region of the brain supplied by the vessel. In the early stages the softened patch is white or haemorrhagic and later becomes yellow. The nerve cells and fibres in the necrotic area degenerate, and in the surrounding tissues there is neuroglial overgrowth with infiltration, especially by compound granular corpuscles. The late result is a neuroglial scar or a cystic cavity. Generalized atheroma without occlusion of a single large vessel leads to diffuse atrophy of the brain with multiple small patches of softening of various ages. The relationship between actual thrombosis of an atheromatous vessel and the occurrence of infarction is complex. If a large artery is sufficiently narrowed by atheroma severe infarction may occur without thrombosis. The development of a thrombus, however, may precipitate symptoms by completing the occlusion of an atheromatous vessel. The patho-genesis of intermittent symptoms is discussed by Denny-Brown (1951, 1960).

Cerebral atheromatosis is chiefly a disease of late middle life and old age, though it may be encountered much earlier, even at the age of 40. The sexes are equally affected, and there is sometimes a familial predisposition.

THE PATHOPHYSIOLOGY OF DISTURBANCES OF THE CEREBRAL CIRCULATION RESULTING FROM ATHEROMA

During recent years much has been learnt about the complexity of the factors influencing the cerebral circulation in patients suffering from atheroma. Since, as we have seen, the cerebral blood flow depends primarily upon the cardiac output it follows that if this, for any reason, is seriously impaired for long enough, symptoms of cerebral ischaemia may result especially if, owing to atheroma, one or more of the arteries concerned in the cerebral circulation is already narrow. Since coronary atheroma is often associated with cerebral atheroma cerebral ischaemia is particularly likely to occur as a result of the hypotension produced by an attack of coronary thrombosis. Shock from any cause may have the same effect in the elderly, for example, a surgical operation, especially one conducted under induced hypotension. Anaemia is also a potent factor as, more rarely, are disorders which increase the viscosity of the blood. These aspects of the subject are stressed by Yates and Hutchinson (1961) who also suggest that intermittent hypotension may also be the result of arterial disease, for example, through interference with the carotid sinus reflex mechan-ism. Whether vasospasm plays any part save in exceptional circumstances is uncertain.

Another factor to which attention has been drawn by Hutchinson and Yates (1956) is the importance of looking at the blood supply to the brain as a whole. Mention has been made above of the importance of the circulus arteriosus in maintaining a stable cerebral circulation. Hutchinson and Yates have shown how, when there is widespread atheroma involving both internal carotid and vertebral arteries, occlusion of a vertebral artery may impair the circulation to one cerebral hemisphere while conversely, internal carotid artery occlusion may lead to infarction of the cerebellum. The possibility of effective anastomosis between the extracranial and the intracranial arteries is also a relevant factor.

It was a long time before students of cerebrovascular disease extended their interest to the internal carotid and vertebral arteries in the neck and only more recently have they traced these vessels down to their origins (Yates and Hutchin-son, 1961). While the common sites for narrowing or occlusion of the internal carotid artery by atheroma are at the sinus and the siphon the introduction of aortography has shown that the common carotid artery may be narrowed by atheroma, as may the vertebral between its origin from the subclavian artery and its entry into its canal in the cervical spine.

But what part does narrowing of one of these arteries in itself play in the pro-duction of cerebral ischaemia? Brice, Dowsett, and Lowe (1964) have studied the haemodynamic effects of carotid artery stenosis and have shown that a much greater degree of narrowing than might have been supposed is necessary sig-nificantly to reduce the blood flow. They conclude that if the minimal area of cross-section is more than 5 mm.² the blood flow will not be reduced even by long stenosis or by several stenoses in series. If the minimal area is between 2 and 5 mm.² the blood flow may be reduced, depending on the shape, on the number of stenoses in series, and, to a less extent, on the length of the stenoses.

How then does atheroma produce cerebral ischaemia in the absence of what Brice and his colleagues have shown to be the critical degree of arterial narrowing? Certain factors extraneous to the blood vessels themselves may sometimes operate, as Hutchinson and Yates showed in their study of the influence of cervical spondylosis on the blood flow through the vertebral arteries, a point to which attention has been drawn by a number of writers, recently Bauer, Sheehan, and Meyer (1961). Head rotation may impair the blood supply through the vertebral arteries especially if these are atheromatous, and on head rotation the internal carotid artery may sometimes be compressed against the transverse process of the atlas. It is usually a transitory impairment of the cerebral circulation which is attributed to these extraneous factors, but we may suspect that they may also be important as a cause of cerebral ischaemia if the head during sleep is maintained in a rotated position for a long time.

But we have still to explain a very common manifestation of cerebral ischaemia, the transient ischaemic attack. These, described in more detail below, are essentially episodes of transient but recurrent ischaemia in the same, often small, area of the brain. One of the first explanations for these put forward was that of Denny-Brown (1951) who suggested that a general fall in cerebral blood flow might be responsible for a transient ischaemic attack in the presence of atheromatous narrowing of certain arteries which made them more vulnerable than the rest to this degree of hypotension. However, Kendell and Marshall (1963) studied the effect of lowering the blood pressure in patients who were subject to transient ischaemic attacks and found that they could not produce focal symptoms before those of a general ischaemia. It seems to follow that the fall in cerebral blood flow is not in general the cause. Recent observations by Fisher (1959) and Ross Russell (1961, 1963) have thrown further light on the matter. Observing patients during transient attacks of monocular blindness they saw small white or yellow bodies passing along the retinal arteries, and it has been established by autopsy examination that these bodies may consist either of platelets (McBrien, Bradley, and Ashton, 1963) or cholesterol esters (David et al., 1963). Gunning et al. (1964) have reported six patients who had attacks of monocular blindness with or without contralateral hemiplegia. In some cases white or yellow bodies were observed in the retinal arteries during the attacks of blindness, and all patients had stenosis of the internal carotid artery with thrombi composed of fibrin, platelets and leucocytes at the site of the stenosis. All this evidence suggests that transient ischaemic attacks may be due to emboli of this kind, which, lodging at a point in the cerebral artery already narrowed by atheroma, produced transient ischaemic symptoms before breaking up and passing on. This seems to leave unexplained why the symptoms should always be of the same kind in a particular case; however, the fact that within cerebral arteries blood flow is usually laminar could explain why recurrent micro-embolism from a single crumbling plaque or mural thrombus always involves the same small peripheral branch. It is, however, unlikely that all transient ischaemic attacks are due to the same cause, and it may well be that in some cases at least, when there is already atheromatous narrowing of a cerebral artery, vasodilatation in surrounding areas may temporarily compete for blood with the affected vessel which, owing to its atheromatous narrowing, is unable to dilate normally.

DIFFUSE SYMPTOMS

Progressive cerebral ischaemia due to atheroma leads to impairment of cerebral function before actual blockage of vessels occurs. The course of the disease is complicated, however, by the occurrence of small or large areas of cerebral softening due usually to cerebral thrombosis.

The onset of the disease is often insidious and its course slowly progressive, or there may be apoplectiform attacks of varying severity leaving residual focal symptoms. The symptoms differ also according to the part of the brain mainly affected. Thus mental symptoms may overshadow motor disturbances, or vice versa, or both may be combined.

Mental symptoms in milder cases consist of a general reduction in intellectual capacity with impairment of memory, especially for recent events and names, and emotional instability. There is a marked tendency to reminiscence, and confabulation may occur. The patient becomes self-centred and hostile to change in all forms. In more severe cases loosely constructed delusions occur and there is often a paranoid trend. Depression is not uncommon and there may be attacks of confusion, which are apt to be precipitated by removal from home and by operations, for example, for cataract or for removal of the prostate. Still greater deterioration leads to a profound dementia.

Epileptiform attacks are common and may consist either of minor attacks, of Jacksonian or uncinate attacks, or of generalized epileptic fits. Various forms of aphasia, agnosia, and apraxia are met with. Corticospinal lesions may take the form of monoplegia, hemiplegia, or double hemiplegia leading to one variety of pseudobulbar palsy. Paraplegia of cerebral origin may occur. Sometimes the patient cannot walk, though he can move his legs freely in bed—an apraxic abasia—or the gait may be the 'marche à petits pas' (atherosclerotic Parkinsonism). The grasp reflex may be encountered in one or both hands and feet, with or without slight corticospinal involvement. Senile tremor is common and athetosis may occur. Generalized chorea is exceptional, but unilateral chorea or hemiballismus due to softening in the region of the subthalamic nucleus is less uncommon. Cerebellar syndromes are very rare but there may be symptoms of ischaemia of the spinal cord. Visual impairment is common as a result of arteriosclerotic retinopathy. Less frequently it is due to softening involving the optic radiations or visual cortex. General arteriosclerosis is usually well marked. The blood pressure is high in the hypertensive group, but little, if at all, raised in patients with simple atheromatosis.

SYNDROMES OF THE CEREBRAL ARTERIES

Obstruction of a cerebral artery gives rise to a clinical picture which depends upon loss of function of the parts of the brain supplied by the vessel. This, of

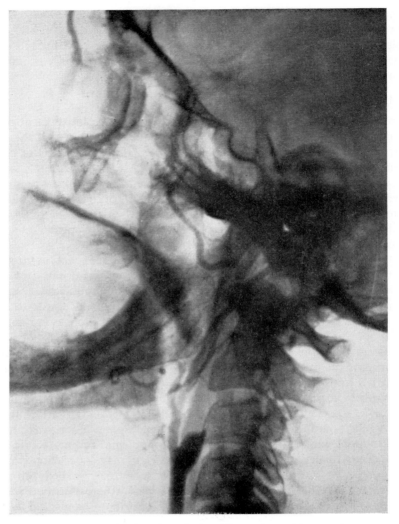

FIG. 56. Angiogram showing thrombosis of internal carotid artery just above
its origin. (Kindly lent by Dr. James Bull.)

course, is influenced by the exact point at which the obstruction occurs, since
blockage at the origin of a vessel may lead to loss of function of a larger region
than is the case when the obstruction is situated more distally or involves only
a single branch. However, as already mentioned, obstruction to a small perforating artery may have more profound and permanent effects (as these are
end-arteries) than may proximal occlusion of a major trunk as the latter can be
compensated for by meningeal arterial anastomoses. Variations in the clinical
picture are also produced by the variability of the distribution of the arteries.
As a result of the importance of the collateral circulation, obstruction of either
the vertebral or the internal carotid artery may intensify symptoms due to
obstruction of the other (Hutchinson and Yates, 1956).

The Internal Carotid Artery

Angiography [FIG. 56] has taught us much about the symptoms of occlusion of the internal carotid artery. There may be no symptoms. At the other extreme the hemiplegia may be complete almost at its onset—the 'completed stroke'. Progressive obliteration of the lumen by atheroma often causes recurrent transitory disturbances due to localized cerebral ischaemia, e.g. epilepsy, aphasia, confusion, or contralateral paraesthesiae or weakness, 'stuttering hemiplegia' terminating in a persistent hemiplegia. There may also be transitory amblyopia in the ipsilateral eye. Transient ischaemic attacks may occur repeatedly within the territory of the internal carotid artery without a stroke resulting. Finally, a stroke may develop slowly over hours or a day or two—the 'stroke-in-evolution'. Unilateral frontal headache may occur with any of these. The symptoms of complete occlusion depend upon the adequacy of the collateral circulation through the circulus arteriosus cerebri and external carotid artery, and may include crossed homonymous hemianopia, temporal hemianopia in the opposite visual field, hemiplegia, and loss of spatial and discriminative sensibility on the opposite side of the body, and, when the lesion is on the left side, aphasia, both receptive and expressive. Symptoms of severe damage to the hemisphere suggest that thrombosis has extended into the middle cerebral artery. The internal carotid pulse may be diminished or lost, and when stenosis is present rather than total occlusion there may be an audible bruit over the vessel. Ophthalmodynamometry and elec-

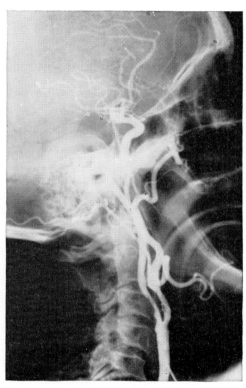

FIG. 57. Left carotid arteriogram demonstrating stenosis at the origin of the internal carotid artery. (From Walton, J. N. (1966) *Essentials of Neurology*, 2nd ed. By kind permission of Pitman Medical Publishing Co. Ltd., London.)

troencephalography may give useful information, and the angiogram is characteristic. Recurrent ischaemic attacks (as already described) of carotid insufficiency are often found to be due to stenosis of the affected artery close to its origin [FIG. 57].

The Anterior Cerebral Artery

This long vessel may undergo occlusion at a number of different points with a corresponding variety of symptoms. The following are the most important of these:

Obstruction at its origin, proximal to Heubner's Artery. This causes hemiplegia on the opposite side together with sensory loss of the cortical type in the paralysed lower limb. When the lesion is on the left side there is in addition some mental deterioration, with expressive aphasia, and apraxia on the left, non-paralysed side. This last symptom is due to interruption in the corpus callosum of fibres running from the left supramarginal gyrus to the right precentral gyrus.

Obstruction of Heubner's Artery. Since this artery supplies part of the frontal lobe, together with the anterior limb of the internal capsule, its obstruction leads to paralysis of the face, tongue, and upper limb on the opposite side, movements at the proximal joints of the limb being more affected than those at the distal joints. In addition, when the lesion is on the left side there is some mental deterioration and expressive aphasia.

Obstruction distal to Heubner's Branch. This leads to hemiplegia on the opposite side, the weakness being most marked in the lower limb. In addition, there is often forced grasping and groping in the affected upper limb.

Obstruction of the Paracentral Artery. This is the branch of the anterior cerebral artery which supplies the paracentral lobule containing the cortical centres for movements of the lower limb. The result of this lesion is a crural spastic monoplegia on the opposite side, with or without sensory loss of the cortical type in the affected lower limb. Angiography may demonstrate obstruction of the anterior cerebral artery.

Obstruction of both Anterior Cerebral Arteries. This syndrome which is a complication of aneurysms on the anterior communicating artery, and which not infrequently follows operation upon aneurysms in this situation, is characterized by profound dementia and apathy with variable long-tract signs. Bilateral grasp reflexes may be present and in the most severe cases the clinical picture resembles that of 'akinetic mutism'.

The Middle Cerebral Artery

Obstruction of the middle cerebral artery at its origin causes hemiplegia with sensory loss on the opposite side. The weakness is most marked in the face, tongue, and upper limb. When the lesion is on the left side there is also expressive aphasia and an impairment of the comprehension of spoken and written speech. Obstruction of the frontal branch which is distributed to the inferior frontal gyrus causes severe expressive aphasia with little or no weakness, except possibly of the face and tongue on the opposite side. Obstruction of the middle cerebral artery distal to this branch causes hemiplegia of the opposite side, the weakness being most marked in the upper limb, but speech disturbances are slight or absent. Obstruction of the parietal and temporal branches, when the lesion is on the left side, causes marked aphasia of the central type, with disturbance of comprehension of heard and written speech, and sometimes jargon aphasia. In addition, there may be a crossed homonymous defect of the visual fields (Lascelles and Burrows, 1965). [Angiogram, FIG. 58.]

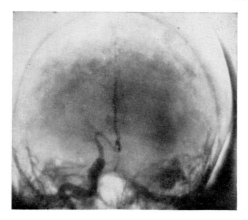

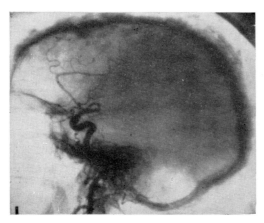

FIG. 58. Angiograms showing obstruction of middle cerebral artery owing to thrombosis in a patient with Paget's osteitis. (Kindly lent by Dr. James Bull.)

The Posterior Cerebral Artery

This artery supplies the visual cortex of the occipital lobe. Its occlusion, therefore, causes crossed homonymous hemianopia. The macular region of the blind fields usually escapes owing to overlapping of the posterior and middle cerebral areas of supply at the occipital pole. If the obstruction is proximal to the supply to the thalamus the thalamic syndrome will be present. Ischaemia of the left occipital lobe causes visual agnosia.

The Basilar Artery

Complete obstruction of the main trunk of the basilar artery is usually rapidly fatal. It leads to impairment of consciousness, small fixed pupils, pseudobulbar palsy, and quadriplegia, but sensation may escape (Kubik and Adams, 1946; Biemond, 1951). Incomplete obstruction of the vertebrobasilar arterial system, however, is much commoner and may lead to a variety of transitory or permanent disorders of brain-stem function, including deafness, vertigo, drop-attacks, ophthalmoplegia, ataxia, nystagmus, and bilateral dysaesthesiae over the body and bilateral corticospinal tract signs (vertebrobasilar insufficiency). Symonds and Mackenzie (1957) suggest that bilateral loss of vision from cerebral infarction is due to embolism or thrombus in the basilar or a vertebral artery. Migraine-like attacks or visual hallucinations may occur. Unilateral obstruction of the paramedian branches of the basilar causes crossed hemiplegia of the Millard-Gubler or Foville type [see p. 25]. If the region deprived of its blood supply extends backwards to involve the lemniscus there is loss of postural sensibility on the paralysed side. Obstruction of one of the lateral branches of the basilar supplying the lateral region of the pons also leads to crossed hemiplegia of the Millard-Gubler or Foville type, with the addition of analgesia and thermo-anaesthesia on the opposite side, but without impairment of postural sensibility. Williams and Wilson (1962) have recently reviewed the syndromes of basilar insufficiency.

The Superior Cerebellar Artery

Obstruction of the superior cerebellar artery causes unilateral symptoms of cerebellar deficiency on the side of the lesion, together with choreiform involuntary movements on the affected side. These are most conspicuous in the upper limb. There are also analgesia and thermo-anaesthesia on the opposite side of the body, since the superior cerebellar artery supplies a small lateral area of the pons containing the trigeminothalamic and spinothalamic tracts.

The Vertebral Artery

The vertebral artery supplies the lateral region of the medulla by the posterior inferior cerebellar artery. Its paramedian branches supply the corticospinal tract, the lemniscus, and the nucleus and emerging fibres of the hypoglossal nerve. The same region of the medulla is supplied at its lowest level by the anterior spinal artery. Obstruction of the paramedian branches of either of these vessels on one side causes crossed hemiplegia with loss of postural sensibility, and wasting and paralysis of the tongue on the side of the lesion.

A new syndrome of the vertebral artery has recently been described—the 'subclavian steal' syndrome (Mannock, Suter, and Hume, 1961) or 'brachio-basilar insufficiency' (North et al., 1962). Occlusion of the first part of the sub-clavian artery before the origin of the vertebral has the effect that exercise of the pulseless arm draws blood *down* the ipsilateral vertebral artery and may cause symptoms of basilar insufficiency, e.g. vertigo, transient blindness, or syncope; or even in one case olfactory hallucinations (Cameron and Wright, 1964).

It has also been suggested that some cases of acute and intense vertigo with vomiting, in which slow resolution of symptoms occurs over a period of several days or weeks and in which deafness may or may not be present, are due to occlusion of the internal auditory artery.

The Lateral Medullary Syndrome

The lateral medullary syndrome of Wallenberg has usually been attributed to obstruction of the posterior inferior cerebellar artery. It is probably more often due to thrombosis of one vertebral artery. In either case there is a characteristic clinical picture which results from infarction of a wedge-shaped area of the lateral aspect of the medulla and the inferior surface of the cerebellum. The onset of thrombosis is associated with severe vertigo, and hiccup and vomiting may occur. There is often dysphagia and, in some cases, pain or paraesthesiae, such as a sensation of hot water running over the face, may be referred to the trigeminal area on the affected side. There is some degree of cerebellar deficiency, with nystagmus, hypotonia, and inco-ordination on the side of the lesion. Ipsilateral paralysis of the soft palate, pharynx, and vocal cord results from involvement of the nucleus ambiguus. Horner's syndrome—myosis, enophthalmos, and ptosis—is present on the affected side. Dissociated sensory loss occurs, though its distribution is somewhat variable. Usually analgesia and thermo-anaesthesia are present on the face on the same side as the lesion and on the trunk and limbs on the opposite side. This is due to involvement of the spinal tract and nucleus of the trigeminal nerve and of the spinothalamic tract respectively. The sensory loss on the face may be confined to the first, or to the first and second, divisions of the nerve, since these regions are represented in the lowest part of the spinal nucleus, which may alone be supplied by the posterior inferior cerebellar artery. Persistent neuralgic pain in the face, on the side of the lesion, and sometimes in the limbs and trunk on the opposite side, is not uncommonly a troublesome sequel of this vascular lesion.

Accessory Investigations

The cerebrospinal fluid is usually normal except after an acute infarction, when the protein may be raised up to 100–200 mg. per 100 ml. for two or three weeks, and the fluid may be xanthochromic at first. There may also be a pleocytosis including a moderate excess of polymorphonuclear cells. Electro-encephalography may yield evidence of focal or diffuse lesions. Williams and Wilson (1962) and Phillips (1964) have drawn attention to the frequency of temporal lobe abnormalities in the EEG in basilar insufficiency. Angiography may be helpful. Carotid angiography is usually free from risk: the dangers of vertebral angiography by direct puncture when the vessel is atheromatous are somewhat greater. There are, however, other methods of performing vertebral angiography, and aortography will show the whole course of the carotid and vertebral arteries below the skull.

DIAGNOSIS

Cerebral atheroma commonly presents in one of four ways, (1) as a focal cerebral lesion of sudden onset, (2) as a focal cerebral lesion of insidious onset, (3) with remittent and recurrent symptoms, and (4) with diffuse and progressive symptoms.

1. *A focal cerebral lesion of sudden onset*, leading, for example, to hemiplegia, may be due to atheromatous occlusion of a large artery. This may be simulated by cerebral haemorrhage due to hypertension, or from a ruptured aneurysm or angioma invading the substance of a cerebral hemisphere. Coma is more likely to be present, and, if present, deeper in cerebral haemorrhage than in cerebral infarction, unless the internal carotid artery is occluded. Hypertension on the whole favours haemorrhage. The cerebrospinal fluid is a valuable guide

since it is likely to contain some red cells, as well as a raised protein, immediately after a cerebral haemorrhage, while if the haemorrhage has also reached the subarachnoid space the blood will be visible to the naked eye in the fluid. Cerebral embolism, which may also produce a focal cerebral lesion suddenly, is uncommon without a demonstrable source (usually in the heart) for the embolus. When there is doubt whether a focal cerebral lesion is ischaemic or haemorrhagic the question can usually be settled by angiography. Achar, Coe, and Marshall (1966) have shown that sonoencephalography is likely to show a shift of midline structures in haemorrhage, but rarely in non-embolic infarction.

An intracranial tumour rarely causes a sudden focal lesion and when it occurs is probably usually due to a vascular disturbance, e.g. haemorrhage, associated with the neoplasm. Transient hemiplegia of sudden onset may occur in migraine, when the diagnosis rests upon its association with the familiar symptoms of migraine and the rapid recovery without residual symptoms or signs. General paresis is an occasional cause of sudden hemiplegia, but the usual physical and serological signs of the disease will be present. Very rarely a single lesion will develop in multiple sclerosis sufficiently suddenly to suggest a vascular lesion. Dissecting aneurysm of the aorta is a cause of sudden cerebral ischaemia. The lesions may be diffuse and will be accompanied by chest pain, and, usually, hypotension.

When it has been established that a lesion is ischaemic, and is associated with local vascular disease, it is usually easy to establish the cause. The diagnosis of atheroma will rest upon the age of the patient, the presence of atheroma elsewhere in the body, particularly the retinal arteries, the absence of any other cause of vascular disease, and in some cases the presence of another disorder known to predispose to atheroma, e.g. diabetes or myxoedema. A syphilitic endarteritis will be associated with the characteristic changes in the cerebrospinal fluid and the serological abnormalities in that and in the blood. There will also be the physical signs of neurosyphilis. Tuberculous endarteritis is the sequel of tuberculous meningitis. The rarer causes of arterial disease, such as thrombo-angiitis obliterans, polyarteritis nodosa, and giant cell (temporal) arteritis can be diagnosed only through their systemic manifestations.

2. *Focal cerebral lesions of insidious onset.* Ischaemic brain disease, especially atheroma of one internal carotid artery, may cause a progressive focal lesion of gradual onset which it may be difficult to distinguish from a neoplasm. Conversely a glioma in an elderly atheromatous subject sometimes progresses so rapidly, and with so little evidence of increased intracranial pressure, that it closely simulates a cerebral vascular lesion. A third condition which may enter into the diagnosis is a chronic subdural haematoma. In such cases the diagnosis can often be made only with the help of accessory methods of investigation, such as electroencephalography, angiography, and pneumoencephalography.

3. *Lesions producing remittent and recurrent symptoms.* Cerebral atheroma may lead to recurrent episodes of disturbance of cerebral function within the territory of a single artery, or successive lesions involving different parts of the brain. These syndromes are unlikely to be confused with any other condition, but occasionally sensory Jacksonian epilepsy due to a glioma may simulate the

former, while multiple metastatic neoplasms may produce symptoms resembling those of multiple vascular lesions. Recurrent epileptic attacks may be the sole manifestation of cerebral atheroma, and other causes of epilepsy of late onset then have to be excluded. The rare 'pulseless disease' (Takayasu's disease) may cause intermittent cerebral ischaemia. This is an inflammatory arteritis of the aortic arch, occurring usually in young women and giving rise to progressive occlusion of those arteries which arise from the aortic arch.

4. *Lesions producing diffuse and progressive symptoms.* The failure of the intellectual powers and impairment of memory, characteristic of diffuse atheromatosis of the smaller cerebral vessels, may simulate dementia due to any other cause [see p. 989]. General paresis is distinguished by the appropriate serological and other tests. In the absence of symptoms of increased intracranial pressure it may be difficult to diagnose an intracranial tumour as the cause of dementia of insidious onset. Pneumoencephalography is often helpful in such cases and in establishing the variety of presensile dementia present. Atherosclerotic Parkinsonism needs to be distinguished from paralysis agitans [see p. 529] and some of the rarer degenerative cerebral diseases of the second half of life may also simulate cerebral atherosclerosis.

PROGNOSIS

The prognosis of cerebral ischaemia due to atheroma depends upon a number of factors, the chief among which are the age of the patient, the adequacy of the collateral circulation, the extent and degree of the atheromatous degeneration within the brain, the condition of the circulation as a whole, and the presence or absence of other metabolic disturbances, such as diabetes, renal disease, &c.

It may be difficult to assess the prognosis of a focal ischaemic lesion during the first two or three days after the onset. When the lesion is within the territory of the internal carotid artery the greater the extent of the area of cerebral damage the worse the outlook. Unconsciousness, and the association of sensory loss and hemiplegia are bad prognostic signs. A small focal lesion in any part of the brain, however, is a less serious affair than evidence of narrowing of one of the main vessels. An elderly patient may live for years after a small focal lesion, even hemiplegia, with no recurrence, but this is exceptional. Adams and Merrett (1961) have reviewed the literature on the prognosis of cerebrovascular disease and themselves studied a series of 736 hemiplegics. Their figures show that the expectation of life after a stroke is greatly shortened, being less than half the normal for people of the same age. They divided their patients into those who recovered in the sense of either becoming fully independent or were able to walk but handicapped by a useless arm, and those who failed to improve appreciably after three months of intensive treatment. They found that a patient's chance of being able to get about and look after himself was little better than that of becoming a relatively helpless invalid. Age, however, did not in itself preclude a good recovery nor did a lesion of the dominant hemisphere. Adams and Hurwitz (1963) have made a useful analysis of the associated defects of cerebral function which were held to be responsible for the failure to respond to treatment. These include defects of comprehension and various forms of apraxia and agnosia.

The clinical picture of diffuse cerebral ischaemia is insidiously progressive with or without focal exacerbations over a period of several years. In the terminal stage the patient is bedridden, with a variable degree of dementia, with or without hemiplegia, pseudobulbar palsy, arteriosclerotic Parkinsonism, or similar physical concomitants. Death occurs either in coma from cerebral infarction, from simple inanition, or from some intercurrent disease.

TREATMENT

When the patient is unconscious, or semiconscious, as the result of an ischaemic stroke he must be treated accordingly [see p. 979]. If it is thought that oedema of the infarcted hemisphere is an important factor there may be a good response to treatment with steroids [see p. 263]. Hemiplegia will require appropriate physiotherapy.

The use of anticoagulants in the treatment of patients who are suffering from cerebral ischaemia secondary to atheroma has recently been reviewed by Carter (1964) and Marshall (1968) in the light of the literature and their own extensive experience. They are agreed that anticoagulants are of no value in the treatment of the completed stroke, but that they may be of value in the treatment of the stroke-in-evolution. There is no doubt about their value in the treatment of transient ischaemic attacks in those patients who do not have a stenotic lesion suitable for surgical treatment. The main danger from anticoagulants lies in mistaking a small cerebral haemorrhage for an infarction. Lumbar puncture should therefore be carried out in every case to make sure there are no red cells in the cerebrospinal fluid, and in doubtful cases, angiography may be necessary. Severe hypertension is a contra-indication to the use of anticoagulants and normally they should not be given to a patient whose blood pressure is higher than 200 systolic and 110 diastolic. The following regime is suitable where an immediate effect is desired, e.g. in the treatment of a patient with a stroke-in-evolution, or when transient ischaemic attacks threaten to develop into a stroke. 125 mg. of heparin should be given intravenously and thereafter 6-hourly for 48 hours. It can if necessary be given intramuscularly but intramuscular injections are painful and less satisfactory. Oral anticoagulant therapy is begun at the same time, 200 mg. of phenindione (*Dindevan*) are given on the first day and 100 mg. on the second, the dosage thereafter being determined by the prothrombin time. There are various methods of estimating this. Marshall says that for anticoagulant therapy to be effective the prothrombin time as measured by the Quick one-stage test must be prolonged to between $2\frac{1}{2}$ and 3 times the normal control or Thrombotest activity reduced to between 10 and 5 per cent. Warfarin appears to be less toxic than phenindione.

The indications for the use of hypotensive drugs are also debatable. If a patient with cerebral ischaemia has hypertension, he will presumably be worse off as the result of lowering his blood pressure unless there is some compensatory improvement in his cerebral blood flow. Where there is spasm, or increased tone, of the cerebral arteries secondary to hypertension, lowering the blood pressure may by reducing this actually improve the blood flow. On the other hand, when the vessels are inelastic as the result of atheroma and medial degeneration, lowering the blood pressure may have the reverse effect. If hypotensive drugs are used in the treatment of patients with symptoms of cerebral ischaemia, therefore, they should be used with caution and withdrawn at once if there is evidence that their use increases the cerebral ischaemia.

Surgical reconstruction of a narrowed common or internal carotid artery may be of value in selected cases (Edwards, Gordon, and Robb, 1960; Edwards and Gordon, 1962). It is essential that the lesion should be diagnosed before irreversible damage is done and that the distal branches of the affected vessel shall not themselves be too much narrowed by atheroma to be unable to transmit the increased blood flow which will result from the operation. Crawford and DeBakey (1963) have surveyed the results of surgery in a large series of reconstructive operations on the external, internal and common carotid, innominate, subclavian and vertebral arteries. Over a thousand lesions were treated and the circulation was restored in 93 per cent. The early and late results were classified in relation to the clinical picture. The operation was most successful when performed prophylactically or for minor or transient ischaemic manifestations, and less successful in the treatment of the stroke-in-evolution and the completed stroke. Out of 536 early results the authors claim that the patient was improved in 123, and became asymptomatic in 284 cases; in 406 late results corresponding figures were 75 improved and 260 asymptomatic.

Little can be done for the patient with diffuse cerebral ischaemia. Since, however, impairment of the blood supply to the brain must reduce its nutrients, including vitamins, high vitamin administration is valuable especially in states of confusion. The treatment of hemiplegia includes the prevention as far as possible of muscular contractures and the re-education of movement. A toe-raising spring may be helpful for the foot. The patient who does not regain the use of his hand will need training in the use of gadgets which make domestic life simpler. In re-training, special attention should be paid to the possible existence of apraxia, agnosia, or some other disorder of function which may be impeding recovery.

There is little evidence to indicate that cerebral vasodilator drugs are of value but cyclandelate, 200 mg. four times daily, has been found to improve cerebral blood flow in some cases and is worthy of a trial. In the presence of hypercholesterolaemia clofibrate, 500 mg. three times a day, may be of theoretical value but rarely gives clinical improvement.

(*References, see page* 305)

CEREBRAL EMBOLISM

AETIOLOGY AND PATHOLOGY

Embolism of a cerebral artery is a complication of a large variety of disorders which possess in common the opportunity for blood clot, or, less frequently, other material, to enter the circulation in such a way that it can reach the brain. Retracing the circulation backwards from the brain we find that the nearest sources of a thrombus are the internal carotid, vertebral and common carotid arteries. In rare cases of thrombosis of the right subclavian artery due to pressure by a cervical rib, the thrombus has extended into the right common carotid and a detached portion has been carried to the brain (Symonds). A clot may come also from an aneurysm of the innominate artery or of the aorta or from mural thrombosis on an atheromatous ulcer in this vessel. A vegetation may become detached from the aortic valves in progressive endocarditis. The left ventricle may be the source of an embolus, following coronary thrombosis, when a clot forms on the endocardium over the infarcted area or when aneurysm of the ventricle results. Vegetations may be detached from the mitral valve in progressive endocarditis, or a clot may form in the left atrium in mitral stenosis of rheumatic origin. This is most likely to occur in auricular fibrillation, and in such cases detachment of the clot may follow the restoration of the normal cardiac rhythm by means of quinidine. It may also occur in auricular flutter, and after valvulotomy.

The source of the thrombus may be in the lung, when thrombosis of a pulmonary vein occurs. Infected emboli from the lungs are the cause of cerebral abscess complicating pulmonary infection, and tumour cells may pass in the same way from the lung to the brain. The lung capillaries constitute a filter which protects the general circulation from emboli of any size derived from the systemic veins. Fat globules, however, may pass through the pulmonary circulation and so reach the brain after fracture of one of the long bones. A patent interatrial septum short-circuits the pulmonary capillary filter and provides a route by which emboli from the systemic veins can in very exceptional circumstances reach the brain—*paradoxical embolism.*

The arteries of the left side of the brain are the site of embolism more frequently than those of the right, and the left middle cerebral is the vessel most often affected. The point at which the embolus lodges depends upon its size. A large clot may be arrested in the internal carotid. A small one may pass to a cortical branch of one of the main arteries. Following the lodgement of an embolus thrombosis usually occurs in the vessel and may spread distally, or less frequently proximally, and infarction occurs in the area of brain deprived of its blood supply [see p. 293]. When the embolus is infected, meningitis or cerebral abscess may subsequently develop, or, when the infection is of low virulence, embolism may be followed by infective softening of the vessel wall and aneurysm formation. Such infective aneurysms may rupture into the subarachnoid space or into the brain [see p. 313].

SYMPTOMS

The onset of the symptoms of cerebral embolism with blood clot is extremely sudden, the lodgement of the embolus occurring more rapidly than either cerebral haemorrhage or thrombosis. Loss of consciousness is not very common, but the patient is usually somewhat dazed. A convulsion may occur at the onset, and there is sometimes headache. The nature of the focal symptoms depends upon the vessel in which the embolus becomes impacted [see p. 294]. After the onset of embolism there may be a gradual increase in the severity of the symptoms due to spasm of the vessel or the development of oedema or the extension of thrombosis proximally along the vessel. On the other hand, the symptoms may diminish in severity owing to the embolus becoming dislodged and passing to a more peripheral part of the vessel.

Fat Embolism. Fat embolism causes symptoms after a latent interval lasting from hours to days following the injury. Restlessness, tachycardia, precordial pain, and dyspnoea are the symptoms of fat embolism of the lungs, and when the fat reaches the brain insomnia, disorientation, and delirium occur, passing into stupor or coma, with signs of cortical irritation or paralysis. The patient is usually pyrexial, petechial haemorrhages may be present, especially on the chest and neck, and fat may be found in the urine.

DIAGNOSIS

See page 299.

PROGNOSIS

The immediate mortality of cerebral embolism is 7–10 per cent. There is always the risk that embolism of other organs may occur and the prognosis of the condition causing the embolism must be taken into consideration. As shock passes off and the oedema of the infarcted area of the brain diminishes, the extent and severity of the symptoms grow less, and the patient is finally left with such disabilities as result from destruction of the region of the brain supplied by the obstructed artery. Epilepsy is a not uncommon sequel.

TREATMENT

Hypotension, if present, should be treated. Wright and McDevitt (1954) stress the prophylactic value of anticoagulants for patients with heart disease who are liable to embolism, otherwise treatment of the cerebral lesion is the same as that of cerebral infarction from any cause. Carter (1957) found anticoagulants of value [see p. 302] but they should not be used when the embolus is due to infective endocarditis. The condition responsible for the embolism must also be dealt with appropriately.

Complete rest for several weeks is essential in order to diminish the risk of further emboli occurring. If embolism occurs in a patient receiving quinidine for auricular fibrillation, this drug must at once be suspended. The treatment of fat embolism is at present symptomatic. Carbon dioxide inhalation has been recommended.

REFERENCES

(Cerebral atheromatosis, Syndromes of the cerebral arteries, Cerebral embolism.)

ACHAR, V. S., COE, R. P. K., and MARSHALL, J. (1966) Echoencephalography in the differential diagnosis of cerebral haemorrhage and infarction, *Lancet*, i, 161.

ADAMS, G. F., and HURWITZ, L. J. (1963) Mental barriers to recovery from strokes, *Lancet*, ii, 533.

ADAMS, G. F., and MERRETT, J. W. (1961) Prognosis and survival in the aftermath of hemiplegia, *Brit. med. J.*, **1**, 309.

ANDERSON, A. G., LOCKHART, R. D., and SOUTER, W. C. (1931) Lateral syndrome of the medulla, *Brain*, **54**, 460.

BAUER, R. B., SHEEHAN, S., and MEYER, J. S. (1961) Arteriographic study of cerebro-vascular disease. II. Cerebral symptoms due to kinking, tortuosity and compression of carotid and vertebral arteries in the neck, *Arch. Neurol. (Chic.)*, **4**, 119.

BIEMOND, A. (1951) Thrombosis of the basilar artery and vascularization of the brain stem, *Brain*, **74**, 300.

BRICE, J. G., DOWSETT, D. J., and LOWE, R. D. (1964) Haemodynamic effects of carotid artery stenosis, *Brit. med. J.*, **2**, 1363.

CAMERON, W. J., and WRIGHT, I. S. (1964) Subclavian steal syndrome with olfactory hallucinations, *Ann. intern. Med.*, **61**, 128.

CARTER, A. B. (1957) The immediate treatment of cerebral embolism, *Quart. J. Med.*, **26**, 335.

CARTER, A. B. (1964) *Cerebral Infarction*, Oxford.

CRAWFORD, E. S., and DE BAKEY, M. E. (1963) *Surgical Treatment of Stroke by Arterial Reconstructive Operation in Clinical Neurosurgery*, ed. MOSBERG, W. H., p. 150, London.

CRITCHLEY, M. (1929) Arteriosclerotic Parkinsonism, *Brain*, **52**, 23.

DAVID, N. J., KLINTWORTH, G. K., FRIEDBERG, S. J., and DILLON, M. (1963) Fatal atheromatous cerebral embolism associated with bright plaques in the retinal arterioles, *Neurology (Minneap.)*, **13**, 709.

DAVISON, C., GOODHART, S. P., and SAVITSKY, N. (1935) The syndrome of the superior cerebellar artery and its branches, *Arch. Neurol. Psychiat. (Chicago)*, **33**, 1143.

DENNY-BROWN, D. (1951) The treatment of recurrent cerebrovascular symptoms and the question of 'vasospasm', *Med. Clin. N. Amer.*, **35**, 1457.

DENNY-BROWN, D. (1960) Recurrent cerebro-vascular episodes, *Arch. Neurol. (Chicago)*, **2**, 194.

EDWARDS, C. H., and GORDON, N. S. (1962) Surgical treatment of narrowing of the internal carotid artery, *Brit. med. J.*, **1**, 1289.

EDWARDS, C. H., GORDON, N. S., and ROB, C. (1960) The surgical treatment of internal carotid artery occlusion, *Quart. J. Med.*, **29**, 67.

FISHER, C. M. (1959) Observations of the fundus oculi in transient monocular blindness, *Neurology (Minneap.)*, **9**, 333.

GUNNING, A. G., PICKERING, G. W., ROBB-SMITH, A. H. T., and RUSSELL, R. (1964) Mural thrombosis of the internal carotid artery and subsequent embolism, *Quart. J. Med.*, **33**, 155.

HILL, A. B., MARSHALL, J., and SHAW, D. A. (1960) A controlled clinical trial of long-term anticoagulant therapy in cerebro-vascular disease, *Quart. J. Med.*, **29**, 597.

HUMPHREY, J. G., and NEWTON, T. H. (1960) Internal carotid occlusion in young adults, *Brain*, **83**, 565.

HUTCHINSON, E. C., and YATES, P. O. (1956) The cervical portion of the vertebral artery: A clinico-pathological study, *Brain*, **79**, 319.

KENDELL, R. E., and MARSHALL, J. (1963) Role of hypotension in the genesis of transient focal cerebral ischaemic attacks, *Brit. med. J.*, **2**, 344.

KUBIK, C. S., and ADAMS, R. D. (1946) Occlusion of the basilar artery—a clinical and pathological study, *Brain*, **69**, 73.

LASCELLES, R. G., and BURROWS, E. H. (1965) Occlusion of the middle cerebral artery, *Brain*, **88**, 85.

McBRIEN, D. J., BRADLEY, R. D., and ASHTON, W. (1963) The nature of retinal emboli in stenosis of the internal carotid artery, *Lancet*, i, 697.

MANNOCK, J. A., SUTER, L. G., and HUME, D. M. (1961) The 'subclavian steal' syndrome, *J. Amer. med. Ass.*, **182**, 254.

MARSHALL, J. (1968) *The Management of Cerebrovascular Disease*, 2nd ed., London.

MERRITT, H., and FINLAND, M. (1930) Vascular lesions of the hindbrain (lateral medullary syndrome), *Brain*, **53**, 290.

MILLIKAN, C. H., SIEKERT, R. G., and SHICK, R. N. (1955). Studies in cerebrovascular disease, 111. Use of anticoagulant drugs in treatment of insufficiency or thrombosis within basilar arterial system, *Proc. Mayo Clin.*, **30**, 116. V. Use of anticoagulant drugs in treatment of intermittent insufficiency of internal carotid system, *Proc. Mayo Clin.*, **30**, 578.

NORTH, R. R., FIELDS, W. S., DE BAKEY, M. E., and CRAWFORD, E. S. (1962) Brachio-basilar insufficiency syndrome, *Neurology (Minneap.)*, **12**, 810.

PHILLIPS, B. M. (1964) Temporal lobe changes associated with the syndromes of basilar-vertebral insufficiency: an electroencephalographic study, *Brit. med. J.*, **2**, 1104.

ROWLANDS, R. A., and WAKELEY, C. P. G. (1941) Fat embolism, *Lancet*, i, 502.

RUSSELL, R. W. R. (1961) Observations on the retinal blood vessels in monocular blindness, *Lancet*, ii, 1422.

RUSSELL, R. W. R. (1963) Atheromatous retinal embolism, *Lancet*, ii, 1354.

STOPFORD, J. S. B. (1930) *Sensation and the Sensory Pathway*, London.

SYMONDS, C., and MACKENZIE, I. (1957) Bilateral loss of vision from cerebral infarction, *Brain*, 80, 415.

TOOLE, J. F., and TUCKER, S. H. (1960) Influence of head position upon cerebral circulation, *Arch. Neurol. (Chicago)*, 2, 616.

WILLIAMS, D., and WILSON, T. G. (1962) The diagnosis of the major and minor syndromes of basilar insufficiency, *Brain*, 85, 741.

WORSTER-DROUGHT, C., and ALLEN, I. M. (1929) Thrombosis of the superior cerebellar artery, including report of case with unusual cerebrospinal fluid reactions, *Lancet*, ii, 1137.

WRIGHT, I. S., and McDEVITT, E. (1954) Cerebral vascular diseases, *Ann. intern. Med.*, 41, 682.

YATES, P. O., and HUTCHINSON, E. C. (1961) Cerebral infarction: the role of stenosis of the extracranial vessels, *Spec. Rep. Ser. med. Res. Coun. (Lond.)*, No. 300, H.M.S.O.

Discussion on fat embolism and the brain, *Proc. roy. Soc. Med.* (1941) 34, 639.

HYPERTENSIVE ENCEPHALOPATHY

Definition. An acute and transitory disturbance of cerebral function which occurs in association with high blood pressure, in acute and chronic glomerulonephritis, malignant hypertension, and eclampsia. The cardinal symptoms are convulsions and focal disturbances, such as amaurosis, aphasia, and hemiplegia.

AETIOLOGY AND PATHOLOGY

The term hypertensive encephalopathy was first used by Oppenheimer and Fishberg (1928) to describe a form of cerebral disturbance occurring in disorders which differ in their pathology but possess a common tendency to cause arterial hypertension. The occurrence of such cerebral episodes in acute and chronic glomerulonephritis and in eclampsia at first suggested that they were the outcome of impaired renal function and they were therefore considered uraemic in nature. This view has been discarded because not only are symptoms of this kind usually absent when renal function is grossly impaired as a result of surgical lesions but they may be conspicuous in hypertensive states in which renal function, as judged by the blood chemistry, is normal. The constant presence of arterial hypertension, however, and especially the fact that the onset of the encephalopathy is not uncommonly preceded by a rapid rise in the blood pressure suggests that the disturbance of function is closely related to the hypertension. Byrom (1954) has shown that it is the result of constriction of the cerebral arterioles. The commonest pathological finding is oedema of the brain, but this is not always present and since oedema of the brain when due to other causes, such as intracranial tumour, does not necessarily lead to symptoms like those of hypertensive encephalopathy, it seems likely that it is itself a by-product of the pathological process and not the cause of the symptoms. Lead encephalopathy in general resembles hypertensive encephalopathy and may be associated with hypertension, and there is experimental evidence that lead produces vasoconstriction by acting directly upon the smooth muscles of the vessels.

The age incidence of hypertensive encephalopathy is that of the causal disorders. Acute glomerulonephritis is commonest in childhood, adolescence, and early adult life; chronic glomerulonephritis in the second and third decade; eclampsia during the early part of the child-bearing period; and malignant hypertension in the thirties and forties, though it may occur in childhood or late middle age.

SYMPTOMS

The onset of symptoms is usually subacute, the patient complaining of headaches of increasing severity, which are often associated with vomiting of a cerebral type. Epileptiform convulsions are common and may be followed either by mental confusion or coma. Impairment of vision, or even complete blindness, may occur. This is cortical in origin, for the retina may be normal and during recovery of vision one homonymous pair of visual half-fields may recover before the other. Other focal cerebral disturbances include aphasia and hemiparesis.

Arterial hypertension is present in every case, but the blood pressure may be not greatly raised in acute nephritis and eclampsia. A rise in an already high blood pressure frequently heralds the encephalopathy. The retinae may be normal or there may be bilateral papilloedema with or without the exudative changes of hypertensive retinopathy, depending upon the causal condition. Evans (1933) drew attention to the occurrence of puffiness of the face, the onset and disappearance of which often coincides with the onset and cessation of the encephalopathic symptoms. Cervical rigidity, tachycardia, and fever sometimes occur. Jellinek et al. (1964) noted that transient blindness of cortical type was common and pointed out that during this stage the EEG often showed diffuse slow activity, loss or impairment of the alpha rhythm and absence of the normal 'following' response to photic stimulation. Both renal function and the composition of the urine may be normal except when the encephalopathy complicates acute or chronic renal damage. The pressure of the cerebrospinal fluid is usually increased and its composition is generally normal.

DIAGNOSIS

Hypertensive encephalopathy must be distinguished from uraemia, cerebral vascular lesions such as haemorrhage and thrombosis, and intracranial tumour. In uraemia convulsive phenomena consist usually of myoclonic twitches rather than of epileptiform attacks and amaurosis is rare. Cerebral vascular lesions do not produce such a diffuse picture of cerebral disturbance and are never as transient as the symptoms of encephalopathy. The diagnosis from intracranial tumour may be very difficult in the presence of papilloedema and a raised pressure of cerebrospinal fluid, since cerebral tumour may occur in a patient who also has hypertension. In doubtful cases ventriculography should be carried out. The examination of the urine and blood pressure will enable convulsions due to encephalopathy complicating acute nephritis in childhood to be distinguished from epilepsy, and in doubtful cases examination of the cerebrospinal fluid will exclude meningitis.

PROGNOSIS

Alarming though the symptoms are, the outlook in hypertensive encephalopathy is on the whole good as to recovery from the cerebral disturbance, though the ultimate outlook depends upon the underlying cause. Most patients recover from encephalopathy complicating acute nephritis and from eclampsia. Even in malignant hypertension the patient may recover from the encephalopathy. Severe and frequent convulsions are a bad sign. Recovery from the amaurosis, aphasia, and other focal symptoms is usually complete in a few days.

TREATMENT

Hypotensive drugs may bring an attack of encephalopathy to an end, and usually produce dramatic relief within hours. Impairment of consciousness is due probably to diffuse cerebral arteriolar spasm with resultant cerebral ischaemia but also to cerebral oedema. Thus reduction of oedema with appropriate drugs (e.g. steroids or powerful diuretics such as frusemide, see p. 263) may be helpful. If the convulsions prove intractable barbiturates or intramuscular paraldehyde are indicated. The treatment appropriate to the causal condition will also be required.

REFERENCES

BYROM, F. B. (1954) The pathogenesis of hypertensive encephalopathy, *Lancet*, i, 201.
ELLIS, A. (1938) Malignant hypertension, *Lancet*, i, 977.
EVANS, H. (1933) Hypertensive encephalopathy in nephritis, *Lancet*, ii, 583.
JELLINEK, E. H., PAINTER, M., PRINEAS, J., and ROSS RUSSELL, R. (1964) Hypertensive encephalopathy with cortical disorders of vision, *Quart. J. Med.*, **33**, 239.
OPPENHEIMER, B. S., and FISHBERG, A. M. (1928) Hypertensive encephalopathy, *Arch. intern. Med.*, **41**, 264.
VOLHARD, F. (1931) In von Bergmann and Staehelin's *Handbuch der inneren Medizin*, vol. vi, p. 561, Berlin.

INTRACRANIAL ANEURYSM

Definition. A localized dilatation of an intracranial artery which may cause symptoms either through localized pressure upon neighbouring structures, especially cranial nerves, or by sudden rupture leading to subarachnoid haemorrhage.

ANEURYSM OF CONGENITAL ORIGIN

'BERRY' OR SO-CALLED 'CONGENITAL' ANEURYSMS

PATHOLOGY

A congenital abnormality is an important factor in the aetiology of intracranial aneurysm. 'Congenital' aneurysms appear to arise, as Turnbull (1914–15) and Forbus (1930) have shown, at a point where there is a deficiency in the media at the point of junction of two of the components of the circulus arteriosus cerebri or at a bifurcation of one of the cerebral arteries. It is now apparent, however, that a medial defect alone is not sufficient to cause aneurysmal formation and that there must be an acquired lesion which breaches the internal elastic lamina at the same point, as the latter alone will withstand more than twice the highest recorded arterial blood pressure. This acquired lesion is atheroma which explains why, despite the ubiquity of congenital medial defects in cerebral arteries, aneurysms usually appear and produce their clinical effects in middle life (Carmichael, 1950). These aneurysms may be single or multiple, as many as eight having been present in the same individual. They are most

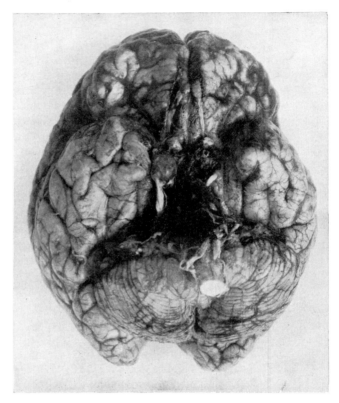

FIG. 59. Congenital aneurysm of right posterior communicating
artery compressing the third nerve

frequently encountered on the intracranial course of the internal carotid artery, on the middle cerebral artery, and at the junction of the anterior communicating with the anterior cerebral arteries, but may occur on any superficial cerebral artery. Only about 10 per cent. are in the posterior fossa. They range in size from smaller than a pin's head to 30 mm. or more in diameter [FIG. 59]. Microscopically the media is extremely narrow and fibrous, and the elastic and muscular elements are absent. 'Congenital' intracranial aneurysms have occurred in more than one member of the same family. They may be found at any age, but more than half first cause symptoms between the ages of 40 and 55 (Fearnsides, 1916) [FIG. 61], and they occur almost equally in the two sexes with perhaps a slight predominance in females. Sooner or later most aneurysms rupture, and the extravasated blood may pass into the subarachnoid space or into the substance of the brain, even reaching the ventricles. Rupture into the subdural space and even externally to the dura has been observed. Subarachnoid haemorrhage accounts for 7 per cent. of all cases of cerebral vascular disease, and occurs about as often as intracerebral haemorrhage.

The effects of rupture of an aneurysm on the brain have recently been studied by Crompton, who stresses the frequency of cerebral infarction (Crompton, 1964 *a* and *b*) and of damage to the hypothalamus (Crompton, 1963). 'Congenital' aneurysm often occurs in the absence of raised blood pressure, though it is likely that a rise of blood pressure in later life may be responsible, if not for the formation of the aneurysm, at least for its rupture.

Other congenital vascular abnormalities, such as congenital heart disease, aneurysm or defects of the media of abdominal arteries leading to intraperitoneal haemorrhage, coarctation of the aorta, and cutaneous naevi, have occasionally been observed in patients suffering from intracranial aneurysm which may also co-exist with an intracranial angioma. Intracranial aneurysms are also commonly found in patients with renal polycystic disease.

SYMPTOMS

The symptoms of congenital intracranial aneurysm differ according to whether the patient is observed (1) before rupture, (2) immediately after rupture, or (3) after recovery from the immediate effects of rupture, and (4) radiography may show abnormalities [FIG. 60].

Symptoms before Rupture of the Aneurysm

It is often impossible to diagnose an intracranial aneurysm before rupture occurs, since it may be too small to produce symptoms by compressing structures in its neighbourhood. However, if such symptoms occur, it is frequently possible to make a correct diagnosis. Unless the aneurysm is very large, symptoms of increased intracranial pressure do not occur at this stage. Some 25 per cent. of patients suffer from recurrent headaches—about half of these from typical migraine. The diagnosis of aneurysm rests upon evidence of focal pressure fairly sharply localized and only slowly, if at all, progressive. The nature of such focal symptoms depends upon the situation of the aneurysm. Aneurysms placed anteriorly in the circulus arteriosus cerebri may compress the optic nerve, leading to unilateral impairment of vision, which may be fluctuating and cause transitory attacks of blindness in one eye, superficially resembling migraine. In such cases optic atrophy and rarely slight papilloedema may be found in the affected eye and exophthalmos may be present. Hemianopia may result from compression of one optic tract, or the chiasm may be compressed (Jefferson, 1937, 1938). Paralysis of the third, fourth, or sixth cranial nerves may occur with or without exophthalmos and pain, sometimes of sudden onset, or anaesthesia in the cutaneous area supplied by the first division of the trigeminal nerve. This is the characteristic picture which may result from an aneurysm of the internal carotid artery within the cavernous sinus (an infraclinoid aneurysm) and if sudden expansion occurs there is pain behind the eye. Aneurysms situated on the cortical course of the middle cerebral artery occasionally cause monoplegia or hemiplegia either through direct pressure if they are very large or through ischaemia in the distribution of their parent vessel, and this is the only situation in which an aneurysm is likely to cause convulsions. Aneurysm of the posterior part of the circulus arteriosus cerebri, for example the posterior communicating artery, usually causes paralysis of the third nerve and possibly hemianopia due to compression of the optic tract. An isolated third nerve palsy is not infrequently produced by pressure from an enlarging aneurysm of the internal carotid artery above the cavernous sinus (a supraclinoid aneurysm). Aneurysm of the posterior cerebral artery may cause crossed hemianopia, owing to coincident thrombosis of the vessel. Aneurysm of the basilar artery usually causes conspicuous localizing signs early. There is often a crossed hemiplegia with paresis of some of the cranial nerves originating from the pons on one side, and of the limbs on the opposite side. A somewhat similar picture is produced by aneurysm of the vertebral artery which, however, is less common. Aneurysms of the cerebellar arteries rarely give rise to localizing signs.

Symptoms immediately following Rupture

Rupture of an aneurysm may prove rapidly fatal. In most cases, however, the patient survives, either to succumb in a few days or to make a more or less complete recovery, with the risk of death from a subsequent leakage. Effort is rarely a precipitating cause of the rupture. Characteristically the patient experiences a sensation of something snapping in the head, followed immediately by an intense throbbing ache.

The symptoms of rupture are those of subarachnoid haemorrhage [see p. 314].

Symptoms persisting after recovery from Rupture

Recovery from the effects of rupture of an intracranial aneurysm may be remarkably complete, though headache is a common sequel. In about 20 per cent. of cases there are persistent symptoms.

If intra-ocular haemorrhages have been severe, recovery of vision may be incomplete, and defects of the visual fields may persist after haemorrhage in the region of the optic chiasma. There may also be some permanent weakness of cranial nerves which have been compressed. If the haemorrhage has invaded the cerebral hemisphere complete recovery from this lesion is not likely to occur. When the frontal lobe has been damaged there may be permanent mental changes which may even necessitate treatment at a mental hospital. Aphasia, hemiparesis, and hemianopia are also occasional sequels. The effects of subarachnoid haemorrhage sometimes persist [see p.318].

Radiography

See page 317.

DIAGNOSIS

See page 317.

PROGNOSIS

See page 318.

TREATMENT

See page 318.

EMBOLIC INTRACRANIAL ANEURYSM

Embolic or 'mycotic' aneurysms are rare. They are due to the impaction in a cerebral vessel of an embolus, bearing organisms of low virulence. The aneurysm is the result of infective softening of the vessel wall. More virulent organisms usually cause cerebral abscess or meningitis. The embolus usually lodges in a cortical branch of one or other middle cerebral artery, the right and left being involved with equal frequency. Less often the main trunk of the middle cerebral artery or the anterior cerebral artery is affected. Embolic

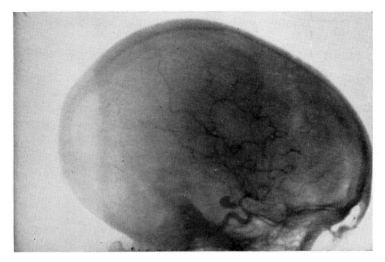

FIG. 60. Aneurysm of posterior communicating artery shown by angiography

aneurysms elsewhere in the intracranial circulation are rare. Subacute bacterial endocarditis is the commonest cause of embolic aneurysm, which may, however, be a complication of other chronic forms of septicaemia and pyaemia, including brucellosis. In most cases the aneurysm subsequently ruptures in the same manner as a congenital aneurysm giving subarachnoid haemorrhage.

The lodgement of the embolus is often the occasion of a 'stroke' and is followed by a hemiplegia or monoplegia. The signs of subacute bacterial endocarditis or of some other pyaemic source for the embolus are usually evident and emboli may occur elsewhere in the body. Treatment of rupture is the same as in subarachnoid haemorrhage due to rupture of a 'berry' aneurysm but in embolic aneurysm the underlying infective condition will also need treatment.

CAROTID CAVERNOUS-SINUS ANEURYSM OR FISTULA

Arteriovenous aneurysm produced by rupture of the internal carotid artery into the cavernous sinus may arise spontaneously or follow head injury with or without fracture of the skull. Hamby (1966) thinks that 'the majority of spontaneous fistulas develop as a result of rupture of pre-existing aneurysms'. However, some cases follow cranial trauma and angiography may fail to demonstrate evidence of any predisposing cause for rupture of the artery. The resulting clinical picture is highly distinctive, consisting of unilateral pulsating exophthalmos, with oedema of the eyelids, conjunctivae, and cornea, and sometimes papilloedema. There is a loud systolic murmur, audible to the patient and on auscultation over the temporal region or even over the whole skull, and suppressible by compression of the ipsilateral carotid artery. There is complete or partial ophthalmoplegia of the affected eye. The other eye may become involved, blood at arterial pressure being carried by the circular sinus to the opposite cavernous sinus. Hamby (1966) discusses the surgical treatment. Common carotid ligation is the method usually employed and, though not without risk it is generally successful. Some fistulae heal spontaneously.

OTHER CAUSES OF INTRACRANIAL ANEURYSM

Other causes of intracranial aneurysm are extremely rare, though examples undoubtedly due to polyarteritis nodosa, to atheroma, and to syphilis have occasionally been described. An atheromatous aneurysm is usually a fusiform dilatation of the internal carotid or basilar artery. The characteristic syphilitic change of the small elastic and muscular arteries, to which group the intracranial vessels belong, is an obliterative endarteritis, a fact which probably explains the rarity of syphilitic intracranial aneurysm. Most of the verified syphilitic aneurysms have been situated upon the basilar artery, which, as Fearnsides suggests, on account of its size is less likely to be obliterated by intimal proliferation and more likely to develop local weakening of its wall than the smaller intracranial vessels. If there is reason to suspect that an intracranial aneurysm may be caused by syphilis, the proper treatment for this condition should be carried out.

(*References, see page* 319)

SUBARACHNOID HAEMORRHAGE

AETIOLOGY

Subarachnoid haemorrhage may occur as the result of any condition in which there is rupture of one or more blood vessels so placed that the extravasated blood can reach the subarachnoid space. The bleeding may be arterial, capillary, or venous, and its site of origin single or multiple. Head injury, including birth injury, may thus cause subarachnoid haemorrhage. Capillary damage leading to haemorrhage may be present in exceptionally acute forms of encephalitis or encephalopathy, and subarachnoid haemorrhage may occur as a symptom of haemorrhagic diseases or during the use of anticoagulants. Rarely it may be the result of an intracranial tumour (angioblastic meningioma, glioma, pituitary adenoma, intracranial metastases (particularly of malignant melanoma, Walton, 1956). It has also been described as a result of an acute hypertensive reaction following the ingestion of cheese in a patient receiving tranylcypromine, one of the group of amine-oxidase inhibitor drugs (Espir and Mitchell, 1963). Subarachnoid haemorrhage from a vein may be encountered in pyaemic states (Alpers and Gaskill, 1944). Intracerebral haemorrhage, due to vascular degeneration associated with high blood pressure, may reach the subarachnoid space either by rupture into the ventricular system or, more rarely, to the surface of the brain, or the haemorrhage which enters the subarachnoid space may also invade the brain from an aneurysm or angioma. The chief causes of intracranial focal subarachnoid haemorrhage are intracranial aneurysm [see p. 309] and angioma [see p. 221], the former being nine or ten times as common as the

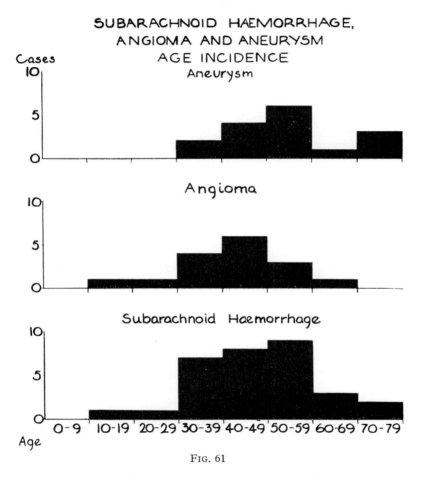

FIG. 61

latter. In a small proportion of cases no cause can be found even at autopsy. Spontaneous spinal subarachnoid haemorrhage—haematorrhachis—usually comes from an angioma of the spinal cord (Henson and Croft, 1956).

Subarachnoid haemorrhage was found in 15 per cent. of 200 patients suffering from cerebral vascular disease: its age incidence, and that of its two principal causes, is shown in FIGURE 61. Females are affected slightly more often than males, and about 50 per cent. of the patients are normotensive.

In addition to blood in the subarachnoid space, secondary haemorrhages may occur in the brain stem, and spasm of the artery on which the aneurysm is situated may lead to oedema or infarction of the part of the brain which it supplies. Infarction may also result from compression, tearing, or distortion of arteries resulting from subarachnoid haematoma formation within sulci (Tomlinson, 1959).

SYMPTOMS

When subarachnoid haemorrhage is due to head injury, acute encephalitis or encephalopathy, or rupture of an intracerebral haemorrhage, it usually constitutes a minor part of the total clinical picture. When it is caused by an aneurysm or an angioma it is usually the most prominent and sometimes the sole obvious disturbance. The following account of its symptomatology will therefore be limited to such cases.

The symptoms of cerebral subarachnoid haemorrhage may be divided into (1) those due to rapidly increasing intracranial pressure with meningeal irritation, (2) focal symptoms, (3) changes in the cerebrospinal fluid, and (4) radiographic evidence.

1. The intensity of the symptoms of increasing intracranial pressure varies according to the rapidity and persistence of the haemorrhage. Loss of consciousness occurs rapidly when the leakage is considerable. Vomiting is not uncommon at the onset; convulsions are exceptional. When coma is deep, the breathing is usually irregular and the pulse slow. The patient may present a picture of profound shock with generalized flaccidity and there may be no cervical rigidity. In less severe cases the patient may not lose consciousness completely, but may pass into a semi-stuporose state, lying in an attitude of general flexion, resenting interference, and confused and irritable when roused. Headache is severe, and the presence of blood in the subarachnoid space produces signs of meningeal irritation, such as cervical rigidity and Kernig's sign. Moderate pyrexia is common at this stage.

Changes are often found in the fundus oculi. Papilloedema is sometimes present, though slight in amount. Unilateral or bilateral retinal haemorrhages occur in some cases and may be accompanied by subhyaloid or vitreous haemorrhages. These have been attributed to the passage of blood from the subarachnoid space of the optic nerves into the eye, but it is more probable that the haemorrhages occur in the eye as the result of acute compression of the central vein of the retina by the blood in the optic sheaths. Fundal changes may be absent when the leaking aneurysm is remote from the optic nerves.

Other signs of subarachnoid haemorrhage include diminution or loss of the tendon reflexes, and of the abdominal reflexes, and extensor plantar responses in the absence of gross muscular weakness. Albuminuria and glycosuria occasionally occur while hyperpyrexia and severe transient arterial hypertension may result from damage to hypothalamic centres.

2. Focal symptoms are due to compression of neighbouring cranial nerves by blood clot or to invasion of the cerebral hemisphere by the haemorrhage or to cerebral infarction. Visual field defect may occur as a result of compression of the optic nerves, chiasma, or tracts. The third, fourth, and sixth cranial nerves are likely to be compressed if an aneurysm is near the cavernous sinus. Haemorrhage from an aneurysm at the junction of the anterior cerebral and anterior communicating arteries is apt to invade the frontal lobe and may cause mental

impairment, hemiparesis, and, if on the left side, expressive aphasia. Leakage from an aneurysm on the cortical course of the middle cerebral may cause epileptiform convulsions, and a monoplegia; and rupture of an aneurysm on the cortical course of the posterior cerebral may cause a crossed homonymous hemianopia as a result of haemorrhage into the substance of the occipital lobe or thrombosis of the artery. Leakage from an aneurysm of the basilar artery may lead to quadriplegia or to one of the various forms of 'crossed paralysis'; and head retraction is likely to be conspicuous when the haemorrhage is derived from an aneurysm in the posterior fossa.

Haemorrhage from an intracranial angioma may pass into the neighbouring brain tissue, or into the subarachnoid space, or into both. Subarachnoid haemorrhage seems more likely to occur from a small cortical angioma which has given rise to no other disturbance than from the massive abnormalities which extend widely and deeply into the white matter. Herpes zoster is an occasional sequel of subarachnoid haemorrhage.

Spinal subarachnoid haemorrhage usually begins with pain in the lower back and lower limbs and sphincter disturbances, with rigidity of the spine and Kernig's sign. Later there may be flaccid weakness of the lower limbs with sensory loss and loss of reflexes. Extension of the haemorrhage to the cerebral subarachnoid space causes headache, cervical rigidity, and other symptoms of intracranial subarachnoid haemorrhage.

3. *The Cerebrospinal Fluid.* Subarachnoid haemorrhage causes characteristic changes in the cerebrospinal fluid, the pressure of which is raised at first. In the first week or more red cells are present, and the supernatant fluid exhibits a yellow coloration which persists for from two to three weeks. The faint coloration of the supernatant fluid which appears within 4–6 hours is due to oxyhaemoglobin while bilirubin first appears within 36–48 hours. The protein content of the fluid is raised, though rarely above 0·1 per cent. Irritation of the meninges by the extravasated blood leads to a pleocytosis consisting usually of mononuclear cells, though rarely polymorphonuclear cells may be present when the substance of the brain has been invaded. In some cases the colloidal gold curve is 'paretic' in type after a severe haemorrhage.

4. *Angiography.* Plain X-rays rarely show evidence of the source of a subarachnoid haemorrhage, though there may be X-ray signs of an angioma [see p. 232] or very rarely an aneurysm may show calcification in its wall. Angiography may be expected to show the causal lesions in about two-thirds of all cases, but bilateral carotid angiography and even vertebral angiography may be called for. Angiography should be carried out [FIG. 60] unless the patient's condition, owing to shock, age, severe atheroma, or hypertension makes surgery impracticable even if the lesion is demonstrated.

DIAGNOSIS

The essence of the clinical picture of subarachnoid haemorrhage is the acute or subacute onset of symptoms of meningeal irritation associated with the presence of blood in the cerebrospinal fluid demonstrated by lumbar puncture. To this extent the diagnosis is usually easy. Meningitis rarely comes on so acutely, and is readily distinguished by examination of the cerebrospinal fluid.

A lumbar puncture, again, enables subarachnoid haemorrhage to be distinguished from other conditions causing coma [but see p. 978]. But the presence of subarachnoid haemorrhage having been established, it is still necessary to decide its origin. Subarachnoid haemorrhage is occasionally found in exceptionally acute forms of encephalitis, but in such states the blood is likely to be present only in small amounts, and there will be evidence of diffuse lesions of the nervous system. Traumatic subarachnoid haemorrhage is usually easily recognized through the history. Intracerebral haemorrhage, due to vascular degeneration associated with hypertension, may reach the subarachnoid space either by rupture of the ventricular system, or, more rarely, to the surface of the brain. Such patients usually exhibit hemiplegia, which is less common in subarachnoid haemorrhage from an intracranial aneurysm, and a raised blood pressure and arterial degeneration which are not necessarily associated with it. When, however, a cerebral aneurysm bleeds both into the subarachnoid space and into the substance of one hemisphere the clinical picture may be indistinguishable from that of a primary intracerebral haemorrhage which has ruptured into the ventricle. In such a case angiography will often settle the diagnosis by demonstrating the presence, or absence, of an aneurysm. Rupture of an embolic aneurysm may lead to a clinical picture indistinguishable from that which occurs when a congenital aneurysm is responsible for the haemorrhage. The former, however, is associated with subacute infective endocarditis, or some other cause of chronic pyaemia, and its embolic origin is often indicated by the sudden development of hemiplegia some time before the onset of the haemorrhage. An angioma is a much less common cause of subarachnoid haemorrhage than an aneurysm, and, again, can usually be demonstrated by angiography. Finally, in about one quarter of all cases of spontaneous subarachnoid haemorrhage, the source of the haemorrhage is not found.

PROGNOSIS

The prognosis of focal subarachnoid haemorrhage depends upon a number of factors—the size and site of the leakage and whether it can be found and treated surgically, the age of the patient and the condition of the cardiovascular system, especially the presence or absence of hypertension and cerebral atherosclerosis. Walton (1956) reviewing the literature and describing patients not treated surgically found an average mortality rate of about 45 per cent. in the first illness. Of these about two-thirds die of the first haemorrhage, and one-third of a recurrence within 8 weeks, most often in the second week. In Walton's own series about 20 per cent. of those who survived an attack died of a recurrence, half in the first 6 months. Of the remainder most were able to pursue some useful activity, but about a third were disabled on account of hemiplegia, epilepsy, headache, or mental symptoms. The prognosis is better in angioma than in aneurysm.

TREATMENT

Angiography should not be carried out on a patient in coma with severe neurological signs, but is essential when the patient is conscious; such patients stand surgery well. Carotid ligation is of value in aneurysms of the posterior communicating artery, though there is a risk that it may cause hemiplegia (McKissock, Richardson, and Walsh, 1960). Direct attack on aneurysms of the middle cerebral artery improves the prognosis (McKissock, Richardson, and Walsh, 1962). Aneurysms at the junction of the anterior cerebral and anterior communicating artery carry a high risk but in Logue's (1956) series surgery improved the prognosis. Some aneurysms in the posterior fossa are amenable to surgery (Dimsdale and Logue, 1959). Unconsciousness will require the usual treatment. Patients not treated surgically should be kept in bed for four weeks, and then allowed to get up gradually, being advised to avoid physical exertion.

REFERENCES

(Intracranial aneurysm, Subarachnoid haemorrhage.)

ALPERS, B. J., and GASKILL, H. S. (1944) The pathological characteristics of embolic or metastatic encephalitis, *J. Neuropath., exp. Neurol.*, **3**, 210.

BIRLEY, J. L. (1928) Traumatic aneurysm of the intracranial portion of the internal carotid artery, *Brain*, **51**, 184.

BULL, J. W. D. (1962) Contribution of radiology to the study of intracranial aneurysms, *Brit. med. J.*, **2**, 1701.

CARMICHAEL, R. (1950) The pathogenesis of non-inflammatory cerebral aneurysms, *J. Path. Bact.*, **62**, 1.

CROMPTON, M. R. (1963) Hypothalamic lesions after rupture of cerebral aneurysms, *Brain*, **86**, 301.

CROMPTON, M. R. (1964 a) Cerebral infarction following the rupture of cerebral berry aneurysms, *Brain*, **87**, 263.

CROMPTON, M. R. (1964 b) The pathogenesis of cerebral infarction following the rupture of cerebral berry aneurysms, *Brain*, **87**, 491.

DANDY, W. E. (1944) *Intracranial Arterial Aneurysms*, Ithaca, N.Y.

DIMSDALE, H., and LOGUE, V. (1959) Ruptured posterior fossa aneurysms and their surgical treatment, *J. Neurol. Neurosurg. Psychiat.*, **22**, 202.

ESPIR, M. L. E., and MITCHELL, L. (1963) Tranylcypromine and intracranial haemorrhage, *Lancet*, ii, 639.

FALCONER, M. A. (1951) The surgical treatment of bleeding intracranial aneurysms, *J. Neurol. Neurosurg. Psychiat.*, **14**, 153.

FEARNSIDES, E. G. (1916) Intracranial aneurysms, *Brain*, **39**, 224.

FORBUS, W. D. (1930) On the origin of miliary aneurysms of the superficial cerebral arteries, *Bull. Johns Hopk. Hosp.*, **47**, 239.

HAMBY, W. B. (1966) *Carotid-cavernous Fistula*, Springfield, Ill.

HENSON, R. A., and CROFT, P. B. (1956) Spontaneous spinal subarachnoid haemorrhage, *Quart. J. Med.*, **25**, 53.

JEFFERSON, G. (1937) Compression of the chiasma, optic nerves and optic tracts by intracranial aneurysms, *Brain*, **60**, 444.

JEFFERSON, G. (1938) On the saccular aneurysms of the internal carotid artery in the cavernous sinus, *Brit. J. Surg.*, **26**, 267.

LOGUE, V. (1956) Surgery in spontaneous subarachnoid haemorrhage. Operative treatment of aneurysms on the anterior cerebral and anterior communicating artery, *Brit. med. J.*, **1**, 473.

McKISSOCK, W., RICHARDSON, A., and WALSH, L. (1960) Posterior communicating aneurysms, *Lancet*. ii. 1203.

McKISSOCK, W., RICHARDSON, A., and WALSH, L. (1962) Middle cerebral aneurysms, *Lancet*, ii, 417.

MAGEE, C. G. (1943) Spontaneous subarachnoid haemorrhage, *Lancet*, ii, 497.

NEVIN, S., and WILLIAMS, D. (1937) The pathogenesis of multiple aneurysms, *Lancet*, ii, 955.

RIDDOCH, G., and GOULDEN, C. (1925) On the relationship between subarachnoid and intraocular haemorrhage, *Brit. J. Ophthal.*, **9**, 209.

SCHMIDT, M. (1930) Intracranial aneurysms, *Brain*, **53**, 489.

STRAUSS, I., GLOBUS, J. H., and GINSBURG, S. W. (1932) Spontaneous subarachnoid hemorrhage, *Arch. Neurol. Psychiat. (Chicago)*, **27**, 1080.

SYMONDS, C. P. (1924–5) Spontaneous subarachnoid haemorrhage, *Quart. J. Med.*, **18**, 93.

TAYLOR, A. B., and WHITFIELD, A. G. W. (1936) Subarachnoid haemorrhage based on observations of eighty-one cases, *Quart. J. Med.*, **29**, 461.

TOMLINSON, B. E. (1959) Brain changes in ruptured intracranial aneurysms, *J. clin. Path.*, **12**, 391.

TURNBULL, H. M. (1914–15) Alterations in arterial structure, and their relation to syphilis, *Quart. J. Med.*, **8**, 201.

TURNBULL, H. M. (1918) Intracranial aneurysms, *Brain*, **41**, 50.

WALTON, J. N. (1956) *Subarachnoid Haemorrhage*, Edinburgh.

WECHSLER, I. S., GROSS, S. W., and COHEN, I. (1951) Arteriography and carotid artery ligation in intracranial aneurysm and vascular malformation, *J. Neurol. Neurosurg. Psychiat.*, **14**, 25.

WOLF, G. A., GOODELL, H., and WOLFF, H. G. (1945) Prognosis of subarachnoid hemorrhage, *J. Amer. med. Ass.*, **129**, 715.

CEREBRAL HAEMORRHAGE

AETIOLOGY AND PATHOLOGY

Intracranial haemorrhage may be venous, capillary, or arterial. Little is known about intracranial venous haemorrhage, but it has been regarded as the cause of acute cerebral lesions during whooping cough and may occasionally occur in pyaemic states (Alpers and Gaskill, 1944). Capillary or petechial haemorrhages are found in a variety of toxic and infective conditions, for example in salvarsan poisoning, in acute inflammatory states, such as the various forms of acute encephalitis, in septicaemia, and in any form of severe anaemia, leukaemia, and in thrombocytopenic purpura. Acute brain purpura due to anaphylaxis or to other forms of acute hypersensitivity reaction is similar. Haemorrhage may occur into a cerebral tumour, for example a glioma, or one of the vessels composing an angioma may bleed, either into the substance of the brain or into the subarachnoid space. Severe trauma, especially if it involves fracture of the skull or penetration of the brain by a missile, is likely to cause haemorrhage, which may be either venous, capillary, or arterial. In a recent series of 108 cases of cerebral haemorrhage Richardson and Einhorn (1963) found that 77 were due to hypertension, 10 were unexplained, 7 were due to neoplasms, 6 to blood disease, 3 to arteritis, 2 to anticoagulants, and 3 resulted from other miscellaneous causes.

Arterial haemorrhage may be extradural, subdural, subarachnoid, or intracerebral. The first three are described elsewhere. The commonest cause of intracerebral arterial haemorrhage is rupture of an atheromatous artery in an individual suffering from high blood pressure. The rise in blood pressure is usually due to primary hypertension, much less frequently to chronic nephritis or congenital cystic kidney. The arterial degeneration is closely bound up with the rise of blood pressure. According to Turnbull, the first change in the arteries in this condition is hypertrophy of the media. The hypertrophied media undergoes degeneration, and atheroma of the intima occurs as a result partly of the raised pressure and partly of the degeneration. The result is a thickened but brittle vessel. Miliary aneurysms have often been described on the cerebral vessels in arteriosclerosis, and Russell (1963) has recently shown that they occur and are much commoner in hypertensive than in normotensive subjects.

There are thus two factors in the causation of arterial cerebral haemorrhage, the degeneration of the vessel and the raised blood pressure. The former in the absence of the latter is likely to lead to thrombosis rather than haemorrhage, while haemorrhage does not necessarily occur even when the blood pressure is very high, unless vascular hypertrophy has given place to degeneration. This account, however, is probably too simple and there are other unknown factors (Stern, 1938). Moreover, cerebral haemorrhage occasionally occurs in the absence of high blood pressure as a result of developmental vascular abnormalities (Elkington, 1935) or in leukaemia or polyarteritis nodosa, and is rarely caused by an infected embolus in bacterial endocarditis.

Most cases of cerebral haemorrhage are found in late middle life. It is comparatively rare in younger hypertensives and the vascular changes of old age more often lead to thrombosis and cerebral softening. Males are more frequently affected than females. A familial incidence is common.

Cerebral haemorrhage may occur in any situation, but it is especially common in the region of the internal capsule. The blood clot may remain encapsulated in the brain or may burst into one lateral ventricle, or, much less frequently, superficially into the subarachnoid space. In 10 per cent. of cases it is in the cerebellum (McKissock, Richardson, and Walsh, 1960).

After a large intracerebral haemorrhage the affected hemisphere is larger than the opposite one and the gyri are flattened. The site of haemorrhage is occupied by a red clot and the surrounding tissues are compressed and may be oedematous. Later the clot is absorbed and may be replaced by a neuroglial scar or by a cavity containing a yellow serous fluid. During absorption of the clot, gliosis takes place in the walls of the cavity with phagocytosis of destroyed neural tissue by compound granular corpuscles. Multiple haemorrhages sometimes occur.

SYMPTOMS

The occurrence of cerebral haemorrhage is always sudden, but the patient may be known to have a high blood pressure and there may have been premonitory symptoms, such as transitory speech disturbances or attacks of weakness of a limb. The actual rupture of the vessel may be brought about by mental excitement or physical effort, or may occur during rest or sleep. Usually the patient complains of sudden severe headache and may vomit. He becomes dazed, and in all but the mildest cases loses consciousness in a few minutes. Convulsions may occur at the onset, but are exceptional. The physical signs produced by a cerebral haemorrhage depend upon its situation and its size.

Haemorrhage in the region of the Internal Capsule

The patient is usually unconscious, but the depth of coma depends upon the size of the haemorrhage and the degree of shock. Slight pyrexia is usually present.

The pulse rate is generally slow—50 to 60—and the pulse full and bounding. The respirations are deep and stertorous, and the respiratory rate may be either slow or quickened or exhibit irregularity, for example Cheyne-Stokes respiration. An unconscious patient is unable to swallow. The head is usually rotated and the eyes are deviated towards the side of the lesion. This is due to paralysis of rotation of the head and of conjugate deviation of the eyes to the opposite side and the consequent unbalanced action of the undamaged cerebral hemisphere. The fundi are likely to show arteriosclerosis of the retinal vessels, but the discs are usually normal, though slight papilloedema is not very uncommon. The pupils may be unequal, but react to light unless the patient is very deeply comatose. A divergent squint is common, and the eyes often exhibit irregular, jerky movements. The corneal reflex is often lost on the side opposite to the lesion and will be lost on both sides when coma is profound. A capsular haemorrhage causes paralysis of the opposite side of the body, but the comatose patient cannot be asked to carry out voluntary movements. It is therefore necessary to resort to indirect methods of demonstrating paralysis.

Flattening of the nasolabial furrow may be evident on the paralysed side, and the cheek is often distended more on the paralysed than on the normal side during expiration. If the patient is not too deeply comatose it may also be observed that he moves the limbs spontaneously on the normal side but not on the paralysed side. Muscular spasticity takes two or three weeks to develop in the paralysed limbs after a capsular haemorrhage. Before this the limbs are flaccid, and this flaccidity is one of the most valuable signs of hemiplegia in a comatose patient. The arm and the leg if lifted up fall to the bed inertly, whereas even in deep coma the normal arm and leg subside much more gradually. Painful stimuli may be used to demonstrate the presence of paralysis. Pricking with a pin even in an unconscious patient usually causes contraction of the muscles of the face and movements of withdrawal of the limb which is pricked. These movements do not occur on the paralysed side. The absence of such movements, however, may also be due to hemianalgesia. This may often be demonstrated by the fact that reflex contraction of the facial muscles occurs when the patient is pricked on one side of the body, the normal side, but not when he is pricked on the analgesic side. The tendon reflexes are variable. They may be much diminished or abolished on the paralysed side; sometimes they are exaggerated. The plantar reflex on the affected side is extensor; on the other side it may be flexor or extensor. The abdominal reflexes are often lost on both sides in coma. Retention or incontinence of urine and faeces is the rule as long as the patient is unconscious.

Pontine Haemorrhage

If the patient is seen soon after the onset of the haemorrhage, the signs may be those of a unilateral lesion of the pons, namely facial paralysis on the side of the lesion with flaccid paralysis of the limbs on the opposite side. Owing to paralysis of conjugate ocular deviation and of rotation of the head to the side of the lesion the patient lies with his head and eyes turned towards the side of the paralysed limbs. Even when the signs at the outset are those of a unilateral lesion of the pons, extension of the haemorrhage soon involves the opposite side, or the signs may be bilateral from the beginning. When both sides of the pons are thus affected there is paralysis of the face and limbs on both sides, with bilateral extensor plantar reflexes. Marked contraction of the pupils, 'pinpoint pupils', the result of bilateral destruction of the ocular sympathetic fibres, is characteristic of a pontine haemorrhage. Moreover, destruction of the pons cuts off the body from the control of the heat-regulating centres in the hypothalamus, and the patient becomes poikilothermic. Since much care is usually taken to keep an unconscious patient warm, his temperature gradually rises and may reach a high level. Absence of nystagmus induced by cold water injected into one or both auditory meati may be useful in distinguishing the condition from cerebral haemorrhage.

Haemorrhage into the Ventricles

It is not uncommon for a haemorrhage in the region of the internal capsule to burst into the lateral ventricle. If the patient is not seen until after this has occurred it may be difficult to differentiate ventricular from pontine haemorrhage. After ventricular haemorrhage coma deepens and signs of a corticospinal lesion are usually present on both sides of the body. There is often a tendency for the upper limbs to adopt a posture of rigid extension. The temperature frequently exhibits a terminal rise, also seen in pontine haemorrhage.

The symptoms of cerebral haemorrhage in other situations are those of a massive focal lesion of sudden onset and are similar to the focal symptoms of a tumour in the same region.

Cerebellar Haemorrhage

Cerebellar haemorrhage is usually sudden, and in some cases consciousness is lost sooner or later. Occipital headache and vomiting are common at the onset. Only a minority of patients show localizing signs: in many of the remainder the clinical picture suggests a cerebrovascular accident without clear evidence as to its site (McKissock, Richardson, and Walsh, 1960). Repeated vomiting and intense vertigo at the onset in a conscious patient who is ataxic and complains of headache but may have no classical 'cerebellar signs' should always suggest this diagnosis as a possibility. Ocular signs such as paralysis of conjugate gaze to the side of the lesion, a sixth nerve palsy or 'skew deviation' are seen in some cases. If the haemorrhage is not evacuated, coma due to brain-stem compression supervenes.

The cerebrospinal fluid after cerebral haemorrhage is under increased pressure and its protein content may be somewhat raised. The presence of blood visible to the naked eye in the fluid indicates usually that the haemorrhage has ruptured into the ventricular system, less frequently that it has come to the surface of the brain and ruptured into the subarachnoid space. Red blood cells may be seen microscopically.

The heart is usually enlarged and the blood pressure raised and the superficial arteries may be thickened and tortuous. Albuminuria may be present, and glycosuria may be a result of the cerebral lesion.

DIAGNOSIS

In the large majority of cases an intracerebral haemorrhage leads to impairment or loss of consciousness, sometimes very rapidly, sometimes more gradually. In such cases it has to be distinguished from other conditions causing coma. This is discussed on page 976. Here it may be said that important diagnostic points are the association of the impairment of consciousness with the physical signs of a focal cerebral lesion of acute or subacute onset, the presence of factors predisposing to a cerebral vascular lesion, particularly hypertension and cerebral atheroma, and the presence of blood, visible either microscopically or macroscopically, in the cerebrospinal fluid.

A cerebral vascular lesion having been diagnosed, it is necessary to decide whether it is haemorrhagic or ischaemic in origin. Ischaemic lesions are either embolic, or due to atheroma or other conditions of arterial degeneration or inflammation, with or without thrombosis. An embolic lesion comes on with great suddenness and presents the neurological picture of obstruction of a particular artery. Moreover, the source of the embolus is usually evident. Ischaemic infarction due to atheroma is usually more gradual than haemorrhage. There may have been previous recurrent episodes with complete or partial recovery, or the onset is insidious over a period of 24 to 48 hours. Exceptionally, however, it is as sudden as a haemorrhage. Unconsciousness is less common and when it occurs usually less profound. The blood pressure is less frequently raised, and there may be evidence of pre-existing disease leading to vascular damage, for example, diabetes.

The cerebrospinal fluid is often helpful. The presence of red blood cells will always suggest haemorrhage, while after infarction the cerebrospinal fluid is likely to be free from red cells but may contain a raised protein.

Primary subarachnoid haemorrhage is distinguished from intracerebral haemorrhage by the prominence of signs of meningeal irritation, i.e. cervical rigidity and Kernig's sign, and the absence of signs of a cerebral lesion. It may, however, be impossible to distinguish on clinical grounds between an intracerebral haemorrhage reaching the subarachnoid space by rupturing into a ventricle, and a subarachnoid haemorrhage from an aneurysm invading one cerebral hemisphere. Angiography, however, should settle the question, and is also useful in doubtful cases in distinguishing between a primary intracerebral haemorrhage and infarction due to atheromatous narrowing, or thrombosis, of a major artery.

An intracranial tumour rarely simulates a cerebral vascular lesion unless it is itself the site of a haemorrhage or of rapidly developing oedema. The true nature of a lesion may be difficult to recognize if there have been no preceding symptoms of increased intracranial pressure. However, the occurrence of what appears to be a cerebral haemorrhage in a patient without hypertension should suggest the possibility of a cerebral tumour, and the need for surgical exploration. The 'congestive attacks' of general paresis may simulate a cerebral haemorrhage closely owing to the rapid onset of hemiplegia with loss of consciousness. Other signs of general paresis, however, are usually present, and examination of the cerebrospinal fluid and the blood Wassermann reaction settles the diagnosis. The same is true of hemiplegia due to meningovascular syphilis.

PROGNOSIS

The immediate problem in the case of cerebral haemorrhage is whether or not the haemorrhage will prove fatal. Death may occur from medullary anaemia as a result of continuance of the bleeding. Even if the bleeding stops, the destruction of brain tissue and rise of intracranial pressure may cause the patient to remain unconscious so long that he dies of exhaustion or from an intercurrent infection, such as pneumonia. When haemorrhage continues, death may occur rapidly, though rarely in less than a few hours, usually during the first two days. The patient may linger in a comatose condition for as long as a week. If the haemorrhage is continuing there is a progressive deepening of the coma, indicated by inability to rouse a formerly responsive patient, and loss of the corneal and pupillary reflexes; the pulse tends to become rapid and irregular; the respiratory rate is often irregular and finally becomes rapid and shallow, and both the temperature and the blood pressure tend to rise.

Bilateral paralysis of limbs is a sign of bad prognostic import, because it indicates either ventricular or pontine haemorrhage, both of which are usually fatal. A visibly blood-stained cerebrospinal fluid usually means a ventricular haemorrhage. If the patient shows no signs of recovery from coma 48 hours after the onset of the haemorrhage the chances of recovery are poor, even though the haemorrhage may have stopped. McKissock, Richardson, and Taylor (1961) in their series of 180 cases had an over-all mortality of 51 per cent. and it was about twice as high in men as in women.

When the patient recovers consciousness he is naturally anxious to know whether he is likely to suffer from permanent disability. This depends upon the situation of the haemorrhage, and the extent of the resulting destruction of brain tissue. It must be remembered that neural shock and oedema of surrounding areas of brain usually cause a more severe depression of function than is actually due to the destructive effect of the lesion. Some improvement may therefore be expected in most cases. The mental efficiency of the patient is rarely as good after a cerebral haemorrhage as before. Apart from lesions grossly impairing functions of intelligence and speech, there is usually diminished power of concentration and memory, together with irritability and emotional instability.

Haemorrhage in the region of the posterior part of the inferior frontal gyrus on the left side may cause for a time total expressive aphasia, but in these cases a very considerable recovery of speech usually occurs in time, and improvement may continue for many months. The speech defect which follows a capsular haemorrhage is a dysarthria and usually improves rapidly. Damage to the cortico-spinal tract by a haemorrhage in the region of the internal capsule causes spastic hemiplegia on the opposite side, the signs of which are described elsewhere [see p. 20]. Some return of power always occurs in the lower limb, so that the patient is likely to be able to walk. If the upper limb exhibits returning power at the end of a month after the onset a considerable degree of recovery of movement at the larger joints will probably occur in it. If, however, there is no improvement at the end of 3 months the paralysis is likely to be permanent. When the posterior part of the capsule is involved, sensory loss and homonymous hemianopia on the side opposite to the lesion may be added to the paralysis. Improvement may occur in respect of these disorders, but is often incomplete. Pain on the paralysed side of the body may occur after a capsular haemorrhage, and is of thalamic origin. If it develops it is likely to be persistent. Involuntary movements sometimes occur after cerebral haemorrhage, but only when paralysis of the limbs is incomplete. They usually appear several weeks or months after the onset, with the return of voluntary power, and are always more marked in the upper than in the lower limb. Simple tremor may develop and is most evident on voluntary movement. Less often there is tremor of the Parkinsonian type which occurs when the limb is at rest. Athetosis also is sometimes seen. All these movements tend to be persistent, though some improvement may occur, especially in the tremor. They are probably due to involvement of the corpus striatum. Choreiform movements may occur as a result of haemorrhage in the region of the subthalamic nucleus. This lesion is often fatal, though improvement and even recovery may take place. Trophic changes are common in the paralysed limbs. There is often cyanosis of the extremities and oedema is not rare. The nails may be brittle. Painful arthritis of the larger joints is seen, especially in older patients.

TREATMENT

Continuing cerebral haemorrhage causes death from medullary anaemia. The objects of treatment are, therefore, to stop the haemorrhage and to reduce the intracranial pressure. The patient should be moved as little as possible, and care should be taken that there is no hindrance to venous return from the head.

Surgical evacuation of the clot is a rational procedure but is rarely practicable. It should, however, be considered when cerebral haemorrhage occurs before middle life, in view of the possibility of haemorrhage from a congenital vascular abnormality which it may be possible to demonstrate by angiography (Small, Holmes, and Connolly, 1953). McKissock, Richardson, and Taylor (1961) have compared surgical and conservative treatment in a series of 180 cases of primary intracerebral haemorrhage. They concluded that with the possible exception of normotensive subjects no group of patients fared better with operation than with conservative treatment. However, there is good evidence to suggest that surgical evacuation of the intracerebellar haematoma in cases of primary cerebellar haemorrhage will often save life and lessen morbidity. Hypotensive therapy appears to be of no value in the acute stage.

Lumbar puncture should be used only when absolutely necessary for diagnostic purposes as it may be dangerous because of the risk of tentorial or cerebellar herniation.

The usual treatment of the unconscious patient should be carried out [see p. 979].

After recovery from the immediate effects of the haemorrhage the patient must be encouraged to make an attempt to use his paralysed limbs. Physiotherapy may help to diminish spasticity and to improve mobility. If the toe drags in walking this may be counteracted by wearing a special shoe with a spring attached below to the toe and above to a gaiter round the calf. When speech is affected speech therapy will often be necessary [see p. 107].

REFERENCES

ALPERS, B. J., and GASKILL, H. S. (1944) The pathological characteristics of embolic or metastatic encephalitis, *J. Neuropath. exp. Neurol.* **3**, 210.

BAGLEY, C., Jr. (1932) Spontaneous cerebral hemorrhage, *Arch. Neurol. Psychiat. (Chicago)*, **27**, 1133.

CHASE, W. H. (1937) Hypertensive apoplexy and its causation, *Arch. Neurol. Psychiat. (Chicago)*, **38**, 1176.

CRAIG, W. McK., and ADSON, A. W. (1936) Spontaneous intracerebral hemorrhage, *Arch. Neurol. Psychiat. (Chicago)*, **35**, 701.

ELKINGTON, J. ST. C. (1935) Cerebral vascular accidents unassociated with cardio-vascular disease, *Lancet*, i, 6.

FIELDS, W. S. (1961) *Pathogenesis and Treatment of Cerebrovascular Disease*, Springfield, Ill.

McKISSOCK, W., RICHARDSON, A., and TAYLOR, J. (1961) Primary intracerebellar haemorrhage, *Lancet*, ii, 221.

McKISSOCK, W., RICHARDSON, A., and WALSH, L. (1960). Spontaneous cerebellar haemorrhage, *Brain*, **83**, 1.

MURPHY, J. P. (1954) *Cerebrovascular Disease*, Chicago.

RICHARDSON, J. C., and EINHORN, R. W. (1963) in *Clinical Neurosurgery*, ed. MOSBERG, WILF, p. 114, London.

RIISHEDE, J. (1957) Cerebral apoplexy, *Acta psychiat. (Kbh.)*, **32**, Supp. 118.

RUSSELL, R. W. R. (1963) Observations on intracranial aneurysms, *Brain*, **86**, 425.

SMALL, J. M., HOLMES, J. M., and CONNOLLY, R. C. (1953) The prognosis and role of surgery in spontaneous intracranial haemorrhage, *Brit. med. J.*, **2**, 1072.

STERN, K. (1938) The pathology of apoplexy, *J. Neurol. Psychiat.*, N.S. **1**, 26.

POLYARTERITIS NODOSA

(Periarteritis Nodosa)

This disorder is now believed to be an allergic reaction to a variety of toxins, including organic arsenicals, sulphonamides, and thiouracil, and possibly bacterial toxins and antisera. It is characterized by multiple focal lesions in the arteries. These begin with necrosis of the media and the internal elastic lamina, which is followed by extension of the inflammation to the adventitia, and periarteritis. Proliferation of the intima produces gradual narrowing of the lumen of the vessels. Secondary aneurysm formation is exceptional. The nervous system is said to be involved in 8 per cent. of cases; and lesions may occur in the meninges, cerebral cortex, medulla, spinal cord, and peripheral nerves, degeneration of which is the result of damage to the nutrient arteries.

Cerebral lesions may lead to headache, convulsions, hemiplegia, mental dullness, and coma. Pupillary changes may be present. The symptoms of involvement of the peripheral nerves are often those of multiple interstitial neuritis ('mono-neuritis multiplex') rather than symmetrical polyneuritis. Pain and muscular weakness may develop in the course of a few hours. Tenderness of the nerve trunks and muscles with muscular wasting and weakness, loss of reflexes, and sensory loss are irregularly distributed according to the distribution of the spinal roots and peripheral nerves affected. The spinal fluid may be under increased pressure and there may be xanthochromia and a polymorphonuclear leucocytosis in the fluid.

Changes are often present in the ocular fundi. There may be choroidal exudate in the form of perivascular hillocks resembling choroidal tubercles. Detachment of the retina may occur, and in the later stages hypertensive retinopathy.

The general symptoms are those of a serious infection, with fever and loss of weight, and focal visceral symptoms depending upon the situation of the lesions, which tend to involve especially the kidneys, heart, liver, and gastro-intestinal tract. The spleen may be enlarged, and radiographically the lungs may show a characteristic infiltration. There is often a leucocytosis in the blood and occasionally an eosinophilia. Asthma is common. Hypertension and albuminuria usually occur in the later stages. The muscles are involved through the affection of their blood vessels and a biopsy of muscle may show the characteristic lesion. Many patients improve when treated with steroid drugs, a few recover after long-term treatment and in some the disease appears to become 'burnt-out' but there is still an appreciable mortality.

REFERENCES

KERNOHAN, J. W., and WOLTMAN, H. W. (1938) Periarteritis nodosa. A clinico-pathologic study with special reference to the nervous system, *Arch. Neurol. Psychiat. (Chicago)*, **39**, 665.

MILLER, H. G., and DALEY, R. (1946) Clinical aspects of polyarteritis nodosa, *Quart. J. Med.*, **15**, 255.

TEMPORAL (GIANT CELL) ARTERITIS

The disorder originally described as temporal, or cranial, arteritis is now recognized to be a generalized vascular disease which attacks elderly patients, being rare before the age of 60 years. The pathological features are those of a subacute inflammation, spreading probably by the vasa vasorum to the media of the arteries with a tendency to spread longitudinally along the vessels in contrast to the lesion in polyarteritis nodosa. The intima becomes hypertrophied, and thrombosis is a common sequel. Stress has been laid upon the presence of giant cells, and the disorder has been described as giant cell arteritis. The characteristic pathological changes have been found in many large and small vessels, including the aorta and the retinal arteries. Biopsy of an affected portion of a superficial temporal artery will establish the diagnosis.

The characteristic physical signs are anorexia, loss of weight, joint and muscle pains, fever and sweating, painful arterial thrombosis, and severe headache. The superficial temporal arteries are intensely tender during the acute stage and may become thrombosed through part or the whole of their length. Papilloedema may occur, and at least half the patients so far reported have had visual disturbances leading in many instances to complete loss of sight. Indeed, in a survey of 80 personal cases Meadows (1966) found that unilateral or bilateral blindness due to central retinal artery occlusion occurred in over half and diplopia in 15 per cent. Sudden unilateral blindness in an elderly patient, even when other evidence of arteritis is unobtrusive, should always raise the possibility of this condition and an erythrocyte sedimentation rate estimation (this is invariably raised in the untreated case) is the single most useful investigation. Treatment with steroid drugs is mandatory as this may be the only means of preserving remaining vision. The disease usually burns itself out in 1–2 years when treatment can gradually be withdrawn. Cerebral symptoms due to involvement of the carotid and vertebral arteries are occasionally seen.

Though the disease may prove fatal, the prognosis is on the whole good. It tends to run a slow course and may last many months and then become arrested, leaving the patient with a variable degree of disability. Treatment with steroids is of value.

REFERENCES

COOKE, W. T., CLOAKE, P. C. P., GOVAN, A. D. T., and COLBECK, J. C. (1946) Temporal arteritis: a generalized vascular disease, *Quart. J. Med.*, **15**, 47.
CROMPTON, M. R. (1959) The visual changes in temporal (giant-cell) arteritis. Report of a case with autopsy findings, *Brain*, **82**, 377.
MEADOWS, S. P. (1966) Temporal or giant-cell arteritis, *Proc. roy. Soc. Med.*, **59**, 329.

THROMBOTIC MICROANGIOPATHY

Thrombotic microangiopathy (thrombotic thrombocytopenic purpura) is a fulminating disorder involving small blood vessels which become inflamed and in which platelet thrombi form resulting in widespread small vessel occlusion in many organs. Fever, haemolytic anaemia, renal damage and variable and fleeting neurological manifestations including confusion, pareses, and convulsions are seen; the response to steroid drugs is variable and most cases are fatal.

REFERENCE

SYMMERS, W. ST. C. (1952) Thrombotic microangiopathic haemolytic anaemias (thrombotic microangiopathy), *Brit. med. J.*, **2**, 897.

THE CEREBRAL VENOUS CIRCULATION

THE VENOUS SINUSES

The intracranial venous sinuses are spaces lying between layers of the dura mater and are lined with endothelium. They receive blood from the veins of the brain and directly or indirectly drain into the internal jugular vein. They communicate with the meningeal veins, and by emissary veins with the veins of the scalp.

The following sinuses are unpaired:

The Superior Sagittal Sinus. The superior sagittal sinus begins anteriorly at the crista galli where it communicates through the foramen caecum with the nasal veins, and passes upwards, backwards, and finally downwards at the convex upper margin of the falx. It ends at the level of the internal occipital protuberance by turning, usually to the right, into the right transverse sinus. Occasionally it turns into the left transverse sinus. It possesses a terminal dilatation—the confluence of the sinuses—from which a communicating channel passes to the junction of the straight sinus and the left transverse sinus. The superior sagittal sinus receives the superior group of superficial cerebral veins and thus drains the upper part of the cerebral hemispheres.

The Inferior Sagittal Sinus. The inferior sagittal sinus lies in the free lower border of the falx for its posterior two-thirds and terminates posteriorly by joining the great cerebral vein to form the straight sinus, which passes between layers of the dura along the line of junction of the falx with the tentorium. Posteriorly it turns to the left at the level of the internal occipital protuberance to become the left transverse sinus.

The following sinuses are paired:

The Transverse Sinuses. The transverse sinuses arise posteriorly, the right from the superior sagittal sinus, the left from the straight sinus, and pass laterally and forwards in the attached border of the tentorium, lying in a groove in the occipital bone. Each then turns downwards on the inner surface of the mastoid process and leaves the skull by the jugular foramen, to enter the internal jugular vein.

The Cavernous Sinuses. The cavernous sinuses lie one on either side of the body of the sphenoid. They begin anteriorly at the inner end of the superior orbital fissure, where they receive the ophthalmic veins, and terminate posteriorly at the apex of the petrous portion of the temporal bone by dividing into the superior and inferior petrosal sinuses. In the lateral wall of the cavernous sinus lie the internal carotid artery with its sympathetic plexus, the third and fourth nerves, the first and second divisions of the fifth nerve, and the sixth nerve.

The Superior Petrosal Sinuses. The superior petrosal sinuses run backwards and laterally along the attached edge of the tentorium, to end in the transverse sinuses.

The Inferior Petrosal Sinuses. The inferior petrosal sinuses run backwards, outwards, and downwards in the posterior fossa, to join the internal jugular veins by passing through the jugular foramina.

The Cerebral Veins. The venous sinuses receive as tributaries the cerebral veins. The superficial cerebral veins are divided into two groups—the superior, which run upwards to the superior sagittal sinus and drain the upper halves of the hemispheres, and the inferior, which drain the lower halves of the hemispheres and run downwards to join the venous sinuses of the base. The most important of the deep cerebral veins is the great cerebral vein of Galen, which drains the choroid plexuses of the third and lateral ventricles and the basal ganglia, and terminates by joining the inferior sagittal sinus to form the straight sinus.

The Diploic Veins. The venous channels in the bones of the skull, the diploic veins, drain either into the venous sinuses or into the superficial veins of the scalp.

(References, see page 335)

THROMBOSIS OF THE INTRACRANIAL VENOUS SINUSES AND VEINS

AETIOLOGY

Thrombosis of the intracranial venous sinuses is usually the result of the extension of infection from neighbouring structures or of direct injury. Rarely it occurs in the absence of any evident local cause in conditions of marasmus or cachexia. These two varieties of sinus thrombosis are rather unsatisfactorily distinguished as 'secondary' and 'primary' respectively.

'Primary' sinus thrombosis is rare and is most frequently seen at the extremes of life, especially during the first year. It occurs in wasted, debilitated infants, especially as a complication of congenital heart disease, and enteritis, and later in life in individuals suffering from severe anaemia, exhausting infections such as enteric fever, or emaciating diseases such as carcinoma and tuberculosis. The principal predisposing factors of 'primary' sinus thrombosis appear to be anaemia, increased coagulability of the blood, slowing of the blood stream as a result of a low blood pressure, and dehydration. It may form part of the picture of thrombophlebitis migrans.

'Secondary' sinus thrombosis may be the result of direct injury of a sinus through fracture of the skull or surgical operation in its vicinity, or puncture of the superior sagittal sinus in infancy for therapeutic purposes. Infection may spread to the sinuses from an area of osteitis of one of the cranial bones. The transverse sinus may thus become infected from mastoiditis, or through the jugular vein from the fauces. Infection may spread from the transverse to the superior sagittal sinus. The latter and the cavernous sinus may be directly infected from frontal sinusitis or from infection of the other nasal air sinuses. Owing to the comparatively free communication between the intracranial venous sinuses and the superficial veins of the face and scalp, cutaneous infections, such as boils, carbuncles, and erysipelas, in these regions, may cause intracranial sinus thrombosis. The cavernous sinus is especially liable to become infected as a result of pyogenic infections in the neighbourhood of the upper lip.

Though sinus thrombosis may be the only manifestation of infection, it may be associated with extradural or subdural abscess, intracerebral abscess, or localized or diffuse leptomeningitis.

Why cerebral thrombophlebitis should occur in pregnancy and the puerperium is still obscure. In over 90 per cent. of the cases of Carroll, Leak, and Lee (1966) it occurred during the puerperium. Toxaemia may predispose to it.

PATHOLOGY

The affected sinus contains a reddish clot, which tends in time to become paler and adherent to the sinus wall. In sinus thrombophlebitis due to pyogenic organisms the clot may become purulent. It may extend into tributary veins or into other sinuses. The internal jugular vein is frequently involved by extension from the transverse sinus. The area of brain drained by the affected sinus exhibits congestive oedema and in some cases softening, and the development of some degree of collateral venous circulation causes congestion of neighbouring veins. Obstruction of a large sinus, such as the superior sagittal, may so impede the absorption of cerebrospinal fluid that hydrocephalus results. Involvement of the Galenic vein causes softening of the central areas of the brain. Extension of infection from the sinus may cause localized or diffuse leptomeningitis or intra-cerebral abscess, while the liberation of organisms or of fragments of infected clot into the general circulation may lead to pyaemia and pyaemic abscesses, especially in the lungs.

The pathology of the condition, as well as its clinical features, have been reviewed recently by Kalbag and Woolf (1967).

SYMPTOMS

The symptoms in intracranial venous sinus thrombosis consist of symptoms of the predisposing condition; symptoms of obstruction to the venous drainage of tissues adjacent to the sinus; in the case of infective thrombo-phlebitis, symptoms of extension of the infection to neighbouring structures and of its dissemination in the blood stream; and in some cases hydrocephalus due to defective absorption of cerebrospinal fluid.

Conditions predisposing to intracranial sinus thrombosis have already been mentioned in the section dealing with aetiology.

The symptoms due to obstructed venous drainage differ according to the sinus affected.

Thrombosis of the Cavernous Sinus

Pain is severe and is located in the eye and forehead on the affected side and is usually associated with hyperalgesia over the cutaneous distribution of the ophthalmic division of the trigeminal nerve. There is conspicuous oedema of the eyelids, the cornea, and the root of the nose, associated with exophthalmos due to congestion of the orbital veins. Papilloedema is sometimes present, in which case vision is markedly reduced and may be lost, but in other cases the optic disc is normal and vision is little impaired. Since the third, fourth, and sixth cranial nerves lie in the lateral wall of the sinus, ocular palsies are usually present and there may be complete internal and external ophthalmoplegia. Cavernous sinus thrombosis is usually unilateral at the outset, but thrombophlebitis readily extends through the circular sinus to the cavernous sinus of the opposite side, the signs then becoming bilateral.

Thrombosis of the Transverse Sinus

Thrombosis of the transverse sinus is almost always the result of an extension of infection from the mastoid. The patient complains of headache and of pain in the ear, which tends to be intensified by moving the head. Vomiting may occur. Venous congestion may be observed in the neighbourhood of the mastoid process and extension of the phlebitis to the jugular vein causes tenderness in the neck. The vein is sometimes, though only exceptionally, palpable as a tender cord. Papilloedema is sometimes present, but is usually slight and may be confined to the eye of the affected side. Focal cerebral symptoms include convulsions and contralateral hemiparesis. Aphasia may be present when the left transverse sinus is affected.

Thrombosis of the Superior Sagittal Sinus

Thrombosis of the superior sagittal sinus usually leads to a considerable rise of intracranial pressure. The earliest symptoms consist of headache, vomiting, delirium, and in some cases head retraction and convulsions. There is marked congestion of the veins of the scalp and sometimes also of the external nasal veins, and in infants the fontanelle is tense. Papilloedema is sometimes present, and squint may occur. Since the superior sagittal sinus receives the superior cortical veins which drain the upper half of the hemispheres, and since the lower limbs are represented in the areas of the precentral gyrus nearest the vertex, thrombosis of this sinus may cause symptoms of bilateral corticospinal lesions, which are most marked in, and may be confined to, the lower limbs. Focal symptoms may be unilateral, e.g. Jacksonian epilepsy and hemiplegia, or even absent. The symptoms may be mainly or exclusively those of hydrocephalus, as in so-called 'otitic hydrocephalus' [see p. 211].

Thrombosis of other Sinuses

Thrombophlebitis may spread from the transverse sinus to the superior petrosal sinus and so reach the cerebral veins draining the lower part of the precentral gyrus causing faciobrachial monoplegia. Thrombophlebitis of the inferior petrosal sinus may explain Gradenigo's syndrome (Symonds, 1944) and involvement of the posterior group of cranial nerves.

Thrombophlebitis in Pregnancy

According to Carroll, Leak, and Lee (1966) the presenting symptoms in order of frequency are severe headache, convulsions, speech disturbances, and drowsiness and confusion.

The cerebrospinal fluid is usually under increased pressure, but may be otherwise normal. In thrombosis of the superior sagittal sinus, however, it is not uncommon to find red blood cells in considerable numbers, with a corresponding rise in the protein content, and even a xanthochromic fluid. The presence of a slight excess of leucocytes, usually both polymorphonuclear and mononuclear, is not uncommon and indicates a localized extension of the infection to the neighbouring leptomeninges.When one transverse sinus is filled with clot the pressure of the cerebrospinal fluid may fail to show the normal rise when the jugular vein on the affected side is compressed alone in Queckenstedt's test, but the sinus may be infected without being obstructed.

Other Investigations

The EEG may show a variety of non-specific changes but may help in the localization of the lesion. Carotid angiography may show venous filling defects.

Intracranial sinus thrombosis of infective origin often leads to *general symptoms* resulting from the passage of organisms into the blood stream. The patient is extremely ill, with a swinging temperature and rapid pulse, and rigors are common. Detachment of fragments of clot with resulting pulmonary embolism is most likely to occur in the case of transverse sinus thrombosis with extension to the jugular vein. This event is indicated by a sudden pain in the chest, associated with dyspnoea and sometimes with haemoptysis, followed by the development of signs of pulmonary consolidation and frequently a pleural rub. Pulmonary abscess may follow. The commonest intracranial extension of the infection is to the leptomeninges, resulting in many cases in a diffuse leptomeningitis, characterized by an increase in the severity of the headache, the development of cervical rigidity, the presence of Kernig's sign and other symptoms of meningitis, together with a marked polymorphonuclear pleocytosis with or without organisms in the cerebrospinal fluid. In many cases, however, thrombophlebitis of cranial sinuses develops insidiously, or after the acute phase of the infection has passed.

DIAGNOSIS

Cavernous sinus thrombosis may occasionally be confused with other lesions in the neighbourhood of the superior orbital fissure. Similar local symptoms may be produced by aneurysm of the cavernous sinus following rupture into it of the internal carotid artery. This, however, as a rule follows trauma, of which a history is obtainable. Pulsation is present in the eye and a bruit is audible to the patient and often to the observer. Symptoms of infection are absent. Compression of the cavernous sinus by intracranial tumour is of gradual onset and is unassociated with symptoms of infection.

Thrombosis of the superior sagittal sinus, when it occurs in infancy, may be difficult to distinguish from other causes of hydrocephalus, to which it often gives rise. The selective paralysis of the lower limbs, when this is present, is the most useful distinctive feature. Examination of the cerebrospinal fluid will enable sinus thrombosis to be distinguished from meningitis.

Transverse sinus thrombosis may be difficult to distinguish from other intracranial complications of mastoiditis, especially extradural, subdural, and intracerebral abscess, with any of which it may coexist. When any of these conditions is suspected, however, the region of the transverse sinus should be explored and the dura and the sinus itself inspected.

PROGNOSIS

Modern chemotherapy has entirely changed the prognosis of infective thrombophlebitis, and recovery may now occur even from cavernous sinus thrombosis, formerly almost always fatal. The outlook is good in transverse sinus thrombosis treated by aural surgery combined with chemotherapy. Hydrocephalus due to thrombosis of the superior sagittal sinus usually responds to treatment. Cranial nerve palsies usually recover. Some permanent loss of function is likely to occur after cortical venous thrombosis and this may be followed by epilepsy as a late sequel. The mortality rate in thrombophlebitis of pregnancy is 33 per cent. and 19 per cent. of the survivors are left with permanent neurological deficits (Carroll, Leak, and Lee, 1966).

TREATMENT

When sinus thrombosis is infective in origin the source of infection must receive appropriate treatment. In the case of transverse sinus thrombosis the jugular vein occasionally needs to be ligatured as a safeguard against pyaemia.

Treatment consists of chemotherapy. The value of anticoagulants is debated: they are most likely to be useful if given in cases of primary thrombophlebitis before venous infarction has occurred. There appear to be no data on the risk that they may cause haemorrhage but in the presence of haemorrhagic infarction this is a real danger. Meningitis may call for appropriate treatment. Otherwise treatment is symptomatic. [For treatment of hydrocephalus see p. 213.]

REFERENCES

(The cerebral venous circulation, Thrombosis of the intracranial venous sinuses and veins.)

BAILEY, O. T., and HASS, G. M. (1937) Dural sinus thrombosis in early life, *Br ain*, **60** 293.

CARROLL, J. D., LEAK, D., and LEE, H. A. (1966) Cerebral thrombophlebitis in pregnancy and the puerperium, *Quart. J. Med.*, **35,** 347.

FRENCKNER, P. (1936) Sinography: a method of radiography in the diagnosis of sinus thrombosis, *Proc. roy. Soc. Med.*, **30,** 413.

HOLMES, G., and SARGENT, P. (1915) Injuries of the superior longitudinal sinus, *Brit. med. J.*, **2,** 493.

KALBAG, R. M., and WOOLF, A· L. (1967) *Cerebral Venous Thrombosis*, London.

LANGWORTHY, H. G. (1916) Anatomic relations of the cavernous sinus to other structures, with consideration of various pathologic processes by which it may become involved, *Ann. Otol. (St. Louis)*, **25,** 554.

MARTIN, J. P., and SHEEHAN, H. L. (1941) Primary thrombosis of cerebral veins (following childbirth), *Brit. med. J.*, **1,** 349.

SYMONDS, C. P. (1937) Hydrocephalic and focal cerebral symptoms in relation to thrombophlebitis of the dural sinuses and cerebral veins, *Brain*, **60,** 531.

SYMONDS, C. P. (1944) Venous thrombosis in the central nervous system, *Proc. roy. Soc. Med.*, **37,** 387.

WEILL, G. (1929) De la thrombo-phlébite du sinus caverneux, *Rev. Oto-neuro-ophtal.*, **7,** 737.

5

NON-PENETRATING INJURIES OF THE BRAIN

AETIOLOGY

DURING recent years head injuries have occurred with increasing frequency, owing to the high speed of modern life. In civil life most head injuries are due to direct violence resulting from motor and industrial accidents. Less frequently they are produced by indirect violence after falls on the feet or buttocks. Penetrating wounds of the brain are comparatively rare. There is no direct parallelism between the severity of an injury to the skull and the extent to which the brain is damaged. Though, naturally, severe fractures of the skull are associated with severe cerebral injury, the brain may be extensively damaged without the skull's being fractured and, on the other hand, fracture of the skull may occur without severe damage to the brain. Compound fractures of the skull, especially fractures involving the base and extending into the nasopharynx, nasal air sinuses, middle ear, and mastoid, assume additional importance as being liable to lead to infection of the intracranial contents and thus to cause meningitis or intracranial abscess. Apart from this risk, however, the crucial question after a head injury is the state of the brain rather than the state of the skull, and this alone will be considered here. For the physics of brain injury, and the characteristics of fractures of the skull and their treatment, see Gurdjian and Webster (1958) and Brock (1960).

PATHOLOGY

The factors operating upon the brain in head injury are multiple and complex, and their results are often equally so. As Gurdjian *et al.* (1966) recently put it, 'compression, acceleration, and deceleration may occur during the traumatic episode. Tissues are injured by compression, tension, and shear. All of these modes of injury may occur simultaneously or in succession in the same accident.' These factors and their effects on the brain are admirably described and discussed by Greenfield and Russell (1963) and by Tomlinson (1964).

Concussion

Concussion was defined by Trotter as 'a condition of widespread paralysis of the functions of the brain which comes on as an immediate consequence of a blow on the head, has a strong tendency to spontaneous recovery, and is not necessarily associated with any gross organic change in the brain substance.' Here the stress is upon reversibility of the process and in clinical terminology, concussion means a reversible impairment of consciousness of comparatively brief duration. It is now clear, however, that this cannot occur without damage to nerve cells and it is doubtful if any physiological or anatomical distinction should be drawn between concussion as just defined and more prolonged states of unconsciousness resulting from head injury. We know that consciousness is dependent upon the integrity of the ascending reticular alerting formation, and there is evidence that 'this system can be reversibly blocked by acceleration concussion' (Ward, 1966). The brain stem, attached above to the massive cerebral hemispheres and passing through an opening in the tentorium may well be especially vulnerable to brief displacements of the cranial contents. Large amounts of acetylcholine have been demonstrated in the cerebrospinal fluid in animals after experimental concussion (Bornstein, 1946) and after head injury in man (Tower and McEachern, 1949).

Cerebral Contusion

Cerebral contusion is a focal or diffuse disturbance of the brain following head injury and characterized by oedema and capillary haemorrhages and chromatolysis of cortical nerve cells. A number of recent workers have shown that in fatal cases of head injury multiple intracerebral haemorrhages are usually found. These are most frequently present at the poles of the hemi-spheres. Microscopical examination shows more widely scattered punctate haemorrhages and widespread cerebral oedema leading to distension of the perivascular sheaths and of the pericellular spaces. Disturbances in the circula-tion of the cerebrospinal fluid play an important part in the production of symptoms. The pressure of the fluid is usually raised but may be subnormal. In the former case there may be increased formation of fluid but diffuse brain oedema is more probably responsible; there may also be diminished absorption owing to blockage of the arachnoid villi by haemorrhage. Rand has shown that in severe cases of head injury changes which include oedema and increased vacuolation are present in the choroid plexuses and ependymal cells. In addition, the circulation of the fluid may be impeded by meningeal adhesions, and rupture of the arachnoid may lead to the formation of encysted subdural collections of fluid, subdural hygroma. Greenfield (1938–9) drew attention to the occurrence of localized severe demyelination which he considered a late result of oedema while Strich (1956) and more recently Tomlinson (1964) have drawn attention to the widespread degeneration of cerebral white matter which may follow severe closed head injury.

Cerebral Laceration

'Cerebral laceration' is the term used when a cerebral contusion is sufficiently severe to cause a visible breach in the continuity of the brain substance. This may occur either immediately beneath the site of the blow or by *contre-coup* on the opposite side of the brain.

Intracranial Haemorrhage

Traumatic intracranial haemorrhage may be either intracranial, subdural, or epidural. Acute subdural haemorrhage is usually the result of a severe lacera-tion, which may either involve the surface of the hemisphere or cause a large cavity filled with blood within its substance. Less often acute subdural haemor-rhage is due to rupture of venous tributaries of the superior sagittal sinus or to laceration of one of the venous sinuses. Epidural haemorrhage is usually due to laceration of the middle meningeal artery or vein by fractured bone, the posterior branches being involved more often than the anterior.

SYMPTOMS

Concussion

After a slight injury the patient may be merely dazed or unconscious for a few seconds only, but his higher mental functions may subsequently be impaired for a period lasting up to several hours, during which he may carry out complicated activities in an automatic fashion, afterwards remembering nothing of these events. This is the period of *post-traumatic amnesia* which is best measured from the injury to the time of the beginning of continuous awareness. This loss of memory may also extend to incidents which occurred before the accident, and is then known as *retrograde amnesia*. For example, a patient who sustains a head injury as a result of an aeroplane crash may remember nothing that happened after he left the ground; or one who has been injured in a motor accident may forget the incidents of a long drive (for further details see p. 981).

In cases of more severe injury unconsciousness is more prolonged, and in addition the patient exhibits impairment of the functions of the brain stem, especially of the medulla. The pupils may be dilated and may fail to react to light, and the cutaneous and tendon reflexes may be lost, the musculature being flaccid. The skin is pale, and bleeds little when injured. The blood pressure is low and the pulse is slow, or, in some cases, rapid and feeble, or imperceptible. Respiration may stop or may be shallow and sighing. Though death may occur in severe cases from medullary paralysis, it is probable that in most fatal cases cerebral contusion is present as well as concussion.

Recovery from concussion is manifested first in an improvement of visceral function; the volume of the pulse increases, respiration becomes deeper, and the pupils again react to light. Vomiting is common at this stage. On recovering consciousness the patient may be delirious, restless, and irritable, and almost always complains of headache. In cases of uncomplicated concussion, however, these symptoms, with the exception possibly of headache, usually disappear within a few days after the injury.

Traumatic Encephalopathy

Brain damage may occur in the absence of concussion. In most cases, however, the patient is rendered unconscious by the injury. In the most severe cases the depth of coma steadily increases, and the patient dies from medullary paralysis within a few hours of the receipt of the injury. In less severe cases the patient, after recovering from concussion, passes into a state of stupor or mental confusion. He is usually drowsy and presents the picture long known as 'cerebral irritation', but better described as traumatic delirium, lying in a flexed attitude, resenting interference, confused and disorientated when roused, and at times noisy and violent. This condition may last for days or even weeks with a corresponding duration of post-traumatic amnesia, and in favourable cases gradually passes away. Or the patient may remain in a state of stupor for many months. Symptoms of a focal lesion of the brain are usually absent, but focal convulsions, hemiparesis, or aphasia may follow a contusion involving the cortex; injury to the basal ganglia may cause mutism and extra-pyramidal syndromes, and damage to the midbrain may cause quadriplegia, tonic convulsions, and in less severe cases ocular palsies, diplopia, and nystagmus; other cranial nerve palsies may be present (see below); and diabetes insipidus is a rare complication.

Though a patient may recover rapidly and completely from a cerebral contusion, persistent disabling symptoms are extremely common. The three cardinal late symptoms are headache, giddiness, and mental disturbances, and they usually develop out of the symptoms of the acute stage. Headache tends to be severe and to occur in paroxysms which may last several hours, often against a background of continuous pain. It is brought on or exacerbated by activities such as stooping, sneezing, physical exertion, and excitement. When the headache is associated with a raised pressure of the cerebrospinal fluid it tends to be increased by lying and relieved by sitting. When the pressure of the fluid is low the reverse is the case. The giddiness is not usually a sense of rotation, but a feeling of instability, though transitory vertigo and staggering or sudden head movement are common.

The commonest mental symptoms are inability to concentrate, fatigability and impairment of memory, together with nervousness and anxiety. These are in fact symptoms of mild dementia of traumatic origin and all grades are encountered between the common milder cases and the less frequent more severe examples.

In the latter the patient passes from the initial stupor into a stage of profound disorientation and confusion with defects of perception and disorganization of speech, and then into a stage resembling Korsakow's psychosis with gross defects of memory for recent events and sometimes confabulation. The final picture depends on many factors, especially the psychological constitution of the patient. Residual mental inefficiency is not uncommon: severe dementia is uncommon but not as rare as has been suggested (Fahy, Irving, and Millac, 1967). Moods of excitement or depression are not infrequent in cyclothymic individuals while after severe head injury with prolonged unconsciousness paranoid and other psychotic manifestations have been reported (Fahy et al., 1967).

'Punch-drunkenness' is a chronic traumatic encephalopathy which may occur in professional boxers. It leads to deterioration of the personality, impairment of memory, dysarthria, tremor, and ataxia (Critchley, 1957; Neubuerger et al., 1959).

Acute Traumatic Cerebral Compression

Cerebral compression leads to progressively deepening unconsciousness, indicated by the failure of the patient to respond to stimuli which have previously been capable of rousing him, and by loss of corneal reflexes. Deepening coma is of special importance when it follows a lucid interval after concussion. Ocular symptoms are important, the pupil on the side of the haemorrhage being first contracted and later dilated and failing to react to light, the same sequence of events subsequently occurring on the opposite side (Hutchinson pupil). These signs are due to tentorial herniation causing pressure upon the trunk of one or both cranial nerves. Papilloedema is usually absent, though the optic discs and fundi may exhibit venous congestion. Symptoms of a progressive lesion of one cerebral hemisphere are frequently present. Focal convulsions indicate irritation of the motor cortex and may be produced either by a laceration or by compression following an extradural haemorrhage, especially from the anterior branches of the middle meningeal artery. Flaccid paralysis of one side of the body associated with a unilateral extensor plantar response indicates compression or laceration of the opposite hemisphere. Medullary symptoms are prominent, especially in the later stages of cerebral compression. The pulse at first is slow and full, later rapid, thready, and irregular. The blood pressure may be subnormal or may exhibit a steady rise. The respirations are at first slow and deep, later irregular, e.g. of the Cheyne-Stokes type, and finally rapid and shallow. The temperature is often somewhat raised. Sugar may be present in the urine.

Cranial Nerve Palsies

Cranial nerve palsies may be due to injury of the brain stem or of the nerves, either in their intracranial or in their extracranial course. Contusion of the mid-brain may leave permanent paresis of ocular movement, usually in the vertical plane, either unilaterally or bilaterally, resulting in diplopia and often associated with nystagmus. Intracranial injuries of the nerves are usually the result of fracture of the base of the skull. The seventh is the nerve most frequently affected and after that the eighth, sixth, second, third, and fourth in this order (Sherren, 1908). The olfactory nerves may be involved with or without fracture passing through the anterior fossa. The effects of injuries of these nerves are described in the sections dealing with the cranial nerves. The facial nerve, or its branches, and branches of the trigeminal may be divided or contused as a result of wounds and blows upon the face. Traumatic cranial nerve palsies are usually permanent, the only exceptions being those which are due to contusion rather than division of intracranial or extracranial nerve trunks.

Cerebrospinal Fluid

Examination of the cerebrospinal fluid may yield information of value, but lumbar puncture is not free from risk after head injury because of the risk of herniation of swollen brain. It should not be performed, therefore, as a routine, and not until the patient has recovered from the immediate effects of the accident; on the first occasion only sufficient fluid for diagnostic purposes should be withdrawn. Blood is present in the fluid immediately after the accident in most cases of cerebral contusion and of more serious injury. The number of red cells present is not always proportionate to the severity of the injury; the protein content of the fluid is proportionate to the number of red cells. The supernatant fluid is xanthochromic. The red cells tend to disappear in four or five days, but the xanthochromia may remain for two or three weeks. The pressure of the fluid should always be determined by manometry, with the patient lying on his side and as far as possible relaxed. In most cases of severe head injury the pressure of the fluid is raised and may be as high as 200 to 300 mm. of fluid. Exceptionally, the pressure is normal or subnormal. In cases of suspected progressive cerebral compression a progressive rise in the pressure of the fluid at successive lumbar punctures affords confirmatory evidence, but the pressure of the fluid must always be considered in relation to clinical observations. In the late stages of cerebral contusion, that is weeks or months after the injury, the pressure is above 200 mm. of fluid in about 50 per cent. of cases, but may be subnormal, a point of importance in determining the appropriate treatment.

Electroencephalography

Suppression of the normal frequencies, widespread abnormally slow waves, and outbursts of high voltage 2 to 3 per second waves are seen in the acute stage. In the chronic post-traumatic state generalized low voltage 2 to 7 per second waves sometimes seen in one or both temporal regions, are the rule and the disturbance is on the whole proportional to the severity of the injury and the persistence of symptoms (Williams, 1941 a and b). However, the EEG may be surprisingly normal after severe brain injury and is often disappointing in predicting which patients will and which will not develop post-traumatic epilepsy (Walton et al., 1964).

Radiography

Radiography during the acute stage may show an unsuspected fracture of the skull, which often proves of greater medico-legal than clinical importance. Sonoencephalography may show a space-occupying lesion. Angiography may demonstrate, and help to locate, an acute haematoma.

Variations from the normal encephalogram have been described in 80 per cent. of cases in the late stages. The commonest abnormality is a slight diffuse enlargement of the lateral ventricles. The shape of the cerebral ventricles may be abnormal [FIG. 62], and there is often an abnormality in the distribution of the air over the cerebral cortex. Air may fail to reach certain areas owing to meningeal adhesions.

Other Investigations

Inspection and palpation of the scalp and skull form part of the routine examination of cases of head injury, the presence of haematomas being noted and the bones carefully examined for depressed fracture. Bleeding from the nasopharynx and ears in the absence of external injury is an important sign of fracture of the base of the skull, and inquiry should always be made as to the discharge of cerebrospinal fluid, which may be recognized by its sugar content. The urinary output should as far as possible be measured from the beginning. Since the body chemistry readily becomes disordered (McLaurin, 1966) it is necessary to make regular determinations of the blood urea, sodium, potassium, chloride, and glucose, and the urinary glucose, sodium, potassium, chloride, and nitrogen.

DIAGNOSIS

Although in most cases the injury to the head is clearly the cause of the patient's symptoms, it is necessary to bear in mind the possibility that a

pre-existing illness, especially a cerebral vascular lesion, may have led to an accident
in which the head has been injured, in which case the symptoms may not be
due to the injury. When this source of confusion has been eliminated it is
necessary to decide the nature of the injury to the brain. If after a head injury
the patient remains unconscious more than a few minutes, or if after recovery
from the concussion he remains confused or exhibits other symptoms of cerebral
disturbance, the conclusion should be drawn that structural damage to the brain

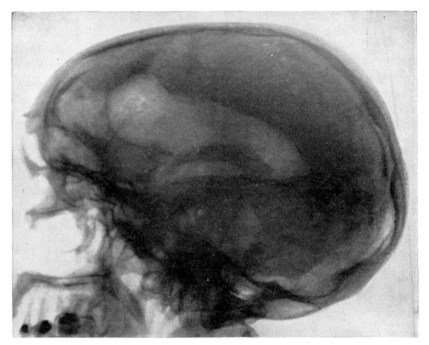

FIG. 62. Ventriculogram showing traction diverticulum in the left frontal region
following a fracture. (Radiogram by Dr. Jupe.)

has occurred, and this may be confirmed by the presence of blood in the cerebrospinal fluid. The symptoms which distinguish acute traumatic cerebral compression from cerebral contusion have already been described. The occurrence
of fat embolism of the brain in a patient already suffering from a head injury
may give rise to difficulty. The existence of a latent interval, pulmonary symptoms and signs, and cutaneous haemorrhages may enable the correct diagnosis
to be made. The onset of meningitis is to be suspected when the patient develops
marked cervical rigidity or Kernig's sign, and is confirmed by the presence of
a polymorphonuclear leucocytosis, with or without pyogenic organisms, in the
cerebrospinal fluid.

When mental confusion and drowsiness increase in severity, or persist for
several weeks, the possibility of subdural haematoma must be considered. When
this is present the symptoms tend to get worse with the passage of time, whereas
in contusion the early symptoms tend to improve. Progressive symptoms in the

later stages, therefore, whether general or focal, render further investigation advisable.

After recovery from the acute symptoms some would attempt to distinguish cerebral contusion from neurosis following the injury. This distinction is sometimes regarded as important in the litigation which frequently follows head injury. Difficulty arises from the facts that focal signs are usually absent in traumatic encephalopathy and that certain mental symptoms are common to both traumatic encephalopathy and anxiety neurosis. In practice it is difficult to make the distinction, and the attempt to do so is often unprofitable and undesirable. The patient must be regarded and treated as a psychophysiological unit.

PROGNOSIS

Concussion is rarely fatal and, when the patient survives the immediate effects of the injury, is followed by complete recovery within a few weeks or months, provided it is not severe or complicated by contusion or more serious injuries.

Traumatic encephalopathy, when severe, may prove fatal, usually within a few hours, from medullary paralysis. Less often the patient lingers in an unconscious condition indefinitely, and death then occurs from exhaustion or pneumonia. Death from traumatic encephalopathy, however, is exceptional—4·8 per cent. in Lewin's (1966 *a*) series of 7,000 patients with non-missile injuries admitted to hospital died. In those who recover from the immediate effects of the injury there are often symptoms, the persistence and disabling character of which appear to be disproportionate to the severity of the injury. Symonds (1928) investigated the outcome in a group of patients, excluding mild and quickly recovering cases. Ten per cent. were totally incapacitated, 43·5 per cent. were able to return to light work, and 46·5 per cent. were able to return to full work. When the patients were divided into two groups according to whether or not the injury had been followed by a stage of confusion, it was found that the prognosis with regard to working capacity was considerably worse in those who had exhibited such confusion than in those who had made a rapid recovery from the immediate effects of the injury. Miller and Stern (1965) reviewed the condition of 100 consecutive cases of severe head injury at a mean interval of 11 years. Approximately half were closed head injuries. Eight patients had died, 21 out of 25 with spastic pareses showed unexpectedly good recovery, 19 had developed epilepsy, 16 had persisting psychiatric symptoms of whom 10 had dementia.

Acute traumatic cerebral compression is fatal in many cases, the outlook being worse when the haemorrhage is subdural than when it is epidural. In most of Vance's cases death occurred within twenty-four hours. In a few the patients lived for from one to two weeks. Extradural haemorrhage is a neurosurgical emergency and although many patients survive and even recover if the clot is removed sufficiently early a significant proportion are left severely disabled.

Prophylactic chemotherapy has much reduced the incidence of meningitis, and lessened its dangers if it occurs. Late results of head injury, which include aphasia, persisting symptoms of injuries to the hypothalamus and midbrain (such as diplopia and diabetes insipidus), cranial nerve palsies, intracranial aerocele, cerebrospinal rhinorrhoea, subdural haematoma, and traumatic epilepsy, are described elsewhere.

TREATMENT

The usual treatment of the unconscious patient should be carried out [see p. 979]. If there is respiratory embarrassment this should be treated by suction or tracheostomy. Oxygen should be administered by nasal tube or tracheostomy catheter. Hypothermia should be used if necessary to control pyrexia and may be useful in other severe cases. Hyperosmolarity of the blood may be due to high dietary protein: if it is hypothalamic in origin it is best treated by forcing fluids or giving a mercurial diuretic. Convulsions, if severe, may need to be controlled by thiopentone. Traumatic cerebral oedema may respond well to intravenous urea but steroid drugs, e.g. dexamethasone, now seem preferable [see p. 263].

The broad outlines of rehabilitation are now well defined, and were set out by Jefferson (1942), Cairns (1942), Symonds (1942), Lewis (1942), and Goldstein (1942). It is essential to ascertain and take into account the personality of the patient before the accident. Explanation of symptoms and reassurance play an important part as soon as consciousness is regained. The present practice is to shorten the stay in bed and to let the patient get up for a short time when he has been free from headache for several days. During the last days in bed increasing mental activity and physical exercises are permitted. After getting up these are increased, beginning with walking, games and light exercises to music, and going on to more strenuous exercises. Supervised occupation should begin as early as possible and occupational therapy should gradually merge into therapeutic occupation. Throughout convalescence the patient's psychology must be kept constantly in mind. Psychological tests are of value for discovering specific disabilities, but the patient's emotional attitude to his difficulties is of equal importance, and explanation and encouragement are necessary throughout. During the later stages of convalescence the patient should be encouraged to go into a town, to the cinema, &c., to test his reactions to noise and bustle. In cases uncomplicated by focal lesions absence from work is likely to last from six weeks to eight months according to the severity of the injury. Persistent disabilities may make it impossible for him to return to his pre-accident occupation. Special disabilities, especially speech disturbances, require prolonged treatment by experts.

TRAUMATIC PNEUMOCEPHALUS

Synonym. Intracranial aerocele.

Definition. The presence of air within the skull as a result of head injury.

AETIOLOGY AND PATHOLOGY

Trauma is by far the commonest cause of the pathological presence of air within the skull, which is usually due to a fracture of the skull affording communication between an air-containing cranial cavity and the interior of the skull. This may occur as the result of a fracture which involves the frontal, ethmoidal, or sphenoidal sinuses or the mastoid air cells or, rarely, after operation on a nasal sinus. Occasionally, however, air enters the skull as a result of erosion of bone from within, for example by intracranial tumour [FIG. 45, p. 233], abscess, or hydrocephalus.

Within the cranial cavity the collection of air may be external to the brain. Both subdural and subarachnoid collections have been described, but as the arachnoid is often torn, it is difficult to discriminate these. The air sometimes penetrates one cerebral hemisphere, in which it becomes encysted.

SYMPTOMS

Cerebrospinal rhinorrhoea, a discharge of cerebrospinal fluid from the nose, is usually an accompaniment of traumatic pneumocephalus. It may, however, occur when the base of the skull is eroded from within by intracranial tumour, abscess, or internal hydrocephalus. The volume of the discharge is variable: it may be small or there may be enough to necessitate the use of a number of handkerchiefs. The discharge is usually influenced by change of posture and may occur, for example, only when the patient sits up. It often affords relief from headache and other symptoms. The presence of sugar in the fluid can be demonstrated by appropriate tests and is a useful diagnostic point. The presence of air within the skull may occasionally be demonstrated by means of a tympanitic note on percussion, more frequently by a succussion splash audible to the patient and to the observer on shaking the patient's head. This last symptom implies the presence of both air and fluid within the cranial cavity.

Air within the skull may lead to focal symptoms, especially when it has invaded one cerebral hemisphere. They may include mental confusion, convulsions, aphasia, hemiparesis, and a grasp reflex. They tend to fluctuate in severity and may be relieved by an attack of cerebrospinal rhinorrhoea. Symptoms of increased intracranial pressure, for example headache and papilloedema, may also be present. In severe cases coma may develop.

X-ray examination of the skull is the most valuable single method of diagnosis, the situation of the air being exactly demonstrated. When fluid is also present within the cavity it may be demarcated from the air by a horizontal line which varies in position in relation to gravity.

DIAGNOSIS

Diagnosis offers little difficulty. All cases of serious head injury should be X-rayed and the presence of air is demonstrated by the radiograms. Isotope ventriculography (R.I.S.A. scan) is valuable in localizing the point of leakage in cerebrospinal rhinorrhoea.

PROGNOSIS

Two factors influence the prognosis in traumatic pneumocephalus, the risks of a focal lesion of the brain associated with increased intracranial pressure and the risks of meningitis due to infection entering the skull through the opening in the bone.

Air in the ventricles and in the subarachnoid space is absorbed in from ten days to a fortnight. It is doubtful, however, whether absorption occurs when the air is encysted by brain tissue. The risk of infection is high and in the large majority of cases of head injury with cerebrospinal rhinorrhoea meningitis supervenes in the absence of operative interference.

TREATMENT

In order to diminish the risks both of further entry of air within the skull and of meningeal infection, the patient should be kept flat and should be told to avoid forcibly blowing his nose. Saline purges are contra-indicated owing to the risks attendant upon lowering the intracranial pressure. Prophylactic chemotherapy should be employed. In Lewin's view 'operative repair is the treatment of choice for all cases of paranasal sinus fracture with cerebral fluid rhinorrhoea, whether this is of early or late onset, of brief or long duration' (Lewin, 1966 b).

SUBDURAL HAEMATOMA

Synonym. Pachymeningitis interna haemorrhagica.

Definition. An encysted collection of blood between the dura mater and the arachnoid, sometimes traumatic, but also occurring in the absence of recognized injury.

PATHOLOGY

Acute subdural haematoma is common in fatal cases of head injury: an extensive but thin layer of haemorrhage may raise the intracranial pressure enough to cause herniation of the uncus, or midbrain haemorrhages.

In chronic subdural haematoma blood slowly accumulates in the subdural space. Its origin is uncertain, but it has been suggested that it is derived from rupture of a vein running from the cerebral cortex to a dural venous sinus. It is possible that the bleeding is maintained by the fact that the blood compresses the veins or venous sinuses, thus causing venous congestion, and by a vicious circle further haemorrhage. Russell and Cairns (1934) in four cases of metastatic carcinoma of the dura complicated by subdural haematoma attributed the bleeding to engorgement and rupture of the capillaries of the areolar layer. In most cases the collection of blood, which may attain a large size, lies over the frontal and parietal lobes, and in nearly half of all cases the haematoma is bilateral. Subdural bleeding in the posterior fossa is rare. The blood is encysted between an outer wall consisting of a layer of highly vascularized granulation tissue slightly adherent to the dura, and a thinner, inner wall of fibrous tissue with a single layer of mesothelium on the side next to the arachnoid. It is mostly fluid, though a coagulum may be present. Subdural hygroma is a collection of cerebrospinal fluid, which eventually becomes xanthochromic, and is indistinguishable before operation from a subdural haematoma.

AETIOLOGY

Males are affected more often than females in the ratio of three to one. Subdural haematoma may occur at any age. It is sometimes seen in infancy, when it has been attributed to birth injury, but is most common in the elderly.

Subdural effusions may, however, develop as a complication of meningitis in infancy. Trauma is the commonest cause. Other causes include chronic alcoholism, liver disease, neurosyphilis, streptococcal infections, blood diseases such as scurvy and thrombocytopenic purpura, treatment with anticoagulants, and carcinoma of the dura.

SYMPTOMS

The symptoms of subdural haematoma may follow an injury immediately. Alternatively there is a latent interval lasting weeks or months, less often more than a year, rarely of many years. During the latent interval the patient may be free from symptoms or may complain of symptoms suggestive of cerebral contusion. After the latent interval there is a gradual onset of headache, drowsiness, and, often, confusion: epilepsy is rare. These symptoms often fluctuate greatly in severity. As is usually the case when the brain is compressed from without, focal cerebral symptoms may be lacking or slight, considering the size of the haematoma. When present they are likely to consist of hemiparesis, with aphasia when the lesion is left-sided. The grasp reflex may be present. Papilloedema is often absent. Transient ocular paralysis may occur. Inequality of the pupils is often present, the larger pupil, together with slight ptosis, being found on the side of the haematoma. The cerebrospinal fluid is usually normal, but the protein may be increased, and the fluid may be xanthochromic. The pressure is usually raised but may be subnormal. There may be a pleocytosis.

In infants the onset occurs during the first year. Enlargement of the head may be the first abnormality to be noticed, but convulsions, irritability, and vomiting are common and pyrexia may be present. The head is found to be enlarged, with a bulging anterior fontanelle and frequently separation of the sutures. The veins of the scalp are often dilated. Papilloedema and retinal and subhyaloid haemorrhages are usually present, leading in the later stages to optic atrophy. The symptoms are therefore those of increased intracranial pressure with cortical irritation, and paralysis of the limbs is usually absent. The cerebrospinal fluid may be blood stained or xanthochromic with considerable excess of protein, and is rarely normal. The diagnosis is established by subdural puncture, carried out at the lateral margin of the anterior fontanelle, xanthochromic or blood-stained fluid being withdrawn from the subdural space.

DIAGNOSIS

The diagnosis of subdural haematoma offers little difficulty when there is a clear history of recent head injury. In the absence of this the signs of a progressive focal lesion may simulate an intracranial tumour, especially when papilloedema is present. The fluctuating character of the drowsiness and confusion, however, may suggest the true diagnosis. In an elderly patient with a history of head injury it may be difficult to distinguish subdural haematoma from a vascular lesion of the brain due to cerebral arteriosclerosis. Chronic alcoholism in its later stages may lead to confusion and drowsiness, and, since it is a predisposing cause of subdural haematoma, and may also lead to accidents which involve head injury may give rise to difficulties in diagnosis. Angiography shows a characteristic displacement of arteries, and ventriculography may demonstrate displacement of the ventricular system to the opposite side. Calcification has occasionally been observed radiographically in a haematoma of very long standing, and Bull (1951) has shown that the floor of the middle fossa may be excavated. The EEG may be helpful. In doubtful cases exploration is necessary.

PROGNOSIS

The prognosis of subdural haematoma is good, provided the diagnosis is made sufficiently early, for operation to be performed before the patient's general condition has seriously deteriorated. In such cases complete recovery is the rule. In other cases, however, the patient fails to respond to drainage of the haematoma. Echlin, Sordillo, and Garvey (1956) report a mortality rate of 39 per cent. in 300 cases. McKissock, Richardson, and Bloom (1960), dividing their cases into acute, subacute, and chronic had a mortality rate of 57 per cent. in the acute, 24 per cent. in the subacute, and 6 per cent. in the chronic group. The prognosis is worst in the aged.

TREATMENT

Treatment consists in the surgical evacuation of the blood clot. The fact that the haematoma is bilateral in nearly 50 per cent. of cases must always be borne in mind.

TRAUMATIC EPILEPSY

AETIOLOGY AND PATHOLOGY

Our knowledge of the factors influencing the development of epileptic attacks after head injury is mainly derived from observation of cases of gunshot wound of the head. Such injuries are not strictly comparable with the head injuries of civil life, since they include a much higher proportion of penetrating wounds and a much smaller proportion of cases of simple concussion and fracture of the base of the skull.

The frequency with which epilepsy follows head injury has been variously estimated at from $4\frac{1}{2}$ per cent. (Sargent) to 25 per cent. (Rawling), 34 per cent. (Ascroft, 1941), and 36 per cent. (Watson, 1947) of cases of gunshot wound of the head. Probably under 5 per cent. represents the average incidence in civil life.

The latent period between the injury and the onset of fits is extremely variable. In a small proportion of cases fits occur immediately after the injury. These usually cease, and if convulsions subsequently develop they do so only after an interval of freedom. There is some evidence (Whitty, 1947; Jennett, 1965) that early attacks predispose to late ones. Apart from these early attacks, attacks may develop within a month or two of the injury, or they may be delayed for many years. A patient of mine, with a retained metallic foreign body, had his first attack twenty-seven years after being wounded. The commonest time of onset is between six and twelve months after the injury (Watson), but figures vary. Jennett (1965) found that half the patients had their first attack within a year of the injury. In Wagstaffe's series (1928) the average interval was about two years. Certainly the majority who become epileptic do so within two years (Miller and Stern, 1965).

The severity of the injury is important in relation to the likelihood of the development of convulsions. Wagstaffe found that when the injury caused penetration of the dura the incidence of epilepsy was 18 per cent., whereas in all cases of less severe injury it was only 2 per cent. This fact acquires significance from Foerster and Penfield's observation (1930) of the part played by scar tissue in the aetiology of traumatic epilepsy. It would appear that epilepsy is most likely to occur when vascularized scar tissue unites the surface of the brain to the dura, and this is obviously most likely to occur when the dura has been penetrated. Jennett (1965) found that late epilepsy was commoner in patients with depressed fracture and that, except in children, it was rare with a duration of post-traumatic amnesia of less than 24 hours. A family history of epilepsy is some-times present, so it is probable that inherited predisposition plays a part in the aetiology of traumatic epilepsy in some cases. The site of the injury in the hemisphere is relatively unimportant, but posterior frontal and parietal lesions seem the most likely to cause epilepsy (Watson, 1947; Russell, 1947).

SYMPTOMS

Traumatic epileptic attacks may be focal or generalized. Focal attacks often occur immediately after the injury. Their character and the nature of the aura, if any, depends upon the situation of the lesion. Even when the early attacks are focal there is a tendency for generalized attacks to occur as time goes on. Patients may also suffer from minor attacks. For the character of these various forms of attack the reader is referred to the section on epilepsy. When the injury has involved the substance of the cerebral hemisphere, corresponding symptoms are likely to be present, and these may be intensified for a short time after each attack. Radiography, especially encephalography, is often of diagnostic value, since air may fail to reach the area of cortex adherent to the dura and it may be possible to demonstrate a 'traction diverticulum', the lateral ventricle being drawn towards the lesion by atrophy of the white matter and by the scar [FIG. 62]. The electroencephalogram may be normal between the attacks (Walter, 1938).

DIAGNOSIS

For the diagnosis of epilepsy see page 935. The traumatic origin of the convulsions can usually only be established when there is a history of injury, and this should be especially inquired for, since the patient may not realize its importance when the attacks do not begin until several years later. It must be remembered that a previous head injury is not necessarily the cause of the attacks, but its aetiological significance is reinforced if the fits have a focal onset, if there are persistent signs of a focal cerebral lesion, and if the radiographic abnormalities already described are present.

PROGNOSIS

The factors which influence the prognosis of idiopathic epilepsy apply equally to traumatic cases, but it appears that when a gross focal lesion of the brain is present the prognosis as to recovery is worse than in epilepsy not thus complicated. The attacks ceased in one-third of Ascroft's cases. The prognosis is best when they begin within two weeks of the injury, worst when the latent interval is over two years.

TREATMENT

Patients with traumatic epilepsy should receive medical treatment on the same lines as cases of idiopathic epilepsy. Only when this fails to yield satisfactory results should operation be considered. The surgical treatment of traumatic epilepsy has been carried out for many years, but has fallen into comparative disrepute. It was revived by Foerster and Penfield (1930) and Penfield and Erickson (1941) claimed good results in selected cases. If it is to be successful the presence of a focal lesion of the brain must be established by the methods already described, and it should be possible to find electrocortico-graphic abnormalities on the exposed cortex in the affected area. Treatment consists in a free excision of the scar tissue.

Other sequels of head injury, which are described in their respective sections, are meningitis, intracranial abscess, diabetes insipidus, and a Parkinsonian syndrome.

REFERENCES

ASCROFT, P. B. (1941) Traumatic epilepsy after gunshot wounds of the head, *Brit. med. J.*, 1, 739.

BIELSCHOWSKY, P. (1928) Störungen des Liquorsystems bei Schädeltraumen, *Z. ges. Neurol. Psychiat.*, 117, 55.

BORNSTEIN, M. B. (1946) Presence and action of acetylcholine in experimental brain trauma, *J. Neurophysiol*, 9, 349.

BROCK, S. (1960) *Injuries of the Brain and Spinal Cord*, London.

BULL, J. W. D. (1951) Diagnostic radiology, in *Modern Trends in Neurology*, 1st series, ed. FEILING, A., London.

CAIRNS, H. (1937) Injuries of the frontal and ethmoidal sinuses with special reference to cerebrospinal rhinorrhoea and aerocele, *J. Laryng.*, 52, 589.

CAIRNS, H. (1941–2) Rehabilitation after injuries to the central nervous system, *Proc. roy. Soc. Med.*, 35, 299.

CRITCHLEY, M. (1957) Medical aspects of boxing, *Brit. med. J.*, 1, 357.

DANDY, W. E. (1925) Pneumocephalus (intracranial pneumatocele or aerocele), *Arch. Surg. (Chicago)*, 12, 949.

DENNY-BROWN, D., and RUSSELL, W. R. (1941) Experimental cerebral concussion, *Brain*, 64, 93.

ECHLIN, F. A., SORDILLO, S. V. R., and GARVEY, T. Q. (1956) Acute, subacute and chronic subdural haematoma, *J. Amer. med. Ass.*, 161, 1345.

FAHY, T. J., IRVING, M. H., and MILLAC, P. (1967) Severe head injuries, *Lancet*, ii, 475.

FOERSTER, O., and PENFIELD, W. (1930) The structural basis of traumatic epilepsy and results of radical operation, *Brain*, 53, 99.

GOLDSTEIN, K. (1942) *After-effects of Brain Injuries in War*, London.

GREENFIELD, J. G. (1938–9) Some observations on cerebral injuries, *Proc. roy. Soc. Med.*, 32, 45.

GREENFIELD, J. G., and RUSSELL, D. S. (1963) Traumatic lesions of the central and peripheral nervous systems, in *Greenfield's Neuropathology*, ed. BLACKWOOD, W., McMENEMEY, W. H., MEYER, A., NORMAN, R. M., and RUSSELL, D. S., 2nd ed., p. 441, London.

GURDJIAN, E. S., LISSNER, H. R., HODGSON, V. R., and PATRICK, L. M. (1966) Mechanism of head injury, in *Clinical Neurosurgery*, p. 112, Baltimore.

GURDJIAN, E. S., and WEBSTER, J. E. (1958) *Head Injuries*, London.

HUNT, F. C. (1930) Internal hemorrhagic pachymeningitis in young children, *Amer. J. Dis. Child.*, **39**, 84.

JEFFERSON, G. (1941–2) Rehabilitation after injuries to the central nervous system, *Proc. roy. Soc. Med.*, **35**, 295.

JENNETT, W. B. (1965) Predicting epilepsy after blunt head injury, *Brit. med. J.*, **1**, 1215.

KAPLAN, A. (1931) Chronic subdural haematoma: a study of eight cases with special reference to the state of the pupil, *Brain*, **54**, 430.

LEWIN, W. (1966 a) Nonsurgical treatment of patients with head injuries, in *Clinical Neurosurgery*, p. 75, Baltimore.

LEWIN, W. (1966 b) Cerebrospinal fluid rhinorrhea in nonmissile head injuries, in *Clinical Neurosurgery*, p. 237, Baltimore.

LEWIS, A. (1941–2) Differential diagnosis and treatment of post-contusional states, *Proc. roy. Soc. Med.*, **35**, 607.

MCKISSOCK, W., RICHARDSON, A., and BLOOM, W. H. (1960) Subdural haematoma, *Lancet*, i, 1365.

MCLAURIN, R. M. (1966) Metabolic changes accompanying head injury, in *Clinical Neurosurgery*, p. 143, Baltimore.

MILLER, H., and STERN, G. (1965) The long-term prognosis of severe head injury, *Lancet*, i, 225.

NEUBUERGER, K. T., SINTON, D. W., and DENST, J. (1959) Cerebral atrophy associated with boxing, *Arch. Neurol. Psychiat. (Chicago)*, **81**, 403.

PENFIELD, W., and ERICKSON, T. C. (1941) *Epilepsy and Cerebral Localization*, London.

RAND, C. W. (1930) Traumatic pneumocephalus, *Arch. Surg. (Chicago)*, **20**, 935.

RAND, C. W. (1931) Histologic studies of the brain in cases of fatal injury to the head, *Arch. Surg. (Chicago)*, **22**, 738.

RAND, C. W., and COURVILLE, C. B. (1936) Histologic studies of the brain in cases of fatal injury to the head, *Arch. Neurol. Psychiat. (Chicago)*, **36**, 1277.

ROWBOTHAM, G. F. (1964) *Acute Injuries of the Head*, 4th ed., Edinburgh.

RUSSELL, D. S., and CAIRNS, H. (1934) Subdural false membrane or haematoma (pachymeningitis interna haemorrhagica) in carcinomatosis and sarcomatosis of the dura mater, *Brain*, **57**, 32.

RUSSELL, W. R. (1947) The anatomy of traumatic epilepsy, *Brain*, **70**, 225.

SHERREN, J. (1908) *Injuries of Nerves and Their Treatment*, London.

SHERWOOD, D. (1930) Chronic subdural hematoma in infants, *Amer. J. Dis. Child.*, **39**, 980.

STRICH, S. J. (1956) Diffuse degeneration of the cerebral white matter in severe dementia following head injury, *J. Neurol. Psychiat.*, **19**, 163.

SYMONDS, C. P. (1928) The differential diagnosis and treatment of cerebral states consequent upon head injuries, *Brit. med. J.*, **2**, 829.

SYMONDS, C. P. (1936–7) Mental disorder following head injury, *Proc. roy. Soc. Med.*, **30**, 1081.

SYMONDS, C. P. (1941–2) Rehabilitation after injuries to the central nervous system, *Proc. roy. Soc. Med.*, **35**, 601.

SYMONDS, C. P. (1960) Concussion and contusion of the brain and their sequelae, in *Injuries of the Brain and Spinal Cord*, ed. BROCK, S., p. 69, London.

TOMLINSON, B. E. (1964) Pathology, in *Acute Injuries of the Head*, 4th ed., ed. ROWBOTHAM, G. F., Edinburgh.

TOWER, D. B., and MCEACHERN, D. (1949) Acetylcholine and neuronal activity; cholinesterase patterns and acetylcholine in cerebrospinal fluids of patients with craniocerebral trauma, *Canad. J. Res.*, **27**, 105.

WAGSTAFFE, W. W. (1928) The incidence of traumatic epilepsy after gunshot wounds of the head, *Lancet*, ii, 861.

WALTER, W. G. (1938) The technique and applications of electro-encephalography, *J. Neurol. Psychiat.*, N.S. **1**, 359.

WALTON, J. N., BARWICK, D. D., and LONGLEY, B. P. (1964) The electroencephalogram in brain injury, in *Acute Injuries of the Head*, 4th ed., ed. ROWBOTHAM, G. F., Edinburgh.

WARD, A. A. (1966) The physiology of concussion, in *Clinical Neurosurgery*, p. 95, Baltimore.

WATSON, C. W. (1947) The incidence of epilepsy following craniocerebral injury, *Res. Publ. Ass. nerv. ment. Dis.*, **26**, 516.

WHITTY, C. W. M. (1947) Early traumatic epilepsy, *Brain*, **70**, 416.

WILLIAMS, D. (1941*a*) The EEG. in acute head injuries, *J. Neurol. Psychiat.*, N.S. **4**, 107.

WILLIAMS, D. (1941*b*) The EEG. in chronic post-traumatic states, *J. Neurol. Psychiat.*, N.S. **4**, 131.

INTRACRANIAL BIRTH INJURIES

AETIOLOGY AND PATHOLOGY

Normal labour involves considerable compression of the foetal head and probably in many cases slight intracranial damage, as is indicated by the presence of red blood cells in the cerebrospinal fluid in a proportion of normal newly-born infants. It is not surprising, therefore, that serious intracranial injury may result from excessive or otherwise abnormal compression due to abnormal presentations or contracted pelvis. The most serious intracranial birth injuries are tears of the dura involving rupture of important venous sinuses. As Holland (1922 *a* and *b*) has shown, the most important aetiological factor is excessive longitudinal stress leading to abnormal tension on the falx, which is anchored postero-inferiorly to the tentorium, as a result of which the tentorium may be torn or the cerebral vein ruptured. Large basal haemorrhages occur in such cases. In Holland's series of 167 fresh foetuses the tentorium was torn in 81 (48 per cent.) and the falx in 5. Subdural haemorrhages occurred in all but 6. Over-riding of the parietal bones may lead to rupture of the superior sagittal sinus or of one or more of its venous tributaries, with the production of a supracortical subdural haemorrhage, which is usually confined to, or predominates upon, one side. Abnormal longitudinal stress is most likely to occur in breech presentations, which are, therefore, fraught with special danger to the child. In such presentations, moreover, the thorax may be subjected to considerable compression, thus leading to intracranial venous congestion, oedema, and petechial haemorrhages. Prematurity appears to predispose to intracranial haemorrhage, perhaps because the intracranial vessels are more delicate in the premature than in the full-term child. Bilateral subependymal haemorrhages may be found in the lateral ventricles and are commonly associated with severe asphyxia. The Schultze method of resuscitation has been blamed for dural tears. False porencephaly may be a later result of supracortical haemorrhage, and it is possible that some cases of congenital hydrocephalus may be late sequels of intracranial birth injury. Other vascular lesions may occur, however. Individual arteries may be compressed in the course of brain distortion. A fall in blood pressure may lead to ischaemia of boundary zones between two arterial territories, and compression of the great cerebral vein may occur (Norman, Urich, and McMenemey, 1957; Norman, 1963). Results of birth injury include ulegyria (atrophic sclerosis), cavitation of the centrum semiovale, and *état marbré* of the basal ganglia.

SYMPTOMS

After a severe intracranial haemorrhage the child may be stillborn. If it is living it is likely to exhibit 'white asphyxia' due to medullary paralysis. If it recovers from this, it may be cyanosed, breathing slowly and irregularly. The pulse may be slow or rapid and feeble. The child cries feebly and is difficult to feed. Generalized rigidity with head retraction is common, and local or general convulsions may occur. A supracortical haemorrhage is likely to lead to hemiplegia. Papilloedema and retinal haemorrhages may be present, and in some cases exophthalmos, inequality of the pupils, squint, and nystagmus occur. The fontanelles may be bulging and non-pulsating. The cerebrospinal fluid is likely to be blood stained and under increased pressure, and when the haemorrhage is supracortical it may be possible to withdraw blood by subdural puncture at the lateral angle of the anterior fontanelle.

In some cases the signs of injury are absent at birth but develop gradually in the course of the first four or five days.

DIAGNOSIS

There is usually little doubt about the diagnosis, though occasionally intracranial injury may be suspected in a child suffering from congenital diplegia. In the latter condition, however, local or general microcephaly is not uncommon; the fontanelle will not bulge; and the cerebrospinal fluid is likely to be normal.

PROGNOSIS

In the majority of cases in which the symptoms are sufficiently severe to enable an intracranial birth injury to be diagnosed, death occurs, if not before or immediately after birth, within three or four days. Infants which survive may suffer from infantile hemiplegia, epilepsy, mental defect, or congenital hydrocephalus. Pachymeningitis interna haemorrhagica of infants is regarded by some as a sequel of intracranial birth injury. Congenital diplegia is probably only very rarely thus produced (Ingram, 1964).

TREATMENT

In mild cases lumbar puncture may be used to lower the intracranial pressure. In severe cases it probably does more harm than good. When the symptoms indicate the presence of a supracortical haemorrhage surgical treatment should be considered.

REFERENCES

BLANCO, L. V., and PAPERINI, H. (1926) Meningeal hemorrhage in the new-born, *J. Amer. med. Ass.*, **87,** 1261.

BYERS, R. K. (1920) Late effects of obstetrical injuries at various levels of the nervous system, *New Engl. J. Med.*, **203, 507.**

CHRISTENSEN, E., and MELCHIOR, J. (1967) *Cerebral Palsy, A Clinical and Neuropathological Study*, Clinics in Developmental Medicine, No. 25, London.

DAVISON, G., and SNAITH, L. M. (1964) Cerebral birth injury, in *Acute Injuries of the Head*, 4th ed., ed. ROWBOTHAM, G. F., Edinburgh.

FORD, F. R., CROTHERS, B., and PUTNAM, M. C. (1927) *Birth Injuries of the Central Nervous System*, London.

HOLLAND, E. (1922 *a*) *The Causation of Foetal Death*, Ministry of Health Reports, No. 7.

HOLLAND, E. (1922 *b*) Cranial stress in the foetus during labour and on the effects of excessive stress on the intracranial contents; with an analysis of eighty-one cases of torn tentorium cerebelli and subdural cerebral haemorrhage, *J. Obstet. Gynaec. Brit. Emp.*, **29,** 549.

INGRAM, T. T. S. (1964) *Paediatric Aspects of Cerebral Palsy*, Edinburgh.

IRVING, F. C. (1930) The obstetrical aspect of intracranial hemorrhage, *New Engl. J. Med.*, **203, 499.**

MUNRO, D. (1930) Symptomatology and immediate treatment of cranial and intracranial injury in the new-born, *New Engl. J. Med.*, **103,** 502.

NORMAN, R. M. (1963) Cerebral birth injury, in *Greenfield's Neuropathology*, ed. BLACKWOOD, W., McMENEMEY, W. H., MEYER, A., NORMAN, R. M., and RUSSELL, D. S., p. 382, London.

NORMAN, R. M., URICH, H., and McMENEMEY, W. H. (1957) Vascular mechanisms of birth injury, *Brain*, **80,** 49.

PATTEN, C. A., and ALPERS, B. J. (1932–3) Cerebral birth conditions with special reference to the factor of hemorrhage, *Amer. J. Psychiat.*, **12,** 751.

SCHWARTZ, P. (1965) Parturitional injury of the newborn as a cause of mental deficiency, in *Medical Aspects of Mental Retardation*, ed. CARTER, C. H., Springfield, Ill.

SHARPE, W. (1923) Intracranial hemorrhage in the new-born, *J. Amer. med. Ass.*, **81,** 620.

SHARPE, W., and MACLAIRE, A. S. (1925) Further observations of intracranial hemorrhage in the new-born, *Surg. Gynec. Obstet.*, **41,** 583.

6

DISEASES OF THE MENINGES

THE ANATOMY OF THE MENINGES

THE brain and spinal cord are covered by three membranes or meninges named, from without inwards, the dura mater, the arachnoid, and the pia mater.

The *dura mater* is thick and fibrous and serves as the internal periosteum of the bones of the skull, to which it is closely applied. The inner surface is covered with a layer of endothelial cells. Sheaths of dura mater extend outwards for a short distance as a covering for the cranial nerves as they pass through their respective foramina. Certain fibrous processes of the dura, or septa, partially separate the cranial cavity into compartments. These are the falx, the tentorium, the falx cerebelli, and the diaphragma sellae. The falx descends from the cranial vault in the midline lying between the cerebral hemispheres in the longitudinal fissure. It is attached anteriorly to the crista galli and posteriorly to the tentorium. At its superior attached border it splits into two layers to contain the superior sagittal sinus, and its lower free border similarly splits to contain the inferior sagittal sinus. The tentorium cerebelli forms a partition between the posterior and middle fossae of the skull, its free border surrounding the midbrain, and its attached border being fixed to the occipital and parietal bones and to the superior border of the petrous portion of the temporal bone. The posterior part of its attached border splits to enclose the transverse sinus, and the anterior part similarly encloses the superior petrosal sinus. The falx cerebelli lies in the midline between the tentorium and the internal occipital protuberance, to both of which it is attached, and its free border separates the cerebellar hemispheres posteriorly. The diaphragma sellae forms a roof to the sella turcica and contains an opening, through which passes the infundibulum.

The *pia mater* is a delicate membrane lined with endothelial cells, which intimately clothes the surface of the brain, dipping into the sulci.

The *arachnoid* is a similar membrane, lying between the dura mater and the pia mater and bridging over the sulci. The space between the arachnoid and the pia mater, which is known as the subarachnoid space, contains the cerebrospinal fluid. Its expansions are known as the subarachnoid cisterns. The cerebello-medullary cistern lies between the inferior surface of the cerebellum and the posterior surface of the medulla. The cisterna pontis, continuous with this, lies anteriorly to the pons and is continued upwards into the cisterna interpeduncularis. This in turn is continued forwards into a cistern lying in front of the optic chiasma—the cisterna chiasmatis. The subarachnoid space and its continuations into the substance of the nervous system—the perivascular spaces—have been described in the section on the cerebrospinal fluid [p. 118]. Between the dura mater and the arachnoid lies a potential space, the subdural space.

The spinal meninges are described in the section on the anatomy of the spinal cord [p. 620].

The dura mater is known as the pachymeninx, the arachnoid and the pia mater as the leptomeninges. Hence infection of the dura mater is described as pachymeningitis, and infection of the pia mater and arachnoid as leptomeningitis or simply as meningitis.

TUMOURS OF THE MENINGES

See Intracranial Tumour, page 214.

CALCIFICATION OF THE FALX

Calcification of the falx is usually discovered accidentally in the routine radiographic examination of the skull. It is best seen in postero-anterior radiograms as a well-defined linear opacity in the midline. The calcification is much less evident in lateral radiograms, in which it appears as scattered opaque flecks, most evident immediately above the crista galli and extending backwards for a variable distance. Little is known as to the cause of the calcification, but it appears to be of no pathological significance.

PACHYMENINGITIS

SYPHILITIC PACHYMENINGITIS

See section on Syphilis, pages 406–8.

PYOGENIC PACHYMENINGITIS

Infection of the dura mater with pyogenic organisms is usually secondary to pyogenic cranial osteitis. The symptoms and treatment are those of subdural abscess [p. 383].

PACHYMENINGITIS INTERNA HAEMORRHAGICA

See section on Subdural Haematoma, page 346.

ACUTE LEPTOMENINGITIS

Definition. Acute inflammation of the leptomeninges.

AETIOLOGY

Infection may reach the leptomeninges by the following routes:

1. *Direct spread from without.* This may occur as a result of fracture of the skull, either in the case of penetrating wounds of the cranial vault or fractures of the base, when organisms may spread to the meninges from the nasopharynx. In the latter case the fracture may be unsuspected until meningitis develops. Other external sources of meningitis are osteitis of the cranial bones, especially

mastoiditis, infection of the nasal air sinuses, especially the frontal sinus, and of the soft tissues of the scalp, and thrombophlebitis of the intracranial venous sinuses. Organisms may be introduced by lumbar puncture.

2. *Direct spread from within* may occur when the meninges are infected secondarily to an intracranial abscess of embolic origin or in tuberculous meningitis secondary to a cerebral tuberculoma.

3. *Infection through the blood stream.* In such cases meningitis follows bacteraemia. It may be the only or the principal manifestation of this, as in so-called 'primary' pneumococcal meningitis, meningococcal meningitis, acute lymphocytic choriomeningitis, and acute aseptic meningitis, or the infection of the meninges may be secondary to focal infection elsewhere in the body, for example, pneumonia, empyema, osteomyelitis, erysipelas, typhoid fever, &c., in which case the bacteraemia may or may not be associated with endocarditis due to the infecting organism. Tuberculous meningitis may thus be part of a general miliary dissemination of tuberculosis.

4. *Meningitis complicating encephalitis and myelitis.* Meningeal inflammation often plays a subordinate part in the picture of encephalitis or myelitis. Polio-myelitis is the best example of such a meningo-encephalomyelitis, and meningeal inflammation similarly occurs in herpes zoster. In such conditions meningeal symptoms may be prominent or slight, but the cerebrospinal fluid yields evidence of meningeal inflammation.

5. *Other forms of meningitis.* Subarachnoid haemorrhage excites an inflam-matory reaction in the leptomeninges, though organisms are absent. Toxic irritation of the meninges also plays a part in acute lead encephalopathy. The term 'serous meningitis' possesses no constant meaning. 'Meningism' occurs as a complication of acute infections, especially in childhood. Symptoms of meningeal irritation are associated with a rise in the pressure of the cerebrospinal fluid. This is secondary to dilution of the blood as a result of which the pressure of the cerebrospinal fluid is increased while its chloride and protein content fall.

Spinal meningitis, that is, meningitis arising in, and at first limited to, the spinal canal, is rare and is usually secondary to osteitis of the vertebral column.

The organisms commonly responsible for meningitis are the *Neisseria meningitidis*, *Diplococcus pneumoniae*, *Haemophilus influenzae*, *Listeria mono-cytogenes* (particularly in neonates), streptococcus, staphylococcus, *Escherichia coli*, all of which cause pyogenic meningitis; the *Mycobacterium tuberculosis*; and various viruses which cause 'lymphocytic meningitis'. Other organisms less frequently the cause of meningitis are *Salmonella typhosa*, *Bacillus anthracis*, *Brucella abortus*, *Pseudomonas aeruginosa*, leptospira and yeasts such as *Crypto-coccus neoformans* (*Torula histolytica*). Mixed infections may occur.

ACUTE PYOGENIC MENINGITIS
PATHOLOGY

Whatever the causative organism the pathological changes in acute pyogenic meningitis are similar in all cases. Whether the organism reaches the meninges by direct spread or through the blood stream, inflammation and its products become rapidly diffused through the whole subarachnoid space of the brain and spinal cord. The space between the pia mater and the arachnoid becomes filled with greenish-yellow pus, which may cover the whole cerebral cortex or may be occasionally confined to the sulci. In cases of cranial osteitis and cerebral abscess the pus may be most evident near the source of the infection. The cortical veins are congested, and the gyri are often flattened owing to internal hydrocephalus. Microscopically the leptomeninges show inflammatory infiltration which in the early stages consists wholly of polymorphonuclear cells, though in the later stages lymphocytes and plasma cells are present [FIG. 63]. The cerebral hemispheres show little change except for perivascular inflammatory infiltration of the cortex. In chronic posterior basic meningitis the inflammation is confined to the base

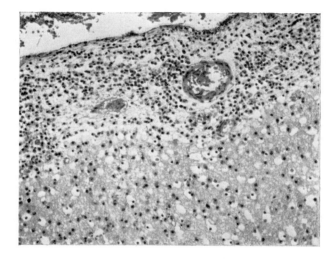

FIG. 63. Pyogenic meningitis

of the brain and consists of chronic thickening of the pia-arachnoid with adhesions, but little or no exudation. Internal hydrocephalus is a common and important complication of acute meningitis. It is most often due to inflammatory adhesions in the cerebellomedullary cistern, obstructing the outflow of cerebrospinal fluid from the fourth ventricle. Another factor in the production of hydrocephalus is the obstruction offered by the inflammatory exudate to the upward passage of the cerebrospinal fluid over the hemispheres, and impairment of its absorption by blockage of the arachnoid villi with inflammatory products. In meningitis the infection may spread to the optic nerves, causing true optic neuritis apart from the papilloedema due to raised intracranial pressure, and to the internal ear, sometimes causing permanent deafness. Other cranial nerves (the third, fourth, sixth, seventh, and eighth) are sometimes involved. Another important complication is endarteritis, particularly often seen in tuberculous and other chronic meningitides and this may give rise to cerebral infarction. Encephalomyelitis may occur as a complication of pyogenic meningitis either in the acute phase or as a late manifestation in a patient in whom the infection has not been completely eradicated by treatment.

SYMPTOMS

All forms of acute meningitis, whatever their cause, possess a number of symptoms in common. The onset may be fulminating, acute, or, less commonly, insidious. Headache, increasing in severity, is usually the initial symptom.

The general symptoms of an infection are usually conspicuous. Fever is the rule, though the degree of pyrexia varies. The temperature is usually between 100° and 102° F., though hyperpyrexia may occur, especially in the terminal stages. The pulse rate is also variable. It is sometimes slow in the early stages, for example between 50 and 60, but always rises as the disease progresses and at the end is usually very rapid and often irregular. The respiratory rate is usually slightly increased, and various forms of irregularity of respiration, especially Cheyne-Stokes breathing, occur in the later stages. Headache is a prominent symptom and is usually very severe, possessing a 'bursting' character. It may be diffuse or mainly frontal, and usually radiates down the neck and into the back, being associated with pain in the spine which radiates to the limbs, especially to the lower limbs. Vomiting may occur, especially in the early stages. Convulsions are common in children but rare in adults. The patient tends to lie in an attitude of general flexion, curled up under the bed-clothes and resenting interference. There may be a high-pitched 'meningeal' cry.

Signs of Meningeal Irritation

The following signs are of special value as indicating meningeal irritation.

Cervical Rigidity. Cervical rigidity is present at an early stage in almost every case of meningitis. It is elicited by the observer's placing his hand beneath the patient's occiput and endeavouring to cause passive flexion of the head so as to bring the chin towards the chest. In a normal individual this can be accomplished with ease and without pain. In meningitis there is a resistance due to spasm of the extensor muscles of the neck, and an attempt to overcome this causes pain.

Head Retraction. Head retraction [FIG. 64] is an extreme degree of cervical rigidity brought about by spasm of the extensor muscles, but it should be noted that cervical rigidity may be demonstrable by the observer before head retraction has developed. Flexion of the neck causes a rise in the tension of the cerebrospinal fluid in the cerebellomedullary cistern. When the meninges are inflamed this is painful, and cervical rigidity and head retraction are examples of reflex spasm of a protective character. Cervical rigidity is usually associated with some rigidity of the spine at lower levels.

Kernig's Sign. Kernig's sign, though slightly less frequently encountered in meningitis than cervical rigidity, is of a somewhat similar nature. An attempt to produce passive extension of the knee with the hip fully flexed evokes spasm of the hamstrings and causes pain. This procedure causes stretching of the spinal nerve roots passing to the lower limb and is painful when the lower end of the subarachnoid space of the spinal cord is distended and the leptomeninges are inflamed.

Other Signs

The mental state of the patient varies according to the stage and progress of the disease. Delirium is common in the early stages, but tends, when the disease is progressive, to give place to drowsiness and stupor, which is followed by coma. Photophobia is frequently present and there is a general hyperaesthesia to all forms of stimuli. The ocular fundi may be normal or may show venous congestion or papilloedema. The last is inconstant. The pupils are often unequal

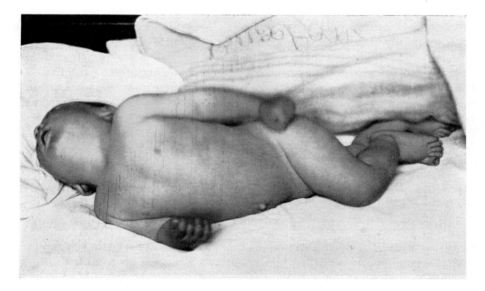

FIG. 64. Head retraction in meningococcal meningitis

and may react sluggishly. In the later stages they tend to be dilated and fixed. Ptosis is common, and squint and diplopia are often present. Any of the ocular muscles may be paralysed, most frequently one or both lateral recti. Facial paresis is not rare. Difficulty in swallowing may occur in the later stages. Muscular power in the limbs is usually well preserved, though slight incoordination and tremor are common and there is considerable muscular hypotonia. A general flaccid paralysis is a terminal event. The tendon reflexes are usually sluggish and often are soon lost; the abdominal reflexes also disappear early; the plantar reflexes are usually flexor at first, though later one or both may become extensor. Sensory loss does not usually occur. True paralysis of sphincter control occurs only late, but the mental state of the patient may lead to retention or incontinence of urine early in the illness and constipation is the rule. *Tache cérébrale* is often elicitable, but is not pathognomonic of meningitis.

Meningitis localized for a time to one hemisphere may cause Jacksonian convulsions, hemiparesis, and even hemianopia. The substance of the brain or spinal cord may be involved exceptionally.

The Cerebrospinal Fluid

The cerebrospinal fluid is under increased pressure. Its appearance depends upon the number of leucocytes present, and ranges from slight turbidity to frank purulence. When the fluid is turbid the deposit is yellow, and when macroscopic pus is present the supernatant fluid is frequently xanthochromic. The spontaneous formation of a fine coagulum is not uncommon. The cells are predominantly polymorphonuclear and these may be present in very large numbers, amounting to many thousands per mm.³ There is frequently a small proportion of large mononuclear cells. The protein is increased, and in frankly purulent fluids may reach a high level—0·5 per cent. or more. The chloride content of the fluid is reduced to 650–680 mg. per 100 ml. on an average. Glucose rapidly disappears from the fluid. Lange's colloidal gold curve is of the meningitic type. Organisms may be demonstrated in the films or on culture, but may be absent in cases of localized inflammation of the meninges. Filterable viruses require special methods to demonstrate them.

DIAGNOSIS

Acute pyogenic leptomeningitis must be distinguished from (1) general infections associated with toxaemia, especially those of which headache is a prominent symptom; (2) meningism; (3) acute cerebral infections, including various forms of encephalitis and intracranial abscess; (4) other forms of meningitis and meningeal irritation.

1. *Acute general infections* which most commonly simulate meningitis are influenza, pneumonia, typhoid fever, and acute rheumatism. These are distinguished from meningitis by the presence of the characteristic local and general symptoms of the infection and by the absence of signs of meningeal irritation, especially cervical rigidity and Kernig's sign. It must be remembered, however, that acute infections may lead to meningism or may be complicated by meningitis, and in either case signs of meningeal irritation will be present. When the diagnosis is in doubt, therefore, lumbar puncture should be performed.

2. *Meningism* is a state of meningeal irritation complicating acute infections. It is usually encountered in association with the acute specific fevers and pneumonia in childhood. Cervical rigidity and Kernig's sign are present, but the cerebrospinal fluid, though under increased pressure, is normal in composition except for a low chloride and protein content.

3. Symptoms of meningeal irritation may be present in the forms of *acute meningo-encephalomyelitis* in childhood and in *acute disseminated encephalomyelitis* complicating the specific fevers, and are almost constant in the early stages of *poliomyelitis*. The diagnosis of these disorders is based upon the presence of signs of involvement of the nervous system, especially the grey matter of the midbrain in meningo-encephalitis and of the corticospinal tracts in the various forms of acute disseminated encephalomyelitis. In acute poliomyelitis the stage of meningeal irritation precedes the development of atrophic paralysis. In meningo-encephalitis and acute disseminated encephalomyelitis the cerebrospinal fluid is not uncommonly normal, and when a leucocytosis is present the cells are mononuclear. In acute poliomyelitis the cerebrospinal fluid

contains an excess of cells, which during the first few days consist of both polymorphonuclear cells and lymphocytes. After the first week lymphocytes alone are found. The presence of large numbers of lymphocytes and of a normal glucose content of the fluid differentiates the condition from acute pyogenic leptomeningitis, and the normal glucose and chloride content distinguish it from tuberculous meningitis. *Intracranial abscess* may simulate meningitis when it gives rise to cervical rigidity, which, however, is usually not severe unless meningitis coexists. In cases of intracranial abscess the cerebrospinal fluid usually contains an excess of cells, though not often more than 100 per mm.³, the majority being lymphocytes. The protein may be disproportionately increased. The chloride and sugar content of the fluid are undiminished and organisms are absent.

4. *Subarachnoid haemorrhage*, since it leads to meningeal irritation, may closely simulate meningitis. Its onset, however, is usually more rapid, and the true diagnosis is readily established by the demonstration of blood in the cerebrospinal fluid. A localized meningitis, sometimes called *serous meningitis*, may occur as a complication of pyogenic infection in the neighbourhood of the meninges, especially of mastoiditis, subdural abscess, and intracranial thrombophlebitis. In such cases the cerebrospinal fluid is usually under increased pressure and exhibits a slight excess of cells, which may be either polymorphonuclear, mononuclear, or mixed. Organisms are absent. Some form of *virus meningitis* should be suspected in cases of meningitis of acute onset running a benign course and in which no focal source of the infection can be detected, and organisms cannot be demonstrated in the cerebrospinal fluid on repeated examination by ordinary methods. *Tuberculous meningitis* usually develops much more insidiously than meningitis due to pyogenic organisms, and symptoms of meningeal irritation, for example cervical rigidity and Kernig's sign, are often slight and may be absent. The cerebrospinal fluid contains an excess of cells, consisting usually of polymorphonuclear and mononuclear cells in varying proportions. The chloride content of the fluid is often subnormal and the glucose content is diminished, usually to between 10 and 40 mg. per 100 ml. Tubercle bacilli may be demonstrable in the fluid or on culture, and there is usually tuberculous infection elsewhere in the body. *Syphilitic meningitis* is occasionally sufficiently acute to lead to confusion with pyogenic meningitis. In such cases the cerebrospinal fluid contains an excess of cells which are usually mononuclear, but in the most acute cases polymorphonuclear cells may also be present. The Wassermann or V.D.R.L. reactions are usually positive in the fluid and also in the blood. A subacute or chronic picture of meningitis with an excess of cells in the cerebrospinal fluid may be due to *brucellosis, cysticercosis*, infection with *Cryptococcus neoformans, Behçet's disease, sarcoidosis*, or *carcinomatosis of the meninges*.

PROGNOSIS

The prognosis of acute pyogenic leptomeningitis depends upon the nature of the invading organism, the number of organisms present in the cerebrospinal fluid, the possibility of removing the source of infection, and the effectiveness of chemotherapy. The introduction of the sulphonamide group of drugs, which pass readily into the cerebrospinal fluid and exert a strong bacteriostatic action there, and of penicillin and streptomycin revolutionized the prognosis of many forms of meningitis. In the past pneumococcal meningitis was almost invariably fatal and streptococcal meningitis was fatal in more than 90 per cent. of cases. Recent work suggests that a recovery rate of 90 per cent. or over may be expected in cases of 'primary' pneumococcal meningitis and meningitis due to *H. influenzae*. In meningitis complicating surgical conditions the mortality rate is still likely to be between 20 and 30 per cent. In uncomplicated meningococcal meningitis treated early the mortality rate is not more than 5–10 per cent. Early and effective treatment of pyogenic meningitis should lead to recovery without residual symptoms. Deafness may be a sequel of meningococcal meningitis, and in any form of pyogenic meningitis permanent damage may lead to mental defect, epilepsy, blindness, or spastic weakness.

TREATMENT

See page 371.

SPECIAL FEATURES OF MENINGOCOCCAL MENINGITIS

AETIOLOGY

Neisseria meningitidis is usually obtainable from the secretions of the eyes, nose, and pharynx of both patients and 'carriers', and in the early stages of the infection it can often be isolated from the patient's blood. Meningococcal meningitis occurs both in epidemics and sporadically. It occurs in the tropics and temperate zone, in which the period of epidemic prevalence is the spring. Epidemics usually begin in December and reach their height in April and May, the number of cases thereafter diminishing, to cease in July. Sporadic cases occur at any time of year.

The disease, although contagious, is only slightly so, and it is exceptional for multiple cases to occur in a single household or for the infection to spread in hospital. The disease is spread by droplet infection, mainly through the agency of 'carriers'. These are usually individuals who have been in contact with a patient and who harbour the meningococcus in the nasopharynx for a period which usually lasts only two or three weeks. Such 'carriers', who greatly outnumber overt cases, may infect other persons without themselves developing the disease, or after a period of apparently good health may develop meningitis. The principal predisposing cause of epidemics is overcrowding, and the disease is thus specially prevalent among children who come into close contact with each other at school, and soldiers who are crowded together. There is some evidence that catarrhal disorders of the nose and throat predispose to the infection. Both sexes are affected with equal frequency, and the age of greatest susceptibility is from infancy to ten years, the highest incidence being in the first year of life. The disease is rare after the age of 40. The incubation period varies from one to seven days and is usually about four days.

The route by which the meningococci, having been implanted in the nasopharynx, reach the meninges is still unsettled. Probably they are carried by the blood stream, though direct spread along the lymphatics of the olfactory nerves cannot be excluded.

PATHOLOGY

The pathology of meningitis is described on page 357. In meningococcal infection the brain may be diffusely invaded, with congestion, oedema, perivascular haemorrhages, capillary thromboses, and acute degenerative changes in nerve cells, or there may be focal areas of encephalomyelitis. In the 'adrenal type', haemorrhage, thrombosis, or toxic or inflammatory changes are found in the adrenals.

SYMPTOMS

Several clinical types of infection are recognized, viz. (1) the average meningitic type, (2) the fulminating cerebral type, (3) the adrenal type, and (4) ameningitic meningococcal septicaemia. The symptoms of the average meningitic type are described on page 359.

The Skin

Several types of rash may occur, the most characteristic being a purpuric eruption which may take the form of petechiae, which are purple at first, fading to a brownish colour, and do not disappear on pressure. They are especially liable to occur on regions subjected to pressure. The purpuric patches may be larger, even reaching the size of half a crown, but these are found only in very severe cases. The purpuric eruption may appear during the first twenty-four hours and is usually present before the third day. It is seen in about one-third of all cases. A maculopapular rash is present somewhat less frequently, usually appearing before the fourth day, first on the trunk and later on the extensor surfaces of the thighs and forearms. Erythematous rashes may occur at any stage of the disease, and facial herpes febrilis appears in between 20 and 30 per cent. of cases.

The Blood

A well-marked leucocytosis occurs in the blood, with a predominant increase of the polymorphonuclear cells. Meningococci can sometimes be cultivated from the blood in the early stages, but rarely after the signs of meningitis have appeared.

The Cerebrospinal Fluid

The changes in the cerebrospinal fluid are those of pyogenic meningitis [see p. 361].

Meningococci can be demonstrated in the fluid in many cases but are often difficult to find. Usually they are present in smears made from the centrifuged deposit on the day of withdrawal. The majority of meningococci are usually intracellular, lying within the polymorphonuclear leucocytes. Some, however, are extracellular, and a large number of extracellular meningococci is believed to be indicative of a severe infection. If meningococci are not demonstrable on the first day they are usually to be found if the fluid is incubated for twenty-four hours or may be obtained from cultures.

It is desirable to examine the cerebrospinal fluid from the cerebral ventricles if internal hydrocephalus develops or if, in spite of improvement in the condition of the spinal fluid, symptoms of infection persist.

Other Symptoms

Slight cardiac dilatation may occur as a result of the toxaemia, the cardiac apex being displaced outwards and the apical first sound soft or muffled. Albuminuria may also occur as in other febrile conditions. A catarrhal inflammation of the upper respiratory tract is also common. Rapid flushing of the skin in response to a light scratch, the symptom known as *tache cérébrale*, is often present, but is not pathognomonic of meningitis.

Complications of Meningococcal Origin

The symptoms already described are those attributable to the meningitis and the bacteraemia which precedes it. We may describe as complications manifestations of the infection which are inconstant and in some instances rare.

Hydrocephalus. Hydrocephalus was once the most important complication of meningococcal meningitis but is now almost unknown. It usually develops late in the course of the disease, rarely during the first two weeks. Its onset is associated with an intensification of the headache, and with persistent vomiting. The mental condition of the patient deteriorates and he becomes drowsy and listless. Memory is impaired. The clinical picture is that of acquired hydrocephalus [see p. 209].

Other Nervous Complications. Symptoms due to invasion of the nervous system by the infection—focal encephalomyelitis—are uncommon. This should be suspected when delirium and restlessness persist in spite of treatment. Aphasia and hemiplegia are sometimes met with and indicate damage to the cerebral hemispheres, while lesions of the spinal cord may cause paraplegia or flaccid paralysis with wasting of a group of muscles. Peripheral neuritis, usually affecting the lower limbs, sometimes occurs.

Deafness. Deafness now occurs in under 5 per cent. of cases. It usually begins early in the illness and may be temporary, but is more often permanent, both ears being usually affected. It is due to involvement of the auditory nerve.

The Eye. Conjunctivitis is a fairly common complication. More severe ocular lesions, such as keratitis, iridochoroiditis, and pseudoglioma of the retina, are fortunately rare. Loss of vision as a result of internal hydrocephalus has been described.

The Heart. Fibrinopurulent pericarditis is a rare complication of severe cases. Bacterial endocarditis is even rarer. When this develops, embolism of the lungs or other parts of the body may occur.

Arthritis. This occurs in from 10 to 15 per cent. of cases in most epidemics. There is a purulent effusion into the joint, from which meningococci can occasionally be cultivated. The knee- and shoulder-joints are most frequently affected, but almost any joint may become involved.

Genito-urinary System. Febrile albuminuria is common. Rarely a true acute nephritis develops, often with haematuria. This is probably due to the meningococcal infection. Pyelitis and cystitis are also sometimes encountered. Epididymitis and orchitis are rare complications.

Non-Meningococcal Complications

Though pneumonia may very rarely be due to the meningococcus, it is more often the result of a secondary infection. Bronchopneumonia is the form usually encountered and is a serious complication. Infection of the urinary tract may occur, especially when frequent catheterization is necessary. It may be difficult to prevent the development of bed sores in very chronic cases.

Other Clinical Types

In the *fulminating cerebral type* the onset is sudden and the patient may rapidly become comatose. Death may occur in a few hours without signs of meningeal irritation and with a clear cerebrospinal fluid. In less acute cases there is slight cervical rigidity and the fluid is turbid and contains meningococci. The rash is purpuric but the patches are not usually large.

In the *adrenal type*—the Waterhouse–Friderichsen syndrome—the characteristic features are grave hypotension and cyanosis, with the biochemical changes characteristic of acute adrenal failure. There is a petechial rash with some larger purpuric elements. The mental condition may remain clear to the end as long as the infection remains bacteraemic and neither meningitis nor encephalitis develops.

Chronic Posterior Basic Meningitis. This is a chronic form of meningococcal meningitis occurring in infants, usually between the ages of 4 months and 2½ years. The onset is usually acute with fever, which, however, tends to subside at the end of the first week. Head retraction is usually well marked and may be associated with opisthotonos. Hydrocephalus develops early, and the later symptoms are similar to those already described under this heading.

Ameningitic Septicaemia. This is a rare but important form of the disease in which the patient suffers from septicaemia proved by blood culture to be due to the meningococcus and persisting in some cases for weeks without meningitis developing. Such cases may terminate in meningitis or recovery may even occur without any infection of the meninges. The characteristic symptoms are intermittent fever, joint pains, and a papular (rarely purpuric) rash. The diagnosis rests upon the blood culture.

PROPHYLAXIS

Since meningococcal meningitis is spread chiefly by droplet infection from carriers, hygienic measures should be taken to ensure adequate ventilation and to avoid overcrowding in institutions and communities exposed to infection. Beds in dormitories should be placed not less than 3 feet apart. The detection of carriers by swabbing the nasopharynx is impracticable on a large scale but may be of value in communities in which infection has occurred. A carrier should be isolated from children and young persons. A single dose of 2 G. of sulphadiazine is said to free carriers from the organism in twenty-four hours.

Sulphonamide has been given prophylactically and it is claimed that 1 G. of sulphadiazine given twice a day for two days to all exposed persons will bring an outbreak to an abrupt end (Kuhns *et al.*, 1943).

LISTERIAL MENINGITIS

Diffuse infection with *Listeria monocytogenes* may be found in aborted, premature, and stillborn children or in neonates dying soon after birth. Listerosis is, however, one of the commonest causes of pyogenic meningitis occurring within the first four weeks of life and cannot be differentiated from other forms of pyogenic meningitis except by culture of the organism, which is, however, readily mistaken for a diphtheroid bacillus. The organism is very sensitive to penicillin and to sulphonamides, chloramphenicol and erythromycin, so that prompt recognition of the condition in neonates is important, as is treatment of genital listerosis in the pregnant female, as treatment may prevent infection of the foetus.

TUBERCULOUS MENINGITIS

AETIOLOGY

Tuberculous meningitis has hitherto usually been regarded as part of a miliary dissemination of tubercle bacilli by the blood stream and this is certainly the commonest cause in children. Rich and McCordock (1933) and MacGregor and Green (1937), however, believe that in most if not in all cases the infection spreads to the meninges from a caseous focus in the brain in contact with either the subarachnoid space or the ventricles. The cerebral focus is infected via the blood stream from a focus, which in children is often in the mediastinal or mesenteric lymph nodes, but may be situated in the bones, joints, lungs, or genito-urinary tract. Tuberculous meningitis may follow an operation upon an infected bone or joint and is sometimes the sequel of one of the specific fevers, especially measles. There is sometimes a history of a fall or other injury. It most frequently occurs in children between the ages of 2 and 5. It is rare during the first year, but may occur at any age. In young children there is usually no history of previous tuberculous infection in the patient, but in Lincoln's (1947) series over 50 per cent. were known to be tuberculous, and the same author found tuberculous contacts in 57 per cent. In adults tuberculous meningitis is usually the terminal event of an illness due to a focal infection in the lungs or elsewhere.

In about one-quarter of all cases the infection used to be due to the bovine bacillus, in the remainder with the human bacillus (MacGregor and Green, 1937) but nowadays the human bacillus is almost always responsible.

PATHOLOGY

In acute cases, macroscopically, the brain is usually pale and the gyri are somewhat flattened. A yellowish gelatinous exudate is found matting together the leptomeninges at the base and extending along the lateral sulci. Miliary tubercles are visible on the leptomeninges, being most conspicuous along the vessels, especially the middle cerebral artery and its branches. Microscopically the tubercles consist of collections of round cells, chiefly mononuclear, often with central caseation [FIG. 65]. Giant cells are rare. The substance of the nervous system shows little inflammatory reaction but marked toxic degeneration of nerve cells. Older caseous tuberculous foci can usually be found in the brain. In some patients treated with streptomycin the basal exudate becomes intensely hard and 'woody', the large arteries passing through it show an arteritis and as a result infarction of the brain may occur (Smith and Daniel, 1947). Hydrocephalus may also develop.

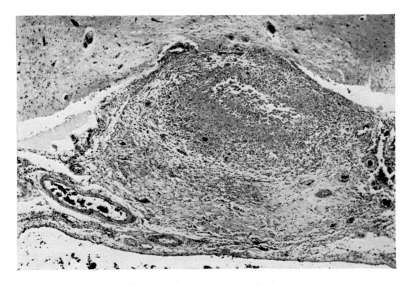

FIG. 65. Tuberculous meningitis

Tuberculous meningitis usually occurs during the active stage of the primary lesion, and in Lincoln's series nearly three-quarters of the patients showed radiological or post-mortem evidence of haematogenous dissemination.

SYMPTOMS

The onset of symptoms is insidious, and there is almost always a prodromal phase of vague ill health. In children lassitude, anorexia, loss of weight, and change of disposition are present. In adults mental changes may be conspicuous, and symptoms of a confusional psychosis may precede those of meningitis. This prodromal phase usually lasts two or three weeks, and is followed by the development of symptoms of meningeal irritation. The pulse, which was previously rapid, becomes slow and irregular. Fever, if previously absent, usually now appears but is rarely high. The temperature, which is often markedly irregular, does not usually rise much above 102° F. Headache and vomiting make their appearance and convulsions may occur. The patient becomes drowsy and at times delirious, but the occurrence of lucid intervals, even up to a late stage of the illness, is a characteristic feature. Signs of meningeal irritation are usually slighter than in pyogenic meningitis. There is usually slight cervical rigidity, but this may be absent and actual head retraction is rare. Kernig's sign is usually present. The patient frequently lies in a flexed attitude, resenting interference, and in the early stages often exhibits photophobia. Children sometimes utter what has been called a 'meningeal cry', a high-pitched scream.

Papilloedema is inconstant and when present develops only in the late stages of the illness. Choroidal tubercles are present in about 25 per cent. of patients and are visible ophthalmoscopically as rather ill-defined rounded or oval yellowish bodies about half the size of the disc. The pupils are usually contracted at first, but later become dilated and fixed. Moderate ptosis is common. Paralysis of any of the oculomotor nerves may occur, leading to strabismus and diplopia. There is frequently facial weakness on one or both sides, and dysphagia develops in the later stages. Voluntary power in the limbs is at first little impaired, though a coarse tremor is usually present on voluntary movement. Hemiplegia occurs in a minority of cases. In the late stages the limbs become paralysed and general extensor rigidity is common. The tendon reflexes are not infrequently diminished or lost in the lower limbs in the early stages, but become exaggerated when rigidity develops. The plantar reflexes, at first flexor, usually later become extensor. Retention of urine in the early stages later gives place to incontinence. Constipation is the rule at first; later faecal incontinence occurs. The *tache cérébrale* is common. The abdomen is retracted.

Tuberculous lesions are usually discoverable outside the nervous system. In one series radiography of the chest showed miliary dissemination in the lungs in 27 per cent., and enlarged hilar glands or active primary complex in 25 per cent.: 13 per cent. showed other lesions in lung, skin, or bone. The Mantoux test is positive in 85 per cent. of cases (Lincoln, 1947).

The Cerebrospinal Fluid

The cerebrospinal fluid is under increased pressure. It is clear, but a fine 'cobweb' clot frequently forms on standing. There is an increase in the number of cells, usually to the number of about 100 per mm.³ but varying from 10 to 1,000. These may be all mononuclear or a mixture of mononuclear and polymorphonuclear, the former predominating. There is a moderate increase in the protein, up to about 0·1–0·4 g. per 100 ml. The chloride content of the fluid is usually much reduced, on an average to 510 mg. per 100 ml. Very rarely, however, it is normal and it now seems that the chloride loss is simply an index of the severity of the vomiting which occurs in most cases. There is a diminution in the glucose content of the fluid, usually to below 50 mg. per 100 ml., and Lange's colloidal gold curve is of the meningitic type. The frequency with which tubercle bacilli are found in the fluid varies in the hands of different workers. Some report that they are almost invariably demonstrable: others find them less often. Consequently, though their presence clinches the diagnosis, their absence is of less significance. The organism should be cultured and its sensitivity to streptomycin tested; guinea-pig inoculation should be used in doubtful cases.

The bromide test, in which serum and cerebrospinal fluid bromide concentrations are measured after 3 days of oral bromide administration or a single intravenous dose of 2–4 G. in 10 ml. of sterile distilled water, is valuable in diagnosis, as in tuberculous meningitis the cerebrospinal fluid:serum ratio approaches unity, whereas in normal individuals it is about 1 : 3 (Taylor, Smith, and Hunter, 1954). The test is also positive in many cases of carcinomatosis of the meninges.

DIAGNOSIS

Now that we possess an effective method of treatment, early diagnosis is of the utmost importance. The general diagnosis of meningitis is discussed on page 361. Owing to the importance of the examination of the cerebrospinal fluid, lumbar puncture should be carried out without delay in any doubtful case, especially in any patient known to be tuberculous who develops symptoms or signs of meningitis. If a patient with meningitis is found to have a mononuclear pleocytosis in the cerebrospinal fluid with a glucose content below 50 mg. per 361 ml., and if no malignant cells are detected by cytological examination of a centrifuged deposit of the fluid, it is wise to treat him for tuberculous meningitis even though there may be no mycobacteria discoverable.

PROGNOSIS

Before the introduction of streptomycin and other antituberculous drugs, tuberculous meningitis was almost invariably fatal in from 1 to 4 weeks after the onset of meningeal symptoms, though recovery was very occasionally reported after tubercle bacilli had been demonstrated in the cerebrospinal fluid.

It is still too early to estimate what proportion of patients it may be possible to cure by means of modern treatment. Hitherto recoveries have been claimed in between 10 per cent. and 50 per cent. in different centres. Cairns and Taylor (1949) reported a fatality rate of 20 out of 49 patients, but recently a detailed review by Miller, Seal, and Taylor (1963) has shown that whereas up to 1952 a mortality of about 30 per cent. was usual, the introduction of isoniazid has transformed the situation so that nowadays over-all mortality should be less than 10 per cent. and recurrence after adequate treatment is rare. As might have been expected, the earlier the patient is submitted to treatment the better the prognosis, and it is generally agreed that when the patient is already comatose when first seen the outlook is almost hopeless. Apart from these, the treated disease may run one of several courses, though the reasons for these variations are not yet understood. In cases which are ultimately fatal the patient may show no response to treatment and deteriorate rapidly and die within the period expected of untreated cases, or there may be a slow progressive deterioration with no period of improvement. Others show a short initial period of improvement, followed by progressive deterioration, others again improve for so long that they appear to be going to recover, when they relapse and progressively deteriorate. Those who survive show an equal variability. Some improve uninterruptedly from the beginning; others only after an initial stationary or deteriorating period. Some recover in spite of a relapse, and some after a long period of deterioration remain in a stationary condition with evidence of gross cerebral lesions. Broadly, among patients treated early by modern methods the mortality-rate should be under 10 per cent. and of those who survive 70 per cent. should be free from sequelae.

THE TREATMENT OF MENINGITIS

The Choice of Chemotherapy

The appropriate treatment of meningitis depends upon the isolation of the organism and tests of its sensitivity to the various available chemotherapeutic agents. The chemotherapy of meningitis is a field in which, owing to the rapidity with which advances are being made, techniques have changed rapidly. This is particularly evident at the moment in the chemotherapy of tuberculous meningitis, where new developments may render older methods out of date. All that can be done in a textbook, therefore, is to provide an up-to-date summary of the methods which, at the time of writing, are generally regarded as the best. A valuable review is given by Garrod and O'Grady (1968) who point out that the policy of administering immediately 10,000 Units (6 mg.) of benzylpenicillin in 10 ml. saline intrathecally as soon as turbid fluid is found on lumbar puncture has much to commend it. Until a bacteriological diagnosis is made they now believe that ampicillin, 150 mg./kg. body weight per day, is the most satisfactory initial systemic treatment.

The principles involved in the specific treatment of meningitis are that the infecting organism shall be sensitive to the chemotherapeutic agent used, and that this shall be used in such a way as to reach the organism in sufficient strength. The application of these principles will be considered in relation to particular varieties of meningitis.

Pyogenic Meningitis other than Meningococcal

Some authorities believe that by giving massive systemic doses of chemo-therapeutic agents most cases of pyogenic meningitis, other than meningococcal, can be satisfactorily treated without intrathecal injections. This may often be true; nevertheless there are undoubtedly cases in which the response to a com-bination of intrathecal and systemic therapy is more rapid than that of systemic therapy alone, and others in which systemic therapy does not completely eradi-cate the infection which may smoulder on in the meninges and involve the substance of the brain or spinal cord. For these reasons there is much to be said for using both routes of administration at least initially.

When a tentative diagnosis of meningitis has been made no treatment should be given until a lumbar puncture has been performed, since the administration of antibiotics at that stage may make it impossible to identify the causal organism. The first step, therefore, is to carry out lumbar puncture, measuring the initial pressure of the cerebrospinal fluid. If the fluid is turbid it may be assumed that the meningitis is pyogenic. Ten ml. in two consecutive portions of 5 ml. each should be removed for examination and culture. Testing the sensitivity of the organism takes time and valuable time may be lost if treatment is delayed until this has been reported upon. If there is clinical evidence that the meningitis is meningo-coccal intrathecal medication may well be unnecessary but many authorities prefer to give a single initial injection of benzylpenicillin intrathecally if the fluid is cloudy, as soon as a sample for bacteriological examination has been obtained. In all other cases of pyogenic meningitis it is wise to begin treatment with an intrathecal injection of benzylpenicillin (penicillin G). The dose for an adult is 10,000 Units (6 mg.) mixed with 10 ml. of saline or of the patient's cerebrospinal fluid, that for a child being calculated in proportion to its weight; 600 mg. of penicillin should also be given intramuscularly. If the infection proves to be pneumococcal, treatment should be continued with four-hourly intramuscular injections of 1·2 G. of penicillin for an adult and daily intrathecal

CHOICE AND DOSAGE OF ANTIBIOTICS

Infecting organism	Antibiotic first choice	Dosage	Route
Meningococcus	Penicillin*	600 mg. 2-hourly	I.M.
	or erythromycin	500 mg. 4–8-hourly	I.V.
H. influenzae	Chloramphenicol	100–200 mg. per kg. of weight daily	I.M.
	or streptomycin	200 mg. per kg. of weight daily	I.M.
	with sulphadiazine		P.O.
	or ampicillin	150 mg. per kg. of weight daily	I.M.
Pneumococcus	Aqueous benzyl-penicillin	600 mg. 2-hourly	I.M.
	or ampicillin	250 mg.–1 G. 4-hourly	I.M.
Str. pyogenes	Penicillin	600 mg. 2-hourly	I.M.
	or chloramphenicol	100 mg. per kg. of weight daily	I.M.
		or 200 mg. per kg. daily	P.O.
	or ampicillin	250 mg.–1 G. 4-hourly	I.M.
Staph. aureus	Aqueous benzyl-penicillin	As for pneumococcus	
	or erythromycin	500 mg. 4–8-hourly	I.V.
	or chloramphenicol	100 mg. per kg. of weight daily	P.O.
	or ampicillin	250 mg.–1 G. 4-hourly	I.M.
E. coli	Streptomycin	40 mg. per kg. of weight daily	I.M.
		+5 mg. daily	I.Th.
	with sulphadiazine	to produce 10–15 mg. per 100 ml. in the blood	P.O.
	or chloramphenicol	As for Str. pyogenes	
	or ampicillin	250 mg.–1 G. 6-hourly	P.O.
Pseudomonas	Polymyxin	2·5 mg. per kg. of weight daily	I.M.
		+2·5 mg. daily	I.Th.
	or streptomycin	40 mg. per kg. of weight daily	I.M.
		+5 mg. daily	I.Th.
	with sulphadiazine	As for E. coli.	

* Sulphadiazine is sufficient for many cases of meningococcal meningitis.
I.V. = intravenously. I.M. = intramuscularly. I.Th. = intrathecally. P.O. = by mouth.
[Modified from Florey, M. E. (1960) The Clinical Application of Antibiotics, Vol. 4, London.]

injections of 10,000 Units (6 mg.) of benzylpenicillin should be given until the infection is well under control (usually for about 1 week). Streptococcal and staphylococcal infections should be treated in the same way, but substituting ampicillin or chloramphenicol, or another drug, for penicillin should the organism be penicillin-resistant. Ampicillin is given in four daily doses to a total of 150 mg./kg. a day. Chloramphenicol is given in quantities of 50 mg. per kilogramme every 24 hours intramuscularly in four divided doses. The intrathecal dose for adults is 3 to 5 mg. daily. Haemophilus influenzae infection should be treated by chloramphenicol intramuscularly and sulphonamides (e.g. sulphadiazine) may also be needed. The treatment of meningitis due to other organisms will depend upon their antibiotic sensitivity [see table above].

How often should intrathecal injections be given in the treatment of pyogenic meningitis? This depends entirely on the condition of the patient. Their chief use is to deal with fulminating infections and to increase the power of the antibiotic when a patient is not responding satisfactorily. They should not be used unnecessarily when all is going well. Among drugs which may be given intrathecally are benzylpenicillin, 10,000 Units (6 mg.) in 10 ml. saline, streptomycin, 5–10 mg., polymyxin, 10,000–50,000 Units, methicillin, 3–5 mg. for children and 10 mg. for adults, ampicillin, 3–5 mg. for children, 10–40 mg. for adults, and gentamicin, 1 mg. (Garrod and O'Grady, 1968). Systemic antibiotic therapy should be continued for at least 96 hours after the cerebrospinal fluid has become sterile and many authorities advise continuing treatment for as long as a week after all clinical evidence of infection has subsided.

In all cases of pyogenic meningitis other than meningococcal careful search should be made for a possible source of infection, especially in the ear and nasal sinuses, and if such is found the possibility of the coexistence of a cerebral abscess should be borne in mind. Arrest of improvement may be due to the development of hydrocephalus.

Meningococcal Meningitis

The meningococcus is sensitive to the sulphonamides and to penicillin, but the response to treatment with sulphonamides has been so good that some authorities give these alone. However, it is probably wise to give penicillin or one of its modern derivatives systemically as well. Sulphadiazine is the drug of choice. Treatment should begin with a loading dose of 6 G. for an adult, 3·5 G. for an adolescent, and 2 G. for an infant. One gramme is given four-hourly as a maintenance dose to an adult with proportionate reductions according to the age of the patient. If necessary part of the loading dose can be given intravenously or intramuscularly. During the administration ample fluids—4 pints daily for an adult—should be given to prevent urinary blockage, and it is also helpful to keep the urine alkaline. The cerebrospinal fluid should be examined at frequent intervals so that progress may be noted or relapse detected. Special measures may be called for to combat adrenal failure.

Tuberculous Meningitis

Each introduction of a new antibiotic effective against the tubercle bacillus has been followed by an improvement in recovery rate from tuberculous meningitis. The routine treatment, therefore, consists of the systemic administration of isoniazid and streptomycin in the following doses for an adult: isoniazid, 100 mg. thrice daily by mouth, and streptomycin, 1 G. daily by intramuscular injection. PAS is also given in a dosage of 18–20 G. daily. Even after clinical recovery treatment should probably be continued for six to twelve months. As in the case of pyogenic infections, some workers believe that tuberculous meningitis can be adequately treated without intrathecal injections. This is true in some cases, but there still appears to be a place for intrathecal injections, particularly in advanced cases and if a patient is not otherwise responding well. The intrathecal dose of streptomycin is from 20 to 50 mg. daily or every other day for ten injections. The routine administration of steroid drugs (e.g. prednisone,

40 mg. daily at first and later 30 mg. or 20 mg. daily) during the first few weeks probably helps to reduce complications such as adhesive arachnoiditis and communicating hydrocephalus and is now recommended in virtually all cases by most authorities. When a rise in cerebrospinal fluid protein and a fall in its pressure suggests that a spinal subarachnoid block is developing, an intrathecal dose of 10 to 25 mg. of hydrocortisone, repeated daily if necessary for a week, is often valuable. Pyridoxine in doses of 40 mg. daily should be given to prevent the development of isoniazid neuropathy, and anticonvulsants are needed in occasional cases. The development of hydrocephalus calls for surgical intervention and sometimes for the administration of streptomycin into the ventricles.

The main index of a good response to treatment is the disappearance of tubercle bacilli from the cerebrospinal fluid. In favourable cases these usually disappear within the first fortnight, but Cairns has reported a patient who recovered though the organism was present in the fluid sporadically up to the twenty-seventh day. Of the chemical constituents the glucose level is the most useful but is of little help after streptomycin has been given intrathecally. The protein content may rise considerably in response to treatment, and a high protein content with a falling cell count has been regarded as a good sign. A high cell count, mainly polymorphonuclear, may be a reaction to the streptomycin. Most patients develop some hydrocephalus, but this is usually compensatory and rarely of the obstructive form calling for surgical interference.

A relapse is indicated by a gradual or sudden deterioration in the condition of the patient who has previously been making good progress. Fever, vomiting, increase in headache, irritability, and apathy are the chief symptoms of a relapse, while the cerebrospinal fluid is likely to show a fall in the glucose content, a rising cell count, and a reappearance of the organism in films or cultures. This calls for a prolongation of intrathecal treatment, or a return to it if it has already been stopped. The development of resistance to streptomycin by the organism is fortunately rare. Details of treatment and of prognosis are given by Miller, Seal, and Taylor (1963).

Toxic effects of the streptomycin include vertigo, which is transitory, and possibly an ataxic gait in the convalescent, which also usually disappears after re-education. Deafness is a more serious complication, since when it occurs it is likely to be permanent.

After an illness involving many months in bed convalescence must necessarily be prolonged, and the after-care should be that of any form of chronic tuberculosis.

General Measures

Good nursing is of the utmost importance and in severe cases the long illness, often with relapses, and the need for repeated lumbar punctures, make heavy demands upon the skill and patience of the nurses. Nasal feeding or the administration of fluids by intravenous drip will be required when swallowing is difficult. Sedatives will usually be needed to control restlessness and in some cases convulsions. Ounsted (1951) stresses the importance of this and the dangers of status epilepticus. Phenobarbitone may be used prophylactically and Ounsted recommends for a child aged one year weighing 24 lb. an initial dose of 30 mg. of soluble phenobarbitone intramuscularly. Fifteen mg. six-hourly may be given thereafter for the next 36 hours by mouth or by injection, then 15 mg. twice daily for the remainder of the acute phase of the illness. Ounsted has found that phenobarbitone, chloral, and inhalant anaesthetics are useful for the actual treatment of convulsions occurring in meningitis and that paraldehyde is difficult to administer to infants and appeared to be relatively ineffective. He obtained the best results with intramuscular amylobarbitone sodium.

The abdomen should be examined daily for distension of the bladder.

REFERENCES

PYOGENIC MENINGITIS

ADAMS, R. D., and KUBIK, C. (1947) The effects of influenzal meningitis on the nervous system, N.Y. St. J. Med., 47, 2676.

BANKS, H. S. (1948) Meningococcosis, Lancet, ii, 635.

BANKS, H. S., and McCARTNEY, J. E. (1942) Meningococcal encephalitis, Lancet, i, 219.

BANKS, H. S., and McCARTNEY, J. E. (1943) Meningococcal adrenal syndromes and lesions, Lancet, i, 771.

EVANS, F. I. (1945) Infection from spinal analgesia, Lancet, i, 115.

GARROD, L. P., and O'GRADY, F. (1968) Bacterial meningitis, Chapter XIX in Antibiotic and Chemotherapy, Edinburgh.

HAGGERTY, R. J., and ZIAI, M. (1960) Acute bacterial meningitis in children, Pediatrics, 25, 742.

HARDING, J. W., and BRUNTON, G. B. (1962) Listeria monocytogenes meningitis in neonates, Lancet, ii, 484.

HOEPRICH, P. D. (1958) Infection due to Listeria monocytogenes, Medicine (Baltimore), 37, 142.

KREMER, M. (1945) Meningitis after spinal analgesia, Brit. med. J., 2, 309.

KUHNS, D. M., NELSON, C. T., FELDMAN, H. A., and KUHN, L. R. (1943) The prophylactic value of sulfadiazine in the control of meningococcic meningitis, J. Amer. med. Ass., 123, 335.

LONG, P. H. (1959) Use of antibiotics in central nervous infections, Res. Publ. Ass. nerv. ment. Dis., 37, 16.

McKENDRICK, G. D. W. (1954) Pyogenic meningitis, Lancet, ii, 510.

McKENDRICK, G. D. W. (1954) Pneumococcal meningitis, Lancet, ii, 512.

OUNSTED, C. (1951) Significance of convulsions in children with purulent meningitis, Lancet, i, 1245.

TUBERCULOUS MENINGITIS

ASHBY, M., and GRANT, H. (1955) Tuberculous meningitis treated with cortisone, Lancet, i, 65.

BULKELEY, W. C. M. (1953) Tuberculous meningitis treated with A.C.T.H. and isoniazid, Brit. med. J., 2, 1127.

CAIRNS, H. (1951) Neurosurgical methods in the treatment of tuberculous meningitis, Arch. Dis. Childh., 26, 373.

CAIRNS, H., SMITH, H. V., and VOLLUM, R. L. (1950) Tuberculous meningitis, J. Amer. med. Ass., 144, 92.

CAIRNS, H., and TAYLOR, M. (1949) Streptomycin in tuberculous meningitis, Lancet, i, 148.

CATHIE, I. A. B. (1949) Streptomycin-streptokinase treatment of tuberculous meningitis, Lancet, i, 441.

ILLINGWORTH, R. S., and WRIGHT, T. (1948) Tubercles of the choroid, Brit. med. J., 2, 365.

LANCET (1959) Treatment of tuberculous meningitis, i, 214.

LORBER, J. (1954) Isoniazid and streptomycin in tuberculous meningitis, Lancet, i, 1149.

Lorber, J. (1960) Treatment of tuberculous meningitis, *Brit. med. J.*, 1, 1309.

MacGregor, A. R., and Green, C. A. (1937) Tuberculosis of the central nervous system, with special reference to tuberculous meningitis, *J. Path. Bact.*, 45, 613.

Miller, F. J. W., Seal, R. M. E., and Taylor, M. D. (1963) *Tuberculosis in Children*, London.

Rich, A. R., and McCordock, H. A. (1933) The pathogenesis of tuberculous meningitis, *Bull. Johns Hopk. Hosp.*, 52, 5.

Smellie, J. M. (1954) The treatment of tuberculous meningitis without intrathecal therapy, *Lancet*, ii, 1091.

Smith, H. V., and Daniel, P. (1947) Some clinical and pathological aspects of tuberculosis of the central nervous system, *Tubercle (Lond.)*, 28, 64.

Smith, H. V., and Vollum, R. L. (1950) Effects of intrathecal tuberculin and streptomycin in tuberculous meningitis, *Lancet*, ii, 275.

Taylor, L. M., Smith, H. V., and Hunter, G. (1954) The blood-cerebrospinal fluid barrier to bromide in the diagnosis of tuberculous meningitis, *Lancet*, i, 700.

LEPTOSPIRAL MENINGITIS

Infection with either *Leptospira icterohaemorrhagica* or *Leptospira canicola* may manifest itself solely or mainly as a meningitis. *L. icterohaemorrhagica* is excreted in the urine of infected rats and is transmitted to human beings who come in contact with media contaminated by rats' urine. Fish-workers, coal-miners, sewer-workers, and farm-labourers are exposed to the risk of infection by their occupations. The other chief source is accidental immersion or bathing in contaminated water, and there is evidence that the meningitic form of Weil's disease is particularly likely to follow infection while bathing (Buzzard and Wylie, 1947). *L. canicola* is transmitted to man from dogs, in which it may cause diarrhoea, but which may harbour the organism while remaining apparently in normal health.

The clinical picture of the meningeal form of both diseases is very similar. The usual symptoms and signs of meningitis are present, often in a benign form, though in Weil's disease the meningitis may be severe. The ocular fundi are often congested and there may be papilloedema. The cerebrospinal fluid is under somewhat increased pressure and contains a considerable excess of cells. It is said that in Weil's disease polymorphonuclear cells predominate at the outset, later giving place to lymphocytes, while in canicola fever a lymphocytosis seems to be a characteristic finding. The number of cells ranges from 50 to over 1,000 per mm.[3] and the protein content of the fluid may be normal or as high as 400 mg. per 100 ml.

Though in either disease meningitis may be associated with the characteristic general symptoms, these may be absent. The most distinctive sign outside the nervous system appears to be ciliary congestion. In canicola fever there may be a morbilliform rash and the spleen may be enlarged. In Weil's disease jaundice may be absent, and there may be no haemorrhages or severe renal damage.

The clinical picture may thus be that of so-called acute aseptic meningitis, and the only clues pointing to the cause may be the ciliary congestion, the occupation of the patient, a history of recent bathing, or of a fall into water. The diagnosis is confirmed by a rising serum-agglutination titre to the infecting organism and by the demonstration by appropriate technique of leptospirae in the blood, urine, or conjunctival secretion.

When the clinical picture is purely or predominantly meningeal the prognosis is good and complete recovery is the rule. Penicillin is often given systemically, but its value is doubtful.

REFERENCES

ALSTON, J. M., and BROOM, J. C. (1958) *Leptospirosis in Man and Animals*, Edinburgh.

BUZZARD, E. M., and WYLIE, J. A. H. (1947) Meningitis leptospirosa, *Lancet*, ii, 417.

DAVIDSON, L. S. P., and SMITH, J. (1939) Weil's disease in the north-east of Scotland, *Brit. med. J.*, **2**, 753.

EDWARDS, G. A., and DOMM, B. M. (1960) Human leptospirosis, *Medicine (Baltimore)*, **39**, 117.

LAURENT, L. J. M., NORRIS, T. ST. M., STARKS, J. M., BROOM, J. C., and ALSTON, J. M. (1948) Four cases of leptospira canicola infection in England, *Lancet*, ii, 48.

MACKAY-DICK, J., and WATTS, R. W. E. (1949) Canicola fever in Germany, *Lancet*, i, 907.

WEETCH, R. S., KOLQUHOUN, J., and BROOM, J. D. (1949) Fatal human case of canicola fever, *Lancet*, i, 906.

ACUTE LYMPHOCYTIC CHORIOMENINGITIS AND ACUTE ASEPTIC MENINGITIS

[See page 464.]

BRUCELLOSIS

Any of the three organisms *Brucella melitensis*, *Brucella abortus*, and *Brucella suis*, may directly or indirectly affect the nervous system. There have now been many recorded cases of meningo-encephalitis due to these organisms. To the naked eye, there are greyish-white 'tubercles' in the meninges, which histologically consist of hyalinized connective tissue infiltrated with chronic inflammatory cells, and in places becoming necrotic. The meninges themselves are invaded by lymphocytes, plasma cells, and a few polymorphonuclear cells.

The clinical picture may consist predominantly of a subacute or chronic meningitis, or there may be symptoms of increased intracranial pressure suggesting a tumour, or the picture may be that of focal areas of encephalitis. Epilepsy, aphasia, mental confusion or deterioration, and spastic weakness of the limbs have all been observed. Myelitis is rare. The cerebrospinal fluid contains an excess of mononuclear cells, usually below 100 per mm.[3] The protein is raised in proportion as a rule, but is sometimes disproportionately high, and the fluid may be xanthochromic. In one reported case it was blood-stained, owing to rupture of a mycotic aneurysm.

Polyneuritis is uncommon.

Headache, fatigability, irritability, and toxic confusional states may occur as symptoms of the toxaemia in the absence of direct involvement of the nervous system.

Brucellosis may lead to spondylitis, and neurological symptoms may be secondary to this, lumbar spondylitis, for example, leading to sciatica.

The clinical picture of meningeal irritation associated with a lymphocytosis of the cerebrospinal fluid may lead to confusion with tuberculous meningitis or meningitis due to *Cryptococcus neoformans*. The diagnosis rests upon the appropriate serological tests for brucellosis, reinforced by the isolation of the organism, which may be obtained from the cerebrospinal fluid.

REFERENCES

DALRYMPLE-CHAMPNEYS, W. (1960) *Brucella Infection and Undulant Fever in Man,* London.
HARRIS, H. J. (1950) *Brucellosis (Undulant Fever),* New York.
HUDDLESON, I. F. (1943) *Brucellosis in Man and Animals,* New York.

MENINGITIS DUE TO *CRYPTOCOCCUS NEOFORMANS (TORULA HISTOLYTICA)*

Cryptococcus neoformans, also known as *Torula histolytica,* is a fungus consisting of a round or oval body surrounded by a thick polysaccharide capsule. It appears to be of world-wide distribution, but most cases have occurred in the more southern parts of the United States and in Australia. It has also been found in Great Britain. Its usual portal of entry appears to be the lung where it forms lesions not unlike those of pulmonary tuberculosis, though rarely undergoing cavitation. The brain, however, is the most important site of infection. There it forms an irregular granulomatous thickening of the meninges which are infiltrated with lymphocytes and occasional plasma cells. Multinucleated giant cells are also present. Capsulated cryptococci are scattered throughout the meninges. To the naked eye the brain shows a diffuse or more localized opacity of the meninges with flattening of the gyri and other evidence of increased intracranial pressure. Other organs besides the nervous system and the lungs may be involved, including the kidneys, spleen, and the lymph nodes. The two latter often present the histological appearances of Hodgkin's disease even though they contain cryptococci. There is, however, evidence that Hodgkin's disease may predispose to the infection with cryptococcus.

Clinically there is an insidious onset of symptoms with a history varying from weeks to years, but usually measured in months. The symptoms of meningitis are usually present, including cervical rigidity and Kernig's sign, but the presence of papilloedema and symptoms of a focal lesion of the nervous system may suggest an intracranial tumour. The cerebrospinal fluid is very variable. It may be clear with only a small excess of cells and protein, or contain a considerable excess of cells, usually lymphocytes and occasionally polymorphonuclears, with or without a high protein. A paretic colloidal gold curve is rather characteristic. Cryptococci may be present in the fluid or may be cultured on Sabouraud's medium: special stains are required to stain the capsule. The condition must be distinguished from other forms of subacute or chronic meningitis, sarcoidosis, and intracranial tumour. The presence of a characteristic pulmonary lesion may be helpful, with fever, hepatosplenomegaly and ulceration of the skin and mucous membranes.

There is recent evidence that amphotericin B given intravenously in a dosage of 0·25 mg., increasing to 1·0 mg./kg. body weight daily by slow infusion, is an effective treatment but is not free from risk. The same drug given intrathecally has been shown to be effective in a recent case (McIntyre, 1967). Steroid drugs, given in combination with amphotericin B, may have an adjuvant value; given alone they cause exacerbation of the condition and have been used as a provocative diagnostic test in doubtful cases, since after the administration of prednisone, 30 mg. daily for 48 hours, the cryptococcus may be found for the first time in the cerebrospinal fluid. Recent work suggests that 5-fluorocytosine, 100–200 mg. per kg. body weight, given by mouth for 6–8 weeks, may be more effective than amphotericin B and is certainly less toxic (Watkins *et al.*, 1969).

REFERENCES

BUTLER, W. T., ALLING, D. W., SPICKARD, A., and UTZ, J. (1964) Diagnostic and prognostic value of clinical and laboratory findings in cryptococcal meningitis, *New Engl. J. Med.*, **270, ** 59.

GREENFIELD, J. G. (1958) in *Neuropathology*, by Greenfield, J. G., Blackwood, W., McMenemey, W. H., Meyer, A., and Norman, R. M., p. 149, London.

McINTYRE, H. B. (1967) Cryptococcal meningitis. A case successfully treated by cisternal administration of amphotericin B with a review of recent literature, *Bull. Los Angeles neurol. Soc.*, **32, ** 213.

ROSE, F. C., GRANT, C., and JEANES, A. L. (1958) Torulosis of the central nervous system in Britain, *Brain*, **81, ** 542.

WATKINS, J. S., GARDNER-MEDWIN, D., INGHAM, H. R., and MURRAY, I. G. (1969) Two cases of cryptococcal meningitis, one treated with 5-fluorocytosine, *Brit. med. J.* (in the press).

7

SUPPURATIVE ENCEPHALITIS:
INTRACRANIAL ABSCESS

PATHOLOGY

INTRACRANIAL abscess may be (1) extradural, (2) subdural, (3) subarachnoid, or (4) intracerebral. (1) Extradural abscess is secondary to osteitis of one of the cranial bones. The infection passes through the bone, but its further advance being arrested by the dura, the accumulating pus strips the dura from the bone. (2) In subdural abscess the infection has penetrated the dura and the pus lies between this membrane and the brain surface. (3) Subarachnoid abscess is a rare form of subdural abscess in which the pus is limited to the subarachnoid space in which it spreads along the surface of the brain. (4) Intracerebral abscess may follow the spread of infection from the surface of the brain, or may be haematogenous. In the former case it usually, but not necessarily, possesses a track communicating with the surface. Intracerebral abscesses are usually single, but may be multilocular, or, less commonly, multiple. The developing intracerebral abscess passes through three stages. The first stage is an acute encephalitis without visible pus formation. In the second stage pus makes its appearance, but the abscess is not well defined from surrounding tissue. In the third stage a definite wall is formed, and the abscess is localized. The localization of the abscess depends upon various factors, of which no doubt the resistance of the patient to the organism is one of the most important. In some cases it does not occur, and the condition remains in the stage of a spreading encephalitis.

Abscesses of otitic origin are usually situated in the middle or posterior part of the temporal lobe or in the cerebellum, the former situation being about twice as common as the latter. An otitic cerebellar abscess usually occupies the antero-superior part of the lateral lobe and is adherent to the posterior part of the petrous bone (Pennybacker, 1948). Much more rarely such abscesses occur in the pons, frontal, or parietal lobes. In otitic cases the brain may become infected as a result of (1) purulent thrombosis of the transverse sinus, or (2) osteomyelitis of the tympanic wall, or (3) by spread along the adventitial spaces of perforating blood vessels (Evans, 1931). The anterior part of the frontal lobe is the seat of abscess following frontal sinusitis. Haematogenous abscesses may occur in any situation, but are nearly always above the tentorium. The left hemisphere is more often affected than the right, and in most cases the abscess lies in the area supplied by the middle cerebral artery and rather superficially.

Microscopically an intracerebral abscess consists of an inner layer of pus cells, outside which is a layer of granulation tissue containing new blood vessels and hyperplastic fibrous tissue. Outside this is a layer of glial reaction, mainly cellular in the early stages, mainly fibrous later. Fat-granule cells, plasma cells, and polymorphonuclear leucocytes are plentiful, especially in the middle layer.

Inflammatory reactions are present in the overlying meninges, and in extradural and subdural abscess granulation tissue is present on the surface of the dura.

AETIOLOGY

The causes of intracranial abscess in approximate order of frequency are: (1) infection of the middle ear, mastoid, and nasal sinuses, (2) pyaemic states, (3) metastasis from intrathoracic suppuration, and (4) head injury. In Evans's (1931) series of 194 cases of brain abscess the numbers for these groups were 121, 24, 22, 8, and other or unknown causes 19 (see also Pennybacker and Sellors, 1948).

1. Infection of the middle ear and mastoid is from four to nine times as common a cause of cerebral abscess as infection of the nasal sinuses, of which the frontal sinus is most often involved, and the sphenoidal sinus next.

2. Intracranial abscess may be the outcome of pyaemia. In bacterial endocarditis the infecting organism is usually of low virulence, and embolism leads to softening of the vessel wall and aneurysm formation more often than to abscess. The latter, however, may occur either in this or in more acute states of pyaemia, such as may constitute the terminal event in acute osteomyelitis or as metastases from boils, carbuncles, cellulitis, &c., especially on the face and scalp.

3. When intracranial abscess is secondary to localized infection elsewhere, the thorax is usually the source, and most cases are complications of bronchiectasis, chronic empyema, or pulmonary abscess. Rarely the primary abscess is elsewhere, for example in the liver or a bone. There is an association between cerebral abscess and cyanotic congenital heart disease (Maronde, 1950; Campbell, 1957; Matson and Salem, 1961).

4. Fracture of the skull is liable to cause abscess when the injury leads to free communication between the surface of the body and the brain, especially when fragments of bone, clothing, or a missile penetrate the latter.

Any of the common pyogenic organisms may be responsible for intracranial abscess, the commonest being streptococcus, *Diplococcus pneumoniae*, and *Staphylococcus aureus*. Friedländer's bacillus and organisms of the *Escherichia coli* group are also found. The causal agent may be a streptothrix, as in actinomycotic abscess, and amoebic abscess of the brain sometimes occurs. In certain parts of South-East Asia, chronic cerebral abscess due to paragonimiasis is relatively common and may be associated with recurrent episodes of low-grade meningitis (Oh, 1969).

SYMPTOMS

Mode of Onset

The history of the development of the symptoms of an intracranial abscess may be of greater diagnostic importance than the physical signs, which are often slight at the stage at which treatment is most likely to be effective.

When abscess follows fracture of the skull it usually develops soon after the injury, though when a missile penetrates the brain there may be a latent interval. These cases, however, offer little difficulty. The history is particularly important when abscess is secondary to otitis media or mastoiditis. In some such cases the onset is acute or subacute. After an exacerbation of a pre-existing otitis media, or a temporary suppression of aural discharge, or the operation of mastoidectomy, the patient rapidly develops headache, vomiting, delirium, and other symptoms to be described. In other cases there is a 'latent interval' which may last months before the *signs* of abscess appear. The existence of *symptoms* during this period may suggest that all is not well. There may be attacks of headache, loss of appetite and weight, constipation, occasional unexplained pyrexia, and a change in temperament leading to depression and irritability.

Abscess of haematogenous origin may develop slowly and insidiously, in which case, unless the primary infective focus is discovered, it may be clinically indistinguishable from an intracranial tumour. It is not uncommon, however, to obtain a history of an acute disturbance of health corresponding to the lodgement of the infected embolus in the brain. This is the rule when the embolus lodges in a large and important vessel, such as the middle cerebral or one of its branches, and the embolic symptoms then tend to be permanent, and to merge into those of the abscess. Even in other cases, however, there is often a history of sudden headache with perhaps some impairment of consciousness, and weakness of a limb, followed by a remission of these symptoms for weeks or months before those of the abscess develop.

The symptoms of intracranial abscess may be conveniently divided into (1) general symptoms of infection, (2) symptoms of increased intracranial pressure, (3) focal symptoms, and (4) changes in the cerebrospinal fluid.

General Symptoms

The severity of the general symptoms is usually proportionate to the acuteness of the abscess, and is therefore most marked in the cases best described as acute suppurative encephalitis. In the acute cases an irregular pyrexia is the rule; in chronic cases the temperature may be intermittently raised but is often subnormal. In both there may be a polymorphonuclear leucocytosis in the blood.

Symptoms of Increased Intracranial Pressure

The incidence of symptoms of increased intracranial pressure differs somewhat in abscess from that found in intracranial tumour. Headache is usually present. In chronic abscess it is paroxysmal, is increased by stooping and exertion, and presents the other features of headache due to increased intracranial pressure. In more acute cases headache may be persistent and very severe. Papilloedema is a late sign and is often absent or slight. When present it is sometimes more marked upon the side of the lesion. Bradycardia is commoner in abscess than in tumour, but is not constant, and when it occurs usually indicates a rapid increase in the severity of the condition. In severe cases delirium, somnolence, stupor, and coma develop. Exceptionally the signs of increased intracranial pressure are slight or lacking, even when a large abscess is present.

Focal Symptoms

Extradural Abscess. This is difficult to diagnose because, unless the abscess is very large, focal symptoms are absent, except for headache radiating from the ear and mastoid process towards the vertex. This is only of significance if the ear and mastoid are receiving adequate drainage, and hence can be excluded as the cause of the headache. Tenderness of the skull to pressure or percussion in front of or above the ear or behind the mastoid may also be present.

Subdural Abscess or Empyema. This condition is almost always a complication of frontal sinusitis but rarely develops as a result of otitis media. A layer of pus forms in the subdural space over one frontal lobe (or rarely over the temporal lobe). The clinical manifestations usually consist of high fever, fits (either focal or generalized) and a rapidly-developing hemiplegia with aphasia if the major hemisphere is involved. Early surgical evacuation of the pus and irrigation of the subdural space with a weak solution of an appropriate antibiotic is imperative; thrombosis of cortical veins is an important complication which may lead to a substantial residual disability even if appropriate treatment is given.

Intracerebral Abscess. 1. *Temporal Lobe Abscess.* An abscess in this position, if situated on the left side in a right-handed individual, may cause aphasia, usually of the nominal type, that is, a difficulty in naming objects. Investigation of this symptom requires care, and a patient who can name familiar objects accurately often shows hesitation, or misnames less familiar articles. Abscess on either side may produce a defect of the visual fields, an especially valuable localizing sign. It usually consists of a homonymous upper quadrantic defect on the opposite side due to involvement of the lower fibres of the optic radiation. Damage to the corticospinal tract is usually slight, and weakness is most marked in the face and tongue. The opposite plantar reflex may be extensor. Oculomotor paralyses may result from pressure upon the third or sixth cranial nerve.

2. *Cerebellar Abscess.* Headache in cerebellar abscess is often predominantly suboccipital. It may radiate down the neck and be associated with some cervical rigidity. The head may be flexed to the side of the lesion or retracted. Signs of cerebellar deficiency vary in severity and may be slight. The most important are—nystagmus, most marked on conjugate deviation to the side of the lesion, the slow phase being centripetal; hypotonia and incoordination in the limbs on the affected side, with an inability to carry out rapid alternating movements as well with the upper limb on the affected side as on the normal side. Pressure upon the brain stem may occur, leading to compression of cranial nerves, especially the sixth and seventh, on the side of the abscess, and slight signs of corticospinal defect on the opposite side. Pass-pointing outwards with the affected hand and a tendency to deviate or fall to the side of the lesion when walking are additional signs which may be present.

3. *Frontal Abscess.* Headache, drowsiness, apathy, and impairment of memory and attention are usually conspicuous, but focal signs are often lacking. A large abscess or much oedema may cause aphasia or hemiparesis. Unilateral anosmia and slight exophthalmos may be present.

4. *Abscesses in other Situations.* These require no special description, the focal symptoms depending upon the position of the abscess, and usually resembling those of tumour in the same situation.

Subarachnoid Abscess. This rather rare condition may be suspected when the signs point to abscess of otitic origin, though neither of the clinical pictures just described is present. Convulsions may occur with a superficial abscess of the cerebral hemisphere. When the signs have pointed to involvement of the cerebellum but no abscess can be found in the cerebellum itself, search should be made for a superficial abscess in the cerebellopontine angle.

The Cerebrospinal Fluid

Examination of the cerebrospinal fluid is often of great diagnostic value, but lumbar puncture may be dangerous in cases of cerebellar abscess. As long as the abscess remains localized, the fluid is clear. Its pressure may be increased. There is usually an excess of cells, though not often more than 100 per mm.[3], the majority of which are lymphocytes, the remainder being polymorphonuclear: the protein is somewhat raised. A protein of perhaps 200 mg. with relatively few cells is particularly suggestive. There is no diminution in the chloride or sugar content, and organisms are absent. The supervention of generalized meningitis upon intracranial abscess leads to a change in the cerebrospinal fluid. The cells increase, and polymorphonuclears predominate, while the chloride content diminishes, and the fluid no longer yields reducing substances. Organisms may be present.

OTHER METHODS OF INVESTIGATION

The EEG may yield valuable evidence as to the site of an abscess demonstrating a striking focus of high amplitude slow delta activity. Sonoencephalography may indicate displacement of the midline as in the case of an intracranial tumour. Isotope encephalography may accurately localize an abscess (Planiol, 1963). Ventriculography may occasionally be necessary for localization but should only be performed immediately before operation. Exploratory puncture may be helpful in localization, and radiography may be carried out after injection of a radio-opaque substance into the cavity.

DIAGNOSIS

Intracranial abscess is rarely encountered without an evident source of infection. It is then usually exposed at an operation for a supposed intracranial tumour. The diagnosis of such cases from tumour is difficult and often impossible. Pyrexia, leucocytosis in the blood, and an excess of cells in the cerebrospinal fluid, however, may suggest the correct diagnosis. When the causal infective focus is obvious, it is necessary to distinguish abscess from other pyogenic intracranial complications. Generalized meningitis, which may co-exist with abscess, is distinguished by the prominence of signs of meningeal irritation, cervical rigidity, in severe cases head retraction, Kernig's sign, and the changes in the cerebrospinal fluid already described. Transverse sinus thrombosis causes little cerebral disturbance, though the resulting congestion may cause slight papilloedema, more marked on the affected side, and slight signs of cortico-spinal tract defect on the opposite side. The signs of pyaemia are usually conspicuous with swinging temperature and rigors. A valuable sign may be demonstrated by Queckenstedt's test. The rise of cerebrospinal fluid pressure may be slight or absent when the jugular vein on the affected side is compressed alone, because the blocked transverse sinus prevents communication of the raised jugular pressure to the cranial cavity. Acute labyrinthitis may be confused with cerebellar abscess, with which it may coexist. In the former vertigo is more, and headache less, intense than in the latter. In the nystagmus due to labyrinthitis the slow phase is always in the same direction, to whichever side the patient directs his gaze. In cerebellar abscess the slow phase is always away from the point of fixation. Evident hypotonia is in favour of a cerebellar lesion. Papilloedema and changes in the cerebrospinal fluid indicate that the infection has passed beyond the internal ear.

PROGNOSIS

Very rarely an intracranial abscess becomes quiescent and is found accidentally at post-mortem, surrounded by a thick layer of gliosis. Recovery by spontaneous drainage may also occur. These occurrences, however, are too exceptional to have any bearing upon prognosis, which may be regarded as uniformly fatal in the absence of surgical interference. Spreading encephalitis, rupture of the abscess into the ventricular system, meningitis, and sinus thrombosis are the usual terminations. Even after surgical drainage these complications may occur, and the mortality rate is high, but with modern surgical methods and antibiotics has fallen to less than 20 per cent. Thoracogenic and otitic cerebellar abscesses are the most serious. Epilepsy is an important sequel, occurring in up to 50 per cent. of cases, usually within 12 months.

TREATMENT

Treatment is surgical, the choice lying between primary excision, and repeated aspiration followed by the instillation of penicillin or other appropriate antibiotics, with secondary excision in reserve if this treatment fails. Excision is attended by the lowest mortality (Jooma, Pennybacker, and Tutton, 1951) but is not always practicable and much depends upon the situation of the lesion. Drugs of the sulphonamide group and antibiotics should be given as for meningitis [see p. 371], but intrathecal penicillin should not be given unless there is also meningitis and then not until the abscess has been dealt with surgically.

REFERENCES

CAMPBELL, M. (1957) Cerebral abscess in cyanotic congenital heart disease, *Lancet*, i, 111.
EVANS, W. (1931) The pathology and aetiology of brain abscess, *Lancet*, i, 1231 and 1289.
GLOBUS, J. H., and HORN, W. L. (1932) Inherent healing properties of abscess of the brain, *Arch. Otolaryng. (Chicago)*, **16**, 603.
JOOMA, O. V., PENNYBACKER, J., and TUTTON, G. K. (1951) Brain abscess, aspiration, drainage or excision?, *J. Neurol. Psychiat.*, **14**, 308.
KERR, F. W. L., KING, R. B., and MEAGHER, J. N. (1958) Brain abscess, *J. Amer. med. Ass.*, **168**, 868.
MARONDE, R. F. (1950) Brain abscess and congenital heart disease, *Ann. intern. Med.*, **33**, 602.
MATSON, D. D., and SALEM, M. (1961) Brain abscess in congenital heart disease, *Pediatrics*, **27**, 772.
NORTHFIELD, D. W. C. (1942) The treatment of brain abscess, *J. Neurol. Psychiat.*, N.S. **5**, 1.
OH, S. J. (1969) Cerebral paragonimiasis, *J. neurol. Sci.*, **8**, 27.

PENNYBACKER, J. (1948) Cerebellar abscess, *J. Neurol. Neurosurg. Psychiat.* N.S. **11**, 1.

PENNYBACKER, J., and SELLORS, T. H. (1948) Treatment of thoracogenic brain abscess, *Lancet*, ii, 90.

PLANIOL, T. (1963) La gamma-encéphalographie, *Rev. Prat. (Paris)*, **13**, 3625.

SCHILLER, F., CAIRNS, H., and RUSSELL, D. S. (1948) Treatment of purulent pachymeningitis and subdural suppuration with particular reference to penicillin, *J. Neurol. Psychiat.*, **11**, 143.

SPERL, M. P., MacCARTY, C. S., and WELLMAN, W. E. (1959) Observations on current therapy of abscess of the brain, *Arch. Neurol. Psychiat. (Chicago)*, **81**, 439.

SYMONDS, C. P. (1926–7) Some points in the diagnosis and localization of cerebral abscess, *Proc. roy. Soc. Med.*, **20**, 1139.

8

NERVOUS COMPLICATIONS
OF MISCELLANEOUS INFECTIONS

ACUTE TOXIC ENCEPHALOPATHY

Synonyms. Acute toxic encephalitis; acute serous encephalitis.

Definition. An acute cerebral disturbance occurring chiefly in children, not uncommonly in small epidemics and characterized pathologically by toxic changes in the nervous system, and clinically by delirium or coma and convulsions, variable pareses of the limbs, and symptoms of meningeal irritation.

PATHOLOGY

The changes in the nervous system distinguish this disorder both from the forms of encephalitis which are caused by the invasion of the nervous system by a virus, and from those in which demyelination is present. Pathologically there is an acute degeneration of the ganglion cells of the brain with hyperaemia and conspicuous perivascular and pericellular oedema, and focal collections of glial cells and round cells. Ring haemorrhages have been described, and 'acute brain purpura', in which multiple punctate haemorrhages with a perivascular distribution are conspicuous in the nervous system, is probably an intense variety of this disorder.

AETIOLOGY

The pathological changes are interpreted as the effect of a toxaemia which varies in the severity of its incidence upon nerve cells and the blood vessels, so producing varying degrees of neural degeneration, oedema, and haemorrhage. In some cases the source of the toxaemia is a focal or generalized pyogenic infection. In others it is unknown and this applies to the small epidemics of the disorder which sometimes attack young children during the summer months. It is not very common in infancy, most cases occurring between the ages of two and ten years.

SYMPTOMS

The onset of the illness is usually acute and may be fulminating. It is sometimes preceded by sore throat or gastro-intestinal disturbance. Severe headache, vomiting, and convulsions are common and the latter may be predominantly unilateral. The child when conscious is usually delirious, but may pass later into coma. There is usually high fever. Meningeal symptoms are often conspicuous. Involvement of the cerebral hemispheres may lead to aphasia, monoplegia, hemiplegia, or double hemiplegia. Optic neuritis may occur; pupillary abnormalities are inconstant. Trismus is sometimes seen and facial paresis is frequently present. The tendon reflexes are not uncommonly diminished or lost, but may be exaggerated, and the plantar reflexes extensor on one or both sides. Retention and incontinence of urine are common when consciousness is clouded or lost. The symptoms may be predominantly meningeal, cerebral, or spinal. The cerebrospinal fluid is usually normal in composition though under increased pressure. Exceptionally there may be a pleocytosis or a rise of protein content. Rarely, chiefly in those cases characterized pathologically by acute haemorrhagic lesions in the brain, haematuria or albuminuria may occur and a purpuric rash has been described.

DIAGNOSIS

The fact that the cerebrospinal fluid is usually normal in composition, and the early involvement of the substance of the nervous system, distinguishes acute toxic encephalopathy from the various forms of meningitis and encephalitis. The diagnosis from poliomyelitis is based upon the absence of a considerable pleocytosis, the presence in many cases of extensor plantar responses, and the absence of muscular wasting. Lead encephalopathy must also be excluded.

PROGNOSIS

The prognosis varies in different groups of reported cases. In some small epidemics almost all the affected individuals have died. In others almost all have recovered. The condition accounted for 6 per cent. of all infants and children coming to autopsy at the Massachusetts General Hospital in one decade (Lyon, Dodge, and Adams, 1961). In fatal cases death usually occurs within two or three days of the onset, coma having supervened within a few hours. In those who survive, the dangers are the persistence of mental defect, aphasia, hemiplegia, or epilepsy. Sometimes the patient recovers consciousness, and hemiparesis clears up in a few days. In other cases improvement is slower but recovery is often surprisingly complete.

TREATMENT

Treatment is symptomatic. Lumbar puncture with free drainage of the cerebrospinal fluid is often helpful. Phenobarbitone, paraldehyde or other sedatives may be required to control the convulsions. Cerebral oedema may be treated by dexamethasone, 2–5 mg. three times daily in the acute stage, depending upon the age of the patient.

REFERENCES

BRAIN, W. R., and HUNTER, D. (1929) Acute meningo-encephalomyelitis of childhood, *Lancet*, i, 221.

BROWN, C. L., and SYMMERS, D. (1925) Acute serous encephalitis; a newly recognized disease of children, *Amer. J. Dis. Child.*, **29**, 174.

GRINKER, R. R., and STONE, T. T. (1928) Acute toxic encephalitis in childhood, *Arch. Neurol. Psychiat. (Chicago)*, **20**, 244.

LOW, A. A. (1930) Acute toxic (non-suppurative) encephalitis in children, *Arch. Neurol. Psychiat. (Chicago)*, **23**, 696.

LYON, G., DODGE, P. R., and ADAMS, R. D. (1961) The acute encephalopathies of obscure origin in infants and children, *Brain*, **84**, 680.

SCARLET FEVER

Nervous complications of scarlet fever are rare. Although focal vascular lesions have been reported, the pathological changes in most cases which have been investigated recently have consisted of acute haemorrhagic encephalitis. Ferraro (1944) suggests that post-scarlatinal encephalitis, like glomerulonephritis, may have an allergic basis. Meningism is not uncommon, symptoms of meningeal irritation coexisting with a normal cerebrospinal fluid. True meningitis occurs less frequently and is usually secondary to otitis or other complications produced by pyogenic organisms. In a few cases the *Streptococcus scarlatinae* has been isolated from the fluid. Hydrocephalus has been reported in a few instances as a sequel of meningitis complicating scarlet fever. Cerebral abscess may occur without otitis. Hemiplegia, however, is the commonest complication resulting from involvement of the nervous system. Rolleston collected 66 cases from the literature. It is usually embolic in origin but may follow cerebral thrombosis or haemorrhage or acute encephalitis. Hypertensive encephalopathy may be responsible for cerebral symptoms. A few cases of localized and multiple neuritis have been reported. Optic neuritis is rare. Chorea is a not uncommon sequel of scarlet fever. Hemiplegia of vascular origin is usually permanent, but symptoms due to hypertensive encephalopathy disappear if the patient recovers.

REFERENCES

FERRARO, A. (1944) Allergic brain changes in post-scarlatinal encephalitis, *J. Neuropath. exp. Neurol.*, **3**, 239.

FORBERS, J. G. (1926) Post-scarlatinal meningitis, *Lancet*, ii, 1207.

MILLER, H. G., STANTON, J. B., and GIBBONS, J. L. (1956) Para-infectious encephalomyelitis and related syndromes, *Quart. J. Med.*, **25**, 427.

NEAL, J. B., and JONES, A. (1927) Streptococcic meningitis following scarlet fever—recovery, *Arch. Pediat.*, **44**, 395.

NEURATH, R. (1912) Die Rolle des Scharlachs in der Ätiologie der Nervenkrankheiten, *Ergebn. inn. Med. Kinderheilk.*, **9**, 103.

ROLLESTON, J. D. (1927–8) Hemiplegia following scarlet fever, *Proc. roy. Soc. Med.*, **21**, 213.

SOUTHARD, E. E., and SIMS, F. R. (1904) A case of cortical hemorrhages following scarlet fever, *J. Amer. med. Ass.*, **43**, 789.

TOOMEY, J. A., DEMBO, L. H., and McCONNELL, G. (1923) Acute hemorrhagic encephalitis: report of a case following scarlet fever, *Amer. J. Dis. Child.*, **25**, 98.

WHOOPING COUGH

The pathogenesis of nervous symptoms in whooping cough is varied. Some are due to focal vascular lesions, especially haemorrhages. Jarke (1896) described multiple patches of softening of the cerebral hemispheres and Askin and Zimmerman (1929) reported a case of encephalitis with focal collections of inflammatory cells. Convulsions are not uncommon in whooping cough, especially in young children. Though they may sometimes be due to transitory metabolic or other functional disturbances, in severe cases the pathological changes of encephalitis have been found but in other cases the changes are those of an encephalopathy, possibly resulting from the mechanical effects of venous congestion due to repeated coughing. Focal symptoms, which include aphasia, unilateral or bilateral hemiplegia, blindness, and deafness, are probably the result of focal vascular lesions or softening. Peripheral nerve palsies are rare and usually late complications. Patients who have severe and frequent convulsions usually die. Of the group with focal lesions approximately one-fifth die, two-fifths are incapacitated by residual symptoms, and two-fifths recover.

REFERENCES

ASKIN, J. A., and ZIMMERMAN, H. M. (1929) Encephalitis accompanying whooping-cough: clinical history and report of postmortem examination, *Amer. J. Dis. Child.*, **38**, 97.

DUBOIS, R., LEY, R. A., and DAGNELIE, J. (1932) Protocoles anatomo-cliniques de huit cas de complications nerveuses de la coqueluche, *J. Neurol. (Brux.)*, **32**, 645.

ELLISON, J. B. (1934) Whooping-cough eclampsia, *Lancet*, i, 227.

FONTEYNE, P., and DAGNELIE, J. (1932). Action de l'endotoxine coquelucheuse sur les centres nerveux (Recherches expérimentales), *J. Neurol. (Brux.)*, **32**, 660.

JARKE, O. (1896) Ein Fall von acuter symmetrischer Gehirnerweichung bei Keuchhusten, *Arch. Kinderheilk.*, **20**, 212.

MIKULOWSKI, V. (1929) Pertussis-encephalitis im Kindesalter, *Jb. Kinderheilk.*, **124**, 103.

MILLER, H. G., STANTON, J. B., and GIBBONS, J. L. (1956) Para-infectious encephalomyelitis and related syndromes, *Quart. J. Med.*, **25**, 427.

TYPHOID FEVER

Mental symptoms are common, those most frequently encountered being acute toxic confusional states during the febrile period and post-typhoid insanities of many forms, the nature of which in individual cases probably depends upon the psychological constitution of the patient. Meningeal symptoms may be due to meningism, the cerebrospinal fluid being normal. Much more rarely true meningitis occurs, due to infection with the *Salmonella typhosa*, the cerebrospinal fluid containing polymorphonuclear cells, together with the causal organism. Suppurative meningitis may also result from infection with other pyogenic organisms, with or without the *Salmonella typhosa*. The substance of the nervous system is less often involved than the meninges, but focal symptoms, especially hemiplegia, with or without aphasia, may occur, and are probably usually vascular in origin, being most frequently due to cerebral thrombosis. Optic neuritis is rare. Cerebral abscess may occur either by extension from otitis media or by metastasis from a focus of pyogenic infection elsewhere. Such abscesses are usually due to a secondary invader, but may be caused by the *Salmonella typhosa*. Occasionally spinal symptoms predominate, yielding a picture of transverse myelitis or of ascending paralysis of the Landry type. Neuritis is a rare sequel, polyneuritis involving the feet and causing tenderness of the toes being the commonest form.

Similar complications may occur in paratyphoid fever, but less frequently than in typhoid.

Meningitis occurring in typhoid fever is usually fatal, and cerebral abscess is a serious complication which usually terminates fatally. Focal vascular lesions do not threaten life to the same extent, but frequently cause permanent disability, e.g. hemiplegia.

REFERENCES

LAROCHE, G., and PEJU, G. (1920) Méningite typhique bénigne au cours d'une septicémie typhique à rechute, *Bull. Soc. méd. Hôp. Paris*, **44**, 150.

MELCHIOR, E. (1911) Über Hirnabscesse und sonstige umschriebene intrakranielle Eiterungen im Verlauf und Gefolge des Typhus abdominalis, *Zbl. GrGeb. Med. Chir.*, **14**, 49.

ROLLESTON, J. D. (1929) *Acute Infectious Diseases*, 2nd ed., London.

SMITHIES, F. (1907) Hemiplegia as a complication in typhoid fever, with report of a case, *J. Amer. med. Ass.*, **49**, 389.

TYPHUS FEVER

Nervous symptoms may occur in typhus fever, and there is abundant evidence that they are usually due to infection of the nervous system by the causative organism. Histologically, microscopical nodules in the walls of the very small blood vessels—typhus nodules—have frequently been observed in the nervous system, where they consist of perivascular collections of glial, endothelial, and other mononuclear cells (Aschoff, Wolbach, Spielmeyer, and others). Thrombosis frequently occurs in the affected vessel. *Rickettsia prowazeki*, the causal organism of typhus, has been seen in the endothelium of the cerebral vessels and sometimes in the typhus nodules.

Headache, delirium, and insomnia, which are common during the febrile stage of the illness, are probably toxic in origin and do not necessarily indicate invasion of the nervous system. Focal nervous symptoms indicative of the latter usually occur during the last few days of the febrile period or within a few days afterwards. Meningeal symptoms may occur, and any part of the nervous system may be involved. Cerebral symptoms may indicate multiple lesions, a disseminated encephalitis, but hemiplegia is the commonest symptom. An acute cerebellar ataxia occurs in a small proportion of cases, and multiple bulbar foci may occur, leading to dysphagia and dysarthria. Lesions are sometimes confined to the spinal cord, yielding the clinical picture of a myelitis. The cranial and peripheral nerves frequently suffer. Optic neuritis may occur. Facial paralysis is particularly common, and deafness may develop. In the peripheral nerves the symptoms may be those of a focal interstitial neuritis, associated with pain and tenderness, or of a polyneuritis.

Changes are frequently present in the cerebrospinal fluid, which is sometimes xanthochromic and may exhibit a lymphocytosis. The albumin content of the fluid is usually little raised, but an excess of globulin, as indicated by a positive Noguchi reaction, is present in 50 per cent. of cases and may persist for from two to eight months after the acute stage.

The occurrence of severe nervous symptoms naturally adds to the gravity of the prognosis. In patients who survive, cerebral symptoms are frequently permanent, and Grodzki (1929) speaks of chronic encephalitis following typhus.

REFERENCES

ARKWRIGHT, J. A., and FELIX, A. (1930) Typhus fever, in *A System of Bacteriology*, vol. vii, ch. xxxiv, p. 393, London.

FELDMANN, P. M. (1926) Über Erkrankungen des zentralen Nervensystems beim Fleckfieber, *Arch. Psychiat. Nervenkr.*, **77**, 357.

GRODZKI, A. B. (1929) Über einige Formen der Flecktyphusenzephalitis, *Münch. med. Wschr.*, **76**, 709.

HIRSCHBERG, N. (1923) Über die Erkrankungen des Nervensystems bei Flecktyphus, *Dtsch. med. Wschr.*, **49**, 817.

HORSFALL, F. J., and TAMM, I. (1965) *Viral and Rickettsial Infections of Man*, 4th ed., Philadelphia.

MORAWETZ, G. (1919) Ein Fall von Fleckfieberencephalitis, *Med. Klin.*, **15**, 637.

ROLLESTON, J. D. (1929) *Acute Infectious Diseases*, 2nd ed., London.

STRONG, R. P., SHATTUCK, G. C., et al. (1920) *Typhus Fever, with Particular Reference to the Serbian Epidemic*, Cambridge, Mass.

MALARIA

Acute nervous symptoms in malaria, cerebral malaria, occur chiefly in infections with the malignant tertian parasite, blackwater fever, and are due to sporulation of the parasite in the cerebral capillaries. Sections of nerve tissue exhibit macroscopically a smoky grey appearance with oedema, hyperaemia, and punctiform haemorrhages. Histologically, the chief abnormality is more or less complete blocking of capillaries with parasitized red cells, leading to thrombosis, oedema, and petechial haemorrhages. The leptomeninges exhibit a perivascular infiltration with small, round cells. Malarial nodules (granulomas) have been observed. These consist of a central capillary filled with parasitized red cells and surrounded by a perivascular necrotic area, with glial proliferation (Thompson and Annecke, 1926).

Acute cerebral malaria is characterized by hyperpyrexia and rapidly developing coma, with or without precedent convulsions. Symptoms of meningeal irritation may occur, especially in children. In such cases the prognosis is always very grave. Focal manifestations include hemiplegia, aphasia, and cerebellar ataxia, which are usually transitory. Paraplegia has been described. Optic neuritis and retinal haemorrhages are often seen, and complete external ophthalmoplegia may occur.

Chronic nervous symptoms in malaria are probably toxic in origin and are usually due to neuritis. Trigeminal neuralgia, facial paralysis, localized neuritis of single nerves of the upper and lower limbs, and polyneuritis may occur.

REFERENCES

AUSTREGESILO, A. (1927) Des troubles nerveux dans quelques maladies tropicales, *Rev. neurol.* **34**, 1.

MANSON-BAHR, P. H. (1966) *Manson's Tropical Diseases*, 18th ed., London.

PERWUSCHIN, G. W. (1924) Malaria und Erkrankungen des Nervensystems, *Z. ges. Neurol. Psychiat.*, **93**, 446.

THOMPSON, J. G., and ANNECKE, S. (1926) Pathology of the central nervous system in malignant tertian malaria, *J. trop. Med. Hyg.*, **29**, 343.

TRYPANOSOMIASIS

African trypanosomiasis is transmitted to man by the bite of the tsetse fly. After an incubation period of about two weeks a local erythematous nodule may form at the site of the bite and this may be followed by insomnia, impaired concentration, formication and deep muscular aching. The parasites may not enter the central nervous system for several years; the onset may then be explosive with convulsions, coma and death within a few days but more often there is a chronic fluctuating illness characterized by progressive drowsiness, apathy, dysarthria and involuntary movements ('sleeping sickness'). The condition is usually fatal within a few months. The cerebrospinal fluid shows a mononuclear pleocytosis and a rise in protein with a 'tabetic' type of colloidal gold curve. Tryparsamide by intravenous injection or pentamidine intramuscularly may be effective in treatment of such cases.

South American trypanosomiasis (Chagas' disease) is acquired as a result of a bite from an affected bug. Meningo-encephalitis may occur, particularly in childhood but diffuse myositis with swelling of the face (pseudomyxoedema) is more common in the adult although central nervous system involvement may result in convulsions and paralysis.

REFERENCE

MANSON-BAHR, P. (1966) *Manson's Tropical Diseases*, 18th ed., London.

INFLUENZA

Nervous symptoms are frequently attributed to influenza, but the diagnosis is usually speculative and, except in cases occurring during epidemics, should always be received with caution. *H. influenzae* is one cause of pyogenic meningitis but clinical influenza is a virus infection. Acute haemorrhagic encephalitis has been ascribed to influenza, and Greenfield reported two cases of acute disseminated encephalomyelitis characterized by perivascular demyelination which followed a febrile illness diagnosed as 'influenza'. Small epidemics of encephalitis and polyneuritis have been observed to coincide with epidemics of influenza. Proof, however, is lacking that these forms of encephalitis are actually due to influenza or even that they complicate this disorder, since a precedent febrile illness, when it occurs, may well be due to invasion by the organism which is responsible for the nervous symptoms. Alternatively and more probably, according to current views, influenza may be one of many specific and non-specific infections which can, from time to time, be followed by a post-infective encephalitis or myelitis, or both, due to an allergic or hypersensitivity phenomenon. Thus, during recent influenza epidemics, especially the pandemic of 1957, cases of acute, sometimes fulminating, encephalomyelitis occurred (Kapila *et al.*, 1958; Thiruvengadam, 1959). In the most acute cases the pathology was that of an acute haemorrhagic encephalomyelitis, and on the whole it seems more likely that these were cases of acute disseminated encephalomyelitis [see p. 489] complicating influenza—a view not incompatible with the isolation of the influenza virus from the brain in some cases.

REFERENCES

DUNBAR, J. M., JAMIESON, W. M., LANGLANDS, H. M., and SMITH, G. H. (1958) Encephalitis and influenza, *Brit. med. J.*, **1**, 913.

FLEWETT, T. H., and HOULD, J. G. (1958) Influenzal encephalopathy and post-influenzal encephalitis, *Lancet*, i, 11.

GREENFIELD, J. G. (1930) Acute disseminated encephalomyelitis as a sequel to 'influenza', *J. Path. Bact.*, **33**, 453.

KAPILA, C. C., KAUL, S., KAPUR, S. C., KALAYANAIN, T. S., and BANERJEE, D. (1958) Neurological and hepatic disorders associated with influenza, *Brit. med. J.*, **2**, 1311.

McCONKEY, B., and DAWS, R. A. (1958) Neurological disorders associated with Asian influenza, *Lancet*, ii, 15.

RIDDOCH, G. (1928–9) Discussion on disseminated encephalomyelitis, *Proc. roy. Soc. Med.*, **22**, 1260.

THIRUVENGADAM, K. V. (1959) Disseminated encephalomyelitis after influenza, *Brit. med. J.*, **2**, 1233.

EPIDEMIC HEPATITIS

Serious nervous complications of epidemic hepatitis are uncommon, though mild cerebral, meningeal, and neuritic symptoms have been observed in epidemics. I have seen one case with unilateral convulsions and hemiplegia, and another with myelitis and neuritis. Byrne and Taylor (1945) report five cases, one with myelitis. The nervous symptoms usually develop four or five days before the jaundice appears. Jaundice, however, may coexist with nervous symptoms in other diseases—with meningitis in spirochaetosis icterohaemorrhagica, and with encephalitis in St. Louis and equine encephalomyelitis. Neurological symptoms due to focal lesions of the nervous system in epidemic hepatitis must be distinguished from those of hepatic failure [see p. 719].

REFERENCES

BYRNE, E. A. J., and TAYLOR, G. F. (1945) An outbreak of jaundice with signs in the nervous system, *Brit. med. J.*, **1**, 477.

NEWMAN, J. L. (1942) Infective hepatitis: the history of an outbreak in the Lavant valley, *Brit. med. J.*, **1**, 61.

SHERLOCK, S. (1963) *Diseases of the Liver and Biliary System*, 3rd ed., Oxford.

WALSHE, J. M. (1951) Observations on the symptomatology and pathogenesis of hepatic coma, *Quart. J. Med.*, **20**, 421.

INFECTIOUS MONONUCLEOSIS

Nervous complications of infectious mononucleosis are uncommon. The clinical picture may be meningitic, encephalitic, myelitic, or polyneuritic. Anosmia, optic neuritis, ophthalmoplegia, and facial palsy have been described. Poliomyelitis may be simulated, or the Guillain-Barré type of polyneuritis. The cerebrospinal fluid may contain an excess of lymphocytes.

Dolgopol and Husson (1949) reviewed the literature and reported a fatal case, dying of respiratory paralysis. There was selective degeneration of the nerve cells of the third and fourth cranial nerves, of the Purkinje cells of the cerebellum, and of the ventral portion of the inferior reticular nucleus, together with recent haemorrhages in the grey matter of the spinal cord. In the polyneuritic type of cases mononuclear cell infiltration of the spinal roots and nerves has been described. In a recent review, Gautier-Smith (1965) has drawn attention to the occurrence of mononeuritis (of cranial or peripheral nerves) in certain cases and gives reasons for supposing that in some cases there is direct viral invasion of the central nervous system, whereas in some of the patients with encephalomyelitis the aetiology of the nervous manifestations is more probably allergic. When the visceral symptoms and blood changes are typical no difficulty in diagnosis arises, but the nervous symptoms may come first, and the diagnosis may then depend upon the positive heterophile antibody test.

REFERENCES

DOLGOPOL, V. B., and HUSSON, G. S. (1949) Infectious mononucleosis with neurologic complications, *Arch. intern. Med.*, **83**, 179.
GAUTIER-SMITH, P. C. (1965) Neurological complications of glandular fever (infectious mononucleosis), *Brain*, **88**, 323.

SARCOIDOSIS

It is now recognized that lesions of Boeck's sarcoidosis may involve any level of the nervous system and the muscles (see Colover, 1948; Jefferson, 1957; and Matthews, 1965). The meninges or peripheral nerves may be infiltrated with endothelioid cells, giant cells, lymphocytes, plasma cells, and mononuclear leucocytes. Associated with the meningo-encephalitis there may be tumour-like masses in the dura mater. Adhesive arachnoiditis may cause hydrocephalus and the hypothalamus may be involved. The eyes may suffer in various ways. There may be papilloedema or retinal lesions, uveitis, and sometimes exophthalmos while paresis of the third or sixth nerves is not uncommon. Facial paralysis on one or both sides, with or without loss of taste, is common, and the glossopharyngeal and vagus nerves may also suffer. The limbs may be the site of polyneuritis or of a focal mononeuritis. An affected peripheral nerve may be palpably thickened. The characteristic lesions of sarcoidosis are likely to be found elsewhere in the body, e.g. the lymph nodes, liver, and spleen and phalanges. The combination of iridocyclitis with parotitis and polyneuritis was the first neurological manifestation of this disorder to be recognized. Crompton and Mac-Dermot (1961) reported three cases of sarcoidosis of muscle without other clinical manifestations of the disease, and presenting with progressive muscular wasting and weakness (sarcoid myopathy).

REFERENCES

COLOVER, J. (1948) Sarcoidosis with involvement of the nervous system, *Brain*, **71**, 451.
CROMPTON, M. R., and MACDERMOT, V. (1961) Sarcoidosis associated with progressive muscular wasting and weakness, *Brain*, **84**, 62.

FEILING, A., and VINER, G. (1921–2) Iridocyclitis-parotitis-polyneuritis: a new clinical syndrome, *J. Neurol. Psychiat.*, **2**, 353.

GARCIN, R. (1960) Les atteintes neurologiques et musculaires dans la maladie de Besnier–Boeck–Schaumann, *Psychiat. Neurol. Neurochir. (Amst.)*, **63**, 285.

JEFFERSON, M. (1957) Sarcoidosis of the nervous system, *Brain*, **80**, 540.

MATTHEWS, W. B. (1965) Sarcoidosis of the nervous system, *J. Neurol. Psychiat.*, **28**, 23.

TOXOPLASMOSIS

Toxoplasmosis is the result of infection with toxoplasma, an organism found in animals, birds, and reptiles and conveyed to man from domestic animals, rats, or mice. The toxoplasma is a crescentic organism 2 to 4 μ wide and 4 to 7 μ long, which is found intracellularly and extracellularly in the central nervous system, retina, heart muscle, kidneys, and endocrine glands. Pathologically it leads to disseminated encephalomyelitis with areas of yellow necrotic softening of the cerebral cortex and a contiguous leptomeningitis. Miliary granulomata are found. The spinal cord may also show softening and necrosis (Wyllie and Fisher, 1950).

Campbell and Clifton (1950) recognize the following clinical types—congenital infantile, acquired infantile, acquired adult, and latent. In the congenital infantile type the cerebral symptoms are present at or soon after birth. The head is large and the eyes are often abnormally small. The fundi show characteristic choroidoretinitis and there may be hemiplegia or diplegia. In the acquired forms the patient is likely to complain of headache and vomiting and joint pains, and may exhibit a rash and fever. Choroidoretinitis is less common than in the congenital form, but papilloedema or optic atrophy may be present together with nerve deafness and the symptoms of a meningo-encephalitis. The spleen may be enlarged and the blood may show an eosinophilia. The cells and protein of the cerebrospinal fluid are likely to be increased and it may be possible to isolate the organism from the fluid. A skin test and various serological tests may be helpful.

So may the characteristic X-ray changes which have been described by Sutton (1951). Calcification is observed in the brain in the form of multiple subcortical flakes and linear or granular areas in the basal ganglia.

REFERENCES

BLACKWOOD, W., McMENEMEY, W. H., MEYER, A., and NORMAN, R. M. (1963) *Greenfield's Neuropathology*, 2nd ed., London.

CAMPBELL, A. M. G., and CLIFTON, F. (1950) Adult toxoplasmosis in one family, *Brain*, **73**, 281.

SUTTON, D. (1951) Intracranial calcification in toxoplasmosis, *Brit. J. Radiol.*, **24**, 31.

WYLLIE, W. G., and FISHER, H. J. W. (1950) Congenital toxoplasmosis, *Quart. J. Med.*, N.S. **19**, 57.

BENIGN MYALGIC ENCEPHALOMYELITIS

Benign myalgic encephalomyelitis is the term applied to a puzzling disorder which has occurred often in small epidemics, especially in institutions, and has been recognized during recent years in many parts of the world. An epidemic in the Royal Free Hospital, London, some years ago led to its being sometimes called the Royal Free Disease. Its puzzling features are the severity of the symptoms in relation to the slightness of the physical signs, its selective incidence upon females, and the absence of any evidence as to its cause. Its mode of spread in institutions is unknown. Sporadic cases undoubtedly occur.

The onset is usually that of a febrile illness, sometimes accompanied by sore throat, upper respiratory or gastro-intestinal symptoms, and often a generalized lymphadenopathy. Jaundice is occasionally seen. In many cases there is no evidence of involvement of the nervous system and the patient recovers completely in a few days. When the nervous system is involved—in 10 out of 48 cases in a recent outbreak in Newcastle (Pool *et al.*, 1961)—psychological disturbances are prominent, particularly depression, disturbances of sleep, and reactions commonly described as hysterical. The limbs are prominently affected with flaccid weakness, muscle pain and tenderness, and paraesthesiae, hyperaesthesia, or relative analgesia of irregular distribution. The tendon jerks may be normal, but are sometimes slightly exaggerated or slightly depressed. The plantar reflexes are usually flexor, but occasionally extensor. Cranial nerve palsies are sometimes observed, but are rare. A characteristic feature of the muscular weakness is the intermittency of muscular contraction, confirmed by electromyography (see below). Objective sensory changes are uncommon.

The cerebrospinal fluid is usually normal, the only abnormalities found on laboratory investigation being the occurrence of an abnormal appearance in the large lymphocytes of the blood. Changes which are believed to be characteristic have been found on electromyography, in particular a characteristic grouping of motor-unit activity with brief silent intervals between groups of two or three motor-unit potentials.

The disease is not fatal and therefore its pathology is unknown. Major persistent disability is rare. A striking feature is the tendency for relapses to occur during the months, and in some cases even years, after the infection. The condition may easily be regarded as hysterical, and indeed some believe that its regular occurrence in closed communities (such as colleges and nurse-training schools) indicate that it is due to a 'mass' hysterical reaction in a community afflicted by an epidemic due to a benign non-neurotropic virus. As Pool *et al.* say, 'the condition should be borne in mind in any patient suffering from a relapsing illness characterised by muscular weakness and by emotional lability'.

REFERENCES

ACHESON, E. D. (1959) The clinical syndrome variously called benign myalgic encephalomyelitis, Iceland disease and epidemic neuromyasthenia, *Amer. J. Med.*, **26**, 569–95.
DIMSDALE, H. (1957) Acute encephalomyelitis of virus origin, in *Modern Trends in Neurology*, ed. WILLIAMS, D. (2nd ser.), p. 177, London.
FIELDS, W. S., and BLATTNER, R. J. (1958) *Viral Encephalitis*, Springfield, Ill.
POOL, J. H., WALTON, J. N., BREWIS, E. G., ULDALL, P. R., WRIGHT, A. E., and GARDNER, P. S. (1961) Benign myalgic encephalomyelitis in Newcastle upon Tyne, *Lancet*, i, 733.
PRICE, J. L. (1961) Myalgic encephalomyelitis, *Lancet*, i, 737.
An Outbreak of Encephalomyelitis in the Royal Free Hospital Group, London, in 1955. By the Medical Staff of the Royal Free Hospital, *Brit. med. J.* (1957), **2**, 895.

BEHÇET'S DISEASE

Behçet's disease is an obscure disorder characterized by ulceration of the mouth and genitalia and involvement of the eyes, particularly with iritis, and running a remittent course characteristically with attacks three or four times a year.

The nervous system may also be involved, the characteristic lesions being disseminated encephalomyelitic lesions with low-grade perivascular inflammatory exudates in the meninges and cortex, but more particularly in the white matter, foci of softening in relation to the blood vessels, and extensive and patchy areas of cortical infarction. The lesions may be widespread, but seem to show a predilection for the upper brain stem. Evans, Pallis, and Spillane (1957) record the isolation of a virus, but even if a virus is the primary cause this does not exclude the possibility that the lesions in the nervous system are allergic in nature, as McMenemey and Laurence (1957) and Kawakita et al. (1967) point out. The relationship of Behçet's syndrome to Reiter's disease is unknown, but in Reiter's disease also ocular lesions may be associated with a meningo-encephalitis or with radiculitic or neuritic symptoms (Oates and Hancock, 1959).

When the nervous system is involved in Behçet's disease headache is often a common symptom. Progressive mental deterioration, Parkinsonism, ophthalmoplegia leading to diplopia, and spastic weakness of the limbs have all been observed. During an active phase the cerebrospinal fluid frequently contains an excess of cells, usually lymphocytes. They rarely number more than a hundred per mm.³, but occasionally much larger numbers have been observed with a high proportion of polymorphonuclears. Aphthous ulceration of the mouth and ulceration of the vagina or scrotum are characteristic. The iritis may lead to hypopyon, and other ocular lesions include conjunctivitis, keratitis, retinitis, retrobulbar neuritis, retinal haemorrhage, and thrombophlebitis. Permanent blindness may occur. Thrombophlebitis of small or large veins elsewhere is said to occur in 25 per cent. of cases. Remissions may occur, but the mortality rate varies from about 21 per cent. in Japan to almost 50 per cent. in Western countries (Kawakita et al., 1967).

Diagnostic difficulty is likely to arise only if the mouth and skin lesions are small or overlooked. Then the neurological manifestations may be confused with tuberculous meningitis, but the fact that in Behçet's syndrome the sugar in the cerebrospinal fluid is normal is stressed by Wadia and Williams (1957). Alternatively the subacute development of spastic weakness of the limbs may suggest multiple sclerosis, but the cell count in the cerebrospinal fluid is likely to be considerably larger than is commonly found in that disease.

No certainly effective treatment is known, but benefit has been claimed in some cases to result from corticotrophin and cortisone.

REFERENCES

EVANS, A. D., PALLIS, C. A., and SPILLANE, J. D. (1957) Involvement of the nervous system in Behçet's syndrome, *Lancet*, ii, 349.
KAWAKITA, H., NISHIMURA, M., SATOH, Y., and SHIBATA, N. (1967) Neurological aspects

of Behçet's disease: a case report and clinico-pathological review of the literature in Japan, *J. neurol. Sci.*, **5**, 417.

McMenemey, W. H., and Laurence, B. J. (1957) Encephalomyelopathy in Behçet's disease, *Lancet*, ii, 353.

Oates, J. K., and Hancock, J. A. H. (1959) Neurological symptoms and lesions occurring in the course of Reiter's disease, *Amer. J. med. Sci.*, **238**, 79.

Pallis, C. A., and Fudge, B. J. (1956) The neurological complications of Behçet's syndrome, *Arch. Neurol. Psychiat. (Chicago)*, **75**, 1.

Viane, A. (1957) La méningo-myélo-encéphalite dans la maladie de Behçet, *Acta neurol. belg.*, **57**, 599.

Wadia, N., and Williams, E. (1957) Behçet's syndrome with neurological complications, *Brain*, **80**, 59.

METAZOAL INFECTIONS

TAENIA SOLIUM (CYSTICERCOSIS)

Cysticercosis is the infestation of man with the encysted larval stage of the human tapeworm, *Taenia solium*, resulting from the ingestion of the ova. The embryos are carried to all parts of the body, but their chief clinical importance lies in their invasion of the nervous system and the muscles. The great majority of cases which have been seen in Great Britain have been the result of infection of British soldiers serving in India. Dixon and Lipscomb (1961) state that the incidence of clinical cysticercosis lies between 1·2 and 2·0 per thousand men serving in India.

In man, the cysts grow for a time, but the larvae die, and the cysts then tend to become calcified. This happens much more frequently in the muscles than in the brain. In the brain, the cysts usually measure about 1 cm. in diameter, and are found in the subarachnoid space, in the cerebral cortex, and to a lesser extent in the white matter. They may be very numerous. A racemose form is encountered particularly in the fourth ventricle basal cisterns, where there is a cluster of grape-like cystic bodies with thin, perhaps translucent, walls containing colourless fluid.

The incubation period between infection and the development of symptoms varies from less than one year to thirty years, the average interval being about five years. The commonest symptom is epilepsy, which occurred in 91·8 per cent. of patients in Dixon and Lipscomb's series. The epilepsy may consist of generalized or focal attacks. It has been pointed out that there is a greater tendency towards variation in the pattern of the attacks, and towards a multiplicity of epileptic manifestations, than occurs in ordinary constitutional epilepsy. All other neurological symptoms are relatively rare, mental disorder occurring in 8·7 per cent. of Dixon and Lipscomb's series, intracranial hypertension in 6·4 per cent., and focal nervous lesions of the brain in 2·7 per cent., and in the spinal cord in 0·2 per cent. Intracranial hypertension may be the result of hydrocephalus produced by the racemose type of cysticercosis, while occasional patients demonstrate the characteristic triad of occipital headache, postural vertigo, and morning vomiting which can result from lesions in the fourth ventricle (Bickerstaff, Small, and Woolf, 1956; Kuper, Mendelow, and Proctor, 1958).

Exceptionally, the clinical picture may be that of a subacute meningo-encephalitis, as in a patient, not known to be suffering from cysticercosis, who after a head injury developed this clinical picture, with bilateral papilloedema and high protein and heavy mononuclear pleocytosis in the cerebrospinal fluid. In chronic cases, there may be a moderate excess of protein and a moderate

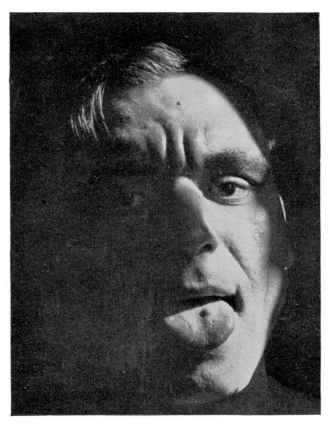

FIG. 66. Cysticercus in tongue
(Kindly lent by Brig. R C. Priest, A.M.S.)

lymphocytic pleocytosis in the fluid, and sometimes a paretic or meningitic colloidal gold curve.

Subcuticular nodules are found in approximately half of all cases, and exceptionally a nodule may be seen in the eye or in the tongue [FIG. 66]. In over 90 per cent. of cases, calcified cysts can be demonstrated by X-raying the muscles [FIG. 67]. Calcification of intracranial cysts occurs in only about one-third of all cases, and then very rarely less than ten years after infection. Biopsy of a subcuticular nodule may be helpful in diagnosis.

According to Dixon and Lipscomb, the annual death rate ranges between 3·3 and 5·8 per thousand cases per annum, death being due usually to status epilepticus or intracranial hypertension. Epilepsy should be treated along the usual lines: this is often successful in diminishing and sometimes in abolishing the attacks. Intracranial hypertension calls for surgical investigation and treatment.

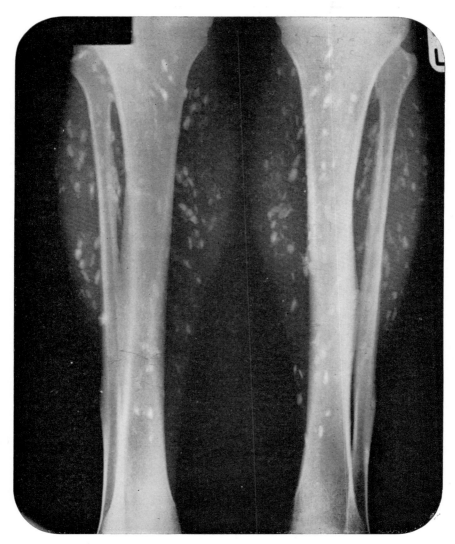

FIG. 67. Calcified cysts in the leg muscles in a patient suffering from cysticercosis with cerebral symptoms

MULTICEPS MULTICEPS (COENURUS CEREBRALIS)

In some countries, especially South Africa, *Multiceps multiceps* is the common tapeworm of dogs, and human infection may lead to the presence of cysts in the ventricles or in the posterior fossa, the clinical picture being predominantly that of intracranial hypertension.

REFERENCES

BICKERSTAFF, E. R., SMALL, J. M., and WOOLF, A. L. (1956) Cysticercosis of the posterior
    fossa, *Brain*, **79**, 622.
DIXON, H. B. F., and LIPSCOMB, F. M. (1961) Cysticercosis: an analysis and follow-up
    of 450 cases, *Spec. Rep. Ser. med. Res. Coun. (Lond.)*, No. 299.
KUPER, S., MENDELOW, H., and PROCTOR, N. S. F. (1958) Internal hydrocephalus caused
    by parasitic cysts, *Brain*, **81**, 235.

TOXOCARA INFECTION

In children who have a history of frequent contact with dogs or cats or of
eating dirt (pica) a syndrome of recurrent wheezy bronchitis or pneumonitis
may be accompanied by fleeting urticarial rashes and convulsions. The condition is due to the ingestion of larvae of the *Toxocara canis* or *Toxocara cati*
which produce a widespread granulomatous reaction in liver, lungs, skeletal
muscle and brain. There is often a striking eosinophilia.

9

SYPHILIS OF THE NERVOUS SYSTEM

AETIOLOGY

SYPHILIS is growing less common and less dangerous as a result of modern chemotherapy. The Registrar General's Annual Statistical Review shows that in England and Wales the mortality from general paresis declined by 94 per cent. between 1916 and 1954 and that from tabes dorsalis by 86·2 per cent. in the same period. Headache and palsies were attributed to syphilis in the Middle Ages, but there was little exact knowledge of neurosyphilis before the nineteenth century. Bayle described general paralysis in 1822, though the term was first used by Delaye in 1824, and the first adequate account of tabes was given by Romberg in 1846, and amplified by Duchenne and Charcot. Argyll Robertson described the pupillary abnormalities which bear his name in 1869. Fournier, also in 1869, described congenital syphilis and introduced the concept of parasyphilis. The discovery of the causal organism in the spirochaete *Treponema pallidum* by Schaudinn and Hoffman in 1903 and the elaboration of the Bordet–Wassermann reaction (1901–7) have rendered it possible to identify conditions as syphilitic, the relationship of which to syphilis was previously a matter of speculation. The Wassermann reaction has recently been supplanted by more modern serological tests of which the V.D.R.L. test is that most commonly used. There are still, however, many unsolved problems in the aetiology and classification of neurosyphilis.

Although the earliest manifestation of acquired syphilitic infection is the primary chancre, it has been proved that spirochaetes may obtain access to the blood and be present in the spleen within ten days of infection and before the chancre appears. There is evidence, which will be described later, that in the secondary stage spirochaetes have reached the nervous system in a large proportion, probably in the majority of persons infected, though they may not then give rise to symptoms. The secondary stage is usually followed by a period of latency, but even within a year, frequently within two or three years, symptoms of the tertiary stage may develop.

On clinical grounds a distinction has long been drawn between two groups of tertiary manifestations of neurosyphilis, one of which has been known as meningovascular or cerebrospinal syphilis, the other, which comprises tabes and general paresis, being distinguished as parenchymatous syphilis, parasyphilis, or metasyphilis. In meningovascular or cerebrospinal syphilis symptoms may occur within a few years of infection, tend to be focal, and on the whole respond well to treatment. Tabes and general paresis, on the other hand, exhibit a longer latent interval, are characterized by diffuse or systematized pathological changes, and respond less satisfactorily to treatment. We are still ignorant of the true basis of this clinical distinction, and the names which have been applied to the two varieties of tertiary neurosyphilis are therefore unsatisfactory. Neither a cerebrospinal distribution nor involvement of the meninges and blood vessels is peculiar to the more benign form, and destruction of the parenchyma of the nervous system is not limited to tabes and general paresis. McIntosh and Fildes (1914) with much cogency put forward the view that in cerebrospinal or meningovascular syphilis the essential lesion is limited to the blood vessels and the mesoblastic tissues and that the parenchyma of the nervous system suffers secondarily, while in tabes and general paresis there is invasion of the nervous tissue itself by spirochaetes in addition to a mesoblastic reaction. This hypothesis justifies the use of meningovascular syphilis as a convenient, though not a strictly accurate, term for the more benign form of tertiary neurosyphilis, and parenchymatous neurosyphilis for tabes and general paresis.

Neurosyphilis occurs in only a small proportion—about 10 per cent.—of persons infected with the *Treponema pallidum*. It has been supposed that certain strains of spirochaetes possess an affinity for the nervous system, while others do not. In favour of this view it has been stated that in some instances a number of individuals infected by the same person have all developed neurosyphilis, that the primary sore and secondary cutaneous manifestations may be slight or absent in persons who subsequently develop neurosyphilis, and that in certain countries where syphilis is rife and other visceral manifestations are common, involvement of the nervous system is rare. Levaditi claims to have separated dermotropic and neurotropic forms of spirochaete by means of experimental inoculation. These arguments have not been accepted as conclusive evidence for the existence of a neurotropic strain of spirochaetes. There is, however, evidence that in populations more recently exposed to syphilitic infection, acute secondary and tertiary manifestations of the infection (meningo-encephalitis, meningovascular manifestations and gumma) are commoner, whereas in those communities long exposed to the disease, such as the North American Indian, neurosyphilis (which some prefer to call quaternary rather than tertiary syphilis) occurs more frequently. Before penicillin intensive methods of treatment of syphilis were blamed as a cause of the subsequent development of neurosyphilis, and it was suggested that such treatment might diminish the patient's natural powers of resistance to the organism or permit the development of resistant strains of spirochaetes in the nervous system. This theory, however, has not received general support, and in any case the early and intensive treatment of infected persons, by diminishing their infectivity, is certainly reducing the prevalence of neurosyphilis.

Various factors have been regarded as predisposing to the development of neurosyphilis, especially alcoholism, other infections, mental strain, and inherited mental instability, but their importance in causation is difficult to assess.

Out of every twelve patients with neurosyphilis approximately five have general paresis, four meningovascular syphilis, and three tabes.

SECONDARY NEUROSYPHILIS

PATHOLOGY

Spirochaetes may reach the nervous system during the primary stage and before the development of the cutaneous exanthem. Nicolau found a lymphocytosis in the cerebrospinal fluid in 9 per cent. of cases at this stage and Cutler *et al.* (1954) positive serological reactions in 1·5 per cent. In the secondary stage abnormalities, which may be transitory, have been found in the fluid in from 36 to 80 per cent. of cases in different series. Cutler *et al.* (1954) found serological abnormalities in 6 per cent. Little is known of the pathology of this stage, as the condition is rarely fatal. In a small number of acute and fatal cases of secondary neurosyphilis the brain has been oedematous, but otherwise histological changes have been almost confined to the leptomeninges. The pia mater and arachnoid have been congested, lost their translucency, and exhibited a diffuse cellular infiltration most marked round the vessels, which have shown endarteritis.

SYMPTOMS

There may be no symptoms referable to the nervous system in spite of the presence of slight changes in the cerebrospinal fluid, or the symptoms may be no more severe than the headache and pains in the back and limbs commonly associated with the secondary stage of syphilis. Exceptionally, symptoms of considerable severity may occur between the onset of the secondary stage and the end of the first year after infection. When the onset of these symptoms is insidious they are indistinguishable from the later manifestations of meningovascular syphilis described in the next section. Very rarely an acute and rapidly fatal meningo-encephalitis may occur during the first year after infection, characterized by generalized convulsions, and quickly deepening coma. Polyneuritis has been described during the first year.

The term 'neuro-relapse' has been applied to the subacute development of nervous symptoms within a few months of the secondary stage in a patient who has received inadequate treatment. The symptoms of a neuro-relapse are commonly more severe than would be likely to occur in an untreated individual, and it appears that partial treatment, while failing to destroy many of the spirochaetes, may either reduce the patient's resistance or render him hypersensitive, so that further multiplication of the spirochaetes may be followed by a severe reaction. Convulsions, coma, severe headache, papilloedema, ocular palsies, aphasia, or hemiplegia may occur in such patients.

The Cerebrospinal Fluid

In patients in the secondary stage who show no symptoms of involvement of the nervous system the changes in the cerebrospinal fluid are usually slight and are present in from one-third to one-half of all cases. They consist of a slight increase in the number of mononuclear cells or of the globulin or of both. The V.D.R.L. reaction is negative in the fluid but may be positive or negative in the blood, according to whether the patient has received treatment. Patients suffering from nervous symptoms are likely to show more marked changes in the fluid, and these are usually proportional to the severity of the symptoms. When clinical evidence of meningitis is present, pressure of the fluid is usually raised and the cell content is increased and may be as high as 1,000 per mm.³ The cells are usually mononuclear, but in the most acute cases polymorphonuclear cells may also be present. Tests for globulin are positive and the V.D.R.L. reaction is usually positive in the fluid. It is usually positive in the blood, but may be negative if the patient has been treated.

For **Diagnosis, Prognosis,** and **Treatment,** see pages 409, 410, and 414.

TERTIARY MENINGOVASCULAR SYPHILIS

CEREBRAL SYPHILIS

PATHOLOGY

The essential lesion in meningovascular syphilis is a vascular and perivascular inflammation [FIG. 68]. The affected vessel exhibits a proliferation and in-

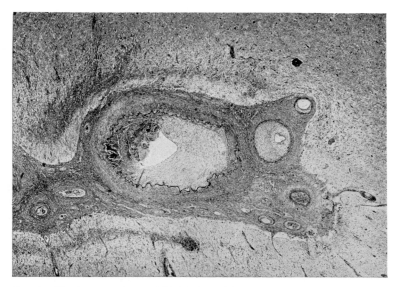

FIG. 68. Meningovascular syphilis. Endarteritis and perivascular inflammation

flammatory infiltration of its wall—endarteritis obliterans—and the perivascular space is infiltrated with lymphocytes, plasma cells, and usually with fibroblasts. The proliferation of the fibroblasts leads to fibrosis, while impairment of blood supply through reduction of the lumen of the vessel, or actual thrombosis, together no doubt with the action of toxins produced by the organism, causes necrosis or caseation of neighbouring tissues. The result is a gumma, which is a granuloma originating in a patch of perivascular inflammation leading to necrosis, surrounded by a zone of fibrotic reaction. Spirochaetes are scanty and difficult to demonstrate in all tertiary syphilitic lesions, but they have been found in the periphery of cerebral gummas. This characteristic reaction of the mesoblastic tissues to the treponemas is the pathological basis of all forms of meningovascular syphilis. Clinical manifestations depend entirely upon the site of the process.

Cranial Pachymeningitis

Syphilitic inflammation of the dura mater of the cranium is comparatively rare. It may be secondary to osteitis of the bones of the vault, or the dura may be involved apart from the bone. Probably many cases described as pachymeningitis in the past were cases of subdural haematoma [see p. 346] occurring in patients with neurosyphilis.

Gummatous Leptomeningitis

Gummatous leptomeningitis is a common manifestation of neurosyphilis. The basal meninges are frequently affected, but the process may be confined to those covering the convexity of the cerebral hemispheres. The arachnoid and pia mater form an adherent thickened membrane, which may contain a gummy exudate and small gummas.

Cerebral Endarteritis

Although endarteritis occurs in all cerebral syphilitic lesions, it assumes especial importance when a main arterial trunk is the site of the process. Progressive occlusion of an artery usually leads finally to thrombosis and causes focal symptoms corresponding to the part of the brain supplied by the vessel.

Gumma

Small cerebral gummas may be multiple and take origin from the meninges. They are usually rounded, greyish in colour, and surrounded by a pink vascular zone. They may be relatively soft from central necrosis, or tough, when fibrosis predominates. Single small gummas are rare and usually occur subcortically.

SYMPTOMS

Meningovascular syphilis may cause symptoms within a few months of infection or at any subsequent period in the patient's life. In most cases, however, symptoms develop within the first five years after infection. Symptoms are very varied on account of the multiplicity and different sites of the lesions. Frequently symptoms of both cerebral and spinal syphilis are present in the same patient.

Asymptomatic Neurosyphilis

In some patients abnormalities are found in the cerebrospinal fluid though the nervous system appears normal. This is known as asymptomatic neurosyphilis. Some workers would include in this group patients with isolated abnormal physical signs such as reflex iridoplegia, without any symptoms of progressive disease, but with an abnormal cerebrospinal fluid.

Cranial Pachymeningitis

This rare condition may give rise to no symptoms apart from headache, but when the dura is adherent to the leptomeninges over the cortex there are likely to be symptoms of cortical irritation, such as focal convulsions and paresis of the limbs. [See p. 346.]

Cerebral Leptomeningitis

The symptoms of gummatous leptomeningitis may be relatively diffuse or sharply focal, for example, limited to one cranial nerve. When the lesions are diffuse the onset of symptoms is usually insidious. Headache is frequently severe, with nocturnal exacerbations, and may be associated with tenderness of the scalp. Papilloedema may occur. Mental changes are common. In mild cases these consist of impairment of memory and intellectual capacity. The patient becomes inefficient at his work and if, as is not uncommon, he exhibits anxiety and nervousness, the condition may be mistaken for neurosis. In more severe cases there is marked apathy, with gross mental deterioration amounting to dementia, or the mental state may resemble that of Korsakow's psychosis. Aphasia may be present, and loss of sphincter control is common. The patient may finally pass into a state of semi-stupor. When the meninges over the convexity of the cerebral hemispheres are involved, convulsions may occur. These may be Jacksonian attacks without loss of consciousness, or generalized attacks in which consciousness is lost. Paresis and incoordination of the limbs on one or both sides are common. Basal meningitis frequently involves the chiasmal region and may thus lead to optic atrophy with defects of the visual fields. Disturbance of the functions of the hypothalamus may cause obesity, diabetes insipidus, transient glycosuria, or narcolepsy. Hydrocephalus occasionally occurs. Reflex iridoplegia is almost constant and cranial nerve palsies are common, the nerves being involved in gummatous inflammation in their passage through the meninges. They may be affected singly or in association with adjacent nerves, and usually unilaterally. The third nerve is most frequently affected, and painless third-nerve palsy as an isolated symptom is not infrequently the cause of the patient's coming for treatment. The paralysis of the intrinsic and extrinsic ocular muscles supplied by the nerve may be incomplete. Its onset is usually rapid. Next in frequency the sixth, seventh, and fifth cranial nerves are liable to be attacked. Thus facial paralysis clinically indistinguishable from Bell's palsy may be syphilitic in origin. When the fifth nerve suffers, sensory disturbances are more common than motor weakness. Neuralgic pain referred to the distribution of one or more of its branches may be associated with either hyperalgesia or analgesia, and sometimes with ophthalmic herpes zoster or neuropathic keratitis. Syphilitic lesions of the eighth nerve may cause vertigo and deafness. The nerves arising from the medulla may be involved, the twelfth suffering more frequently than the tenth and eleventh, but any of the three may be affected either alone or in combination with the others.

Cerebral Endarteritis

Any cerebral artery may be the site of syphilitic endarteritis. Before occlusion is complete there are frequently premonitory motor or sensory symptoms due to ischaemia of the region supplied by the vessel. Finally, thrombosis leads to symptoms of infarction which are described elsewhere [p. 293]. The middle cerebral artery or its branches and the posterior cerebral are most frequently the site of syphilitic thrombosis, but the anterior cerebral or the arteries of the brain stem may be involved.

Hemiplegia is the commonest manifestation of cerebral thrombosis due to syphilis and may occur as a result of occlusion, either of the middle cerebral artery itself or of one of its basal branches supplying the internal capsule. Hemiplegia usually occurs within two or three years of infection. Its onset is rapid and associated with headache, but not with loss of consciousness. Syphilitic hemiplegia is rarely bilateral.

Parkinsonism is a very rare manifestation of cerebral syphilis, but has occasionally been described in association with symptoms of syphilitic inflammation of the midbrain.

Cerebral Gumma

A large gumma causes the symptoms of an intracranial tumour, situated usually subcortically in one cerebral hemisphere. The syphilitic origin of the tumour can only be inferred from the history of infection, the presence of signs of syphilis elsewhere, and a positive V.D.R.L. reaction in the blood or cerebrospinal fluid. Cerebral gumma is very rare, however, whereas both intracranial neoplasm and syphilitic infection are common, and may be present in the same individual. A positive V.D.R.L. reaction, therefore, must not be interpreted as indicating that a space-occupying lesion within the skull is necessarily, or even probably, a gumma.

The Cerebrospinal Fluid

In meningovascular syphilis the V.D.R.L. reaction is positive in the blood in 60 or 70 per cent. of cases. The treponema immobilization test is even more specific, a positive result invariably being indicative of syphilitic infection. The pressure of the cerebrospinal fluid may be either normal or increased. There is usually an excess of cells ranging between 20 and 100 per mm.^{3}, though the latter number may be exceeded. The cells are mononuclear. The protein content of the fluid is usually increased and lies between 0·05 and 0·15 per 100 ml. An increase in the globulin is almost invariably present, and the V.D.R.L. reaction is positive in from 90 to 100 per cent. of cases when 1 ml. of fluid is used. In cases of syphilitic cerebral thrombosis the V.D.R.L. reaction may be positive in the blood and negative in the fluid. Lange's colloidal gold test yields either a 'paretic' curve, e.g. 5542210000, or a 'luetic' curve—1355421000.

DIAGNOSIS

Cerebral syphilis is so protean in its manifestations that its diagnosis covers a large field of neurology. Fortunately, serological tests come to the aid of clinical observation. It is rare that the V.D.R.L. reaction is negative in the cerebrospinal fluid in active cerebral syphilis, and still more rare to find the reaction negative in both the cerebrospinal fluid and the blood. Any suspicion of syphilis should, therefore, lead to the examination of both.

The mental changes associated with cerebral syphilis require to be distinguished from other mental disorders and in their milder forms from neurosis. A clue to their true nature is usually afforded by the presence of abnormalities in the nervous system, especially in the pupils and their reactions.

When meningovascular syphilis is associated with papilloedema it may be confused with other conditions causing increased intracranial pressure, especially intracranial tumour. The symptoms in syphilis, however, rarely suggest a single focal lesion, and if such are present a tumour should not be too readily excluded, even if the V.D.R.L. reaction is positive, since it is not very rare for a tumour to develop in a patient suffering from syphilis.

When either focal or generalized epileptiform attacks appear for the first time in adult life care must always be taken to exclude syphilis as a cause.

Cerebral thrombosis of syphilitic origin usually occurs at an earlier age than thrombosis due to atheroma, but otherwise it can be distinguished from the latter only when a history of infection or other signs of syphilis are present, or, in their absence, by serological tests.

Meningovascular syphilis, since it frequently causes multiple cerebral lesions, may be confused with encephalitis and multiple sclerosis. In encephalitis lethargica a history of the acute attack may be obtainable, though less frequently today than previously. The reaction of the pupils on convergence is more often impaired than that to light, whereas in cerebral syphilis the opposite is the case, and Parkinsonian symptoms of varying severity are frequently present in encephalitis lethargica. In multiple sclerosis it is very rare for the pupillary reflexes to be affected, while nystagmus and incoordination of the limbs in the absence of sensory loss are rare in syphilis. In multiple sclerosis the tendon jerks are exaggerated, in neurosyphilis they are more often diminished or lost.

PROGNOSIS

The prognosis of cerebral syphilis is on the whole good, and excellent results are often obtained from energetic treatment. When severe mental symptoms have occurred, however, although there may be marked improvement, the patient is likely to be left with some impairment of intellectual efficiency and emotional stability. The results of vascular occlusion are permanent, and though some improvement may follow the disappearance of shock following the onset of the lesion, there is likely to be little further change for the better in hemiplegia, and the hemianopia resulting from posterior cerebral thrombosis persists unaltered. Relapses are not uncommon, especially in patients who have abandoned treatment. They are unlikely to occur in those who are thoroughly treated and kept under regular observation.

TREATMENT

See page 414.

SPINAL SYPHILIS

PATHOLOGY

The histological character of the lesions of meningovascular syphilis has already been described.

Spinal Pachymeningitis

Syphilitic inflammation of the spinal dura mater may follow spread of infection from syphilitic osteitis of the spine or may occur independently of disease of the bone. The cervical region is usually involved—pachymeningitis cervicalis hypertrophica—but it is probable that this condition is sometimes non-syphilitic. The dura mater is thickened and adherent to the arachnoid and pia. The vessels entering the cord are involved in the inflammation, and the cord becomes sclerosed, and may contain a central cavity. Destruction of the long tracts is followed by ascending and descending degeneration.

Meningomyelitis

As in cerebral syphilis the meninges and blood vessels are both involved, though frequently not equally severely. When leptomeningitis predominates, degenerative changes in the cord itself may be superficial, as in syphilitic amyotrophy. When the vessels also suffer severely, lesions of the substance of the cord are more extensive. Though the lesions are chronic, thrombosis of an important vessel may precipitate acute changes leading to an acute or subacute transverse lesion of the cord. In such cases the leptomeninges are adherent to the cord, which is visibly softened. Microscopically the vessels show endarteritis and perivascular cellular infiltration, and the meninges are also infiltrated. Within the cord there is degeneration of the myelin sheaths and sometimes also of the axis cylinders. The ganglion cells exhibit chromatolysis, and ascending and descending degeneration are to be found. Syphilitic myelitis usually involves the dorsal region of the cord and, though the leptomeninges may be extensively infiltrated, the area of softening of the cord is usually limited to two or three segments.

Erb's Syphilitic Spinal Paralysis

Progressive spastic paraplegia developing in syphilitics during middle life was first described by Erb. This condition is probably no more than a manifestation of syphilitic meningomyelitis.

Spinal Endarteritis

As in the brain, endarteritis of one of the spinal arteries or of its branches may be followed by thrombosis leading to a circumscribed area of softening within the cord, corresponding to the area of supply of the obstructed vessel.

Radiculitis

One or more of the spinal dorsal roots may be involved in syphilitic inflammation spreading inwards from the meninges.

SYMPTOMS

Cervical Pachymeningitis

The earliest symptom is pain due to strangulation of the dorsal roots, which radiates round the neck, over the shoulders, and down the upper limbs. The pains are followed by progressive atrophy of the muscles supplied by the corresponding ventral roots. Finally, compression and ischaemia of the cord lead to progressive spastic paraplegia with sensory loss below the level of the lesion.

Meningomyelitis

Myelitis is frequently an early symptom of meningovascular syphilis and not uncommonly occurs within three years of infection. The dorsal region of the cord is usually affected but when the cervical region is involved, and the course of the illness is subacute, pain in the neck and upper limbs may be followed by amyotrophy and sensory loss in the upper extremities due to root involvement. Motor symptoms resulting from a dorsal lesion are generally preceded by pains in the back, spreading round the chest and abdomen. Weakness of the lower limbs develops between a few days and several weeks after the onset of the pains. In some cases complete flaccid paraplegia rapidly develops, with retention of urine and impairment or loss of all forms of sensibility below the level of the lesion. Sometimes the onset is more gradual and the functions of the cord are less severely affected. In such cases the patient develops spastic paraplegia-in-extension; control over the bladder is less severely impaired and sensory loss may be slight. In the flaccid form of paraplegia the reflexes in the lower limbs may at first be lost; extensor plantar responses shortly appear, however, and as spinal shock passes off, severe flexor spasms are likely to develop.

Erb's Syphilitic Spinal Paralysis

This syndrome differs only from other forms of syphilitic myelitis in its more gradual onset and more slowly progressive course, the early involvement of bladder control, and the comparatively slight sensory loss.

Spinal Endarteritis

Endarteritis and arterial thrombosis play an important part in syphilitic myelitis. Exceptionally thrombosis of a branch of the anterior or posterior spinal arteries comparable with syphilitic cerebral thrombosis occurs. When a lateral branch of the anterior spinal artery is the site of thrombosis there is a sudden onset of weakness, followed by wasting of the muscles innervated by the affected spinal segment. The spinothalamic tract on the same side is frequently damaged, with the production of relative hemi-analgesia and hemi-thermo-anaesthesia on the opposite side of the body, with an upper level a few segments below that involved in the lesion. When thrombosis of one posterior spinal artery occurs this is usually limited to a few segments. All forms of sensibility are likely to be impaired in the corresponding cutaneous segments owing to destruction of the posterior horn of grey matter. The posterior columns and the corticospinal tract on the same side are also the site of softening, as a result of which postural sensibility and appreciation of passive movement and of vibration are lost below the level of the lesion on the same side, and there is also spastic paralysis below the lesion on the side affected.

Radiculitis

Syphilitic radiculitis usually affects the dorsal roots and causes pain of a corresponding segmental distribution associated with either hyperalgesia or analgesia. Herpes zoster is a not uncommon complication of this lesion. When the ventral roots are also affected, weakness and wasting develop in the muscles which they supply.

The Cerebrospinal Fluid

In chronic spinal syphilis the changes in the cerebrospinal fluid are the same as those found in cerebral syphilis; see page 409. After a subacute lesion, such as meningomyelitis, there is frequently a considerable excess of protein and of mononuclear cells, and both in this condition and in syphilitic pachymeningitis leptomeningeal adhesions may lead to obstruction of the subarachnoid space, in which case the fluid will exhibit the changes characteristic of spinal block [see p. 129]. There is usually an excess of cells, however, and the V.D.R.L. reaction is positive. A vascular lesion of the spinal cord may be associated with a normal spinal fluid, but the V.D.R.L. reaction is usually positive in the blood.

DIAGNOSIS

Spinal syphilis has to be differentiated from other conditions causing paraplegia or irritation of dorsal spinal roots, especially from spinal tumour and from multiple sclerosis. The diagnosis is not as a rule difficult. A history of infection is usually obtainable. Signs of cerebral syphilis, especially irregularity of the pupils and impairment of their reaction to light, are frequently present and characteristic changes, especially a positive V.D.R.L. reaction, are found in the cerebrospinal fluid.

PROGNOSIS

Spinal syphilis usually responds well to treatment, the determining factor in prognosis being the extent to which irreparable damage has already been done to the spinal cord. Even when myelitis has led to complete paraplegia, improvement is likely to occur as shock passes off and oedema of the cord disappears. Complete recovery, however, is not to be expected. The prognosis is naturally worse in patients who have developed urinary infection or other serious complications. In amyotrophy the progress of the muscular wasting can frequently be arrested and slight improvement may occur, but much of the disability will be permanent. Root pains can usually be relieved, but are sometimes intractable.

TREATMENT OF MENINGOVASCULAR SYPHILIS

Before treatment is begun, the blood V.D.R.L. reaction should be examined and a complete investigation of the cerebrospinal fluid should be carried out for comparison with future findings. The object of treatment is the destruction of all the spirochaetes in the body. Until the introduction of penicillin few were sanguine enough to believe that this could be accomplished, at least unless treatment was begun within a few weeks of infection. It may now be practicable, if penicillin can reach all the organisms. Before the introduction of penicillin the most important spirochaeticidal drugs were bismuth and the arsenobenzene derivatives. The action of the first was gradual, that of arsenic more intense but less enduring. The best therapeutic results were therefore obtained by using them in combination. Iodide was also valuable in promoting the absorption of inflammatory products. However, although some venereologists continue to use these preparations their use is diminishing and most workers rely on penicillin and when necessary, other modern antibiotics.

Penicillin

Experience has shown that the smaller doses of penicillin at first given were inadequate and the dose now employed is 600 mg. daily. The optimal frequency of doses is not yet settled. Dattner *et al.* (1947) gave an intramuscular injection every 3 hours, Nicol and Whelen (1947) only once a day. Most workers are now agreed that a single daily injection of 600 mg. of procaine penicillin for 20 days is all that is required. However, occasional untoward reactions to penicillin continue to occur (Beerman *et al.*, 1962). Chloramphenicol and chlortetracycline are also effective. There is no evidence that fever is of value as an adjuvant to penicillin. Erythromycin, 500 mg. four times daily for 10–15 days, is now probably the drug of choice in patients unable to tolerate penicillin (Thomas, 1964).

THE ROUTINE OF TREATMENT

It is generally agreed that penicillin is the foundation of treatment. To diminish the risk of Herxheimer reactions some authorities have advised beginning with small doses of penicillin which are then gradually increased but there is now general agreement that this is no longer necessary. After the initial course of 12 G., no other treatment should be necessary for six months, when the blood V.D.R.L. reaction and the cerebrospinal fluid are re-examined. The first favourable change in the fluid is a fall in the cell count, the protein falls next, sometimes after an initial rise, and changes in the colloidal gold curve and V.D.R.L. reaction occur last. If the fluid shows improvement at the end of six months and the patient's clinical condition is satisfactory he can safely be left without treatment for a further six months, when the blood and cerebrospinal fluid are examined again. The progress made will decide whether further penicillin is necessary. If not, the blood V.D.R.L. reaction should be examined every six months and the cerebrospinal fluid once a year. The object to be aimed at is primarily the relief of symptoms and the arrest of the progress of the disease. The latter can only be regarded as having been achieved when the cerebrospinal fluid is normal, with a negative V.D.R.L. reaction, and the V.D.R.L. reaction in the blood is also negative. When this has taken place the patient should be thoroughly examined clinically and the blood V.D.R.L. reaction tested once a year for five years, but it is unnecessary to examine the cerebrospinal fluid again unless fresh symptoms appear. Sometimes, however, patients in whom the clinical course of the disease appears to be arrested continue to manifest a positive V.D.R.L. reaction in the blood or in the cerebrospinal fluid or in both. Such patients may benefit from further penicillin or perhaps from induced pyrexia produced by three or four intravenous injections of graduated doses of *E. coli* vaccine (Pyrifer) or by inoculation with benign tertian malaria. If, in spite of treatment for two or three years, the patient remains 'V.D.R.L.-fast' and his clinical condition is satisfactory, further treatment is inadvisable.

GENERAL PARESIS

Synonyms. Dementia paralytica; general paralysis of the insane (G.P.I.).

AETIOLOGY

General paresis was recognized as a clinical entity about a hundred years ago, though, as its name 'general paralysis of the insane' implies, it was at first regarded as a form of paralysis supervening in persons who had already become insane. In the latter half of the last century its relationship to syphilitic infection was established, though syphilis was then regarded as predisposing to general paresis rather than as actually causing it, hence it was termed a 'parasyphilitic' or 'metasyphilitic' disorder. Noguchi, however, in 1911, first demonstrated the presence of spirochaetes in the brains of sufferers from general paresis.

Many hypotheses have been proposed in explanation of the marked difference in the clinical features of general paresis and cerebral meningovascular syphilis, notably the rapidly progressive course of the former and its failure to respond to treatment which effects improvement in the latter. The most satisfactory explanation is that put forward by McIntosh and Fildes, according to whom the nerve cells of the brain in meningovascular syphilis suffer secondarily as a result of infection of the mesoblastic tissues, especially the blood vessels, whereas in general paresis spirochaetes penetrate through the blood vessels and reach the nerve cells, which their toxins directly affect. Not only is the resulting degeneration of the nervous elements irreparable, but the spirochaetes lying within the brain substance are beyond the reach of the older spirochaeticidal drugs which cannot pass through the blood vessels. This theory leaves unexplained the different distribution of the spirochaetes in meningovascular syphilis and in general paresis, the invasion of the nervous tissues in the latter presumably being due to constitutional or immunological factors which are not yet understood.

General paresis is the disorder present in about five out of twelve sufferers from neurosyphilis. Males are more liable to it than females in the proportion of four to one. It usually develops between 10 and 15 years after infection, though the interval may be much shorter, and exceptionally 30 or more years may elapse. It is rare, however, that the incubation period is more than 20 years. It has been stated that its duration is inversely proportional to the age at which infection occurs. The first symptoms usually appear between the ages of 40 and 50 but a congenital form is known to occur rarely [see p. 431].

In many tropical and subtropical countries where syphilis is rife general paresis is almost unknown amongst the natives. This, however, cannot be due to a peculiarity in the infecting organism, since Europeans who acquire the infection from the natives are liable to develop it.

Alcoholism, mental strain, physical trauma, and an inherited neuropathic constitution have all been regarded as predisposing to the development of general paresis, but the influence of these factors is difficult to assess. Kretschmer has pointed out that the majority of sufferers come of a cyclothymic stock which is associated with a pyknic (i.e. short, thickset) physique.

PATHOLOGY

Macroscopically the brain is shrunken, the gyri being unusually well defined, and there is a compensatory hydrocephalus, both external and internal, but the atrophy is confined to the anterior two-thirds of the hemispheres. The pia-arachnoid is usually more opaque than normal, and the walls of the ventricles present a granular appearance due to ependymitis. Haemorrhagic pachy-meningitis is sometimes present.

Microscopical changes [FIG. 69] are predominantly cortical and are found in the meninges, blood vessels, and neurones. The leptomeninges show a diffuse infiltration with lymphocytes and plasma cells. Similar cells occupy the perivas-cular spaces of the small vessels and capillaries of the cerebral cortex, and there is usually evidence of new formation of capillaries. The ganglion cells of the cortex show a varying degree of degeneration, going on to complete disappear-ance. These changes are most marked in the molecular layer and the layers of

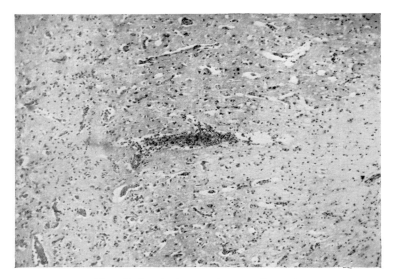

FIG. 69. Cerebral cortex in general paresis

small and medium-sized pyramidal cells. The deeper layers, including the large pyramidal cells, show slighter or sometimes more acute alterations. Demyelination of the fibres of the cortex, especially of the tangential fibres, is also present, frequently with a focal distribution. There is a proliferation of the glia, with the formation of both fibroglia and of giant glial cells. The micro-glia is also hypertrophied. Iron is present in large amounts both in the peri-vascular spaces and in the microglia.

These cortical changes are always diffuse, but the frontal and temporal regions usually suffer most severely. Similar changes are to be found in the basal ganglia and in the cortex of the cerebellum. It has been pointed out that there appears to be no relationship between the severity of the cortical degeneration and the degree of infiltration of the overlying leptomeninges. Spirochaetes are demon-strable in the cortex in some 50 per cent. of cases, especially in the frontal region, and have sometimes been found within ganglion cells. In the 'Lissauer type' of general paresis, localized cortical atrophy, a 'spongy state' and patchy demyelina-tion of the white matter are found. The pathological changes of tabes may co-exist with general paresis. Aortitis is almost invariably present.

SYMPTOMS

Mental Symptoms

The earliest symptoms are usually mental, and in the early stages they are frequently so slight as to be apparent only to those who know the patient well. It is important, therefore, always to obtain a history from a relative or friend. The earliest mental change is usually an impairment of intellectual efficiency. The patient is unable to do his work as well as formerly. He loses the power to concentrate, and his memory becomes untrustworthy. His business inefficiency, however, is apparent to others, but not to himself, though exceptionally anxiety may be prominent, and together with the other symptoms described may lead to a mistaken diagnosis of neurosis. As the condition progresses, the patient's behaviour becomes more abnormal, and he is apt to become careless about his dress and personal appearance, and about money, as a result of which he may throw large sums away in extravagance or in ill-judged speculations. Alcoholic excess and sexual aberrations are common at this stage. The commonest early mental changes are thus symptoms of dementia [see also p. 990], and this form of the disorder is sometimes described as the 'simple dementing type'.

The form taken by the mental disorder, however, doubtless depends upon the patient's mental constitution, and thus other clinical pictures occur. The grandiose form, though frequently regarded as typical, is less common than simple dementia. Patients of this type are euphoric, and develop delusions in which they figure as exceptional persons endowed with superhuman strength, immense wealth, or other magnificent attributes. They readily act on these delusions, and may order large quantities of goods or write their physician a cheque for a million pounds, and they see no discrepancy between their imaginary attributes and their debilitated and unfortunate actual condition. Other emotional states may dominate the picture, leading to so-called depressed, agitated, maniacal, and circular types. Sometimes the condition closely resembles Korsakow's psychosis. As the patient becomes worse, however, the symptoms of dementia become more prominent, and in the terminal stage there is little evidence of any mental activity, and the sufferer, bedridden, incontinent, and dirty, leads a vegetative existence.

Speech exhibits a degradation parallel with that of other mental activities and suffers both in its receptive and expressive functions. Difficulty in naming objects is common. Echolalia may occur.

Physical Symptoms

Epileptiform attacks occur in approximately 50 per cent. of cases. They may take the form of localized convulsions, without loss of consciousness; generalized attacks, in which consciousness is lost; or petit mal, in which brief impairment or loss of consciousness occurs without a convulsion. Status epilepticus sometimes occurs.

Apoplectiform attacks, so-called 'congestive attacks', sometimes occur and such an episode may bring the patient under observation. The resulting symptoms, of which hemiplegia is the commonest, but which include aphasia, apraxia, and hemianopia, are always transitory and the associated loss of consciousness is usually brief. Recovery from an apoplectiform attack is often complete in a week or two.

Although in most cases physical abnormalities are present when the patient first comes under observation, it is important to recognize that they may be absent when mental changes are conspicuous. The expression is often vacant or fatuously smiling, sometimes somewhat mask-like. The pupils are usually contracted and irregular and react sluggishly to light. Typical Argyll Robertson pupils are often found. Optic atrophy is not uncommon, but is rarely severe enough to cause marked loss of visual acuity.

Voluntary power becomes progressively impaired, and weakness is usually associated with tremor, which is most conspicuous on voluntary movement, and is best seen in the facial muscles, especially the lips and the tongue, and in the outstretched fingers. The slow slurred speech is highly characteristic. In addition, incoordination usually develops during the later stages, rendering the gait unsteady, and the movements of the upper limbs ataxic.

Owing to bilateral degeneration of the corticospinal tracts, the tendon reflexes are usually exaggerated, the abdominal reflexes diminished or lost, and the plantar reflexes extensor. The association of tabes with general paresis—so-called 'taboparesis'—however, is not uncommon, and in such cases the tendon reflexes are lost. Except in taboparesis, when the sensory changes characteristic of tabes are present, sensation is unimpaired in general paresis. A loss of control over the sphincters is common at a comparatively early stage, but is then the outcome of the mental deterioration and not of a disorder of innervation at lower levels.

Syphilitic aortitis is common, but rarely causes symptoms. There is usually a progressive loss of body-weight.

The Cerebrospinal Fluid

The cerebrospinal fluid exhibits characteristic changes of great diagnostic importance. The pressure is frequently somewhat increased. There is usually an excess of cells, which are mononuclear, but the cell count rarely exceeds 100 per mm.³ The protein content is also increased and usually lies between 0·05 and 0·10 per 100 ml. Marked increase of globulin is found and the globulin content of the fluid may be as high as one-third of the protein content (Hewitt). Of the total globulin, more than 25 per cent. may be found to be γ-globulin. Lange's colloidal gold curve is of the paretic type, e.g. 5554311000 or even 5555555444. Exceptionally, though the curve remains of this type, precipitation is not quite complete, and the highest figure is 4. The V.D.R.L. reaction is positive in the cerebrospinal fluid in 100 per cent. of cases, and in the blood in from 90 to 100 per cent. The treponema immobilization test is even more specific, being invariably positive in the fluid in the untreated case.

DIAGNOSIS

The constancy of serological abnormalities in the blood and cerebrospinal fluid in general paresis is of the utmost diagnostic importance, as it frequently confirms a diagnosis which on clinical grounds alone might be doubtful. In all cases, therefore, in which general paresis is a possibility these tests should be carried out.

The mental symptoms in the early stage may simulate neurosis or manic-depressive psychosis. Neither of these conditions, however, is associated with signs of organic disease in the nervous system.

General paresis must be distinguished from the presenile and senile dementias. In arteriosclerotic dementia the pupils may be contracted and tremor and extensor plantar responses may be present. In such cases the diagnosis can be made only after an examination of the blood and cerebrospinal fluid.

Alcoholic dementia—'alcoholic pseudoparesis'—may closely simulate general paresis and may be distinguishable only by serological tests.

It is often difficult to distinguish general paresis from meningovascular syphilis when this condition is associated with severe mental changes, since the V.D.R.L. reaction may be positive in both blood and cerebrospinal fluid in both conditions. When the colloidal gold curve in the fluid is of the luetic type this is a point in favour of meningovascular syphilis, but a paretic curve is not pathognomonic of general paresis.

PROGNOSIS

Before the introduction of malarial treatment general paresis was invariably fatal, and it was exceptional for a patient to survive more than three years. Exceptionally the disease ran a rapid course and proved fatal within a year. Remissions, which, however, are only temporary, occur spontaneously in from 10 to 20 per cent. of cases. Malarial treatment considerably improved the outlook, but penicillin is even more effective. Arrest can usually be achieved, hence the earlier the stage at which the diagnosis is made and treatment is begun, the better the outlook.

TREATMENT

Penicillin

Penicillin is the treatment of choice; some workers still prefer to supplement it with malaria, especially for advanced cases in mental hospitals. My own experience suggests that penicillin is as effective as the two in combination, and my practice is to use penicillin as for meningovascular syphilis [see p. 414], and malaria only in resistant cases. The further routine of investigation is the same as for meningovascular syphilis.

Malarial Therapy

The introduction of infection with malaria by Wagner-Jauregg in 1917 was a great advance in the treatment of general paresis. Histologically, after treatment with malaria spirochaetes disappear from the brain and the inflammatory exudate diminishes. Some observers have described the development of miliary gummas, which they interpret as indicating increased immunity.

The parasite of benign tertian malaria (*P. vivax*) is usually employed, and unless the source of infection is reliable, the donor's blood should first be examined microscopically to exclude the risk of infection with the malignant parasite

(*P. falciparum*), which is dangerous. The patient may be inoculated by the bite of an infected mosquito, and such mosquitoes can be obtained in England through the Ministry of Health. When case-to-case transmission is used the donor's blood is withdrawn from a vein at the elbow, preferably during the decline of the fever, from 1 to 5 ml. being received into a syringe which contains a few drops of 5 per cent. sodium citrate solution to prevent clotting. If the donor and recipient are in the same building the blood requires no further treatment, but should be injected without further delay. The injection is usually made subcutaneously; but intramuscular, intracutaneous, and intravenous routes may be employed, the last-named yielding the shortest incubation period.

The incubation period is extremely variable, ranging from two or three days to seven weeks. Usually after subcutaneous injection it is about ten days. The patient is allowed to have a number of rigors, usually ten, unless it becomes necessary to terminate the infection earlier. The infection is terminated by the administration of the appropriate antimalarial drugs.

Slight jaundice is not uncommon during the malaria. Occasionally severe cardiac failure occurs. This requires appropriate treatment and is an indication for terminating the infection. Digitalis may be given prophylactically during the treatment. Exceptionally also malaria may lead to an exacerbation of the mental symptoms or to the development of severe mental confusion, agitation, or, occasionally, acute mania. Malarial therapy is unsuitable for very debilitated and for senile patients and for those with marked cardiovascular disease.

Other methods of inducing artificial pyrexia are sometimes used.

Early cases of general paresis, especially those characterized by simple dementia, can usually be treated at home, if suitable nursing is available, or in a general hospital. Those with more severe mental symptoms will require to be treated in a mental hospital. Adequate medical supervision is necessary for a long time in those who do well, and patients who return to positions of responsibility must be carefully watched, and the cerebrospinal fluid examined annually for evidence of deterioration. A relapse may be treated in the same way as the first attack, but the results are usually not as good as after the first treatment.

TABES DORSALIS

Synonym. Locomotor ataxia.

AETIOLOGY

Tabes was first recognized as a clinical entity by Romberg and Duchenne. Its association with syphilis was first suspected by Fournier, and was established by the introduction of the Wassermann reaction and the discovery of spirochaetes in the brain and spinal cord of affected individuals by Noguchi and by Marinesco and Minea. Tabes, like general paresis, differs from meningovascular syphilis in respect of the systematized character of the spinal lesions and in the less satisfactory response of advanced cases to treatment. The various theories which have been brought forward to explain this difference are discussed in connexion with general paresis.

As in the case of general paresis, it is not uncommon to find that tabetic patients deny having had a primary chancre and the secondary manifestations of syphilis. These indications of infection may, therefore, be absent or so slight as to pass unnoticed. Tabes affects males much more frequently than females in the ratio of at least 4 to 1, and is the disorder present in 3 out of 12 cases of neurosyphilis. Although trauma has sometimes been blamed for precipitating the onset of symptoms, it is unlikely that it has this effect, but the patient in whom tabes is already developing may be able to compensate for his ataxia until he is

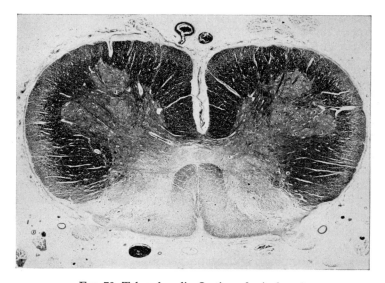

FIG. 70. Tabes dorsalis. Section of spinal cord

confined to bed by an injury, when he temporarily loses this power, as a result of which incoordination is conspicuous when he gets up. Tabetic symptoms usually appear between 8 and 12 years after infection. Exceptionally they may develop within 3 years, or their onset may be delayed until after 20 years or even longer. The age of onset usually lies between 35 and 50 years.

PATHOLOGY

Macroscopically there is evidence of atrophy of the dorsal spinal roots, especially of those in the lower thoracic and lumbosacral regions. The posterior columns of the spinal cord are flat or even sunken; hence the name tabes dorsalis or dorsal wasting. On section of the cord the posterior columns appear grey and translucent, in contrast to the normal appearance of the rest of the white matter.

Microscopically the essential lesion is a degeneration of the exogenous fibres of the cord, that is, of the central processes of the dorsal root ganglion cells, which themselves are usually little affected. Since the only exogenous fibres which possess a long course within the cord are situated in the posterior columns, these exhibit a selective degeneration and their demyelination is conspicuous, stained by stains for myelin [FIG. 70]. The endogenous fibres in the cornu-commissural zone, the region of the posterior columns lying just posterior to the grey commissure, usually escape. The incoming fibres earliest affected are those which in the thoracic region constitute the middle-root zone of the posterior columns or the bandelette of Pierret. Since the lower thoracic and lumbosacral roots are first attacked and their fibres entering the posterior columns shift towards the midline as they ascend the cord, the fasciculus gracilis suffers earlier than the fasciculus cuneatus in the cervical region. The latter, however, is affected later. There is secondary neuroglial proliferation in the posterior columns and the overlying pia mater is somewhat thickened. Exceptionally degeneration of anterior horn cells may occur in certain segments, in which case there is atrophy of the fibres of the corresponding ventral roots.

Many theories have been proposed in explanation of the selective character of the degenerative lesions of tabes in the spinal cord. The view of the older pathologists, and that adopted by Spielmeyer, is that tabes is due to a primary degeneration of the exogenous fibres within the cord. Obersteiner and Redlich believe that degeneration is due to compression of the dorsal root fibres by meningeal constriction at a point at which they pass through the pia mater. Hassin (1929) considers that proliferation of the arachnoid leads to the retention of lymph within the tissue spaces of the cord. Nageotte and Richter believe that the essential lesion is syphilitic inflammation of the radicular nerve, while others incriminate action of syphilitic toxins upon the dorsal roots. No satisfactory explanation has been given as to why a primary degeneration of the exogenous fibres of the cord should occur, and theories which place the lesion in the radicular nerve fail to explain the escape of the motor fibres. On the whole, Obersteiner and Redlich's theory appears the most plausible.

Optic atrophy is common and occurs in two forms, the degeneration of the nerve fibres being either primary or secondary to syphilitic inflammation of the interstitial tissues [see p. 149]. The Argyll Robertson pupil has been variously explained [see p. 90]. Sensory fibres of the cranial nerves, especially the trigeminal and glossopharyngeal, like those of the dorsal roots, may exhibit degeneration as they approach the brain stem, and degenerative changes have also been described in the afferent fibres of the sympathetic. The pathological changes of meningovascular syphilis may be associated with tabes, and those of general paresis may also be found.

Tabes is the most frequent cause of arthropathy—Charcot's joints. According to Moritz (1928), the earliest change in the joint is a hyperplasia of the cartilage. Later, destruction of the cartilage and erosion of the epiphyses occur and are often associated with the development of osteophytic outgrowths. There is an increase in the volume of the synovial fluid, and subluxation of an affected joint is not uncommon. Trauma frequently plays a part in the production of arthropathy. Syphilitic aortitis is a common complication of tabes.

SYMPTOMS

The principal symptoms of tabes are readily interpreted as a result of the degeneration of the afferent fibres of the dorsal roots. Pains and paraesthesiae are attributable to an irritable state of the degenerating sensory fibres. Sensory loss, i.e. analgesia and impairment of postural sensibility and appreciation of vibration, are due to interruption of the corresponding sensory fibres. Ataxia is due in part to impairment of appreciation of posture and passive movement, in part to interruption of afferent fibres conveying impulses concerned in co-ordination which do not reach consciousness. Diminution and loss of the tendon reflexes are due to interruption of their reflex arcs on the afferent side. Impotence and sphincter disturbances are the result of a similar loss of afferent impulses concerned in sexual function, and in the evacuation of the bladder and rectum.

Mode of Onset

The onset of tabes is usually gradual and insidious, but exceptionally it is rapid and the patient may become grossly ataxic within three months. Usually sensory symptoms, especially pain, precede ataxia by months or years, but ataxia may develop early, and a distinction between pre-ataxic and ataxic stages, though useful, is not universally applicable. Frequently the early sensory symptoms are so slight that the patient does not come for treatment until a more serious symptom develops. Hence the symptom which brings him to the doctor may be pain, ataxia, vomiting, impotence, disorder of micturition, failing vision, diplopia, or even arthropathy.

Sensory Symptoms

Pain is the most characteristic early symptom and usually takes the form of so-called 'lightning pains'. These pains, which are stabbing in character, occur in brief paroxysms in the lower limbs and may be very severe. As a rule they do not radiate longitudinally along the limb, but are localized to one spot, where the patient experiences a sensation as though a sharp object were being driven into the limb. Each attack lasts only a few seconds, but attacks may recur repeatedly in the same place, or may shift from place to place in the limb. A fresh attack of lightning pains may be precipitated by a change in the weather. They are usually worse when the patient is constipated. A pyogenic infection, such as an alveolar abscess, may lead to a severe exacerbation. It is not uncommon to find hyperalgesia, and vasodilatation of the skin in the region to which the pains are referred, and in severe cases ecchymosis may occur. Similar severe paroxysmal pains may occur in the upper limbs or in the distribution of the trigeminal nerve. Other forms of pain may be experienced, such as burning or tearing pains in the feet, pain in the distribution of the sciatic nerve, and a constricting pain around the chest or abdomen—'root pains' or 'girdle pains'.

Paraesthesiae are not uncommon, especially in the lower limbs. The patient may complain that the feet feel numb or cold, and a sensation as of walking on wool is a common complaint. The skin of the trunk and lower limbs is frequently hypersensitive to touch and to heat and cold. The patient may be aware that certain parts of the body are anaesthetic. Thus he may be unable to feel the chair upon which he sits, and he may notice that he is unaware when his bladder is full, and that he is unconscious of the act of defaecation. Giddiness may occur as a result of impairment of postural sensibility in the lower limbs.

Objective Sensory Changes

The forms of sensibility which are first impaired are usually those which are mediated by the posterior columns. In particular, appreciation of vibration suffers early, and usually before recognition of posture and passive movement. As a rule these forms of sensibility are affected in the lower limbs before the upper, though exceptionally the upper limbs suffer first—so-called 'cervical tabes'.

Painful sensibility is also early impaired, the deep tissues becoming insensitive to pain before the skin. Forcible compression of the muscles and the tendo calcaneus evokes no pain, and painful sensibility is frequently lost in the testicles. Cutaneous painful sensibility is not uniformly impaired, but is usually first lost in certain situations, namely, the side of the nose, the ulnar border of the arm and forearm, the region of the trunk between the nipples and the costal margin, the outer border of the leg and dorsum and sole of the foot, and the region surrounding the anus. In these regions, even when pin-prick is appreciated as painful, there is often a long delay, which may reach several seconds, between the application of the stimulus and its perception. Cutaneous sensibility to light touch, heat, and cold is usually unimpaired until a late stage, but finally there may be a diffuse loss of all forms of sensibility, extending over the whole of the body.

Ataxia

Ataxia is due partly to loss of postural sensibility and partly to loss of 'unconscious' afferent impulses concerned in the regulation of posture and movement. The importance of the latter factor is well seen in patients who exhibit considerable ataxia of the lower limbs without detectable impairment of postural sensibility or of appreciation of passive movement. Ataxia usually begins in the lower limbs and at first is evident only as slight unsteadiness in walking and turning. Since the patient is able to some extent to compensate by means of vision for the deficit of afferent impulses from his lower limbs, his ataxia becomes worse in the dark or when he closes his eyes, whence arises the characteristic symptom of falling into the basin when the eyes are closed in washing the face. As the ataxia increases, movements of the lower limbs become increasingly incoordinate. The patient walks with a wide base; the feet are lifted too high and brought down to the ground too violently. Walking becomes impossible without a stick, and finally he can only walk if he is supported on both sides. The ataxia is equally evident when the patient is lying in bed and can be elicited by asking him to place one heel upon the opposite knee. Voluntary movement of the lower limbs against resistance is jerky and irregular, and when the patient is lying at rest irregular, jerky, involuntary movements can often be observed, especially in the feet and toes.

In the early stages ataxia of the lower limbs is best demonstrated by asking the patient to stand with the toes and heels together and the eyes closed, and watching whether he sways—Romberg's test—or by asking him to walk along a line placing one heel in front of the opposite toe.

In severe cases the trunk muscles also become ataxic and the patient may then be unable to sit up in bed without support. Ataxia of the upper limbs is manifest in the clumsiness with which fine movements of the fingers are performed and in special tests, such as the finger–nose test. The defective maintenance of posture may often be demonstrated in the outstretched fingers by asking the patient to close his eyes. When the posture of the fingers is no longer controlled by vision they slowly droop, and irregular, so-called 'piano-playing', movements may occur.

Muscle Tone

Deficiency of the afferent impulses from the muscles upon which muscle tone depends leads to muscular hypotonia, as a result of which exaggerated passive movements of the joints become possible, for example, an extreme degree of flexion of the hip with the knee extended.

The Reflexes of the Limbs and Trunk

Degeneration of the afferent fibres concerned in the tendon reflexes leads to their diminution and ultimately to their disappearance. The ankle-jerks are thus affected before the knee-jerks, and it is not uncommon to find the reflexes unequal on the two sides. The tendon-jerks of the upper limbs are usually diminished at an early stage, but are finally lost only after those of the lower limbs have disappeared. The plantar reflexes usually remain elicitable and are flexor, except in those rare cases in which corticospinal tract degeneration is present, when they are extensor. The abdominal reflexes are also obtainable, and are frequently unusually brisk.

Sphincter Disturbances

Disturbances in bladder control may occur early when the sacral roots are early involved. When the lumbar roots suffer first, considerable ataxia of the lower limbs may precede bladder symptoms. The patient may complain either of difficulty of micturition or of incontinence. The bladder is large and atonic, and catheterization not uncommonly reveals the presence of several ounces of residual urine, and complete retention may occur. Infection of the urinary tract develops sooner or later when the bladder is incompletely emptied, and ascending pyelonephritis may prove fatal. Constipation is the rule, but faecal incontinence may occur, especially when the patient is unconscious of the act of defaecation. Impotence is sometimes an early symptom; in other cases it is absent, although the patient is ataxic.

Ocular Symptoms

Pupillary abnormalities are present in a large proportion of patients when they come under observation and in more than 90 per cent. at some time in the course of the disease. The pupils are usually contracted and frequently irregular. Exceptionally they are moderately or even widely dilated, especially in congenital neurosyphilis. Somewhat more frequently one is moderately dilated and the other contracted. The pupillary reaction to light is at first impaired and later lost, while that on accommodation-convergence is retained. The iris is pale and atrophic. The complete Argyll Robertson pupil, however, is often a late manifestation, and in the early stages it is commoner to find that the reaction of the pupil to light is present but reduced in amplitude, exhibits a latent period which is longer than normal, and is ill-sustained. The light reflex is often brisker in one eye than in the other, and the consensual reaction may be brisker than the direct. Rarely the pupil dilates in response to light. The contracted pupil fails to dilate in response to a scratch upon the skin of the neck, and both the myosis and the loss of this reflex are probably due to degeneration of the fibres of the oculosympathetic. A moderate degree of ptosis, probably also due to oculo-sympathetic paralysis, is common, and the compensatory action of the frontalis muscle by wrinkling the brow contributes to the characteristic facies. Diplopia is a common symptom and is usually due to defective balance of the ocular muscles. In the early stages it is often transitory, but nuclear ophthalmoplegia or permanent paralysis of the third or sixth nerve may develop. A bizarre dissociation of ocular movement may occur if one eye is allowed to fix an object while the vision of the other is obscured.

Optic atrophy is of the 'primary' variety [see p. 148]. The optic disc is small and pale, the physiological cup is preserved, and the lamina cribrosa is often visible. The fundal vessels are usually reduced in calibre. Optic atrophy in tabes may be slight and non-progressive, giving rise to no subjective impair-ment of visual acuity and being discovered only on routine examination. When, however, the patient complains of failing vision the atrophy is likely to be pro-gressive and to terminate in blindness. Usually visual acuity deteriorates first in the periphery of the visual fields; less often there is a central scotoma. It is an old observation that when optic atrophy develops early, ataxia of the lower limbs does not usually become severe, and the development of the whole disorder is arrested.

Other Cranial Nerves

Pain and analgesia in the distribution of the trigeminal nerve have already been described. Loss of smell and taste occasionally occurs. Degeneration of the eighth nerve may lead to deafness, and involvement of the vestibular fibres may cause vertigo. Exceptionally, degeneration of part of the nucleus ambiguus causes bilateral paralysis of the abductors of the larynx, and paralysis of the accessory and hypoglossal nerves is occasionally observed.

Trophic Changes

Arthropathies—Charcot's joints—are not uncommon. Their complete aetio-logy is not understood, though symptoms not infrequently appear after an injury. The onset of the joint change is frequently rapid, and there is considerable swelling, with increase in the synovial fluid. The skin may appear hot, but pain is almost invariably absent. Later, osteophytic outgrowths frequently develop around the joint, which thus becomes much increased in size, and considerable disorganization with subluxation may occur. Radiograms show as a rule marked erosion of the joint surfaces with formation of new bone at the articular margins or from the adjacent part of the shaft [FIG. 71]. The knee is most frequently affected, and after that the hip. The shoulder, tarsal joints, elbow, ankle, small joints of the fingers and toes and spine are involved in approximately this order of frequency. The long bones are brittle, and fractures may occur as a result of slight trauma.

The commonest trophic change in the skin is the perforating ulcer, which is usually seen beneath the pad of the great toe or at other pressure-points on the sole [FIG. 72]. The first stage is an epithelial thickening resembling a corn, and, either spontaneously or as a result of attempts to cut it away, an indolent ulcer develops. Sometimes a sinus extends deeply as far as the underlying bone, and considerable bony disorganization and deformity may result. Other trophic

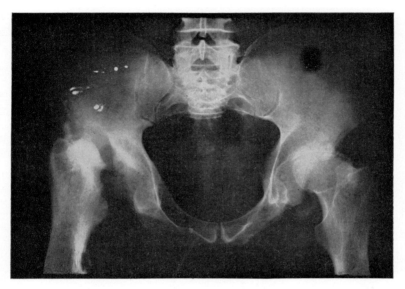

FIG. 71. Radiogram of bilateral Charcot hips in a tabetic patient

changes include the cutaneous ecchymoses already described, brittleness and falling out of the hair, and even exceptionally of the teeth. Herpes zoster may occur, as in other conditions in which there is a lesion of the spinal dorsal roots.

Tabetic Crises

Paroxysmal painful disorders of function of various viscera occur in tabes, and have received the name of crises. The gastric crisis is the commonest of these disturbances. It is characterized by attacks of epigastric pain associated with severe vomiting, and may last from a few hours to several days. Laryngeal crises consist of attacks of dyspnoea associated with cough, and inspiratory and expiratory stridor and appear to be associated with laryngeal paralyses. Rectal crises, characterized by tenesmus, and vesical crises, characterized by pain in the bladder or penis, and strangury, may also occur, and renal and other crises have been described. The common feature of most tabetic crises appears to be increased motility of a hollow viscus, which is probably the result of a disorder of autonomic afferent impulses.

The Cerebrospinal Fluid

The pressure is frequently somewhat above normal. There is usually an excess of cells, which are mononuclear and do not often exceed 70 per mm.[3] The protein may be normal or slightly increased. There is an excess of globulin in 90 per cent. of cases. The colloidal gold curve is usually of the 'luetic' type. A 'paretic' curve, even in the absence of symptoms of general paresis, should suggest the possibility that this may develop later. The Wassermann reaction is positive in

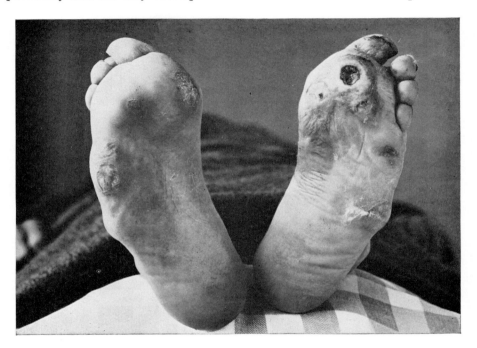

FIG. 72. Perforating ulcers in tabes dorsalis

both blood and cerebrospinal fluid in 65 per cent. of cases, positive in the fluid alone in 10 per cent., in the blood alone in 5 per cent., and negative in both in 20 per cent. The treponema immobilization test is, however, positive in the fluid in about 60 per cent. of the cases but is almost invariably positive in the blood (Duperrat and Cayol, 1962). For this reason the Wassermann reaction is now being largely supplanted by the T.P.I. and V.D.R.L. tests. The Wassermann reaction may be negative in the fluid in spite of an excess of cells, protein, and globulin, and a negative reaction in both blood and fluid or indeed a completely normal fluid may be found in a patient in whom the disease is progressive.

Complications

Symptoms of meningovascular syphilis, including muscular wasting, may coexist with those of tabes, though this is unusual. General paresis may be associated with tabes. A tabetic patient may, after a lapse of years, develop general paresis, or the symptoms of tabes may be present in an individual who comes under observation on account of symptoms of this disorder. Apart from general paresis, psychotic reactions, often with a paranoid trend, may occur in long-standing cases of tabes. Syphilitic aortitis is often present, but rarely gives rise to symptoms. However, there is some evidence that even after the apparently successful treatment of neurosyphilis with full doses of penicillin, cardiovascular manifestations of syphilis, and particularly signs of aortitis, may appear several years later. Chronic gastric ulcer occurs more often than can be explained by chance, and the symptoms may be mistaken for gastric crises.

DIAGNOSIS

When the patient has reached the ataxic stage, diagnosis usually presents little difficulty, for the characteristic physical signs are by then well developed, and the matter is clinched by investigation of the blood and cerebrospinal fluid. In multiple sclerosis ataxia of the lower limbs is associated with spasticity, exaggerated tendon reflexes, and extensor plantar responses. Friedreich's ataxia resembles tabes in the association of ataxia of the lower limbs with diminution or loss of the ankle-jerks, but this disorder usually begins at an early age and is differentiated from tabes clinically by the presence of nystagmus, dysarthria, extensor plantar responses, scoliosis, and pes cavus. Polyneuritis may simulate tabes when there is pronounced ataxia of the lower limbs. In alcoholic polyneuritis the pupillary reactions may be sluggish, the tendon reflexes are diminished or lost, the lower limbs are frequently ataxic, pains occur in the limbs, and there is an impairment of postural sensibility. In this condition, however, weakness of the peripheral muscles of the limbs is conspicuous and wrist- and foot-drop are often present, and the deep tissues, especially the muscles, are tender on pressure and not, as in tabes, analgesic. However, some cases of diabetic polyneuropathy may experience pain in the limbs and on examination there may be pupillary changes, areflexia and peripheral impairment of pain sensation ('diabetic pseudotabes') and even if the patient has been diabetic for some time the positive coincidental association of tabes dorsalis may have to be excluded by serological tests and motor-nerve conduction velocity measurements which are usually abnormal in diabetic neuropathy and normal in tabes.

When ataxia is absent the prominence of some other symptom may lead to a mistake in diagnosis, for example, pains in the limbs may be attributed to arthritis, root pains in the trunk to lesions of underlying viscera, gastric crises to ulceration of the stomach or duodenum, disturbances of the vesical sphincter to enlarged prostate or lesions of the bladder, arthropathy to arthritis, facial pain to trigeminal neuralgia, and optic atrophy to toxic amblyopia. These mistakes can be avoided only by systematic examination of the nervous system, special stress being laid upon the pupillary reflexes and upon diminution, absence, or inequality of the tendon reflexes in the lower limbs, especially the ankle-jerks. In doubtful cases the blood and cerebrospinal fluid should be examined. It must always be borne in mind that tabes may coexist with other disorders. All patients suspected of gastric crisis should have a barium meal, as the failure to diagnose a gastric ulcer in a tabetic may be more disastrous for the patient than to mistake a gastric crisis for an organic lesion of the stomach.

PROGNOSIS

Tabes is extremely variable in its rate of progress and in the extent to which it responds to treatment. A rapidly progressive course with the development of ataxia in a few months is rare. Usually the duration of the pre-ataxic stage lies between two and five years. In some cases ataxia never develops to a serious extent, and one encounters abortive forms with signs such as Argyll Robertson pupils and absent knee- and ankle-jerks, but no symptoms. The rate at which ataxia is likely to increase can be roughly assessed from the duration of the pre-ataxic stage. The longer this is, the slower is likely to be the subsequent progress of the disorder. The response to treatment is equally variable. Sometimes considerable improvement occurs and the disorder appears to be arrested. Other patients go downhill rapidly or slowly in spite of all treatment. Optic atrophy is not necessarily progressive, but when the patient complains of failing vision it often terminates in blindness. Early treatment may be expected to arrest its progress in about 50 per cent. of cases. Gastric crises often respond satisfactorily to the general treatment of tabes, and perforating ulcers which are not too far advanced can usually be induced to heal. No improvement can be expected in the bony changes associated with arthropathy. Improvement frequently occurs in sphincter control, and impotence, though often permanent, is not necessarily so, for sexual power may return after treatment. In fatal cases death usually occurs from infection of the urinary tract, from syphilitic infection of the heart and aorta, or from some intercurrent disease.

TREATMENT

General Treatment

The tabetic patient should be urged to avoid excessive fatigue and indulgence in alcohol. Special attention should be paid to the care of the bowels on account of the liability of the tabetic to constipation, which intensifies the pains.

Vigorous antisyphilitic treatment must be carried out along the lines indicated for meningovascular syphilis. Malaria, employed as in the treatment of general paresis, is a valuable adjunct to treatment in suitable cases. It should be reserved for patients in whom the course of the disorder is rapidly progressive in spite of the usual antisyphilitic treatment and for those in whom particular symptoms, such as severe pains, prove otherwise intractable. Taboparesis should be treated as for general paresis.

Treatment of Special Symptoms

Pain. Tabetic pains are usually ameliorated by simple analgesics. When they are severe, however, they can only be relieved by morphine, which is debarred on account of the risk of addiction. Induced pyrexia is valuable in some cases, typhoid vaccine being injected intravenously. Cortisone has been found useful by Moore (1953) and Bertini (1958) has used intrathecal prednisone. Several authors advocate injections of vitamin B_{12} in doses of 1000 mg. Relief may also be obtained from X-ray irradiation of the spinal cord and dorsal roots or from chordotomy.

Ataxia. Co-ordination of the limbs may be improved by suitable re-educational exercises on the lines of those first suggested by Frenkel.

The Bladder. Precipitancy of micturition may be relieved by propantheline, 15 mg. three times daily, or similar remedies. The atonic bladder should not be treated surgically unless either there is impairment of renal function or there is an infection of the urinary tract which has failed to respond to chemotherapy. The choice will then lie between suprapubic cystostomy, and transurethral division of the internal sphincter. Catheterization should always be carried out to determine whether there is any residual urine. The patient should be instructed to pass urine at four-hourly intervals whether he feels the need to micturate or not. Even when the bladder has become overdistended it is probably best treated in this way, with the addition of drugs of the acetylcholine group such as carbamylcholine. Catheterization should not be carried out unnecessarily, and surgical intervention should be postponed as long as possible.

Crises. Patients subject to gastric crises should take a bland, non-irritating diet, together with alkalies. A crisis can frequently be cut short by an injection of pethidine hydrochloride, 100 mg. If this fails, morphine and atropine may be tried. In severe cases benefit has followed section of the lower thoracic spinal dorsal roots, and the corresponding sympathetic rami, though the results of this operation are uncertain. When pain is severe bilateral upper cervical chordotomy may be necessary.

Laryngeal crises are best treated by the inhalation of amyl nitrite or by spraying the larynx with a 1 per cent. solution of procaine.

Perforating Ulcer. Tabetic patients should wear well-fitting boots and should be warned against cutting their corns, on account of the risk that a perforating ulcer may follow a slight injury. When an ulcer has developed, the foot must be rested, and the thickened epidermis should be softened by repeated hot fomentations and carefully pared away with a sharp razor. Dattner recommends mercury ointment.

Arthropathy. The object of treatment is to relieve the strain on the damaged joint. The knee and ankle may be supported by a leather corset strengthened with steel. When the hip or knee is affected a Thomas walking caliper will be required. Spinal arthropathy necessitates a leather corset or spinal brace. When there is much fluid in the joint this may be aspirated. Excision of an arthropathic joint should not be attempted, since, on account of the existing trophic disorder, the result is likely to be unsatisfactory.

Optic Atrophy. In the past the best results have been obtained with malaria or artificial pyrexia. Penicillin is probably equally effective, and should first be tried in every case, malaria being given in addition if the visual acuity continues to deteriorate. Surgery is of no value (Bruetsch, 1948).

CONGENITAL NEUROSYPHILIS

Active neurosyphilis occurs in from 8 to 10 per cent. of congenitally syphilitic children, males being affected slightly more often than females (Jeans and Cooke,

1930). Neither in its pathological nor in its clinical features does congenital neuro-syphilis differ in any essential respects from the acquired form except for the fact that fixed dilated pupils rather than those of the typical Argyll Robertson type are more common in the congenital variety. Both meningovascular and parenchyma-tous neurosyphilis occur. The intra-uterine infection of the nervous system with the spirochaete may lead to actual developmental arrest so that the cerebral hemi-spheres are unusually small. Gross disappearance of Purkinje cells with gliosis of the cerebellar cortex is rather characteristic of juvenile general paresis.

SYMPTOMS

The meningovascular form is much commoner than the parenchymatous. Both mental deficiency and convulsions are common. Slight hydrocephalus is not rare, but the head does not attain the large size seen in idiopathic congenital hydrocephalus. Syphilitic hydrocephalus appears always to be of the communica-ting type. Pupillary abnormalities are the most frequent disorders found within the region of the cranial nerves. The pupils are often large, irregular, and unequal and the reaction to light is sluggish or absent. Optic atrophy is often present and may arise in several ways. It may be secondary to choroidoretinitis or the result of involvement of the optic nerves or chiasma in basal syphilitic meningitis, or associated with congenital general paresis or tabes. Facial weakness is fre-quently seen. Deafness, a common manifestation of congenital syphilis, is due in most cases to a lesion within the temporal bone and not to involvement of the eighth nerve in its intracranial course. Destruction of the corticospinal fibres may lead to diplegia or hemiplegia. Moderate degrees of infantilism are not uncommon. I have seen extreme infantilism of the Lorain type associated with optic atrophy as a result of basal meningitis in congenital syphilis. Narcolepsy and diabetes insipidus are rare manifestations.

Parenchymatous neurosyphilis is rare. Stewart (1933) estimates that general paresis occurs in 1 per cent. of congenital syphilitics. The child may be mentally defective from birth, but symptoms usually develop during the first half of the second decade of life. The symptoms are similar to those of the acquired form, though the mental symptoms are usually less florid and are those of acquired mental subnormality. Grandiose delusions, if present, are puerile in type; for example, a boy stated that he owned all the sweet shops in the country. The course of the disorder is somewhat slower than in the adult, and the untreated patient may live for ten or more years.

Congenital tabes usually develops somewhat later in life than congenital general paresis, and may not make its appearance until early adult life but tabo-paresis may occur in adolescence. Optic atrophy is common in both, and in both the pupils are often widely dilated and fixed.

The V.D.R.L. reaction of the blood is usually positive and the treponema immobilization test is always so when congenital neurosyphilis is progressive, but the V.D.R.L. test is sometimes negative in latent or arrested cases. The cerebro-spinal fluid usually shows the changes associated with the same forms of the acquired disorder, but in some cases of congenital meningovascular syphilis the V.D.R.L. reaction may be negative in the cerebrospinal fluid, although other changes, such as an increase in the globulin and a pleocytosis, are present.

DIAGNOSIS

The diagnosis is usually easy when it is considered, since other signs of congenital syphilis are generally present, and is confirmed by the serological reactions of the child and its parents. However, juvenile general paresis or taboparesis, when presenting, as it may with fits, dementia and even akinetic mutism, with or without areflexia and sphincter disturbance may be mistaken for encephalitis or polyradiculitis.

PROGNOSIS

The response to treatment is disappointing in patients who come under observation on account of the presence of nervous symptoms, especially in congenital general paresis and tabes. Hence it is important that the cerebrospinal fluid should be examined in all congenitally syphilitic children at an early age, in order that latent neurosyphilis may be detected.

TREATMENT

Treatment should be carried out on the same lines as for acquired syphilis.

REFERENCES

BEERMAN, H., NICHOLAS, L., SCHAMBERG, I. L., and GREENBERG, M. S. (1962) Syphilis: review of the recent literature, 1960–1, *Arch. intern. Med.*, **109**, 323.

BERTINI, F. (1958) Terapia cortisonica a scopo antalgico nella tabe dorsale, *Gazz. med. ital.*, **117**, 417.

BOGAERT, L. VAN, and VERBRUGGE, J. (1928) The pathogenesis and the surgical treatment of gastric crisis of tabes: neuroramisectomy, *Surg. Gynec. Obstet.*, **47**, 543.

BRUETSCH, W. L. (1948) Surgical treatment of syphilitic primary atrophy of the optic nerves (syphilitic optochiasmatic arachnoiditis), *Arch. Ophthal.*, **38**, 735.

CLARK, E. G., and DANBOLT, N. (1964) The Oslo study of the natural course of untreated syphilis, *Med. Clin. N. Amer.*, **48**, 613.

CURTIS, A. C., KRUSE, W. T., and NORTON, D. H. (1950) Neurosyphilis. IV. Post-treatment evaluation 4–5 years following penicillin and penicillin plus malaria, *Amer. J. Syph.*, **24**, 554.

CUTLER, J. C., BAUER, T. J., PRICE, E. V., and SCHWIMMER, B. H. (1954) Comparison of spinal fluid findings among syphilitic and nonsyphilitic individuals, *Amer. J. Syph.*, **38**, 447.

DATTNER, B. (1948 *a*) Neurosyphilis and the latest methods of treatment, *Med. Clin. N. Amer.*, **32**, 707.

DATTNER, B. (1948 *b*) Treatment of neurosyphilis with penicillin alone, *Amer. J. Syph.*, **32**, 399.

DATTNER, B., KAUFMAN, S. S., and THOMAS, E. W. (1947) Penicillin in treatment of neurosyphilis, *Arch. Neurol. Psychiat. (Chicago)*, **58**, 426.

DATTNER, B., THOMAS, E. W., and WEXLER, S. (1944) *The Management of Neurosyphilis*, New York.

DUPERRAT, B., and CAYOL, J. (1962) Le test de Nelson dans les tabès, *Bull. Soc. Méd. Paris*, **113**, 556.

FOIX, C., CRUSEM, L., and NACHT, S. (1926) Sur l'anatomo-pathologie de la syphilis médullaire en général et en particulier des paraplégies syphilitiques progressives, *Ann. Méd.*, **20**, 81.

GALBRAITH, A. J. (1938) Some problems in the histopathology of general paralysis of the insane, *Brit. J. vener. Dis.*, **14**, 197–216.

GILLESPIE, E. J., and BROWN, B. C. (1964) New laboratory methods in the diagnosis of syphilis and other treponematoses, *Med. Clin. N. Amer.*, **48**, 731.

GOLDMAN, D. (1945) Treatment of neurosyphilis with penicillin, *J. Amer. med. Ass.*, **128**, 274.

GREENFIELD, J. G., and CARMICHAEL, E. A. (1925) *The Cerebrospinal Fluid in Clinical Diagnosis*, London.

HAHN, R. D. (1951) The treatment of neurosyphilis with penicillin and with penicillin plus malaria, *Amer. J. Syph.*, **35**, 433.

HAHN, R. D., CUTLER, J. C., CURTIS, A. C., GAMMON, G., HEYMAN, A., JOHNWICK, E., STOKES, J. H., SOLOMON, H., THOMAS, E., TIMBERLAKE, W., WEBSTER, B., and GLEESON, G. (1956) Penicillin treatment of asymptomatic central nervous system syphilis, I and II, *Arch. Derm.*, **74**, 355, 367.

HASSIN, G. B. (1929) Tabes dorsalis, *Arch. Neurol. Psychiat. (Chicago)*, **21**, 311.

HOFF, H., and KAUDERS, O. (1926) Über die Malariabehandlung der Tabes dorsalis, *Z. ges. Neurol. Psychiat.*, **104**, 306.

HURIEZ, C., AGACHE, P., and SOUILLART, F. (1963) Panorama actuel des syphilis viscérales, *Vie méd.*, **44**, 369.

JAUREGG, W. (1929) La malariathérapie de la paralysie générale et des affections syphilitiques du système nerveux, *Rev. neurol.*, **36**, 889.

JEANS, P. C., and COOKE, J. V. (1930) *Prepubescent Syphilis* (Clin. Pediatrics, xvii), New York.

KENNEY, J. A., and CURTIS, A. C. (1953) The treatment of syphilitic optic atrophy by penicillin with and without therapeutic malaria, *Amer. J. Syph.*, **37**, 449.

LÉRI, A. (1925) Sur certaines pseudo-scléroses latérales amyotrophiques syphilitiques, *Rev. neurol.*, **32**, 827.

LEYMANN, C. A. (1938) *Artificial Fever Produced by Physical Means. Its Development and Application*, London.

LHERMITTE, J. (1933) La syphilis diencéphalique et les syndromes végétatifs qu'elle conditionne — étude clinique, *Ann. Méd.*, **33**, 272.

MARTIN, J. P. (1925) Amyotrophic meningo-myelitis, *Brain*, **48**, 153.

MARTIN, J. P. (1948) Treatment of neurosyphilis with penicillin, *Brit. med. J.*, **1**, 922.

MCINTOSH, J., and FILDES, P. (1914–15) A comparison of the lesions of syphilis and 'parasyphilis', together with evidence in favour of the identity of these two conditions, *Brain*, **37**, 141.

MCINTOSH, J., and FILDES, P. (1914) The demonstration of *Spirochœta pallida* in chronic parenchymatous encephalitis (dementia paralytica), *Brain*, **37**, 401.

MEAGHER, E. T. (1929) *General Paralysis and its Treatment by Induced Malaria* (Board of Control), London.

MERRITT, H. H., ADAMS, R. D., and SOLOMON, H. C. (1946) *Neurosyphilis*, New York.

MERRITT, H. H., and MOORE, M. (1935) Acute syphilitic meningitis, *Medicine (Baltimore)*, **14**, 119.

MONTGOMERY, C. H., and KNOX, J. M. (1959) Antibiotics other than penicillin in the treatment of syphilis, *New Engl. J. Med.*, **261**, 277.

MOORE, J. E. (1932) The syphilitic optic atrophies, *Medicine (Baltimore)*, **11**, 263.

MOORE, J. E. (1953) The effect of adrenocortical hormones on the lightning pains and visceral crises of tabes dorsalis, *Amer. J. Syph.*, **37**, 226.

MORITZ, A. R. (1928) Tabische Arthropathie, *Virchows Arch. path. Anat.*, **267**, 746.

NELSON, R. A., and DUNCAN, L. (1945) Acute syphilitic meningitis treated with penicillin, *Amer. J. Syph.*, **29**, 141.

NICOL, W. D. (1948) Neurosyphilis, *Postgrad. med. J.*, **24**, 25.

NICOL, W. D., and WHELEN, M. (1947) Penicillin in the treatment of neurosyphilis, *Proc. roy. Soc. Med.*, **40**, 684.

NIELSEN, A., and IDSOE, O. (1962) *Evaluation of the Fluorescent Treponemal Antibody Test (FTA)*, W.H.O. Monograph No. 102.

RIMBAUD, P. (1958) Le traitement des syphilis sérologiques asymptomatiques, *Sem. méd. (Paris)*, **34**, 1209.

ROSE, A. S., and CARMEN, L. R. (1951) Clinical follow-up studies of 130 cases of long-standing paretic neurosyphilis treated with penicillin, *Amer. J. Syph.*, **35**, 278.

RUDOLF, G. DE M. (1927) *Therapeutic Malaria*, London. (Contains nearly 400 references.)

SPITZER, H. (1926) Zur Pathogenese der Tabes dorsalis, *Arb. neurol. Inst. Univ. Wien*, **28**, 227.

STERN, R. O. (1932) Certain pathological aspects of neurosyphilis, *Brain*, **55**, 145.

STEWART, R. M. (1933) Juvenile types of general paralysis, *J. ment. Sci.*, **79**, 602.

THOMAS, E. W. (1964) Some aspects of neurosyphilis, *Med. Clin. N. Amer.*, **48**, 699.

VEDSMAND, H. (1927) La thrombose des artères de la moelle épinière, *Acta Psychiat. (Kbh.)*, **2**, 371.

WILKINSON, A. E. (1963) The fluorescent treponemal antibody test in the serological diagnosis of syphilis, *Proc. roy. Soc. Med.*, **56**, 478.

WILSON, S. A. K., and COBB, S. (1924–5) Mesencephalitis syphilitica, *J. Neurol. Psychopath.*, **5**, 44.

10

VIRUS INFECTIONS OF THE NERVOUS SYSTEM

GENERAL CONSIDERATIONS

THE NATURE OF VIRUSES

THE term 'neurotropic virus' is used to describe minute filterable pathogenic agents which attack the nervous system. The first neurotropic virus, the causal organism of rabies, was discovered by Pasteur in 1884, and poliomyelitis was shown to be due to a neurotropic virus in 1909. During recent years the causal organisms of a number of other nervous diseases, both in man and in animals, have been found to be neurotropic viruses. These include in man a number of varieties of encephalitis of which the most important are the Japanese type B, the St. Louis type, Russian Far Eastern and spring-summer encephalitis, Murray Valley encephalitis and the Eastern, Western, and Venezuelan forms of equine encephalitis, herpes simplex encephalitis and acute lymphocytic choriomeningitis. Three other diseases, encephalitis lethargica, inclusion-body encephalitis, and herpes zoster, though they have never been transmitted to animals, are regarded as almost certainly due to neurotropic viruses. Other viruses not normally neurotropic sometimes attack the nervous system, especially those of mumps and the presumed viral agent of infectious mononucleosis.

The neurotropic viruses possess a number of characteristics in common. They are invisible, except in some cases with the electron microscope, and usually pass through filter candles. In size they range from 125 mμ in the case of rabies and lymphocytic choriomeningitis to 10–25 mμ in the case of poliomyelitis and equine encephalitis. They require special media for artificial cultivation, but survive for long periods in glycerol and in the dry state. They are destroyed by heat at relatively low temperatures, but they are resistant to cold. They are more susceptible to oxidizing agents, such as hydrogen peroxide and potassium permanganate, than to ordinary disinfectants. The blood serum of the convalescent organism possesses the power of neutralizing a certain amount of the virus, but each virus is a specific antigen.

Much interest has been aroused in recent years by the concept of 'slow virus' infections. Kuru, a progressive and fatal disorder of the nervous system seen in the eastern highlands of New Guinea, has now been transmitted to the chimpanzee and shows close affinities with the chronic neurological disorder of sheep known as scrapie which has an incubation period, following the inoculation of infected material, of at least 9 months. Both disorders are due to filterable agents, almost certainly viruses, the scrapie agent measuring between 17 and 27·5 mμ (Gajdusek, 1965; Gibbs et al., 1965). In cases of progressive multifocal leuco-encephalopathy, occurring usually as a complication of systematic reticulosis, viruses of the polyoma group have been identified in cerebral lesions with the electron microscope (Howatson *et al.*, 1965; Webb, 1967) while cytomegalic inclusion disease is another disorder of the central nervous system which is almost certainly due to slow virus infection, though the causal agent has not yet been identified.

The links between human and animal disease are nowhere closer than in the realm of the neurotropic viruses. Rabies is always acquired by man from an infected animal. Acute lymphocytic choriomeningitis is endemic among mice, which may be the source of human infection. Another neurotropic virus known as B virus, transmitted to man from monkeys, has caused two fatal cases of acute ascending myelitis. The following varieties of encephalitis are known to be arthropod-borne—the Eastern, Western, and Venezuelan forms of equine encephalitis, Japanese B, St. Louis (mosquito-borne), Russian Far Eastern and spring-summer, Murray Valley, and louping-ill (tick-borne). Various animals and birds may act as intermediate hosts. The enteric group of viruses or enteroviruses invade the body via the alimentary canal and include poliomyelitis, and the Coxsackie and Echo groups. Viruses among animals are responsible for Borna disease of horses, dog distemper, and fox encephalitis.

Pathological Changes in the Nervous System

The viruses appear to be obligatory intracellular parasites. They damage the nervous system, therefore, by directly attacking the ganglion cells. In very acute lesions there is necrosis of these cells. When the process is less acute, diffuse and focal microglial proliferation occurs and in some diseases inclusion bodies are found in the nerve cells. In many cases mesodermal changes such as perivascular cuffing and meningeal infiltration are a reaction to the inflammation, but some viruses invade both glial and mesodermal elements. The affinity of the neurotropic viruses is for the grey matter of the nervous system, hence they have been called polioclastic. There is no evidence that any of the primarily demyelinating diseases of the nervous system is directly due to a neurotropic virus.

REFERENCES

FIELDS, W. S., and BLATTNER, R. J. (1958) *Viral Encephalitis*, Springfield, Ill.
GAJDUSEK, D. C. (1965) Kuru in New Guinea and the origin of the NINDB study of slow, latent and temperate virus infections of the nervous system in man, in *Slow, Latent and Temperate Virus Infections*, NINDB Monograph No. 2, p. 3, Washington.
GEAR, J. (1949) Virus diseases of the central nervous system, *J. Neurol. Neurosurg. Psychiat.*, **12**, 66.
GIBBS, C. J., JR., GAJDUSEK, D. C., and MORRIS, J. A. (1965) Viral characteristics of the scrapie agent in mice, in *Slow, Latent and Temperate Virus Infections*, NINDB Monograph No. 2, p. 195, Washington.
HORSFALL, F. L., and TAMM, I. (1965) *Viral and Rickettsial Infections of Man*, 4th ed., Philadelphia.
HOWATSON, A. F., NAGAI, M., and ZURHEIN, G. M. (1965) Polyoma-like lesions in human demyelinating brain disease, *Canad. med. Ass. J.*, **93**, 379.
OLITSKY, P. K., and CASALS, J. (1952) *Viral and Rickettsial Infections of Man*, ed. RIVERS, T. M., 2nd ed., Philadelphia.
RHODES, A. J., and VAN ROOYEN, C. E. (1953) *Textbook of Virology*, 2nd ed., Baltimore.
WEBB, H. E. (1967) Viruses and the neuroglia with special reference to scrapie, kuru and disseminated sclerosis, *Proc. roy. Soc. Med.*, **60**, 698.

EPIDEMIC ENCEPHALITIS LETHARGICA

Synonyms. Epidemic encephalitis, type A; 'sleepy sickness'.

Definition. An epidemic disease probably due to a neurotropic virus with an acute, subacute, or insidious onset and in most cases a chronic course, and characterized pathologically by inflammatory and degenerative changes, especially in the grey matter of the midbrain, and clinically in the acute stage by disturbance of the sleep rhythm, especially lethargy, and pupillary abnormalities, and in the chronic stage by the Parkinsonian syndrome.

AETIOLOGY

Encephalitis lethargica was first described by von Economo in May 1917, and about the same time by Cruchet, Moutier, and Calmette. It seems to have made its first appearance in 1915, though some authorities believe that epidemics of it can be recognized in medical history. During the next decade widespread epidemics occurred, but now an illness with the characteristic clinical features is rare. It affects the sexes equally and no age is exempt, though it is commonest in early adult life. There is a seasonal incidence, most cases occurring as a rule in the first quarter of the year. The occurrence of outbreaks in institutions and the occasional appearance of case-to-case infection indicate that the disease is contagious, though only feebly so. There is no evidence for its transmission by non-human agencies. Numerous attempts by bacteriologists to isolate a causative organism have failed, but there is little doubt that it is due to a filterable virus. Outbreaks of epidemic hiccup have coincided with epidemics of encephalitis lethargica, and it is possible that both are due to the same organism.

PATHOLOGY

The macroscopic changes in the nervous system are slight, consisting, in the acute stage, of congestion, oedema, and sometimes petechial haemorrhages. Microscopically [FIGS. 73 and 74] perivascular changes are conspicuous in the early stages. The smaller vessels are engorged and many exhibit perivascular cuffs or sleeves of inflammatory cells, chiefly lymphocytes and plasma cells. In addition the nerve tissue is diffusely infiltrated with mononuclear cells, and the nerve cells themselves show degenerative changes. In the chronic stages the mesodermal elements show little evidence of reaction, but degeneration of nerve cells continues. In the acute stage the brunt of the infection falls upon the grey matter of the upper part of the midbrain, the region of the oculomotor nuclei, and the substantia nigra. The basal ganglia and the pons and medulla are affected next in frequency. No part of the nervous system is exempt, and the spinal cord may be diffusely affected. In the chronic stage also the degenerative changes are diffuse. The substantia nigra usually suffers severely, but the grey matter of the cerebral cortex and basal ganglia is also involved. The Parkinsonian syndrome, a common feature of chronic encephalitis lethargica, has been attributed to the destruction of the cells of the substantia nigra, but in view of the widespread changes elsewhere in such cases it is difficult to relate the Parkinsonian syndrome to a lesion localized in one situation [see pp. 518 and 522].

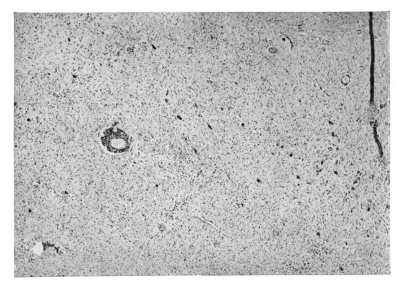

FIG. 73. Encephalitis lethargica. Substantia nigra showing perivascular and diffuse inflammatory infiltration. H & E, ×36

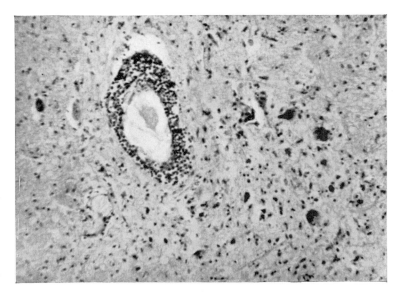

FIG. 74. The same. H & E, ×145

SYMPTOMS

The symptoms of encephalitis lethargica have changed remarkably in the fifty years during which it has been under observation. When it first appeared it was an acute disease, often with a fulminating onset. After several years the acute stage became less severe and the chronic stage more prominent. At the present day it is doubtful if acute cases occur, and fresh cases of encephalitic Parkinsonism are probably the outcome of infection acquired in the past, possibly even thirty or more years ago. Some authorities believe that the disease has died out, although sporadic cases showing some features of the condition are rarely seen. If it is true that the disease no longer exists, then no new cases of post-encephalitic Parkinsonism are likely to be seen in the future. It will be convenient to consider separately the symptoms of the acute and those of the chronic stages.

Symptoms of the Acute Stage

The onset may be sudden or gradual. In the earlier epidemics it was often fulminating and characterized by headache, vertigo, delirium, convulsive and apoplectic phenomena, and severe pain in the trunk or limbs. Later the onset became more gradual. The three most constant symptoms of the acute stage were headache, disturbance of sleep rhythm, and visual abnormalities, such as blurred vision or diplopia. The headache was usually not severe and was occasionally accompanied by vomiting or by pain in the back or limbs. The characteristic disturbance of sleep rhythm was lethargy by day with insomnia or restlessness at night. The lethargy was sufficiently constant, especially in the early cases, to contribute the epithet 'lethargica' to the name of the disease. The patient could always be roused, except when lethargy passed into coma. Neither lethargy by day nor insomnia by night was present in all cases. Either dominated the picture throughout the 24 hours. Delirium and fever occurred only in the more severe cases.

Visual disturbances were important on account of their frequency. Papilloedema and optic atrophy were very rare. Pupillary disturbances were common. The pupils were often irregular and unequal. The reaction on accommodation was more often lost than that to light. The Argyll Robertson pupil was rare. Ptosis was frequent but usually slight. External ophthalmoplegia was common, and was probably often due to neuritis of the oculomotor nerve trunks. The sixth was most often affected. Nuclear and supranuclear ophthalmoplegias were less common, but all forms of conjugate ocular palsy have been seen. The blurred vision of which the patient so often complained was due to paresis of accommodation or of an external ocular muscle. Diplopia was frequent.

Facial weakness was common, and was almost always transitory. Vertigo was also common, and probably due to involvement of the vestibular tracts, the same lesion possibly causing the fine nystagmus which was often present. Bulbar symptoms were rare, and so too were aphasia and hemiplegia, though slight corticospinal tract damage, indicated by unilateral or bilateral extensor plantar responses without gross weakness, was frequently encountered.

Extrapyramidal disturbances so typical of the chronic stage could appear also in the acute. A Parkinsonian facies was often seen, but the muscles were usually hypotonic and rarely rigid. Rigidity, when present, was catatonic: true Parkinsonian rigidity was never present in the acute stage. Choreiform movements closely simulating Sydenham's chorea were not uncommon between 1916 and 1922. The same was true of myoclonic muscular contractions, of which hiccup was perhaps a special form. These consisted of shock-like muscular twitches varying in frequency from 8 or 10 to 80 contractions a minute and were especially common in the abdominal wall. They did not as a rule cause displacement of the limb segments. Sometimes muscles in different parts of the body exhibited a synchronous myoclonus. Myoclonus was sometimes associated with severe pain in the affected muscles. Hiccup could occur in the acute stage of encephalitis, with or without myoclonus elsewhere. Static and intention tremor were sometimes seen.

Spontaneous pains in the trunk and limbs occurred especially during the early years. Sensory loss was very uncommon, but the thalamic syndrome, with over-reaction to painful stimuli on one half of the body, was occasionally observed.

The cerebellum and spinal cord were rarely involved, though muscular wasting and the clinical picture of transverse myelitis were occasionally encountered, and a polyneuritic form of the disease was described.

The tendon reflexes were often diminished in the acute stage. Diminution of the abdominal reflexes was usually associated with other signs of corticospinal tract lesion. There was usually no sphincter disturbance unless the patient was comatose, when retention or incontinence of urine and faeces might occur.

Signs of meningeal irritation, such as cervical rigidity and Kernig's sign, were very rare. The cerebrospinal fluid was usually normal, though a slight excess of cells, almost always lymphocytes, could be found. The protein and globulin were sometimes increased; the chloride content of the fluid was normal. There was no constant abnormality of the colloidal gold curve.

After passing through the acute stage the disease sometimes became arrested or persisted as a chronic and slowly progressive disorder. Complete arrest was rare, but even when it occurred the patient was likely to show some of the residual features about to be described, though in a non-progressive form. The chronic progressive form of the disease could follow an acute attack, or else it developed insidiously, without being preceded by any recognizable acute symptoms. It was at first thought that the disabilities of function which followed encephalitis lethargica were not indications that the infection itself persisted. On pathological grounds it is now regarded as probable that in these cases the infection persisted in a chronic form in some ways comparable with the tertiary stage of syphilis.

Symptoms of the Chronic Stage

Parkinsonism. This is described in CHAPTER 12, pages 522–34.

Sleep Disturbances. Lethargy or insomnia, or both, frequently outlasted the acute attack, the form of disorder of sleep present in the acute attack usually persisting as a chronic symptom.

Mental Symptoms. Though gross mental disturbances have been reported in only 27 per cent. of cases, if less severe degrees of impairment of mental efficiency were included this figure would be much higher. In adults, in milder cases, nervousness, fatigability, inability to concentrate, anxiety, and depression often persisted for long periods. Changes of emotional disposition were common in children, who often became restless and unstable and exhibited abnormalities of behaviour ranging from mere naughtiness to stealing, cruelty, acts of violence, and sexual offences, which often brought them into the hands of the police.

Ocular Abnormalities. Gross ocular abnormalities, such as nystagmus, squint, and true diplopia, persisted in only a small proportion of cases, but the patient often complained of dimness or mistiness of vision, which was due to defective muscle balance or weakness of accommodation. These symptoms were usually associated with slight inequality of the pupils and an impairment of pupillary reactions on accommodation, and less frequently to light. Oculogyral spasm, one of the most striking ocular sequels of encephalitis, is described in the section on Parkinsonism.

Involuntary Movements. 1. *Choreiform movements* were at one time relatively common during the acute stage of the disease. They were rare during the chronic stage, but were occasionally observed.

2. *Bradykinesias.* This term was applied to slow, regular, rhythmical movements of large amplitude, involving the limbs alone or the limbs and trunk.

Other involuntary movements included (3) myoclonic movements, (4) tremor, and (5) tics, often consisting of complex co-ordinated rhythmical movements of the jaw, lips, tongue, and palate, and (6) torticollis.

Respiratory Disturbances. Respiratory disturbances occurring during the chronic stage of encephalitis consisted of disorders of the respiratory rate and rhythm, and respiratory tics.

Metabolic and Endocrine Disorders. Metabolic and endocrine disorders, probably due to involvement of the hypothalamus, were rare. Obesity, often associated with genital atrophy, was the commonest of these sequels. Polyuria associated with polydipsia occasionally occurred, though the urinary output did not often much exceed 2 litres a day. Symptoms of hyperthyroidism with enlargement of the thyroid were also occasionally encountered.

Epileptiform Convulsions. Epileptiform convulsions have been known to follow encephalitis lethargica, as they may other infective conditions of the nervous system, but it is probable that this occurs only in patients who suffer from a predisposition to epilepsy.

DIAGNOSIS

Encephalitis lethargica was distinguished from other forms of encephalitis by the characteristic disturbance of sleep rhythm, the prominence of the ocular symptoms, and the rarity of paralysis of the limbs; and from meningitis by the absence of cervical rigidity and Kernig's sign and frequently of an excess of cells in the cerebrospinal fluid. When, however, this contained a mononuclear pleocytosis, the disease could be distinguished from tuberculous meningitis by the normal sugar and chloride content of the fluid. Poliomyelitis differs from encephalitis lethargica in the presence of signs of meningeal irritation and a mixed-cell pleocytosis in the cerebrospinal fluid in the early stages, and later by the development of flaccid paralysis. For the diagnosis of encephalitis from other conditions causing coma see page 976, and for that of encephalitic Parkinsonism see pages 528–9.

PROGNOSIS

When it first made its appearance epidemic encephalitis lethargica was an extremely acute disease. Today, if it occurs at all, the acute stage may pass unnoticed.

The mean death-rate in one large series of over 2,000 cases was 38·2 per cent. Most patients who died in the acute stage did so during the first month of the illness, and fourteen days was the commonest length of a fatal attack. The mortality rate during the acute stage was highest in the first year of life and after the age of 70, and lowest between the ages of 20 and 30.

Complete recovery occurred in only about 25 per cent. of cases. The remainder who survived the acute stage were more or less severely disabled, most of them being incapacitated from carrying on their usual occupations. Even after apparent recovery from an acute attack occurred, the patient could suffer from relapses with the recurrence of similar symptoms at intervals of a year or two or could pass into the chronic stage, an event which could occur after an interval of as long as twenty years or more after the acute attack.

The prognosis in Parkinsonism is described in CHAPTER 12, page 529.

TREATMENT

The Matheson Commission reported upon seventy-five methods of treating encephalitis lethargica, none of which proved to influence the course of the infection, though some were of value for the relief of symptoms. All treatment was therefore symptomatic.

Treatment in the chronic stage was also very disappointing, and all attempts to arrest or retard the progress of the infection must be regarded as ineffective.

Parkinsonism. See CHAPTER 12, page 532.

The treatment of mental sequelae of encephalitis in adults followed the usual lines. Children suffering from mental abnormality often required institutional treatment.

REFERENCES

EAVES, E. C., and CROLL, M. M. (1930) The pituitary and hypothalamic region in chronic epidemic encephalitis, *Brain*, **53,** 56.

EBAUGH, F. G. (1923) Neuropsychiatric sequelae of acute epidemic encephalitis in children, *Amer. J. Dis. Child.*, **25,** 89.

VON ECONOMO, C. (transl. NEWMAN, K. O.) (1931) *Encephalitis Lethargica: Its Sequelae and Treatment*, London.

HALL, A. J. (1924) *Epidemic Encephalitis*, Bristol.

HALL, A. J. (1931) Chronic epidemic encephalitis with special reference to the ocular attacks, *Brit. med. J.*, **2**, 833.

HALL, A. J., and YATES, A. G. (1926) Clinical report. Report of sub-committee on the Sheffield outbreak of epidemic encephalitis in 1924, *Spec. Rep. Ser. med. Res. Coun. (Lond.)*, No. 108, p. 29.

HOLT, W. L., Jr. (1937) Epidemic encephalitis. A follow-up study of two hundred and sixty-six cases, *Arch. Neurol. Psychiat. (Chicago)*, **38**, 1135.

LEVADITI, C. (1929) Etiology of epidemic encephalitis, its relation to herpes, epidemic poliomyelitis, and post-vaccinal encephalopathy, *Arch. Neurol. Psychiat. (Chicago)*, **22**, 767.

LEVY, G. (1922) *Contributions à l'étude des manifestations tardives de l'encéphalite épidémique*, Paris.

MACNALTY, A. S. (1927) *Epidemic Diseases of the Central Nervous System*, London.

PARSONS, A. C. (1928) Report of an enquiry into the after-histories of persons attacked by encephalitis lethargica, *Min. Hlth Rep. publ. Hlth*, No. 49, London.

REIMOLD, W. (1925) Über die myoklonische Form der Encephalitis, *Z. ges. Neurol. Psychiat.*, **95**, 21.

RISER, M., and MERIEL, P. (1931) Les 'séquelles' neurologiques de l'encéphalite épidémique, *Rev. Oto-neuro-ophtal.*, **9**, 297, 323.

TURNER, W. A., and CRITCHLEY, M. (1925) Respiratory disorders in epidemic encephalitis, *Brain*, **48**, 72.

TURNER, W. A., and CRITCHLEY, M. (1927-8) The prognosis and the late results of post-encephalitic respiratory disorders, *J. Neurol. Psychopath.*, **8**, 191.

WIMMER, A. (1924) *Chronic Epidemic Encephalitis*, London.

Epidemic Encephalitis. Report of a survey by the Matheson Commission, New York, 1929.

Epidemic Encephalitis. Second report by the Matheson Commission, New York, 1932.

EPIDEMIC ENCEPHALITIS: JAPANESE TYPE B, ST. LOUIS TYPE AND MURRAY VALLEY TYPE

Definition. These three varieties of epidemic encephalitis, one occurring in Japan and other Asian countries, another in the United States of America, and the third in Australia, have been shown to be due to neurotropic viruses. These viruses are distinct because no cross-immunity exists between them, but the epidemiology and the pathological and clinical features of the three diseases are so similar that they can conveniently be considered together.

AETIOLOGY

These diseases are all caused by arthropod-borne so-called arboviruses which measure 15–40 μ in diameter. Of the large group of arboviruses, relatively few are encephalitogenic. The reservoir of these viruses in nature is probably in mammals, birds, or arthropods and the virus is usually transmitted to man by the bite of a mosquito or tick.

The Japanese encephalitis type B is caused by a virus which was first transmitted to monkeys by Hayashi. Kawamura and his fellow workers transmitted the virus to mice and monkeys and proved that it was filterable (Inada, 1937 *a*, 1937 *b*). These workers also showed that it was immunologically distinct from the virus of the St. Louis epidemic. This was proved to be a filterable virus and transmitted to monkeys and mice by Muckenfuss, Armstrong, and McCordock (1933) and Webster and Fite (1935). Russian autumnal encephalitis is now generally regarded as identical with Japanese type B encephalitis while the Murray Valley type (Australian X disease) which occurs in Australia and New Guinea is clinically indistinguishable from the Japanese variety and is due to a very similar but nevertheless distinctive virus. Also closely related are the so-called Russian tick-borne complex including Russian spring-summer encephalitis and louping-ill (in which the reservoir of infection is in the sheep).

EPIDEMIOLOGY

Eight epidemics of encephalitis occurred in Japan in various summers between 1871 and 1919, since when outbreaks have occurred every few years, and in 1935 there were 5,000 cases. The St. Louis epidemic occurred in 1933 when there were over 1,000 cases in the neighbourhood during the late summer. There were smaller outbreaks in other cities in the United States, including one in Toledo in 1934. In St. Louis relatively more cases occurred in the county than in the city. Multiple cases in the same family were not common. The incubation period appeared usually to be between 9 and 14 days. There was a marked preponderance of susceptibility among the elderly and aged, and a relatively small incidence in children but children are more commonly affected by the Japanese and Murray Valley types. Though mosquitoes have been demonstrated to be carriers both in the United States and in Japan, there is also evidence that the disease may be spread by human carriers and that the route of infection is the nose, from which the virus travels to the brain by the olfactory nerves. It has been shown that mosquitoes may infect patients with the viruses of St. Louis and Western equine encephalitis at the same time (Hammon, 1941).

PATHOLOGY

The pathological picture in the three diseases is identical except that Japanese observers have described small patches of softening in the brain which were not observed in the American epidemics and in the Japanese B and Murray Valley types selective damage to Purkinje cells is seen. All levels of the nervous system may be affected, and severe inflammation is always observed in the brain stem, the basal ganglia, and the white matter of the hemispheres. The inflammatory changes are diffuse, involving the basilar part of the pons, the entire width of the medulla, the cortex and white matter of the cerebellum, the basal ganglia, and also the cerebral cortex (Löwenberg and Zbinden, 1936; Robertson, 1952). The brain shows ganglion-cell degeneration, diffuse, microglial and macroglial proliferation, and perivascular cuffing. Perivascular microglial nodes are common. Intranuclear inclusion bodies have been found in the cells of the tubular epithelium of the kidney.

SYMPTOMS

Several workers classify cases as (1) abortive, (2) mild, and (3) severe, including the fulminating cases. Abortive cases, with fever, headache, malaise and recovery in a few days are occasionally seen in epidemics but are uncommon. The onset of the disease is usually acute with high fever, 104° to 105° F., headache and stiffness of the neck, and within a few hours many patients develop mental confusion and tremor of the lips, tongue, and hands. Rigidity may involve the upper limbs or the whole body. Drowsiness is common but the patient may be hyper-excitable. In severe cases coma develops early. The optic discs are usually normal as are the pupils and their reactions. Nystagmus, facial palsy, mono-paresis and spastic tetraparesis are not infrequent.

The cerebrospinal fluid is usually clear and under increased pressure. There is an excess of cells, usually between 50 and 500, predominantly lymphocytes. The globulin content is increased but the sugar is normal. The blood usually exhibits a moderate or striking polymorphonuclear leucocytosis.

DIAGNOSIS

See diagnosis of encephalitis lethargica, page 442.

PROGNOSIS

In the St. Louis epidemic the mortality rate was 20 per cent. In the Japanese and Murray Valley epidemics it has been much higher, usually 50 to 60 per cent. The mortality rate increases after the age of 50. In favourable cases recovery is often rapid and complete. Many patients in the St. Louis epidemic had ap-parently recovered completely in from 10 to 14 days, but the disease sometimes ran a protracted course. A study by Bredeck *et al.* (1938) of survivors of the 1933 St. Louis epidemic showed that 66 per cent. had made a complete recovery and only 6·3 per cent. were physically unfit for work. Finley (1958) has made similar observations in a follow-up of 350 cases.

PROPHYLAXIS AND TREATMENT

Prophylaxis consists of measures to eliminate insect vectors. Attempts to pre-pare specific protective vaccines have to date been unsuccessful. No specific treatment is known, and it is therefore purely symptomatic.

REFERENCES

BECKMANN, J. W. (1935) Neurologic aspects of the epidemic of encephalitis in St. Louis, *Arch. Neurol. Psychiat. (Chicago)*, **33**, 732.
BREDECK, J. F., BROUN, G. O., HEMPELMANN, T. C., McFADDEN, J. F., and SPECTOR, H. I. (1938) Follow-up studies of the 1933 St. Louis epidemic of encephalitis, *J. Amer. med. Ass.*, **111**, 15.
FINLEY, K. H. (1958) in *Viral Encephalitis*, ed. FIELDS, W. S., and BLATTNER, R. J., Springfield, Ill.
HAMMON, W. M. (1941) Encephalitis in Yakima valley: mixed St. Louis and Western equine types, *J. Amer. med. Ass.*, **117**, 161.
HEMPELMANN, T. C. (1933) Encephalitis in St. Louis, *Amer. J. publ. Hlth*, **23**, 1149.
HORSFALL, F. L., JR., and TAMM, I. (1965) *Viral and Rickettsial Infections of Man*, 4th ed., Philadelphia.
INADA, R. (1937 a) Recherches sur l'encéphalite épidémique du Japon, *Presse méd.*, **45**, 99.
INADA, R. (1937 b) Du mode d'infection dans l'encéphalite épidémique, *Presse méd.*, **45**, 386.
KAWAKITA, Y. (1939) Cultivation *in vitro* of the virus of Japanese encephalitis, *Jap. J. exp. Med.*, **17**, 211.
LÖWENBERG, K., and ZBINDEN, T. (1936) Epidemic encephalitis (St. Louis type) in Toledo, Ohio, *Arch. Neurol. Psychiat. (Chicago)*, **36**, 1155.

MUCKENFUSS, R. S., ARMSTRONG, C., and McCORDOCK, H. A. (1933) Encephalitis: studies on experimental transmission, *Publ. Hlth Rep. (Wash.)*, **48**, 1341.

RIVERS, T. M., and HORSFALL, F. L., JR. (1959) *Viral and Rickettsial Infections of Man*, 3rd ed., Philadelphia.

ROBERTSON, E. G. (1952) Murray Valley encephalitis: pathological aspects, *Med. J. Aust.*, i, 107.

ROBERTSON, E. G., and McLORINAN, H. (1952) Murray Valley encephalitis: clinical aspects, *Med. J. Aust.*, i, 103.

WEBSTER, L. T., and FITE, G. L. (1935) Experimental studies on encephalitis, *J. exp. Med.*, **61**, 103.

WOLSTENHOLME, G. E. W., and CAMERON, M. P. (1960) *Virus Meningoencephalitis*, Ciba Foundation Study Group No. 7, London.

EQUINE ENCEPHALOMYELITIS

Equine encephalomyelitis has been known in the United States for many years. In 1931 a neurotropic virus was first identified as the cause of an outbreak among mules in California, and a few years later a virus was isolated from an epizootic occurring in the Eastern states. These viruses, though similar, are immunologically distinct, and are known as the Western and Eastern strains; like those responsible for the disorders considered above they belong to the arbovirus group. Numerous cases of human infection with these viruses have been observed, and in 1941 an epidemic of infection with the Western virus affected at least 1,700 persons in Minnesota and North Dakota with 150 deaths. It has been proved that various species of bird constitute a reservoir of infection, that a wood-tick also harbours the virus, and that mosquitoes can transmit it to man.

Pathological changes differ somewhat in the two forms. In the Western type the vessels of the nervous system are always much congested, and petechial haemorrhages may or may not be present. Both neutrophil and mononuclear inflammatory cells are present in the perivascular spaces and as focal or diffuse infiltrations. Small, discrete patches of demyelination are scattered irregularly throughout the entire brain. The nervous elements appear to suffer secondarily to these changes. The spinal cord may show disseminated involvement, mainly in the central grey matter. The meninges show little change as a rule.

In the Eastern variety, on the other hand, there is widespread involvement of nerve cells, ranging from early nuclear changes to complete disappearance. Polymorphonuclear infiltration of the brain is conspicuous and there is an inflammatory infiltration of the meninges, lymphocytes predominating.

The clinical features of the two diseases also differ. In the Western form the onset is sudden, with generalized headache, nausea, elevation of temperature, and lethargy. Focal signs of nervous involvement are usually absent, but there are stiffness of the neck, muscular weakness, and diminution of tendon reflexes. The spinal fluid shows a moderate, predominantly mononuclear, pleocytosis. The mortality rate is about 10 per cent. Most patients make a complete recovery in a week or two, but mental defect, epilepsy, and spastic palsies have been observed as sequels, especially in young children (see Finley, 1958).

In the Eastern form, which chiefly attacks children, the onset is very abrupt with severe general symptoms; lethargy soon appears, passing into stupor or coma. Cervical rigidity and Kernig's sign are present. Aphasia, diplopia, and paralyses indicate damage to the brain. The spinal fluid contains many cells, often more than 1,000 per mm.[3], and polymorphonuclears may predominate. There is a mortality rate of 65 per cent., and severe sequels are common in those who survive.

Prophylaxis is directed to the destruction of mosquitoes and protection from their bites. Treatment is symptomatic.

REFERENCES

BAKER, A. B., and NORAN, H. H. (1942) Western variety of equine encephalitis in man, *Arch. Neurol. Psychiat. (Chicago)*, **47**, 565.

DAVID, W. A. (1940) A study of birds as hosts for the virus of Eastern equine encephalo-myelitis, *Amer. J. Hyg.*, **32**, 45.

FINLEY, K. H. (1958) in *Viral Encephalitis*, ed. FIELDS, W. S., and BLATTNER, R. J., Springfield, Ill.

FOTHERGILL, N. D., DINGLE, J. H., FARBER, S., and CONNERLEY, M. L. (1938) Human encephalitis caused by the virus of the Eastern variety of equine encephalomyelitis, *New Engl. J. Med.*, **219**, 411.

HAMMON, W. H. (1941) Encephalitis in Yakima Valley: mixed St. Louis and Western equine types, *J. Amer. med. Ass.*, **117**, 161.

NORAN, H. H., and BAKER, A. B. (1943) Sequels of equine encephalitis, *Arch. Neurol. Psychiat. (Chicago)*, **49**, 398.

SYVERTON, J. T., and BERRY, G. P. (1941) Hereditary transmission of the Western type of equine encephalitis by the wood tick, Dermacentor Andersoni Stiles, *J. exp. Med.*, **73**, 507.

FORMS OF ENCEPHALITIS DUE OR PROBABLY DUE TO VIRUSES

Acute Polioclastic Encephalitis

Greenfield (1950) reports a few cases of this description, characterized by inflammatory and perivascular and tissue infiltration of the nervous system with variable changes in the nerve cells. The symptoms are those of encephalitis as described in previous sections. The cerebrospinal fluid may be normal or show an excess of cells. Pette and Döring (1939) have described a few cases of pan-encephalitis in which both grey and white matter suffer.

Subacute Inclusion Body Encephalitis (Subacute Sclerosing Panen-cephalitis)

This form, first observed by Dawson, has been recognized only comparatively recently and has been described by Brain, Greenfield, and Russell (1948), Greenfield (1950), Foley and Williams (1953) amongst others. The condition described in 1945 by van Bogaert as subacute sclerosing leuco-encephalitis is now believed to be identical as inclusion bodies were eventually found in some of van Bogaert's pathological material from his cases. The distinctive patho-logical lesion is widespread degeneration of ganglion cells, many of which show acidophilic hyaline inclusion bodies in the nucleus and cytoplasm, together with astrocytic gliosis. Most cases occur in the first decade of life but in recent years the disease has been recognized in adolescents and young adults. No specific virus has yet been isolated consistently from such cases but Connelly *et al.* (1967) have found that antibody titres to measles virus rise in the serum during the course of the illness and suggest that it may be a rare manifestation of measles infection. Dayan *et al.* (1967) and Lennette *et al.* (1968) have demonstrated myxovirus-like particles in the brains of affected patients, and Saunders *et al.* (1969) have found lymphocyte transformation in response to measles antigen in such a case.

The disease runs a slowly progressive course of from two to eighteen months in which three stages can be recognized. First the mood changes and there is some intellectual deterioration, sometimes accompanied by epileptic attacks or more often by recurrent myoclonic jerking. This is followed by progressive dementia leading to akinetic mutism often with complex involuntary movements. The third stage is one of decortication. The cerebrospinal fluid may show a paretic colloidal gold curve, and characteristic EEG changes have been described taking the form of complex generalized slow-wave complexes, recurring repetitively and often in time with the myoclonic jerks and separated by intervals of comparative electrical silence in the record.

The disease usually terminates fatally, but may become arrested and occasional cases of possible spontaneous recovery have been reported. No treatment is known to be of value.

Encephalitis due to Herpes Simplex

Encephalitis due to herpes simplex may occur in young infants as part of a generally disseminated infection with haemorrhages and enlargement of the liver and spleen, or as a cerebral disorder. Convulsions, rigidity, involuntary movements, paralyses, and coma may occur. Van Bogaert (1959) states that this condition is probably an acute disseminated encephalitis not due to direct damage to the brain by the herpes virus.

It has recently become apparent that in many patients of all ages who develop an acute and explosive cerebral illness with coma, hyperpyrexia and features suggesting a massive lesion of one temporal lobe (most patients show a hemiplegia from shortly after the onset and may have fits) a herpes simplex encephalitis may be responsible. Often in such cases intracerebral haemorrhage or cerebral abscess are suspected (Gostling, 1967). Pathologically massive necrosis, often largely confined to one temporal lobe, but involving both white and grey matter is found and there may be inclusion bodies in astrocytes or neurones while virus may be cultured from the necrotic tissue. Massive doses of dexamethasone, 5 mg. four times daily, may reduce oedema and some workers advocate subtemporal decompression. Most cases are fatal but antiviral chemotherapy may yet transform the prognosis, and intravenous idoxuridine, 200 mg./kg. body weight by intravenous infusion, has recently been recommended (Marshall, 1967). Very rarely it seems that a similar clinical picture may result from Coxsackie B5 virus infection (Heathfield *et al.*, 1967).

REFERENCES

BOGAERT, L. VAN (1945) Une leuco-encéphalite sclèrosante subaiguë, *J. Neurol. Neurosurg. Psychiat.*, **8**, 101.

BOGAERT, L. VAN (1959) Acute encephalitis in childhood, *Brit. med. J.*, **1**, 1201.

BRAIN, W. R., GREENFIELD, J. G., and RUSSELL, D. S. (1948) Subacute inclusion encephalitis (Dawson type), *Brain*, **71**, 365.

COBB, W., and HILL, D. (1950) Electroencephalogram in subacute progressive encephalitis, *Brain*, **73**, 392.

CONNELLY, J. H., ALLEN, I. V., HURWITZ, L. J., and MILLAR, J. H. D. (1967) Measles-virus antibody and antigen in subacute sclerosing panencephalitis, *Lancet*, i, 542.

DAYAN, A. D., GOSTLING, J. V. T., GREAVES, J. L., STEVENS, D. W., and WOODHOUSE, M. A. (1967) Evidence of a pseudomyovirus in the brain in subacute sclerosing leucoencephalitis, *Lancet*, i, 980.

FOLEY, J., and WILLIAMS, D. (1953) Inclusion encephalitis and its relation to subacute sclerosing leuco-encephalitis, *Quart. J. Med.*, **22**, 157.

GOSTLING, J. V. T. (1967) Herpetic encephalitis, *Proc. roy. Soc. Med.*, **60**, 693.

GREENFIELD, J. G. (1950) Encephalitis and encephalomyelitis in England and Wales during the last decade, *Brain*, **73**, 141.

HAYMAKER, W., SMITH, M. G., BOGAERT, L. VAN, and DE CHENAN, L. (1958) Inclusion body encephalitis, in *Viral Encephalitis*, ed. FIELDS, W. S., and BLATTNER, R. J., Springfield, Ill.

HEATHFIELD, K. W. G., PILSWORTH, R., WALL, B. J., and CORSELLIS, J. A. N. (1967) Coxsachie B5 infections in Essex, 1965, with particular reference to the nervous system, *Quart. J. Med.*, **36**, 579.

LENNETTE, E. H., MAGOFFIN, R. L., and FREEMAN, J. N. (1968) Immunological evidence of measles virus as an etiologic agent in subacute sclerosing panencephalitis, *Neurology (Minneap.)* **18**, 21.

MARSHALL, W. J. S. (1967) Herpes simplex encephalitis treated with idoxuridine and external decompression, *Lancet*, ii, 579.

PETTE, H., and DÖRING, G. (1939) Über einheimische Panencephalomyelitis vom Charakter der Encephalitis japonica, *Deutsch. Z. Nervenheilk.*, **149**, 7.

SAUNDERS, M., KNOWLES, M., CHAMBERS, M. E., CASPARY, E. A., GARDNER-MEDWIN, D., and WALKER, P. (1969) Cellular and humoral responses to measles in subacute sclerosing panencephalitis, *Lancet*, i, 72.

POLIOMYELITIS

Synonyms. Infantile paralysis; Heine-Medin disease.

Definition. An acute infective disease due to a virus with a predilection for the cells of the anterior horns of the grey matter of the spinal cord and the motor nuclei of the brain stem, destruction of which causes muscular paralysis and atrophy.

PATHOLOGY

In the acute stage naked-eye examination yields evidence of a general reaction to the infection in parenchymatous degeneration of the liver and kidneys, and a general enlargement of the lymphoid tissue of the body, including the lymph nodes of the alimentary canal. The spinal cord is congested, soft, and oedematous, and minute haemorrhages may be visible in the grey matter.

Histologically the changes in the nervous system are usually most marked in the grey matter of the spinal cord and medulla. The basal ganglia and cerebral cortex are little affected. In the cord the changes consist of degeneration of the anterior horn cells and an inflammatory reaction with small haemorrhages in the grey matter. The ganglion cells of the anterior horns show changes of all degrees of severity from slight chromatolysis to complete destruction with neuronophagia. The inflammatory reaction consists of perivascular cuffing, mainly with lympho-cytes but with a smaller number of polymorphonuclear cells, and a diffuse infiltration of the grey matter, with similar cells and cells of neuroglial origin

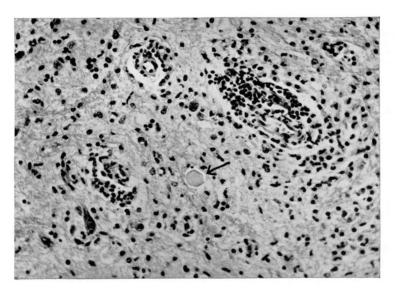

FIG. 75. Poliomyelitis. Anterior horn showing inflammatory infiltration and advanced chromatolysis of neurone (arrow). H & E, ×215

[FIG. 75]. The white matter of the cord shows some perivascular infiltration. The meninges share in the inflammatory reaction, exhibiting infiltration with lymphocytes and endothelial cells.

Cortical lesions are similar but are more focal, and inflammatory changes have also been observed in the spinal dorsal roots and in the peripheral nerves. In rare cases the brunt of the infection falls upon the brain stem (polioencepha-litis). Focal necroses are found in the liver, and an inflammatory hyperplasia in the lymphoid tissue. The virus has been demonstrated in the walls of the pharynx, the small and large intestines and the mesenteric lymph nodes, and the nervous system.

Recovery from the acute stage is attended by restoration to normal of ganglion cells which have not been too severely damaged. Others disappear completely, and sections therefore show a paucity of cells in the anterior horns in the affected regions with secondary degeneration in the corresponding ventral roots and peripheral nerves. The muscles supplied by these segments show varying degrees of atrophy with a relative increase of the connective tissue and fat.

AETIOLOGY

Our knowledge of the causative organism of poliomyelitis dates from the observation of Landsteiner and Popper in 1909, that the disease could be transmitted to monkeys, and it has since been shown to be a filterable virus. A comprehensive review of the present state of our knowledge of the bacteriology and epidemiology has been published by W.H.O. (1954). Three strains of virus have now been isolated, known as 'Brunhilde' (Type 1), 'Lansing' (Type 2), and 'Leon' (Type 3). The virus was first grown in tissue culture by Enders, Weller, and Robbins (1949). It is said to measure 15–25 mμ in at least one diameter. The virus can be obtained from the nasopharyngeal mucous membranes of patients in the acute stage, healthy contacts, and convalescents, and also from the stools. Monkeys can be successfully inoculated by direct intracerebral injection or by injection subcutaneously, intraperitoneally, into the lymph nodes, or into a nerve trunk, but it is now believed that the usual route of infection in man is the alimentary tract, and it has been suggested that the virus reaches the nervous system from here by way of the autonomic nerves (Howe and Bodian, 1941 a, 1941 b, 1942). Fairbrother and Hurst's work (1930) has shown that the virus travels readily along the axis cylinders both in the peripheral nerves and in the central nervous system. But recent work has suggested that the blood stream may be more important for the diffusion of the virus than used to be thought (Horstmann, 1952). A low level of antibody in the serum may be sufficient to prevent the virus spreading from the bowel via the blood stream (Bodian, 1952). It is possible that exceptionally the pharynx or tonsils may be the portal of entry or the raw tonsillar bed after tonsillectomy (Aycock and Luther, 1929). There is good evidence also that physical exertion during the stage of incubation may predispose to paralysis, particularly of those muscles which have been most used and paralysis may also develop in a limb which has been traumatized as by an injection. For these reasons prophylactic inoculations and tonsillectomy are generally abandoned during an epidemic and violent physical exercise is unwise in those unprotected individuals who have been exposed to infection (Russell, 1956). The virus is highly resistant to chemical agents, but sensitive to heat and to desiccation.

EPIDEMIOLOGY

In Great Britain poliomyelitis occurs for the most part sporadically, but considerable epidemics have occurred. The United States is subject from time to time to severe epidemics, and Wickman studied epidemics in Norway and Sweden. This worker found ample evidence that the transmission of the disease could often be traced to an apparently healthy individual who had been in contact with a paralytic case but never himself developed the disease. Such healthy carriers and abortive cases, in which recovery occurs before the paralytic stage is reached, greatly outnumber the paralytic cases and are probably mainly responsible for the spread of the infection, though there is evidence that the disease can be acquired from a paralytic case. There is evidence that most members of a household have been infected by the time a paralytic case appears, though multiple paralytic cases in a household occur in less than 10 per cent.

of infected families. For every person with symptoms there may be 10 to 100 infected individuals with no obvious illness. The virus has been demonstrated in the pharyngeal secretions and in the faeces of patients, in sewage, and in flies caught in the neighbourhood of infected cases. Aycock and Eaton have shown that the peak of incidence of poliomyelitis occurs at the same time as that of typhoid fever. Personal contact and the faecal contamination of food appear to be the principal modes of transmission.

The seasonal incidence in the late summer and early autumn may be explained by these facts. Infants under the age of 1 year are rarely attacked. In a country where hygiene is poor most sufferers are between the ages of 2 and 4. After the age of 5 susceptibility rapidly diminishes, and after the age of 25 the disease is rare. During and after the Second World War in the U.S.A. and in Great Britain the age incidence rose steadily. In Massachusetts in 1907, 7 per cent. of those affected were over the age of 15, in 1945, 25 per cent.; and cases in adults became commoner (Horstmann, 1948). Males suffer somewhat more frequently than females. The incubation period appears to be usually from 7 to 14 days but may be as long as 5 weeks.

The last 10 years has seen a dramatic and sharp decline in the incidence of the disease in all countries in which campaigns of prophylactic inoculations have been carried out using first injections of the Salk (Salk, 1960) and British vaccines and more recently the Sabin type oral attenuated live vaccine (Sabin, 1959). It seems probable that within the next decade the disease will disappear.

SYMPTOMS

There are four possible ways in which a person may react to infection by the virus of poliomyelitis. (1) There is evidence that exposure to the virus leads in a large majority of cases to development of immunity without any symptoms of illness. This may be termed subclinical or inapparent infection. (2) Most workers believe that there are patients in whom the symptoms are never more than those of a mild general infection without involvement of the nervous system. These may be termed abortive cases. (3) A majority of patients, in some epidemics as many as 75 per cent., develop general symptoms, and at this stage may exhibit an excess of cells in the cerebrospinal fluid yet never develop paralysis. Evidently, though the nervous system is invaded, the anterior horn cells are not attacked. The infection is overcome in the pre-paralytic stage and these are called non-paralytic cases. (4) Only in a minority does the infection run its full course and cause paralysis.

(1) Patients with subclinical infections exhibit no symptoms. (2) Symptoms of patients of the abortive type are indistinguishable from those of any other general infection unless the virus can be demonstrated in the nasopharynx or stools. There remain to be considered the symptoms of (3) the pre-paralytic stage and (4) the stage of paralysis.

The Pre-paralytic Stage

In this stage two phases can often be recognized. The first symptoms of infection are fever, malaise, headache, drowsiness or insomnia, sweating, flushing, faucial congestion, and often gastro-intestinal disturbances such as anorexia, vomiting, and diarrhoea. This phase, 'the minor illness', which lasts one or two days, sometimes followed by temporary improvement with remission of fever for 48 hours, or it may merge into the second phase, 'the major illness', in which headache is more severe and associated with pain in the back and limbs, together with hyperaesthesia often of both the superficial and deep tissues. The symptoms of these closely resemble those of other forms of viral meningitis.

Delirium may occur. The patient is often tremulous, and cervical rigidity and Kernig's sign may be observed. In the absence of such marked signs of meningeal irritation the 'spinal sign' is of diagnostic value. In adults, infants, and children too ill to be taken from bed this is elicited by means of passive flexion of the spine when the patient is lying on his side, resistance being encountered on account of pain in the back. Flexion of the spine, even when assisted by passive movement, is prevented by pain. Convulsions may occur in infants in either of the first two phases.

In non-paralytic cases the patient recovers after exhibiting in mild or more severe form either or both of the phases of the pre-paralytic stage.

The Cerebrospinal Fluid

In the second phase the cerebrospinal fluid shows changes which are the outcome of meningeal irritation. The pressure is increased and there is an excess of cells, usually 50 to 250 per mm.^{3} During the first few days both polymorphonuclear cells and lymphocytes are present, but after the first week lymphocytes alone are found. The protein and globulin show a moderate increase, but the glucose and chloride content of the fluid is normal. During the second week the protein may rise to between 100 and 200 mg.

The Paralytic Stage

Spinal Form. The onset of paralysis, which is often ushered in by muscular fasciculation, usually follows rapidly upon the pre-paralytic stage, and is attended by considerable pain in the limbs and tenderness of the muscles on pressure. Exceptionally the pre-paralytic phase may last for a week or even two. The paralysis may be widespread or localized. In severe cases the muscles of the neck, trunk, and all four limbs may be powerless, except for a feeble movement here and there. When the paralysis is less extensive its asymmetry and patchy character are conspicuous features, and some muscles may be severely affected on one side of the body and escape injury on the other. Usually the maximum of damage is done within the first 24 hours, but sometimes the paralysis is progressive. In the ascending form it gradually spreads upwards from the legs, and endangers life through respiratory paralysis. A descending form is described. Sometimes the infection merely smoulders on, in which case fresh weakness may appear a week or more after the onset of the paralysis. The lower limbs are more often affected than the upper. In the former the quadriceps and the muscles below the knee suffer most, especially the peronei and the anterior tibial group. In the latter the small muscles of the hands are frequently involved. During this stage careful watch should be kept upon movement of the intercostals and the diaphragm.

Fortunately it is the rule that only a proportion of the muscles affected at the outset remain permanently paralysed. The disease produces temporary loss of function in many anterior horn cells which ultimately recover. Improvement usually begins at the end of the first week after onset of the paralysis. In common with other causes of lower motor neurone paralysis, poliomyelitis leads to wasting of, and loss of cutaneous and tendon reflexes carried out by, the affected muscles, though the tendon reflexes may be exaggerated for a brief period at the onset. Complete paralysis of the muscles around a joint may permit subluxation to occur. When opposing muscle groups are unequally affected, contractures are apt to occur in the stronger muscles, causing limitation of movement at the joint. In the upper limb this most often happens in the adductors of the shoulder after paralysis of the deltoid; in the lower limb, in the calf muscles, after paralysis of the peronei and anterior tibial group. Talipes equinovarus results from contracture of the calf. Asymmetrical palsy of the spinal muscles causes scoliosis. The affected limbs are blue and cold and may be the site of oedema or chilblains. Fasciculation may continue for years in partially paralysed muscles. Bone growth is retarded in the paralysed limbs, and the bones show rarefaction radiographically.

Rarely the inflammation extends to the white matter of the lateral columns of the cord. Involvement of the spinothalamic tracts causes impaired appreciation of pain, heat, and cold, and damage to the corticospinal tracts leads to spastic paralysis. Such an extension in the cervical enlargement produces spastic paraplegia associated with muscular wasting of the upper limbs. Except in such cases sphincter disturbance is rare and sensory loss is absent.

Brain Stem Form (Polioencephalitis). In a small percentage of cases the brunt of the infection falls upon the brain stem, leading to facial, pharyngeal, laryngeal, lingual, or very rarely ocular paralysis. Tremor and nystagmus may be present and there is grave danger of involvement of the cardiac and respiratory centres. It is of great practical importance to distinguish embarrassment of respiration caused by the accumulation of saliva and mucus in pharyngeal paralysis from true paralysis of the muscles of respiration.

DIAGNOSIS

Diagnosis is rarely possible in the stage of constitutional disturbance, except in an epidemic. Even then suspicion cannot be confirmed until changes in the cerebrospinal fluid indicate that the nervous system is invaded. At this stage in sporadic cases the disease has to be distinguished from other causes of meningeal irritation. In the acute pyogenic forms of meningitis the glucose content of the spinal fluid is reduced, and the cells are exclusively polymorphonuclear. Mumps meningitis, which is also associated with a lymphocytic pleocytosis in the spinal fluid, is not likely to cause confusion if parotitis is present. Tuberculous meningitis may be difficult to distinguish. In this condition the onset is usually more gradual and the child is pale rather than flushed as in poliomyelitis. The diagnosis, however, rests upon the examination of the spinal fluid, which in both may contain an excess of cells, both polymorphonuclear and lymphocytes, and an excess of protein. In poliomyelitis the sugar and chloride content of the fluid are normal; in tuberculous meningitis the sugar is invariably, the chloride sometimes, diminished. Tubercle bacilli if present are, of course, conclusive.

The spinal form of the disease in the paralytic stage is usually easy to diagnose. When the pain and tenderness are severe it may be confused with acute rheumatism, syphilitic epiphysitis, and acute osteomyelitis. In these, however, the tenderness is more localized than in poliomyelitis and in the first two is related to the joint; in the last the lesion is often near a joint. Moreover, in none of these are the tendon reflexes lost as in poliomyelitis. The V.D.R.L. reaction is usually positive in cases of the syphilitic lesion.

In adults poliomyelitis may need to be distinguished from acute transverse myelitis, but in this condition flaccid paralysis of the legs is associated with extensor plantar reflexes, sensory loss, and loss of sphincter control.

When the patient is seen years after the acute attack the presence of muscular wasting may suggest motor neurone disease, syringomyelia, or myopathy. The fact that the wasting is not progressive, however, excludes all these alternatives. The absence of fasciculation also helps to distinguish it from the first named, and the absence of sensory loss from the second, while the wasting is usually too patchy and asymmetrical to simulate myopathy very closely.

The bulbar form must be distinguished from other forms of encephalitis. In encephalitis complicating the exanthemata and vaccination the primary cause is usually obvious, and the long tracts, both motor and sensory, are likely to be involved.

PROGNOSIS

The mortality varies in different epidemics and may be as high as 25 per cent. The mortality rate is highest in the first year of life and in those who are attacked after the fifth year. The cause of death is usually respiratory paralysis due to direct involvement of the respiratory centres in the bulbar form or to paralysis of the intercostals and diaphragm, which is most liable to occur in the ascending form of the disease.

When the progress of the paralysis has ceased, it is safe to predict that considerable recovery will occur. Favourable indications are the presence of voluntary movement, of reflex responsiveness, and of a reaction to faradism which persists three weeks after the onset of the paralysis. Improvement once begun may be expected to continue for at least a year and in some cases for even longer. The nature and extent of the remaining disability will, of course, depend upon the distribution of the residual paralysis. Second attacks, though very rare, are well authenticated.

Motor neurone disease is a rare sequel of acute anterior poliomyelitis, which it may follow after many years, the progressive wasting usually beginning in the region originally affected.

TREATMENT

General Management

Immediate and complete rest should be insisted on in every suspected case, however mild, since there is evidence that physical activity in the pre-paralytic stage increases the risk of severe paralysis (Russell, 1949).

Four categories of paralytic case require to be distinguished because in each form the treatment needed is different. These are (1) the patient with neither respiratory nor bulbar paralysis, (2) the patient with respiratory paralysis, (3) the patient with bulbar paralysis, and (4) the patient with both respiratory and bulbar paralysis.

The Treatment of a Patient without Respiratory and Bulbar Paralysis

During the acute stage plenty of fluid should be given. Lumbar puncture may be needed for diagnostic purposes and may help to relieve headache and backache. Aspirin in doses of 300–600 mg. and sedatives, such as phenobarbitone, will be required for the relief of pain and restlessness. Hypertonic saline baths diminish the hyperaesthesia. Gentle passive movements are the only form of physical treatment which is permissible at this stage. Antibiotics are of no value except as a prophylactic against pneumonia in patients with respiratory paralysis, and serotherapy is valueless because as soon as the virus has reached the nervous system it is beyond the reach of antibodies.

For purposes of treatment the course of the disease after the onset of paralysis is divided into: (1) An acute stage, during which pain and tenderness of the muscles persist. This usually lasts for three or four weeks. (2) A convalescent stage, during which improvement in muscular power continues. This may last from six months to two years. (3) A chronic stage in those left with permanent paralysis after the maximum recovery has occurred.

The principal object in the treatment of the muscular paralysis in the acute stage is to prevent stretching of the paralysed muscles and contracture of their antagonists. If great care is not taken over this, damage may be done in a few days which it will take months to repair. The patient should be nursed on a firm bed and the limbs kept in the positions in which the paralysed muscles are relaxed by means of sandbags and pillows.

During the stage of convalescence prolonged rest in bed will be necessary in severe cases, the limbs being kept in position by suitable splints if necessary. Rigid splinting is undesirable, and unnecessary at this stage. Passive movements should be carried out from the beginning so far as the patient will tolerate them. Except when the trunk muscles are severely paralysed the patient should as soon as possible be allowed to stand for a few minutes daily, but paralysis of the spinal muscles requires prolonged recumbency or suitable spinal supports if severe spinal deformity is to be prevented. During convalescence active exercises are of great importance. They may need to be assisted or carried out in baths or in the Guthrie-Smith sling-suspension apparatus. Passive movements, massage, and galvanism are also necessary. Affected parts should be put through a full range of movement at least once, and if possible twice, a day. Adequate instrumental support for the spine and limbs may be required and falls within the province of the orthopaedic surgeon. In the later stages contractures and deformities may require tenotomy or other surgical treatment, but these may often be avoided by adequate care during the acute stage.

In the chronic stage when oedema, cyanosis, and chilblains are troublesome in the feet, lumbar sympathectomy may be helpful in improving the circulation.

Treatment of Respiratory Paralysis

A patient suffering from respiratory paralysis needs to be treated by some method of artificial respiration which may be required for weeks, or even for months. Such artificial respiration may be effected by means of negative pressure operating through some device which sucks the thoracic cage outwards, or by positive pressure which inflates the lungs by raising the pressure within the trachea. For uncomplicated respiratory paralysis a negative pressure method is the more suitable. The cuirass type of respirator (Kelleher *et al.*, 1952) which operates through the application of negative pressure directly to the chest and abdomen, though of great value and convenience in certain cases, is not so efficient as the box type of respirator as regards the ventilation produced. Some form of box respirator, therefore, which encloses the whole patient except for his head, is the most suitable for general purposes. The use of these respirators has been discussed by Bourdillon *et al.* (1950) and by Russell (1956). It requires considerable skill and experience. The authors point out that while the dangers of respirator treatment may be appreciable it is important to use the apparatus at the earliest detectable signs of involvement of the respiratory motor neurones. Since the vital capacity of most people is about eight times as great as their tidal air when at rest, a patient at rest will not show distress from failure of respiratory muscles until a very large fraction of their power is lost. In determining the first onset of respiratory weakness a rough estimate can be formed by finding out how many numbers the patient can count verbally in one expiration. But if the apparatus is available, some kind of spirometer is much more accurate. By means of early measurements of vital capacity it is possible to detect the first signs of respiratory involvement, and tidal air measurements are indicated as a rough guide to the correct setting of respiratory pressures so as to avoid under- or over-ventilation. Under-ventilation is perhaps more dangerous and an oximeter may be of great value for the detection of this. The indications for, and the technique of, respiratory treatment are also discussed by Russell (1956).

Treatment of Bulbar Paralysis

Russell (1956) has done much to clarify the treatment of bulbar paralysis in poliomyelitis. When bulbar paralysis occurs in the absence of respiratory paralysis the danger to the patient arises from his inability to prevent fluids, or secretions in the pharynx, from being sucked into the lungs with inspiration. Vomiting, for example, with the patient lying on his back, is likely to be followed by fatal inhalation of vomitus. The dysphagia also leads to difficulty in feeding. The proper posture of the patient is all-important. He should be nursed in the semi-prone position, being turned from one side to the other every few hours, while the foot of the cot or bed should be raised to make an angle of 15 degrees with the horizontal. This posture should be relaxed for nursing or other purposes only for short periods under close supervision. Tracheostomy in such cases is rarely necessary except in the presence of bilateral abductor paralysis of the vocal cords. A mechanical sucker is required to remove pharyngeal secretions. After about 24 hours of starvation feeding should be carried out by an oesophageal catheter, preferably passed through the nose.

The Treatment of Respiratory Paralysis Combined with Bulbar Paralysis

The combination of respiratory paralysis with bulbar paralysis constitutes an extremely difficult problem for treatment. If the patient is treated in a breathing-machine for his respiratory paralysis this introduces the danger that the suction created by the machine will aspirate pharyngeal secretions forcibly into the lungs. There are three possible solutions of the problem, to maintain postural drainage while the patient is in the respirator, or to combine respirator treatment with tracheostomy, or to treat the patient by a combination of tracheostomy and positive pressure artificial respiration, as was used successfully in an epidemic in Denmark by Lassen (1953) and in Britain by Smith, Spalding, and Russell (1954).

Intermittent positive pressure respiration, using a variety of different automatic devices, is now the standard treatment for these cases throughout the world. The advantage of the positive pressure method is that the use of a cuffed intratracheal tube effectively blocks the trachea to the downward passage of the pharyngeal secretions and so protects the lungs.

Whatever method is used for the treatment of respiratory or bulbar paralysis, or the two combined, necessitates a team of experienced doctors, nurses, and physiotherapists. A doctor accustomed to the use of the bronchoscope will be required to remove accumulated secretions from the bronchi and so prevent pulmonary collapse. X-ray of the chest may be required. Prophylactic penicillin should be given, or other antibiotics as may be appropriate. Acute gastric dilatation is a serious complication and when it occurs a stomach tube should be passed and an attempt made to empty the stomach by gastric suction. Retention of urine should be treated by an indwelling catheter which should be changed every few days and appropriate antibiotics will be required to keep the urine sterile. Purgatives are theoretically contra-indicated in the acute stage and constipation of a few days need cause no anxiety. After that an enema should be used if necessary.

PROPHYLAXIS

Since the nasopharyngeal secretions, the urine, and the faeces of the patient may contain the virus barrier nursing should be adopted. Virus is present in the stools 3 weeks after the onset in 50 per cent. of patients and 5–6 weeks after the onset in 25 per cent. It is not easy to say how long the patient remains infectious, but he should be isolated for at least 6 weeks.

During an epidemic it is desirable as a rule that residential schools should not be closed. For reasons given in the section on epidemiology it is uncertain whether closure of a school will modify the spread of the disease among those already exposed to it, and there is a risk that this course will tend to disseminate the infection among younger and therefore more susceptible children. When a case occurs in a residential house in a boarding school, the house should be isolated. Children in an affected household should be isolated from other children for three weeks after the isolation of the patient. Operations on the ear, nose, and throat and inoculations should not be carried out during an epidemic, and dental extractions should be avoided if possible.

The protective value of the Salk vaccine was well established between 1950 and 1960. Three doses, which give 90 per cent. protection, were given as a routine, and a fourth was often added later in special circumstances. Immunity induced by injection did not prevent colonization of the gut by wild virus; hence an immune person could still be a carrier. On the other hand, attenuated live vaccine, given orally, by multiplying in the gut blocks the entry of wild virus. Its capacity to confer immunity is now established and the Sabin type vaccine, given as one or two drops on a sugar lump, appears to confer almost total immunity for three years or more. In children and young adults, 'booster' doses at regular intervals are recommended.

REFERENCES

AFFELDT, J. E. (1954) Recent advances in the treatment of poliomyelitis, *J. Amer. med. Ass.*, **156**, 12.

AYCOCK, W. L., and LUTHER, E. H. (1929) The occurrence of poliomyelitis following tonsillectomy, *New Engl. J. Med.*, **200**, 164.

BODIAN, D. (1952) A reconsideration of the pathogenesis of poliomyelitis, *Amer. J. Hyg.*, **55**, 414.

BOURDILLON, R. B., DAVIES-JONES, E., STOTT, F. D., and TAYLOR, L. M. (1950) Respiratory studies in paralytic poliomyelitis, *Brit. med. J.*, **2**, 539.

COX, H. R., CABASSO, V. J., MARKHAM, F. S., MOSES, M. J., MAYER, A. W., ROCA-GARCIA, M., and RUEGSEGGER, J. M. (1959) Immunological response to trivalent oral poliomyelitis vaccine, *Brit. med. J.*, **2**, 591.

DANE, D. S., DICK, G. W. A., McALISTER, J. J., and NELSON, R. T. (1960) Epidemic control of poliomyelitis with inactive virus vaccines, *Lancet*, i, 835.

ENDERS, J. F., WELLER, T. H., and ROBBINS, F. C. (1949) Cultivation of the Lansing strain of poliomyelitis virus in tissue culture, *Science*, **109**, 85.

FAIRBROTHER, R. W., and HURST, E. W. (1930) The pathogenesis of, and propagation of the virus in, experimental poliomyelitis, *J. Path. Bact.*, **33**, 17.

HALE, J. H., DORAISINGHAM, M., KANAGARATNAM, K., LEONG, K. W., and MONTEIRO, E. S. (1959) Large scale use of Sabin type 2 attenuated poliomyelitis vaccine in Singapore during a type 1 poliomyelitis epidemic, *Brit. med. J.*, **1**, 1541.

HORSTMANN, D. M. (1948) Problems in the epidemiology of poliomyelitis, *Lancet*, i, 273.

HORSTMANN, D. (1952) Poliomyelitis virus in blood of orally infected monkeys and chimpanzees, *Proc. Soc. exp. Biol. (N.Y.)*, **79**, 417.

HOWE, H. A., and BODIAN, D. (1941 *a*) The pathology of early, arrested and nonparalytic poliomyelitis, *Bull. Johns Hopk. Hosp.*, **69**, 135.

HOWE, H. A., and BODIAN, D. (1941 *b*) Poliomyelitis in the chimpanzee: a clinical-pathological study, *Bull. Johns Hopk. Hosp.*, **69**, 149.

HOWE, H. A., and BODIAN, D. (1942) *Neural Mechanisms in Poliomyelitis*, New York.

HURST, E. W. (1930) A further contribution to the pathogenesis of experimental poliomyelitis: inoculation into the sciatic nerve, *J. Path. Bact.*, **33**, 1133.

HURST, E. W. (1932) Further observations on the pathogenesis of experimental poliomyelitis: intrathecal inoculation of the virus, *J. Path. Bact.*, **35**, 41.

KELLEHER, W. H., WILSON, A. B. K., RUSSELL, W. R., and STOTT, F. D. (1952) Notes on cuirass respirators, *Brit. med. J.*, **2**, 413.

KOPROWSKI, H. (1960) Historical aspects of the development of live virus vaccine in poliomyelitis, *Brit. med. J.*, **2**, 85.

KRAMER, S. D., HOSKWITH, B., and GROSSMAN, L. H. (1939) Detection of virus of poliomyelitis in nose and throat and gastro-intestinal tract of human beings and monkeys, *J. exp. Med.*, **59**, 49.

LANCET (1960) Live poliovirus vaccine, Editorial, i, 1057.

LASSEN, H. C. A. (1953) A preliminary report on the 1952 epidemic of poliomyelitis in Copenhagen, *Lancet*, i, 37.

MORGAN, I. M. (1948) Mechanisms of immunity in poliomyelitis, *Proc. First Internat. Poliomyelitis Conference*, New York.

MURPHY, D. P., DRINKER, C. K., and DRINKER, P. (1931) The treatment of respiratory arrest in the Drinker respirator, *Arch. intern. Med.*, **47**, 424.

NATIONAL ADVISORY COMMITTEE FOR EVALUATION OF GAMMA GLOBULIN. Summary of Report (1954) *J. Amer. med. Ass.*, **154**, 1087.

NEAL, J. B. (1932) *Report of International Committee for the Study of Infantile Paralysis*, Baltimore.

PAUL, J. R., TRASK, J. W., BISHOP, M. B., MELNICK, J. L., and CASEY, A. E. (1941) The detection of poliomyelitis virus in flies, *Science*, **94**, 395.

RUSSELL, W. R. (1949) Paralytic poliomyelitis, *Brit. med. J.*, **1**, 465.

RUSSELL, W. R. (1956) *Poliomyelitis*, 2nd ed., London.

SABIN, A. B. (1959) Present position of immunization against poliomyelitis with live virus vaccines, *Brit. med. J.*, **1**, 663.

SALK, J. E. (1960) Persistence of immunity after administration of formalin-treated poliovirus vaccine, *Lancet*, ii, 715.

SEDDON, H. J. (1947) The early treatment of poliomyelitis, *Brit. med. J.*, **2**, 319.

SMITH, A. C., SPALDING, J. M. K., and RUSSELL, W. R. (1954) Artificial respiration by intermittent positive pressure in poliomyelitis and other diseases, *Lancet*, i, 939.

TRASK, J. D., VIGNEC, A. J., and PAUL, J. R. (1938) Poliomyelitis virus in human stools, *J. Amer. med. Ass.*, **111**, 6.

WORLD HEALTH ORGANIZATION EXPERT COMMITTEE ON POLIOMYELITIS, First Report (1954) *Wld Hlth Org. techn. Rep. Ser.*, No. 81.

RABIES

Synonym. Hydrophobia.

Definition. An infection of the nervous system due to a filterable neurotropic virus communicated to man by the bite of an infected animal. The resulting encephalitis, which is almost always fatal, is distinguished by the characteristic pharyngeal spasm evoked by the attempt to drink.

AETIOLOGY

Rabies is due to a filterable virus which possesses a predilection for the nervous system. It is communicated to man by the bite of an infected animal which carries the virus in its saliva. Most cases of human infection are due to dog bites, though bites of jackals, cats, and wolves are occasionally responsible. The bites of rabid horses and cattle hardly ever communicate the disease. An epidemic in Trinidad has been attributed to vampire bats which are believed to carry the infection from cattle to man. The virus of rabies has been isolated from a fatal case occurring in a human epidemic of encephalitis in Japan. The risk of infection is influenced by the severity of the bite and is much diminished when the individual is bitten through clothes, which to some extent free the animal's teeth from saliva. The virus, having entered the body, is transmitted only along the nerve trunks, moving in both directions.

PATHOLOGY

The pathological changes in the nervous system exhibit the general characteristics associated with infection with a neurotropic virus. Severe degenerative changes are found in the ganglion cells of the cerebrospinal and sympathetic ganglia. The small vessels show narrowing of the lumen and enlargement of the endothelial cells, with marked perivascular round-cell infiltration. The ganglion-cell degeneration is more diffuse than the inflammatory reaction, and the ganglion cells of the cortex may be extensively affected. There is considerable reaction of oligodendroglia and microglia, and collections of inflammatory and glial cells are known as Babes' nodes. The Negri body is of diagnostic importance. It is an acidophil inclusion body contained within the cytoplasm or protoplasmic processes of the ganglion cells. Negri bodies are most constantly present in the ganglion cells of the hippocampus major, but may also be found in the pyramidal cells of the cortex, the Purkinje cells of the cerebellum, and the ganglion cells elsewhere. Negri bodies are not constantly present in human rabies nor in the experimental infection of animals with the *virus fixé*.

The pathological picture in the so-called 'neuroparalytic accidents' occurring during the prophylactic treatment of rabies is different [see p. 481].

SYMPTOMS

Rabies in Animals

The first symptoms of rabies in the dog are a change in behaviour associated with perversion of appetite. The animal will gnaw and swallow paper, sticks, earth, and other unusual substances. This stage is followed by excitement, in which it will snap at and bite other animals. There is a flow of saliva from the mouth, and the bark often becomes high-pitched. After one or two days paralysis develops, beginning first in the hind limbs and spreading to the forelimbs and jaw. Muscular spasms may occur affecting the whole body. Emaciation is marked and death is almost invariable.

In other animals, especially rodents and herbivora, the stage of excitement does not occur and the symptoms are paralytic from the beginning, and this paralytic form of the disease occurs in a small proportion of dogs.

Rabies in Man

The incubation period in man depends upon the distance of the infected lesion from the central nervous system. When the bite is on the head it is about 27 days, when on the arm 32 days, when on the leg 64 days, but these periods are liable to wide variations. During the incubation period there are no symptoms. Local pain in the bitten limb is often the first symptom to appear. The first general symptoms are depression, often associated with apprehension, and disturbed sleep. The next symptom is pharyngeal spasm brought on by the attempt to drink and rapidly extending to involve both the ordinary and the accessory muscles of respiration, and later all the muscles of the body, often producing opisthotonos. When this stage is at its height not only the attempt to drink but the sound and even the thought of water will bring on the spasm, which may also be excited by other external stimuli, even a current of air. Salivation is excessive, and vomiting is common. A horror of water develops and hallucinations may appear. Even so, the human patient does not as a rule exhibit the impulse to bite characteristic of the rabid dog. Later the symptoms of excitement and the spasm diminish and may give place to a terminal paralysis. Fever is usually present, and a terminal hyperpyrexia may occur. Death may take place during the spasmodic stage from respiratory or cardiac failure, or the patient may die in coma in the stage of paralysis.

Rarely the spasms and mental excitement are absent and the symptoms are paralytic from the beginning, as is the case in certain species of animal. An epidemic of paralytic rabies occurred in Trinidad in 1931. In such cases the clinical picture is that of an ascending paralysis beginning in the lower limbs and associated with loss of sphincter control. The upper limbs may or may not be affected and sensory loss is inconstant. Finally, bulbar paralysis leads to dysphagia, and death occurs from paralysis of the respiratory muscles.

DIAGNOSIS

The diagnosis of typical rabies is usually easy on account of the history of the bite and the presence of the distinctive pharyngeal spasm. The condition must be distinguished from tetanus, the incubation period of which is shorter. The symptoms of tetanus unmodified by the injection of serum usually begin within 14 days of the injury and almost invariably within 3 weeks. Trismus is an early symptom and pharyngeal spasm is usually absent.

Hysteria may simulate hydrophobia in a patient who has been bitten by a dog which is supposed to be rabid. In hysteria, however, true pharyngeal spasm does not occur and the condition is amenable to sedatives combined with suggestion.

The paralytic form of rabies should offer no difficulty in diagnosis, when there is a history of a bite, but in cases such as those in Trinidad, when the mode of infection is obscure, the diagnosis may be established only by means of animal inoculation.

PROGNOSIS

The risk of contracting rabies is estimated at about 5 per cent. of individuals bitten by animals supposed to be rabid. Adequate prophylactic treatment reduces this incidence to about 1·5 per cent. Those who develop rabies invariably die.

PROPHYLAXIS AND TREATMENT

The prophylactic treatment of rabies introduced by Pasteur is still carried out, though it has been modified in various details. It consists of successive doses of a vaccine derived from animals which have been infected with the *virus fixé*. The vaccine may consist of living or dead virus from the cord or brain of infected animals and may be given alone or combined with antiserum. A vaccine free from brain tissue and prepared in duck embryos has recently been introduced in the United States and is given in a course of 14 daily injections to the individual exposed to infection. The indications for vaccine treatment are set out in the report of the W.H.O. Committee (1950). The administration should be begun as early as possible after the bite. The long incubation period of rabies permits the development of an acquired immunity after infection. The prophylactic vaccine treatment of rabies is thus analogous to the vaccination of individuals after exposure to smallpox. The risk of producing acute or subacute demyelination of the nervous system by the treatment [p. 481] should be borne in mind and treatment interrupted if this is suspected. Though complications have been most frequent following the use of the earlier forms of vaccine, a case of transverse myelitis following the use of the duck embryo vaccine has been described (Prussin and Katabi, 1964). The bite itself should be treated, though cauterization has little influence in preventing the development of the disease. When rabies has developed, treatment is purely symptomatic, its principal object being to diminish the spasms. Muscle-relaxing drugs may be used combined with artificial respiration. The paralytic form of the disease will require the usual treatment of paraplegia.

REFERENCES

GIBBS, F. A., GIBBS, E. L., CARPENTER, P. R., and SPIES, H. W. (1961) Comparison of rabies vaccines grown on duck embryo and on nervous tissue, *New Engl. J. Med.*, **265**, 1002.

HILDRETH, E. A. (1963) Prevention of rabies, or the decline of Sirius, *Ann. intern. Med.*, **58**, 883.

HURST, E. W., and PAWAN, J. L. (1931) An outbreak of rabies in Trinidad without history of bites and with the symptoms of acute ascending myelitis, *Lancet*, ii, 622.

HURST, E. W., and PAWAN, J. L. (1932) A further account of the Trinidad outbreak of acute rabic myelitis. Histology of the experimental disease, *J. Path. Bact.*, **35**, 301.

KNUTTI, R. E. (1929) Acute ascending paralysis and myelitis due to the virus of rabies, *J. Amer. med. Ass.*, **93**, 754.

KORITSCHONER, (1923) Ueber die Ueberimpfung des Enzephalitisvirus auf Hunde, *Wien. klin. Wschr.*, **36**, 385.

PRUSSIN, G., and KATABI, G. (1964) Dorsolumbar myelitis following antirabies vaccination with duck embryo vaccine, *Ann. intern. Med.*, **60**, 114.

SCHÜKRI, I., and SPATZ, H. (1925) Über die anatomischen Veränderungen bei der menschlichen Lyssa und ihre Beziehungen zu denen der Encephalitis epidemica, *Z. ges. Neurol. Psychiat.*, **97**, 627.

VIETS, H. R. (1926) A case of hydrophobia with Negri bodies in the brain, *Arch. Neurol. Psychiat.* (*Chicago*), **15**, 735.

WORLD HEALTH ORGANIZATION EXPERT COMMITTEE ON RABIES (1950) *Wld Hlth Org. techn. Rep. Ser.*, No. 28.

WORLD HEALTH ORGANIZATION EXPERT COMMITTEE ON RABIES (1966) *Wld Hlth Org. techn. Rep. Ser.*, No. 321.

VIRUS MENINGITIS

Synonyms. Acute benign lymphocytic meningitis; epidemic serous meningitis; acute aseptic meningitis.

AETIOLOGY

There is no clearcut distinction between encephalitis and meningitis, as is shown by the term meningo-encephalitis. Nevertheless, a number of virus infections may present the clinical picture of an acute meningitis with a pleocytosis in the cerebrospinal fluid, and little or no evidence of involvement of the substance of the nervous system. These viruses include those of acute lymphocytic choriomeningitis, mumps, infectious mononucleosis, some of the Coxsackie and Echo viruses, poliomyelitis, psittacosis, and louping-ill.

Recent observations suggest that benign lymphocytic meningitis accounts for about 50 per cent. of all cases of infectious meningitis seen in hospital. Mumps is one of the commonest causes in Britain, being found in 26 per cent. of a recent series of cases in Glasgow in which Echo 9 virus accounted for 61 per cent. and other enteroviruses for 13 per cent.; lymphocytic choriomeningitis was uncommon in this series (Grist, 1967).

Some of the commoner of these will now be discussed separately.

ACUTE LYMPHOCYTIC CHORIOMENINGITIS

The disorder occurs sporadically and also in small epidemics. Children are usually affected, but it may occur in adults also. The work of Armstrong and Lillie (1934), Findlay, Alcock, and Stern (1936), and others has shown that it is caused by a filterable virus, which has been recovered from the cerebrospinal fluid of patients and transmitted to mice and monkeys. Mice are subject to the disease in the wild state and may be the source of the human disease, which has been encountered in Europe, North America, New Zealand, and Malaya.

PATHOLOGY

Animals infected experimentally show intense lymphocytic infiltration of the leptomeninges, the ependyma of the ventricles, and the choroid plexuses. Viets and Warren (1937) report similar changes in a fatal case together with degeneration of the ganglion cells of the brain, which in the midbrain showed cytoplasmic inclusion bodies. Perivascular infiltration with round cells was seen in both the brain and the spinal cord.

SYMPTOMS

The onset is acute, and symptoms of meningeal irritation usually develop rapidly but there may be prodromal manifestations of a general infection followed by a remission before nervous symptoms occur. The symptoms resemble those of acute pyogenic meningitis [see p. 359]. Papilloedema may occur, and squint and nystagmus are common. Apart from the occasional occurrence of facial paralysis, the other cranial nerves are normal. Paraplegia and retention of urine have been described, but symptoms of invasion of the substance of the nervous system are rare. There is usually high fever at the onset, and as a rule the temperature falls by lysis in about a week. Pneumonitis—'atypical pneumonia'—may occur (Smadel et al., 1942), and it is probable that a general infection without meningitis is the commonest form of the disease (Farmer and Janeway, 1942).

The cerebrospinal fluid is under increased pressure and may be clear, turbid, or, exceptionally, purulent. The albumin and globulin are increased and a 'cobweb clot' has occurred in some cases. There is an excess of cells ranging from 50 to 1,500 per mm.^{3}; about half show over 1,000 at some stage. These may be mainly mononuclear from the onset, but in a minority of cases polymorphonuclear cells predominate at the beginning, giving place to mononuclear cells in the course of the first week. The chloride and sugar of the fluid are usually little, if at all, depressed. The pleocytosis in the cerebrospinal fluid is often remarkably persistent, and in some of my own cases a considerable excess of mononuclear cells has been present for many weeks after the disappearance of symptoms, when the patient has apparently been in normal health.

DIAGNOSIS

For the diagnosis of meningitis see page 361.

Acute lymphocytic choriomeningitis is most likely to be confused with tuberculous meningitis, and since the absence of tubercle bacilli from the cerebrospinal fluid cannot be held to exclude the latter, the two conditions may be difficult to distinguish. A low chloride and sugar content in the fluid, however, is against the benign disorder. The acuteness of the onset of symptoms in acute lymphocytic choriomeningitis may help to distinguish this condition from the tuberculous form, and the white cell count in the blood and Paul–Bunnell test from meningitis due to infectious mononucleosis. Mumps meningitis is very similar, and cannot be distinguished clinically in the absence of parotitis or orchitis. It may be possible to transmit the disease to mice or hamsters from the cerebrospinal fluid or to demonstrate antibodies in the blood. Serum complement-fixing antibodies may be found within 2 weeks, neutralizing antibodies within 6–8 weeks.

PROGNOSIS

The prognosis is good and complete recovery is the rule. Relapses occasionally occur. Paraplegia, however, may be permanent and diffuse arachnoiditis has been described as a sequel.

TREATMENT

Treatment is purely symptomatic; appropriate analgesics should be given for the relief of headache; chemotherapy is of no value.

REFERENCES

ADAIR, C. V., GOULD, R. L., and SMADEL, J. E (1953) Aseptic meningitis: a disease of diverse etiology, *Ann. intern. Med.*, **39**, 675.

ARMSTRONG, C., and LILLIE, R. D. (1934) Experimental lymphocytic choriomeningitis of monkeys and mice, *Publ. Hlth Rep. (Wash.)*, **49**, 1019.

BAIRD, R. D., and RIVERS, T. M. (1938) Relation of lymphocytic choriomeningitis to acute aseptic meningitis (Wallgren), *Amer. J. publ. Hlth*, **28**, 47.

FARMER, T. W., and JANEWAY, C. A. (1942) Infections with the virus of lymphocytic choriomeningitis, *Medicine (Baltimore)*, **21**, 1.

FINDLAY, G. M., ALCOCK, N. S., and STERN, R. O. (1936) The virus aetiology of one form of lymphocytic meningitis, *Lancet*, i, 650.

GRIST, N. R. (1967) Acute viral infections of the nervous system, *Proc. roy. Soc. Med.*, **60**, 696.

KREIS, B. (1937) *La maladie d'Armstrong: chorio-méningite lymphocytaire*, Paris.

MACCALLUM, F. O., and FINDLAY, G. M. (1939) Lymphocytic choriomeningitis. Isolation of the virus from the nasopharynx, *Lancet*, i, 1370.

MACCALLUM, F. O., FINDLAY, G. M., and SCOTT, T. M. (1939) Pseudo-lymphocytic choriomeningitis, *Brit. J. exp. Path.*, **20**, 260.

SMADEL, J. E., GREEN, R. H., PALTAUF, R. M., and GONZALES, T. A. (1942) Lymphocytic choriomeningitis: two human fatalities following an unusual febrile illness, *Proc. Soc. exp. Biol. (N.Y.)*, **49**, 683.

VIETS, H. R., and WARREN, S. (1937) Acute lymphocytic meningitis, *J. Amer. med. Ass.*, **108**, 357.

NERVOUS COMPLICATIONS OF MUMPS

AETIOLOGY

The experimental work of Gordon lent support to the view that mumps is due to infection with a filterable virus which possesses potential neurotropic propensities. Gordon was able to produce meningitis in monkeys by the intra-cerebral injection of a filtrate of the saliva of patients suffering from mumps. Since the commonest nervous complication of mumps is meningitis, it seemed probable that this was due to an infection of the meninges with the mumps virus and this has now been recovered from the cerebrospinal fluid. The much rarer lesions of the substance of the nervous system may be due to a spread of this infection from the meninges to the neuraxis, but are probably more usually the result of an acute encephalomyelitis similar to that complicating other specific fevers. The recent observation of Johnson et al. (1967) that the inoculation of mumps virus into suckling hamsters produced hydrocephalus and aqueduct stenosis may eventually prove to be of importance in relation to the aetiology of similar lesions in man.

PATHOLOGY

Little is known about the pathology of the nervous complications of mumps. After experimental infection of monkeys, hyperaemia of the brain and meninges, with lymphocytic infiltration of the latter, is found. In one case of encephalitis complicating mumps Bien (1913) observed in addition to leptomeningitis an area of demyelination in the corona radiata, and Miller, Stanton, and Gibbons (1956) reviewing the literature, state that the pathological changes in the substance of the nervous system are those of a perivenous encephalitis.

SYMPTOMS

Nervous symptoms may occur at the onset or during the first stage of the disease, but usually develop somewhat later, in the adult male immediately before the appearance of orchitis. They may occur without parotitis but with orchitis or may be the sole manifestation of the infection. The symptoms are usually those of an acute meningitis [see p. 359], but encephalitis may occur and in rare cases aphasia and hemiplegia have been described. Optic neuritis and optic atrophy are rare complications. Deafness, either unilateral or bilateral, is commoner.

A small number of cases of polyneuritis occurring in association with mumps has been recorded, usually developing two or three weeks after the onset of the primary symptoms. In all the reported cases there has been a flaccid paralysis of all four limbs, and in some cases cranial nerve paralyses have occurred, most frequently facial paralysis. Localized neuritis is also sometimes encountered, for example, unilateral facial paralysis.

The cerebrospinal fluid usually exhibits a marked lymphocytosis in cases of meningitis. Monod first pointed out that this is frequently present in mumps in the absence of any meningeal symptoms, and it may also occur in contacts who never develop other symptoms of the disease. Serological tests have been developed (Enders and Cohen, 1942; Kane, Cohen, and Levens, 1945).

DIAGNOSIS

The parotitis usually renders the diagnosis easy. In cases of meningitis associated with lymphocytosis of the cerebrospinal fluid for which no cause can be found, inquiry should always be made whether symptoms of parotitis or orchitis have been present, as this may not have been mentioned spontaneously. Serological tests of antibodies in paired sera are often successful in establishing the diagnosis.

PROGNOSIS

Recovery from mumps meningitis is the rule, but the condition is occasionally fatal. Polyneuritis patients usually recover, though slowly, and recovery may be incomplete. The mortality rate of encephalomyelitis is about 20 per cent.

TREATMENT

Treatment is purely symptomatic. Specific mumps immune globulin may be used to protect susceptible adolescents and adults during an epidemic and active immunization with a vaccine may confer temporary immunity.

REFERENCES

BIEN, G. (1913) Encephalitis und Mumps, *Jb. Kinderheilk.*, **78, 619.**
COLLENS, W. S., and RABINOWITZ, M. A. (1928) Mumps polyneuritis; quadriplegia with bilateral facial paralysis, *Arch. intern. Med.*, **41,** 61.
DOPTER, C. (1910) La méningite ourlienne, *Paris méd.*, **1,** 35.
ENDERS, J. F., and COHEN, S. (1942) Detection of antibodies by complement-fixation in sera of man and monkey convalescent from mumps, *Proc. Soc. exp. Biol.*, **1,** 180.
FINKLESTEIN, H. (1938) Meningo-encephalitis in mumps, *J. Amer. med. Ass.*, **111,** 17.
GORDON, M. H. (1927) Experimental production of the meningo-encephalitis of mumps, *Lancet*, i, 652.
GRIST, N. R. (1967) Acute viral infections of the nervous system, *Proc. roy. Soc. Med.*, **60,** 696.
HARRIS, W., and BETHELL, H. (1938) Meningo-encephalitis and orchitis as the only symptoms of mumps, *Lancet*, ii, 422.
JOHNSON, R. T., JOHNSON, K. P., and EDMONDS, C. J. (1967) Virus-induced hydrocephalus: development of aqueductal stenosis in hamsters after mumps infection, *Science*, **157,** 1066.
KANE, L. W., COHEN, S., and LEVENS, J. H. (1945) Immunity in mumps, *J. exp. Med.*, **81,** 93.
LENNETTE, E. H., CAPLAN, G. E., and MAGOFFIN, R. L. (1960) Mumps virus infection simulating paralytic poliomyelitis, *Pediatrics*, **25,** 788.
MILLER, H. G., STANTON, J. B., and GIBBONS, J. L. (1956) Para-infectious encephalomyelitis and related syndromes, *Quart. J. Med.*, **25,** 427.
PITRES, A., and MARCHAND, L. (1922) Polynévrite post-ourlienne quadriplégique à forme pseudo-tabétique, *Progr. méd. (Paris)*, **35,** 397.
TOCMANN, S. L. (1921) Quelques considérations générales sur l'histoire de l'affection ourlienne en général et de la méningite ourlienne en particulier: lois essentielles de cette méningite, *Thèse de Paris*, No. 159.

THE COXSACKIE VIRUSES

Following the isolation in Coxsackie, New York, of a virus which could produce paralysis in mice, the term Coxsackie or C. viruses has been applied to a group which now includes a number of viruses. In infant mice some strains attack the muscles, and some the nervous system also. In man the chief clinical manifestations so far recognized are: (1) Aseptic meningitis. The cerebrospinal fluid does not usually contain more than 100 cells per mm.[3], and the percentage of polymorphonuclears ranges from 10 to 50. The febrile period lasts on an average five days, and recovery is complete as a rule. However, there is now good evidence that the Coxsackie A7 virus, which closely resembles that of polio-myelitis, may on occasion cause paralysis which is generally less severe than that of poliomyelitis. However, this infection can occur in individuals immunized against poliomyelitis. In a recent series of hospital cases diagnosed neurologically over an 8-year period, paralysis was found in 70 per cent. of poliovirus infections and in 19 per cent. of Coxsackie A7 virus infections (Grist, 1966). (2) Epidemic myalgia or pleurodynia. It is now established that the clinical picture of Born-holm disease may be caused by one of the Coxsackie viruses. Epidemic myalgia and acute aseptic meningitis may both occur in the same patient. (3) Herpangina. This is a febrile illness with pharyngitis characterized by vesicular or ulcerative lesions. Vomiting and abdominal pain may be present. (4) Encephalomyo-carditis of the new-born.

The diagnosis depends upon the isolation of one of the Coxsackie viruses from the faeces or oropharyngeal swabs, and the appearance of or an increase in neutralizing antibodies against the virus in the patient's serum at appropriate intervals.

C. virus has often been recovered from the faeces of patients suffering from poliomyelitis, but there is no evidence that either virus influences the patient's reaction to the other.

No specific treatment is known.

REFERENCES

GIUNCHI, G. (1960) Clinical aspects of Coxsackie viruses, in *Virus Meningo-encephalitis*, ed. WOLSTENHOLME, G. E. W., and CAMERON, M. P., London.

GRIST, N. R. (1966) *Tenth Symposium of the European Association against Poliomyelitis and Allied Diseases*, p. 275, Brussels.

HUMMELEN, K., KIRK, D., and OSTAPICK, M. (1954) Aseptic meningitis caused by Cox-sackie virus and isolation of virus from cerebrospinal fluid, *J. Amer. med. Ass.*, **156,** 676.

MELWICK, J. L., and CURWEN, E. C. (1952) in *Viral and Rickettsial Infections in Man*, ed. RIVERS, T. M., p. 338, London.

THE ECHO VIRUSES

There are at present twenty-eight distinct antigenic types of the Echo viruses (enteric cytopathic human orphan). They infect the gastro-intestinal tract and are excreted mainly in the stools. They cause a febrile illness, sometimes with a rash. Some types cause an acute aseptic meningitis, and it has been suggested that they can cause a poliomyelitis-like illness but it now seems more probable that in such cases paralysis is caused by a concomitant infection with poliovirus or Coxsackie A7 virus as enterovirus infections are commonly multiple. In the meningitic cases there may be more than 500 cells per mm.^{3}, usually mainly mononuclear. The virus may be isolated from the fluid or stools. Antibodies may be present in the blood.

REFERENCES

GRIST, N. R. (1961) Echo viruses, in *Virus Meningo-encephalitis*, ed. WOLSTENHOLME, G. E. W., and CAMERON, M. P., p. 17, London.
KAHLMETER, O. (1961) Clinical aspects of Echo viruses, in *Virus Meningo-encephalitis*, ed. WOLSTENHOLME, G. E. W., and CAMERON, M. P., p. 24, London.

HERPES ZOSTER

Synonym. Shingles.

Definition. An acute infection involving primarily the first sensory neurone and the corresponding area of skin.

PATHOLOGY

The pathological changes in the nervous system are those of an acute inflammation at some point in the course of the first sensory neurone. The dorsal root ganglia and the corresponding sensory ganglia of the cranial nerves are the commonest sites of the lesion, but the posterior horn of the grey matter of the spinal cord, the dorsal root, and the peripheral nerves may also be involved. One or more successive metameric segments may be affected, but it is very rare for the lesion to be bilateral. The microscopical changes in the acute stage consist of haemorrhages and infiltration with mononuclear and occasional polymorphonuclear leucocytes, especially in the form of perivascular cuffs, and degenerative changes in the nerve cells. Fibrosis and secondary degeneration follow in severe cases. Inflammatory changes are present in the neighbouring leptomeninges. In a fatal case of zoster meningo-encephalitis, chromatolysis of ganglion cells, and perivascular infiltration were found at all levels of the nervous system up to the cerebral cortex (Biggart and Fisher, 1938). The cutaneous lesions show inflammatory infiltration of the epidermis and dermis, with vesicle formation produced by serous exudation beneath the stratum corneum. Acidophil nuclear inclusion bodies have been described in the cells of the vesicle epithelium.

AETIOLOGY

These pathological changes are clearly infective, and the infective character of zoster is borne out by numerous facts. It often occurs in epidemics with a seasonal incidence, most cases occurring in the early summer and late autumn. The contagiousness of the infection is well established. It is closely related to varicella, and there is reason to believe that in the majority of cases, if not in all, zoster and varicella are due to the same organism. Either may give rise to the other in contacts, though varicella follows exposure to zoster much more frequently than the reverse. It has been suggested that herpes zoster may be due to reactivation of varicella virus which is latent in the tissues (Gajdusek, 1965). The zoster-varicella virus is entirely distinct from that responsible for simple or febrile herpes. It has been observed with the electron microscope and is described as circular and between 196 and 218 mμ in size (Nagler and Rake, 1948; Farrant and O'Connor, 1949).

Zoster may occur without any evident predisposing cause, or as a complication of some other disease or toxic state, especially when this causes damage to the first sensory neurone. These two groups are distinguished as 'idiopathic' and 'symptomatic' zoster, but the evidence indicates that both are due to the same virus. 'Symptomatic' zoster may be precipitated by intoxication with arsenic, bismuth, carbon monoxide, and other poisons, and may occur in the course of infections such as pneumonia and tuberculosis or toxic states such as uraemia. It may complicate any lesion of the dorsal roots and may therefore follow fracture-dislocation of the spine, secondary carcinoma of the vertebral column, meningococcal and other forms of meningitis, subarachnoid haemorrhage, syphilitic radiculitis, and spinal tumour. It occasionally follows quite a slight injury.

Zoster may occur at any age, but is rare in infancy and more frequent in the second half of life than in the first. It is most often seen in patients over 50.

The incubation period is from seven to twenty-four days, and is usually about a fortnight.

SYMPTOMS

General Symptoms

The eruption is often preceded by a disturbance of the general health and sometimes by fever, and there is enlargement of the lymph nodes draining the affected area of skin. The general symptoms are usually slight but may be severe in the aged.

Zoster of the Limbs and Trunk

The first local symptom is usually pain in the segment or segments involved, which is burning or shooting in character and is often associated with hyperalgesia of the area of skin supplied by the affected nerve roots. Three or four days after the onset of pain the eruption appears as a series of localized papules which develop into vesicles grouped together upon an erythematous base [FIG. 76]. The eruption, like the other symptoms, possesses a segmental distribution. After a few days the eruption fades, the vesicles drying into crusts which separate, leaving small permanent scars in the skin. The subsidence of the eruption may be associated with some loss of sensibility in the affected segments. The skin may become partially or completely analgesic, though the pain may persist, the association of pain with sensory loss being sometimes described as anaesthesia dolorosa. Thermal and postural sensibility may also be impaired. Pain may persist for weeks or months or indefinitely after the eruption, and this 'post-herpetic neuralgia' is the more likely to occur the older the patient. Severe itching is sometimes a troublesome sequel.

Segmental Complications of Zoster

In addition to involving the first sensory neurone and the skin, zoster may cause a disturbance of function of other structures innervated by the spinal segment affected. Muscular wasting of segmental distribution is a rare accompaniment of zoster and is probably due to an extension of the infection from the posterior to the anterior horns of grey matter in the spinal cord. Thus I have seen atrophic paralysis of the muscles supplied by the fifth cervical segment and also paralysis of the abdominal wall, the latter leading to pseudohernia. These palsies are sometimes permanent but often recover slowly over a period of several months. Visceral manifestations of zoster may also occur. Arthritis is rare, but I have seen two cases. It has been described only in the joints of the

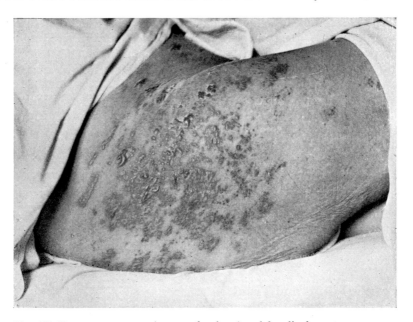

FIG. 76. Herpes zoster eruption over lumbar 1 and 2 radicular cutaneous areas

hand and wrist as a complication of zoster involving the upper limb. There is severe pain and peri-articular swelling with much limitation of movement, which is likely to be permanent. Radiographically the bones show only rarefaction. Other visceral manifestations of zoster which have been reported include zoster of the pleura, and urinary bladder, and symptoms resembling those of duodenal ulceration.

Ophthalmic Zoster

When the zoster virus invades the trigeminal ganglion the eruption appears in some part of the cutaneous distribution of the trigeminal nerve, being usually confined to one division. When the ophthalmic division is involved the cornea may be attacked, usually only when the eruption appears on the part of the nose supplied by the nasociliary branch, as Jonathan Hutchinson pointed out. The corneal lesion takes the form of small, round infiltrations in the more superficial layers of the substantia propria of the cornea. Other orbital structures may be involved, the most serious complication, fortunately a rare one, being optic neuritis, followed by atrophy and leading to blindness. Oculomotor paralyses may occur, the third nerve being more often affected than the fourth and sixth. Trigeminal zoster, like zoster elsewhere, may be either idiopathic or symptomatic. In the latter case it may follow any intracranial lesion of the fifth nerve, even alcoholic injection of the trigeminal ganglion.

Geniculate Zoster

Zoster of the geniculate ganglion was the explanation proposed by Ramsay Hunt (1915) of cases in which the vesicles are found in the auricle and less often on the anterior pillar of the fauces. There is pain in the ear and mastoid region radiating to the anterior pillar of the fauces and to the vertex. There may be a serosanguineous discharge from the ear. Taste may be lost in the anterior two-thirds of the tongue on the same side, the region innervated by the geniculate ganglion through the chorda tympani. Almost invariably the infection spreads to the trunk of the facial nerve and leads to facial paralysis, often associated with clonic facial spasm. The eighth nerve may become involved, with resulting deafness or vestibular disturbances and facial sensory loss on the same side is not uncommon. It is now doubted whether the geniculate ganglion is involved in all such cases (Denny-Brown, Adams, and Fitzgerald, 1944; O'Neill, 1945) and there is some evidence to indicate that the seat of infection in such cases is more often in the brain stem.

Meningitis, Encephalitis, and Myelitis

Some degree of meningeal inflammation is the rule in zoster and is indicated by an excess of mononuclear cells and a raised protein content in the cerebrospinal fluid, which is almost constantly present. Less frequently clinical signs of meningitis may be observed, headache and cervical rigidity complicating zoster of the trigeminal ganglion, and pains in the lower limbs and Kernig's sign being associated with dorsal and lumbar zoster. Extension of the infection to the substance of the brain or the white matter of the spinal cord is rare. Nevertheless, zoster encephalitis and myelitis have been observed and actual necrosis of the cord resembling subacute necrotizing myelopathy has been observed in a fatal case (Rose et al., 1964). In the latter myoclonus is not uncommon and intractable hiccup may occur. The corticospinal tract may be invaded, causing spastic weakness of the lower limb on the same side as the eruption.

Generalized Zoster

Besides the segmental eruption, the patient may exhibit scattered vesicles. These may be few in number—'aberrant vesicles'—or a widespread eruption resembling varicella. Usually the generalized rash appears within three or four days of the outbreak of zoster, but the interval may be longer.

DIAGNOSIS

The diagnosis of herpes zoster offers little difficulty, as in no other condition is there a vesicular eruption associated with pain and hyperalgesia of a segmental distribution. Herpes febrilis is less painful, is usually situated in the proximity of a mucous membrane, is often bilateral, and leaves neither residual pain nor scarring. Post-herpetic neuralgia is distinguished from other types of root pain by the history of the eruption, the scars of which can usually be found. Diagnosis is impossible in the pre-eruptive stage, but the possibility of zoster should be suggested by root pains of sudden onset less than four days before examination.

PROGNOSIS

The majority of sufferers from zoster recover without residual symptoms, except for scarring of the skin. One attack usually confers permanent immunity but second or repeated attacks sometimes occur especially in the symptomatic form. Severe secondary infection of the vesicles is a rare complication. Zoster of the cornea may be followed by corneal ulceration, and the occurrence of optic atrophy has already been mentioned. Recovery from facial paralysis following geniculate zoster is often incomplete. Zoster encephalitis is very uncommon, but at least two cases have been reported. The most troublesome sequel of zoster is persistent intractable pain, which may endure for years in elderly patients.

TREATMENT

In most cases the treatment of zoster is simple. Dusting powder and a dry dressing or collodion are all that are needed for the cutaneous eruption. Powerful analgesics are usually required. Dihydrocodeine or paracetamol may be sufficient in some cases but more often stronger remedies such as pethidine are required in the acute stage, particularly in ophthalmic cases. Chloramphenicol has been used but it is too early to assess its value. Some authors recommend liver injections. Persistent post-herpetic pain is a very troublesome complication which is very liable to occur in the elderly and aged. In severe cases analgesics are almost useless. It makes life a burden and may lead the patient to the verge of suicide. Morphine is contra-indicated owing to the risk of habit formation. Deep X-ray irradiation of the spinal cord and nerve roots or of the trigeminal ganglion has been tried and is occasionally successful but rarely has a lasting effect. Surgical division of sensory nerves or roots and alcohol or phenol injection of the Gasserian ganglion have also been advocated but relief is often temporary. Recent work suggests that the local application for up to twenty minutes three times a day of an electrical vibrator to the painful area or else repeated freezing of the skin segment involved with an ethyl chloride spray, if continued for several weeks or months, may give lasting relief. Often dihydrocodeine and chlorpromazine three or four times daily must be given for as long as the local treatment is continued. The accompanying depression which is almost invariably present in severe cases must usually be treated with amine-oxidase inhibitors or with amitriptyline or imipramine in appropriate dosage. Frequently it is best to admit the patient to hospital initially to teach him to use the vibrator or the cooling spray, depending upon which is the more effective in the individual case.

REFERENCES

AITKEN, R. S., and BRAIN, R. T. (1933) Facial palsy and infection with zoster virus, *Lancet*, i, 19.

BIGGART, J. H., and FISHER, J. A. (1938) Meningo-encephalitis complicating herpes zoster, *Lancet*, ii, 944.

BRAIN, W. R. (1931) Zoster, varicella and encephalitis, *Brit. med. J.*, **1**, 81.

CHAUFFARD, A., and RENDU, H. (1907) Méningite zonateuse tardive dans un cas de zona ophtalmique, *Bull. Soc. méd. Hôp. Paris*, **24**, 141.

DENNY-BROWN, D., ADAMS, R. D., and FITZGERALD, P. J. (1944) Pathologic features of herpes zoster: a note on 'geniculate herpes', *Arch. Neurol. Psychiat. (Chicago)*, **51**, 216.

FARRANT, J. L., and O'CONNOR, J. L. (1949) Elementary bodies of varicella and herpes zoster, *Nature (Lond.)*, **163**, 260.

GAJDUSEK, D. C. (1965) in *Slow, Latent and Temperate Virus Infections*, N.I.N.D.B. Monograph No. 2, p. 3, Bethesda, S. Ca.

GRÜTER, W. (1924) Das Herpesvirus, seine ätiologische und klinische Bedeutung, *Münch. med. Wschr.*, **71**, 1058.

HEAD, H., and CAMPBELL, A. W. (1900) The pathology of herpes zoster and its bearing on sensory localisation, *Brain*, **23**, 353.

HUNT, J. R. (1915) The sensory field of the facial nerve: a further contribution to the symptomatology of the geniculate ganglion, *Brain*, **38**, 418.

KUNDRATITZ, K. (1927) Zur Frage der gemeinsamen Atiologie der Varizellen und des Herpes zoster, *Wien. med. Wschr.*, **77**, 771.

LEVADITI, C. (1926) *L'herpès et le zona*, Paris.

LIDSKY, M. D., KLASS, D. W., McKENZIE, B. F., and GOLDSTEIN, N. P. (1962) Herpes zoster encephalitis. Case report with electroencephalographic and cerebrospinal fluid studies, *Ann. intern. Med.*, **56**, 779.

NAGLER, F. P. O., and RAKE, G. (1948) The use of the electron microscope in the diagnosis of variola, vaccinia and varicella, *J. Bact.*, **55**, 45.

NETTER, A., and URBAIN, A. (1926) Les relations de zona et de la varicelle. Étude sérologique de 100 cas de zona, *C.R. Soc. Biol. (Paris)*, **94**, 98.

O'NEILL, H. (1945) Herpes zoster auris ('geniculate' ganglionitis), *Arch. Otolaryng. (Chicago)*, **42**, 309.

PATON, L. (1926) The trigeminal and its ocular lesions, *Brit. J. Ophthal.*, **42**, 305.

PETTE, H. (1930) Infection and the nervous system, *Arch. Neurol. Psychiat. (Chicago)*, **24**, 1064.

ROSE, F. C., BRETT, E. M., and BURSTON, J. (1964) Zoster encephalomyelitis, *Arch. Neurol. (Chicago)*, **11**, 155.

RUSSELL, W. R., ESPIR, M. L. E., and MORGANSTERN, F. S. (1957) Treatment of postherpetic neuralgia, *Lancet*, i, 242.

SCHIFF, C. I., and BRAIN, W. R. (1930) Acute meningo-encephalitis associated with herpes zoster, *Lancet*, ii, 70.

TAVERNER, D. (1960) Alleviation of post-herpetic neuralgia, *Lancet*, ii, 671.

WOHLWILL, F. (1924) Zur pathologischen Anatomie des Nervensystems beim Herpes zoster (Auf Grund von zehn Sektionsfällen.), *Z. ges. Neurol. Psychiat.*, **89**, 171.

11

DEMYELINATING DISEASES OF THE NERVOUS SYSTEM

CLASSIFICATION

A LARGE and important group of diseases of the nervous system possess, as a common pathological feature, foci in which the myelin sheaths of the nerve fibres are destroyed. These foci, which are mainly situated in the white matter, vary in size, shape, and distribution and also in the acuteness of the pathological process of which they are the result, but they are sufficiently similar in the different diseases to justify the application to the whole group of the name *demyelinating diseases of the nervous system*. However, it must be remembered that the axis cylinders often suffer as well as their myelin sheaths and it is not certain that myelin destruction is always the primary change: it may be part of a more diffuse process. Moreover, as Lumsden (1961) points out, 'we mostly use the word "myelin" for a complex structural unit consisting of a formed sheath of myelin with satellite nutrient cells'. Not only does it not follow, but it is unlikely, that destruction of myelin is always the result of the same process. Myelin has been the subject of much recent study (see Lumsden, 1957; Finean, 1961; Wright, 1961; Thompson, 1961; and Robertson, 1965). Much new information has been gleaned, not only from the electron microscopy of myelin but also from biochemical and tissue culture studies (Field, 1967).

Apart from the fact that all but the most acute forms of demyelinating disease are sometimes familial, and that the most acute forms often follow acute infections, especially the exanthemata caused by viruses such as measles, smallpox, and vaccination, little is known as to the aetiology of this group of disorders. An aetiological classification is therefore impossible.

The attempt to classify them upon a pathological basis encounters the difficulty that although a large number of pathological varieties have been distinguished, they merge into one another to form an almost continuous series. A purely clinical classification is equally unsatisfactory in that it fails to accommodate transitional forms exhibiting features common to two clinical varieties, which can usually clearly be distinguished. The best available classification is a clinico-pathological one, which is based upon the recognition that to a large extent clinical and pathological features can be correlated. Such a classification must be provisional and must be qualified by the recognition of transitional forms. Increased knowledge may well show that clinico-pathological distinctions do not correspond to aetiological differences, but that they are the outcome of differences in respect of the acuteness of the pathological process, which may be influenced by the heredity of the patient, his age, the nature of the precipitating factors, and, possibly also, by processes concerned in immunity. We do not yet know even whether these diseases are due to an infection, an intoxication, or, as has been suggested in some cases, an allergic process, or whether they should be classed as deficiency or metabolic disorders. It is uncertain, therefore, when a demyelinating disorder affects the brain and spinal cord, whether encephalitis or encephalopathy, myelitis or myelopathy is the more appropriate term. Encephalitis and myelitis are employed here as being less cumbersome and better known. The following is a convenient clinico-pathological classification:

Variety	Synonyms	Incidence	Distribution of lesion	Course
Acute disseminated encephalomyelitis following acute infections, e.g. measles, chickenpox, smallpox, vaccination against smallpox and rabies.	Acute perivascular myelinoclasis.	Sporadic, very rarely familial: usually in children or adolescents.	Patchy in brain and spinal cord, tending especially to a perivenous distribution; rarely in optic nerves.	Acute or sub-acute and self-limited.
Acute haemorrhagic leuco-encephalitis.	Acute necrotizing haemorrhagic leuco-encephalopathy.	Sporadic, in all age groups.	Patchy in white matter of brain, generally perivascular.	Explosive, often fatal within 24–48 hours.
Disseminated myelitis with optic neuritis.	Neuromyelitis optica. Ophthalmoneuromyelitis (Devic's disease).	Sporadic (once reported in twins), any age from 12 onwards.	Massive in optic nerves and chiasma and spinal cord which may undergo softening and cavitation.	Acute or subacute in onset; sometimes self-limited, sometimes relapsing and progressive.
Multiple sclerosis.	Insular sclerosis. Disseminated sclerosis.	Sporadic, occasionally familial; usually in the first half of adult life.	Patchy in brain, optic nerves, and spinal cord, the lesions being multiple and successive.	Progressive, ranging from acute to extremely chronic with a conspicuous tendency to remissions and relapses.
Diffuse sclerosis.	Encephalitis periaxialis diffusa (Schilder's disease). Centrolobar sclerosis. Encephaloleucopathia scleroticans. Progressive degenerative subcortical encephalopathy. Leucodystrophy. Leuco-encephalopathia myeloclastica primitiva. Encephalomyelomalacia chronica diffusa. Concentric demyelination (Baló's disease). Infantile varieties: (Krabbe's disease) (Scholz's disease) (Pelizaeus-Merzbacher disease).	Sporadic and familial, usually in infancy and adolescence, less often in adult life.	Diffuse and massive, usually symmetrical, cerebral much more than spinal.	Acute, subacute, and chronic, steadily progressive or intermittent.
Central pontine myelinolysis.	No synonyms at present.	Sporadic in alcoholic and malnourished patients.	Central in pons.	Subacute, progressive.

In addition to arising spontaneously, as just described, demyelination may be produced either in the course of treatment or experimentally by a wide variety of toxic substances, including arsphenamine, sulphonamide, spinal anaesthetics, carbon monoxide, saponin, and potassium cyanide. Hurst (1941) considers that demyelination must be mediated by enzymatic processes, but we do not know whether it arises from specific poisoning of a particular enzyme or is a type of reaction of nervous tissue to poisons of different kinds or is derived and spreads from a central focus within the white matter. The enzymatic theory is discussed by Lumsden (1950) in connexion with experimental cyanide leuco-encephalopathy in rats.

It should also be noted that there are clinicopathological grounds for suggesting that there is a resemblance between the experimental allergic encephalitis which may be induced experimentally in animals on the one hand and human acute disseminated encephalomyelitis on the other. A relatively specific encephalitogenic factor has been isolated from human brain (Field, Caspary, and Ball, 1963). Rose and Pearson (1963) have recently reviewed experimental work on demyelination.

REFERENCES

FERRARO, A. (1937) Primary demyelinating processes of the central nervous system, *Arch. Neurol Psychiat.* (*Chicago*), **37**, 100.

FIELD, E. J. (1967) Experimental allergic demyelination and multiple sclerosis, *J. roy. Coll. Physcns., Lond.*, **1**, 56.

FIELD, E. J., CASPARY, E. A., and BALL, E. J. (1963) Some biological properties of a highly active encephalitogenic factor isolated from human brain, *Lancet*, ii, 11.

FINEAN, J. B. (1961) Electron microscopy of the myelin, *Proc. roy. Soc. Med.*, **54**, 19.

GRINKER, R. R., and BASSOE, P. (1931) Disseminated encephalomyelitis, *Arch. Neurol. Psychiat.* (*Chicago*), **25**, 723.

HURST, E. W. (1941) Demyelination: a clinico-pathological and experimental study, *Med. J. Aust.*, ii, 661.

LUMSDEN, C. E. (1950) Cyanide leucoencephalopathy in rats and observations on the vascular and ferment hypotheses of demyelinating diseases, *J. Neurol. Neurosurg. Psychiat.*, **13**, 1.

LUMSDEN, C. E. (1957) Aspects of the chemistry of myelin and the sheath cell complex, *and* Cell structure and cell physiology in relation to myelin, *Modern Trends in Neurology*, ed. WILLIAMS, D., pp. 130, 148. London.

LUMSDEN, C. E. (1961) Consideration of multiple sclerosis in relation to the auto-immunity process, *Proc. roy. Soc. Med.*, **54**, 11.

ROBERTSON, J. D. (1965) in *The Living Cell*, p. 45, *Scientific American*, San Francisco.

ROSE, A. S., and PEARSON, C. M., eds. (1963) *Mechanisms of Demyelination*, New York.

THOMPSON, R. H. S. (1961) Myelinolytic mechanisms, *Proc. roy. Soc. Med.*, **54**, 30.

WRIGHT, G. P. (1961) The metabolism of myelin, *Proc. roy. Soc. Med.*, **54**, 26.

See also Multiple sclerosis and the demyelinating diseases, *Res. Publ. Ass. nerv. ment. Dis.* (1958), **28**.

ACUTE DISSEMINATED ENCEPHALOMYELITIS

Synonym. Acute perivascular myelinoclasis.

Definition. An acute disorder characterized by demyelination of the nervous system, usually with a perivascular distribution, and by symptoms of damage to the brain and spinal cord, especially in the white matter, occurring in the course of infection with the causal virus of one of the exanthemata, such as measles, German measles, smallpox, mumps, chickenpox, as a sequel to vaccination against smallpox and rabies or banal infection, or spontaneously.

PATHOLOGY

Naked-eye changes consist merely of congestion and oedema of the nervous system. Microscopically [FIG. 77] there is marked perivascular infiltration of the

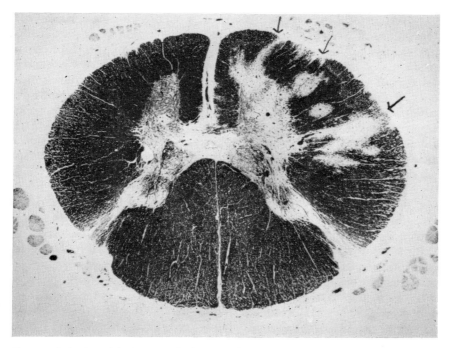

FIG. 77. Spinal cord in post-vaccinal encephalomyelitis. The arrows indicate patches of demyelination. (By courtesy of Dr. Urich.)

brain and spinal cord with lymphocytes and plasma cells both within the perivascular spaces and still more conspicuously at a greater distance from the vessels. In the white matter the most striking feature is the presence of zones of demyelination, that is, loss of the myelin sheaths of the neurones, around the vessels, especially the veins. The grey matter also shows degeneration and infiltration. The most intense changes are often found in the cerebral white matter and/or in the lumbar and upper sacral regions of the spinal cord, and in the pons. In the midbrain the substantia nigra is the structure most affected. Inflammatory changes may be present throughout the whole length of the nervous system. Meningeal infiltration is relatively slight. Herkenrath (1935) reported a case of recovery from post-vaccinal encephalitis followed by death from another cause 18 months later. The nervous system showed no abnormality except for some fat-laden scavenger cells in the perivascular spaces of the cerebellum, pons, medulla, and spinal cord. It was inferred that the process which results in perivascular demyelination is capable of complete reversal resulting in clinical and anatomical recovery.

AETIOLOGY

The most obvious explanation of the aetiology of this form of encephalomyelitis is that the changes in the nervous system are the direct result of its invasion by the virus of the exanthem, which has occasionally been found in the nervous system after the development of encephalitis. This view, however, now has few adherents, since it has not been possible to produce experimentally the pathological picture of acute perivascular myelinoclasis by means of the virus in question, and inoculation of the nervous system with vaccinial virus and with rabies virus does not cause demyelination. Moreover, it seems unlikely that an identical pathological picture would be produced by so many different viruses. An alternative view proposed is that the encephalitis is due to some other virus common to all the patients and aroused into activity by the exanthem. This would explain the common pathological features and also perhaps the increased incidence of this form of encephalitis during recent years. It would also explain the occasional spontaneous cases of acute perivascular myelinoclasis arising unpreceded by an exanthem. Nevertheless no such demyelinating virus has been shown to exist, and all known neurotropic viruses produce quite different pathological changes, so that many will agree with Hurst (1935) that there is no evidence that acute disseminated encephalomyelitis is due to a virus.

A third hypothesis postulates some unusual process intervening between the original infection and the change in the nervous system. Thus Glanzmann (1927) believed that the encephalitis is the outcome of an allergic or hyperergic process, the nervous system having in some way become sensitized to the original virus. Van Bogaert (1932, 1933) considered that the involvement of the nervous system is due to a lack of the normal defensive reaction of the skin, and explained the occasional occurrence of multiple cases in one family as a result of inherited deficiency of the capacity for developing immunity. Finley (1937, 1938), on the basis of the incubation period, linked the encephalitis with the general eruption and a coincident allergic reaction in the brain. Much experimental work has been done since Rivers and Schwentker showed that a demyelinating encephalitis could be produced in monkeys by repeated injections of brain material with adjuvants (Bailey and Gardner, 1940; Kabat, Wolf, and Bezer, 1947; Morgan, 1947; Morison, 1947; Wolf, Kabat, and Bezer, 1947; Lumsden, 1949 a and b; Kies and Alvord, 1959; Waksman, 1959; Field, Caspary, and Ball, 1963). It has been claimed that such encephalitis, which pathologically appears to resemble post-exanthematous encephalitis, is allergic, but this cannot yet be regarded as finally proved. This question is discussed by Lumsden (1961) and Field (1961). Whatever the nature of the process, the occurrence and pathological nature of a demyelinating encephalomyelitis in man after antirabic inoculation with a vaccine containing brain tissue provides evidence that man is susceptible to the same type of disorder [see p. 481].

REFERENCES

BAILEY, G. H., and GARDNER, R. E. (1940) The tissue specificity of brain and medullated nerves as shown by passive anaphylaxis in guinea-pigs, *J. exp. Med.*, **72,** 499.

BOGAERT, L. VAN (1932) Essai d'interprétation des manifestations nerveuses observées au cours de la vaccination, de la maladie sérique et des maladies éruptives, *Rev. neurol. (Paris)*, **39,** 1.

BOGAERT, L. VAN (1933) Les manifestations nerveuses au cours des maladies éruptives, *Rev. neurol. (Paris)*, **40,** 150.

FIELD, E. J. (1961) Experimental allergic encephalomyelitis, *Proc. roy. Soc. Med.*, **54,** 15.

FIELD, E. J., CASPARY, E. A., and BALL, E. J. (1963) Some biological properties of a highly active encephalitogenic factor isolated from human brain, *Lancet*, ii, 11.

FINLEY, H. K. (1937) Perivenous changes in acute encephalitis associated with vaccination, variola and measles, *Arch. Neurol. Psychiat. (Chicago)*, **37,** 505.

FINLEY, H. K. (1938) Pathogenesis of encephalitis occurring with vaccination, variola and measles, *Arch. Neurol. Psychiat. (Chicago)*, **39,** 1047.

GLANZMANN, E. (1927) Die nervösen Komplikationen der Varizellen, Variola und Vakzine, *Schweiz. med. Wschr.*, **8,** 145.

HERKENRATH, B. (1935) Pathologisch-anatomisch gesicherte Ausheilung eines Falles von Encephalitis post vaccinationem, *Z. ges. Neurol. Psychiat.*, **152,** 293.

HURST, E. W. (1935) The neurotropic virus diseases, *Lancet*, ii, 697, 758.

KABAT, E. A., WOLF, A., and BEZER, A. E. (1947) The rapid production of a demyelinating encephalomyelitis in Rhesus monkeys by injection of heterologous and homologous brain tissue with adjuvants, *J. exp. Med.*, **85,** 117.

KIES, M. W., and ALVORD, E. C. JR. (1959) *Allergic Encephalomyelitis*, Springfield, Ill.

LUMSDEN, C. E. (1949 *a*) Experimental 'allergic' encephalomyelitis, *Brain*, **72,** 198.

LUMSDEN, C. E. (1949 *b*) Experimental 'allergic' encephalomyelitis: II. On the nature of the encephalitogenic agent, *Brain*, **72,** 517.

LUMSDEN, C. E. (1961) Consideration of multiple sclerosis in relation to the auto-immunity process, *Proc. roy. Soc. Med.*, **54,** 11.

MORGAN, I. M. (1947) Allergic encephalomyelitis in monkeys in response to injection of normal monkey nervous tissue, *J. exp. Med.*, **85,** 131.

MORISON, L. R. (1947) Disseminated encephalomyelitis experimentally produced by the use of homologous antigen, *Arch. Neurol. Psychiat. (Chicago)*, **58,** 391.

WAKSMAN, B. H. (1959) *Experimental Allergic Encephalomyelitis and the 'Auto-allergic' Diseases*, Basle.

WOLF, A., KABAT, E. A., and BEZER, A. E. (1947) The pathology of acute disseminated encephalomyelitis produced experimentally in the rhesus monkey and its resemblance to human demyelinating disease, *J. Neuropath. exp. Neurol.*, **6,** 333.

ENCEPHALOMYELITIS FOLLOWING VACCINATION AGAINST RABIES

It now appears to be established that the nervous complications of antirabic inoculation, whose incidence varies from 1 in 1,000 to 1 in 4,000 persons treated, are due to sensitization to the brain tissue contained in the vaccine and are therefore comparable with the experimental encephalomyelitis induced with brain substance in animals. The pathological changes are those of an acute disseminated encephalomyelitis (Uchimura and Shiraki, 1957). The clinical picture may be encephalitic, myelitic, or polyradiculitic. Retrobulbar neuritis, either unilateral or bilateral may occur in these cases. The death rate in the encephalitic and myelitic types of case is said to be 30 per cent. The incidence of these complications may be reduced by using a vaccine made from rabies virus grown on duck embryos [see p. 463]. Lumsden (1961) in an analysis of the pathological findings in 9 fatal cases found that the changes were in certain respects different from those of multiple sclerosis on the one hand and from acute 'spontaneous' disseminated encephalomyelitis on the other.

REFERENCES

BASSOE, P., and GRINKER, R. R. (1930) Human rabies and rabies vaccine encephalomyelitis, *Arch. Neurol. Psychiat. (Chicago)*, **23**, 1138.

HURST, E. W. (1932) The effects of the injection of normal brain emulsion into rabbits with special reference to the paralytic accidents of antirabic treatment, *J. Hyg. (Lond.)*, **32**, 33.

LUMSDEN, C. E. (1961) The pathology and pathogenesis of multiple sclerosis, in *Scientific Aspects of Neurology*, ed. GARLAND, H., Edinburgh.

UCHIMURA, I., and SHIRAKI, H. (1957) A contribution to the classification and the pathogenesis of demyelinating encephalomyelitis, *J. Neuropath. exp. Neurol.*, **16**, 139.

POST-VACCINAL ENCEPHALOMYELITIS

AETIOLOGY

See page 480.

PATHOLOGY

See page 479 and FIGURE 77.

EPIDEMIOLOGY

Nervous complications, for example hemiplegia, have been known to follow vaccination since 1860, but appear to have been isolated occurrences until 1922, since when epidemics of post-vaccinal encephalomyelitis have occurred. Ninety-three cases were reported in England between November 1922 and November 1927, and 124 cases had been observed in Holland prior to the latter date. Cases have been observed elsewhere in Europe and the United States, though they have been much rarer than in the countries mentioned. Post-vaccinal encephalomyelitis is a rare complication of vaccination. In Holland it has been estimated that one case occurred in over 5,000 persons vaccinated. It follows primary vaccination much more frequently than revaccination, the incidence in Holland being approximately one case in 2,300 primary vaccinations and one case in 50,000 revaccinations. It is practically unknown in infants vaccinated under the age of 1 year and most cases have occurred in children of school age. Though no age is exempt, it is rare after 30. Both sexes are affected equally.

The condition has occurred in epidemics which have coincided with an increase in the number of persons vaccinated owing to the prevalence of smallpox. In the English outbreak of 1923 the 51 cases reported were distributed across the country from Exeter in the south-west to Morpeth in the north-east, with an extension to London and the home counties. In the 1962 epidemic of smallpox in South Wales, Spillane and Wells (1964) record that of 800,000 individuals vaccinated, some 39 individuals (24 primary vaccinations, 15 revaccinations) suffered neurological complications. There were 11 cases of post-vaccinal encephalomyelitis, 3 of encephalopathy (convulsions and focal neurological signs in infants), 7 cases of meningism, 3 of epilepsy, 6 with focal lesions of brain or cord, 5 with polyneuritis and 2 with brachial neuritis, while 2 patients with myasthenia gravis relapsed. De Vries (1965) also draws attention to the importance of encephalopathy as a cause of convulsions and coma in infancy, occurring as a sequel of vaccinations or other infections and points out that the pathological changes are different from those of encephalomyelitis. There is no evidence of spread of encephalomyelitis by contagion or by any other method of dissemination from one place to another, but it has been noticed that there are often proportionately more cases in small communities and rural areas than in large towns. In several cases two members of the same family who had been vaccinated at the same time both developed encephalomyelitis. The source of vaccine lymph does not appear to be of any aetiological significance.

SYMPTOMS

Incubation Period

In most cases the symptoms of encephalomyelitis develop between the tenth and the twelfth days after vaccination, though the onset has occurred as early as the second day or as late as the twenty-fifth. There is evidence that when the disorder follows revaccination the incubation period is less than when it occurs after primary vaccination.

Symptoms

The onset is usually rapid and is characterized by headache, vomiting, drowsiness, fever, and in some cases convulsions. When fully developed, the clinical picture is usually that of meningeal irritation associated with widespread disturbance of function of the brain and spinal cord. In severe cases drowsiness passes into stupor and coma. Cervical rigidity and Kernig's sign are often present. The ocular fundi are usually normal, but transient papilloedema has occasionally been observed. The incidence of ocular abnormalities is variable. In some cases impairment of the pupillary reflexes and ocular palsies have been present. In others they have not been noted. Trismus has frequently been described, and more than one case has been mistaken for tetanus on account of this symptom. Flaccid paralysis of some or all of the limbs often develops, associated with loss of tendon reflexes and extensor plantar responses. Retention or incontinence of urine and faeces is the rule in severe cases. Sensory loss is inconstant, but may be marked when the spinal cord is severely affected. The cerebrospinal fluid is frequently normal, though under increased pressure. An excess of mononuclear cells and of protein may be found. The cutaneous site of vaccination shows the usual inflammatory changes corresponding to the stage at which the patient comes under observation. Not uncommonly there is a severe local reaction, and in a few cases a generalized vaccinial rash has been observed.

DIAGNOSIS

The diagnosis rarely presents any difficulty, since there is a history of recent vaccination and the cutaneous lesions are still visible. Apart from this, the clinical picture cannot be distinguished from other forms of acute disseminated encephalomyelitis occurring spontaneously or complicating the exanthemata.

The severe involvement of the substance of the nervous system indicated by flaccid paralysis distinguishes the condition from meningitis, while the presence of signs of meningeal irritation and the subsequent occurrence of convulsions, trismus, and paralysis of the limbs, together with the inconstancy of ocular abnormalities, distinguish it from epidemic encephalitis lethargica. Post-vaccinal encephalomyelitis is distinguished from poliomyelitis by the fact that the paralyses, though flaccid, are not associated with wasting of the muscles, and by the presence of extensor plantar responses and in some cases of sensory loss. In poliomyelitis, moreover, the mental state of the patient is usually little affected.

PROGNOSIS

The mortality rate is high, ranging from 30 per cent. to over 50 per cent. in different epidemics. In most fatal cases the patient dies in coma from medullary paralysis within a few days of the onset of the illness. Less frequently death is due to bronchopneumonia or infection of the urinary tract. If recovery occurs it is usually remarkably complete and residual symptoms are exceptional. In some cases, however, there may be some persistent loss of power or sensory loss or, in the case of young children, mental defect.

PROPHYLAXIS

With the object of preventing post-vaccinal encephalomyelitis as far as possible, the Minister of Health has made a number of recommendations contained in the Vaccination Order 1929, and the Memorandum on Vaccination against Smallpox (1956). Since the main incidence of post-vaccinal encephalomyelitis falls upon previously unvaccinated adolescents, the opinion was expressed that 'as long as the smallpox prevalent in this country retains its present mild character, it is not generally expedient to press for the vaccination of persons of these ages who have not previously been vaccinated, unless they have been in personal contact with a case of smallpox or directly exposed to smallpox infection'. In all ordinary cases of vaccination or revaccination the operation should be carried out in one insertion, preferably by the multiple pressure technique But where the maximal protection against smallpox is desired, the number of insertions may be increased to two and the scratch technique may be used to reduce the risk of failure.

TREATMENT

See page 490.

REFERENCES

BASTIAANSE, F. S. VAN B. (1925) Encéphalite consécutive à la vaccination antivariolique, *Bull. Acad. Méd. (Paris)*, **94,** 815.
LUCKSCH, F. (1924) Blatternimpfung und Encephalitis, *Med. Klin.*, **20,** 1170.
LUCKSCH, F. (1925) Die Vakzineencephalitis, *Med. Klin.*, **21,** 1377.
LUCKSCH, F. (1925) Gibt es beim Menschen eine Vakzine-Enzephalitis? *Zbl. Bakt.*, *I. Abt. Orig.*, **96,** 309.
LUCKSCH, F. (1926) Über Impfschäden des Zentralnervensystems, *Dtsch. Z. ges. gerichtl. Med.*, **7,** 203.
LUCKSCH, F. (1927) Enzephalitis nach Vakzination oder Vakzineenzephalitis, *Zbl. Bakt.*, *I. Abt. Orig.*, **103,** 227.

McINTOSH, J., and SCARFF, R. W. (1927–8) The histology of some virus infections of the central nervous system, *Proc. roy. Soc. Med.*, **21**, 705.

MINISTRY OF HEALTH. *Reports of the Committee on Vaccination*, London, 1928 and 1930.

PERDRAU, J. R. (1928) The histology of post-vaccinal encephalitis, *J. Path. Bact.*, **31**, 17.

PETTE, H. (1930) Infektion und Nervensystem, *Dtsch. Z. Nervenheilk.*, **110**, 221 (abs. *Arch. Neurol. Psychiat. (Chicago)*, **24**, 1064).

SPILLANE, J. D., and WELLS, C. E. C. (1964) The neurology of Jennerian vaccination, *Brain*, **87**, 1.

TURNBULL, H. M., and McINTOSH, J. (1926) Encephalomyelitis following vaccination, *Brit. J. exp. Path.*, **7**, 181.

DE VRIES, E. (1965) The acute encephalopathic reaction in infants, *Psychiat. Neurol. Neurochir. (Amst.)*, **68**, 85.

WIERSMA, D. (1929) Remarks on the etiology of encephalitis after vaccination, *Acta psychiat. (Kbh.)*, **4**, 75.

ENCEPHALOMYELITIS COMPLICATING SMALLPOX

The occurrence of nervous symptoms as a complication of smallpox has been known for many years, but is a rare event, having been observed in only approximately 2·5 cases per 1,000 persons suffering from smallpox. The investigations of Troup and Hurst (1930) and of McIntosh and Scarff (1928) showed that the pathological changes in the nervous system are indistinguishable from those of post-vaccinal encephalomyelitis. In some cases bulbar symptoms, especially dysarthria, have been prominent, and these are sometimes accompanied by paralysis of the limbs. In other cases bulbar symptoms are absent and paraplegia occurs, with or without sphincter disturbances and impairment of sensibility. Mental changes are sometimes present. In many cases recovery occurs and is strikingly complete, but the patient may die during the acute attack or subsequently from urinary infection or other complications of paraplegia. For treatment see page 490.

REFERENCES

MARSDEN, J. P., and HURST, E. W. (1932) Acute perivascular myelinoclasis ('acute disseminated encephalomyelitis') in smallpox, *Brain*, **55**, 181.

McINTOSH, J., and SCARFF, R. W. (1927–8) The histology of some virus infections of the central nervous system, *Proc. roy. Soc. Med.*, **21**, 705.

TROUP, A. G., and HURST, E. W. (1930) Disseminated encephalomyelitis following smallpox, *Lancet*, i, 566.

TURNBULL, H. M., and McINTOSH, J. (1926) Encephalomyelitis following vaccination, *Brit. J. exp. Path.*, **7**, 181.

ENCEPHALOMYELITIS COMPLICATING MEASLES

According to Miller, Stanton, and Gibbons (1956) neurological complications occur in less than 1 in 1,000 cases: 95 per cent. are encephalitic or encephalomyelitic, less than 3 per cent. myelitic, and less than 2 per cent. polyradiculitic. The pathological picture ranges from congestion, perivascular infiltration, and occasional haemorrhages in the more acute cases to typical perivenous demyelination in the later stages. Aetiology and pathology are further discussed on pages 479–80.

SYMPTOMS

Nervous complications of measles have been known for over a century, but appear to have become more common during recent years. The onset of symptoms is usually four to six days after the beginning of the illness when the fever has fallen and the rash is fading. Ford (1928) reviewed the literature and distinguished a number of clinical types. It is probable that acute perivascular myelinoclasis is not the pathological basis of all the nervous complications of measles.

1. The nervous symptoms may be relatively mild and transient and present a clinical picture resembling 'meningism' or 'serous meningitis'. In such cases headache, stupor, signs of meningeal irritation, and sometimes convulsions occur, but focal lesions of the substance of the nervous system are absent.

2. Multiple focal or diffuse lesions of the nervous system may occur, involving the cerebral cortex, basal ganglia, brain stem, cerebellum, optic nerves, and spinal cord in various combinations.

3. There may be a single focal cerebral lesion, hemiplegia and aphasia being the commonest.

4. The symptoms may be predominantly those of cerebellar deficiency.

5. The spinal cord may be mainly affected, the clinical picture being an acute ascending paralysis leading to paraplegia, with or without concurrent involvement of the brain. I have seen neuromyelitis optica exactly simulated.

6. Other nervous symptoms are rare, the clinical picture of polyradiculitis being the most important. The cerebrospinal fluid may be normal or may show a moderate increase in lymphocytes and protein.

7. There is increasing evidence to suggest that subacute sclerosing panencephalitis may be a late but rare sequel of measles infection [p. 448].

DIAGNOSIS

The diagnosis is usually easy, since the measles rash is generally present when the nervous symptoms develop. If the attack of measles has passed unnoticed the disorder cannot be distinguished from other forms of acute disseminated encephalomyelitis.

PROGNOSIS

The mortality rate is 10 to 20 per cent. in different series, and probably about 50 per cent. are left with residual symptoms, of which the most important are hemiplegia, ataxia, mental defect or change of personality, and epilepsy. Coma and convulsions are bad prognostic signs.

TREATMENT

See page 490.

REFERENCES

FERRARO, A., and SCHEFFER, I. H. (1931) Encephalitis and encephalomyelitis in measles, *Arch. Neurol. Psychiat.* (*Chicago*), **25**, 748.
FERRARO, A., and SCHEFFER, I. H. (1932) Toxic encephalopathy in measles, *Arch. Neurol. Psychiat.* (*Chicago*), **27**, 1209.

FORD, F. R. (1928) The nervous complications of measles with a summary of the litera-
    ture and publication of 12 additional case reports, *Bull. Johns Hopk. Hosp.*, **43**, 140.
GREENFIELD, J. G. (1928–9) The encephalomyelitis of measles, *Proc. roy. Soc. Med.*, **22**,
    297.
GREENFIELD, J. G. (1929) The pathology of measles encephalomyelitis, *Brain*, **52**, 171.
MALAMUD, N. (1937) Encephalomyelitis complicating measles, *Arch. Neurol. Psychiat.
    (Chicago)*, **38**, 1025.
MILLER, H. G., STANTON, J. B., and GIBBONS, J. L. (1956) Para-infectious encephalo-
    myelitis and related syndromes, *Quart. J. Med.*, **25**, 427.
MUSSER, J. H., and HAUSER, G. H. (1928) Encephalitis as a complication of measles,
    J. Amer. med. Ass., **90**, 1267.
WOHLWILL, F. (1928) Über Encephalomyelitis bei Masern, *Z. ges. Neurol. Psychiat.*,
    112, 20.
ZIMMERMANN, H. M., and YANNET, H. (1930) Encephalomyelitis complicating measles,
    Arch. Neurol. Psychiat. (Chicago), **24**, 1000.

ENCEPHALOMYELITIS COMPLICATING RUBELLA

Nervous complications of rubella are very rare, but the available evidence suggests that in general both the pathological and clinical pictures are similar to those of measles. Meningeal symptoms have been reported in a few cases and both ascending paralysis of the Landry type and polyneuritis have been encountered. When encephalitis does occur it is usually mild.

REFERENCES

BRIGGS, J. F. (1935) Meningoencephalitis following rubella, *J. Pediat.*, **7**, 609.
MERRITT, H. H., and KOSKOFF, Y. D. (1936) Encephalomyelitis following German
    measles, *Amer. J. med. Sci.*, **191**, 690.
MILLER, H. G., STANTON, J. B., and GIBBONS, J. L. (1956) Para-infectious encephalo-
    myelitis and related syndromes, *Quart. J. Med.*, **25**, 427.
SKINNER, H. O. (1935) Encephalitis complicating German measles, *J. Amer. med. Ass.*,
    105, 24.

ENCEPHALOMYELITIS COMPLICATING CHICKENPOX

Encephalitis and myelitis are rare complications of chickenpox, but more than 80 cases have been reported during recent years.

PATHOLOGY

Owing to the benign nature of the disorder there have been few opportunities of studying its pathology. Although perivascular infiltration and demyelination have been described in two cases, areas thus affected were very circumscribed in both, and other changes distinct from the pathological picture of the demyelinating diseases of the nervous system have been observed, particularly degeneration of ganglion cells. Van Bogaert (1930) reported circumscribed foci in the white matter and a more diffuse affection of the grey matter of the cerebrum and cerebellum, lesions resembling young plaques of multiple sclerosis. Miget (1933) reported a case in which inflammatory infiltration of the leptomeninges was the most conspicuous feature. On the whole, however, the pathological picture appears to be the same as that found in measles encephalomyelitis.

AETIOLOGY

See pages 480–1.

SYMPTOMS

Symptoms of involvement of the nervous system develop in such cases between the fifth and the twentieth day after the appearance of the rash, usually during the first half of the second week. Encephalitis is said to occur in 90 per cent. of cases, myelitis in 3 per cent., and polyradiculitis in 7 per cent. The onset is acute, and is characterized by fever, headache, vomiting, and giddiness, and sometimes by delirium. The disturbance may be mainly meningeal, mainly cerebral, or mainly spinal but in addition some cases present with what appears to be an almost 'pure' cerebellar ataxia. The meningeal form is characterized by the usual symptoms of meningitis with little or no evidence of involvement of the substance of the nervous system. In the 'cerebellar' cases, incoordination is the commonest symptom, occurring with or without involuntary movements. The ataxia is often so gross as to render the child incapable of walking. Tremor and choreic or choreo-athetoid movements occur in some cases. Signs of cortico-spinal tract lesions may be present, but diplegia and hemiplegia are rare. Ophthalmoplegia has been observed. The spinal lesion usually produces the picture of a transverse myelitis at the dorsal level of the cord. The spinal fluid may be normal, or may show an excess of protein and cells, usually mononuclear.

DIAGNOSIS

The cause of the nervous symptoms is evident when the diagnosis of chicken-pox has already been made. If, however, this has passed unnoticed, the encephalomyelitis cannot be distinguished from other forms of acute disseminated encephalomyelitis, except that the involvement of the cerebellum appears to be peculiarly frequent in encephalitis complicating chickenpox.

PROGNOSIS

The prognosis is good, both as to life and as to recovery of function. The mortality rate in encephalitic cases is 10 per cent. and sequelae are rare in those who survive.

TREATMENT

See page 490.

REFERENCES

BÉRODE, P. (1932), *Les Complications nerveuses de la varicelle (à propos des formes méningées)*, Thèse de Paris.
BOGAERT, L. VAN (1930) Contribution clinique et anatomique à l'étude des manifestations
BRAIN, W. R. (1931) Zoster, varicella, and encephalitis, *Brit. med. J.*, 1, 81.
DE TONI, G. (1924) Sulla meningite da varicella, *Policlinico, Sez. prat.*, 31, 1434.
GLANZMANN, E. (1927) Die nervösen Komplikationen der Varizellen, Variola und Vakzine, *Schweiz. med. Wschr.*, 8, 145.
GORDON, M. B. (1924) Acute hemorrhagic nephritis and acute hemorrhagic encephalitis following varicella, *Amer. J. Dis. Child.*, 28, 589.
KRABBE, K. H. (1925) Varicella myelitis, *Brain*, 48, 535.

MIGET, A. (1933) Les complications nerveuses de la varicelle, *Médecine*, **14**, 137.

MILLER, H. G., STANTON, J. B., and GIBBONS, J. L. (1956). Para-infectious encephalo-myelitis and related syndromes, *Quart. J. Med.*, **25**, 427.

ROTEM, C. E. (1961) Complications of chicken-pox, *Brit. med. J.*, **1**, 944.
neurologiques et psychiatriques de l'infection varicelleuse, *J. Neurol.(Brux.)*, **30**, 623.

WILSON, R. E., and FORD, F. R. (1927) The nervous complications of variola, vaccinia and varicella, with report of cases, *Bull. Johns Hopk. Hosp.*, **40**, 337.

ZIMMERMANN, H. M., and YANNET, H. (1931) Nonsuppurative encephalomyelitis accompanying chickenpox, *Arch. Neurol. Psychiat. (Chicago)*, **26**, 322.

SPONTANEOUS ACUTE DISSEMINATED ENCEPHALOMYELITIS

A form of acute disseminated encephalomyelitis clinically and pathologically identical with that which follows the above-mentioned exanthems may occur spontaneously or as a complication of a febrile illness of an 'influenzal' type. Miller and Evans (1953) support the view that acute disseminated encephalo-myelitis represents a non-specific allergic reaction of the nervous system to various antigens, chiefly of bacterial or virus origin, in which case the 'spon-taneous' form of the disease may be a reaction to a banal infection, particularly, perhaps, of the upper respiratory tract, or rarely of an inoculation or the administration of antiserum.

The symptoms of spontaneous acute disseminated encephalomyelitis are indistinguishable from those of encephalomyelitis following one of the exan-thems, for example, vaccination [see p. 482]. It appears that the condition recently referred to as acute cerebellar ataxia of infancy and childhood may well be a form of encephalomyelitis predominantly involving the cerebellum. Brum-lik and Means (1969) have pointed out that whereas many such cases occur in infancy a similar acute cerebellar ataxia of encephalitic type is also seen in adults; in some cases the condition may be post-infectious but in others it is associated with ECHO or Coxsackie virus infection.

DIAGNOSIS

The diagnosis of encephalomyelitis rests upon the occurrence of a febrile illness with evidence of subacute lesions of the white matter of the brain or spinal cord or both, usually in multiple foci, and with or without signs of meningeal irritation [see also p. 483]. The main difficulty lies in distinguishing acute disseminated encephalomyelitis from the acute lesions of multiple sclerosis.

McAlpine, Lumsden, and Acheson (1965) have considered the differential diagnosis between acute disseminated encephalomyelitis and acute multiple sclerosis. They point out that whereas in the acute stage distinction between the two conditions may be impossible on clinical grounds, an acute attack of encephalomyelitis or myelitis may resolve completely and that subsequently the patient may remain free from relapse for many years. Pette (1928) first suggested that no clinical or pathological distinction could be made between the two conditions and this 'unitary' theory was later supported by Ferraro (1958) and Miller and Schapira (1959).

Van Bogaert (1950) pointed out that some cases diagnosed clinically as cases of acute encephalomyelitis are in every respect similar to those cases which occur after specific infectious fevers; others run a course typical of multiple sclerosis, while others recover and remain well. The encephalitic form is particularly common in children and young adults and may affect principally the cerebral hemispheres, brain stem or cerebellum, while the myelitic form may occur at any age (McAlpine, Lumsden, and Acheson, 1965).

After the acute stage has subsided, if the patient is found to have residual physical signs, the diagnosis from multiple sclerosis may be extremely difficult. It must be based upon the history of the onset and development of symptoms in the acute stage and the absence of any extension of the physical signs after the first few weeks of the illness.

PROGNOSIS

Although fresh lesions may occur within two or three weeks of the onset, acute disseminated encephalomyelitis is usually a self-limited disease, and relapses are uncommon, but Miller and Evans (1953) point out that recurrences may occur, especially when the nervous disorder follows a non-specific minor infection, usually of the upper respiratory tract, in which the development of lasting immunity is known to be exceptional, and in which repeated antigenic insults furnish a possible pathogenetic mechanism. In all acute demyelinating disorders a substantial degree of recovery of function can be expected, but if the initial disorder has been severe some residual disability is likely, and this may be added to if recurrences occur.

TREATMENT

When hyperpyrexia occurs in such cases, tepid sponging or other methods of cooling may be necessary. In comatose patients, tube-feeding, parenteral fluids, careful nursing care and even tracheostomy with or without assisted respiration may be required. Miller (1953) and Miller and Gibbons (1953) recommended corticotrophin(ACTH), 80 Units daily, in the acute phase and it is now generally agreed that this drug is beneficial in limiting the spread of the inflammatory process. Appropriate antibiotics are often needed to control secondary infections and anticonvulsants may also be required in selected cases to control convulsions.

REFERENCES

BOGAERT, L. VAN (1950) Post-infectious encephalomyelitis and multiple sclerosis, *J. Neuropath.*, 9, 219.

BRUMLIK, J., and MEANS, E. D. (1969) Tremorine-tremor, shivering and acute cerebellar ataxia in the adult and child—a comparative study, *Brain*, 92, 157.

FERRARO, A. (1958) Studies on multiple sclerosis, *J. Neuropath.*, 17, 278.

McALPINE, D., LUMSDEN, C. E., and ACHESON, E. D. (1965) *Multiple Sclerosis: a Reappraisal*, Edinburgh.

MILLER, H. G. (1953) Acute disseminated encephalomyelitis treated with A.C.T.H., *Brit. med. J.*, 1, 177.

MILLER, H. G., and EVANS, M. J. (1953) Prognosis in acute disseminated encephalomyelitis; with a note on neuromyelitis optica, *Quart. J. Med.*, N.S. 22, 347.

MILLER, H. G., and GIBBONS, J. L. (1953) Acute disseminated encephalomyelitis and acute multiple sclerosis; results of treatment with ACTH, *Brit. med. J.*, 2, 1345.

MILLER, H. G., and SCHAPIRA, K. (1959) Aetiological aspects of multiple sclerosis, *Brit. med. J.*, **1**, 737.

PETTE, H. (1928) Klinische und anatomische Studien über die Pathogenese der multiplen Sklerose, *Dtsch. med. Wschr.*, **84**, 2061.

ACUTE HAEMORRHAGIC LEUCO-ENCEPHALITIS

Acute haemorrhagic leuco-encephalitis was first described by Hurst (1941) and subsequently by Henson and Russell in 1942. It is characterized pathologically by macroscopic oedema of the brain with numerous minute haemorrhages and microscopically by severe damage to the vessel walls, perivascular necrosis, perivascular and focal demyelination, intense polymorphonuclear exudation, and microglial reaction. Clinically there is a febrile illness characterized by headache, vomiting, deepening stupor with or without hemiparesis, and a leucocytosis in the blood. Hurst suggested, and Greenfield (1950) accepts, the view that the haemorrhagic lesions and the non-haemorrhagic areas of necrosis or demyelination represent different degrees of injury by a single noxious agent, and Russell (1955) agrees that acute haemorrhagic leuco-encephalitis is simply a hyperacute and explosive form of acute disseminated encephalomyelitis.

REFERENCES

GREENFIELD, J. G. (1950) Encephalitis and encephalomyelitis in England and Wales during the last decade, *Brain*, **73**, 141.

HENSON, R. A., and RUSSELL, D. S. (1942) Acute haemorrhagic leuco-encephalitis, *J. Path. Bact.*, **54**, 227.

HURST, E. W. (1941) Acute haemorrhagic leuco-encephalitis, a previously undefined entity, *Med. J. Aust.*, **2**, 1.

RUSSELL, D. S. (1955) The nosological unity of acute haemorrhagic leuco-encephalitis and acute disseminated encephalomyelitis, *Brain*, **78**, 369.

DISSEMINATED MYELITIS WITH OPTIC NEURITIS

Synonyms. Acute disseminated myelitis; diffuse myelitis with optic neuritis; neuromyelitis optica; ophthalmoneuromyelitis; Devic's disease.

Definition. A form of subacute encephalomyelitis characterized by massive demyelination of the optic nerves and spinal cord, sometimes running a self-limited and sometimes a progressive course.

PATHOLOGY

Both optic nerves and spinal cord exhibit massive demyelination. Loss of myelin sheaths is found in the optic nerves and chiasma, and in the spinal cord may be limited to a few segments, usually in the lower cervical and upper dorsal region, or may be more diffuse, extending through the greater part of the cord's length. In severe cases cavitation may occur. Marked perivascular infiltration is not only present in the demyelinated areas but may be found throughout the nervous system. The infiltrating cells are principally mononuclear, but poly-morphonuclear cells may also be present. In the demyelinated areas there is a great multiplication of vessels surrounded by many fat-granule cells and also neuroglial cells, though with little formation of new neuroglial fibres. To the naked eye the affected areas are swollen, congested, and softened.

AETIOLOGY

The cause of Devic's disease is unknown. It is rare and affects both sexes at all ages from 12 to 60. McAlpine (1938) has reported its occurrence in identical twins. While in the past the condition has generally been regarded as an inde-pendent clinical and pathological entity, McAlpine, Lumsden, and Acheson (1965) point out that there is a growing body of opinion which favours the view that it is simply a form of multiple sclerosis. Even in Japan where it has proved to be very common, Okinaka et al. (1960) have reached a similar conclusion.

SYMPTOMS

The clinical features have been reviewed by Stansbury (1949) and Scott (1952), who point out that the illness often begins with a sore throat, cold in the head, or febrile disturbance. Either the ocular or the spinal lesion may develop first, and these events may be separated by days or weeks, or both may occur simul-taneously. Usually one eye is first affected, to be followed by the other after an interval varying from a few hours to several weeks. Rarely the onset of the myelitis intervenes between the affection of the two eyes.

The ocular lesion may be a true optic neuritis or a retrobulbar neuritis, depending upon whether it is situated sufficiently anteriorly to involve the optic discs. In the former case papilloedema is present, though the swelling is usually slight; in the latter the discs are normal. The characteristic field defect is a bilateral central scotoma. In severe cases blindness may be complete or almost so. Homonymous field defects have been described. The two eyes are often unequally affected. Pain in the eyes is often severe and is accentuated by moving them and by pressure upon the globes.

The spinal cord lesion, the onset of which may be associated with severe pain in the back and limbs, leads to the usual symptoms of transverse myelitis, with paralysis of the upper motor neurone type and loss of some or all forms of sensibility below the level of the lesion and loss of sphincter control. When, as frequently happens, the cervical region of the cord is involved a quadriplegia results.

The cerebrospinal fluid may show no abnormality or there may be an increase of protein and globulin and an excess of cells, which are usually mononuclear, though occasionally polymorphonuclear cells have been described. There is no characteristic colloidal gold curve.

It is probable that the disorder may abort after the development of optic neuritis and before the spinal symptoms appear and that the reverse may also occur, so that some cases of acute bilateral optic neuritis or retrobulbar neuritis without other symptoms or with only mild spinal disturbances, and also cases of acute transverse myelitis without optic neuritis, may belong to this group.

DIAGNOSIS

The presence of bilateral optic neuritis before symptoms of the lesion of the spinal cord appear, may suggest a diagnosis of intracranial tumour. In optic neuritis, however, the papilloedema is slight in proportion to the severity of the loss of vision and the characteristic field defect is bilateral central scotomas, in contrast to the peripheral constriction of the fields associated with papilloedema in increased intracranial pressure. Moreover, in cases of optic neuritis headache and vomiting are absent, though pain in the eyes may be severe. Syphilitic myelitis can be distinguished by serological tests.

PROGNOSIS

The mortality rate in the past was about 50 per cent., death occurring either from respiratory paralysis as a result of the upward spread of the myelitis, or from infections of the skin or urinary tract complicating the paraplegia. If the patient survived, recovery was often remarkably complete. Cases occurring in the last 20 years have seemed often to be less severe and assisted respiration has greatly improved the outcome. Complete blindness may be followed by a considerable return of vision, though some degree of optic atrophy is likely to persist. Similarly, the functions of the spinal cord may be largely, if not completely, restored. Recovery, once achieved, may be permanent, but progressive and relapsing cases occur. These underline the close relationship of the disorder to multiple sclerosis. In a recent follow-up study of 12 cases Scott (1961) has confirmed that the ultimate outlook in many cases is good.

TREATMENT

Corticotrophin (ACTH) 80 Units daily at first, with subsequent reduction to 40 Units daily, continuing until progressive clinical improvement is manifest and giving thereafter smaller maintenance doses for several weeks, is now generally recommended. The usual measures for the care of the skin, urinary and intestinal tracts, and musculature, which are required in paraplegia, will be necessary and assisted respiration may be required in severe cases with ascending paralysis.

REFERENCES

BRAIN, W. R. (1929–30) Critical review: disseminated sclerosis, *Quart. J. Med.*, **23**, 343.
GOULDEN, C. (1914) Optic neuritis and myelitis, *Trans. ophthal. Soc. U.K.*, **34**, 229.
HASSIN, G. B. (1937) Neuroptic myelitis versus multiple sclerosis, *Arch. Neurol. Psychiat. (Chicago)*, **37**, 1083.
HOLMES, G. (1927) Discussion on diffuse myelitis associated with optic neuritis, *Brain*, **50**, 702.
LEJONNE, P., and LHERMITTE, J. (1909) De la nature inflammatoire de certaines scléroses en plaques, *Encéphale*, iv, i, 220.
MCALPINE, D. (1938) Familial neuromyelitis optica: its occurrence in identical twins, *Brain*, **61**, 430.
MCALPINE, D., LUMSDEN, C. E., and ACHESON, E. D. (1965) *Multiple Sclerosis: a Reappraisal*, Edinburgh.
OKINAKA, S., MCALPINE, D., MIYAGAWA, K., SUWA, N., KUROIWA, Y., SHIRAKI, H., ARAKI, S., and KURLAND, L. T. (1960) Multiple sclerosis in Northern and Southern Japan, *Wld Neurol.*, **1**, 22.

Scott, G. I. (1952) Neuromyelitis optica, *Amer. J. Ophthal.*, **35**, 755.

Scott, G. I. (1961) Ophthalmic aspects of demyelinating diseases, *Proc. roy. Soc. Med.*, **54**, 38.

Stansbury, F. C. (1949) Neuromyelitis optica (Devic's disease), *Arch. Ophthal. (Chicago)*, **42**, 292, 465.

Symonds, C. P. (1924) The pathological anatomy of disseminated sclerosis, *Brain*, **47**, 36.

MULTIPLE SCLEROSIS

Synonyms. Disseminated sclerosis; insular sclerosis.

Definition. A disease of unknown aetiology characterized pathologically by the widespread occurrence in the nervous system of patches of demyelination followed by gliosis. In many cases the early manifestations of the disease are followed by conspicuous improvement, so that remissions and relapses are a striking feature of the disorder, the course of which may thus be prolonged for many years. The early symptoms are often those of focal lesions of the nervous system, while the later clinical picture is one of progressive dissemination tending to produce the classical features of ataxic paraplegia.

PATHOLOGY

The first pathological accounts of the disease were given by Cruveilhier in 1835 and Carswell in 1838. The pathological 'unit' in multiple sclerosis is a circumscribed patch of nervous tissue in which the pathological process begins with destruction of the myelin sheaths of the nerve fibres and to a much less extent of the axis cylinders, and ends with the formation of a 'sclerotic plaque' [FIG. 78]. These patches predominantly affect the white matter of the brain and spinal cord. They are sometimes found in the grey matter of the cerebral cortex and in the cranial and spinal nerve roots, rarely in the grey matter of the spinal cord. Many writers have stressed the perivascular distribution of some of the patches, though Dawson (1916) pointed out that 'the changes appear within but do not coincide with the area of distribution of the arteries'. Putnam (1937) emphasized the relationship of the patches to the cerebral venules, but Dow and Berglund (1942) reported many exceptions to this; and stated that thrombosis of a vein within a plaque, stressed by Putnam, is rare. The optic nerves and chiasma, the neighbourhood of the cerebral ventricles, and the subpial region of the spinal cord are favourite sites.

To the naked eye the sclerotic plaque appears slightly sunken, greyish, and more translucent than normal nervous tissue. In the acute stage the blood vessels are dilated, and the perivascular spaces contain fat-granule cells and frequently also lymphocytes and plasma cells. The myelin of the nerve sheaths is undergoing degeneration, and the axis cylinders show diffuse or irregular swellings and other abnormalities. Even at this stage, as Greenfield and King (1936) pointed out, there is a conspicuous proliferation of the fibroglia. In late patches the destroyed myelin has been removed; the axis cylinders are reduced in number, and some of those persisting show abnormalities, and there is a thick condensation of the original glial meshwork.

There has been much discussion as to whether the pathological picture described by Marsden and Hurst (1932) as acute focal myelinoclasis (acute disseminated encephalomyelitis) is distinct from multiple sclerosis. Many writers, especially Anton and Wohlwill (1912), Redlich (1927), and Spielmeyer (1923), believed that acute disseminated encephalomyelitis was pathologically distinguishable from acute multiple sclerosis. Others, such as Fraenkel and Jakob (1913), Ferraro (1937, 1958), and Alvord (1966) believe that the two are identical pathologically.

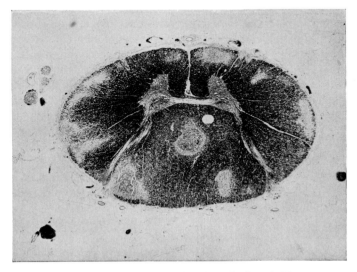

FIG. 78. Disseminated sclerosis: spinal cord, T. 9

Van Bogaert (1950) and Greenfield and Norman (1965) agree that whereas the pathological changes are essentially similar in the acute phase of the two disorders there are certain fine points of distinction and the chronic lesions of multiple sclerosis are virtually distinctive. As Lumsden (1965) has pointed out, the pathological changes in fatal cases of multiple sclerosis are usually of such long-standing that the methods of classical morbid anatomical study make it virtually impossible to determine the character of the earliest pathological changes which occur in such patients. Thus massive and widespread demyelination may well be the end-result of various disease states of diverse aetiology.

AETIOLOGY

General Considerations

Earlier pathologists regarded the gliosis as the primary change, hence the name multiple 'sclerosis'. The modern view is that the glial overgrowth is either a scar reaction to the earlier inflammatory and demyelinating process, or that it is simultaneously evoked by the same agent which causes the destruction of the myelin sheaths. A large variety of aetiological theories have been proposed. The disease has been attributed to infection by a spirochaete (Steiner and others). The isolation of a filterable virus by Margulis, Soloviev, and Shubladze (1946) is unconfirmed and the negative evidence against infection so far outweighs the positive though the finding of certain 'slow virus' infections in man and animals, including kuru, multifocal leuco-encephalopathy and scrapie [see CHAPTER 10] has revived interest in the possibility that multiple sclerosis might be a similar infection (Poskanzer, Schapira, and Miller, 1963). Field (1966) showed that inoculation of brain biopsy material from a case of multiple sclerosis produced in white mice, after passage, a few cases of scrapie but points out that his results were open to several different interpretations and that so far the electron microscope has failed to demonstrate viral particles in the nervous system of patients with multiple sclerosis or in animals with scrapie.

Much has been published concerning the possible relationship between experimental allergic encephalomyelitis in animals and multiple sclerosis in man and Miller and Schapira (1959), Lumsden (1961), and Alvord (1966) have given reasons for supposing that this disease may be due to an auto-immune process in the central nervous system. The altered reactivity of the meninges to PPD (purified protein derivative of tuberculin) demonstrated in such cases by Smith, Espir, Whitty, and Russell (1957) was later shown to be non-specific (Marshall and O'Grady, 1959) and theories relating the aetiology of the disease to thrombosis in cerebral venules (Putnam, 1937), to the ingestion of heavy metals such as copper and to excess fat in the diet have won few adherents. The position, therefore, remains uncertain.

The Role of Inherited Predisposition

Multiple cases of multiple sclerosis in the same family sometimes occur. Curtius in 1933 collected 84 references to this in the literature and the subject has been studied by Pratt, Compston, and McAlpine (1951) and by McAlpine, Lumsden, and Acheson (1965). In most instances two siblings are affected. Affection of two successive generations is less common but conjugal cases rarely occur (Schapira, Poskanzer, and Miller, 1963).

McAlpine, Lumsden, and Acheson (1965) conclude that the risk that multiple sclerosis will develop in a first-degree relative of an affected individual is at least 15 times that in the general population. No definite pattern of inheritance emerges but on the whole it seems likely that environmental factors are more important than genetic predisposition.

Precipitating Factors

A large variety of events may immediately precede the onset of the illness and have often been regarded as precipitating factors though their mode of operation is unknown. They include influenza and infections of the upper respiratory tract, the specific fevers, superficial sepsis, surgical operations, and the extraction of teeth. Recent investigation casts doubt on the danger of surgical operations (Miller, 1961) but relapses have been noted to occur after vaccination against smallpox (Miller, Cendrowski, and Schapira, 1967). Millar et al. (1959) believe that pregnancy does not influence the relapse rate. Trauma requires special consideration. McAlpine and Compston (1952) obtained a history of trauma preceding the onset of symptoms by less than 3 months in 14·4 per cent. of cases, but in only 5·2 per cent. of controls, and there is some evidence for a relation between the site of the trauma and the site of the first symptom (Miller, 1964). Trauma may thus precipitate the onset of the disease or a relapse: we cannot yet say whether it initiates it, in the sense that apart from the trauma the disease would never have occurred.

Distribution, Age, and Sex

Multiple sclerosis is most prevalent in Northern Europe and Switzerland. It is less common in North America and is rare in tropical countries. McAlpine and Compston (1952) estimate its prevalence in England and Wales at about 1 in 2,400 and in Scotland at 1 in 1,570. In Switzerland it is about the same. A recent estimate for the United States (Limburg, 1950) is about 1 in 3,000. The epidemiology of the disease is discussed by Allison (1961). There is undoubtedly a correlation with latitude: the higher the latitude, the higher the incidence. Acheson (1965) concludes that the disease is neither a disorder of affluence nor one associated with malnutrition or atmospheric pollution. It is a disorder associated with particular localities rather than with race. No particular factors other than latitude have been found to characterize 'high risk' and 'low risk' areas. Their limits are too wide to suggest a relationship to trace elements and whatever harmful (or protective) factors are associated with these areas they do not appear to be freely transportable to other parts of the globe. The 'latent period' of the disease, related to the stage of life spent in a certain locality is prolonged and may extend over several decades so that the critical period which probably determines the later development of the disease is probably in childhood or adolescence.

The disease principally attacks young adults. In two-thirds of all cases it begins between 20 and 40, rather more often in the third than the fourth decade. Its occurrence below the age of 10 is doubtful, but it is occasionally seen in children between the ages of 12 and 15. During recent years the proportion of patients in whom the disease begins after the age of 50 has increased, but onset after 60 is almost unknown. In most published series males have been reported more often than females, but in England the reverse is the case, female patients outnumbering males in the ratio of 3 to 2.

SYMPTOMS

The Clinical Picture

The natural history of the disease produces a very varied clinical picture. In the early stages it is often that of a single focal lesion, acute or, during a remission, quiescent. As time goes on, the cumulative effects of earlier lesions constitute a persistent background of incapacity upon which fresh disabilities due to new lesions are superimposed. The early stages thus usually show long and often remarkably complete remissions, while later the patient's condition fluctuates only to the small extent that fresh lesions temporarily regress. However, occasional severe cases beginning in early adult life and more indolent chronic cases of onset in middle life run a progressive course from the outset, without remission.

Mode of Onset

The onset of the illness is usually the rapid development, within a few hours or a day or two, of symptoms of a single focal lesion of the white matter of the nervous system. Much less often symptoms appear insidiously. In a series of 100 consecutive patients the first symptom noticed was as follows:

	Weakness or loss of control over limbs	*No.*
Involving both lower limbs	. . . . .	18
Involving one lower limb	. . . . .	14
Involving one upper limb .	. . . . .	9
Involving one upper and one lower limb	. . .	7
Involving all four limbs	. . . . . .	2
		— 50

	Visual symptoms	
'Blindness' in one eye	. . . . . .	16
Double vision .	. . . . . .	8
'Dimness' of vision .	. . . . .	4
Homonymous field defect .	. . . .	1
		— 29

	Sensory symptoms	
Numbness and other painless paraesthesiae .	. .	11

	Miscellaneous symptoms	
Vertigo .	. . . .	2
Tremor .	. . . .	2
Multiple symptoms .	. . . . . .	2
Ptosis .	. . . .	1
Loss of taste .	. . . .	1
Epilepsy .	. . . .	1
Impotence .	. . . .	1
		— 10

Thus weakness of one or both lower limbs is the first symptom in about one-third of all cases, and a disturbance of vision in almost one-third more. Sensory symptoms which cause no disability are often forgotten and probably occur more frequently than in 11 per cent. Patients who are carefully questioned at the time of onset often describe symptoms of multiple small lesions occurring within a period of a few weeks. Weakness of the lower limbs is the commonest presenting symptom in patients in whom the disease develops insidiously, and in those in whom it begins after the age of 35.

Rarely the onset is fulminating, with an acute encephalitic, myelitic, or encephalomyelitic picture [see p. 502].

Motor Symptoms

Motor Weakness. Loss of power in the lower limbs is first manifest as fatigability or a feeling of heaviness, and later as spastic paraplegia. Sometimes sudden weakness of one upper limb occurs, often associated with loss of postural sensibility in the fingers—the 'useless hand' of Oppenheim. Facial weakness and hemiplegia occur occasionally.

Muscular wasting is very rare owing to the infrequency of involvement of the anterior horn cells in the patches, but very occasional cases with amyotrophy, often in the small hand muscles, have been described.

Incoordination. This is frequently present. In the upper limbs it usually takes the form of *intention tremor*, a tremor occurring only on voluntary movement and increasing in intensity the greater the accuracy demanded of the movement. In touching the nose with the finger the tremor increases in amplitude as the finger approaches the nose. The same phenomenon is shown if the patient be asked to touch his own nose and the observer's finger alternately, and also in lifting a glass of water to the lips. In certain exceptionally severe cases cerebellar ataxia is so severe that the wild 'flinging' movements of the limbs which occur on attempted volitional activity make it virtually impossible for the patient to use the limbs for any purpose. In the lower limbs incoordination is evident in an ataxic gait. Tremor of the head is common in the late stages when evidence of cerebellar involvement is prominent.

Dysarthria. Dysarthria may be due either to spastic weakness or to ataxia of the muscles of articulation or to a combination of these factors. In the early stages articulation may be slurred, later it may become explosive and almost unintelligible. The 'syllabic' or 'scanning' speech, sometimes regarded as typical, is exceptional and only occurs when cerebellar ataxia dominates the clinical picture. Transitory aphasia is rare.

Sensory Symptoms

Paraesthesiae occur at some period of the disease in most cases, commonly in the form of numbness and formication over one side of the face or one upper or both lower limbs. Impairment of position and joint sense and of the finer discriminative aspects of sensibility due to a lesion in the posterior columns of the spinal cord is often accompanied by sensations of apparent swelling of the limb and by feelings suggesting that tight strings or bandages have been applied to the trunk or extremities. When there is a patch in the posterior columns of the cervical cord a sensation resembling an electric shock may radiate through the body on flexing the cervical spine ('Lhermitte's sign'). Pain is uncommon except in the back, but typical trigeminal neuralgia, which is sometimes bilateral, is occasionally encountered. Objective sensory loss is present in at least 50 per cent. of cases. Defect of postural sensibility and of appreciation of vibration is the commonest disturbance, but cutaneous sensibility may also be impaired. Inability to recognize objects placed in the hand may occur as the result of a plaque in the fasciculus cuneatus in the cervical region. There may be a sharply defined upper level of sensory loss on the trunk suggestive of a spinal tumour.

Ocular Symptoms

Acute unilateral retrobulbar neuritis is one of the most important early symptoms of the disease. It occurs most often between the ages of 20 and 30. The vision of one eye becomes misty and in 24 or 48 hours is reduced to a perception of hand movement or of light only. The eye is painful on movement and tender on pressure, and there is a central scotoma larger for red and green than for white. The optic disc is usually normal in appearance during the acute stage, but if the lesion is near the disc papillitis may occur, though the swelling is usually slight. In a few weeks vision improves, but the residual damage to the nerve manifests itself in some degree of optic atrophy—pallor of the disc, especially in its temporal half—and often a persistent though smaller central scotoma. Permanent blindness is very rare. Simultaneous retrobulbar or optic neuritis in both eyes is uncommon in multiple sclerosis but undoubtedly occurs. The lesions of the optic nerves may be so insidious as to produce the characteristic temporal pallor of the disc, which is found in over 50 per cent. of cases, without the patient's being aware of any impairment of vision. Lesions of the optic chiasma and optic tracts are uncommon, and when they occur cause distinctive defects of the visual fields.

Nystagmus. This is present in at least 70 per cent. of cases. It is usually absent on central fixation and appears on conjugate deviation both laterally and vertically. The slow phase is towards the central fixation point and the quick phase away from it. A rotary element is sometimes present, especially on vertical fixation. Nystagmus on central fixation is rarely seen in multiple sclerosis.

Ocular Paralysis. Paralysis of conjugate ocular deviation may occur as the result of a plaque in the midbrain or pons, but is uncommon: paresis of single ocular muscles occurs in about 6 per cent. of cases; but diplopia without objective ocular palsy is commoner (34 per cent. of cases). Dissociation of lateral conjugate deviation may occur, the adducting eye being less completely deviated than the abducting. When this occurs (Harris' sign, a form of 'internuclear ophthalmoplegia') nystagmus is often apparent only in the abducting eye (so-called 'ataxic' nystagmus). This has been ascribed to a lesion of the medial longitudinal fasciculus. I have seen paresis of both medial recti. Ptosis is rare, retraction of the upper lids slightly commoner.

Pupillary Abnormalities. The pupillary reactions are usually normal. Loss of the reaction to light with preservation of that to accommodation is occasionally observed and is more frequently unilateral than in syphilis. Total ophthalmoplegia interna may occur. Paresis of the ocular sympathetic leading to ptosis, enophthalmos, and myosis may be seen as the result of a brain stem lesion.

Auditory and Vestibular Symptoms

Deafness is rare, but vertigo is a common and early symptom, usually as a mild sense of instability. Sometimes severe vertigo with vomiting and coarse nystagmus occurs in attacks lasting for several days, but is usually accompanied by other signs indicating the presence of a pontine plaque involving vestibular nuclei and other contiguous structures.

Mental Symptoms

Some reduction in the intellectual efficiency of the patient is not uncommon, but emotional changes are more frequent. The characteristic sense of mental and physical well-being—euphoria—is well known. On the other hand, depression and irritability are sometimes conspicuous. Some loss of control over emotional movements, leading to involuntary laughter and tears, is common, especially in the later stages of the illness. Delusional states and a terminal dementia are sometimes met with.

Reflex Changes

The length of the corticospinal tracts exposes them to a great chance of injury by some of the multiple lesions, hence the reflex signs of corticospinal tract damage are frequent. The tendon reflexes are exaggerated. The abdominal reflexes are absent in at least two-thirds of all cases and may be lost at an early stage, and extensor plantar reflexes occur in from 80 to 90 per cent. of cases in the later stages.

Other Symptoms

Sphincter control is frequently impaired. In the early stages urgency or precipitancy of micturition is common. Later, retention or reflex evacuation of both urine and faeces may occur. Occasionally acute retention of urine is the first symptom. Impotence is common.

Pyrexia may develop during acute exacerbations of the disease, which is consequently sometimes described by the patient as having begun with an attack of 'influenza'. Headache sometimes occurs.

There are convulsions in a small proportion of cases which may confuse the diagnosis unless their occasional occurrence is remembered. They may be terminal.

Trophic changes are rare, but I have occasionally seen cyanosis of the extremities with extreme dryness of the skin and brittleness of the nails.

Cerebrospinal Fluid

Some abnormality is found in the cerebrospinal fluid in at least half of all cases. An excess of mononuclear cells is found in about 10 per cent. An abnormal colloidal gold curve was regarded in the past as the most characteristic change. This is usually of the 'paretic', less often of the 'luetic', type, one or the other occurring in from 50 to 75 per cent. of cases. The protein is usually normal or only slightly raised but there may be an abnormally high gamma globulin estimated by paper electrophoresis (Schapira and Park, 1961). Prineas, Teasdale, Latner, and Miller (1966) used a simple zinc sulphate precipitation method for estimating spinal fluid gamma globulin and found this to be raised to above 29 per cent. of the total protein content in 44 per cent. of patients with multiple sclerosis. Except for neurosyphilis and certain encephalitides, this figure was exceeded in less than 5 per cent. of patients with other neurological diseases.

Symptom Groups

The extreme variability of the clinical picture justifies the recognition of 'forms' of the disease due to the predominant involvement of different parts of the nervous system.

1. The classical triad of Charcot, nystagmus, intention tremor, and scanning speech, is comparatively rare, and occurs in under 10 per cent. of cases.

2. The generalized form, common among younger patients, is characterized by pallor of the optic discs, nystagmus, slight intention tremor, ataxia, weakness and spasticity of the lower limbs, and defective sphincter control.

3. Onset with ocular symptoms. Retrobulbar neuritis or a transient episode of diplopia may be the only symptom for many years.

4. Hemiplegia is rarely the first symptom and is usually transitory.

5. Spinal forms. (a) *Progressive spastic paraplegia* may occur with few if any other physical signs, especially in middle-aged patients. (b) *Unilateral spinal lesions* occur chiefly in the cervical cord. The posterior and lateral columns are usually involved. A partial Brown-Séquard syndrome developing in a young person is not uncommon in this disease and usually remits within a few months. (c) *Sacral form*. A plaque in the conus medullaris may lead to incontinence of urine and faeces, impotence, and anaesthesia in the region of the sacral cutaneous supply.

6. Cerebellar, vestibular, pontine, and bulbar forms are self-explanatory.

7. Acute form. Occasionally the disease may run an acute or subacute course terminating fatally in three or four months or followed by partial recovery and subsequently exhibiting the usual relapses and remissions. In such acute cases fever may be present. Headache, vomiting, and giddiness are common at the onset, and delirium occurs in severe cases. The symptoms may be predominantly cerebral, predominantly spinal, or both brain and cord may be diffusely affected. There is a tendency for the affection to extend to hitherto unaffected parts of the nervous system after a lapse of days or even weeks. The symptoms of the cerebral type include mental changes, convulsions, aphasia, hemiplegia, hemianopia, nystagmus, and ataxia of the upper limbs. However, aphasia and hemianopia are signs of exceptional rarity in this disease. Optic neuritis may occur, usually bilaterally. Cranial nerve palsies are comparatively uncommon, except for facial paresis, and diplopia is uncommon in the acute form as is unilateral facial sensory loss. Symptoms of meningeal irritation are usually absent. In the spinal type pains in the back and limbs or with a girdle distribution are common. Paraesthesiae may occur. Paraplegia of varying severity is usually present, associated with sensory loss, which may be confined either to postural sensibility and passive movement, or to appreciation of pain, heat, and cold. A partial or complete Brown-Séquard syndrome is not rare. Bladder disturbances are present in the more severe cases of paraplegia. The tendon reflexes may be exaggerated, but are not uncommonly diminished or lost in the acute stage of 'spinal shock'. The plantars are frequently extensor. The cerebrospinal fluid frequently shows no abnormality, but may exhibit a rise in protein, or pleocytosis.

DIAGNOSIS

Multiple sclerosis must be distinguished from *diffuse sclerosis*, which has a more restricted age-range and often occurs in childhood. It is usually steadily progressive and by symmetrically destroying the white matter of the cerebral hemispheres leads to blindness, spastic tetraplegia, and dementia.

In *acute disseminated myelitis with optic neuritis*, or *neuromyelitis optica*, the symptoms of optic or retrobulbar neuritis are associated with those of transverse myelitis, both developing within a few weeks. These lesions are not usually contemporaneous in multiple sclerosis. Acute bilateral optic or retrobulbar neuritis may occur without myelitis, and also runs a benign course. Although both eyes may be successively the site of optic or retrobulbar neuritis in multiple sclerosis, it is rare for them both to be affected simultaneously in this disease.

Meningovascular Syphilis. Multiple sclerosis is distinguished from meningo-vascular syphilis by the rarity of pupillary changes and of diminution of the knee- and ankle-jerks in the former and the absence of a positive V.D.R.L. reaction and treponema immobilization test, which are present in the blood and spinal fluid in most cases of the latter. Moreover, nystagmus is rare in cerebral syphilis and true intention tremor unknown.

Tabes may to some extent be simulated by the ataxic gait of multiple sclerosis, but in the latter this is usually associated with spasticity, the knee- and ankle-jerks being exaggerated and the plantar reflexes extensor, while the pupillary reflexes are normal.

Friedreich's ataxia causes, in common with many cases of multiple sclerosis, nystagmus, absent abdominal reflexes, ataxia of the lower limbs, loss of postural sensibility, and extensor plantar responses. In this disease, however, we find diminution or loss of the ankle-jerks, and later of the knee-jerks, scoliosis, and pes cavus, while the frequent onset in childhood, slow progressive course, and occurrence of multiple cases in one family are distinctive.

Other Familial Ataxias. Some forms of familial ataxia have been described of which individual cases have been indistinguishable from multiple sclerosis, e.g. the Drew family described by Ferguson and Critchley. Differential points, however, are the familial incidence, the onset either earlier or later than is usual in multiple sclerosis, the steadily progressive course, and the occurrence of symptoms, e.g. marked ocular palsies, extrapyramidal signs, and extensive sensory loss, which are unusual in multiple sclerosis.

Subacute combined degeneration may lead to confusion as a cause of 'ataxic paraplegia'. It begins, however, later in life than do most cases of multiple sclerosis; paraesthesiae appear early and persist; the tendon reflexes in the lower limbs are often lost, and gastric achylia, megalocytic anaemia, and a low serum B_{12} activity are distinctive features.

Spinal Tumour. Multiple sclerosis may closely simulate spinal tumour when it gives rise to progressive spastic paraplegia, with or without sensory loss up to a segmental level, and without evident physical signs above the spinal cord. Such symptoms in a case of spinal tumour are, however, often associated with obstruction of the spinal subarachnoid space, demonstrable by Queckenstedt's test. In any case of doubt, however, myelography is an essential investigation.

Cervical spondylosis with myelopathy may lead to ataxic weakness of the upper limbs and spastic paraplegia, and so be confused with multiple sclerosis. Plain X-rays of the cervical spine and, if necessary, myelography, will usually settle the diagnosis. However, the two conditions are so common that they not infrequently coexist.

Hysteria can be confused with multiple sclerosis only through neglect to make a thorough examination of the nervous system. Such early symptoms as giddiness, paraesthesiae, and paresis may superficially suggest hysteria, but these are rarely present without some sign of organic disease, and pallor of the optic discs, absent abdominal reflexes, and extensor plantar responses are unequivocal evidence of such a condition. It is not rare, however, for a patient to develop hysterical symptoms in addition to those of an organic disease such as multiple sclerosis.

PROGNOSIS

. The extremely variable course renders prognosis difficult. The disease in its acute form may terminate fatally in three months or less, or the patient may still be able to work 50 years after the onset. One patient of mine was still doing her housework 39 years after her first symptom. When retrobulbar neuritis is the first symptom the next may not follow for many years. Among my own patients there have been remissions of 13, 15, 17, and 19 years after an attack of retrobulbar neuritis, and of 20 and 25 years after another symptom, before the disease has recurred. It is conceivable that a remission may last a lifetime and the patient recover permanently from his first attack (McAlpine, Lumsden, and Acheson, 1965). McAlpine and Compston (1952) in their study of the course of the disease found the average number of fresh 'attacks' to be about 0·4 per year for patients of both sexes. In some cases the disease is progressive from the beginning, in others only after several remissions. The average duration of life in fatal cases is about 20 years (Allison, 1950; McAlpine and Compston, 1952). McAlpine, Lumsden, and Acheson (1965) and others have stressed that benign forms of the disease are not infrequent. In a patient whose disability is slight within 5 years of the onset, the outlook is reasonably good. They found that 32 per cent. of a series of 241 such cases were not disabled in the tenth year or more of the disease.

The end is distressing. An account of it is given by a sufferer who was also a graphic writer, W. N. P. Barbellion, in *The Diary of a Disappointed Man* and *Enjoying Life*. Ataxia, weakness, and spasticity confine the patient to bed and prevent him from carrying out the simplest actions for himself. Swallowing becomes difficult and speech almost unintelligible. Urinary or cutaneous infection or pneumonia finally releases the sufferer. In rare cases the last event is an acute exacerbation of the disease itself, taking the form of an acute myelitis or encephalomyelitis.

TREATMENT

There is no specific treatment. The general management of the patient requires tact and judgement. Fatigue is to be avoided, but short of this every effort should be made to keep him at his usual occupation as long as possible. Ventrolateral thalamotomy may abolish severe intention tremor but should only be used in carefully selected cases as it may cause confusion and hasten intellectual deterioration if there is any evidence of incipient dementia. In the later stages encouragement and suggestion, and vigorous physiotherapy including active and passive movements and re-educational walking exercises may long postpone the bedridden state. Even though pregnancy may not influence the relapse rate it may accelerate deterioration in a moderately advanced case. There is no convincing evidence of the value of maintenance therapy with prednisolone (Miller, Newell, and Ridley, 1961). There is a clinical impression that cortico-trophin may be helpful during an acute exacerbation. The value of this treatment and the conflicting evidence with regard to its efficacy have been reviewed in detail by McAlpine, Lumsden, and Acheson (1965). It is now apparent that short courses of treatment, 80 Units daily for 1–2 weeks then every other day for 1–2 weeks and later twice weekly injections for 4–6 weeks, may promote remis-sion in acute relapses and may even be beneficial in some cases showing slow deterioration; but long-term maintenance treatment has been shown to be of no value (Millar *et al.*, 1967). Spasticity may be relieved by drugs such as diazepam, 2–5 mg. three or four times daily, while in selected cases intrathecal phenol injections are useful for the relief of flexor spasms. Propantheline, 15 mg., may control urgency and incontinence of urine. Calipers and other mechanical aids are of value in appropriate cases. In the late stages the skin, bladder, and rectum will require special attention, as in paraplegia from any cause. In such patients investigation will often reveal residual urine and impaired renal efficiency.

REFERENCES

ACHESON, E. D. (1965) The epidemiology of multiple sclerosis, in *Multiple Sclerosis: a Reappraisal*, Edinburgh.

ADIE, W. J. (1932) The aetiology and symptomatology of disseminated sclerosis, *Brit. med. J.*, **2**, 997.

ALLISON, R. S. (1950) Survival in disseminated sclerosis, *Brain*, **73**, 103.

ALLISON, R. S. (1961) Epidemiology of disseminated sclerosis, *Proc. roy. Soc. Med.*, **54**, 1.

ALVORD, E. C., JR. (1966) The relationship of hypersensitivity to infection, inflammation and immunity, *J. neuropath. exp. Neurol.*, **25**, 1.

ANTON, G., and WOHLWILL, F. (1912) Multiple nicht-eitrige Encephalomyelitis und multiple Sklerose, *Z. ges. Neurol. Psychiat.*, Orig. **12**, 31.

BOGAERT, L. VAN (1950) Post-infectious and multiple sclerosis, *J. neuropath. exp. Neurol.*, **9**, 219.

BRAIN, W. R. (1929–30) Critical review. Disseminated sclerosis, *Quart. J. Med.*, **23**, 343.

COURNAND, A. (1930) *La Sclérose en plaques aiguë: contribution à l'étude des encéphalo-myélites aiguës disséminées*, Paris.

CURTIUS, F. (1933) *Multiple Sklerose und Erbanlage*, Leipzig.

DATTNER, B. (1937) Zur Pathogenese der multiplen Sklerose, *Wien. klin. Wschr.*, **50**, 87.

DAWSON, J. W. (1916) The histology of disseminated sclerosis, *Trans. roy. Soc. Edinb.*, **50**, 517.

DOW, R. S., and BERGLUND, G. (1942) Vascular pattern of lesions of disseminated sclerosis, *Arch. Neurol. Psychiat. (Chicago)*, **47**, 1.

FERRARO, A. (1937) Primary demyelinating processes of the central nervous system, *Arch. Neurol. Psychiat. (Chicago)*, **37**, 1, 100.

FERRARO, A. (1958) Studies on multiple sclerosis, *J. Neuropath. exp. Neurol.*, **17**, 278.

FIELD, E. J. (1966) Transmission experiments with multiple sclerosis: an interim report, *Brit. med. J.*, **2**, 564.

FRAENKEL, M., and JAKOB, A. (1913) Zur Pathologie der multiplen Sklerose mit beson-derer Berücksichtigung der akuten Formen, *Z. ges. Neurol. Psychiat.*, **14**, 565.

GREENFIELD, J. G., and KING, L. S. (1936) Histopathology of the cerebral lesions in dis-seminated sclerosis, *Brain*, **59**, 445.

GREENFIELD, J. G., and NORMAN, R. M. (1965) Demyelinating diseases, in *Greenfield's Neuropathology*, 2nd ed., London.

LIMBURG, C. C. (1950) The geographic distribution of multiple sclerosis and its estimated prevalence in the U.S., *Res. Publ. Ass. nerv. ment. Dis.*, **28**, 15.

LUMSDEN, C. E. (1961) Consideration of multiple sclerosis in relation to the auto-immunity process, *Proc. roy. Soc. Med.*, **54**, 11.

LUMSDEN, C. E. (1965) The clinical pathology of multiple sclerosis, in *Multiple Sclerosis: a Reappraisal*, Edinburgh.

MANDELBROTE, B. M., STANIER, M. W., THOMPSON, R. H. S., and THRUSTON, M. N. (1948) Studies on copper metabolism in demyelinating diseases of the nervous system, *Brain*, **71**, 212.

MARGULIS, M. S., SOLOVIEV, V. D., and SHUBLADZE, A. K. (1946) Aetiology and patho-genesis of acute sporadic encephalomyelitis and multiple sclerosis, *J. Neurol. Neurosurg. Psychiat.*, **9**, 63.

MARSDEN, J. P., and HURST, E. W. (1932) Acute perivascular myelinoclasis ('acute dis-seminated encephalomyelitis') in small-pox, *Brain*, **55**, 181.

McALPINE, D. (1931) Acute disseminated encephalomyelitis: its sequelae and its rela-tionship to disseminated sclerosis, *Lancet*, i, 846.

McALPINE, D., and COMPSTON, N. (1952) Some aspects of the natural history of dis-seminated sclerosis, *Quart. J. Med.*, N.S. **21**, 135.

McALPINE, D., COMPSTON, N., and LUMSDEN, C. E. (1955) *Multiple Sclerosis*, Edinburgh.

McALPINE, D., LUMSDEN, C. E., and ACHESON, D. (1965) *Multiple Sclerosis: a Reap-praisal*, Edinburgh.

MARSHALL, J., and O'GRADY, F. (1959) The non-specificity of the intrathecal reaction to tuberculin in multiple sclerosis, *J. Neurol. Psychiat.*, **22**, 277.

MILLAR, J. H. D., ALLISON, R. S., CHEESEMAN, E. A., and MERRETT, J. D. (1959) Pregnancy as a factor influencing relapse in disseminated sclerosis, *Brain*, **82**, 417.

MILLAR, J. H. D., VAS, C. J., NORONHA, M. J., LIVERSEDGE, L. A., and RAWSON, M. D. (1967) Long-term treatment of multiple sclerosis with corticotrophin, *Lancet*, ii, 429.

MILLER, H. (1961) Aetiological factors in disseminated sclerosis, *Proc. roy. Soc. Med.*, **54**, 7.

MILLER, H. (1964) Trauma and multiple sclerosis, *Lancet*, i, 848.

MILLER, H., CENDROWSKI, W., and SCHAPIRA, K. (1967) Multiple sclerosis and vaccina-tion, *Brit. med. J.*, **2**, 210.

MILLER, H., NEWELL, D. J., and RIDLEY, A. (1961) Multiple sclerosis. Trials of main-tenance treatment with prednisolone and soluble aspirin, *Lancet*, i, 127.

MILLER, H., and SCHAPIRA, K. (1959) Aetiological aspects of multiple sclerosis, *Brit. med. J.*, **1**, 737, 811.

PETTE, H. (1928) Über die Pathogenese der multiplen Sklerose, *Dtsch. Z. Nervenheilk.*, **105**, 76.

PETTE, H. (1929) Infektion und Nervensystem, *Dtsch. Z. Nervenheilk.*, **110**, 221.

POSKANZER, D., MILLER, H., and SCHAPIRA, K. (1963) Epidemiology of multiple sclerosis in the counties of Northumberland and Durham, *J. Neurol. Psychiat.*, **26**, 368.

POSKANZER, D. C., SCHAPIRA, K., and MILLER, H. (1963) Multiple sclerosis and polio-myelitis, *Lancet*, ii, 917.

PRATT, R. T. C., COMPSTON, N. D., and McALPINE, D. (1951) The familial incidence of disseminated sclerosis and its significance, *Brain*, **74**, 191.

PRINEAS, J., TEASDALE, G., LATNER, A. L., and MILLER, H. (1966) Spinal fluid gamma-globulin and multiple sclerosis, *Brit. med. J.*, **2**, 922.

PUTNAM, T. J. (1937) Evidences of vascular occlusion in multiple sclerosis and 'encepha-lomyelitis', *Arch. Neurol. Psychiat. (Chicago)*, **37**, 1298.

REDLICH, E. (1927) Über ein gehäuftes Auftreten von Krankheitsfällen mit den Er-scheinungen der Encephalomyelitis disseminata, *Mschr. Psychiat. Neurol.*, **64**, 152.

REFSUM, S. (1961) Possible genetic factors in disseminated sclerosis, *Proc. roy. Soc. Med.*, **54**, 35.

SCHAPIRA, K., POSKANZER, D. C., and MILLER, H. (1963) Familial and conjugal multiple sclerosis, *Brain*, **86**, 315.

SCHAPIRA, K., and PARK, D. C. (1961) Gamma globulin studies in multiple sclerosis and their application to the problem of diagnosis, *J. Neurol. Neurosurg. Psychiat.*, **24**, 121.

SMITH, H. V., ESPIR, M. L. E., WHITTY, C. W. M., and RUSSELL, W. R. (1957) Abnormal immunological reactions in disseminated sclerosis, *J. Neurol. Psychiat.*, **20**, 1.

SPIELMEYER, W. (1923) Der anatomische Befund bei einem zweiten Fall von Pelizaeus-Merzbacherscher Krankheit, *Z. ges. Neurol. Psychiat.*, **32**, 203.

TURNBULL, H. M. (1928) Encephalomyelitis in virus diseases and exanthemata, *Brit. med. J.*, **2**, 331.

See also Multiple sclerosis and the demyelinating diseases. *Res. Publ. Ass. nerv. ment. Dis.*, **28**, 1950.

CENTRAL PONTINE MYELINOLYSIS

In 1959 Adams, Victor, and Mancall described four patients in whom autopsy studies revealed a single sharply outlined focus of myelin destruction in the rostral part of the pons, involving all fibre tracts indiscriminately but largely sparing nerve fibres and axis cylinders. The process appeared to begin centrally in the pons and to spread centrifugally. In two of their patients the clinical picture was one of a rapidly evolving flaccid paraplegia with facial and tongue weakness, dysphagia and anarthria; the clinical picture in the other two cases was less dramatic. Three of the patients were alcoholics, the other was severely malnourished. While the condition is provisionally classified at present in the demyelinating diseases it seems probable that it is of metabolic or nutritional origin.

REFERENCE

ADAMS, R. D., VICTOR, M., and MANCALL, E. L. (1959) Central pontine myelinolysis, *Arch. Neurol. Psychiat. (Chicago)*, **81**, 154.

DIFFUSE SCLEROSIS

Classification and Synonyms. See page 477.

Definition. A group of progressive diseases usually occurring early in life and characterized pathologically by widespread demyelination of the white matter of the cerebral hemispheres, and clinically in typical cases by visual failure, mental deterioration, and spastic paralysis. Both sporadic and familial cases are encountered. The aetiology of these disorders is unknown and there is no general agreement as to their classification. At present their resemblances to one another appear to outweigh their differences and they are therefore included under a common title. For a discussion of the problems involved in their classification see page 476. The many different disorders falling into this group are now frequently referred to as the leucodystrophies.

PATHOLOGY

There is usually considerable atrophy of the brain, and it may be tougher than normal. On section, the white matter of the cerebral hemispheres exhibits a slightly translucent and somewhat hyaline appearance, varying in colour from grey to yellow or brown. The abnormal areas, which may be gelatinous or much firmer than normal brain, are sharply demarcated from healthy cerebral tissue, especially from the cortex, though occasionally this suffers also. The white matter of the occipital lobes is usually most severely affected [FIG. 79]. The white matter of the cerebellum may be involved as well as that of the cerebral hemispheres. Microscopically, the primary change appears to be a degeneration of the myelin sheaths and later of the axis cylinders of the white matter of the affected areas. In some cases this alteration has been described as possessing a perivascular distribution at the onset. Neuroglial overgrowth is conspicuous, especially in the neighbourhood of the blood vessels. There is a diffuse infiltration of the

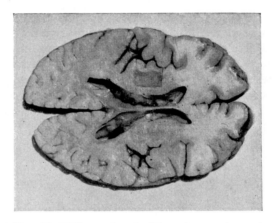

FIG. 79. Diffuse sclerosis. Note the massive and symmetrical demyelination of the white matter of the posterior two-thirds of the cerebral hemispheres

brain with compound granular corpuscles, and these are present in large numbers in the perivascular sheaths, which usually also contain small, round cells resembling lymphocytes.

Greenfield (1958) on the basis of pathological detail distinguished four varieties: (1) The sudanophilic type, in which the process of myelin breakdown resembles that found in multiple sclerosis. This form may begin in childhood, when it is often familial, or in adult life when it is usually not (Schilder's disease). (2) The Pelizaeus–Merzbacher type (aplasia axialis extracorticalis congenita), a slowly progressive form, usually familial, and often appearing during early childhood. There is widespread absence or poverty of myelin, but little evidence of breakdown. (3) Krabbe type, a familial form occurring usually during the first year of life. A distinctive feature is the occurrence of perivascular and more widespread collections of epithelioid and 'globoid' cells. Greenfield's fourth type, metachromatic leuco-encephalopathy, is now classified with the lipidoses.

The vexed question of classification of this obscure group of disorders and the biochemical differences (largely concerned with variations in the concentration of specific brain lipids in the white matter) between them which are beginning to emerge have been discussed recently by Greenfield and Norman (1965). Many authors now separate off Schilder's disease from other forms of sudanophilic diffuse sclerosis while spongy degeneration of the white matter (Canavan, 1931) is also recognized as a distinctive disorder (van Bogaert, 1963; Buchanan and Davis, 1965).

The pathological change usually begins symmetrically in both occipital lobes and spreads forwards in the white matter of the hemispheres, ultimately involving the corpus callosum and reaching as far forwards as the frontal and temporal poles, but there are exceptions to this. The frontal lobes may suffer more than the occipital, and the changes may be asymmetrical, even predominantly unilateral. Concentrically arranged rings of demyelination with relatively normal white matter between them have been described (Baló) but it is now believed that this uncommon pathological feature is more often observed in severe cases of multiple sclerosis. The white matter of the internal capsules and brain stem may be similarly involved, but the subsulcine and arcuate fibres usually escape. Involvement of the basal ganglia is inconstant. Small clear-cut areas of demyelination resembling those of multiple sclerosis have been found in the brain stem, even in cases which otherwise show characteristic pathological changes of diffuse sclerosis.

AETIOLOGY

The only known facts about the aetiology of the diffuse scleroses are statistical. In half the cases the onset occurs before the age of 14 and in 40 per cent. before 10. These 40 per cent. are approximately equally divided between the first and second quinquennia. In a small number of patients the disease begins later in life, even up to old age. Males are affected more often than females in childhood, but the sexes suffer with equal frequency after adolescence. Although most reported cases have been sporadic, the number of familial examples is increasing. Bielschowsky and Henneberg (1928) believe that encephalitis periaxialis diffusa (Schilder's disease) is a sporadically occurring inflammatory condition, and is therefore to be distinguished from the familial and degenerative diffuse scleroses. Many writers, however, regard these two conditions, whatever their aetiology, as allied if not identical. There is no evidence, beyond a doubtful interpretation of perivascular round-cell infiltration, in favour of their inflammatory nature. The early infantile examples have been attributed to a failure of development of the myelin sheaths, later cases to a failure to maintain their nutrition. This in turn has been ascribed to a defect of the oligodendrocytes (Greenfield, 1932–3), a disturbance of the power of the glial cells to regulate lipid metabolism (Scholz, 1925), and the presence of abnormal lipids in the blood (Bielschowsky and Henneberg). Einarson, Neel, and Strömgren (1942, 1944) believe that diffuse sclerosis is the result of a complex interplay of factors in which infection, allergy, and a constitutional defect of the interfascicular glia may all play a part, leading to the diffusion of a myelinolytic agent into the brain. A vascular disturbance of the white matter has also been blamed. Innes has pointed out the resemblance between 'sway-back', a pre- and post-natal disease of lambs, and Schilder's disease. The cause of 'sway-back' is obscure, but it can be prevented by giving copper to the ewes (Innes, 1939).

Current opinion favours the view that Schilder's disease may well prove a demyelinating disorder sharing certain affinities with multiple sclerosis whereas most of the other leucodystrophies (sudanophilic, familial, globoid body and other forms) will more probably be shown to be due to single or multiple enzyme defects concerned with the metabolism of those lipids from which myelin is formed. Thus, as is now accepted in the case of metachromatic leucodystrophy, it is probable that many of these heterogeneous disorders will eventually be reclassified with the cerebral lipidoses, the important difference being that most of the conditions under discussion are essentially disorders of myelin formation and breakdown whereas most of the 'classical' lipidoses appear to affect predominantly the nerve cell.

SYMPTOMS

The onset of symptoms is sometimes rapid, sometimes insidious. Headache and giddiness may occur, but fever is exceptional. Visual impairment is one of the earliest symptoms, but may be preceded by mental deterioration, epileptiform attacks, aphasia, or weakness and incoordination of the limbs. Visual failure is usually due to destruction of the optic radiations. When one occipital lobe is first involved, the first visual field defect is homonymous hemianopia on the opposite side, the remaining halves of the visual fields being subsequently gradually lost as the opposite occipital lobe becomes involved. More often both sides are involved symmetrically. In either case the end result is blindness. Sometimes visual impairment is due to demyelination of the optic nerves leading to retrobulbar or optic neuritis with bilateral central scotomas. In such cases there may be papillitis during the acute stage followed by optic atrophy. Papillitis is found in about 25 per cent. of patients. Unless the optic nerves are thus involved the pupillary reactions are likely to be normal. Diplopia is not uncommon and is usually due to lateral rectus paralysis. Third-nerve palsy occurs much less frequently. Nystagmus is common. Loss of smell and taste, deafness, and tinnitus have been described.

Progressive spastic weakness of the extremities gradually develops. One side of the body may be thus affected before the other, but a spastic tetraplegia is the final state. Sensory loss is not uncommon and is usually of the cortical type, with loss of postural sensibility, appreciation of passive movement, and tactile discrimination, leading to astereognosis. When the internal capsules are involved, analgesia involving one or both halves of the body is added. General incoordination is common in the early stages. Aphasia may occur, but later tends to be masked by spastic dysarthria. Mental changes are usually conspicuous and are those of a progressive dementia. Epileptiform attacks, which may be either generalized or Jacksonian, may occur at any stage of the disease. The cerebrospinal fluid is usually normal, but slight mononuclear pleocytosis and an increase of protein content have been described.

DIAGNOSIS

In a typical case the early onset of blindness unattributable to a lesion of the optic nerves, together with progressive mental failure and spastic paralysis, constitutes a highly distinctive clinical picture. When the symptoms of diffuse sclerosis are for a time predominantly unilateral and especially when papilloedema occurs, it may be confused with intracranial tumour. The EEG is often of considerable value in diagnosis from subacute encephalitis and lipidosis; it usually shows only diffuse slow activity and very rarely do recordings demonstrate changes in any way comparable to the recurrent bizarre complexes of subacute encephalitis or the irregular spike and wave discharges seen in cerebral lipidosis. Slowing of motor conduction velocity in peripheral nerves in the Krabbe or globoid body type of diffuse sclerosis may indicate that peripheral nerves as well as the brain are involved in the disease process. Encephalography may help in the diagnosis by yielding evidence of cerebral atrophy, and the ultimate development in diffuse sclerosis of extensive involvement of both cerebral hemispheres will enable a tumour to be excluded. Diffuse sclerosis may also simulate multiple sclerosis, but many cases of the former occur at an age when the latter is either unknown or very rare. Further, the severe visual impairment without involvement of the optic nerves which is characteristic of diffuse sclerosis does not occur in multiple sclerosis, in which also epileptiform attacks are very uncommon, and mental deterioration is only rarely severe.

PROGNOSIS

The disease is invariably progressive and almost always terminates fatally, although exceptionally temporary remissions occur, and it may possibly sometimes become arrested. It may run an acute course, leading to death within one or two months, and few patients survive more than three years after the onset of the symptoms. Very rarely life may be prolonged for a number of years.

TREATMENT

The cause of the disease being unknown, treatment is empirical and none is known to arrest its course. The usual anticonvulsant drugs should be employed to control the convulsions.

REFERENCES

BATTEN, F. E., and WILKINSON, D. (1914) Unusual type of hereditary disease of the nervous system. (Pelizaeus-Merzbacher) Aplasia axialis extra-corticalis congenita, *Brain*, **36**, 341.

BIELSCHOWSKY, F. (1927) Die Bedeutung des Infektes für die diffuse Sklerose, *Jb. Psychiat. Neurol.*, **33**, 12.

BIELSCHOWSKY, M., and HENNEBERG, R. (1928) Über familiäre diffuse Sklerose. (Leukodystrophia Cerebri Progressiva Hereditaria.), *Jb. Psychiat. Neurol.*, **36**, 131.

BOGAERT, L. VAN (1963) Familial spongy degeneration of the brain, *Acta psychiat. (Kbh.)*, **39**, 107.

BUCHANAN, D. S., and DAVIS, R. L. (1965) Spongy degeneration of the nervous system, *Neurology (Minneap.)*, **15**, 207.

CANAVAN, M. M. (1931) Schilder's encephalitis periaxialis diffusa: report of a case in a child aged sixteen and one half months, *Arch. Neurol. Psychiat. (Chicago)*, **25**, 299.

COLLIER, J., and GREENFIELD, J. G. (1924) The encephalitis periaxialis of Schilder, *Brain*, **47**, 489.

EINARSON, L., and NEEL, A. V. (1942) On the problem of diffuse brain sclerosis with special reference to the familial forms, *Acta Jutlandica, Aarsskrift for Aarhus Universitet*, **14**, 2.

EINARSON, L., NEEL, A. V., and STRÖMGREN, E. (1944) On the problem of diffuse brain sclerosis with special reference to the familial forms, *Acta Jutlandica, Aarsskrift for Aarhus Universitet*, **16**, 1.

FERRARO, A. (1937) Primary demyelinating processes of the central nervous system, *Arch. Neurol. Psychiat. (Chicago)*, **37**, 1100.

FOLCH-PI, J., and BAUER, H. (1963) *Brain Lipids and Lipoproteins and the Leucodystrophies*, Amsterdam.

GERSTL, B., MALAMUD, N., HAYMAN, R. B., and BOND, P. R. (1965) Morphological and neurochemical study of Pelizaeus-Merzbacher disease, *J. Neurol. Neurosurg. Psychiat.*, **28**, 540.

GLOBUS, J. H., and STRAUSS, I. (1928) Progressive degenerative subcortical encephalopathy, *Arch. Neurol. Psychiat. (Chicago)*, **20**, 1190.

GREENFIELD, J. G. (1932–3) A form of progressive cerebral sclerosis in infants associated with primary degeneration of the interfascicular glia, *Proc. roy. Soc. Med.*, **26**, 690.

GREENFIELD, J. G. (1933) A form of progressive cerebral sclerosis in infants associated with primary degeneration of the interfascicular glia, *Volume Jubilaire en l'honneur du Professeur G. Marinesco*, p. 257, Bucarest.

GREENFIELD, J. G. (1958) Demyelinating diseases, in *Neuropathology*, 1st ed., ed. GREENFIELD, J. G., BLACKWOOD, W., McMENEMY, W. H., MEYER, A., and NORMAN, R. M., London.

GREENFIELD, J. G., and NORMAN, R. M. (1965) Demyelinating diseases, in *Greenfield's Neuropathology*, 2nd ed., ed. BLACKWOOD, W., McMENEMEY, W. H., MEYER, A., NORMAN, R. M., and RUSSELL, D. S., London.

INNES, J. R. M. (1934–5) The pathology of 'swayback'—a congenital demyelinating disease of lambs with affinities to Schilder's encephalitis, Univ. of Camb. Institute of Animal Pathology, Fourth Report.

INNES, J. R. M. (1939) Swayback: a demyelinating disease of lambs with affinities to Schilder's encephalitis and its prevention by copper, *J. Neurol. Psychiat.*, N.S. **2**, 323.

KRABBE, K. (1916) A new familial infantile form of diffuse brain-sclerosis, *Brain*, **39**, 74.

LEVADITI, C. (1930) Les ultravirus provocateurs des ectodermoses neurotropes, *Ann. Inst. Pasteur*, **45**, 673.

NORMAN, R. M., TINGEY, A. H., VALENTINE, J. C., and HISLOP, H. J. (1967) Sudanophil leucodystrophy: a study of inter-sib variation in the form taken by the demyelinating process, *J. Neurol. Psychiat.*, **30**, 75.

RUSSELL, D. S., and TALLERMAN, K. H. (1937) Familial progressive diffuse cerebral sclerosis of infants, *Arch. Dis. Childh.*, **12**, 71.

SCHILDER, P. (1912) Zur Kenntnis der sogenannten diffusen Sklerose, *Z. ges. Neurol. Psychiat.*, **10**, 1.

SCHOLZ, W. (1925). Klinische, pathologisch-anatomische und erbbiologische Untersuchungen bei familiärer, diffuser Hirnsklerose im Kindesalter, *Z. ges. Neurol. Psychiat.*, **99**, 651.

STEWART, T. G., GREENFIELD, J. G., and BLANDY, M. A. (1927) Encephalitis periaxialis diffusa. Report of three cases with pathological examinations, *Brain*, **50**, 1.

SYMONDS, C. P. (1928) A contribution to the clinical study of Schilder's encephalitis, *Brain*, **51**, 24.

SYMONDS, C. P. (1932–3) Discussion on encephalitis periaxialis diffusa (Schilder), *Proc. roy. Soc. Med.*, **26**, 301.

12

EXTRAPYRAMIDAL SYNDROMES

THE CORPUS STRIATUM

ANATOMY AND CONNEXIONS OF THE CORPUS STRIATUM

THE corpus striatum is, phylogenetically, the oldest part of the cerebrum. It lies deep in the substance of the cerebral hemisphere between the lateral ventricle and the insula. It consists of the caudate nucleus and the lentiform nucleus, the latter being divided into the putamen and the globus pallidus [FIGS. 4 and 80].

The Caudate Nucleus. The caudate nucleus is a pear-shaped mass of grey matter. Its head, the most anterior part of the corpus striatum, is on the lateral side of the anterior horn of the lateral ventricle, into which it bulges. Its tail runs backwards in the floor of the lateral ventricle, and then forwards and downwards in the roof of the descending horn.

The Putamen. This is separated from the insula by a narrow zone of grey matter, the claustrum, and another of white matter, the external capsule.

The Globus Pallidus. This lies medial to the putamen. It is separated from the thalamus and the caudate nucleus by the internal capsule, which also separates the head of the caudate from the anterior part of the putamen.

The caudate nucleus and putamen develop from the same mass of grey matter and show the same histological structure. They contain two types of ganglion cell, a small number of large cells among more frequent small ones. The globus pallidus contains only one type of ganglion cell. On account of their common origin and identical structure the caudate and putamen are grouped together by some writers as 'the striatum', the globus pallidus being distinguished as 'the pallidum'.

The corpus striatum contains numerous fibres which may be divided into (1) afferent, (2) internuncial, and (3) efferent [FIG. 80].

1. Afferent fibres reach it from the cerebral cortex, from the thalamus, and from the midbrain. They are distributed chiefly to the caudate nucleus and putamen.

2. Internuncial fibres unite the caudate and the putamen, and also connect these fibres with the globus pallidus. It is thought that the afferent fibres terminate in relation with the small ganglion cells, and that the fibres connecting the striatum with the pallidum originate in the large ganglion cells.

3. Efferent fibres run from the striatum to the substantia nigra and from the globus pallidus by the ansa lenticularis to the thalamus, the red nucleus, the substantia nigra, and the subthalamic nucleus or corpus Luysii.

The Red Nucleus. The red nucleus lies in the tegmentum of the midbrain at the level of the superior colliculi. In addition to fibres from the corpus striatum it receives impulses from the opposite dentate nucleus of the cerebellum by the superior peduncle. It is divided into a large-celled and a small-celled portion. From the former the rubrospinal tract takes origin, and crossing the midline

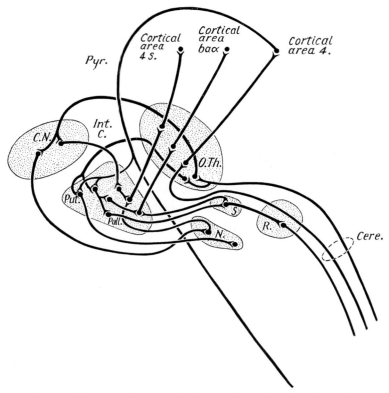

FIG. 80. Diagram of the principal connexions of the basal ganglia

Abbreviations: Pyr., corticospinal tract; Int. C., internal capsule; C.N., caudate nucleus; Put., putamen; Pall., globus pallidus; O. Th., optic thalamus; S., subthalamic nucleus; N., substantia nigra; R., red nucleus; Cere., ascending cerebellar pathways

in the ventral tegmental decussation descends through the brain stem to the spinal cord. The small-celled portion gives rise to fibres which ascend to the frontal lobe.

The Substantia Nigra. The substantia nigra is a grey mass lying between the crus cerebri and tegmentum of the midbrain at the level of the superior colliculi. It consists of a zona compacta lying dorsally and containing large melanin-bearing ganglion cells to which it owes its dark colour, and a zona reticulata lying under this and resembling in structure the globus pallidus. Besides incoming fibres from the corpus striatum it is said to receive a direct connexion from the cortex of the frontal lobe, and it sends fibres to the red nucleus, to the subthalamic nucleus, and to lower regions of the brain stem.

The Subthalamic Nucleus. The subthalamic nucleus (corpus Luysii) is a small mass of grey matter on the dorsal aspect of the crus cerebri, to the lateral side of the substantia nigra. Besides receiving fibres from the globus pallidus, it communicates with the red nucleus and with the substantia nigra.

To sum up, the extrapyramidal pathways descend from the cortex to the striatum and thence to the substantia nigra, and also to the latter direct. There is also a thalamo-pallido-rubral system. All three connect with the tegmental and pontine reticular substance and olives, from which the main spinal connexions arise.

DISORDERS OF THE CORPUS STRIATUM AND THEIR INTERPRETATION

The interpretation of disorders of the corpus striatum has proved very difficult, and much still remains to be learned. Indeed the study of pathological changes in the basal ganglia and of clinico-pathological correlations in this group of disorders are probably less advanced than almost any other field of dynamic neuropathology. The best way to approach the subject seems to be first to describe the symptoms produced by striatal disorders, then to see how far these can be correlated with lesions in these situations. This can be attempted both by ascertaining what pathological lesions are present in patients presenting certain symptoms, and conversely what symptoms are present in patients who are found to have limited pathological lesions. Finally, an attempt may be made in the light of such facts and animal experiment, to build up a picture of the functions of the corpus striatum and to explain why the characteristic symptoms are produced by damage to it.

SYMPTOMS OF STRIATAL DISORDERS

In any consideration of the symptoms of striatal disorder, it is important to note at the outset that such symptoms are in a sense artificial abstractions from a larger whole. This is so for two reasons, first, because one individual symptom tends to merge into others, however clear-cut it may be in an individual patient. For example, there are intermediate forms between chorea and athetosis and between athetosis and dystonia. Similarly, Parkinsonian rigidity tends to merge into other types of muscular hypertonia. Hence a particular symptom of striatal disorder is to be regarded as part of a spectrum rather than as a completely isolated entity. The second reason is that although in some patients a symptom of striatal disease may remain virtually unchanged for years, in many others, suffering from a progressive disorder, the clinical picture itself changes in the course of time, moving as it were along the spectrum from one group of symptoms to another.

Athetosis

Athetosis is a term meaning instability of posture, and it is applied to a disturbance of both posture and voluntary movement resulting in involuntary movements. It may be unilateral or bilateral. In the upper limb, when, for example, the arm is outstretched, there is a characteristic alternation between two postures. The first is characterized by exaggerated flexion of the wrist and hyperextension of the fingers, particularly at the metacarpophalangeal joints, the forearm tending to be pronated. This is apt to change into a posture of flexion of the fingers, often with the thumb flexed beneath the remaining digits, and the wrist flexed and somewhat supinated. Rather characteristically, the change from extension to flexion occurs successively in one digit after another. The athetotic movements are less marked in the lower limb, where the characteristic picture is one of plantar flexion of the ankle and dorsiflexion of the great toe. Voluntary movement is impeded, and, in the upper limb particularly, wild excursions may occur at shoulder and elbow when it is attempted. The lips, jaw, and tongue are involved, particularly when the disorder is bilateral, and this leads to facial grimaces and dysarthria.

Chorea

As already mentioned, there is no sharp distinction between athetosis and chorea. Typical chorea, however, consists of a series of continuous involuntary movements involving the face, tongue and limbs, chiefly in their distal joints, and even the trunk and respiratory muscles. Choreic movements are rapid and are sometimes described as 'pseudo-purposive'. This means that they resemble fragmentary and disordered forms of emotional and voluntary movement, continually interrupted, and never proceeding to completion. As in athetosis, voluntary movement is grossly disturbed in the more severe forms of chorea by the involuntary movements. Associated movements are exaggerated in chorea. When a choreic patient is made to clench his fists, his whole body partakes in movements which are an exaggerated and disorganized form of the associated movements which normally accompany great muscular effort. The disorganization consists of a loss of reciprocal relaxation, and a loss or incoordination of the synergic muscular contractions necessary for orderly movement. Chorea is characterized by muscular hypotonia and impairment of the ability to maintain a posture. Many patients show a combination of the predominantly peripheral and relatively rapid movements of chorea with the slower, more proximal writhing movements of athetosis and are then said to demonstrate choreo-athetosis.

Hemiballismus

Hemiballismus is a somewhat uncommon form of involuntary movement related to chorea. It is limited to one side of the body, and differs from chorea chiefly in the greater involvement of the proximal joints of the limbs and a prominent tendency to rotation of the limbs. The wild 'flinging' and continuous character of the movement in severe cases may produce virtual exhaustion of the patient and excoriation of skin due to repeated trauma to the affected limbs.

Dystonia

Whereas in one direction athetosis merges into chorea, in the other direction it merges into dystonia. Dystonia is the term applied to the persistent maintenance of a posture by exaggerated muscle tone, the posture being usually not one intermediate between flexion and extension, as is the case in Parkinsonism, but an extreme degree of one or the other, usually extension in the lower limb and either extension or flexion in the upper limb. Dystonia frequently begins with an exaggerated plantar-flexion and inversion of the foot, or hyperextension of the fingers. In extreme cases, as Denny-Brown (1960, 1962) points out, the extremity becomes set in one of the postures of athetosis. The facial muscles and tongue may be involved. The disorder may be unilateral or bilateral, and the asymmetrical distribution of the hypertonia may lead to torsion of the trunk and torticollis [FIG. 83, p. 539]. Spasmodic torticollis in fact merges into torsion dystonia of the neck. Denny-Brown points out that the EMG in dystonia is indistinguishable from that of Parkinsonian rigidity.

Rigidity

Rigidity is the muscular disorder characteristic of Parkinsonism. It is often described as a plastic rigidity, and it is characterized by a relatively constant resistance to passive stretching of the muscles, and approximately equal distribution to the flexors and extensors. It is usually evident in the flexors of the wrist and fingers, and pronators of the forearm. Denny-Brown points out that the plastic rigidity of Parkinsonism can be made to disappear if the limb is completely supported and the patient instructed to relax. In such a state of relaxation unimpeded passive movement is possible in either direction at any joint within a small range of 5 to 10 degrees. Movement of larger range, however, immediately sets up a contraction in the stretched muscle, demonstrating that the rigidity is a stretch reflex in each muscle concerned. Denny-Brown states that 'the plastic quality of Parkinsonian rigidity, that distinguishes it from spasticity, is due to a tendency of motor units recruited into a contraction by stretching, to drop out again one by one as others are recruited. . . . When a spastic muscle is stretched more and more motor units respond, and resistance to stretch mounts to a peak. At this point many units suddenly cease responding, and resistance to further stretch melts away ("lengthening reaction"). In plastic rigidity the lengthening reaction affects one motor unit after another from the beginning of stretch, so that resistance to stretch remains approximately constant.' So-called 'cog-wheel rigidity' is merely due to the combination of rigidity and tremor, the resistance to passive movement waxing and waning with the phases of contraction and relaxation of the muscle produced by the tremor.

Tremor

Tremor is a rhythmical alternating contraction of opposing muscle groups. Tremor is commonly associated with rigidity in Parkinsonism, but may occur independently of it. Parkinsonian tremor commonly occurs when the limb is at rest and is temporarily abolished by voluntary movement, but there are exceptions to this, and the tremor may persist during voluntary movement. Denny-Brown (1960) has analysed the relationship between tremor, rigidity, and dystonia electromyographically. He concludes that 'plastic rigidity, Parkinsonian tremor, and dystonia are different aspects of a conflict of released proprioceptive reactions. The conflict is resolved more slowly in plastic rigidity, more rapidly and rhythmically in tremor, and not at all in intense dystonia.'

Abbe-Fessard et al. (1966) discuss the evidence, drawn from observations on man and monkeys, that a rhythmical activity capable of producing tremor originates in the thalamus. In Parkinsonian patients stereotaxic exploration has demonstrated thalamic rhythms corresponding to the tremor. It is suggested that the lesion responsible for Parkinsonism may release such rhythms from inhibition.

THE RELATIONSHIP OF SYMPTOMS TO LESIONS OF THE CORPUS STRIATUM

The precise correlation of particular striatal symptoms with pathological changes in particular regions is difficult. Many such disorders are diffuse and progressive, and it is therefore often not easy to say at autopsy which symptoms were due to particular parts of the pathological disorder. On the other hand, acute lesions of the corpus striatum may also be diffuse, and tend to produce immediately clinical pictures otherwise associated only with very advanced stages of the slowly progressive disorders. We must be content, therefore, with certain established correlations which so far fill in only part of the picture.

Athetosis

The pathological evidence suggests that the lesion responsible for athetosis is situated in the outer segment of the putamen as in the *état marbré* responsible for congenital double athetosis.

Chorea

It is probable that experimental work in the past has not sufficiently distinguished between chorea and hemiballismus. True chorea appears to result from a lesion of the corpus striatum involving particularly the caudate nucleus. Hemiballismus appears almost always to be due to damage to the opposite subthalamic nucleus or to lesions which isolate it from the globus pallidus (Martin, 1957).

Dystonia

The close relationship between dystonia and athetosis has already been noted, so it is not surprising that the causative lesions are in a similar situation. The putamen is involved in both, but in dystonia the thalamus and cerebral cortex may be involved as well.

Parkinsonian Tremor and Rigidity

These two symptoms will be considered together, since they are closely related both clinically and physiologically, and it is not at present possible to distinguish their pathological basis. Indeed, the pathological basis of the Parkinsonian syndrome is still under dispute. The whole subject is discussed by Denny-Brown (1960, 1962). The older view attributed Parkinsonism to lesions of the globus pallidus. The importance of the substantia nigra, which suffers severely in encephalitis lethargica, was then stressed (Greenfield, 1958). Denny-Brown himself now re-emphasizes the lesions of the globus pallidus. It is pointed out that in paralysis agitans degeneration in the cells of the substantia nigra is slight, and in acute cases of encephalitis lethargica there may be gross destruction of the substantia nigra without symptoms of Parkinsonism.

The high incidence of Lewy bodies in 'idiopathic' Parkinsonism and of

Alzheimer-type neurofibrillary tangles, in the post-encephalitic cases, in the melanin-containing cells of the brain stem is stressed by Alvord (1958) who is confident that the Parkinsonian syndrome embraces at least two distinctive pathological entities. It is agreed that the cells of the globus pallidus may show little change in post-encephalitic Parkinsonism, but Denny-Brown stresses the importance of the loss of small thinly-medullated fibres entering the external putamen from the external capsule, and the external lamina of the globus pallidus from the internal capsule.

Massive Lesions of the Corpus Striatum

An important light is thrown upon the functions of the corpus striatum by the clinical pictures which result from massive bilateral lesions of the putamen and caudate nucleus, and the globus pallidus respectively. Denny-Brown, reviewing this question, notes that the characteristic effect of the former is muscular rigidity with the upper limbs in flexion and the lower in extension, particularly evident when the patient is suspended in the air. The effect of symmetrical necrosis of the globus pallidus, commonly the result of carbon monoxide poisoning, is an akinetic mute state with generalized rigidity of all four limbs in a semi-flexed attitude.

THE PHYSIOLOGICAL NATURE OF DISORDERS OF THE CORPUS STRIATUM

The physiology of the extrapyramidal motor system has recently been reviewed by Jung and Hassler (1960). They begin by pointing out that the subject is difficult because 'extrapyramidal system' is defined anatomically and in a negative sense, since the functions of the corticospinal tracts are by definition excluded. Then our knowledge of extrapyramidal functions is mainly derived from neurological observations on man, and, finally, to consider a motor system in isolation from sensory control is to substitute a fiction for the reality. However, these authors agree with Denny-Brown that the corpus striatum plays a fundamental part in the regulation of posture, and they point out that since man differs from animals in his assumption of the erect posture, it is to be expected that the neural centres concerned with posture and locomotion will have distinctive functions in man, which they do not possess in quadrupedal animals. Denny-Brown sees many of the symptoms of lesions of the corpus striatum in relation to the righting reflexes, and draws attention to the way in which in extrapyramidal syndromes the posture of the patient and the involuntary movements can sometimes be modified by changing the position of his body in space, or removing it from contact with a surface. He also interprets some symptoms of striatal disease in terms of the grasping and avoiding reactions, which he has discussed elsewhere. The involuntary movements that result from diffuse partial lesions of the putamen and globus pallidus are to be regarded as different aspects of incomplete control of the labyrinthine and body-righting reflexes, and the cortical mechanisms that normally modify them. These reactions exemplify the principle that for every cerebral cortical function that is lost, a corresponding coarser type of subcortical reaction is released. The distortion of posture and movement known as athetosis is the result of a lesion of the putamen, but, as the lesion becomes increasingly severe, involuntary movements give place to a fixed posture (dystonia). Chorea is to be regarded as a disorder of subordinate centres, which normally regulate and reinforce corticospinal activity. Parkinsonism, due to impairment of function of the globus pallidus (according to Denny-Brown) or substantia nigra (according to Jung and Hassler) is characterized by a combination of impairment of certain important motor functions, and release phenomena, such as rigidity and tremor. There is evidence, cited by Jung and Hassler, that there is a disorder of the gamma innervation in Parkinsonism. They say that 'during many movements gamma innervation precedes the alpha innervation, the former having a kind of "starter function"; it is precisely this function, however, which is missing in Parkinsonism, in which the greatest difficulty is in the initiation of a movement (akinesia). The finding of excessive spinal motoneurone excitability, as demonstrated by facilitation of the H-reflex, in patients with Parkinsonian rigidity, as recently reviewed by Yap (1967), suggests that alpha motoneurones are hyperexcitable; the opposite may well be the case with gamma neurones. This accounts for the loss of a considerable number of involuntary movements, such as the spontaneous synergic and associated movements. The impairment of voluntary motor activity in general (bradykinesia) may also be explained by this deficiency of the central mechanism triggering the so-called "external loop".' The nature of Parkinsonian rigidity and tremor has been discussed above.

Any account of the functions of the basal ganglia must take into account the recent discovery of the effects of surgical lesions of the globus pallidus and ventrolateral nucleus of the thalamus. There is now ample evidence that a lesion in either of these situations will diminish or abolish the tremor and rigidity of Parkinsonism on the opposite side of the body, and may have a similar beneficial effect upon dystonia and hemiballismus, though athetosis is influenced very much less. It is difficult to reconcile the view that Parkinsonism is due to a lesion of the globus pallidus with the fact that it benefits from surgical lesions of that structure. On the other hand, the following hypothesis, which receives support from the views of Martin (1959, 1960, 1963, 1967) and Jung and Hassler, seems best to explain the known facts, though there are still considerable gaps in our knowledge. The basal ganglia include the caudate nucleus, the putamen, the globus pallidus, the substantia nigra, the subthalamic nucleus, and the red nucleus, and have close functional relationships with the cerebellum and the cerebral cortex. The basal ganglia play an important part in postural regulation, and are concerned with maintaining that background of involuntary activity which underlies all voluntary action. The globus pallidus constitutes the final coordinating pathway of the basal ganglionic mechanisms. Its activity is influenced and regulated by impulses derived from other parts of the system, notably the caudate nucleus, the putamen, the substantia nigra, and the subthalamic nucleus. If it be accepted that Parkinsonism results from a lesion of the substantia nigra, it may be concluded that the functions of that body are concerned, in the words of Jung and Hassler, with 'supranuclear control of the gamma neurons of the anterior horn and an inhibition of myotatic reflexes'. Failure to control myotatic reflexes leads to plastic rigidity, and failure of the 'starter function' of the substantia nigra in voluntary motor activity impairs 'phasic muscle innervation, the rapid onset of a movement, associated movements, and many automatic movements'. The development of tremor is attributed to loss of inhibitory activity of the substantia nigra over 'synchronising and de-synchronising reticulospinal influences' [see p. 517].

The subthalamic nucleus appears to be concerned with stabilization of the limbs on the opposite side of the body in relation to their posture at rest and also in voluntary movement. Destruction of this nucleus therefore leads to uncontrolled movements, and incoordination of postural mechanisms. A disorder of a somewhat similar type occurs in chorea, when the caudate nucleus and possibly some parts of the putamen are damaged, while lesions of the outer part of the putamen cause a different type of involuntary movement, athetosis, and release mechanisms concerned with body posture which show themselves in lesser degree in the postures adopted in athetosis, and in more severe forms in dystonia.

If all these extrapyramidal syndromes are due to a disturbance of what is normally a delicate physiological balance of these intricate systems, it may be presumed that the benefit which results from pallidectomy is due to the fact that, the globus pallidus being the main efferent nucleus, its destruction blocks the outgoing pathway of the whole basal ganglionic system, and ventrolateral thalamotomy has the same effect because the main efferent pathway from the globus pallidus runs to the ventrolateral nucleus of the thalamus. We are left with the unanswered question as to why these operations, if they in fact put the whole basal ganglionic mechanism out of action, leave the patient with no corresponding disability.

Various workers have claimed that different types of involuntary movement have benefited from surgical interruption of the corticospinal pathways either at the cortex or at a subcortical level, and it has even been suggested that corticospinal fibres may be damaged in their pathway through the internal capsule in the course of operations on the globus pallidus or thalamus. Physiologically, these observations are no doubt to be explained by the close relationship between voluntary movement and its background of involuntary postural and associated mechanisms, so that in so far as these are activated by voluntary movement, the symptoms of their disorder will be at any rate diminished by damage to the corticospinal pathways.

Finally, it must also be mentioned that recent biochemical studies have underlined the important part played by certain catecholamines in the functioning of the basal ganglia. The caudate nucleus and putamen, which contain little or no noradrenaline, are rich in dopamine, and Hornykiewicz (1963) and others have shown, in post-mortem studies on the brains of patients with Parkinsonism, that dopamine and its principal metabolite, homovanillic acid, may be reduced to 10 per cent. or less of their normal concentration in the basal ganglia and substantia nigra of such cases.

REFERENCES

ABBE-FESSARD, D., GUIOT, G., LAMARRE, Y., and ARFEL, G. (1966) Activation of thalamocortical projections related to tremorogenic processes, in *The Thalamus*, ed. PURPURA, D. P., and YAHR, M. D., p. 237, New York.

ALVORD, E. C., JR. (1958) Pathology of Parkinsonism, in *Pathogenesis and Treatment of Parkinsonism*, ed. FIELDS, W. S., Springfield, Ill.

DENNY-BROWN, D. (1960) Diseases of the basal ganglia, *Lancet*, ii, 1099, 1155.

DENNY-BROWN, D. (1962) *The Basal Ganglia: and Their Relation to Disorders of Movement*, Oxford.

GREENFIELD, J. G. (1958) in *Neurology*, by GREENFIELD, J. G., BLACKWOOD, W., McMENEMEY, W. H., MEYER, A., and NORMAN, R. M., p. 530, London.

HORNYKIEWICZ, O. (1963) Die topische Lokalisation und das Verhallen von Noradrenaline und Dopamin im der Substantia der normallen und Parkinson Kranken Menschen, *Wien. Klin. Wschr.*, 75, 309.

JUNG, R., and HASSLER, R. (1960) The extrapyramidal motor system, in *Handbook of Physiology*, vol. 2, p. 863, Washington.

MARTIN, J. P. (1957) Hemichorea (hemiballismus) without lesions in the corpus Luysii, *Brain*, 80, 1.

MARTIN, J. P. (1959) Remarks on the functions of the basal ganglia, *Lancet*, i, 999.

MARTIN, J. P. (1960) Further remarks on the function of the basal ganglia, *Lancet*, i, 1362.

MARTIN, J. P. (1963) The basal ganglia and locomotion, *Ann. roy. Coll. Surg. Engl.*, 32, 219.

MARTIN, J. P. (1967) *The Basal Ganglia and Posture*, London.

YAP, C.-B. (1967) Spinal segmental and long-loop reflexes on spinal motorneurone excitability in spasticity and rigidity, *Brain*, 90, 887.

THE PARKINSONIAN SYNDROME

Definition. The Parkinsonian syndrome, named after James Parkinson, who first described paralysis agitans in 1817, is a disturbance of motor function characterized chiefly by slowing and enfeeblement of emotional and voluntary movement, muscular rigidity, and tremor. Parkinsonism may be produced by a number of different pathological states and is usually ascribed to lesions involving the corpus striatum or the substantia nigra.

AETIOLOGY AND PATHOLOGY

Jakob and Ramsay Hunt considered that loss of the large ganglion cells of the corpus striatum was the essential cause of Parkinsonism, though the former placed the lesion principally in the caudate nucleus and putamen and the latter in the globus pallidus. A number of workers have demonstrated that in Parkinsonism due to encephalitis lethargica there are constant changes in the substantia nigra, but that the corpus striatum may be normal.

The histological changes depend upon the nature of the causal pathological process. Greenfield and Bosanquet (1953) and Greenfield (1958) review the pathology of idiopathic and encephalitic Parkinsonism, with special reference to the substantia nigra and the locus caeruleus. They describe five types of cell change: (1) saccular distension with lipochrome granules, (2) vacuolation, and (3) binucleated cells—all changes found in post-encephalitic Parkinsonism, (4) Lewy's spherical concentric hyaline inclusions, found in idiopathic Parkinsonism, and (5) neurofibrillary tangles, found in post-encephalitic cases. Yet these distinctions may not be absolute. Multifocal cerebral softening due to vascular occlusion is the basis of Parkinsonism due to cerebral arteriosclerosis. Drugs of the phenothiazine group, used chiefly in the treatment of psychiatric disorders, have been found to produce a variety of extrapyramidal syndromes, chiefly Parkinsonian (Ayd, 1961), although distressing and irreversible dyskinesias of the lips and tongue have also been reported (Hunter, Earl, and Janz, 1964). A Parkinsonian syndrome may also be due to poisoning with carbon monoxide or with manganese and has been observed to follow severe head injury. It has been observed to follow injury to a limb, the symptoms beginning in the injured limb. The so-called 'punch-drunk' syndrome, occurring as a result of repeated head injury in professional boxers often shows certain clinical affinities with Parkinsonism. It is rarely due to neurosyphilis.

In a recent series of 100 consecutive cases of Parkinsonism of all types there were 42 males and 58 females, but Kurland (1958) reports a slight excess of males. The ages of onset were:

10–19	20–29	30–39	40–49	50–59	60–69	70+
3	0	2	18	33	29	12

(3 indeterminate)

The death rate in North America is between 1·7 and 1·9 per 100,000 (Kurland).

SYMPTOMS

A general description of the symptoms of the Parkinsonian syndrome will first be given, and the distinctive features of the various forms of the disorder will then be considered separately. Their pathogenesis is discussed on page 518.

Facies and Attitude

The Parkinsonian facies is characteristic. The palpebral fissures are usually wider than normal, and blinking is infrequent. The eyes have a staring appearance, due partly to these features and partly to the fact that spontaneous ocular movements are lacking or seldom occur. The facial muscles exhibit an unnatural immobility [FIG. 81]. The attitude of the limbs and trunk is one of moderate flexion. The spine is usually somewhat flexed, but is occasionally extended. There is little rotatory movement of the cervical spine. The limbs are moderately flexed and adducted, but the wrist is usually slightly extended. The fingers are flexed at the metacarpophalangeal, and extended or only slightly flexed at the interphalangeal, joints, and adducted. The thumb is usually adducted, and extended at the metacarpo- and interphalangeal joints.

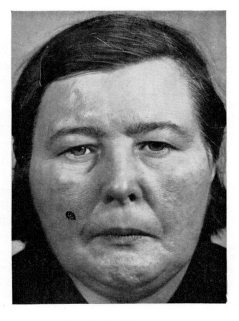

FIG. 81. Parkinsonism

Disorders of Movement (Akinesia and Bradykinesia)

Voluntary movement exhibits some impairment of power, but more striking is the slowness with which it is performed. It is important to recognize that, in many cases, signs may initially be present on one side of the body and not on the other ('hemiplegic' Parkinsonism). In general, the movements which are carried out by small muscles suffer most. Hence the patient shows weakness of the ocular movements, especially convergence; of the facial movements, associated with tremor of the eyelids on closure of the eyes; and of movements concerned in mastication, deglutition, and articulation. The speech in severe cases is slurred, quiet and monotonous, owing to defective pronunciation of consonants and lack of variation in pitch. Rarely palilalia occurs and occasionally in severe cases phonation and articulation is so impaired by muscular rigidity and akinesia that the patient is virtually mute. Movements of the small muscles of the hands are also markedly affected, with resulting clumsiness and inability to perform fine movements, such as those used in needlework, dealing cards, and taking money from a pocket. Characteristically the range of movement, as in opposition of the thumb and individual fingers is greatly reduced. Micrographia is common; the writing becomes progressively smaller and may trail away to nothing. Certain associated and synergic movements suffer conspicuously. Swinging of the arms in walking is early diminished and later lost, and the synergic extension of the wrist, which is normally associated with flexion of the fingers, is also impaired. Thoracic expansion in inspiration is reduced, but the contraction of the diaphragm may be increased in compensation.

Emotional movements of the face are also reduced in amplitude, slow in developing, and unduly protracted.

Muscular Rigidity

Muscular rigidity does not always develop *pari passu* with the disorders of movement just described, which not uncommonly somewhat precede it. It differs from the hypertonia associated with corticospinal lesions in that it is present to an equal extent in opposing muscle-groups, for example, the flexors and extensors of the elbow; it is uniform throughout the whole angle of movement at a joint. When tremor is also present the rigidity exhibits an interrupted character when tested by passive movement, the muscles yielding to tension in a series of jerks, hence the term 'cog-wheel rigidity'. When tremor is absent the rigidity is smooth and is of the so-called 'plastic' or 'lead-pipe' variety. Parkinsonian rigidity, like other Parkinsonian symptoms, is often unequal on the two sides of the body. In spite of the rigidity full passive movement is usually possible at all joints. Occasionally, however, contractures occur which limit such movement. This happens most frequently in the hands and the feet. The fingers may be so strongly flexed that a pad has to be used to prevent the nails being driven into the palm. Similar flexor deformity of the toes may occur, and talipes equinovarus may be produced.

Gait

The Parkinsonian gait is in part at least the outcome of the patient's attitude and rigidity. It is usually slow, shuffling, and composed of small steps (*marche à petits pas*). The patient is often unable to stop quickly when pushed forwards or backwards—propulsion and retropulsion. When propulsion occurs spontaneously during walking, the patient exhibits a 'festinating' gait, hurrying with small steps in a bent attitude as if trying to catch up his centre of gravity. Some patients find their gait arrested, especially if they try to change direction, or when attempting to begin to walk (akinesia). A striking feature of Parkinsonism is the frequent ability of the patient to carry out rapid movements requiring considerable exertion better than slower and less energetic movements. Thus a patient who can walk only very slowly may be able to run quite fast. This phenomenon has been called 'kinesia paradoxa'.

Tremor

Tremor is the characteristic involuntary movement of Parkinsonism. Tremor, rigidity, and slowness and weakness of movement are, however, to a large extent independent variables. Tremor may be the first symptom, as it frequently is in paralysis agitans, and may precede rigidity by months or years. In post-encephalitic Parkinsonism rigidity more often precedes tremor. Tremor usually begins in one upper limb and later involves the lower limb on the same side, the other side being affected in the same order after a further interval. The head is involved late, if at all.

The tremor consists of rhythmic alternating movements of opposing muscle-groups [FIG. 82]. In the upper limb the hand is most affected. Movements of the fingers occur at the metacarpophalangeal joints and may be combined with movements of the thumb—the 'pill-rolling movement'. Movements at the wrist may be flexion and extension, lateral displacement, or pronation and supination. Often the tremor shifts from one to another group of muscles while the patient is under observation. Little movement usually occurs at the joints above the wrist. In the lower limb tremor is most marked at the ankle, at which flexion and extension occur. Either flexion and extension or a rotatory tremor of the head may occur. When the mandibular muscles are involved, rhythmical opening and closure of the mouth are observed, and in the tongue the tremor takes the form of protrusion and withdrawal.

The rate of the tremor lies between four and eight movements a second, being slower in paralysis agitans than in post-encephalitic Parkinsonism. It is present when the patient is at rest ('static' tremor), and is often temporarily or wholly suppressed when the limb is voluntarily moved. Rarely, however, it is present throughout movement ('action' tremor). It can often be inhibited for a time by conscious effort, but is liable to break from this control with increased intensity. It is increased by emotional excitement and almost always disappears during sleep.

Sensory Symptoms

There is no loss of sensibility in Parkinsonism. Pain, however, is common, especially in the later stages, when most patients complain of cramp-like pains in the limbs and spine due to the muscular rigidity and the changes induced in the joints and ligaments by the abnormal posture. Extreme restlessness is also a common symptom, the patient suffering great discomfort unless his position is changed every few minutes.

The Reflexes

Parkinsonism does not involve any essential changes in the reflexes, though rigidity may render the tendon-jerks difficult to elicit and reduced in amplitude. However, in the early stages the reflexes may actually be increased in limbs

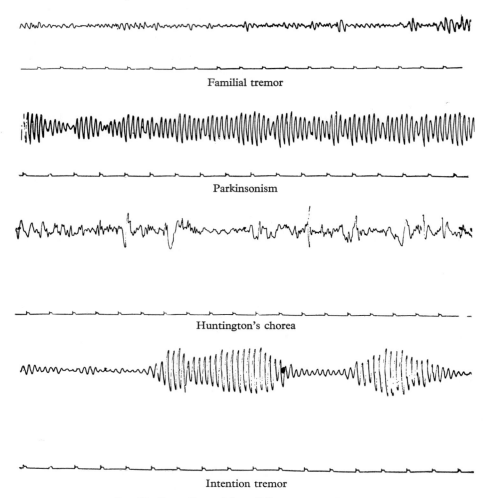

Familial tremor

Parkinsonism

Huntington's chorea

Intention tremor

FIG. 82. Recordings of four different types of tremor.

The intervals on the time marker are one second.
(By courtesy of Dr. John Marshall.)

showing early rigidity and in a case of 'hemiplegic' Parkinsonism this may give rise to diagnostic difficulty. The plantar reflexes are usually flexor, but it is not unknown for one or both to be extensor, due either to involvement of the corticospinal tracts by the encephalitic or arteriosclerotic lesion responsible for the Parkinsonism or to associated cervical spondylosis leading to myelopathy. Cases of presenile dementia with Parkinsonian features and with evidence of pyramidal tract dysfunction, often classified in the past, probably incorrectly, as examples of Jakob-Creutzfeld disease, also occur.

Autonomic Symptoms

Derangement of the autonomic nervous system is probably responsible for a group of symptoms which often cause much discomfort. Flushing of the skin may occur accompanied by uncomfortable sensations of heat and sometimes by sweating. These symptoms may be limited to, or more marked upon, one side of the body. Oedema and cyanosis of a limb are rare. Parkinsonian patients usually tolerate cold much better than heat, and will often sit out of doors, lightly clad, in the coldest weather without feeling cold. This fact, combined with their immobility, renders such patients particularly liable to suffer episodes of hypothermia, particularly if confined to bed in an unheated room in cold weather. Excessive salivation is also a feature in many cases. There is usually a gradual loss of weight.

Mental State

Parkinsonism is not necessarily accompanied by any mental change, and the sufferer's intellectual capacity and emotional reactions may continue unimpaired behind the mask in which his disorder fixes his features. But when the syndrome is a manifestation of a diffuse pathological process, such as cerebral arteriosclerosis or encephalitis lethargica, involvement of other parts of the brain may cause associated mental deterioration, leading to various degrees of dementia, or a loss of emotional responsiveness, or profound depression with a suicidal tendency. It must also be borne in mind that Parkinsonian features may be present in certain forms of presenile dementia, and such cases are often familial. In the island of Guam, a familial Parkinsonism-dementia complex, often associated with features of motor neurone disease, is common and is due to progressive degenerative changes which are widespread in the cerebral hemispheres, brain stem and spinal cord (Hirano, Malamud, and Kurland, 1961).

FORMS OF PARKINSONISM

PARALYSIS AGITANS

Synonyms. Parkinson's disease; shaking palsy.

PATHOLOGY

See page 522.

AETIOLOGY

The disease appears to be a primary degeneration, and it is doubtful whether external factors have any aetiological significance, though there is some rather indefinite evidence that injury to a limb may determine the site of onset of the symptoms. Males are affected about twice as frequently as females. Paralysis agitans is a disease of late middle life and begins in most cases between the ages of 50 and 60. In women its onset not uncommonly occurs within a year or two of the menopause and in men at about 60. It rarely begins before 40 or after 65, but in the rare juvenile form the onset may be as early as the second decade (Hunt, 1917). Exceptionally it is hereditary or familial—in 16 per cent. of cases according to Kurland (1958).

SYMPTOMS

In the majority of cases tremor is the first symptom. Less frequently weakness, stiffness, and slowness of movements are complained of before tremor. The tremor usually begins in one hand—as a rule the right—the leg on the same side being next involved. After a further interval it spreads to the opposite hand and later to the opposite leg. It may be confined to one side of the body for several years, but both upper limbs may be affected before the lower limbs. The characteristics of the tremor, rigidity, and other symptoms have already been described. The pupils are often rather contracted but usually react normally.

PROGNOSIS

The disease is always progressive, though cases differ considerably in the rate of progress. The symptoms may be confined to one limb for months or years, and the spread to other limbs when it occurs may be slow or fairly rapid. The prognosis in cases in which tremor in one upper limb is the only manifestation of the disease during the first two or three years is very much better than in the average case. The development of rigidity may diminish the tremor, but greatly reduces the patient's activities. Even so he may survive in a helpless condition for many years. The average duration of the disease is about ten years, but it is not uncommon for patients to live considerably longer. Death occurs usually from complications such as pneumonia or bed-sores. Occasionally there is a terminal stage of lethargy passing into coma.

PARKINSONISM FOLLOWING ENCEPHALITIS LETHARGICA

PATHOLOGY

See pages 518 and 522.

AETIOLOGY

See pages 438 and 522.

SYMPTOMS

It was common to observe some Parkinsonian symptoms in the acute attack of encephalitis and in many cases Parkinsonism developed insidiously during the subsequent twelve months. The interval, however, may be as long as twenty years; or there may be no history of an acute attack obtainable. Since the greatest incidence of the disease is in early adult life, for 20 years after the epidemic most cases of encephalitic Parkinsonism occurred before the age of 40. Now this is no longer true and the age of onset may be as late as 60. With the virtual disappearance of encephalitis lethargica it now seems that this form of the disease is also gradually disappearing.

Stiffness, slowness of movement, and weakness usually precede tremor. These symptoms are usually more marked upon, and may be confined to, one side of the body. Sometimes they are even more restricted and involve only one upper limb, or one upper limb and the same side of the face. In the early stages the upper limb is usually more affected than the lower. Rigidity is usually more conspicuous than tremor throughout the course of the illness. The pupillary reactions to accommodation or to light or to both are usually impaired, and mental apathy or depression is usually conspicuous. There is often an excess of sebaceous secretion over the face, and of saliva which characteristically drips from the open mouth.

Oculogyral Spasm

Spasm of conjugate ocular muscles was a not infrequent complication of Parkinsonism following encephalitis lethargica, but is now rarely seen except in hospitals with many sufferers from encephalitis, but it is also one of the dystonic symptoms produced by drugs of the phenothiazine group. The attacks last from a few seconds to hours. The eyes are usually deviated upwards, with lids retracted, less often laterally, and rarely downwards or obliquely. There may be an associated spasmodic deviation of the head in the same direction. Occasionally the eyes become fixed when the gaze is directed forwards, or in a position of convergence. During the attack the patient's attempts to move the eyes in other directions result in only a very feeble, jerky displacement from the position of spasmodic deviation.

Other Encephalitic Symptoms

Other encephalitic symptoms may be associated with the Parkinsonism, especially torticollis or other dystonic attitudes of the trunk and limbs. Bizarre contractures of the extremities are not infrequently seen in severe post-encephalitic cases but are rare in paralysis agitans.

PROGNOSIS

In most cases Parkinsonism following encephalitis is a progressive condition running a much shorter course than paralysis agitans. In a few cases the disorder seems to become arrested and this happens most often when the symptoms are predominantly unilateral. In severe cases the patient may become quite incapacitated within a year of the onset of symptoms, but at present milder chronic cases are the rule and the disorder often reaches a stationary condition. Death is due to pneumonia, bed-sores, or a general cachexia terminating in coma.

ARTERIOSCLEROTIC PARKINSONISM

Parkinsonian features may make their appearance in the course of cerebral arteriosclerosis, but the resulting clinical picture is not only very variable in itself but is also frequently complicated by the presence of other symptoms of vascular lesions. Thus a Parkinsonian syndrome may exist alone, or in association with pseudobulbar palsy, corticospinal lesions, dementia, or signs of a lesion of the midbrain.

The majority of cases are due to the decrescent type of arteriosclerosis with low blood pressure, and are, therefore, found in late middle and old age. However, a number of patients with severe hypertension and with consequent multiple small softenings in the cerebral hemispheres and brain stem may develop a slow shuffling gait, facial immobility, emotional lability (pathological over-emotionalism) with rigidity of the limbs, hyperreflexia and extensor plantar responses. These patients often develop other signs of pseudobulbar palsy. The age-incidence is generally later than that of paralysis agitans, though in severely hypertensive patients it may occur earlier in life. The onset is usually insidious, but in some cases follows a 'stroke'; and a series of mild 'strokes' may each be followed by an increase in the severity of the symptoms.

Of the true Parkinsonian symptoms, the expressionless facies, bodily attitude, slowness and weakness of movement, and the festinating gait are the commonest. The rigidity is often atypical, being variable in degree and predominating in the flexors of the elbows and in the extensors of the knees. Parkinsonian tremor is rare in these cases. Catatonia is not uncommon. It seems probable that the symptoms are in part due to lesions at a higher level than the corpus striatum, interrupting corticostriate fibres.

The course of the disorder is more rapid than that of paralysis agitans. When the blood pressure is high, a fatal cerebral haemorrhage may occur. Progressive dementia, dysphagia and eventual incontinence render nursing difficult, and the patient succumbs in a few years.

THE DIAGNOSIS OF PARKINSONISM

It is necessary to distinguish the Parkinsonian syndrome from other conditions which may simulate it. The most striking Parkinsonian symptoms being tremor and muscular rigidity, Parkinsonism is most likely to be confused with conditions causing one or other of these symptoms.

Other Causes of Tremor

Senile Tremor. Tremor is not uncommon in old age. It differs from Parkinsonian tremor in being finer and more rapid. At first it is absent when the limbs are at rest and occurs only on voluntary movement ('action' tremor). Later it may be present during rest also. It is most marked in the upper limbs, but is more frequently present in the head than Parkinsonian tremor. The rhythmical to-and-fro 'titubating' movements of the head are characteristic. It is not associated with muscular weakness or rigidity.

Benign or 'Essential' Familial Tremor. This is a form of tremor which may occur in several members of the same family, sometimes in successive generations. It may begin in childhood and usually develops during the first twenty-five years of life. It may be fine and rapid or slower and coarser, is usually absent at rest in the early stages and tends to be increased by voluntary movement and emotion. It is thus classified as an action tremor; senile tremor may be regarded as a similar disorder of sporadic occurrence in late life. It may be generalized or involve especially the hands, lips, and tongue. As a rule it persists and worsens slightly throughout life and no other nervous abnormality occurs. In rare instances paralysis agitans has been observed in a member of a family afflicted with familial tremor. A curious feature of benign familial tremor is that it is almost specifically, though temporarily, relieved by ethyl alcohol.

Hysterical Tremor. Two forms of hysterical tremor are encountered: a fine tremor, localized to one limb or generalized, and resembling the shaking of extreme fear, of which it is probably a perpetuation; and a coarse, irregular shaking, intensified by voluntary movement. In common with other hysterical symptoms, hysterical tremor is characterized by its irregularity, variability from time to time, and by a tendency to diminish when the patient's attention is distracted and to increase when it is directed to the affected part of the body. The tremor of acute anxiety states is similar but less florid and variable.

Tremor in Hyperthyroidism. This is a fine, rapid tremor usually confined to the outstretched arms and sometimes more marked on one side than the other. The associated exophthalmos, thyroid enlargement, tachycardia, and flushed and sweating skin usually render diagnosis easy.

Toxic Tremor. Tremor may be a symptom of intoxication with various poisons, especially mercury, cocaine, and alcohol. The tremor of cocaine addiction and chronic alcoholism is fine and is unlikely to be confused with Parkinsonian tremor. The tremor of chronic mercurial poisoning and delirium tremens is somewhat coarser, but has not the rhythmical character of Parkinsonian tremor. In all these cases the cause is usually easily discoverable, and in delirium tremens the acute onset and characteristic mental symptoms are distinctive.

Multiple Sclerosis. In multiple sclerosis intention tremor is common as it is in other conditions causing cerebellar ataxia. It is absent when the limb is at rest and develops only during voluntary movement, increasing as the limb approaches its objective. In this respect it is the opposite of Parkinsonian tremor, which is present at rest and diminishes on movement. Static tremor is rare in multiple sclerosis, and is most often seen in the head. It disappears when the patient is lying with the neck muscles relaxed. In this disease there are usually nystagmus and signs of corticospinal lesions, which, apart from the character of the tremor, distinguish it from Parkinsonism.

Hereditary Ataxia

Intention tremor similar to that observed in multiple sclerosis is a common feature of several types of inherited cerebellar degeneration. Static tremor, showing certain resemblances to that of Parkinsonism is, however, seen in patients with olivo-ponto-cerebellar degeneration in which, however, the associated features of dementia, cerebellar ataxia and corticospinal tract degeneration are distinctive.

General Paresis. Tremor affecting especially the face, tongue, and hands is an early symptom of general paresis. This is a fine tremor, increased on voluntary movement. The mental changes, Argyll Robertson pupils, signs of corticospinal tract lesions, and positive V.D.R.L. reaction in the blood and spinal fluid will distinguish the condition from Parkinsonism.

Other States of Rigidity

Hysterical Rigidity. This is characterized by the fact that the degree of the rigidity is proportional to the observer's efforts to move the limb. In

Parkinsonism the rigidity is, by contrast, a definite quantum which always yields to the exercise of slightly greater force.

Spasticity due to Corticospinal Tract Lesions. This is distinguished by the selective distribution of the rigidity to certain muscle groups, usually the flexors in the upper and the extensors in the lower limbs. Moreover, it tends to be maximal at the beginning of a passive movement and to diminish as the movement proceeds. Parkinsonian rigidity is uniform both in its distribution and throughout the angle of joint movement. In paraplegia-in-flexion hypertonia occurs in the flexors of the lower limbs, but in this condition, as in paraplegia-in-extension, the plantar reflexes are extensor, whereas they are flexor in un-complicated Parkinsonism.

Multiple Arthritis. Rigidity due to joint disease occasionally simulates Parkinsonism, especially when the vertebral joints are affected. The flexion of the spine and immobility of the head may at first glance be deceptive. Pain in such cases, however, is usually severe at some stage of the disease, and it is easy to demonstrate that the rigidity is bony and not muscular in origin.

TREATMENT

Though the treatment of Parkinsonism is palliative rather than curative, much can be done to relieve the patient's discomfort.

The sufferer from Parkinsonism should be encouraged to lead an active life as long as possible but should avoid fatigue. A 'zip' fastener on the trousers is a convenience. Massage and passive movements are valuable for their temporary effect in diminishing the rigidity, but more as a means of postponing the development of contractures. Re-educational walking exercises under the supervision of a skilled physiotherapist are often valuable. A walking-stick is an invaluable aid in many cases and in patients with severe akinesia a frame walking aid which encourages the patient to lean forwards and to initiate those walking reflexes which are impaired by the disease process may be very helpful. For many years the only drugs available to diminish the rigidity were those of the belladonna group, and these also reduce salivation and sweating. Traditional remedies such as hyoscine hydrobromide, belladonna and stramonium, which undoubtedly reduce rigidity and salivation, have now been supplanted by synthetic anti-spasmodic drugs. On the whole the most useful are benzhexol (*Artane*), beginning with 2 mg. three times a day, and ethopropazine (*Lysivane*), beginning with 50–200 mg. a day and increasing the dose in accordance with the patient's tolerance, or orphenadrine hydrochloride (*Disipal*), 50–100 mg. up to three times a day. It is often necessary to try several preparations, since the drug which suits one patient may not suit another. Benztropine (*Cogentin*), 1–2 mg. at night, and methixene (*Tremonil*), 5–10 mg. three times a day, may be a little more successful than other remedies in controlling tremor but no drug is really effective in this respect; in Tennyson's words, 'What drugs can make a wither'd palsy cease to shake?'. All of the drugs mentioned may produce dryness of the mouth, constipation, and blurring of vision. The latter may be helped by adding pilocarpine, 10 mg. three times daily. Confusion is an even more important side-effect, particularly in elderly patients and may be accompanied by disturbing visual and auditory hallucinations. Retention of urine may also occur. Such side-effects may even necessitate withdrawal of all drugs in a few cases. Most patients are best treated by a combination of up to two drugs (e.g. *Artane* and *Cogentin*; or *Disipal* and *Tremonil*). Amphetamine is sometimes of value in diminishing the rigidity and oculogyric spasms and improving the mental state. When the patient becomes bedridden much care will be needed to prevent the development of bed-sores and to maintain adequate nutrition.

The recent introduction of *l*-DOPA as a means of treating the condition may well prove to be a major advance. The drug is not yet generally available but preliminary reports (Cotzias *et al.*, 1967) suggest that this substance, when given in an initial dosage of 1 G. daily, increasing, depending on tolerance and response, up to 5 G. daily or more, is sometimes dramatically successful in relieving akinesia or bradykinesia in many cases, though it has little effect upon tremor. Side-effects of the drug include nausea, granulocytopenia, and involuntary movements of choreo-athetotic type.

Surgery

The operations of pallidectomy and ventrolateral thalamotomy, or both combined, now have an established place in the treatment of Parkinsonism. In general, surgery is most suitable for idiopathic Parkinsonism with unilateral symptoms in a patient under the age of 65. Severe akinesia, generalized cerebral atheroma, and hypertension are contra-indications (Cooper, 1961; Gillingham *et al.*, 1960). Various stereotaxic techniques are used by different neurosurgeons; chemopallidectomy (injection of alcohol) has now been largely supplanted by methods involving thermocoagulation or freezing (cryothalamotomy). Increasing experience has indicated that tremor can be greatly reduced or abolished and rigidity reduced by these methods but akinesia, speech disturbance, and salivation are uninfluenced. Dementia is a complete contra-indication to surgery. Bilateral operations carried out simultaneously, or with an interval of a few months between the two procedures, are now practicable, even in patients of 70 years or older who are in good general condition, but confusion and permanent intellectual impairment are more common after bilateral procedures and patients must still be carefully selected for surgical treatment which is only one method of treatment in such cases and does not as a rule supplant the use of appropriate drugs (Hankinson, 1960; Cooper, 1965; Selby, 1967).

REFERENCES

AYD, F. J., JR. (1961) A survey of drug-induced extrapyramidal reactions, *J. Amer. med. Ass.*, **175**, 1054.

BOGAERT, L. VAN (1930) Contribution clinique et anatomique à l'étude de la paralysie agitante, juvénile primitive, *Rev. neurol. (Paris)*, **2**, 315.

BUCY, P. C. (1951) The surgical treatment of extrapyramidal diseases, *J. Neurol. Neurosurg. Psychiat.*, **14**, 108.

COOPER, I. S. (1961) *Parkinsonism, Its Medical and Surgical Treatment*, Springfield, Ill.

COOPER, I. S. (1965) The surgical treatment of Parkinsonism, *Ann. Rev. Med.*, **16**, 309.

COTZIAS, G. C., VAN WOERT, M. H., and SCHIFFER, L. M. (1967) Aromatic amino acids and modification of Parkinsonism, *New Engl. J. Med.*, **276**, 374.

CRITCHLEY, M. (1929) Arteriosclerotic Parkinsonism, *Brain*, **52**, 23.

CRITCHLEY, M. (1949) Observations on essential (heredofamilial) tremor, *Brain*, **72**, 113.

DENNY-BROWN, D. (1962) *The Basal Ganglia and Their Relation to Disorders of Movement*, Oxford.

FOERSTER, O. (1921) Zur Analyse und Pathophysiologie der striären Bewegungsstörungen, *Z. ges. Neurol. Psychiat.*, **73**, 1.

GILLINGHAM, F. J., WATSON, W. S., DONALDSON, A. A., and NAUGHTON, J. A. L. (1960) The surgical treatment of Parkinsonism, *Brit. med. J.*, **2**, 1395.

GREENFIELD, J. G. (1958) in *Neuropathology*, by GREENFIELD, J. G., MCMENEMEY, W. H., MEYER, A., and NORMAN, R. M., p. 530, London.

GREENFIELD, J. G., and BOSANQUET, F. D. (1953) The brain-stem lesions in Parkinsonism, *J. Neurol. Neurosurg. Psychiat.*, **16**, 213.

HALL, A. J. (1931) Chronic epidemic encephalitis, with special reference to the ocular attacks, *Brit. med. J.*, **2**, 833.

HANKINSON, J. (1960) The surgical treatment of Parkinson's disease, *Postgrad. med. J.*, **36**, 242.

HIRANO, A., MALAMUD, N., and KURLAND, L. T. (1961) Parkinsonism-dementia complex—an endemic disease on the island of Guam, II, Pathological features, *Brain*, **84**, 662.

HUNT, J. R. (1917) Progressive atrophy of the globus pallidus, *Brain*, **40**, 58.

HUNTER, R., EARL, C. J., and JANZ, D. (1964) A syndrome of abnormal movements and dementia in leucotomized patients treated with phenothiazines, *J. Neurol. Psychiat.*, **27**, 219.

JAKOB, A. (1925) The anatomy, clinical syndromes and physiology of the extrapyramidal system, *Arch. Neurol. Psychiat. (Chicago)*, **13**, 596.

KESCHNER, M., and SLOANE, P. (1931) Encephalitic, idiopathic and arteriosclerotic Parkinsonism, *Arch. Neurol. Psychiat. (Chicago)*, **25**, 1011.

KLIPPEL, M., and LHERMITTE, J. (1925) Les syndromes sous-corticaux, *Nouveau traite de médecine*, fasc. xix. 149.

KURLAND, L. T. (1958) in *The Pathology and Treatment of Parkinsonism*, ed. FIELDS, W. S., p. 5, Springfield, Ill.

LARSSON, T., and SJÖGREN, T. (1960) Essential tremor, *Acta psychiat. (Kbh.)*, **36**, Suppl. 144.

LOTMAR, F. (1928) Zur traumatischen Entstehung der Paralysis agitans, *Nervenarzt*, **1**, 6.

POLLOCK, M., and HORNABROOK, R. W. (1966) The prevalence, natural history and dementia of Parkinson's disease, *Brain*, **89**, 429.

SELBY, G. (1967) Stereotactic surgery for the relief of Parkinson's disease, *J. neurol. Sci.*, **5**, 315, 343.

WALKER, G. F. (1937) Parkinsonism following peripheral trauma, *Brit. med. J.*, **2**, 65.

WILSON'S DISEASE

Synonyms. Tetanoid chorea (Gowers); pseudosclerosis (Westphal); progressive lenticular degeneration; hepatolenticular degeneration.

Definition. A progressive disease of early life which is due to an autosomal recessive gene and is characterized by a disorder of copper metabolism leading to degeneration of certain regions of the brain, especially the corpus striatum, and cirrhosis of the liver, and clinically by increasing muscular rigidity, tremor and progressive dementia. Although pseudosclerosis, which was first investigated by Alzheimer, Westphal, and others between 1883 and 1898, and progressive lenticular degeneration, described by Wilson in 1912, were at one time thought to be different diseases and are still so regarded by some authorities, they are now more usually considered to be identical and are both included under the title Wilson's disease.

PATHOLOGY

The pathological change in the nervous system consists of a degeneration of ganglion cells with neuroglial overgrowth, but without evidence of inflammation or vascular abnormality. Alzheimer's type 2 cells are present. This change is most marked in the putamen of the lentiform nucleus which in severe and un-treated cases may show cavitation. The caudate nucleus is usually similarly affected, though to a lesser extent, but the globus pallidus is less frequently involved. Similar alterations are often present in other parts of the nervous system; for example, in the cerebral cortex, the thalamus, the red nucleus, and the cerebellum. Macroscopically the most conspicuous abnormality is found in the lentiform nucleus. In about half the recorded cases visible softening and cavitation of both lentiform nuclei have been observed. In other cases the nucleus has appeared shrunken and occasionally its naked-eye appearance is normal.

In the liver the changes are those of a multilobular cirrhosis which possesses no distinctive characteristics, and is often associated with enlargement of the spleen. The typical Kayser–Fleischer ring around the edge of the cornea has been shown to be due to copper deposition.

AETIOLOGY

Much recent work has been done on the metabolism of patients with Wilson's disease. It has been shown that there is an increased excretion of amino acids in the urine, not only in patients but also in their asymptomatic siblings (Matthews, Milne, and Bell, 1952; Denny-Brown, 1953). An abnormal concentration of copper has been found in the liver and in the brain, and an increased excretion in the urine (Mandelbrote et al., 1948; Cumings, 1951). Matthews (1954), using radio-copper, found an increased absorption, and that copper exists in an abnormal form in the plasma. The copper-carrying protein in the plasma, caerulo-plasmin, is reduced to 10 per cent. of normal. It seems that failure to synthesize this protein is the basic genetically-determined abnormality which is responsible for the disease (Walshe, 1967). The loosely combined copper is normal or some-what increased in amount. Hence copper is deposited in the tissues and excreted in increased quantities in the urine.

Hepatolenticular degeneration is a disease of adolescence and early adult life, which usually produces clinical manifestations first between the ages of 10 and 25 years.

SYMPTOMS

Nervous Symptoms

In most cases choreiform movements of the face and hands or flapping tremor are the first symptoms. These movements may occur when the limbs are apparently at rest and yet be abolished by complete relaxation or support. They are increased by voluntary movement. Athetoid and writhing move-ments of the trunk and limbs have, however, been observed, and one patient in the terminal stage exhibited violent muscular spasms resembling tetanus. In general, plastic rigidity followed by tremor or athetoid movements characterize the younger patients while tremor precedes rigidity in those in whom the onset is over the age of 20.

Rigidity in distribution and general character resembles the rigidity of Parkinsonism. The limbs become fixed, usually in a position of flexion, and contractures ultimately develop, but in younger patients the terminal state is a bilateral hemiplegic dystonia.

Voluntary movement is impaired, and articulation and deglutition are early and severely affected. Speech may become unintelligible or the patient may even lose entirely the power of articulation. The facies exhibits, as in Parkinsonism, a vacant, expressionless appearance, or a vacuous smile. Loss of emotional control is usually present, and involuntary laughing and crying may occur. There seems always to be some degree of mental deterioration amounting to a mild dementia. There is no essential change in the tendon-jerks or the abdominal reflexes, though muscular rigidity may render them difficult to elicit. The plantar reflexes are flexor and there is no disturbance of sensibility.

Corneal Pigmentation (The Kayser–Fleischer Ring)

Corneal pigmentation was first observed by Kayser and Fleischer. Although it has been described in only a proportion of cases, it is present with sufficient frequency to render it of diagnostic value. It may be invisible in daylight and is best seen with the slit lamp and corneal microscope. Indeed, slit-lamp examination reveals that it is present in virtually all cases. It consists of a zone of golden-brown granular pigmentation about 2 mm. in diameter on the posterior surface of the cornea towards the limbus. It is due to the deposit of copper, and may be present before any nervous symptoms have developed.

Symptoms of Cirrhosis of the Liver

Although these may be inconspicuous, in some cases they prove fatal before the patient develops any nervous symptoms. In the early stages pyrexial attacks, with slight jaundice, may occur; later the liver may be enlarged, and ascites, haematemesis, and other symptoms of portal obstruction may be present.

Biochemical Changes

Biochemical tests of value include a low serum copper (normal 86–112 μg. per 100 ml.) a low caeruloplasmin in the blood (normal 27–38 mg. per 100 ml.), and a high urinary copper (normal 24-hour excretion 0–26 μg.) especially if increased after treatment with BAL or penicillamine. Both total and α amino acids are increased in the urine and figures up to 500–600 mg. of α amino acids a day may be found. Patients do not incorporate radioactive copper, ^{67}Cu, normally with caeruloplasmin. Some biochemical abnormalities may be present in clinically normal heterozygotes.

DIAGNOSIS

There are few disorders with which Wilson's disease is likely to be confused. No other disease is characterized by the familial occurrence of tremor and rigidity with liver damage in the second decade of life. Corneal pigmentation and symptoms of cirrhosis of the liver, when present, are pathognomonic. Sporadic cases may simulate other disorders in which the corpus striatum is damaged. Double athetosis, which is characterized by muscular rigidity and choreo-athetoid movements, is usually congenital. Symptoms are therefore present from an early age, and some improvement may occur.

Other rare familial degenerative disorders of the corpus striatum, without liver damage, cause progressive rigidity, spasmodic laughing, dysarthria, and dementia beginning in childhood, e.g. Hallervorden-Spatz disease and progressive pallidal degeneration.

When Wilson's disease is suspected in one member of a family, all the sibs should be examined for evidence of nervous abnormalities, cirrhosis of the liver, corneal pigmentation, and biochemical change. Any of these symptoms, if present, will not only render it possible to anticipate the development of the disorder in other members of the family but will afford support for the diagnosis in the patient already affected.

PROGNOSIS

The course of the disease may be acute, subacute, or chronic, but it is invariably fatal if not treated. In the shortest illness on record death occurred five weeks after the onset of symptoms. Before effective treatment was available 50 per cent. of patients died in from one to six years. It is now recognized, however, that the duration of the disorder may sometimes be longer than was at one time supposed, and Hall (1921) collected from the literature 11 cases in which the patients survived from fourteen to thirty years. The prognosis has, however, been transformed by treatment with D-penicillamine.

TREATMENT

Different experiences of the therapeutic value of dimercaprol (BAL) which promotes the excretion of copper, have been reported. Denny-Brown (1953) has observed improvement and gives details of dosage. Oral potassium sulphide reduces the absorption of copper from the alimentary canal. Though dimercaprol and chelating agents such as calcium EDTA (*Versene*) were found to be of some value, both have now been supplanted by D-penicillamine, which is given in a dosage of 1·5–2 G. daily indefinitely. This drug has transformed the prognosis; if given early enough neurological signs and symptoms regress and the affected children grow and develop normally and are symptom-free as long as maintenance treatment is continued.

REFERENCES

BICKEL, H., NEALE, F. C., and HALL, G. (1957) A clinical and biochemical study of hepato-lenticular degeneration (Wilson's disease), *Quart. J. Med.*, **26, 527.**
BICKEL, H., NEALE, F. C., and HALL, G. (1959) in *Heavy Metals and the Brain*, Oxford.
CUMINGS, J. N. (1948) The copper and iron content in the brain and liver in the normal and in hepatolenticular degeneration, *Brain*, **71, 410.**
CUMINGS, J. N. (1951) The effects of B.A.L. in hepatolenticular degeneration, *Brain*, **74, 10.**

DENNY-BROWN, D. (1953) Abnormal copper metabolism and hepatolenticular degeneration, *Res. Publ. Ass. nerv. ment. Dis.*, **32**, 190.

GREENFIELD, J. G., POYNTON, F. J., and WALSHE, F. M. R. (1923–4) On progressive lenticular degeneration. (Hepato-lenticular degeneration.), *Quart. J. Med.*, **17**, 385.

HALL, H. C. (1921) *La dégénérescence hépato-lenticulaire*, Paris.

LANGE, J. (1961) Experiences in long-term treatment of Wilson's disease with penicillamine, in *Wilson's Disease*, ed. WALSHE, J. M., and CUMINGS, J. N., p. 267, Oxford.

MANDELBROTE, B. M., STANIER, M. W., THOMPSON, R. H. S., and THRUSTON, M. N. (1948) Studies on copper metabolism in demyelinating diseases of the central nervous system, *Brain*, **71**, 212.

MATTHEWS, W. B. (1954) The absorption and excretion of radio-copper in hepatolenticular degeneration (Wilson's disease), *J. Neurol. Neurosurg. Psychiat.*, **17**, 242.

MATTHEWS, W. B., MILNE, M. D., and BELL, M. (1952) The metabolic disorder in hepatolenticular degeneration, *Quart. J. Med.*, **21**, 425.

RICHMOND, J., ROSENOER, V. M., TOMPSETT, S. L., DRAPER, I., and SIMPSON, J. A. (1964) Hepato-lenticular degeneration (Wilson's disease) treated by penicillamine, *Brain*, **87**, 619.

WALSHE, J. M. (1967) The physiology of copper in man and its relation to Wilson's disease, *Brain*, **90**, 149.

WALSHE, J. M., and CUMINGS, J. N., eds. (1961) *Wilson's Disease. Some Current Concepts*, Oxford.

WILSON, S. A. K. (1911–12) Progressive lenticular degeneration: a familial nervous disease associated with cirrhosis of the liver, *Brain*, **34**, 295.

WILSON, S. A. K. (1913–14) An experimental research into the anatomy and physiology of the corpus striatum, *Brain*, **36**, 427.

TORSION DYSTONIA

Synonym. Dystonia musculorum deformans (Oppenheim).

Definition. A syndrome characterized by involuntary movements producing torsion of the limbs and the vertebral column, which may occur as a symptom of more than one pathological state.

AETIOLOGY AND PATHOLOGY

Torsion dystonia is a rare syndrome which was first described by Schwalbe in 1908 in three siblings. Mendel in 1919 collected 30 cases from the literature. It is frequently, though not invariably, familial, and appears to be particularly prevalent among Russian Jews. Pathological investigations have been carried out in a few cases. The caudate nucleus and putamen suffer most. In Thomalla's and Wimmer's cases cirrhosis of the liver was found, together with degenerative changes in the lentiform nuclei, while in addition in Thomalla's case similar changes were found in the subthalamic nucleus and in Wimmer's case in the thalamus, hypothalamus, and dentate nucleus of the cerebellum. The characteristic lesion is an *état marbré*. On the other hand, Levy and Wimmer have shown that torsion dystonia may occur as a sequel of encephalitis lethargica. It is evidently a syndrome which may be produced by a variety of disorders, some familial examples being probably due to a cerebral degeneration allied to, if not identical with, Wilson's disease. Its pathogenesis is discussed on page 520. Zeman and Dyken (1967) suggest that whereas clinical features resembling those of dystonia musculorum deformans (so-called symptomatic dystonia) can be seen in cases of Wilson's disease and cerebral palsy, there is a specific dystonic disorder of dominant inheritance (due to a gene with low penetrance) in which no specific pathological changes have yet been discovered.

SYMPTOMS

In the familial cases the onset usually occurs in childhood or adolescence, and the abnormality is frequently first noticed when the patient walks. In Schwalbe's family the disorder began with spasmodic plantar-flexion of the feet, rendering it impossible to place the heel on the ground. The resultant bizarre gait, when first observed in an otherwise healthy child, is often misconstrued as being hysterical. The involuntary movements in the upper limbs consist of rotation or torsion round the long axes and are associated with similar torsion movements of the vertebral column, especially in the lumbar region [FIG. 83]. There are frequently lordosis and scoliosis, which are conspicuous when the patient walks, but tend to disappear when he lies down. Other forms of involuntary movement, such as tremor and myoclonic muscular contractions, have been described. Muscular tone is variable, being exaggerated during the spasms which may be extremely painful, and sometimes diminished in the intervals between them. Signs of a lesion of the corticospinal tracts are absent. There

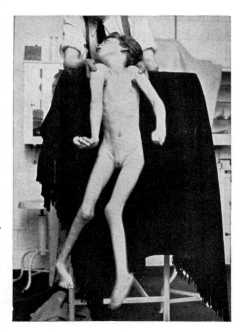

FIG. 83. A case of torsion dystonia

is no muscular wasting except as a result of cachexia in the terminal stages. The reflexes are normal, and sensibility is unimpaired. Mental changes are absent, and speech is usually unaffected.

DIAGNOSIS

Torsion dystonia must be distinguished from other forms of involuntary movement, especially from athetosis and from chorea. In athetosis the movements, which are of a slow, writhing character, involve the peripheral parts of the limbs, rather than the proximal as in torsion spasm. Double athetosis, moreover, is usually congenital, and hence the movements develop at an earlier age than torsion spasm. Choreic movements, like athetosis, involve the peripheral parts of the limbs to a greater extent than torsion dystonia. In chorea, however, movements of rotation of the limbs and trunk occur, but they are quicker and briefer than the corresponding movements of torsion spasm. Dystonic movements may develop in the affected limbs after an interval of some years in occasional cases of infantile hemiplegia. Hysteria may cause bizarre involuntary movements resembling torsion dystonia, and Schwalbe considered that the movements in his patients were neurotic. Hysterical involuntary movements, however, rarely involve the trunk and the proximal parts of the limbs, and in hysteria the emotional attitude of the patient to the disorder and the presence of other hysterical symptoms usually settle the diagnosis.

PROGNOSIS

When dystonic features develop as a manifestation of Wilson's disease, cerebral palsy, and infantile hemiplegia the prognosis is that of the underlying disease. In occasional cases of unknown aetiology recovery has been described. In the 'idiopathic' disorder the condition may remain static for some years but in most cases there is slow progressive deterioration and death eventually occurs as a result of the combined effects of cachexia and respiratory or urinary infection.

TREATMENT

An attempt should be made to ameliorate the involuntary movements by means of rest and re-educational exercises. Sedative drugs, such as diazepam, 2–5 mg. three or four times daily, may help to diminish their severity, and drugs of the belladonna group may be tried as for Parkinsonism. Good results are now claimed for pallidectomy and thalamotomy (Cooper, 1965).

REFERENCES

COOPER, I. S. (1965) Clinical and physiologic implications of thalamic surgery for disorders of sensory communication, Part 2 (Intention tremor, dystonia, Wilson's disease and torticollis), *J. neurol. Sci.*, **2**, 520.

KAUFMAN, M. R., SAVITSKY, N., and FREID, J. R. (1928) Dystonia musculorum deformans of encephalitic etiology, *Arch. Neurol. Psychiat. (Chicago)*, **20**, 824.

LARSSON, T., and SJÖGREN, T. (1966) Dystonia musculorum deformans. A genetic and population study of 121 cases, *Acta neurol. scand.*, **42**, Suppl. 17.

LÉVY, G. (1922) *Contribution à l'étude des manifestations tardives de l'encéphalite épidémique*, Paris.

MENDEL, K. (1919) Torsiondystonie, *Mschr. Psychiat. Neurol.*, **46**, 309.

PUTNAM, T. J. (1933) Treatment of athetosis and dystonia by section of extrapyramidal motor tracts, *Arch. Neurol. Psychiat. (Chicago)*, **29**, 504.

SCHWALBE, M. W. (1908) *Eine eigentümliche tonische Krampfform mit hysterischen Symptomen*, Berlin.

THÉVENARD, ANDRÉ (1926) *Les dystonies d'attitude*, Thèse, Paris.

THOMALLA, C. (1918) Ein Fall von Torsionsspasmus mit Sektionsbefund und seine Beziehungen zur Athétose double, Wilsonschen Krankheit und Pseudosklerose, *Z. ges. Neurol. Psychiat.*, Orig. **41**, 311.

WIMMER, A. (1924) *Chronic Epidemic Encephalitis*, London.

WIMMER, A. (1925) Études sur les syndromes extra-pyramidaux, *Rev. neurol. (Paris)*, **2**, 281.

ZEMAN, W., and DYKEN, P. (1967) Dystonia musculorum deformans. Clinical, genetic and pathoanatomical studies, *Psychiat. Neurol. Neurochir. (Amst.)*, **70**, 77.

ZIEHEN (1911) Demonstrat. eines Patienten mit tonischer Torsionsneurose, *Neurol. Zbl.*, **30**, 109.

SPASMODIC TORTICOLLIS

Synonym. Wry neck.

Definition. A rotated attitude of the head, brought about by clonic or tonic contraction of the cervical muscles and occurring as a symptom both of organic disease of the nervous system and of hysteria. Torticollis of organic origin is a fragmentary form of torsion spasm. Retrocollis is a similar disorder, in which the neck is extended.

AETIOLOGY AND PATHOLOGY

In the past, confusion as to the nature of torticollis has arisen from a failure to distinguish hysterical torticollis from torticollis occurring as a symptom of organic disease. Since torticollis can be effected voluntarily, it may occur as an hysterical symptom, being then a form of tic. The hysterical nature of the symptoms in such cases is proved by the fact that it is often possible to discover and remove its cause by psychological methods. There is abundant evidence, however, that torticollis may occur as a result of organic disease of the nervous system, and in such cases there are grounds for regarding it as a limited form of torsion dystonia. It may occur as a sequel to encephalitis lethargica, with or without Parkinsonism, or as a part of other extrapyramidal syndromes. Since torticollis as an isolated symptom is not fatal, pathological investigations are scanty. Cassirer, however, has reported a case in which degenerative changes were present in the corpus striatum and were associated with cirrhosis of the liver, and Foerster (1933) one in which bilateral focal lesions of the corpus striatum were present. Physiologically, torticollis is a disturbance of the normal posture of the head. The rotated posture of the head which follows unilateral labyrinthectomy and lesions of the eighth nerve indicates the importance of the labyrinth in the maintenance of the posture of the head, and torticollis is probably due to a lesion involving the higher centres concerned in this function, most frequently in the neighbourhood of the corpus striatum. Both sexes are affected, and the onset usually occurs during adult life. The disorder may be familial.

SYMPTOMS

The development of torticollis is usually insidious but may be sudden, especially when it is a symptom of hysteria. The rotation of the head is brought about by contraction of the cervical muscles, and though both the superficial and deep muscles of the neck are involved, the muscular contraction is evident to the observer only in the sternomastoid, trapezius, and splenius. The precise posture of the head varies in different cases. Contraction of the sternomastoid alone causes rotation to the opposite side, with flexion of the neck to the side of the contracted muscle. Rotation, however, may occur without lateral flexion, or the head may be flexed to the side to which it is rotated, in such cases contraction of the sternomastoid on one side being associated with contraction of the splenius and trapezius on the opposite side. The muscles involved become hypertrophied. The disturbance may be predominantly tonic, leading to a sustained posture, or may consist of repeated clonic jerks, as is particularly common in hysterical cases. It may be possible to modify the abnormal posture by altering the position of the patient in relation to gravity, for example, from the erect to the supine, or from the supine to the prone position. There may or may not be resistance to passive movement of the head in the direction opposite to the abnormal position. In a few cases torticollis has been associated with paralysis of rotation to the opposite side. There may be spasm of the facial muscles and platysma on the side to which the head is rotated, or spasmodic torsion movements of the upper limb or whole body. The patient not infrequently finds that he can inhibit the torticollis by exerting slight pressure with his finger upon the jaw on the side to which the head is rotated, and the movement ceases during sleep. Pain may occur in the cervical muscles. The reflexes and sensation are normal. Long-continued torticollis may cause cervical spondylosis.

Retrocollis is due to a bilateral contraction of the splenius and trapezius.

DIAGNOSIS

The distinction between hysterical torticollis and torticollis of organic origin may be difficult. Hysteria should be suspected when the symptom develops suddenly in circumstances of mental stress, and also when it can be controlled by relaxation and suggestion. A complete examination of the nervous system must be made to exclude signs of organic nervous disease.

Spasmodic torticollis is distinguished by the age of onset from congenital torticollis, which may be due either to fibrosis of one sternomastoid following a haematoma in the muscle, or to a congenital deficiency of one-half of a cervical vertebra. It is necessary also to exclude as causes of torticollis myositis of the cervical muscles, caries of the cervical spine, adenitis of the cervical lymph nodes, and impaired ocular-muscle balance.

PROGNOSIS

Torticollis is almost always an intractable disorder, but when it is due to hysteria great improvement and even cure may be effected by psychotherapy. Sufficiently radical surgical treatment using radiculectomy and neurectomy has given good results in a considerable proportion of cases of organic origin, though the spasm may recur after operation.

TREATMENT

Hysterical torticollis should be treated by psychotherapy along the same lines as other hysterical symptoms (Paterson, 1945), and the patient should be taught to practise muscular relaxation. Sedative and tranquillizing drugs such as chlordiazepoxide (*Librium*), 10 mg. three or four times daily, or diazepam (*Valium*), 2–5 mg. three times a day, may be of some value. Mechanical support to the head may give considerable relief. Torticollis of organic origin is unlikely to respond to medical measures. Surgical treatment, therefore, should not be too long delayed. A number of operations have been recommended. Finney and Hughson (1925) divided the accessory nerves and the dorsal divisions of the upper three or four cervical nerves at their points of emergence from the vertebrae. Dandy (1930) combined division of the accessory nerves with interruption of the upper three cervical sensory and motor roots within the spinal canal, and Foerster performed intradural section of both the ventral and dorsal roots of the upper three cervical segments.

Sorensen and Hamby (1966) have reviewed the results obtained in 71 cases treated surgically and found that patients subjected to anterior cervical rhizotomy and subarachnoid section of the spinal accessory nerve did best. In intractable cases simultaneous bilateral lesions produced in ventrolateral thalamic nuclei by stereotaxic methods may be beneficial but the results of this treatment are variable (Cooper, 1965).

REFERENCES

COOPER, I. S. (1965) Clinical and physiologic implications of thalamic surgery for disorders of sensory communication, Part 2 (Intentional tremor, dystonia, Wilson's disease and torticollis), *J. Neurol. Sci.*, **2**, 520.

DANDY, W. E. (1930) An operation for the treatment of spasmodic torticollis, *Arch. Surg.* (*Chicago*), **20**, 1021.

FINNEY, J. M. T., and HUGHSON, W. (1925) Spasmodic torticollis, *Ann. Surg.*, **81**, 255.

FOERSTER, O. (1925) Operative Behandlung des Torticollis spasticus, *Zbl. Chir.*, **53**, 2804.

FOERSTER, O. (1933) Mobile spasm of the neck muscles and its pathological basis, *J. comp. Neurol.*, **58**, 725.

PATERSON, M. (1945) Spasmodic torticollis: results of psychotherapy in 21 cases, *Lancet*, ii, 556.

SCHALTENBRAND, G. (1937) Klinik und Behandlung des Torticollis spasticus, *Dtsch. Z. Nervenheilk.*, **145**, 36.

SORENSEN, B. F., and HAMBY, W. B. (1966) Spasmodic torticollis. Results in surgically-treated patients, *Neurology (Minneap.)*, **16**, 867.

ATHETOSIS

Definition. Athetosis, or 'mobile spasm', is the term applied to a form of involuntary movement which in some respects resembles chorea, as is recognized by the use of the term 'choreo-athetosis' to describe an intermediate condition. Athetoid movements, however, are slower, coarser, and more writhing than choreic movements. Athetosis is due to a variety of pathological states which damage the basal ganglia.

AETIOLOGY AND PATHOLOGY

The same difficulties are encountered in localizing the lesion responsible for athetosis as in the case of chorea. Nevertheless, there is considerable evidence that it is usually situated in the putamen. Bilateral athetosis is occasionally familial.

Bilateral Athetosis

Bilateral athetosis may be congenital, when it may be due to the *état marbré* of the corpus striatum described by Oppenheim and Vogt (1911). Rarely bilateral athetosis may develop during adolescence as a progressive disorder terminating in generalized rigidity, as a result of degeneration of the corpus striatum described by C. and O. Vogt (1919) as *état dysmyélinique*. The common pathological factor, according to Denny-Brown (1946), the *état marbré* or status marmoratus, is a disorder of glial formation leading to hypermyelination, involving to a varying extent the cortex, basal ganglia, and other structures, and underlying dystonia musculorum deformans, double athetosis, and some cases of congenital diplegia. Athetosis may rarely occur as a symptom of hepato-lenticular degeneration, and very rarely bilateral athetosis may develop in adult life.

Unilateral Athetosis

Unilateral athetosis may also be congenital, being then usually associated with infantile hemiplegia. The brain in such cases may exhibit the Bielschowsky type of cerebral hemiatrophy, in which there is an elective necrosis of the third cortical layer of the precentral gyrus, atrophy of the thalamus, and a condition of the striatum described by the Vogts as *état fibreux*, or false porencephaly, may be present. Unilateral athetosis may also occur as a result of focal lesions involving the corpus striatum at any age, due, for example, to acute encephalitis or a cerebral vascular lesion complicating the specific fevers in childhood, but it is also seen in late middle life and old age, as a result of focal cerebral softening secondary to atheroma.

SYMPTOMS

Congenital athetosis is not usually noticed until the child is several months old, when abnormal postures or movements attract the mother's attention. In the early months of life many such children are hypotonic ('floppy infants') and may be suspected of suffering from the flaccid or hypotonic form of cerebral palsy. Athetosis caused by an acute inflammatory or vascular lesion of the brain may develop rapidly within a few days of the lesion, or insidiously after an interval of several weeks, or even years.

Typical athetosis possesses the following features. One or both halves of the body may be involved. The muscles innervated by the cranial nerves are always much more severely affected when the athetosis is bilateral than when it is unilateral. In bilateral athetosis the patient exhibits frequent grimaces resembling caricatures of normal facial expressions of all kinds. Involuntary laughing and crying are common. The tongue is the site of writhing movements of protrusion and withdrawal, and the patient is often unable to maintain it protruded unless it is held between the teeth. The involuntary movement of the articulatory and pharyngeal muscles leads to dysarthria and dysphagia. The head may be rotated to one or other side, or extended. In unilateral athetosis the facial movements usually consist of little more than an exaggeration of normal expressions. In the upper limbs the peripheral segments exhibit the involuntary movements to a greater extent than the proximal segments. The limb is usually adducted and internally rotated at the shoulder and semiflexed at the elbow. The characteristic posture of the hand is one of marked flexion of the wrist, with flexion at the metacarpophalangeal and extension at the interphalangeal joints, the posture produced by contraction of the interossei, and the thumb is usually adducted, and extended at the two distal joints. This posture is disturbed by slow, writhing movements of flexion and extension at the wrist and at the metacarpophalangeal joints, the fingers remaining extended at the interphalangeal joints, with varying degrees of adduction and abduction. Movements may also occur at the shoulder and elbow, leading sometimes to retraction and internal rotation at the shoulder and extension at the elbow. In severe cases of unilateral athetosis the patient characteristically grasps the affected upper limb with the normal hand, to restrain the movement. He may even sit upon the affected hand or trap it behind his back in a chair in order to restrain the movement. Except in the mildest cases the movements completely interfere with the voluntary use of the limb. The movements of the lower limb are usually less severe than those of the upper, and again are most marked in the distal segments. The foot is usually maintained in the position of talipes equinovarus, often with marked dorsiflexion of the great toe. Athetotic movements are always exaggerated by an attempt to use the limbs in voluntary movement and by nervousness and excitement. They diminish when the patient lies down and disappear during sleep. Though the tone of the muscles is exaggerated during the movements, they are usually found to be hypotonic in the intervals if sufficient relaxation can be obtained. In severe cases, especially of unilateral athetosis, muscular contractures usually develop and the peripheral segments of the limbs become fixed in their characteristic postures.

Double athetosis may be associated with spastic diplegia. The mental state of the patient is usually an amentia which may be mild or severe but some patients with severe athetosis may be normal intellectually.

DIAGNOSIS

The involuntary movements are so distinctive that diagnosis is easy. Choreic movements are more rapid and jerky: those of dystonia slower and to a greater extent around the long axis of the limbs and trunk. Athetosis, in fact, is midway between chorea and dystonia. The age and mode of onset distinguish the cause as either congenital abnormality, progressive degeneration, or acute focal lesion.

PROGNOSIS AND TREATMENT

The medical treatment of athetosis is disappointing. Benzhexol (*Artane*) and sedatives such as phenobarbitone, chlordiazepoxide (*Librium*) and diazepam (*Valium*) may slightly diminish the movements, and some improvement may follow re-educational exercises, such as the relaxation exercises advocated by Phelps (1941, 1942), perseveringly carried out over a long period. Extensive section of the dorsal roots innervating the upper limb has been advocated. Horsley and others have abolished the movements by excising an area of the precentral gyrus corresponding to the affected limb (Bucy and Buchanan, 1932; Bucy, 1951). Putnam's operation of division of the extrapyramidal tracts in the anterior column of the spinal cord above the cervical enlargement may greatly improve the patient's control over the limbs. Evidence as to the value of pallidectomy is conflicting: Cooper (1955) found it produced alleviation, but Paxton and Dow (1958) found it of no value for congenital athetosis and most authorities now agree that these are the least rewarding cases for stereotaxic surgery.

REFERENCES

BUCY, P. C. (1951) The surgical treatment of extrapyramidal diseases, *J. Neurol. Neurosurg. Psychiat.*, **14**, 108.

BUCY, P. C., and BUCHANAN, D. N. (1932) Athetosis, *Brain*, **55**, 479.

CARPENTER, M. B. (1950) Athetosis and the basal ganglia: Review of the literature and study of forty-two cases, *Arch. Neurol. Psychiat.* (*Chicago*), **63**, 875.

COOPER, I. S. (1955) Relief of juvenile involuntary movement disorders by chemopallidectomy, *J. Amer. med. Ass.*, **164**, 1297.

DENNY-BROWN, D. (1946) *Diseases of the Basal Ganglia and Subthalamic Nuclei*, New York.

DENNY-BROWN, D. (1962) *The Basal Ganglia and Their Relation to Disorders of Movement*, Oxford.

OPPENHEIM, H., and VOGT, C. (1911) Nature et localisation de la paralysie pseudo-bulbaire congénitale et infantile, *J. Psychol. Neurol. (Lpz.)*, **18**, 293.

PAXTON, H. D., and Dow, R. S. (1958) Two years' experience of chemopallidectomy, *J. Amer. med. Ass.*, **168**, 755.

PHELPS, W. M. (1941) The management of cerebral palsies, *J. Amer. med. Ass.*, **117**, 1621.

PHELPS, W. M. (1942) Evidences of improvement in cases of athetosis treated by re-education, *Res. Publ. Ass. nerv. ment. Dis.*, **21**, 529.

PUTNAM, T. J. (1933) Treatment of athetosis and dystonia by section of extrapyramidal motor tracts, *Arch. Neurol. Psychiat.* (*Chicago*), **29**, 504.

VOGT, C. (1924–5) Sur l'état marbré du striatum, *Jb. Psychiat. Neurol.*, **31**, 256.

VOGT, C., and VOGT, O. (1919) Erster Versuch einer pathologisch-anatomischen Einteilungsträrer Motilitätsstörungen nebst Bemerkskungen über seine allgemeine wissenschaftliche Bedeutung, *J. Psychol. Neurol. (Lpz.)*, **24**, 1.

CHOREA

SYDENHAM'S CHOREA

Synonym. St. Vitus' Dance.

Definition. An acute toxi-infective disorder of the nervous system, usually due to acute rheumatism, occurring in childhood and adolescence and characterized by involuntary movements as its most prominent symptom.

PATHOLOGY

Cases of chorea which have come to autopsy have often shown diffuse changes in the brain. Macroscopically, oedema and congestion have been observed. Microscopically, the changes have usually been most marked in the corpus striatum, substantia nigra, and subthalamic nucleus, but cortical abnormalities have also been present. Vasodilatation is conspicuous, but perivascular infiltration with lymphocytes and plasma cells, though sometimes present, is exceptional. There is a diffuse degeneration of ganglion cells, and sometimes perivascular patches of degeneration with compound granular cell infiltration and neuroglial reaction have been described. Encephalitic changes have been described in acute rheumatism (Winkelman and Eckel, 1932; Bruetsch and Bahr, 1939).

AETIOLOGY

The large majority of cases of chorea in childhood are due to acute rheumatism, as is shown by the frequency with which other rheumatic manifestations are present or subsequently develop. Other infections may, however, be the cause, especially scarlet fever and diphtheria; and choreiform movements may be encountered as a symptom of encephalitis lethargica, or as a rare complication of chickenpox.

Heredity may play some part in aetiology, since some families appear to be unusually susceptible to acute rheumatism, and there may be a family history either of chorea or of some other rheumatic manifestation. Left-handedness is also sometimes a predisposing cause. There is a much larger incidence of left-handedness among sufferers from chorea than among the general population, and even when the patient is not left-handed other members of the family may exhibit the peculiarity.

The white race is more susceptible than the coloured races, and females suffer more than males in the proportion of about three to one. Chorea is rare before the age of 5 and after 20; four-fifths of all cases occur between the ages of 5 and 15.

Mental stress may play a part in the aetiology. Overwork at school may be a predisposing factor, and it is not uncommon for the onset of the attack to be ascribed to a fright. In a small number of cases chorea occurs during pregnancy —chorea gravidarum. That psychical factors may be in part responsible for this is suggested by the fact that it is relatively commoner in illegitimate pregnancies. There is often, however, a rheumatic history in such cases, and other rheumatic manifestations may be present. Chorea gravidarum usually occurs during the first pregnancy and may recur in subsequent pregnancies. It rarely occurs for the first time in a multipara or after the age of 25. Thyrotoxicosis is a rare cause.

SYMPTOMS

Mode of Onset

The onset of chorea is usually insidious, the first complaint being often that the child is clumsy and drops things. When the movements are noticed it is described as restless, fidgety, or unable to keep still. Sometimes the onset is more abrupt and is then often ascribed to a fright.

Involuntary Movements

Involuntary movements are the most prominent symptom of chorea. Choreic movements are best described as quasi-purposive. They are movements of a high order, and although they achieve no purpose, they often resemble fragments of purposive movements following one another in a disorderly fashion. In the face the movements are always bilateral. Frowning, raising the eyebrows, pursing the lips, smiling, and bizarre movements of the mouth and tongue occur. The protruded tongue may be held between the teeth to prevent its sudden withdrawal. The eyes may be rolled from one side to the other, the head turning in the same direction.

In mild cases the speech is not affected; in severe cases there is considerable dysarthria, articulation being slurred and words sometimes being jerked out explosively. In severe cases also mastication and swallowing may be so much disturbed that the patient requires to be artificially fed.

In the upper limb movements occur at all joints. At one moment the elbow may be flexed and the fingers grasping the bedclothes; at the next the arm may be flung out in full extension. Respiration is often jerky and irregular and is frequently impeded by movements involving the abdominal wall and movements of rotation or flexion of the spine. Movements of the lower limbs are usually less conspicuous and are most evident at the periphery. Choreic movements are intensified by voluntary effort and by excitement. They disappear during sleep.

Associated Movements

In chorea the involuntary muscular contractions normally associated with strong voluntary movement are exaggerated, and at the same time incoordinate. When the patient clenches his fist, vigorous associated movements may occur in the face, trunk, and limbs. Yet observation shows that even the synergic extension of the wrist associated with strong flexion of the fingers is not normally carried out. Contraction of the flexors may conflict with, and even overpower, that of the extensors, while the radial and ulnar extensors may not contract synchronously, so that the hand deviates from side to side. This disturbance of associated movement is an early sign of chorea which may precede active involuntary movements, and can be elicited in suspected cases by asking the patient to clench his fists over the observer's fingers, while protruding the tongue.

Voluntary Movement

In mild cases voluntary power is little impaired, though the movements have an abrupt character. For example, if the patient be asked to stretch out the arms, he does so with a sudden movement as though he were flinging his hands away from him. In severe cases the involuntary movements cause considerable incoordination, and voluntary power may thus be impaired. Muscular weakness may be very marked, as in so-called paralytic chorea, though complete paralysis never develops. It is not uncommon to find that chorea is predominantly unilateral in which case a diagnosis of hemiplegia due to an intracranial lesion may initially be entertained unless the hypotonia and involuntary movements are recognized.

Hypotonia and Posture

Hypotonia is invariably present in chorea, and is best demonstrated by passively extending the wrists and ankles, when a considerable degree of hyperextension can be obtained. The so-called choreic posture of the hand, in which the thumb and fingers are hyperextended at the metacarpophalangeal joints and the wrist is flexed, is merely a manifestation of muscular hypotonia, being an exaggeration of the normal attitude resulting from loss of tone in the antagonistic muscles. The upper limbs characteristically are hyperpronated when outstretched and held above the head.

Reflexes

The cutaneous reflexes in chorea are often exceptionally brisk; the plantar reflexes are flexor. When hypotonia is extreme, the tendon reflexes may be difficult to elicit, but they are usually obtainable and sometimes show a characteristic and repetitive prolongation of the muscular contraction (the 'pendular' reflex).

Sensory changes do not occur, and there is no disturbance of the sphincters.

Mental State

Most choreic children exhibit some emotional instability, but they are often above the average in intelligence. In severe cases there may be a persistent state of excitement associated with insomnia—so-called *maniacal chorea*.

The Heart

Since in most cases chorea is due to acute rheumatism it is not surprising that cardiac abnormalities are common. They are not, however, constant. When the heart is involved for the first time during the attack of chorea, the pulse rate is quickened, there is usually slight cardiac dilatation indicated by outward displacement of the apex beat, the apical first sound is somewhat muffled, and there is often a soft systolic murmur in the mitral area. These signs point to myocarditis. When the heart has been affected in previous attacks of rheumatism, signs of valvular damage are more likely to be present. Pericarditis, arthritis, and rheumatic nodules are rarely associated with chorea. Pyrexia is usually absent, unless chorea is complicated by mental excitement or by other manifestations of acute rheumatism.

DIAGNOSIS

The diagnosis of chorea is usually simple, since the involuntary movements are distinctive. It is most likely to be confused with habit spasm, in which, however, the same movements are repeated again and again. In athetosis the movements are slower than in chorea and have been well described as mobile spasm. Moreover, in most cases, athetosis in childhood is congenital in origin or is noticed before the age of 5, when chorea is very rare. Hysterical involuntary movements may simulate chorea. These usually occur after the age of 15, and in females, and are an imitation of a case of true chorea. The imitation, however, is never exact. The movements are usually more jerky than those of chorea, and are sometimes rhythmical. There is neither exaggeration nor disorganization of associated movements, and the face usually escapes.

Paralytic chorea may simulate other forms of paralysis in childhood. It is distinguished from hemiplegia by the fact that the upper limb alone is paretic, and by the absence of signs of a corticospinal lesion, especially an extensor plantar reflex. The absence of wasting and of changes in the electrical reaction of the muscles distinguishes it from poliomyelitis. A further diagnostic point is that even in the weak limb slight involuntary movements are present, and they may also be observed elsewhere in the body. Choreiform movements occurring in cerebral palsy are accompanied by other signs of brain damage.

In maniacal chorea the mental state may overshadow the physical symptoms, but the history of precedent involuntary movements or the presence of signs of rheumatic endocarditis may enable the correct diagnosis to be made.

Chorea having been diagnosed, the cause can usually be easily ascertained. Many patients will show other evidences of the rheumatic infection. Even if these are absent, rheumatism is the most likely cause if there is no history of some other infection. Confusion has arisen in the past from cases of encephalitis lethargica characterized by choreiform movements, though these have not been observed for many years. In such cases the characteristic lethargy is often absent, and the movements are often associated with insomnia and mental excitement. Ocular symptoms, however, may be present, especially an impairment of the pupillary reflexes, and possibly diplopia, and an excess of mononuclear cells may be found in the cerebrospinal fluid. Chorea has also been described as a rare manifestation of systemic lupus erythematosus, while in adult life a choreiform syndrome has been observed in cases of chronic liver disease.

Huntington's chorea is distinguished by its onset in later life, usually after the age of 30, by its hereditary character, and its association with progressive dementia.

PROGNOSIS

Death from chorea is rare and occurs in only 2 per cent. of cases. It has been suggested that chorea gravidarum carries a less favourable prognosis (Matthews, 1963) but this no longer appears to be the case (Lewis and Parsons, 1966). Most patients recover in from two to three months, rarely in less than six weeks. Recurrences occur in about one-third of all cases: a patient may have two, three, four, or even more attacks. The average intervals between attacks is about one year; it is rarely more than two years. The presence of other rheumatic manifestations, e.g. valvular lesions, does not appear to influence recovery from chorea, but the occurrence of repeated attacks of chorea predisposes to the development of rheumatic carditis and endocarditis. Chorea, as such, leaves no serious sequels, though some mental instability may persist for a long time, and slight involuntary movements may be perpetuated as a habit.

TREATMENT

All patients suffering from chorea should be kept in bed for at least four weeks, and should then be allowed to get up only if the movements are considerably diminished in severity. The presence of cardiac complications will probably necessitate a longer stay in bed, and the condition of the heart must be considered independently. Isolation of the patient is beneficial, and if possible the child should be nursed in a room by itself. In the hospital ward isolation may be obtained by the use of screens round the bed. Excitement is to be avoided, but in all but the most severe cases some quiet occupation should be provided. When the movements are very severe it may be difficult to keep the patient in bed, and more convenient to nurse him upon a mattress placed upon the floor. Special attention must be devoted to the care of the skin, and bony points which are liable to be abraded by being rubbed against the bedclothes in movements should be protected. The diet should be ample. If dysphagia is very severe it may be necessary to feed the patient by means of a tube. Salicylates and corticosteroid drugs are now known to have no influence upon the disease process. Traditional sedatives such as phenobarbitone, 30 mg. three or four times daily, are sufficient in some cases but many patients are dramatically improved with chlorpromazine, 25–50 mg. three or four times daily (Lewis and Parsons, 1966).

During convalescence attention should be paid to re-education of the movements of the limbs. This is best promoted at first by occupations requiring fine manipulation, such as knitting, sewing, bead-threading, drawing, and painting.

These, however, are of little value unless carried out under supervision. When the child is up, and if the cardiac condition permits, remedial exercises may be added.

The influence of infected tonsils upon chorea and other rheumatic manifestations is difficult to assess. The tonsils should only be removed when there is a history of repeated sore throats and their condition clearly warrants the operation. This should not be performed until the child is convalescent from chorea, but the fact that some movements persist is not a contra-indication.

REFERENCES

BRAIN, W. R. (1928) Posture of the hand in chorea and other states of muscular hypotonia, *Lancet*, i, 439.

BRUETSCH, W. L., and BAHR, M. A. (1939) Chronic rheumatic brain disease as a factor in the causation of mental illness, *J. Indiana med. Ass.*, **32**, 4.

LEWIS, B. V., and PARSONS, M. (1966) Chorea gravidarum, *Lancet*, i, 284.

LHERMITTE, J., and PAGNIEZ, P. (1930) Anatomie et physiologie pathologiques de la chorée de Sydenham, *Encéphale*, **25**, 24.

MATTHEWS, W. B. (1963) *Practical Neurology*, Oxford.

MEYJES, F. E. P. (1931) Zur Lokalisation und Pathophysiologie der choreatischen Bewegung, *Z. ges. Neurol. Psychiat.*, **133**, 1.

VON MAYENDORF, N. (1929–30) Chorea und Linsenkern, *Mschr. Psychiat. Neurol.*, **74**, 273.

WINKELMAN, N. W., and ECKEL, J. L. (1932) The brain in acute rheumatic fever, *Arch. Neurol. Psychiat. (Chicago)*, **28**, 844.

HUNTINGTON'S CHOREA

Definition. A hereditary disorder characterized pathologically by degeneration of the ganglion cells of the forebrain and corpus striatum, and clinically by choreiform movements and progressive dementia, which usually begin during early middle life.

PATHOLOGY

The brain is small and of diminished weight, the reduction being chiefly, if not entirely, in the forebrain, which shows evidence of marked atrophy affecting the gyri and especially the corpus striatum. The ganglion cells in both the caudate nucleus and in the putamen are reduced in numbers and sometimes almost absent. According to Dunlap (1927), the putamen is more affected than the caudate nucleus and suffers most severely in its second and third fourths. This observer found no loss of cells and no evidence of primary disease in the globus pallidus. Such shrinkage in size as occurred in the latter appears to be due to destruction of fibres coming from the caudate nucleus and putamen. The degenerative changes are accompanied by an extensive proliferation of neuroglia. The ganglion cells of the cortex are small and shrunken in appearance, and the white matter of the cerebral hemispheres is reduced in amount, possibly more than the grey.

AETIOLOGY

Huntington's chorea is uncommon in Great Britain but is not uncommon in the United States of America. Though sporadic cases are occasionally encountered, the only known cause is heredity, and the disorder is inherited as a Mendelian dominant. According to Davenport and Muncey (1917) its ancestral source in the United States can be traced to three brothers who migrated there in the seventeenth century. Of a thousand cases in certain districts practically all could be traced to six individuals. Both sexes are affected and transmit the disease with equal frequency. The age of onset of symptoms is usually between 30 and 45, but may be either later or earlier. Exceptionally members of affected sibships have developed the disease in childhood. Much attention has been paid recently to the possibility that a specific biochemical abnormality may be present in cases of this disease. Suggestions that it may be due to a disorder of magnesium metabolism have not been confirmed (Fleming, Barker, and Stewart, 1967).

SYMPTOMS

The first symptom is usually involuntary movements, which develop insidiously. They are most conspicuous in the face and upper limbs, and are usually more rapid and jerky than the movements of Sydenham's chorea. As the disorder progresses they lead to dysarthria and ataxia of the upper limbs and of the gait. Mental changes gradually develop, usually a few years after the onset of the involuntary movements. They consist of a progressive dementia. Most patients become inert, apathetic, and irritable. Delusions may occur, and outbursts of excitement are not uncommon. Suicide is exceptional.

As Davenport and Muncey have shown, the clinical picture does not always exhibit the classical features just described. Dementia may precede involuntary movements or the latter may never appear. An example of this was reported by Curran (1930). Alternatively, involuntary movements may not be followed by dementia. Exceptionally Parkinsonian rigidity (the 'rigid' form) takes the place of the involuntary movements (Campbell *et al.*, 1961). The onset of symptoms in childhood has already been mentioned, and in such cases diffuse extrapyramidal rigidity, fits and pseudobulbar palsy may be the presenting features.

DIAGNOSIS

In typical cases with a family history the diagnosis is easy. In sporadic cases progressive dementia developing in middle life in association with involuntary movements which somewhat resemble tremor may lead to a diagnosis of general paresis. This, however, can easily be excluded by the absence of iridoplegia and by the negative serological reactions. Cerebral arteriosclerosis, which may lead to both dementia and choreiform involuntary movements, does not usually develop until late middle life or old age. In advanced cases air encephalography often shows a characteristic dilatation of the lateral ventricles with absence of the usual indentation due to the body of the caudate nucleus but by the time this appearance is present the diagnosis is usually self-evident.

PROGNOSIS

Save in rare cases, the disorder is progressive and terminates fatally, usually in from ten to fifteen years, though it may be much more acute, and on the other hand survival for twenty or thirty years is not uncommon.

On account of the dominant heredity, half the children of an affected person may be expected to develop and to be capable of transmitting the disease. Those who remain free from it will not transmit it, but, unfortunately, since symptoms usually do not develop until middle life, it is impossible in the case of children of an affected parent to decide whether they will transmit the disorder until they have passed the usual age of marriage. When, however, the parent has reached the age of 60 without developing symptoms, it may be assumed that his children are unlikely to develop, and hence to transmit, the disease.

TREATMENT

The onset of the mental deterioration frequently necessitates institutional care. No form of treatment is known to arrest the progress of the dementia. Chlorpromazine or thiopropazate (*Dartalan*) may help to control the involuntary movements. Stereotaxic surgery has been tried in some cases but may accelerate the development of dementia and is therefore contra-indicated as a rule except in rare cases in which there is no trace of intellectual impairment and no evidence of ventricular dilatation on air encephalography.

REFERENCES

BELL, J. (1934) Huntington's chorea, *Treasury of Human Inheritance*, vol. iv, pt. 1, London.

CAMPBELL, A. M. G., CORNER, B., NORMAN, R. M., and URICH, H. (1961) The rigid form of Huntington's disease, *J. Neurol. Neurosurg. Psychiat.*, **24**, 71.

CURRAN, D. (1929–30) Huntington's chorea without choreiform movements, *J. Neurol. Psychopath.*, **10**, 305.

DAVENPORT, C. B., and MUNCEY, E. B. (1916–17) Huntington's chorea in relation to heredity and eugenics, *Amer. J. Insan.*, **73**, 195 (also *Proc. nat. Acad. Sci. (Wash.)*, 1915, **1**, 283).

DAVISON, C., GOODHART, S. P., and SHLIONSKY, H. (1932) Chronic progressive chorea, *Arch. Neurol. Psychiat. (Chicago)*, **27**, 906.

DUNLAP, C. B. (1927) Pathologic changes in Huntington's chorea, *Arch. Neurol. Psychiat. (Chicago)*, **18**, 867.

FLEMING, L. W., BARKER, M. G., and STEWART, W. K. (1967) Plasma and erythrocyte magnesium in Huntington's chorea, *J. Neurol. Neurosurg. Psychiat.*, **30**, 374.

KEHRER, F. (1925–6) Bemerkungen zu der Arbeit von J. L. Entres: 'Genealogische Studien zur Differentialdiagnose zwischen Wilsonscher Krankheit und Huntingtonscher Chorea', *Z. ges. Neurol. Psychiat.*, **100** 476.

ROSENTHAL, C. (1927) Zur Symptomatologie und Frühdiagnostik der Huntingtonschen Krankheit, *Z. ges. Neurol. Psychiat.*, **111**, 254.

STONE, C. S. (1931) Huntington's chorea; a sociological and genealogical study of a new family, *Ment. Hyg. (N.Y.)*, **15**, 350.

SENILE CHOREA

Choreiform movements may follow vascular lesions of the brain in middle life and old age. Their onset is usually sudden, and they are generally unilateral. When this is the case they differ only in degree from hemiballismus. Chronic progressive chorea occasionally occurs in the absence of hereditary predisposition. The large and small cells of the caudate nucleus and putamen degenerate but the cerebral cortex is spared (Alcock, 1936). It is difficult to distinguish this from the sporadic occurrence of Huntington's chorea, though it has been stated that the age of onset of senile chorea is usually later than that of Huntington's variety, and that mental symptoms are less likely to occur. Otherwise the symptoms and prognosis are those of Huntington's chorea. Chlorpromazine is a useful drug in the management of these sporadic cases.

HEMIBALLISMUS

Hemiballismus is the term applied to involuntary movements which affect the limbs unilaterally, though the face may be involved on both sides. Hemiballismus differs from chorea in that the movements affect the proximal parts of the limbs to a greater extent, and hence lead to wide excursions, and they are practically continuous except during sleep. The lesion responsible is usually situated in the subthalamic nucleus (corpus Luysii) of the opposite side, but lesions have been observed elsewhere, especially in the corpus striatum and in the pathways connecting it to the subthalamic nucleus (see Whittier, 1947; Meyers, Sweeney, and Schwidde, 1950; Martin, 1957).

Spontaneous cessation of the movements is rare, and many patients die from exhaustion. Surgical measures which have been found to give relief include extirpation of the precentral cortex, linear cortico-subcortical section, and midbrain pyramidotomy (Meyers, Sweeney, and Schwidde, 1950) but these operations have now been replaced by stereotaxic thalamotomy (Martin and McCaul, 1959).

FACIAL DYSKINESIA

A Parkinsonian syndrome and choreiform movement may develop in patients receiving long-term treatment with phenothiazine drugs for psychiatric conditions but usually improve when these drugs are withdrawn. However, distressing facial dyskinetic movements with grimacing, chewing, and intermittent protrusion of the tongue are more disturbing complications of such treatment and are unfortunately irreversible (Hunter, Earl, and Janz, 1964; Evans, 1965).

PALATAL MYOCLONUS

Palatal myoclonus is a condition in which rhythmical movements of the soft palate, occurring 60–180 times a minute develop insidiously. They interfere with speech, swallowing, and respiration and usually persist during sleep. Often pathological examination reveals hypertrophy of the olivary nuclei; the condition appears to be due to a disorder within the olivocerebellar modulatory projection on to the rostral brain stem; the aetiology is unknown (Herrmann and Brown, 1967).

REFERENCES

ALCOCK, N. S. (1936) A note on the pathology of senile chorea (non-hereditary), *Brain*, **59**, 376.

EVANS, J. H. (1965) Persistent oral dyskinesia in treatment with phenothiazine derivatives, *Lancet*, i, 458.

HERRMANN, C., JR., and BROWN, J. W. (1967) Palatal myoclonus; a reappraisal, *J. neurol. Sci.*, **5**, 473.

HUNTER, R., EARL, C. J., and JANZ, D. (1964) A syndrome of abnormal movements and dementia in leucotomized patients treated with phenothiazines, *J. Neurol. Psychiat.*, **27**, 219.

MARTIN, J. P. (1927) Hemichorea resulting from a local lesion of the brain (the syndrome of the body of Luys), *Brain*, **50**, 637.

MARTIN, J. P. (1928) A contribution to the study of chorea. The symptoms which result from injury of the corpus Luysii, *Lancet*, ii, 315.

MARTIN, J. P. (1957) Hemichorea (hemiballismus) without lesions in the corpus Luysii, *Brain*, **80**, 1.

MARTIN, J. P., and McCAUL, I. R. (1959) Acute hemiballismus treated by ventrolateral thalamotomy, *Brain*, **82**, 104.

MEYERS, R., SWEENEY, D. B., and SCHWIDDE, J. T. (1950) Hemiballismus. Aetiology and surgical treatment, *J. Neurol. Neurosurg. Psychiat.*, **13**, 115.

WHITTIER, J. R. (1947) Ballism and the subthalamic nucleus, *Arch. Neurol. Psychiat. (Chicago)*, **58**, 672.

13

CONGENITAL AND DEGENERATIVE DISORDERS

CEREBRAL PALSY

The inclusive term 'cerebral palsy' has been used by Ingram (1964) to identify a group of chronic non-progressive disorders occurring in young children in which disease of the brain causes impairment of motor function. The impairment of motor function may be the result of paresis, including movement or incoordination, but motor disorders which are transient or are the result of progressive disease of the brain or attributable to abnormalities of the spinal cord are excluded.

The classification of conditions which fall into this group remains a matter of dispute but, modified from Ingram (1964), the following is suggested as being reasonably satisfactory in the present state of knowledge:

Diplegia (including hypotonic, dystonic, and rigid or spastic forms)
Hemiplegia
Bilateral hemiplegia
Ataxia (cerebellar diplegia)
Dyskinesia (dystonic, choreoid, athetoid forms)

To these groups may be added the disputed category of so-called 'minimal cerebral palsy' or 'minimal cerebral dysfunction' (Bax and MacKeith, 1963). The dyskinetic forms of cerebral palsy have been considered in CHAPTER 12.

REFERENCES

BAX, M., and MACKEITH, R. (1963) Minimal cerebral dysfunction, *Little Club Clinics in Developmental Medicine*, No. 10, London.
HOLT, K. S. (1965) *Assessment of Cerebral Palsy*, London.
INGRAM, T. T. S. (1964) *Paediatric Aspects of Cerebral Palsy*, Edinburgh.

CONGENITAL DIPLEGIA

Synonyms. Congenital spastic paralysis; Little's disease; atrophic lobar sclerosis.

Definition. The term 'congenital diplegia' is now used to include a group of cases characterized by bilateral and symmetrical disturbances of motility, which are present from birth and which subsequently remain stationary or show a tendency towards improvement. Though commonly the lesion involves chiefly the corticospinal tracts, causing weakness and spasticity which are most conspicuous in the lower limbs, mental defect, involuntary movements, and ataxia may be present either in association with spastic weakness or as the sole manifestations of the cerebral or cerebellar lesion.

AETIOLOGY AND PATHOLOGY

It is estimated that 'spastics' constitute between 1 and 2 per 1,000 of the school population and 0·5 per 1,000 of the adult population in England and Wales (Ministry of Health, 1953).

There has been much discussion concerning the aetiology of congenital diplegia, and five principal theories have been put forward. The view that most cases were due to injury to the brain at birth through meningeal haemorrhage was one of the earliest to gain acceptance. It was later thought that asphyxia at birth might cause the condition in the absence of meningeal haemorrhage. Since a proportion of diplegic infants are premature, the condition has been ascribed to an arrest of myelination of the nervous system following premature birth. During the present century the view has been gaining ground that the damage responsible for the diplegia occurs comparatively early in foetal life and that an arrest in development or an actual degeneration of certain parts of the nervous system occurs in utero. Finally, congenital diplegia has been ascribed to gross maldevelopment of the brain. Stewart (1942–3) points out that the pathological lesions are so diverse that no single cause can be implicated. However, abnormal pregnancy, labour and delivery certainly occur in a high proportion of cases resulting in the birth of diplegic infants (Ingram, 1964).

Although the attribution of congenital diplegia to meningeal haemorrhage at birth appears plausible at first sight, there are serious objections to it. The pathology of cerebral birth injury has now been thoroughly investigated, and it is recognized that meningeal haemorrhage is usually unilateral, and when bilateral is rarely symmetrical. Though it may sometimes be responsible for congenital hemiplegia, it is unlikely to cause a symmetrical disturbance of function similar to that found in diplegia. Moreover, in many cases of diplegia labour is easy.

It seems unlikely also that asphyxia at birth can cause diplegia, since many infants survive it without injury and again many diplegics are not exposed to it.

It is equally difficult to accept prematurity as a common cause, since most premature infants develop perfectly normally, and many diplegic infants are born at full term. There is some evidence that mothers of diplegic patients are older and relatively infertile when compared to mothers in the general population.

Pathological investigations support the view first put forward by Freud and Collier that in most cases of diplegia the arrest of development or the onset of degeneration occurs in utero. The commonest pathological finding is a condition which has received the name 'atrophic lobar sclerosis'. This is characterized by a symmetrical atrophy of both cerebral hemispheres with the destruction of nerve cells and glial proliferation. To the naked eye atrophy is apparent, and may be either diffuse or more or less localized. The gyral pattern of the hemispheres is usually normal but is sometimes primitive. The atrophied gyri are firmer than normal. According to Buzzard and Greenfield the condition is one of neuroglial overgrowth associated with degeneration of the neurones, a process affecting primarily the deeper layers of the cortex and spreading to the underlying white matter and to the superficial layers of the cortex. It is possible that the neuroglial hyperplasia is secondary to the neuronal degeneration. The cause of the latter is unknown, but it has been suggested by Patten that an interference with myelination may come about in foetal life, owing to some maternal abnormality. Stewart (1942–3) suggested that maternal mal-nutrition may be important. Denny-Brown, on the other hand, regards it as a primary glial disorder leading to hypermyelination.

Gross maldevelopment of the brain is probably a rare cause of congenital diplegia, but in some cases the gyri have exhibited a primitive foetal pattern and the cortical ganglion cells have been primitive and confined to one layer. The corpus callosum may be absent. Bilateral true porencephaly is due to abnormal cerebral development, which leaves a free communication between the lateral ventricle and the surface of the hemisphere, but this condition, involving as it does the lower part of the hemispheres, is more likely to cause double hemiplegia with marked spasticity and weakness of the upper limbs than diplegia, in which the upper limbs are less severely affected than the lower.

Microcephaly, which is present in 35 per cent. of cases, is the result of the cerebral hypoplasia and not its cause, the size and shape of the skull depending upon those of the brain.

Exceptionally congenital diplegia appears in several sibs, and this is some-times the case with double athetosis. Congenital syphilis is a rare cause of diplegia.

SYMPTOMS

The symptoms depend upon the distribution of the degenerative changes in the brain. These may predominate in the prefrontal region which is concerned especially with psychical functions, in the precentral gyri, or in the sub-ordinate centres concerned in motility and its co-ordination. Thus one function may be affected almost alone, with the production of types of congenital diplegia characterized by the predominance of (1) mental deficiency, (2) spastic weakness, (3) involuntary movements, and (4) cerebellar deficiency. Mixed varieties, how-ever, are common.

Frequently nothing abnormal is noticed about the child at birth and for some time afterwards, though diplegic infants are often difficult to feed. In some cases microcephaly and muscular rigidity are so marked that attention is drawn to them early. Usually the child is only regarded as abnormal when it fails to reach one of the landmarks of normal development at the expected time. Thus it may be observed that it fails to take notice of its surroundings, that it does not begin to raise its head when 3 months old, sit up at 6 months, and begin to walk and talk at the end of the first year of life. Diplegic children, too, are usually late in acquiring control of the sphincters.

Mental Defect

Mental defect may be the predominant symptom and then may occur in the absence of any gross disturbance of motility, except such clumsiness as results from an inability to learn to control the limbs. In other cases mental defect is associated with diplegia. It ranges through all the degrees arbitrarily characterized as idiocy, imbecility, and feeble-mindedness, up to slight backwardness. Frequently the diplegic child appears to be more defective mentally than is actually the case, since its slowness in learning to walk, and its clumsiness in using its hands retard its mental development. Such children, though developing late, may ultimately achieve a high degree of intelligence in spite of severe motor disabilities.

Weakness and Spasticity

These symptoms, which are mainly attributable to defective development of, or damage to, the corticospinal and extrapyramidal tracts, are usually remarkably symmetrical on the two sides. Rarely one side is more affected than the other. The lower limbs are always more severely affected than the upper. The severity of the symptoms of corticospinal defect varies greatly in different cases. When at its slightest, power and tone may be almost normal, the sole indications of the lesion being exaggerated knee- and ankle-jerks, extensor plantar responses, and slight contractures of the calf muscles, leading to a moderate degree of talipes equinovarus. A somewhat more severe lesion causes a spastic paraplegia of the type originally described by Little in 1862, in which weakness and spasticity are confined to the lower limbs and the muscles of the lower trunk. The lower limbs are rigid in a position of plantar flexion of the ankle, extension at the knee, and adduction and internal rotation at the hip, and contractures develop in the spastic muscles. Voluntary power is often fairly strong, though much hampered by the spasticity. The gait is characteristic, since the plantar flexion of the feet causes the child to walk on the toes, while owing to adduction of the hips the knees may rub together, or may be actually crossed, the so-called 'scissors gait'. The tendon reflexes in the lower limbs are much exaggerated, and the plantar reflexes are extensor. The abdominal reflexes are frequently brisk in spite of the severity of the corticospinal lesion. Spinal deformities, such as lordosis and scoliosis, are common.

In the most severe cases the upper limbs and bulbar muscles suffer from spastic weakness as well as the lower limbs. In the upper limbs the rigidity is usually most marked in the flexor muscles, and the involvement of the bulbar muscles leads to spastic dysarthria and in severe cases to dysphagia. Dribbling of saliva is common.

Involuntary Movements

Involuntary movements may be athetotic or choreiform, or may present some of the features of both, being then described as choreo-athetoid. The characteristics of these involuntary movements are described elsewhere; see pages 515 and 516. In double athetosis athetotic or choreiform movements are present on both sides of the body and are increased by voluntary and emotional movements. The involuntary movements are most evident in the slighter cases, being replaced by hypertonia in the most severe examples of the disorder. The face is expressionless in repose, but involuntary laughing and crying frequently occur. There are gross disturbances of articulation, phonation, mastication, and deglutition, and voluntary movement of the limbs is slow and clumsy. In typical double athetosis there is no clinical evidence of damage to the corticospinal tracts and the plantar reflexes are flexor, but it is not uncommon to find athetotic or choreiform movements associated with spastic diplegia of the type described in the previous section.

Cerebellar Diplegia

In this rare form of diplegia there is marked hypoplasia of the cerebellum, and the symptoms are those of cerebellar deficiency, especially nystagmus, hypotonia, and ataxia (see Walsh, 1963). In many such cases in early infancy hypotonia dominates the clinical picture; cerebellar diplegia is thus one cause of flaccid diplegia in infancy although in some other cases demonstrating hypotonia and flaccidity the typical involuntary movements of chorea and/or athetosis make their appearance in the second year of life.

Other Symptoms

Primary optic atrophy may be associated, though rarely, with any of the forms of diplegia already described. The child may be blind from birth, and I have known more than one case in which it was brought under observation on this account. Squint and nystagmus are common in diplegic children, and epilepsy occurs in a small proportion of cases. A moderate degree of skeletal infantilism is usually present, and puberty is not uncommonly delayed.

DIAGNOSIS

In most cases diagnosis is easy, since the symptoms have clearly been present since birth. The presence of muscular rigidity readily distinguishes spastic diplegia from benign congenital hypotonia and progressive spinal muscular atrophy of infants, in both of which conditions the muscles are flaccid. Difficulty may, however, be experienced in distinguishing these conditions from flaccid diplegia (due to cerebellar diplegia or incipient choreo-athetosis) during the first twelve to eighteen months of life. It is important to distinguish congenital diplegia from progressive degenerative disorders of the brain developing in early life, such as cerebromacular degeneration and diffuse sclerosis, both of which lead to bilateral spastic weakness. The distinction is based upon the fact that in these two disorders the child is normal at birth and develops normally during the early months of its life, and symptoms, when they develop, become progressively worse, whereas in congenital diplegia the child is abnormal from the beginning and its condition remains stationary or slowly improves. This aspect of differential diagnosis has important genetic implications as cerebral palsy is rarely familial while the degenerative disorders are usually inherited and may affect other sibs.

PROGNOSIS

The prognosis of congenital diplegia depends upon its severity and especially upon the degree of mental defect present. In the most severe cases the child rarely survives more than a year or two, usually succumbing to pneumonia. Even when the disability is only moderately severe, many affected individuals fail to survive beyond the early years of adult life. Although some patients remain stationary, there is usually a very slow improvement in the motor symptoms, both in the group characterized by spastic weakness and in that in which involuntary movements predominate, but this depends chiefly upon the mental state of the patient, and little improvement can be expected when a severe mental defect is present. In favourable cases it may be expected that a child will learn to walk, even though it may not do so until it is 5 or 6 years old.

TREATMENT

Treatment consists essentially of the education of movement, e.g. by the methods of Phelps [see p. 545], combined with the removal as far as possible of the obstacles which result from contractures and deformities. Much, therefore, depends upon the patience and care which are available for the education of the patient. Every effort must be made to help the child to learn to walk, and by means of simple games and occupations involving manipulative skill it must gradually be taught control over the movements of the upper limbs. Intensive physiotherapy is undoubtedly of value in many cases. Contractures must be dealt with by tenotomy, and in addition severe abductor spasm may be relieved by dividing the obturator nerve. Drugs such as chlordiazepoxide (*Librium*) and diazepam (*Valium*) have some value in reducing spasticity and in occasional cases intrathecal phenol injections are indicated for the relief of severe spasticity with flexor spasms. Various surgical procedures directed towards the relief of spasticity and deformity have been utilized in selected cases. These operations, however, should only be carried out in children whose mental capacity and voluntary power will enable them to profit by them. Epilepsy must be treated in the usual way.

REFERENCES

BAKER, R. C., and GRAVES, G. O. (1931) Cerebellar agenesis, *Arch. Neurol. Psychiat. (Chicago)*, **25,** 548.

COLLIER, J. (1924) Pathogenesis of cerebral diplegia, *Brain,* **47,** 1.

COLLIER, J. S. (1899) Cerebral diplegia, *Brain,* **22,** 373.

FORD, F. R., CROTHERS, B., and PUTNAM, M. C. (1927) *Birth Injuries of the Central Nervous System,* London.

FREUD, S. (1897) Die infantile Cerebrallähmung, *Spec. Path. Ther. Nothnagel,* **9,** Th. II, Abt. 2. Wien.

HOLT, K. S. (1965) *Assessment of Cerebral Palsy,* London.

INGRAM, T. T. S. (1964) *Paediatric Aspects of Cerebral Palsy,* Edinburgh.

LeCOUNT, E. R., and SEMERAK, C. B. (1925) Porencephaly, *Arch. Neurol. Psychiat. (Chicago),* **14,** 365.

MINISTRY OF HEALTH (1953) Welfare of Handicapped Persons, Circular 26/53.

NAVILLE, F. (1923) Les diplégies congénitales et les troubles dysthyroïdiens dans les classes d'enfants anormaux de Genève, *Schweiz. Arch. Neurol. Psychiat.* **13,** 559.

PATTEN, C. A. (1931) Cerebral birth conditions with special reference to cerebral diplegia, *Arch. Neurol. Psychiat. (Chicago),* **25,** 453.

STEWART, R. M. (1942–3) Observations on the pathology of cerebral diplegia, *Proc. roy. Soc. Med.,* **36,** 25.

WALSH, E. G. (1963) Cerebellum, posture and cerebral palsy, *Little Club Clinics in Developmental Medicine,* No. 8, London.

CONGENITAL AND INFANTILE HEMIPLEGIA

Definition. 'Congenital hemiplegia' is self-explanatory; 'infantile hemiplegia' is the term applied to hemiplegia which develops during the first few years of life. Like hemiplegia in adult life, it is a symptom of a large variety of pathological states.

AETIOLOGY

The causation of hemiplegia in childhood is in many cases obscure, and pathological investigations of acute examples comparatively few. The most convenient classification is, therefore, one based upon the clinical features and associations of the hemiplegia, and we may recognize the following varieties: (1) congenital hemiplegia, (2) hemiplegia complicating known infections, (3) hemiplegia of acute onset in the absence of any evident predisposing cause, (4) hemiplegia of slow onset.

1. Congenital hemiplegia is rare. There is a history of difficult labour in a large proportion of such cases, and the commonest cause is probably a vascular lesion occurring during birth. Norman, Urich, and McMenemey (1957) have discussed the factors which may lead to these, viz. a fall in systemic blood pressure, arterial compression owing to displacement of the cranial contents, and obstruction of the great cerebral vein. Less often the condition may be due to a congenital cerebral deformity, such as true porencephaly, aplasia of the cerebral hemisphere, intracranial angioma, or a cerebral vascular lesion or encephalitis occurring during foetal life. Congenital double hemiplegia is distinguished from congenital diplegia by the more severe affection of the upper limbs.

2. Hemiplegia may occur as a complication of many acute infective disorders of childhood, but is much commoner in some than in others. Whooping cough is one of the commonest causes. Less frequently it occurs in association with measles, scarlet fever, diphtheria, chickenpox, smallpox, vaccinia, pneumonia, otitis media, septicaemia due to pyogenic organisms, typhoid fever, typhus, dysentery, mumps, chorea, encephalitis lethargica. The relationship of the hemiplegia to the infection which it complicates is often obscure. In many cases the cerebral lesion is a vascular one. Thus meningeal and intracerebral haemorrhage have frequently been described in whooping cough, and arterial thrombosis and embolism have been observed in diphtheria. Cerebral thrombosis, too, appears to be the commonest cause of hemiplegia in typhoid and typhus fevers and either cerebral venous thrombosis or cerebral abscess or meningitis may cause hemiplegia in cases of otitis media. In scarlet fever so-called 'acute haemorrhagic encephalitis' has been reported, while in smallpox, chickenpox, vaccinia, and measles the lesion in most cases is a demyelinating encephalitis, which is regarded by some as due to the infecting organism and by others as caused by a secondary infection. Acute poliomyelitis was once held to be responsible for the majority of cases of infantile hemiplegia of acute onset, but there is little evidence in favour of regarding it as a common cause of this condition. Actually hemiplegia is a rare occurrence in epidemics of poliomyelitis. Congenital syphilis and tuberculous meningitis are equally rare causes.

3. Cases of hemiplegia occurring in early childhood without any obvious predisposing cause are slightly more frequent than those which fall within the preceding group. In some cases the hemiplegia is probably a manifestation of an encephalitis or toxic encephalopathy of unknown origin. In the majority, however, it is probably due to a vascular lesion, for example haemorrhage or thrombosis, especially haemorrhage from an angioma or aneurysm, or subdural haematoma. Bickerstaff (1964) suggests that in many cases the condition is due to internal carotid artery thrombosis, perhaps as a result of carotid arteritis, resulting, for instance, from infected lymph nodes in the neck.

Infantile hemiplegia usually develops during the first three years of life and rarely after the age of 6.

4. Hemiplegia of slow onset is very rare in childhood. The causes include intracranial tumour, arising either in one cerebral hemisphere or in the pons, cerebral tuberculoma, and diffuse sclerosis.

PATHOLOGY

The pathological changes, as might be expected, are very varied. Cases which are examined shortly after the onset of the hemiplegia frequently show focal vascular lesions, including meningeal and intracerebral haemorrhage and arterial thrombosis. Ischaemic lesions within the fields of individual arteries or in the boundary zones between two arteries have been described. Wiesel has described destructive changes in the cerebral arteries leading to necrosis of the media and atheroma in children who died of acute infective diseases. In some cases the pathological picture has been so-called 'acute haemorrhagic encephalitis', and a form of encephalitis characterized by perivascular demyelination occurs in smallpox, chickenpox, vaccinia, and measles. In brains examined long after the onset of the hemiplegia the changes commonly found are meningeal thickening, localized atrophic sclerosis, cysts, and pseudoporencephaly. The Sturge-Weber syndrome [see p. 222] is one rare cause of infantile hemiplegia but the associated facial naevus and the characteristic intracranial calcification are distinctive.

SYMPTOMS

Congenital hemiplegia is usually detected at an early age, because it is observed that the child does not move the affected arm and leg normally, or because these limbs feel rigid.

Infantile hemiplegia usually develops suddenly. When it occurs as a complication of an existing infective disease hemiplegia does not usually develop until some days after the onset of the infection, usually during the second week and sometimes not until the patient is convalescent. Convulsions occur at the onset in a large proportion of cases. Consciousness is lost and the convulsive movements frequently predominate upon and may be confined to the side which subsequently becomes paralysed. Usually a series of attacks occurs during twenty-four hours and the patient remains comatose for a variable period, sometimes for several days after the convulsions stop. Headache, vomiting, delirium, and pyrexia frequently usher in the attacks. During the stage of coma the limbs on the affected side are found to be completely flaccid and the plantar reflex is extensor. When the patient recovers consciousness he is hemiplegic, and when the right side of the body is paralysed, usually aphasic also, and sometimes there is intellectual impairment. In less severe cases hemiplegia may develop without convulsions and without loss of consciousness. The cerebrospinal fluid may be normal or may show an increase in the protein content, red blood cells, or a leucocytosis, depending upon the nature of the cerebral lesion. In a patient with an intracranial angioma there may be a systolic bruit over the cranium or of the carotid artery in the neck.

In favourable cases improvement occurs, and in a few weeks or months recovery may be complete. When the hemiplegia does not recover, flaccidity gives place to spasticity in the course of a few weeks and the condition of the limbs on the paralysed side comes to resemble that found in congenital hemiplegia. The upper limb is severely affected as well as the lower and usually becomes spastic in an attitude of flexion, less often in extension. The signs of hemiplegia are described elsewhere [see p. 20]. Owing to the early age of onset the development of the paralysed limbs is retarded and they remain smaller than those of the normal side. Contractures readily develop in both upper and lower limbs. When the paralysis is incomplete, involuntary movements of an athetoid or choreic character may develop on the affected side and dystonic features are seen to develop in occasional cases many years after the onset. Epilepsy is much commoner in infantile hemiplegia than in cerebral diplegia and occurs in over 50 per cent. of cases. The convulsions usually begin with tonic spasm or clonic movements of the paralysed side, but rapidly become generalized and are attended by loss of consciousness.

DIAGNOSIS

Congenital hemiplegia is readily recognized: hemiplegia acquired in childhood must be distinguished from paralytic chorea, which is preceded by involuntary movements, and acute poliomyelitis which is rarely limited to one upper and lower limb and which is characterized by loss of tendon reflexes and muscular wasting. When the child is seen during the acute stage of a cerebral disturbance the subsequent development of hemiplegia cannot always be anticipated, but the occurrence of repeated convulsions, especially if these are predominantly unilateral, should suggest this possibility.

Hemiplegia of gradual onset is rare in childhood and is usually due to intracranial tumour or tuberculoma. Angiography, air encephalography, or ventriculography may be helpful in difficult cases.

PROGNOSIS

Little improvement is likely to occur in congenital hemiplegia, but in mild cases careful education may enable the child to make some use of the paralysed limbs. It is exceptional for the lesion responsible for acquired infantile hemiplegia to prove fatal, but, if the child shows no signs of returning consciousness 48 hours after the onset of the convulsions, the outlook for recovery is bad. The more severe the symptoms of the acute stage, the more likely are mental defect, aphasia, and hemiplegia to be persistent. Nevertheless, there are exceptions to this rule, and for several weeks after the acute stage there is no sure method of deciding to what extent recovery of function will occur. Some patients recover completely, but a considerable proportion remain intellectually impaired and hemiplegic, and of these more than half become epileptic. The hope of considerable improvement should not be abandoned until at least a year has elapsed after the onset of the illness. Even after this lapse of time some increase of power and co-ordination may occur in the paralysed limbs in response to treatment. Almost invariably the affected children eventually walk and in general lower limb function improves considerably but often little effective movement returns in the arm and hand.

TREATMENT

When the patient is unconscious the usual measures will be called for [see p. 979]. Otherwise treatment in the acute stage depends upon the cause. Cerebral oedema may require treatment with steroid drugs, and hyperpyrexia with hypothermia. The after-treatment of hemiplegia, both of the congenital and of the acquired forms, includes massage and passive movements to diminish the risk of contractures, and the correction of the latter by tenotomy when they develop. When any voluntary power remains, re-educational exercises should be instituted. Small doses of phenobarbitone should be given daily over a period of several years in the hope of preventing the development of epilepsy. Aphasia, when present, must be treated by attempting to re-educate the child's powers of speech. In some severe cases with severe hemiplegia, intractable epilepsy and behaviour disorder the operation of hemispherectomy has been advocated and has resulted in marked reduction in the fits, improved behaviour and intellectual performance and no significant increase in weakness of the affected limbs (Krynauw, 1950; McKissock, 1953). Unfortunately, follow-up studies of such cases have suggested that, except in cases of the Sturge-Weber syndrome [see p. 222], improvement after the operation is only temporary.

REFERENCES

BICKERSTAFF, E. R. (1964) Aetiology of acute hemiplegia in childhood, *Brit. med. J.*, **2**, 82.

FORD, F. R., CROTHERS, B., and PUTNAM, M. C. (1927) *Birth Injuries of the Central Nervous System*, London.

FORD, F. R., and SCHAFFER, A. J. (1927) The etiology of infantile acquired hemiplegia, *Arch. Neurol. Psychiat.* (*Chicago*), **18**, 323.

KRYNAUW, R. W. (1950) Infantile hemiplegia treated by removing one cerebral hemisphere, *J. Neurol. Psychiat.*, **12**, 243.

LeCOUNT, E. R., and SEMERAK, C. B. (1925) Porencephaly, *Arch. Neurol. Psychiat.* (*Chicago*), **14**, 365.

McKISSOCK, W. (1953) Infantile hemiplegia, *Proc. roy. Soc. Med.*, **46**, 431.

MARIE, P. (1885) Hémiplégie cérébrale infantile et maladies infectieuses, *Progr. méd.* (*Paris*), **2**, 167.

NORMAN, R. M., URICH, H., and McMENEMEY, W. H. (1957) Vascular mechanisms of birth injury, *Brain*, **80**, 49.

MINIMAL CEREBRAL DYSFUNCTION

It has been suggested that this is a condition of cerebral abnormality which, though not sufficient to cause easily identifiable syndromes of cerebral palsy, is severe enough to cause minor motor dysfunctions, epilepsy, learning difficulties or abnormalities of behaviour (Bax and MacKeith, 1963). Certainly there are some children who show no evidence of a lesion in the primary motor or sensory pathways but who have disorders of skilled movement (praxis), of the recognition and interpretation of sensory information (gnosis) or of speech and related faculties. Some such are the so-called 'clumsy children' described by Gubbay *et al.* (1965) who showed marked clumsiness of movement without paralysis, incoordination, or sensory loss. Improvement with increasing maturity was the rule but educational difficulties were striking initially in these cases.

REFERENCES

BAX, M., and MACKEITH, R. (1963) Minimal cerebral dysfunction, *Little Club Clinics in Developmental Medicine*, No. 10, London.
GUBBAY, S., ELLIS, E., WALTON, J. N., and COURT, S. D. M. (1965) Clumsy children, *Brain*, **88**, 295.

ERYTHROBLASTOSIS FOETALIS

Erythroblastosis foetalis is a familial disorder. The cause is believed to be the presence of red-cell antigens of the Rhesus group in the blood of the foetus, inherited from a Rh positive father which excites anti-Rh agglutinins in the blood of a Rh negative mother. This is believed to be due to the passage of the infant's red cells across the placental barrier. It is only pregnancies which occur later than the one in which the mother is sensitized that give rise to abnormal children.

The pathological changes consist of general bile-staining of the tissues. There is active blood formation in the liver, spleen, which is enlarged, kidneys, and hyperplastic bone marrow. The liver may be otherwise normal, or may show a centrolobar necrosis. In the brain the bile pigmentation is heaviest in the lentiform and caudate nuclei ('kernicterus'), less marked in other nuclear masses and in the cortex. The ganglion cells in these regions degenerate. Lathe (1955) reviews the evidence that the damage is due to the indirect-reacting plasma bile pigment.

The infant is usually jaundiced at birth and the jaundice rapidly deepens. Bile is present, however, in the stools as well as in the urine. Anaemia and erythroblastaemia are present. The bleeding time is prolonged, and spontaneous haemorrhages occur. Convulsions, rigidity, and coma mark the damage to the brain. In case of doubt a positive Coombs test will establish the diagnosis.

The mortality rate is high if the condition is untreated, but about 25 per cent. survive, usually with nerve deafness, mental defect, epilepsy and extrapyramidal symptoms, such as chorea and athetosis. When the blood-forming organs alone are affected complete recovery may occur, but how far this is the case after the brain has been damaged is unknown. The treatment is exchange transfusion with Rh-negative whole blood. Cappell (1948) reported complete recovery in 30 infants treated thus within twelve hours of birth. The neurological sequelae of kernicterus have been reviewed by Evans and Polani (1950) and by Byers, Paine, and Crothers (1955).

REFERENCES

BYERS, R. K., PAINE, R. S., and CROTHERS, B. (1955) Extra-pyramidal cerebral palsy with hearing loss following erythroblastosis, *Pediatrics*, **15**, 248.
CAPPELL, D. F. (1948) Advances in knowledge of the Rh factor, *Brit. med. J.*, **2**, 323.
EVANS, P. R., and POLANI, P. E. (1950) The neurological sequelae of Rh sensitisation, *Quart. J. Med.*, **19**, 129.
LATHE, G. H. (1955) Exchange transfusion as a means of removing bilirubin in haemolytic disease of the newborn, *Brit. med. J.*, **1**, 192.
PARSONS, L. G. (1947) Haemolytic disease of the new-born, *Lancet*, i, 534.
ROBERTS, G. F. (1947) *The Rhesus Factor*, London.
ZIMMERMAN, H. M., and YANNET, H. (1933) Kernikterus: jaundice of the nuclear masses of the brain, *Amer. J. Dis. Child.*, **45**, 740.
ZIMMERMAN, H. M., and YANNET, H. (1935) Cerebral sequelae of icterus gravis neonatorum and their relation to kernikterus, *Amer. J. Dis. Child.*, **49**, 418.

NEUROLOGICAL MANIFESTATIONS OF THE LIPIDOSES

Much remains obscure about the group of diseases characterized by disordered lipid metabolism, but it is clear that the nervous system may be involved in any of them. In the varieties of *cerebromacular degeneration* it appears to suffer alone; in *Niemann–Pick* and *Gaucher's* diseases and in the *Hand–Schüller–Christian* syndrome—xanthomatosis—as part of a more general disturbance. According to Thannhauser (1940) the following are the main differences between the last three. In Niemann-Pick disease, which is familial, the histiocytes and reticulocytes of all organs are involved and the cortical ganglion cells are ballooned. The Niemann–Pick cells, which are large, pale, and ovoid or round, contain sphingomyelin. In Gaucher's disease, which is also familial, the characteristic cell is opaque and homogeneous and often has many nuclei. It contains kerasin, a cerebroside, which does not stain with Sudan III or Scarlet R. The ganglion cells of the cerebral cortex, basal ganglia, and cerebellum are distended with this (Oberling and Worniger, 1927). In the Hand–Schüller–Christian syndrome the abnormal cells contain cholesterol and other lipids.

All these disorders are rare, but examples would probably be more often found if lipidosis was more often thought of as a cause of obscure deterioration of the nervous system in children. It has recently been shown that metachromatic leuco-encephalopathy, originally described by Brain and Greenfield (1950), is a lipidosis due to the accumulation of aryl-sulphatide which results from a genetically-determined deficiency of the enzyme sulphatase (Norman et al., 1960; Jervis, 1960; Austin et al., 1965).

CEREBROMACULAR DEGENERATION

Synonyms. Tay-Sachs disease; amaurotic family idiocy.

Definition. A disease of early life, frequently occurring in several members of the same family, characterized pathologically by widespread deposit of lipids, mainly gangliosides, in the ganglion cells of the brain and retina, and clinically by progressive mental failure, blindness, and paralysis.

PATHOLOGY

Several forms of cerebromacular degeneration have been described, differing mainly in the age of onset. The infantile form, described as amaurotic family idiocy by Warren Tay (1881) and Bernard Sachs (1887), develops during the first year of life. A late infantile form of Bielschowsky (1914) begins during the second and third year, and a juvenile form of Spielmeyer-Vogt (1906) and a late juvenile form (Kufs, 1925) develop between the ages of 3 and 10, and 15 and 25 respectively.

Although there are corresponding differences in the pathological picture, it would seem that the underlying pathological process is the same. Macroscopically, the brain usually shows moderate general atrophy, although megalencephaly has been described and when this is the case there is usually ventricular dilatation, massive demyelination, and cystic degeneration of the white matter (Crome, 1964). Microscopically, the characteristic pathological change is found in the ganglion cells. According to Schaffer (1925) the first alteration is a swelling of the hyaloplasm, which subsequently undergoes a granular degeneration with the formation of lipids and lipochrome. The nucleus is often eccentric, and the dendrites are frequently swollen. The ganglion cells of the cortex and of the thalamus suffer severely. The cerebellum is usually more affected in the late infantile and juvenile forms than in the infantile form. The ganglion cells of the spinal cord may show similar changes. The white matter shows tract degeneration. An overgrowth of neuroglia occurs secondarily to the ganglion cell degeneration. The retina shows changes similar to those found elsewhere in the nervous system. The ganglion cells show degeneration. In the forms of later onset there is degeneration of the external layers of the retina with proliferation of the neuroglia and of the pigment epithelial cells. These changes are most evident in the region of the macula.

AETIOLOGY

The disease is frequently familial and occurs in several sibs. Though it depends upon an inherited predisposition, there is no history of the disorder in previous generations. It is probably inherited as a Mendelian recessive factor.

The infantile form is confined to the Jewish race, but this is not true of the late infantile and juvenile forms.

The cause of the peculiar degeneration of the ganglion cells is unknown, though it seems likely that it is due to the progressive accumulation of abnormal lipid material. Attempts have been made to relate amaurotic family idiocy to Niemann–Pick disease, which is characterized by widespread intracellular deposition of lipids throughout the body, and, like the infantile form of amaurotic family idiocy, has a familial incidence in Jewish children during the first year of life. Schaffer, however, points out that amaurotic family idiocy is essentially a degeneration of an ectodermal tissue, whereas in Niemann–Pick disease meso-dermal tissues take part in the reaction, and the brain probably suffers secondarily to a general disturbance of lipid metabolism. Diezel (1960) agrees that the two conditions are distinctive and so, too, is gargoylism (Hurler's disease) [see p. 574] in which changes which seem similar histologically are observed.

SYMPTOMS

The age of onset of the various forms has already been stated. The symptoms are essentially the same in all forms, consisting of progressive mental deteriora-tion, visual failure, fits, and paralysis.

In the infantile form the child is normal at birth and symptoms usually appear between the third and sixth months. The child becomes listless and apathetic and ceases to take notice of its surroundings. It fails to raise its head and to sit up. Convulsions may occur and myoclonic jerking in response to 'startle' (i.e. sudden noises) is commonly seen. The retina and optic disc are atrophied, and there is a cherry-red spot visible at the macula, which at this age is patho-gnomonic. This is due to severe atrophy of the macular region of the retina, which renders the vascular choroid visible. Progressive flaccid paralysis of all four limbs develops, and finally the child is completely blind and paralysed, and fails to respond to external stimuli, except occasionally by a simple reflex muscu-lar contraction. The retinal atrophy leads to impairment of the reaction of the pupils to light, and squint and nystagmus may be present.

In the late infantile and juvenile forms the red spot at the macula is usually absent and may be replaced by fine pigmentation (Batten-Mayou type of degeneration). Convulsions appear to be commoner in cases of later onset, and flaccidity if replaced by spasticity and contractures. The gradual development of Parkinsonian symptoms in some such cases has been noted.

DIAGNOSIS

No other condition exactly simulates the infantile form of the disease and the red spot at the macula settles the diagnosis. Similar nervous symptoms, including the red spot at the macula, have been described in Niemann–Pick disease, but in this condition the liver and spleen are enlarged. Gaucher's disease may cause dementia and diplegia in infancy or later in childhood, but in this disease also the spleen is enlarged. The juvenile form of cerebromacular degeneration may simulate diffuse cerebral sclerosis (Schilder's disease), which is also charac-terized by progressive blindness, paralysis, and mental deterioration. In this condition, however, the blindness is usually due to degeneration of the optic radiations, and optic atrophy is rare. The electroencephalogram may be very helpful as it often shows irregular, generalized spike and wave discharges, which are not seen in diffuse sclerosis (Cobb, Martin, and Pampiglione, 1952). Brain biopsy is now being used increasingly for diagnosis.

PROGNOSIS

The disease is inevitably progressive, and the younger the patient at the onset the more rapid the downward course. In the infantile form death occurs in from one to two years, the terminal stages being characterized by wasting and anaemia. In the juvenile form the patient may live for ten or fifteen years. Accurate diagnosis, which may be achieved by means of biochemical analysis and histo-logical examination of a brain biopsy sample, is of value not only in relation to forecasting the outcome of the illness but also for genetic counselling as in this condition there is a 1 in 4 chance that a subsequent child born to the same parents will be affected.

TREATMENT

No treatment is known to influence the disease.

REFERENCES

AUSTIN, J., ARMSTRONG, D., and SHEARER, L. (1965) Metachromatic form of diffuse cerebral sclerosis, *Arch. Neurol. (Chic.)*, **13**, 593.

BIELSCHOWSKY, M. (1928) Amaurotische Idiotie und lipoidzellige Splenohepatomegatie, *J. Psychol. Neurol. (Lpz.)*, **36**, 103.

BIRD, A. (1948) The lipidoses and the central nervous system, *Brain*, **71**, 434.

BOGAERT, L. VAN (1953) Thésaurismoses dites phosphatidiques au point de vue clinique, histopathologique et clinique, *Rep. Vth Int. Neur. Cong.*, **1**, 261.

BRAIN, W. R., and GREENFIELD, J. G. (1950) Late infantile metachromatic leuco-encephalopathy with primary degeneration of the interfascicular oligodendroglia, *Brain*, **73**, 291.

COBB, W., MARTIN, F., and PAMPIGLIONE, G. (1952) Cerebral lipidosis: an electro-encephalographic study, *Brain*, **75**, 343.

CROME, L. (1964) Neuropathological changes in diseases caused by inborn errors of metabolism, in *Neurometabolic Disorders in Childhood*, ed. HOLT, K. S., and MILNER, J., Edinburgh.

DIEZEL, P. B. (1960) Lipidoses of the central nervous system, in *Modern Scientific Aspects of Neurology*, ed. CUMINGS, J. N., London.

GREENFIELD, J. G., and HOLMES, G. (1925) The histology of juvenile amaurotic idiocy, *Brain*, **48**, 183.

HASSIN, G. B. (1924) A study of the histopathology of amaurotic family idiocy, *Arch. Neurol. Psychiat. (Chicago)*, **12**, 640.

HASSIN, G. B. (1930) Niemann-Pick's disease, *Arch. Neurol. Psychiat. (Chicago)*, **24**, 61.

JERVIS, G. A. (1960) Infantile metachromatic leucoencephalopathy, *J. Neuropath.*, **19**, 323.

KLENK, E. (1953) On the chemistry of the so-called phospholipid-storage diseases of the nervous tissue, *Rep. Vth. Neur. Cong.*, **1**, 253.

LEINER, J. H., and GOODHART, S. P. (1927) The infantile type of family amaurotic idiocy, *Arch. Neurol. Psychiat. (Chicago)*, **17**, 616.

MARINESCO, G. (1930–1) Nouvelles contributions à l'étude de la forme tardive de l'idiotie amaurotique (type Bielschowsky) et à son mécanisme biochimique, *J. Psychol. Neurol. (Lpz.)*, **41**, 1.

NORMAN, R. M., URICH, H., and TINGEY, A. H. (1960) Metachromatic leuco-encephalo-pathy: a form of lipidosis, *Brain*, **83**, 369.

OBERLING, C., and WORNIGER, P. (1927) La maladie de Gaucher chez le nourrisson, *Rev. franç. Pédiat.*, **3**, 475.

RICHARDSON, M. E., and BORNHOFEN, J. H. (1968) Early childhood cerebral lipidosis with prominent myoclonus, *Arch. Neurol. (Chic.)*, **18**, 34.

SACHS, B. (1929) Amaurotic family idiocy and general lipoid degeneration, *Arch. Neurol. Psychiat. (Chicago)*, **12**, 247.

SCHAFFER, C. (1925) General significance of Tay-Sachs disease, *Arch. Neurol. Psychiat. (Chicago)*, **14**, 731.

THANNHAUSER, S. J. (1940) *Lipidoses: Diseases of the Cellular Lipid Metabolism*, New York.

HAND–SCHÜLLER–CHRISTIAN SYNDROME

Synonyms. Diabetic exophthalmic dysostosis; xanthomatosis.

Definition. A rare disorder usually occurring in childhood and characterized by widespread xanthomatous deposits, leading to diabetes insipidus, exophthalmos, and progressive erosion of bones, especially of the membranous bones of the skull, and probably related to eosinophilic granuloma, and Letterer-Siwe disease.

AETIOLOGY

This rare disease was first described by Hand in 1893 then by Schüller (1915) and subsequently Christian (1919). The essential feature is a tissue infiltration by xanthomatous masses rich in cholesterol. These are now generally regarded as the products of a disturbance of lipid metabolism. Hence the disease, like Niemann–Pick disease and Gaucher's disease, is a lipidosis, though the actual lipid material which accumulates differs in all three. The cause of the metabolic abnormality is unknown. The diabetes insipidus is due to invasion of the tuber cinereum and hypophysis by xanthomatous material.

Multiple cases in the same family have been recorded only twice. Males are affected two or three times as often as females. In three-fourths of all cases the disease begins during the first decade of life, but it may start as late as the second decade.

PATHOLOGY

The xanthomatous infiltration is extremely widespread. The reticulo-endothelial cells stuffed with lipid material are known as 'foam' cells. Bones are diffusely affected, especially the membranous bones of the skull. The pelvic bones are also a common site. The hypophysis and tuber cinereum are commonly invaded by the xanthomatous material, and the exophthalmos is produced by xanthomatous masses situated in the orbital fat. Plaques of demyelination containing 'foam' cells have been described in the nervous system by Davison (1933) and Chiari (1933). Xanthomatosis may also be present in the liver, spleen, lymph nodes, lungs, and pleura.

SYMPTOMATOLOGY

Diabetes insipidus leading to polyuria and polydipsia is often the earliest symptom, and may occur at a time when there is no radiological evidence of bony change in the skull. It is present in three out of four cases. Exophthalmos is slightly less frequent. Retardation of growth and mental development has been observed in about half of the cases, and adiposogenital dystrophy is sometimes seen. Gingivitis and falling out of the teeth may occur, and there may be a persistent discharge from the ears. The colour of the skin may alter owing to xanthomatous deposits, and the liver, spleen, and lymph nodes may be enlarged. The total fat of the blood may be above normal, but the blood cholesterol, calcium, and phosphorus have been found normal.

Radiographs of the skull may show large areas of defect in the membranous bones, especially towards the base in the frontal, temporal, and parietal regions. The sella turcica is often, but not invariably, normal. Other bones, especially those of the pelvis, femora, vertebrae, scapulae, and ribs, may also exhibit decalcification. Radiographs of the lungs may show a diffuse mottling resembling miliary tuberculosis with increased density of the hilar shadows.

DIAGNOSIS

The diagnosis will hardly give rise to difficulty except in those cases in which diabetes insipidus develops before there is any radiographic change in the skull, and in the absence of exophthalmos. In such cases an area of bone destruction will often be found somewhere in the body, particularly in the pelvis. Biopsy may be helpful.

PROGNOSIS

The disorder appears usually to be progressive and to terminate fatally, but owing to the small number of cases in the literature it is uncertain whether this is invariably the case.

TREATMENT

The polyuria responds considerably to posterior pituitary extract (*Pitressin*) given as snuff or by injecting the tannate in oil, and a temporary improvement in symptoms often follows X-ray irradiation and the use of corticosteroids.

REFERENCES

CHIARI, H. (1933) Über Veränderungen im Zentralnervensystem bei generalisierter Xanthomatose vom Typus Schüller-Christian, *Virchows Arch. path. Anat.*, **288**, 527.

CHRISTIAN, H. A. (1919) Defects in membranous bones, exophthalmos, and diabetes insipidus, *Contr. Med. Biol. Res.*, **1**, 390. New York.

DAVISON, C. (1933) Xanthomatosis and the central nervous system, *Arch. Neurol. Psychiat. (Chicago)*, **30**, 75.

HAUSMAN, L., and BROMBERG, W. (1929) Diabetic exophthalmic dysostosis, *Arch. Neurol. Psychiat. (Chicago)*, **21**, 1402.

HEATH, P. (1931) Xanthomatosis or lipoid histiocytosis; report of ocular observations in 2 cases of Christian's syndrome: correlation with other ocular syndromes, *Arch. Ophthal. (Chicago)*, **5**, 29.

MORISON, J. M. W. (1934) Schüller's disease, *Brit. J. Radiol.*, N.S. **7**, 213.

SCHÜLLER, A. (1915–16) Über eigenartige Schädeldefekte im Jugendalter, *Fortschr. Röntgenstr.*, **23**, 12.

SCHÜLLER, A. (1926) Dysostosis hypophysaria, *Brit. J. Radiol.*, **31**, 156.

THANNHAUSER, S. J. (1940) *Lipidoses: Diseases of the Cellular Lipid Metabolism*, New York.

GAUCHER'S DISEASE
Definition

A condition characterized by enlargement of the liver and spleen due to the accumulation of kerasin in cells of the reticulo-endothelial system; the nervous system is involved in some cases.

Pathology

Reticulo-endothelial cells in the liver, spleen, lymph nodes and bone marrow are distended by granular material; in the brain nerve cells may be similarly distended and globular swellings may be found on dendritic processes.

Aetiology

The condition is due to an autosomal recessive gene and is an inborn error of lipid metabolism.

Symptoms and Signs

In the comparatively small proportion of acute infantile cases showing central nervous system involvement, progressive apathy, ataxia, oculomotor palsies, trismus and signs of pseudobulbar palsy may occur consecutively and eventually spasticity of the limbs and decerebrate rigidity may appear. Convulsions occur in some cases. In most cases the illness ends fatally by about the end of the first year of life. In adults the condition is characterized by enlargement of the liver and spleen without evidence of central nervous system involvement. No effective treatment is known.

Diagnosis

There may be characteristic areas of rarefaction and condensation in the long bones shown radiologically. Liver or bone-marrow biopsy will reveal the characteristic cells.

REFERENCES

BARLOW, C. (1957) Neuropathological findings in a case of Gaucher's disease, *J. Neuropath. exp. Neurol.*, **16**, 239.
BOGAERT, L. VAN (1957) *Cerebral Lipidoses*, Springfield, Ill.
DIEZEL, P. B. (1960) Lipidoses of the central nervous system, in *Modern Scientific Aspects of Neurology*, ed. CUMINGS, J. N., London.

NIEMANN–PICK DISEASE
Definition

Seen usually in patients of Jewish extraction, this condition is characterized by progressive enlargement of the liver and spleen and, in occasional cases, by evidence of central nervous system involvement.

Pathology

Reticulo-endothelial cells in liver, spleen, adrenals, pancreas and often in the heart and vascular endothelium show a foamy appearance due to distension with sphingomyelin. Similar foamy cells, presumably of mesodermal origin, may be seen in the brain but in cases with cerebral involvement ganglion cells are also distended with lipid.

Aetiology

The condition is due to an autosomal recessive gene.

Clinical Features

The condition becomes manifest as a rule within the first few months of life with progressive hepatic and splenic enlargement, cutaneous pigmentation and progressive anaemia. When the brain is involved progressive dementia occurs and is followed by flaccid paresis of the limbs, areflexia, deafness, and blindness. A cherry-red spot may be seen at the macula. Most patients die within 3 years of onset and no effective treatment is known.

Diagnosis

Circulating lymphocytes may show characteristic vacuoles and splenic puncture will reveal the typical cells.

REFERENCES

CROCKER, A. C., and FARBER, S. (1958) Niemann-Pick disease: a review of 19 patients, *Medicine (Baltimore)*, **37**, 1.

DIEZEL, P. B. (1960) Lipidoses of the central nervous system, in *Modern Scientific Aspects of Neurology*, ed. CUMINGS, J. N., London.

GARGOYLISM

Synonym

Hurler's syndrome, lipochondrodystrophy.

Definition

A disorder of infancy and childhood due to the accumulation of gangliosides in the brain and the deposition of mucopolysaccharides, glycogen and lipids in the cells of other organs. It is characterized by dwarfism, deformities of the face and bones, visceral abnormalities and mental deterioration.

Pathology

The brain usually shows atrophy of the cortex and white matter and ventricular dilatation. The nerve cells are distended with gangliosides and in other organs reticulo-endothelial cells may be similarly distended but in addition supporting and connective tissues show marked deposition of mucopolysaccharides showing resemblances to chondroitin sulphate.

Aetiology

Most cases are due to an autosomal recessive gene but in some families the disorder appears to be sex-linked.

Clinical Features

Defective bodily growth, mental backwardness, a grotesque facial appearance with flattening and broadening of the nose, a large head with a short neck, progressive opacification of the corneae and deformities of the hands and feet are characteristically seen. Eventually spastic weakness of the limbs followed by paralysis occurs and death is usual at or before the tenth year of life. Enlargement of the liver and spleen is usual, cardiac murmurs and eventual cardiac failure are frequently observed and some patients show a white papulonodular skin eruption while others are excessively hirsute.

Diagnosis

Characteristic radiological changes are observed in long bones, in the skull and the vertebral bodies. Often there is wedging of one or more lumbar vertebral bodies with an anterior hook-like projection and the epiphyses of long bones are widened and irregular. Sulphated mucopolysaccharides (chondroitin and heparitin sulphates) can usually be detected in the urine while typical granules may be found in leucocytes in the circulating blood.

REFERENCES

DIEZEL, P. B. (1960) Lipidoses of the central nervous system, in *Modern Scientific Aspects of Neurology*, ed. CUMINGS, J. N., London.
MCKUSICK, V. (1956) *Heritable Disorders of Connective Tissue*, St. Louis, Mo.
TERRY, K., and LINKER, A. (1964) Four forms of Hurler's syndrome, *Proc. Soc. exp. Biol. (N.Y.)*, **115**, 394.

METACHROMATIC LEUCO-ENCEPHALOPATHY

Definition

A progressive disorder of infancy and childhood characterized clinically by progressive dementia and spastic paralysis, and pathologically by the presence of metachromatic deposits in the nerve cells and white matter of the central and peripheral nervous systems.

Pathology

The brain is frequently large and heavy for the age of the child and there is diffuse demyelination in the white matter, without sparing of the arcuate fibres. There is usually an almost total degeneration of the interfascicular oligodendroglia. Metachromatic material (staining brown rather than blue with cresyl violet and thionine) and giving a positive P.A.S. reaction, is seen not only within nerve cells but also in the white matter of the brain and in the peripheral nerves. Metachromatic material may also be found in the cells of the renal tubules and in the ganglion cells of the bowel wall. Originally believed to be a form of diffuse sclerosis (Brain and Greenfield, 1950) the condition is now known to be a lipidosis due to an accumulation of cerebroside sulphatides.

Aetiology

The condition is due to an autosomal recessive gene and has recently been shown to be due to a deficiency of arylsulphatase A (Austin *et al.*, 1966).

Clinical Features

The affected children often develop normally up to the second or third year of life. Difficulty in walking and clumsiness in upper limb movement then appear and convulsions occur occasionally. Progressive spastic (or occasionally flaccid) paralysis is accompanied by mental deterioration. Bulbar paralysis eventually supervenes in most cases and death generally occurs within one or two years of the onset. No effective treatment is known but accurate diagnosis is essential in order to advise the parents upon the prospect that subsequent children may be affected.

Diagnosis

The finding of metachromatically-staining granules in centrifuged deposits of urine may be diagnostic in the earlier stages. The cerebrospinal fluid usually shows an increase in its protein content but no other specific abnormality. There may be a progressive slowing of motor nerve conduction velocity in peripheral nerves (Fullerton, 1964). Some authors have advised full-thickness rectal biopsy while others prefer appendicectomy with histological examination of the specimen, seeking for metachromatic deposits. Sural nerve biopsy is also recommended in cases showing clinical or electrical evidence of peripheral neuropathy. The diagnosis may be finally confirmed by brain biopsy.

REFERENCES

AUSTIN, J., ARMSTRONG, D., SHEARER, L., and MCAFEE, D. (1966) Metachromatic form of diffuse cerebral sclerosis. VI. A rapid test for sulphatase A deficiency in the urine, *Arch. Neurol. (Chic.)*, **14**, 259.

BRAIN, W. R., and GREENFIELD, J. G. (1950) Late infantile metachromatic leucoencephalopathy with primary degeneration of the interfascicular oligodendroglia, *Brain*, **73**, 291.

FULLERTON, P. M. (1964) Peripheral nerve conduction in metachromatic leucoencephalopathy (sulphatide lipidosis), *J. Neurol. Psychiat.*, **27**, 100.

NORMAN, R. M., and TINGEY, A. H. (1960) Metachromatic leucoencephalopathy, a form of lipidosis, *Brain*, **83**, 369.

REFSUM'S DISEASE

Synonym

Heredopathia atactica polyneuritiformis.

Definition

A progressive degenerative disorder of the central nervous system, beginning often in childhood but sometimes in adult life, and characterized by atypical retinitis pigmentosa, cerebellar ataxia and a peripheral neuropathy.

Aetiology

The condition appears to be due to an autosomal recessive gene and is characterized by the storage of 3, 7, 11, 15-tetramethyl hexadecanoic acid (phytanic acid) in the liver, kidney, and peripheral nerves. The condition thus appears to be due to an inborn error of metabolism, due to storage in the tissues of an abnormal fatty acid and it is therefore classified provisionally with the lipidoses.

Pathology

The most striking changes are in the peripheral nerves which show thickening due to the proliferation of connective tissue in concentric layers. The retina shows loss of ganglion cells and degenerative changes in the nuclear layers.

Clinical Features

Refsum (1946) first described the condition in five members of two families in each of which the affected individuals resulted from a consanguineous marriage. Most patients show slow progressive visual deterioration, ataxia and evidence of a progressive polyneuropathy with loss of tendon reflexes, peripheral sensory impairment and palpable hypertrophy of peripheral nerves. The eyes show optic atrophy and pigmentary retinal degeneration without the typical vascular changes of retinitis pigmentosa. Less constant features are fixed pupils, nerve deafness, cataracts, icthyotic skin changes, bony abnormalities, and cardio-myopathy. The condition runs a variable but usually indolent course with slow deterioration occurring over a period of many years. A diet devoid of phytanic acid has been shown to be of some value in arresting the progress of the disease (Eldjarn et al., 1966).

Diagnosis

The diagnosis rests upon the typical clinical features, the isolation of phytanic acid from the urine, and the characteristic rise in cerebrospinal fluid protein content. Nerve biopsy may be confirmatory.

REFERENCES

ELDJARN, L., TRY, K., STOKKE, O., MUNTHE-KAAS, A. W., REFSUM, S., STEINBERG, D., AUIGUN, J., and MIZE, C. (1966) Dietary effects on serum-phytanic acid levels and on clinical manifestations in heredopathia atactica polyneuritiformis, *Lancet*, i, 691.

NEVIN, N. C., CUMINGS, J. N., and McKEOWN, F. (1967) Refsum's syndrome. Heredo-pathia atactica polyneuritiformis, *Brain*, **90**, 419.

RAKE, M., and SAUNDERS, M. (1966) Refsum's disease; a disorder of lipid metabolism, *J. Neurol. Neurosurg. Psychiat.*, **29**, 417.

REFSUM, S. (1946) Heredopathia atactica polyneuritiformis, *Acta psychiat. (Kbh.)*, Suppl. 38.

RICHTERICH, R., VAN MECHELEN, D., and ROSSI, E. (1965) Refsum's disease. An inborn error of lipid metabolism with storage of 3, 7, 11, 15-tetramethyl hexadecanoic acid, *Amer. J. Med.*, **39**, 230.

INFANTILE NEUROAXONAL DYSTROPHY

This rare disorder, which also seems to be due to an autosomal recessive gene, was first described by Seitelberger in 1952. Pathologically it is characterized by the accumulation of large axonal swellings in the grey matter of the brain and spinal cord and by degeneration of the globus pallidus, cerebellum and long spinal tracts. Optic atrophy and partial denervation of skeletal muscles may also occur.

The condition usually begins between the ages of one and three years with arrest of development and motor weakness progressing to paralysis due to a combination of pyramidal tract and lower motor neurone dysfunction; there may be loss of pain sensation in the legs. Convulsions are rare but progressive optic atrophy leads to blindness and most patients die before the end of the first decade.

The EEG usually shows diffuse fast activity, the EMG confirms the presence of denervation and the serum lactate dehydrogenase activity may be raised. Certain features of the condition resemble those of experimental tocopherol deficiency in animals but no specific biochemical abnormality has yet been detected in these cases, while no effective treatment has yet been introduced.

REFERENCES

Cowen, D., and Olmstead, E. V. (1963) Infantile neuroaxonal dystrophy, *J. Neuropath.*, **22**, 175.

Huttenlocher, P. R., and Gilles, F. H. (1967) Infantile neuroaxonal dystrophy. Clinical, pathological and histochemical findings in a family with 3 affected siblings, *Neurology (Minneap.)*, **17**, 1174.

Seitelberger, F. (1952) Eine unbekannte Form von infantiler lipoidopercher Krankheit des Gehirns, *Proceedings of the First International Congress of Neuropathology*, Vol. 3, p. 323, Turin.

SUBACUTE NECROTIZING ENCEPHALOMYELOPATHY

This rare condition, first described by Leigh in 1951, is inherited by an autosomal recessive mechanism and its clinical and pathological features strongly suggest that it is due to an inherited enzyme defect. In the past the diagnosis has usually been made only at post-mortem but recently a number of cases have been diagnosed during life and have been found to show raised blood pyruvate levels. Pathologically the brains of affected individuals show widespread cellular necrosis with capillary proliferation in the optic nerves and chiasm, basal ganglia, and brain stem. The appearances are similar to those of Wernicke's encephalopathy, but the distribution of the lesions is somewhat different, the corpora mamillaria usually being spared. Clinically the affected children show failure to thrive, poverty of movement, hypotonia and spasticity, loss of tendon reflexes, nystagmus, and optic atrophy; convulsions sometimes occur and the condition is usually fatal in six to twelve months. In some cases there has been apparent temporary arrest of the disease process following treatment with lipoic acid.

REFERENCES

Crome, L. (1964) Neuropathological changes in diseases caused by inborn errors of metabolism, in *Neurometabolic Disorders in Childhood*, ed. Holt, K. S., and Milner, J., Edinburgh.

Greenhouse, A. H., and Schneck, S. A. (1968) Subacute necrotizing encephalomyelopathy. A reappraisal of the thiamine deficiency hypothesis, *Neurology (Minneap.)*, **18**, 1.

LEIGH, D. (1951) Subacute necrotizing encephalomyelopathy in an infant, *J. Neurol. Neurosurg. Psychiat.*, **14**, 216.

WORSLEY, H. E., BROOKFIELD, R. W., ELWOOD, J. S., NOBLE, R. L., and TAYLOR, W. H. (1965) Lactic acidosis with necrotizing encephalopathy in two sibs, *Arch. Dis. Childh.*, **40**, 492.

EPILOIA

Synonyms. Tuberose sclerosis; Bourneville's disease; Brushfield–Wyatt disease.

Definition. A rare congenital disorder characterized pathologically by sclerotic masses in the cerebral cortex, adenoma sebaceum, and tumours in various organs, and clinically by mental deficiency and epilepsy.

PATHOLOGY

Macroscopically the brain may exhibit microgyria and macrogyria, and absence of the corpus callosum has been described. The characteristic sclerotic patches to which the disease owes its name were first described by Bourneville and Brissaud in 1880. They are found in the cortex of the cerebral hemispheres, and are rare in the cerebellum. They are hard to the touch, and white in appearance, ranging in size from $\frac{1}{2}$ to 2 cm. in diameter. Microscopically they are composed of glial fibres, and contain in addition large cells, some of which are believed to be abnormal ganglion cells, while others are thought to be derived from spongioblasts. Tumour-like masses are also found in the cerebral ventricles, and these appear to be derived from the ependyma. Occasionally a large tumour, glioblastoma or astrocytoma, has been observed. Circular laminated bodies resembling corpora amylacea have been found scattered throughout the cerebral cortex, cerebellum, choroid plexus, and the tumours themselves, and cystic degeneration is found in the cerebral hemispheres and cerebellum, leading to small cavities which may be traversed by fine fibrils. The ganglion cells of the cerebral cortex are reduced in number, and are often atypical. The retinal tumours, phakomas, are composed of neuroglia. Adenoma sebaceum described by Balzer in 1885 and Pringle in 1890 consists of a hyperplasia of sebaceous glands embedded in a vascular matrix. Tumours in other situations include rhabdomyoma of the heart, teratoma, and adenosarcoma of the kidney, and tumours have also been described in the thyroid, thymus, breast, and duodenum. Other associated abnormalities which are sometimes present include hydromyelia and spina bifida, and congenital malformations of the heart. The bones may show osteoporosis, cyst formation, and periosteal deposits which are visible radiologically (Holt and Dickerson, 1952).

AETIOLOGY

Beyond the fact that tuberose sclerosis is due to a congenital dysplasia probably occurring at an early stage in embryonic life, little is known about its aetiology. It is occasionally familial, two or more sibs being affected. The first-born appear more liable to develop it than later children. Males are affected more often than females. The disorder is almost confined to the white races and is found especially among the poorer classes. Penrose suggests that it is probably due to a single dominant gene, which is subject to modification by autosomal genetic factors. It appears to be closely related to the syndrome of neurofibroblastomatosis.

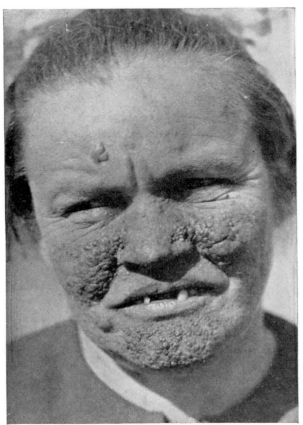

FIG. 84. Epiloia: showing adenoma sebaceum
(Kindly lent by Dr. R. M. Stewart.)

SYMPTOMS

Typical sufferers from tuberose sclerosis are mentally defective, being usually imbeciles of a low grade, and are epileptic. The convulsions begin as a rule during the first year of life. Both petit mal and major attacks occur, and Jacksonian convulsions have been described. Status epilepticus may supervene. In spite of the diffuse distribution of the cerebral lesions spastic paralysis and contractures are rare. A single large tumour will cause the general and focal symptoms of an intracranial neoplasm. The mental deterioration is progressive and consists of intellectual defect associated with a primitive type of psychosis.

Adenoma sebaceum, which is not invariably present, manifests itself at about the fourth or fifth year of life as a pale pink, slightly raised rash, consisting of discrete spots, which fade on pressure, and appear first in the nasolabial folds, spreading over the face in a 'butterfly' pattern, sparing the upper lip [FIG. 84].

A few scattered nodules may also appear on the forehead and neck, but rarely below the clavicles. After the second dentition the adenomas tend to coalesce and darken in colour to a deep red or brown hue. Exceptionally the cutaneous lesion does not make its appearance until puberty or early adult life. Tumours in other situations occasionally grow large enough to cause symptoms. The retinal phakomas, described by van der Hoeve in 1923, are flat, white, round or oval areas about half the size of the optic disc. Abortive forms of the disease occur. Adenoma sebaceum or epilepsy, or both, may occur without mental defect. The ventricular tumours may show in pneumoencephalograms.

DIAGNOSIS

Tuberose sclerosis can be distinguished from other causes of mental deficiency associated with epilepsy only by the presence of adenoma sebaceum or of tumours elsewhere. The pneumoencephalographic appearance of the cerebral ventricles and retinal phakomas may, however, be diagnostic in the absence of skin changes.

PROGNOSIS

Most patients die between the ages of 5 and 15 years, though exceptionally an individual may survive to between 30 and 40. Death, if not due to inter-current disease, usually occurs from status epilepticus and has sometimes been due to a renal tumour.

TREATMENT

The mental deficiency usually necessitates institutional treatment, and the treatment appropriate for epilepsy should be carried out.

REFERENCES

BIELSCHOWSKY, M. (1923–4). Zur Histopathologie und Pathogenese der tuberösen Sklerose, *J. Psychol. Neurol. (Lpz.)*, **30**, 167.

BRAIN, W. R., and GREENFIELD, J. G. (1937) Epiloia, in *British Encyclopaedia of Medical Practice*, Vol. 5, p. 117, London.

BRUSHFIELD, T., and WYATT, W. (1926) Epiloia, parts I and II. *Brit. J. Child. Dis.*, **23**, 178 and 254.

CRITCHLEY, M., and EARL, C. J. C. (1932) Tuberose sclerosis and allied conditions, *Brain*, **55**, 311.

FERRARO, A., and DOOLITTLE, G. J. (1936) Tuberous sclerosis, *Psychiat. Quart.*, **10**, 365.

HOLT, J., and DICKERSON, W. (1952) Osseous lesions of tuberous sclerosis, *Radiology*, **58**, 1.

KESSEL, F. K. (1949) Some radiologic and neurosurgical aspects of tuberous sclerosis, *Acta psychiat. (Kbh.)*, **24**, 499.

NEUROFIBROMATOSIS

Synonyms. Neurofibroblastomatosis; von Recklinghausen's disease.

Definition. A disease of congenital origin, characterized by cutaneous pigmentation and the formation of tumours in various tissues. The commonest of these are cutaneous fibromas, mollusca fibrosa, and perineurial fibroblastomas (neurofibromas), but meningeal fibroblastomas (meningiomas) and gliomas may also occur. Combinations of these abnormalities have been designated as separate syndromes. Thus Worster-Drought, Carnegie Dickson, and McMenemey (1937) recognize the following:

1. Central type (*a*) meningeal and perineurial—syndrome of Wishart (1822) which is rare. (*b*) Meningeal only—syndrome of Schultze (1880) which is the rarest. (*c*) Perineurial only—syndrome of Knoblauch (1843) which is the commonest.

2. Peripheral type. The peripheral neurofibromatosis of von Recklinghausen (1882) first described by Tilesius in 1793. The central and peripheral types may also occur in combination. The disorder appears to be closely related to epiloia.

PATHOLOGY

The neurofibromas are tumours usually situated upon peripheral nerves and composed of bundles of long spindle cells. There has been much controversy as to the nature of the cells of which neurofibromas are composed. Russell and Rubinstein (1959) distinguish on histological grounds schwannomas, derived from cells of the neurilemma (sheath of Schwann), and neurofibromas, which they believe to be also of Schwannian origin and not derived from fibroblasts. Both may be found on the peripheral nerves and also upon the cranial nerves, most frequently upon the vestibulocochlear nerve, but also upon others, especially the optic and trigeminal, and they may occur upon spinal nerve roots, usually the dorsal, or upon the cauda equina. Schwannomas particularly may be solitary. The cutaneous fibromas, or mollusca fibrosa, are formed from the connective tissue elements of the cutaneous nerves. The bone changes associated with neurofibromatosis may consist either of hyperostosis or of rarefaction, with or without cyst formation. According to Thannhauser (1944) the bone lesions in neurofibromatosis and in the osteitis fibrosa cystica of von Recklinghausen are identical. Nerve elements are absent, but there are characteristic whorls of spindle cells.

Neurofibromas may become sarcomatous. Abnormalities may be present in parts of the nervous system other than the peripheral nerves. Patches of gliosis and ependymal overgrowth may occur in the brain and spinal cord, syringomyelia, and even occasionally malignant tumours—glioma and ependymoma—may develop. Glioma of the optic chiasma may be associated with neurofibromatosis, and meningeal fibroblastomas are sometimes present. Neurofibromatosis is occasionally associated with other congenital abnormalities, such as spina bifida, cerebral meningocele, buphthalmos, syndactyly, and haemangiectatic naevi.

AETIOLOGY

The disease appears to be due to a congenital abnormality of the ectoderm. It is hereditary, behaving in inheritance as a Mendelian dominant. Some members of affected families may show only cutaneous pigmentation, while others exhibit a more extensive clinical picture. Bilateral acoustic neurofibromas sometimes occur in many members of a sibship in successive generations.

SYMPTOMS

Some of the symptoms of neurofibromatosis are always present at birth, for example, cutaneous pigmentation. Others may be absent or may appear later, as a result of slow growth of the neurofibromas or of the reaction of other tissues to these tumours. In some cases, however, the disorder is little, if at all progressive, and may be discovered accidentally. Except in those cases in which gross congenital abnormalities are present, the patient does not usually come under observation on account of symptoms until after the age of 20.

Cutaneous Pigmentation

This is almost invariably present. It consists of brownish spots, *café au lait* in colour, varying in size from a pin's head to areas the size of the palm. Unlike the *café au lait* spots of Albright's syndrome (polyostotic fibrous dysplasia) the patches of pigmentation in neurofibromatosis usually show a regular outline without deep indentations. Occasionally a sheet of diffuse pigmentation may be present on one or both sides of the trunk, corresponding to the cutaneous distribution of several spinal segments. Cutaneous pigmentation is always most evident on the trunk and may be absent from the exposed parts. [See Fig. 85.]

Cutaneous Fibromas

Cutaneous fibromas or mollusca fibrosa are soft, pinkish swellings, which may be sessile or pedunculated, and vary in size from a pin's head to an orange. They are frequently present in large numbers, and are situated chiefly upon the trunk, but some are usually to be found on the face.

Neurofibromas

Neurofibromas are most readily discovered upon the superficial cutaneous nerves, especially those of the extremities and of the sides of the neck. The tumours are to be felt as movable, bead-like nodules. They may give rise to pain and are occasionally tender on pressure; sometimes they appear to grow within the sheath of a nerve, when pressure may produce pain along the nerve trunk and paraesthesiae in the appropriate dermatome.

Plexiform Neuroma

'Plexiform neuroma' is the term applied to a diffuse neurofibromatosis of nerve trunks, which is often associated with an overgrowth of the skin and subcutaneous tissues. In this way large folds of skin may be formed, or there may be a diffuse enlargement of the subcutaneous tissues of a limb, with or without underlying bony abnormality. The commonest sites are the temple, the upper lid, and the back of the neck. The cutaneous hyperplasia has received the names of dermatolysis, pachydermatocele, and elephantiasis neuromatosa. It is probable that the famous 'Elephant Man' described by Treves was an example of this disorder. A similar hyperplasia may occur in one half of the tongue and in the gums on one side.

Acoustic neuroma is described on pages 220 and 254.

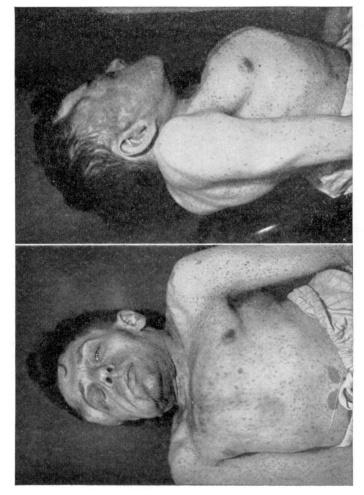

FIG. 85. A case of neurofibromatosis with cutaneous pigmentation, hyperostosis of the skull, right-sided buphthalmos, plexiform neuroma of the right side of the face, and kyphoscoliosis (elephantiasis neuromatosa).

Osseous Manifestations

Kyphoscoliosis is frequently present in neurofibromatosis and may be so severe as to cause compression of the spinal cord. This occurred in the patient shown in FIGURE 85. Even in the absence of intrathecal neurofibromas related to the nerve roots a characteristic concave 'scalloping' of the posterior borders of the vertebral bodies may be seen in radiographs of the spine. There may be marked hyperostosis of the bones of the face, with enlargement and rarefaction of the calvarium. These changes may be mainly unilateral. The long bones of the limbs may undergo subperiosteal hyperostosis, and their shafts may be curved.

Retinal Manifestations

Phakomas, which are flat, white or grey, oval or circular masses, about half the size of the optic disc, may occur in the retina (van der Hoeve, 1923).

Visceral Neurofibromas

Neurofibromas have been described on the mucous membranes and in various viscera, including the suprarenals. The vagus and sympathetic nerves may also be affected.

Complications

Compression of the spinal cord may occur as a result of severe kyphoscoliosis or of a neurofibroma, or the scoliosis may lead to root pains. Neurofibromas within the skull may give rise to symptoms of increased intracranial pressure, and of focal compression of the brain. Intracranial glioma or meningioma may be present. A sarcomatous change in a neurofibroma manifests itself as a rapid increase in the size of the tumour, with compression and invasion of the neighbouring structures. Epilepsy, acromegaly, adiposogenital dystrophy, infantilism of the Lorain type, phaeochromocytoma of the adrenal, and Addison's disease have all been encountered as complications. Optic atrophy may occur either as an associated finding or as a result of a glioma of an optic nerve or of the chiasm.

DIAGNOSIS

The association of cutaneous pigmentation with neurofibromas and frequently with other associated abnormalities constitutes a unique clinical picture. Difficulties in diagnosis are likely to arise only when some of these clinical features are absent or inconspicuous. Thus a patient may come under observation presenting symptoms of an intracranial tumour, spinal compression, scoliosis with root pains, hyperostosis, or localized elephantiasis. A careful examination of the skin of the whole body for pigmentation, cutaneous and neural fibromas, will usually enable a correct diagnosis to be made, but a similar pigmentation of the skin is sometimes associated with other abnormalities, especially syringomyelia.

PROGNOSIS

The disorder is not always progressive, but the presence of any symptoms in a child or adolescent should lead to a guarded prognosis, as the disorder may later reach its fully developed form. Pregnancy especially may lead to an exacerbation. Frequently the disease does not shorten life nor lead to marked discomfort. In severe cases death may occur from one of the complications described above, from tuberculosis, or after a terminal phase of cachexia.

TREATMENT

Treatment is often palliative. Painful subcutaneous neurofibromas may be treated by X-ray irradiation or by excision. Suitable operative treatment may be required for associated intracranial or intraspinal tumours, or when a peripheral neurofibroma compresses a mixed nerve or becomes sarcomatous.

REFERENCES

BIELSCHOWSKY, M., and ROSE, M. (1927) Zur Kenntnis der zentralen Veränderungen bei Recklinghausenscher Krankheit, *J. Psychol. Neurol. (Lpz.)*, **35**, 42.

CROME, L. (1962) Central neurofibromatosis, *Arch. Dis. Child.*, **37**, 640.

FORD, F. R. (1966) *Diseases of the Nervous System in Infancy, Childhood and Adolescence*, 5th ed., p. 995, Springfield, Ill.

HOEVE, J. VAN DER (1923) Augengeschwülste bei der tuberösen Hirnsklerose (Bourneville) und verwandten Krankheiten, *Arch. Ophthal.*, **111**, 1.

KIENBÖCK, R., and RÖSLER, H. (1932) *Neurofibromatose*, Leipzig.

LEHMAN, E. P. (1926) Recklinghausen's neurofibromatosis and the skeleton, *Arch. Derm. Syph. (Chicago)*, **14**, 178.

PENFIELD, W., and YOUNG, A. W. (1930) The nature of von Recklinghausen's disease and the tumors associated with it, *Arch. Neurol. Psychiat. (Chicago)*, **23**, 320.

RUSSELL, W. S., and RUBINSTEIN, L. J. (1959) *Pathology of Tumours of the Nervous System*, pp. 236 et seq., London.

THANNHAUSER, S. J. (1944) Neurofibromatosis (von Recklinghausen) and osteitis fibrosa cystica localisata et disseminata (von Recklinghausen), *Medicine (Baltimore)*, **23**, 105.

WEBER, F. P. (1929–30) Periosteal neurofibromatosis, with a short consideration of the whole subject of neurofibromatosis, *Quart. J. Med.*, **23**, 151.

WORSTER-DROUGHT, C., DICKSON, W. E. C., and McMENEMEY, W. H. (1937) Multiple meningeal and perineural tumours with analogous changes in the glia and ependyma, *Brain*, **60**, 85.

THE HEREDITARY ATAXIAS

Definition. The term 'hereditary ataxia', though by no means completely descriptive, is a convenient one to apply to a group of closely related disorders, usually hereditary or familial, and characterized pathologically by degeneration of some or all of the following parts of the nervous system—the optic nerves, the cerebellum, the olives, and the long ascending and descending tracts of the spinal cord. These localized degenerations occur in various combinations, with corresponding symptoms. Probably these disorders are closely related also to peroneal muscular atrophy, hypertrophic interstitial polyneuropathy, and hereditary sensory neuropathy with any of which they may, in occasional families, be combined. The age of onset ranges from childhood to middle life, and the course of the disease is slowly progressive. A number of varieties have been described, differing in the distribution of the symptoms. Friedreich's ataxia is relatively common. Some forms of hereditary ataxia are confined to a single family. Each variety tends to breed true, but does not always do so, and more than one form may occur in the same family. The existence of transitional forms lends support to the view that all varieties are due to the same underlying abnormality, which varies in its incidence upon different parts of the nervous system. It is impossible to describe in detail all the forms of hereditary ataxia which have been reported. The principal case reports have been reviewed by Pratt (1967). The following are the most important:

1. Hereditary spastic paraplegia.
2. Friedreich's ataxia.
3. The Roussy-Lévy syndrome.
4. The varieties described by Sanger-Brown and Marie.
5. Various forms of progressive cerebellar degeneration.

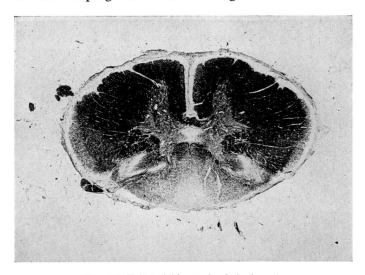

FIG. 86. Friedreich's ataxia. Spinal cord

PATHOLOGY

The pathology of the different varieties of hereditary ataxia will be described in more detail in the appropriate sections. They present the following features in common.

There is a degeneration of the ectodermal elements of the nervous system. The nerve fibres are usually affected more severely than the ganglion cells, but in the later stages these also suffer, though it is difficult to say whether their degeneration is primary or secondary to the degeneration of their axons. The cerebellum and spinal cord are usually smaller than normal and occasionally show evidence of congenital abnormalities. The brunt of the degenerative process usually falls either on the spinal cord or on the cerebellum. Exceptionally both are involved. In the spinal forms some degenerative changes are usually to be found in all the long ascending and descending tracts, though a predominant incidence upon certain tracts determines the nature of the clinical picture. Thus the corticospinal tracts are most affected in hereditary spastic paraplegia; the corticospinal tracts, the posterior columns, the posterior spinocerebellar tracts, and the ganglion cells of the dorsal nucleus in Friedreich's ataxia [FIG. 86]; while the changes are most marked in the anterior columns in the cerebellar ataxias. Degeneration is manifest in loss of myelin and destruction of axons, with a reactionary gliosis.

AETIOLOGY

An inherited abnormality is the primary cause of the hereditary ataxias, but as in the case of other inherited disorders sporadic cases are not much less common than familial ones. Males and females are affected with approximately equal frequency, and the disease may be transmitted either by affected or by normal individuals. When it develops early in life it usually acts as a barrier to marriage in those individuals who survive to a marriageable age, and in such families transmission necessarily occurs more frequently through normal than through affected individuals. Hereditary ataxia and paraplegia may be inherited either as a dominant or a recessive factor (Bell, 1939; Sjögren, 1943). Haldane (1941) believes that partial sex-linkage can be demonstrated in families with a recessive mode of inheritance. Nothing is known as to the cause of the germinal mutation by which it originates. Acute infections have sometimes been regarded as precipitating factors. These are so common that little importance can be attached to them, though it is possible that they may accelerate degeneration in the nervous system in an individual already predisposed to it by heredity.

CLINICAL VARIETIES
HEREDITARY SPASTIC PARAPLEGIA

This disorder usually affects several sibs, with or without a history of cases in previous generations. Sporadic cases occur. Males suffer more frequently than females. The onset of symptoms is usually in childhood, between the ages of 3 and 15 years, rarely in middle age.

PATHOLOGY

The maximal degeneration is found in the corticospinal tracts of the spinal cord, especially from the upper thoracic region downwards. This is associated with slighter degenerative changes in the posterior columns, especially the fasciculus gracilis, and in the large corticospinal cells of the precentral gyrus.

SYMPTOMS

Symptoms are those of a progressive destruction of the corticospinal tracts beginning in the lower limbs. Attention is first attracted to the child on account of its stiff and clumsy gait. The lower limbs are found to be weak and spastic, with exaggerated tendon reflexes and extensor plantar responses. The abdominal reflexes are diminished or lost, and pes cavus is usually present. Later the upper limbs are similarly affected, and finally the muscles innervated from the brain stem, with the production of spastic dysarthria and dysphagia and loss of emotional control. The sphincters are usually slightly affected in the later stages. In spite of degeneration in the posterior columns, no loss of superficial or deep sensibility can usually be detected. Primary optic atrophy and retinal pigmentation have been described. Mentality is usually normal. Tyrer and Sutherland (1961) describe electrocardiographic changes.

PROGNOSIS

The disease runs a slowly progressive course, weakness and contracture finally confining the patient to bed. However, despite the alarming evidence of spasticity and the clonus and grossly exaggerated lower limb reflexes it is remarkable that patients often manage to walk for 30 years or more after the onset. Death occurs after many years, usually from an intercurrent infection.

FRIEDREICH'S ATAXIA

The mode of inheritance of this disorder has already been discussed. It is usually familial and hereditary (generally recessive but rarely dominant), but sporadic cases occur. The age of onset, interpreted as the age at which symptoms first bring the patient under observation, is usually between 5 and 15 years, though abnormalities such as pes cavus may be discovered in apparently normal members of affected families in early childhood. Exceptionally, symptoms first appear between the ages of 20 and 30, rarely after 30.

PATHOLOGY

The spinal cord is unusually small, but the cerebellum is usually normal. Histologically [FIG. 86], the degeneration is most marked in the posterior columns, especially in the fasciculus gracilis. It is most intense in the lower parts of the cord and diminishes towards the medulla. Next to the posterior columns, the lateral columns suffer most, especially the corticospinal tracts and the posterior spinocerebellar tracts, together with the cells of the dorsal nucleus, from which the latter are derived. The anterior spinocerebellar tracts usually escape. There is a reactionary gliosis in the degenerated regions. The dorsal root fibres also exhibit degeneration, though their ganglion cells may be little affected. Exceptionally there is some degeneration of the anterior horn cells with resulting muscular weakness and atrophy, often in distal limb muscles.

The heart may show a diffuse change, enlargement being caused by thickening of the muscle, and a diffuse fibrosis. Microscopically there is fatty degeneration of the muscle fibres with slight chronic inflammatory infiltration and fibrosis (Russell).

SYMPTOMS

As might be deduced from the pathological changes, the cardinal symptoms of Friedreich's ataxia are: ataxia, most marked in the lower limbs, with signs of destruction of the corticospinal tracts, loss of deep reflexes, and, to a variable extent, impairment of sensibility, especially deep sensibility (vibration sense and position and joint sense). In addition, pes cavus and scoliosis are present, and nystagmus and dysarthria indicate a disturbance of cerebellar function at the level of the cranial nerves.

Symptoms appear first in the lower limbs, and it is the ataxic gait which usually first attracts attention. The patient walks on a broad base and tends to reel or stagger. In severe cases he is unable to walk without support on both sides. Standing is similarly affected, and he sways and may be unable to stand without support. The unsteadiness of stance is sometimes intensified by closing the eyes. Ataxia of the lower limbs is usually less evident in movement of the limbs individually when the patient is lying in bed. In the later stages movements of the upper limbs also become ataxic, and intention-tremor is present. Slight involuntary movements, which have sometimes been described as choreiform or myoclonic, are often present in the later stages. These are probably the result of defective co-ordination. Irregular oscillations of the head are common. Nystagmus is present in 70 per cent. of cases, and it is usually most marked on lateral ocular deviation. Speech is invariably dysarthric in the later stages, the dysarthria being of the variety associated with cerebellar disease. Speech is usually slow, monotonous, and slurred, and may be explosive or scanning. It is frequently accompanied by vigorous grimaces and associated movements of the facial musculature. Corticospinal tract degeneration leads to weakness, most marked in the lower limbs, with loss of the abdominal reflexes and extensor plantar responses. The tendon reflexes tend to be lost owing to interruption of the reflex arcs on the afferent side. The ankle-jerks are lost before the knee-jerks, and the latter may be exaggerated, owing to the corticospinal lesion, when the former are diminished. The limbs may be either hypotonic or slightly spastic, depending upon the relative severity of loss of afferent impulses from the muscles, which tends to diminish muscle tone, and of the corticospinal tract lesion, which tends to increase it. Sensory changes are inconstant and may be absent. Shooting pains occasionally occur in the limbs. Postural sense and appreciation of passive movement are not infrequently impaired, especially in the lower limbs. In some cases all forms of sensibility are affected. The sphincters are usually unaffected, though incontinence of urine, and more rarely of faeces, may occur in the late stages. Pes cavus and scoliosis are present in almost all cases, the former being usually associated with a slight contracture of the muscles of the calf. Pes cavus is usually attributed to occurrence of corticospinal tract degeneration at an early age, but Tyrer and Sutherland (1961) suggest that it is due to unbalanced action of the tibialis posterior muscle. However, the fact that it may be seen in otherwise unaffected sibs suggests that it may even be due to an associated hereditary abnormality of bony development. The scoliosis is probably due to interruption of afferent impulses regulating posture from the spinal muscles.

Optic atrophy occasionally occurs, and retinal pigmentation has been described. Other rare ocular symptoms include ptosis, abnormalities of the pupillary reflexes, and ophthalmoplegia. Deafness sometimes occurs. Muscular atrophy is a rare complication and is most frequently seen in the hands, leading to claw-hand, which Roth (1948) suggests indicates a relationship to peroneal muscular atrophy. Associated congenital abnormalities include spina bifida occulta and infantilism.

The mental condition of sufferers from Friedreich's ataxia is frequently normal, but a mild dementia is not uncommon in the later stages, leading to impaired intelligence and irritability. The cerebrospinal fluid is normal.

The cardiac changes may lead to heart failure, heart block, and electro-cardiographic abnormalities (Evans and Wright, 1942; Tyrer and Sutherland, 1961). Diabetes mellitus may occur (Tyrer and Sutherland, 1961).

PROGNOSIS

Friedreich's disease is in most cases slowly but steadily progressive. Occasionally, however, it appears to become arrested, and abortive cases are encountered, for example as accidental discoveries in apparently healthy members of affected families, in whom the disorder does not progress. Few patients, however, live for more than twenty years after the onset of symptoms, and death usually occurs from an intercurrent infection or from heart failure.

THE ROUSSY-LÉVY SYNDROME

This syndrome (hereditary areflexia with amyotrophy) shows certain affinities with Friedreich's ataxia on the one hand and with peroneal muscular atrophy on the other. The affected patients show mild ataxia, pes cavus, loss of the ankle- and knee-jerks, and peripheral amyotrophy in the upper and lower limbs. The course of the illness is slow with long periods of apparent arrest and the prognosis is therefore much better than that of Friedreich's disease.

SANGER-BROWN'S AND MARIE'S ATAXIA

Sanger-Brown in 1892 described a variety of hereditary ataxia affecting 24 individuals in five successive generations of the same family. Pathological examination showed degeneration of the cells of the dorsal nucleus, of the posterior columns, and of the posterior spinocerebellar tracts. There was little or no cortico-spinal tract degeneration, and changes in the cerebellum were slight or absent.

The age of onset lay between 16 and 35 years, the first symptom being ataxia of the lower limbs. The condition differed from Friedreich's ataxia in the presence of optic atrophy, ptosis, diplopia, and, occasionally, of complete internal and external ophthalmoplegia, and exaggerated tendon reflexes and ankle clonus, whereas nystagmus and pes cavus were absent.

A very similar disorder was reported by Neff in four generations of a single family, thirteen individuals being affected. This disorder differed from the ataxia of Sanger-Brown in that the onset of symptoms was delayed until between the ages of 50 and 65, and in some cases even later. Four affected members of Neff's family developed dementia.

Marie, in 1893, under the title of 'hereditary cerebellar ataxia', described a group of patients suffering from signs of cerebellar deficiency and corticospinal tract degeneration with, in some cases, optic atrophy. The onset of symptoms occurred during adolescence, and multiple cases were observed in the same family. Pathological examination of cases exhibiting the clinical features described by Marie has usually shown a slight degree of atrophy of the cerebellum, while in the spinal cord degeneration was most marked in the ascending cerebellar tracts, and the anterolateral columns, the corticospinal tracts and posterior columns being little affected. It is doubtful, however, whether this form of cerebellar ataxia can be considered either a clinical or a pathological entity. It is probably a mixed group containing some cases of Friedreich's ataxia together with cases allied to the Sanger-Brown variety. Greenfield (1954) considers that 'hereditary spastic ataxia' covers many families in these groups.

PROGRESSIVE CEREBELLAR DEGENERATION

Although not all forms of progressive cerebellar degeneration have been shown to be familial or hereditary, they exhibit a sufficient clinical and pathological similarity to justify their consideration together. The following are the more important varieties that have been described:

Primary parenchymatous degeneration of the cerebellum (Holmes).
Olivopontocerebellar atrophy (Dejerine and Thomas).
Olivorubrocerebellar atrophy (Lhermitte and Lejonne).
Delayed cortical cerebellar atrophy (Rossi, Marie, Foix, and Alajouanine).

As their names imply, these forms of cerebellar degeneration differ in the precise localization of the degenerative process and its incidence upon the brain stem. Their relationship is discussed by Critchley and Greenfield (1948).

Primary Parenchymatous Degeneration of the Cerebellum

Under this title Homes described four cases occurring in a single family. One case was investigated pathologically. The cerebellum, pons, and medulla were abnormally small, especially the cerebellum, which on microscopical examination showed atrophy of all three cortical layers. This was associated with atrophy and gliosis of the olive and of the olivocerebellar fibres in the medulla and inferior cerebellar peduncle. The midbrain, pons, and spinal cord were normal. The symptoms, the onset of which occurred in early middle life, between the ages of 33 and 40, were those of progressive cerebellar deficiency. Speech became explosive, and nystagmus and ataxia of the upper and lower limbs were present. Vision and the optic nerves were normal; the tendon reflexes were brisk and there was no sensory disturbance.

Olivopontocerebellar Atrophy

This form of cerebellar atrophy was described by Dejerine and Thomas in 1900. It is only exceptionally familial, in most cases being sporadic.

The pathological changes consist of atrophy of the ganglion cells of the olives, and of the grey matter of the pons, with degeneration of the middle cerebellar penduncles and to a lesser extent of the inferior cerebellar peduncles. The cerebellum suffers mainly as a result of atrophy of its afferent fibres by these routes. The Purkinje and other ganglion cells of the cerebellar cortex are affected secondarily. It is the olive and the neocerebellum which undergo degeneration. The central nuclei of the cerebellum are relatively unaffected, but in *olivorubrocerebellar atrophy* these degenerate, together with the superior peduncles, and degeneration can be traced as far as the red nuclei.

The onset of symptoms occurs in late middle life up to the age of 60. The symptoms are those of a slowly progressive cerebellar deficiency, namely, dysarthria, ataxia and tremor of the limbs, ataxic gait, and muscular hypotonia. Nystagmus is usually absent. Voluntary power is well preserved and the reflexes are usually normal, except that the ankle-jerks may be lost. Parkinsonian features may develop, and mental deterioration (dementia) may occur in the later stages. In some cases, spasticity, exaggerated reflexes, and extensor plantar responses rather than hypotonia occur and there is a static tremor superficially resembling that of Parkinson's disease.

Delayed Cortical Cerebellar Atrophy

This disorder occurs sporadically. Greenfield (1954) considers that it is indistinguishable from the Holmes type of cerebellar degeneration (above).

DIAGNOSIS

The diagnosis of the hereditary ataxias rests upon the onset, in most cases before the age of 20, of progressive symptoms, of which ataxia is usually the most conspicuous, and which frequently include symptoms of bilateral corticospinal tract degeneration, sensory loss, pes cavus and scoliosis, and sometimes optic atrophy. When the disorder is familial or hereditary and the history of its incidence can be obtained it is usually easy to make a correct diagnosis. Sporadic cases, however, may give rise to difficulty. Hereditary spastic paraplegia must be distinguished from congenital diplegia by the fact that the patient is normal at birth, and the disorder is progressive, whereas in diplegia the symptoms are congenital, and tend to improve, and are not uncommonly associated with mental deficiency and with epilepsy. Friedreich's ataxia must be distinguished from multiple sclerosis and from tabes. It frequently begins before the age of 15, when the onset of multiple sclerosis is rare. Both disorders are characterized by nystagmus, ataxia, and extensor plantar responses, but scoliosis, pes cavus, and loss of the knee- and ankle-jerks are peculiar to Friedreich's disease. The distinction of Friedreich's disease from tabes is based upon the absence in the latter of pes cavus, scoliosis, dysarthria, and extensor plantar responses, and the presence of Argyll Robertson pupils and, in most cases, of positive serological reactions in the blood and cerebrospinal fluid. The diagnosis of a sporadic case of the ataxia described by Ferguson and Critchley (1929) from multiple sclerosis may be extremely difficult, if not impossible. The most helpful points of distinction are the occurrence in the ataxia of external ophthalmoplegia, especially weakness of upward deviation of the eyes and the absence of the remissions so characteristic of multiple sclerosis.

The progressive hereditary cerebellar degenerations of late middle life are to be distinguished from sporadic spinocerebellar degeneration arising as a complication of carcinoma in the lung or elsewhere; from tumours, by the absence of increased intracranial pressure; from tabes, by the usual preservation of the tendon reflexes, and the absence of sensory loss and of pupillary abnormalities; and from subacute combined degeneration, by the absence of paraesthesiae, sensory loss, and gastric achylia.

TREATMENT

No treatment which can influence the course of the degeneration is known. Although the patient will ultimately become bedridden, this should be postponed as long as possible. Re-educational exercises may do much to keep the ataxia under control. In Friedreich's ataxia the pes cavus may require surgical treatment or appropriate boots. In the later stages care must be taken to avoid as far as possible exposing the patient to the risk of respiratory infections.

ATAXIA TELANGIECTASIA

This rare disorder, which is probably of autosomal recessive inheritance and which has been called the Louis-Bar syndrome, is characterized by cerebellar ataxia with onset in infancy and with inability to walk by the age of 10 years. Telangiectasiae are seen in the bulbar conjunctivae and, later, on the skin. Most patients show a deficiency in serum γ-globulin resulting in a diminished resistance to respiratory infections, one of which eventually proves fatal. Pathologically the Purkinje and granular cells of the cerebellum are selectively involved. Boder and Sedgwick (1963) have reviewed 101 cases and Strich (1966) describes the pathological findings in 3 cases.

REFERENCES

BELL, J. (1939) Hereditary ataxia and spastic paraplegia, *Treasury of Human Inheritance*, vol. iv, pt. 3, London.

BODER, E., and SEDGWICK, R. P. (1963) Ataxia-telangiectasia: a review of 101 cases, *Little Club Clinics in Developmental Medicine*, **8**, 110.

BROWN, S. (1892) On hereditary ataxy, with a series of twenty-one cases, *Brain*, **15**, 250.

BRUGSCH, H. G., and HAUPTMANN, A. (1944) Familial occurrence of Friedreich's ataxia with Charcot-Marie-Tooth's neural muscular atrophy, *Bull. New Engl. med. Cent.*, **6**, 42.

COURVILLE, C. B., and FRIEDMAN, A. P. (1940) Chronic progressive degeneration of the superior cerebellar cortex (parenchymatous cortical cerebellar atrophy), *Bull. Los Angeles neurol. Soc.*, **5**, 171.

CRITCHLEY, M. (1931) Goulstonian lectures. The neurology of old age, *Lancet*, i, 1119, 1221, 1331.

CRITCHLEY, M., and GREENFIELD, J. G. (1948) Olivo-ponto-cerebellar atrophy, *Brain*, **71**, 343.

DEJERINE, J., and THOMAS, A. (1900) L'atrophie olivo-ponto-cérébelleuse, *N. Iconogr. Salpêt.*, **13**, 330.

EVANS, W., and WRIGHT, G. (1942) The electrocardiogram in Friedreich's disease, *Brit. Heart J.*, **4**, 91.

FERGUSON, F. R., and CRITCHLEY, M. (1929) A clinical study of an heredofamilial disease resembling disseminated sclerosis, *Brain*, **52**, 203.

FORD, F. R. (1966) *Diseases of the Nervous System in Infancy, Childhood and Adolescence*, 5th ed., Springfield, Ill.

FRIEDREICH, N. (1863) Ueber degenerative Atrophie der spinalen Hinterstränge, *Virchows Arch. path. Anat.*, **26**, 391.

FRIEDREICH, N. (1876) Ueber Ataxie mit besonderer Berücksichtigung der hereditären Formen, *Virchows Arch. path. Anat.*, **68**, 145.

GREENFIELD, J. G. (1954) *The Spinocerebellar Degenerations*, Oxford.

HALDANE, J. B. S. (1941) Partial sex-linkage of recessive spastic paraplegia, *J. Genet.*, **41**, 141.

HALL, G. W., and MACKAY, R. P. (1937) Forms of familial ataxia resembling multiple sclerosis, *Arch. Neurol. Psychiat. (Chicago)*, **38**, 19.

HOLMES, G. (1907) A form of familial degeneration of the cerebellum, *Brain*, **30**, 466.

HOLMES, G. (1907) An attempt to classify cerebellar disease, with a note on Marie's hereditary cerebellar ataxia, *Brain*, **30**, 455.

LEJONNE, P., and LHERMITTE, J. (1909) Atrophie olivo-rubro-cérébelleuse, *N. Iconogr. Salpêt.*, **22**, 605.

LEJONNE, P., and LHERMITTE, J. (1909) Atrophie olivo- et rubro-cérébelleuse, *Rev. neurol. (Paris)*, **17**, 109.

MARIE, P., FOIX, C., and ALAJOUANINE, T. (1922) De l'atrophie cérébelleuse tardive à prédominance corticale, *Rev. neurol. (Paris)*, **29**, 849, 1082.

MARINESCO, G., and TRETIAKOFF, C. (1920) Étude histo-pathologique des centre nerveux dans trois cas de maladie de Friedreich, *Rev. neurol. (Paris)*, **27**, 113.

MATHIEU, P., and BERTRAND, I. (1929) Études anatomo-cliniques sur les atrophies cérébelleuses, *Rev. neurol. (Paris)*, **36**, 721.

PRATT, R. T. C. (1967) *The Genetics of Neurological Disorders*, London.

RABINOWITSCH, V. (1929) Zur Pathogenese der Friedreichschen Krankheit, *Z. ges. Neurol. Psychiat.*, **122**, 462.

ROSSI, I. (1907) Atrophie parenchymateuse primitive du cervelet à localisation corticale, *N. Iconogr. Salpêt.*, **20**, 66.

ROTH, M. (1948) On a possible relationship between hereditary ataxia and peroneal muscular atrophy, *Brain*, **71**, 416.

ROUSSY, G., and LÉVY, G. (1926) Sept cas d'une maladie familiale particulière, *Rev. neurol.*, **1**, 427.

SCHAFFER, K. (1922) Zur Pathologie und pathologischen Histologie der spastischen Heredodegeneration (hereditäre spastische Spinalparalyse), *Dtsch. Z. Nervenheilk.*, **73**, 101.

SJÖGREN, T. (1943) Klinische und erbbiologische Untersuchungen über die Heredoataxien, *Acta psychiat. (Kbh.)*, Supp. xxvii.

STRICH, S. J. (1966) Pathological findings in three cases of ataxia-telangiectasia, *J. Neurol. Neurosurg. Psychiat.*, **29**, 487.

TYRER, J. H., and SUTHERLAND, J. M. (1961) The primary spino-cerebellar atrophies and their associated defects with a study of the foot deformity, *Brain*, **84**, 289.

WINKLER, C. (1923) A case of olivo-pontine cerebellar atrophy, and our conceptions of neo- and palaeo-cerebellum, *Schweiz. Arch. Neurol. Psychiat.*, **13**, 684.

MOTOR NEURONE DISEASE

Synonyms. Amyotrophic lateral sclerosis; progressive muscular atrophy; progressive bulbar palsy; chronic poliomyelitis; motor system disease.

Definition. A disease characterized pathologically by degenerative changes, which are most marked in the anterior horn cells of the spinal cord, the motor nuclei of the medulla, and the corticospinal tracts, and clinically by progressive wasting of the muscles, especially those of the upper limbs and those innervated from the medulla, combined with symptoms of corticospinal tract degeneration. The term 'progressive muscular atrophy' is associated especially with the names of Aran (1850) and Duchenne (1847). Charcot (1869) distinguished two varieties —progressive muscular atrophy of Aran and Duchenne, characterized only by lower motor neurone lesions, and a form in which these were associated with symptoms of corticospinal tract lesions and which he called 'amyotrophic lateral sclerosis'. These two varieties are now usually regarded as nosologically similar. When the lower motor neurone lesions predominate, or, as more rarely happens, occur alone, the term 'progressive muscular atrophy' is still generally applied to the disease, and when the muscles innervated from the medulla are predominantly involved it has been termed 'progressive bulbar palsy'. Some authors then use the term 'amyotrophic lateral sclerosis' for those cases in which signs of corticospinal tract disease predominate in the early stages and in which it may initially be difficult or impossible to find evidence of lower motor neurone involvement. In most cases, however, the symptoms of upper and lower motor neurone lesions are mixed, except in the lower limbs, where the latter are frequently absent until the terminal stages. Greenfield (1958) prefers the term amyotrophic lateral sclerosis to motor neurone disease on the grounds that the pathological changes in the spinal cord are not limited to the motor neurones and many American authors use this term as an inclusive one, embracing all varieties of the disease. Motor neurone disease, however, is a better inclusive term.

PATHOLOGY

The Spinal Cord

Naked-eye changes in the spinal cord are slight, but on section the grey matter of the anterior horns appears smaller than normal, and the ventral roots are

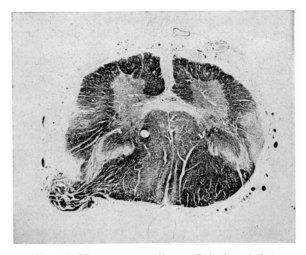

FIG. 87. Motor neurone disease. Spinal cord, L.1

wasted. Microscopically there is severe degeneration of the ganglion cells of the anterior horns. This change is usually most marked in the cervical enlargement of the cord, but is always widespread, and its severity is not invariably proportional to the clinical condition. The ganglion cells exhibit chromatolysis, which is at first perinuclear. The neurofibrils disappear, and there is frequently a granular deposit of lipochrome. The total number of ganglion cells is much reduced. As a rule all groups within the anterior horn suffer equally. There are exceptions to this, however, but there is no general agreement as to whether some are more susceptible than others. The degeneration is associated with a slight secondary gliosis, and occasionally slight perivascular infiltration with round cells has been observed.

The Weigert-Pal stain or other suitable myelin stains reveal degeneration of the white matter of the spinal cord, which is most marked in, and often confined to, the anterolateral columns [FIG. 87]. The corticospinal fibres suffer most, both the direct and the crossed corticospinal tracts being affected. Corticospinal tract degeneration is never equally severe at all levels. It is not uncommon to find an advanced change in the lower thoracic and lumbosacral regions, while the upper thoracic region is but slightly affected, and severe changes are found again in the cervical enlargement, extending up to the medulla. The spinocerebellar tracts usually show degeneration, especially the anterior, and the severity of this change varies in different segments. The rubrospinal, vestibulospinal, and tectospinal tracts are also degenerated to a variable extent, and despite the well-known fact that sensory symptoms and signs are absent, slight degeneration is occasionally present in the posterior columns. The endogenous fibres of the spinal cord which lie close to the grey matter are degenerated in the anterolateral columns, but not in the posterior columns (Smith, 1960).

The Medulla

The ganglion cells of the medullary motor nuclei show degenerative changes which are in all respects similar to those of the anterior horn cells of the spinal cord. These alterations are most marked in the hypoglossal nucleus, the dorsal nucleus of the vagus, the nucleus ambiguus, and the trigeminal motor nucleus. The facial nucleus is usually less severely affected. Similar changes have been observed in the sensory nuclei. There is a marked degeneration in the pyramids of the medulla. Bertrand and van Bogaert (1925) described a case in which corticospinal tract degeneration was severe in the medulla and negligible in the pons and cerebral peduncles. Degeneration has also been described in the inferior cerebellar peduncle, the medial longitudinal fasciculus, the medial and lateral lemnisci, and the reticular formation. The third and fourth nerve nuclei in the midbrain almost invariably escape.

The Cerebral Hemispheres

Naked-eye changes are usually inconspicuous, but slight atrophy of the ascending frontal gyri has been described. Microscopical changes are most marked in the cerebral cortex anterior to the central sulcus. The typical lesion in subacute cases is a lipochrome degeneration of the ganglion cells in the frontal and precentral regions. This change is most marked in the third and fifth cortical layers, the latter of which contains the large corticospinal motor cells of Betz. Degeneration has also been observed in the tangential fibres of the cortex. Some glial overgrowth is usually present in the regions which are the site of atrophy. Degenerative changes are also found in the middle-third of the corpus callosum and in the corticospinal fibres in the posterior limb of the internal capsule.

Peripheral Nerves and Muscles

The ventral roots and peripheral nerves exhibit degeneration, with atrophy of their myelin sheaths. The muscles show characteristic changes of denervation atrophy in that large (or sometimes small and scattered) groups of uniformly atrophic but otherwise normal-appearing muscle fibres are seen lying alongside other groups which are normal or even larger than normal. In long-standing cases there may be so-called 'secondary myopathic change' (Drachman et al., 1967) with some random variation in fibre size, central nuclei and degeneration or necrosis of individual fibres similar to that seen in myopathic disorders; this change appears to be due to the interplay of denervation and re-innervation (through collateral sprouting of surviving neurones) and to the trauma to which a weakened muscle is regularly subjected.

AETIOLOGY

Motor neurone disease is a disease of late middle life, usually beginning between the ages of 50 and 70, occasionally as early as the third decade or as late as the eighth. It is very rare in early life, but it has been known to occur in childhood, usually during the second decade. Most cases are sporadic, but familial occurrence, though very rare, is not unknown, and in such cases the onset may occur either in middle life or in childhood. Amyotrophic lateral sclerosis is endemic on the island of Guam and shows there a high familial incidence; it is still uncertain whether this condition, with which the so-called Parkinsonism-dementia complex is often associated, is a genetically determined disorder of dominant inheritance or whether it could be the result of combined genetic and environmental (such as a slow virus) factors (Kurland, 1957; Hirano, Kurland, and Sayre, 1967). This disorder is probably different from the sporadic form of motor neurone disease which is commonly observed in Europe and in America though it may be clinically indistinguishable. When genetically determined motor neurone disease is seen, as happens rarely, in races other than the Chanarro Indians of Guam, it tends to give a somewhat atypical clinical picture (benign proximal forms and chronic bulbar palsy have each been described) and the family history may suggest either dominant or recessive inheritance. Males are affected more often than females in the proportion of two to one.

The condition has been regarded by some workers as inflammatory, and hence has been called 'chronic poliomyelitis', but this hypothesis is not borne out by the histological appearances. Inflammatory infiltration is rare and scanty, and when it occurs probably should be regarded as a reaction to degeneration. Some authorities regard motor neurone disease as due to a toxin which possesses a predilection for the anterior horn cells. Bertrand and van Bogaert make the interesting suggestion that the primary disturbance is damage to the grey matter of the spinal cord, the process spreading across the synapses to involve the endogenous associated fibres and the corticospinal fibres. This hypothesis affords an explanation of the patchy segmental distribution of the corticospinal degeneration, which on this account can hardly be regarded as secondary to degeneration of the Betz cells of the motor cortex. If the disease is indeed toxic in origin, the nature of the toxin is unknown. Exceptionally, motor neurone disease has been observed to supervene in an individual who many years previously suffered from acute anterior poliomyelitis. This association is so rare that it may be coincidental. It is conceivable, however, that the injury of the anterior horn cells due to acute poliomyelitis may render them liable to degenerate later if exposed to other toxins or may shorten their active life. This observation may give some support to the view that the condition is the result of a premature senescence of motor neurones but, in truth, while there has been much speculation, and some have invoked such processes as heavy metal poisoning, ischaemia, and an association with carcinoma (Brain *et al.*, 1965; Vejajiva, Foster, and Miller, 1967), the cause of the condition remains obscure. There is no conclusive evidence that trauma plays any part in aetiology, but it is an old observation that weakness and wasting may first appear in the muscles which are most used by the patient in his occupation, or have been the site of an injury: the significance of this relationship is as yet undetermined.

SYMPTOMS

Mode of Onset

The disease is usually chronic, but may run a subacute course. Correspondingly the onset is generally insidious, but may be more rapid. The nature of the earliest symptoms depends upon which region of the nervous system is first affected. Commonly the first abnormality is observed in the hands, where the patient may be conscious of weakness, stiffness, or clumsiness of movements of the fingers, or his attention may be drawn to the wasting, or he may perceive fascicular twitching. When the shoulder girdle and upper arm muscles are first affected the first symptom is weakness of movements of the shoulder. When degeneration begins in the bulbar motor nuclei the first symptom to be noticed is usually dysarthria or dysphagia. Less frequently the disease begins with spastic paraplegia, or wasting of one or both lower limbs. Cramp-like pains in the limbs are often an early symptom.

Symptoms of Lower Motor Neurone Degeneration

Degeneration of the anterior horn cells, and of the motor cells of the medulla, leads to weakness and wasting of the muscles which they innervate. Fasciculation is also a conspicuous symptom, and occurs in those muscles which are supplied by ganglion cells undergoing active degeneration. It may be limited to a few groups of muscles, or be much more widespread, and its extent is an indication of the diffuseness of the degenerative process. Very rarely, widespread weakness and wasting may occur in the absence of fasciculation. When fasciculation is not immediately evident it can often be evoked by sharply tapping the muscle. Contractures are usually slight. As a rule muscular wasting begins in the hands, the muscles of the thenar eminences being first affected. Not uncommonly one hand may begin to waste some months or even a year before the other. In other cases the onset is symmetrical. The wasting tends to spread to the muscles innervated by the segment of the spinal cord adjacent to that first affected. Hence, after the hands the forearm muscles are involved, the flexors usually suffering before the extensors. The weakness and atrophy of the hand muscles lead to clumsiness of the finger movements, and some degree of claw-hand usually develops [FIG. 88]. This deformity is not, however, as a rule severe, since the long flexors and extensors of the fingers, by which it is maintained, are soon themselves affected.

Next in frequency the muscles of the shoulder girdle and upper arm are first involved, those innervated by the fifth cervical spinal segment, especially the deltoids, being earliest affected. Those supplied by the sixth cervical segment, namely, the triceps, latissimus dorsi, the sternal part of the pectoralis major and serratus anterior, are usually involved much later, and the upper part of the trapezius also escapes until a late stage. The muscles innervated by the medulla may be the first to suffer or they may be affected simultaneously with, or shortly after, the upper limbs. The tongue is then usually the first to waste and becomes shrunken and wrinkled and shows conspicuous fasciculation [FIG. 89]. The orbicularis oris also suffers early, but the orbicularis oculi and other facial muscles are affected later, and less severely. It has been suggested that the orbicularis oris may be innervated by part of the hypoglossal nucleus, fibres from which join the facial nerve, and its affection *pari passu* with the tongue has been thus explained. Functionally the lips and tongue are closely related, but doubt has been cast upon the anatomical association of the nuclei. The palate is usually involved shortly after the tongue, together with the extrinsic muscles of

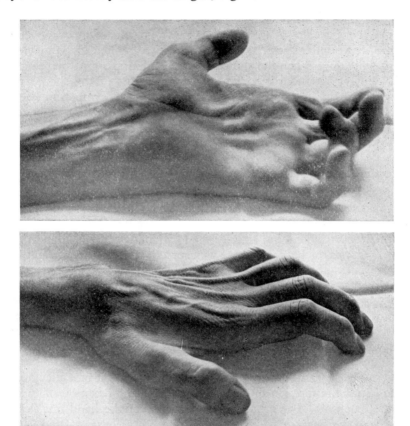

FIG. 88. A case of motor neurone disease. Wasting of the muscles of the hand.
Note the prominence of the flexor tendons in the palm

the pharynx and larynx. The intrinsic laryngeal muscles usually escape until late. The mandibular muscles usually suffer less severely than the tongue and orbicularis oris. Owing to weakness of the muscles concerned, pursing of the lips and whistling become impossible, and in the later stages saliva runs from the open lips. Protrusion of the tongue is at first weak and later lost. Speech suffers from paresis of the lips, tongue, and palate. The capacity to pronounce labials and dentals is early impaired, and later gutturals. Speech becomes slurred and finally unintelligible. Phonation, however, suffers late, if at all. Swallowing becomes increasingly difficult, and food tends to regurgitate through the nose. Patients usually find semi-solids easier to swallow than either solids or fluids.

Exceptionally the extensor muscles of the cervical spine suffer early, and when this occurs the head falls forwards. Early involvement of the muscles of the lower limbs is rare. The anterior tibial group and peronei are usually first affected and bilateral foot-drop results. This mode of onset may closely simulate polyneuritis, especially when, as occasionally happens, the motor symptoms are associated with muscular pain. It has, therefore, sometimes been called the 'pseudopoly-neuritic' form.

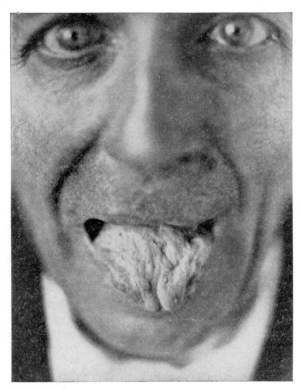

FIG. 89. A case of motor neurone disease. Wasting of the tongue.

In whatever part of the body muscular wasting begins, in most cases it sooner or later becomes generalized, though progressive bulbar palsy may prove fatal before wasting has had time to develop to a severe extent elsewhere. In the final stages weakness of the trunk muscles renders it impossible for the patient to sit up in bed, and paresis of the respiratory muscles leads to increasing dyspnoea.

Electrodiagnostic Findings

Strength duration curves will demonstrate evidence of partial or total de-nervation in the affected muscles.

Motor nerve conduction velocity is normal, if the temperature of the limb is controlled, up to a late stage of the disease, as surviving neurones conduct at a normal rate but the amplitude of the compound muscle potential evoked by supramaximal stimulation of its motor nerve may be reduced.

Electromyography shows fibrillation potentials on mechanical stimulation by the exploring needle, spontaneous fibrillation and fasciculation potentials when the needle is stationary in the relaxed muscle and a duration and amplitude of action-potentials greater than normal; even in cases of moderate weakness there may be a marked reduction in the number of spikes on maximal contraction (Kugelberg, 1949) and synchronization of the activity recorded by two separate electrodes within the same muscle (Buchthal and Pinelli, 1953).

Symptoms of Upper Motor Neurone Degeneration

Save in those rare cases in which the degeneration is confined to the lower motor neurones the clinical picture is complicated by the symptoms of the upper motor neurone lesions which may be present from the beginning or develop after muscular wasting. Since lower motor neurone lesions are rarely present at an early stage in the lower limbs, these usually for a long time present an uncomplicated picture of corticospinal tract degeneration, with weakness and spasticity, which rarely become severe. In the upper limbs the effect of the addition of an upper to a lower motor neurone lesion is to cause a degree of weakness which is disproportionately great in comparison with the severity and extent of the wasting, and the tendon reflexes are exaggerated in spite of the wasting. It is in the muscles innervated from the medulla that the effects of corticospinal tract degeneration are of the greatest importance. Here we may encounter lower motor neurone degeneration only—progressive bulbar palsy; upper motor neurone degeneration only—'pseudobulbar palsy'; or a combination of the two, which is the most frequent occurrence. A lesion of both corticospinal tracts above the medulla, so-called 'pseudobulbar palsy', causes weakness and spasticity of the bulbar muscles and hence leads to dysarthria and dysphagia. The paretic or paralysed muscles are not wasted and hypotonic, as in progressive bulbar palsy, but spastic. The tongue may appear somewhat smaller than normal on account of the spastic contraction of its muscles, but is not wrinkled and exhibits no fasciculation. The jaw-jerk, palatal and pharyngeal reflexes are exaggerated, and sneezing and coughing may be excited reflexly with abnormal readiness. The dysarthria resembles that which results from a lower motor neurone lesion of the muscles of articulation. Pseudobulbar palsy, when severe, also leads to an impairment of voluntary control over emotional reactions, as a result of which paroxysmal attacks of involuntary laughing and crying occur. These may take the form of an exaggeration or prolongation of a normal emotional response. Thus a patient laughs because he is amused, but having begun to laugh, is unable to stop. On the other hand, the emotional response may be quite inappropriate, such as uncontrollable laughter on hearing bad news, and then fails to correspond to, or express, the patient's emotional state. When pseudobulbar palsy and progressive bulbar palsy are associated in the same individual, dysarthria and dysphagia are intensified, impairment of emotional control may be present, and an exaggerated jaw-jerk is obtained, in spite of manifest wasting of the bulbar muscles.

The Reflexes

The condition of the reflexes in a given case depends upon the relative preponderance of upper and lower motor neurone degeneration. The palatal and pharyngeal reflexes tend to be lost in the later stages owing to interruption of the reflex arcs concerned. Owing to the presence of corticospinal tract degeneration the abdominal reflexes are eventually diminished or lost, and the plantar reflexes extensor. The deep reflexes, that is, the jaw-jerk and the tendon reflexes of the limbs, vary between exaggeration and abolition. Degeneration of the lower motor neurones causes impairment, and finally loss, of the reflexes effected by the muscles innervated. Corticospinal degeneration, however, leads to exaggeration of the deep reflexes. Hence it is not uncommon to find exaggerated tendon-jerks in the upper limbs in spite of considerable muscular atrophy, an association which led to the term 'tonic muscular atrophy' being applied to such cases. Since in the lower limbs muscular wasting is usually late in developing, the knee- and ankle-jerks are generally exaggerated and the plantar responses become extensor. The abdominal reflexes are often preserved until comparatively late in the course of the disease, despite the evidence of severe upper motor neurone involvement, in contrast to the situation which usually obtains in multiple sclerosis.

Other Symptoms

In the early stages the sphincters are not as a rule severely affected, though slight precipitancy or difficulty of micturition is not uncommon. Later retention or incontinence may rarely occur. Impotence often develops early. There is no sensory impairment.

When the sympathetic ganglion cells in the lateral horns of the grey matter of the upper dorsal region undergo degeneration, symptoms of oculosympathetic paralysis will be present.

The subcutaneous fat tends to disappear *pari passu* with the muscular wasting, and marked emaciation characterizes the later stages. Mental changes are absent and, although psychosis has occasionally been described, this is probably a coincidence or merely the reaction to a serious and disabling disease. Impairment of emotional control is a disorder of emotional expression and not of the underlying mental state.

DIAGNOSIS

Motor neurone disease requires to be distinguished from other conditions leading to muscular wasting, especially in the upper limbs, and from other causes of bulbar palsy.

In syringomyelia muscular wasting of the upper limbs is associated with spastic weakness of the lower limbs. Fasciculation, however, is rarely as striking in the wasted muscles as in motor neurone disease, and the characteristic dissociated sensory loss, if not present at the outset, develops at an early stage.

In syphilitic amyotrophy the onset of the weakness and wasting is often accompanied by pain of considerable severity and of radicular distribution. Signs of corticospinal tract degeneration are usually lacking; pupillary abnormalities may be present; the serological reactions are usually positive in either the blood or the cerebrospinal fluid, in which other abnormalities characteristic of syphilis may also be found.

Tumour of the spinal cord involving the cervical enlargement is likely to cause muscular wasting in one or both upper limbs, together with spastic paraplegia, but sensory loss is rarely absent, and the changes characteristic of spinal block are usually to be found in the cerebrospinal fluid.

Cervical spondylosis may closely simulate motor neurone disease when it causes muscular wasting and fasciculation in the upper limbs, and spastic weakness in the lower limbs without sensory loss. The course, however, is usually much slower than that of motor neurone disease, and the characteristic X-ray changes are present.

Spinal radiculitis ('neuralgic amyotrophy') causes wasting and weakness of muscles. The fifth cervical nerve is that most frequently affected. The onset is usually acute and associated with considerable pain in the neck and shoulder. The condition is not progressive, and any change is in the direction of improvement.

Cervical rib may be confused with progressive muscular atrophy. One or both hands may be wasted. Muscular fasciculation, however, is absent, and pain along the ulnar border of the hand and forearm is usually a prominent symptom, being frequently associated with relative anaesthesia and analgesia in this region, and vascular anomalies. Moreover, cervical rib can be demonstrated radiographically, though it must be remembered that in the costoclavicular syndrome the same symptoms may be caused by pressure upon a normal first rib. However, digital pressure in the root of the neck will usually reproduce the patient's pain and paraesthesiae.

Lesions of peripheral nerves give rise to little difficulty as a rule, since the distribution of the muscular wasting is at once recognizable as corresponding to the supply of the nerve, and in the case of the median and ulnar nerves is usually associated with sensory abnormalities possessing an equally distinctive distribution. However, a lesion of the deep branch of one ulnar nerve, resulting in wasting of small hand muscles without sensory loss may cause difficulty, but nerve conduction velocity measurements (increased terminal latency) are usually diagnostic.

Polymyositis is usually too acute to give rise to difficulties, and can also be distinguished electromyographically and by muscle biopsy. Various myopathies of late onset, however, may be confused with motor neurone disease when there is little or no evidence of upper motor neurone involvement. Their diagnosis is discussed on page 883.

The muscular dystrophies also are unlikely to be confused with amyotrophic lateral sclerosis, since they usually develop at a much earlier age. Dystrophia myotonica, however, is a disorder of adult life, but this condition is readily distinguished on account of the peculiar distribution of the wasting, with its predilection for the sternomastoids and the tibialis anterior, the presence of myotonia, the absence of fasciculation, and the association with cataract either in the patient or his ancestors.

Peroneal muscular atrophy is distinguished by the peculiar distribution of the wasting, which begins in the periphery of the limbs, but generally in the lower before the upper, and is associated with sensory impairment. This disease, moreover, is usually familial, and the first symptoms generally appear in childhood.

Arthritis of the hands and fingers generally leads to considerable wasting of the muscles of the hands. The history of pain in the joints and the presence of articular or periarticular swelling, with limitation of joint movement, render the correct diagnosis easy.

Pseudobulbar palsy may be due to vascular lesions involving the corticospinal tracts at any point above the medulla. When these are sudden in onset the condition is unlikely to be confused with amyotrophic lateral sclerosis. When the onset is insidious, the distinction must be based upon the absence of muscular wasting and the presence of arterial degeneration. Myasthenia is distinguished by the characteristic fatigability, the response to edrophonium hydrochloride (*Tensilon*), and the absence of wasting and fasciculation.

In syringobulbia the presence of the characteristic dissociated sensory loss over the face is a distinctive feature.

It may sometimes be difficult or impossible to distinguish motor neurone disease of unusually early onset from benign spinal muscular atrophy of adolescence or early adult life (*vide infra*) save by the age of onset and benign course of the latter disorder.

PROGNOSIS

Motor neurone disease is a progressive disease, but its rate of progress shows considerable variations. In the minority of cases the patient goes rapidly downhill, muscular weakness, wasting, and fasciculation early becoming widespread, and death may occur within a year. In the cases in which the onset is slower the prognosis is influenced by several factors. Those in which the degeneration is for a long time confined to the lower motor neurones do best. Early involvement of the bulbar muscles makes the outlook worse, especially when progressive bulbar palsy is combined with pseudobulbar palsy. In general, patients with progressive bulbar palsy survive about 2–3 years, those with amyotrophic lateral sclerosis 3–5 years, and those with progressive muscular atrophy 3–10 years from the onset of symptoms, but there are many exceptions to this general guide. The prognosis is reviewed by Vejajiva, Foster, and Miller (1967). Temporary remissions may occur, during which for a time the disease ceases to progress.

TREATMENT

The cause of the disease being in most cases undiscoverable, treatment is limited to dealing with symptoms. Every effort should be made, however, to ascertain whether the patient has been exposed to any form of chronic intoxication. Syphilis may be excluded by the usual serological tests. The patient should avoid fatigue and exposure to cold, but should be encouraged to continue at a light occupation as long as possible. Regular moderate exercise to maintain power in innervated muscles is probably beneficial provided the patient does not exhaust himself. Prostigmine, 15 mg. orally, two, three or four times daily with atropine, 0·6 mg., or propantheline, 15 mg. twice daily, to overcome its side-effects, may have a temporary beneficial effect upon speech and swallowing in patients with bulbar weakness, and diazepam, 2–5 mg. three times daily, may diminish spasticity. Antibiotics may be needed for respiratory and urinary infection. In the late stages tracheostomy may be necessary if dysphagia and choking attacks become severe and the usual attention should be given to the bladder and skin. Tube-feeding or gastrostomy are occasionally required to give appropriate nutriments. Some patients are helped by calipers and toe-springs if foot-drop is troublesome and later a wheel-chair may be necessary. Unfortunately no drug is known which has any influence upon the disease process.

REFERENCES

ARAN, F. A. (1850) Recherches sur une maladie non encore décrite du système musculaire, *Arch. gén. Méd.*, **24**, 5.

BERTRAND, I., and BOGAERT, L. VAN (1925) Rapport sur la sclérose latérale amyotrophique, *Rev. neurol. (Paris)*, **32**, 779.

BRAIN, LORD, CROFT, P. B., and WILKINSON, M. (1965) Motor neurone disease as a manifestation of neoplasms (with a note on the course of classical motor neurone disease), *Brain*, **88**, 479.

BUCHTHAL, F., and PINELLI, P. (1953) Action potentials in muscular atrophy of neurogenic origin, *Neurology (Minneap.)*, **3**, 591.

CHARCOT, J. M., and JOFFROY, A. (1869) Deux cas d'atrophie musculaire progressive avec lésions de la substance grise et des faisceaux antéro-latéraux de la moelle épinière, *Arch. Physiol. norm. Path.*, **2**, 354, 629, 744.

DAVISON, C. (1942) Amyotrophic lateral sclerosis, *Arch. Neurol. Psychiat. (Chicago)*, **46**, 1039.

DRACHMAN, D. B., MURPHY, S. R., NIGAM, M. P., and HILLS, J. R. (1967) 'Myopathic' changes in chronically denervated muscle, *Arch. Neurol. (Chic.)*, **16**, 14.

DUCHENNE, G. B. (1853) Étude comparée des lésions anatomiques dans l'atrophie musculaire progressive et dans la paralysie générale, *Un. méd.*, **7**, 202.

DUCHENNE, G. B. (1860) Paralysie musculaire progressive de la langue, du voile du palais et des lèvres, *Arch. gén. Méd.*, **2**, 283.

DUCHENNE, G. B. (1861) Atrophie musculaire graisseuse progressive, in *Électrisation localisée*, 2nd ed., p. 437, Paris.

GREENFIELD, J. G. (1958) in *Neuropathology*, by GREENFIELD, J. G., BLACKWOOD, W., MCMENEMEY, W. H., MEYER, A., and NORMAN, R. M., p. 545, London.

HIRANO, A., KURLAND, L. T., and SAYRE, G. P. (1967) Familial amyotrophic lateral sclerosis, *Arch. Neurol. (Chic.)*, **16**, 232.

KUGELBERG, E. (1949) Electromyography in muscular dystrophies, *J. Neurol. Neurosurg. Psychiat.*, **12**, 129.

KURLAND, L. T. (1957) Epidemiological investigations of amyotrophic lateral sclerosis, *Proc. Mayo Clin.*, **32**, 449.

LIVERSEDGE, L. A. (1969) The spinal muscular atrophies, in *Disorders of Voluntary Muscle*, 2nd ed., ed. WALTON, J. N., London.

MARINESCO, G. (1925) Contribution à l'histo-chimie et à la pathogénie de la maladie de Charcot, *Rev. neurol. (Paris)*, **32**, 513.

SMITH, M. A. (1960) Nerve fibre degeneration in the brain in amyotrophic lateral sclerosis, *J. Neurol. Neurosurg. Psychiat.*, **23**, 269.

VEJAJIVA, A., FOSTER, J. B., and MILLER, H. (1967) Motor neuron disease; a clinical study, *J. neurol. Sci.*, **4**, 299.

SPASTIC PSEUDOSCLEROSIS (CREUTZFELD-JAKOB DISEASE)

The term *spastic pseudosclerosis* was first applied by Jakob (1920) to a group of cases described by Creutzfeld (1920) and himself, in which mental deterioration was associated with symptoms of both corticospinal and extrapyramidal disease. It is convenient for the present to retain it for this group, though as the work of Lhermitte and McAlpine (1926) and Davison (1932) shows it is not certain that it corresponds to a nosological entity.

There has been a tendency for some years to utilize this title in referring to patients who show a slowly-progressive syndrome characterized by clinical features of Parkinsonism, dementia with evidence of corticospinal tract dysfunction and with or without 'lower motor neurone' type wasting of muscles of the extremities due to fall-out of anterior horn cells. In fact this latter disorder, which may be familial and which also occurs sporadically in Europe and in the United States shows certain similarities to the so-called Parkinsonism-dementia complex which is endemic in the island of Guam [see p. 527]. It is different from the rapidly-progressive form of presenile dementia which Creutzfeld and Jakob first described.

Clinically the course of this sporadic form of the Parkinsonism-dementia complex, which may be called spastic pseudosclerosis, or cortico-striato-nigral degeneration, is usually rapid, the patient surviving only for two or three years. The symptoms are progressive dementia, dysarthria, spastic weakness of the limbs, extrapyramidal symptoms, such as rigidity of the Parkinsonian type, tremor or athetosis, and muscular wasting.

Recently, however, Foley and Denny-Brown (1955) and Brownwell and Oppenheimer (1965) have described a condition which corresponds more closely to that which Creutzfeld and Jakob originally described and have entitled it subacute progressive or presenile polioencephalopathy. The condition usually begins in middle age with ataxia, dementia, abnormal movements (often myoclonus), and stupor, with death occurring within a few months. Pathologically these cases show degenerative changes with some cell loss but marked astrocytic hyperplasia in the cerebral cortex, striatum, and thalamus and marked cell loss in the granular layer of the cerebellum.

REFERENCES

BROWNWELL, B., and OPPENHEIMER, D. R. (1965) An ataxic form of subacute presenile polioencephalopathy (Creutzfeld-Jakob disease), *J. Neurol. Psychiat.*, **28**, 350.

CREUTZFELD, H. G. (1921) Über eine eigenartige herdförmige Erkrankung des Zentralnervensystems, *Z. ges. Neurol. Psychiat.*, **57**, 1.

DAVISON, C. (1932) Spastic pseudo-sclerosis (cortico-pallido-spinal degeneration), *Brain*, **55**, 247.

FOLEY, J., and DENNY-BROWN, D. (1955) Subacute progressive encephalopathy with bulbar myoclonus, *J. Neuropath.*, **16**, 133.

JAKOB, A. (1920) Über eigenartige Erkrankungen des Zentralnervensystems mit bemerkenswerten anatomischen Befunden. Spastische Pseudosklerose — Encephalomyelopathie mit disseminierten Degenerationsherden, *Z. ges. Neurol. Psychiat.*, **64**, 146.

JAKOB, A. (1923) *Spastische Pseudosklerose; die extrapyramidalen Erkrankungen*, p. 215, Berlin.

LHERMITTE, J., and McALPINE, D. (1926) A clinical and pathological résumé of combined disease of the pyramidal and extra-pyramidal system with especial reference to a new syndrome, *Brain*, **49**, 157.

SUBACUTE SPONGIFORM ENCEPHALOPATHY

This somewhat rare disorder was first described by Jones and Nevin (1954), and has been reviewed with a report of additional cases by Nevin et al. (1960). It is a subacute disorder chiefly occurring between the ages of 50 and 70. The characteristic lesion is a spongy state affecting chiefly the cerebral cortex, and causing destruction and loss of nerve cells in all layers without obvious pattern. Nevin et al. think it probable that the lesions are vascular in origin, though the nature of the vascular dysfunction is obscure. The progressive symptoms include visual failure, motor paralysis, speech disturbances, progressive dementia, generalized convulsions, and myoclonic fits. Characteristic EEG changes include sharp waves associated with the myoclonus, obliteration of normal rhythms, and widespread high-voltage slow activity. The disease terminates fatally in from a few months to a year. The cause is unknown and no treatment has proved to be effective. The condition seems to be closely related to acute forms of Creutzfeld-Jakob disease (*vide supra*).

REFERENCES

Jones, D. P., and Nevin, S. (1954) Rapidly progressive cerebral degeneration (Subacute vascular encephalopathy) with mental disorder, focal disturbances and myoclonic epilepsy, *J. Neurol. Neurosurg. Psychiat.*, **7**, 148.
Nevin, S., McMenemey, W. H., Behrman, S., and Jones, D. P. (1960) Subacute spongiform encephalopathy—a subacute form of encephalopathy attributable to vascular dysfunction (Spongiform cerebral atrophy), *Brain*, **83**, 519.

PERONEAL MUSCULAR ATROPHY

Synonyms. Neural progressive muscular atrophy; Charcot-Marie-Tooth disease.

Definition. A hereditary form of progressive muscular atrophy first described in 1886 by Charcot and Marie and later in the same year by Tooth. Wasting usually begins in the small muscles of the feet and later in those of the hands, and never advances beyond the peripheral parts of the limbs. The muscular atrophy is secondary to degeneration of the motor nerves, though whether this begins in the nerves or in the spinal cord is uncertain.

PATHOLOGY

According to Buzzard and Greenfield (1921) the most constant pathological change is an interstitial neuritis of branches of the common peroneal nerve. Alajouanine et al. (1967) found marked proliferation of endoneurial connective tissue with secondary demyelination in lumbar roots. In most cases, though not invariably, changes are also found in the spinal cord, especially degeneration of the ganglion cells of the anterior horns in the cervical and lumbar enlargements and of the cells of the dorsal nucleus, together with degeneration of the posterior columns. Degeneration of the pyramidal tracts has been reported in some cases but it is inconstant and underlines the relationship of this disorder to other conditions in the hereditary ataxia group. It appears likely that the changes in the spinal cord are secondary to the affection of the peripheral nerves or roots. The muscular atrophy has usually been regarded as neurogenic, but Haase and Shy (1960) have reported myopathic changes with or without those of neurogenic atrophy. It now seems probable, however, that these were merely the so-called 'secondary myopathic changes' which are known to occur in muscle in long-standing cases of neurogenic atrophy of varying aetiology.

AETIOLOGY

Although sporadic cases occur, the disease is usually hereditary and a number of pedigrees of affected families have been published. Herringham (1889) reported one in which 20 cases occurred in the course of five generations, the disease being transmitted as a sex-linked recessive, males only being affected. In many affected families, however, it has behaved as a Mendelian dominant, affecting and being transmitted by, both sexes while in yet others it has seemed to be of autosomal recessive inheritance. Males are affected more frequently than females, possibly on account of the occurrence of families with a sex-linked transmission.

In most cases the onset of symptoms is during the second half of the first decade of life, but has been known to occur up to the age of 40.

SYMPTOMS

The first symptoms are muscular wasting and weakness, which usually begin in the peronei, extensor digitorum longus, or the small muscles of the foot, symmetrically on the two sides. Paralysis of the peronei leads to talipes equino-varus, but when the wasting begins in the intrinsic muscles of the feet pes cavus results. Not uncommonly it is the deformity of the feet and the resulting laborious 'steppage' gait which bring the patient under observation. Wasting does not usually appear in the hands until a number of years after its onset in the feet. Occasionally, however, both upper and lower extremities are affected simultaneously; exceptionally the hands suffer first. The muscular atrophy, which is not uncommonly associated with fasciculation, tends to spread very slowly proximally, not involving the muscles longitudinally but transversely. It does not extend above the elbows nor above the junction of the middle and lower thirds of the thigh. This peculiar ascending distribution of the wasting leads to a striking appearance of the limbs. When the lower part of the calf is wasted the 'fat bottle' calf is produced, and wasting of the lower third of the thigh leads to the so-called 'inverted champagne bottle' limb. The muscles of the head and trunk almost invariably escape, though wasting of the spinati and pectoralis major has been described. However, it would now appear that the rare syndrome of so-called 'scapuloperoneal muscular atrophy' is sometimes myopathic but more often neuropathic; the neuropathic variety is more severe than, and probably should be regarded as different from, classical peroneal muscular atrophy (Kaeser, 1965). Contractures occur, but are usually slight in proportion to the degree of wasting [FIG. 90].

Electromyography typically shows signs of denervation in the affected muscles and large discrete motor unit action potentials are generally present suggesting that the lesion responsible lies proximally in the motor neurones. There is usually marked slowing of motor nerve conduction velocity and evoked sensory potentials are often lost (Dyck, Lambert, and Mulder, 1963).

The tendon reflexes are variable. They are usually diminished or lost in the wasted muscles in proportion to the degree of wasting, but loss of the tendon reflexes may precede atrophy. The plantar reflexes are usually lost eventually.

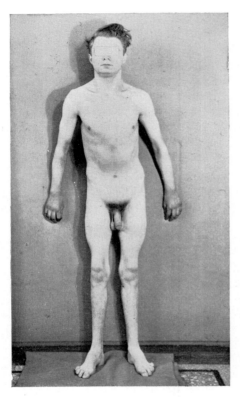

FIG. 90. A case of peroneal muscular atrophy, with wasting stopping sharply at the junction of the middle and lower thirds of the thighs

Sensibility may be unaffected, but there is generally loss of vibration sense at the ankles, often some impairment of appreciation of light touch, pain, and temperature over the periphery of the limbs. Deep sensibility is less often affected. Charcot and Marie, in their original paper, described vasomotor changes in the extremities, and perforating ulcers may occur probably due to the presence of an associated hereditary sensory neuropathy (England and Denny-Brown, 1952). The function of the sphincters remains normal.

The cranial nerves are usually normal, but optic atrophy has been described in a few cases and so, too, has inequality of the pupils, which is possibly due to implication of the ocular sympathetic fibres. Very occasionally the pupils are of the Argyll Robertson type (Alajouanine et al., 1967). Trigeminal neuralgia and anaesthesia rarely occur.

Symonds and Shaw (1926) have described an abortive form of the disease characterized by claw-foot and absence of the tendon reflexes in the lower limbs. This may occur in some members of a sibship, other members of which exhibit the disorder in its fully developed form. It has also been observed as the sole manifestation of the disorder in a family, while in certain families slowing of motor nerve conduction has been observed in some members who were apparently unaffected clinically at the time of examination (Dyck et al., 1963).

DIAGNOSIS

The onset of the muscular wasting in the lower limbs, and its peculiar ascent from the periphery are distinctive features which usually render the diagnosis easy. In the muscular dystrophies affected muscles waste longitudinally and selectively and the distribution of the wasting is characteristic of the various forms. In Welander's hereditary distal myopathy (1951) the age of onset is later than in peroneal atrophy, and there is no sensory loss. Dystrophia myotonica is distinguished by the presence of myotonia and by the distribution of the wasting, especially its selection of the sternomastoids and the quadriceps. Progressive muscular atrophy usually begins in adult life, and the feet are rarely the site of wasting. Friedreich's ataxia, like peroneal atrophy, is a hereditary disorder which gives rise to pes cavus, but nystagmus, ataxia, and extensor plantar responses are peculiar to the former in which, moreover, muscular wasting is rare. Polyneuritis may cause wasting of the peripheral muscles of both upper and lower limbs, but it is rare in childhood and usually leads also to pain and tenderness of the muscles and more marked sensory impairment than occurs in peroneal atrophy.

PROGNOSIS

The disorder runs a very slow course and arrest may occur at any stage. Since the wasting always remains confined to the limbs, the disease does not shorten life and many patients have been reported alive 45 or 50 years after the onset of symptoms. In the case reported by Alajouanine *et al.* (1967) the patient, whose condition was first diagnosed by Charcot, lived an active life for 60 years and eventually died at the age of 80. In spite of the deformities the degree of disability is often surprisingly slight.

TREATMENT

No treatment will arrest the course of the disorder. Massage and appropriate exercises will help to maintain the nutrition of the muscles and to enable the patient to make the best use of his available resources. Appropriate surgical boots and below-knee calipers with toe-springs will usually be required.

REFERENCES

ALAJOUANINE, T., CASTAIGNE, P., CAMBIER, J., and ESCOUROLLE, R. (1967) Maladie de Charcot-Marie. Étude anatomo-clinique, *Presse méd.*, 75, 2745.
BUZZARD, E. F., and GREENFIELD, J. G. (1921) *Pathology of the Nervous System*, London.
CHARCOT, J. M., and MARIE, P. (1886) Sur une forme particulière d'atrophie musculaire progressive souvent familiale, *Rev. Médecine*, 6, 97.
DYCK, P. J., LAMBERT, E. H., and MULDER, D. W. (1963) Charcot-Marie-Tooth disease. Nerve conduction and clinical studies of a large sibship, *Neurology (Minneap.)*, 13, 1.
EISENBUD, A., and GROSSMAN, M. (1927) Peroneal form of progressive muscular atrophy, *Arch. Neurol. Psychiat. (Chicago)*, 18, 766.
ENGLAND, A. C., and DENNY-BROWN, D. (1952) Severe sensory changes, and trophic disorder, in peroneal muscular atrophy (Charcot-Marie-Tooth type), *Arch. Neurol. Psychiat. (Chicago)*, 67, 1.
HAASE, G. R., and SHY, G. M. (1960) Pathological changes in muscle biopsies from patients with peroneal muscular atrophy, *Brain*, 83, 631.
HERRINGHAM, W. P. (1888–9) Muscular atrophy of the peroneal type affecting many members of a family, *Brain*, 11, 230.
KAESER, H. E. (1965) Scapuloperoneal muscular atrophy, *Brain*, 88, 407.
SYMONDS, C. P., and SHAW, M. E. (1926) Familial claw-foot with absent tendon-jerks: a 'forme fruste' of the Charcot-Marie-Tooth disease, *Brain*, 49, 387.

Tooth, H. H. (1886) *The Peroneal Type of Progressive Muscular Atrophy*, Cambridge thesis, London.
Welander, L. (1951) Myopathia distalis tarda hereditaria, *Acta med. scand.*, Suppl. 265.

INFANTILE SPINAL MUSCULAR ATROPHY AND RELATED DISORDERS

There has been considerable discussion as to the relationship between two muscular disorders of infancy, namely amyotonia congenita, or myatonia of Oppenheim (1900) on the one hand, and progressive spinal muscular atrophy of infancy on the other; the latter condition was first described by Werdnig (1890) and Hoffmann (1891). Spiller (1913), on clinical grounds, cast doubt upon the distinction of these diseases, and Greenfield and Stern (1927) pointed out that they were pathologically indistinguishable. But it is now believed that in such cases the diagnosis of amyotonia congenita had been wrongly made and that the progressive disorder which terminates fatally is always Werdnig-Hoffmann disease.

Confusion appears to have arisen from the fact that in the past infants showing severe hypotonia and weakness from the moment of birth were usually diagnosed as examples of amyotonia congenita whereas the diagnosis of Werdnig-Hoffmann disease was reserved for the cases in which weakness and hypotonia developed during the first year of life. In fact, as Walton (1956) and Paine (1963) pointed out, the syndrome of diffuse muscular hypotonia and weakness developing early in infancy is one of multiple aetiology and the inclusive term 'amyotonia congenita', which has been utilized to identify the syndrome, is better discarded since in every case an attempt should be made to identify the pathological basis of the disorder. Thus in many such cases with severe weakness and hypotonia, even when present from birth, the condition proves to be one of progressive spinal muscular atrophy; in others the hypotonia is symptomatic, being secondary to mental defect, flaccid cerebral diplegia or to a variety of metabolic or nutritional disorders; there is, however, a small group of cases in which no cause for the hypotonia is discovered and in which slow improvement usually occurs—for the present these cases may be regarded as suffering from 'benign congenital hypotonia', but even this is almost certainly a disorder of multiple aetiology.

PROGRESSIVE SPINAL MUSCULAR ATROPHY OF INFANCY
PATHOLOGY

There is atrophy and chromatolytic degeneration of the ganglion cells of the anterior horns of the spinal cord and, to a variable extent, of the cranial nerve nuclei. The ventral roots are small and largely demyelinated. The peripheral nerves exhibit a high proportion of small finely myelinated fibres, and the muscles show simple 'grouped' or neurogenic atrophy with a number of very small fibres and a considerable amount of fat replacement in chronic cases. The diaphragm, however, is generally normal.

AETIOLOGY

The cause of this condition is unknown, but it may occur in more than one member of the same family. Cases have not been described in successive generations. The condition is due to an autosomal recessive gene and this affects one in four offspring of either sex of two heterozygous carriers. Unfortunately no method of detecting carriers is available and it is not uncommon to find that two or three successive children of healthy parents may be affected. Although cases have been reported following acute infections it is doubtful if these play a part in aetiology.

SYMPTOMS

Affected children may be normal at birth and often do not begin to exhibit the symptoms of the disorder until they are a few months old. In other cases severe generalized weakness and hypotonia are present from birth, suggesting that the disease process may have begun in foetal life. In occasional cases muscular weakness first appears later in childhood and runs a more benign course than is usual when the onset is in infancy. Muscular weakness usually begins in the muscles of the back, and the pelvic and shoulder girdles, whence it spreads to the proximal, and later to the distal, muscles of the limbs. The affected muscles waste rapidly: though the wasting may be obscured by subcutaneous fat, it may be shown by X-rays. Muscular fasciculation is present and may be seen in the tongue. The intercostal muscles usually become affected and the bulbar muscles may suffer also, but the diaphragm usually escapes until the later stages. The tendon reflexes are lost. Sensibility is unimpaired, and muscle biopsy shows the features of a neurogenic atrophy while electromyography reveals as a rule spontaneous fibrillation and discrete isolated motor unit action potentials of normal or increased size on volition.

DIAGNOSIS

The condition must be distinguished from benign congenital hypotonia which is present at birth, is characterized by generalized muscular hypotonia with less wasting, preservation of the tendon reflexes, absence of complete paralysis, and of involvement of the intercostals, and in which there is a tendency to improvement; and from congenital myopathy, in which also there may be improvement. Muscle biopsy is generally distinctive in each case. Congenital diplegia and other causes of symptomatic hypotonia are usually easily recognized.

PROGNOSIS

The condition, as its name implies, is generally progressive, and often terminates fatally in a few months, though the disease may remain stationary for years and then progress again. Severe contractures, scoliosis, and other skeletal deformities are usual in chronic cases. Greenfield, Cornman, and Shy (1958) describe this in a patient aged 31, but this is most exceptional. However, the experience of recent years shows that arrest of the disease occurs more often than is generally realized and may take place when the patient is already severely disabled or else at a comparatively early stage. Discordance in the age of onset and in the severity of the condition may be seen in different members of the same family (Dubowitz, 1964; Gardner-Medwin, Hudgson, and Walton, 1967).

TREATMENT

No drug treatment of any value is known but physical exercise, active and passive movement under supervision, and care to avoid contractures and to maintain normal posture are essential in the less severe cases.

BENIGN SPINAL MUSCULAR ATROPHY OF CHILDHOOD AND ADOLESCENCE

In 1956 Kugelberg and Welander described 12 patients occurring in six families, all of whom were suffering from a heredofamilial form of muscular atrophy simulating muscular dystrophy and suggested that this condition, which appeared to be of autosomal recessive inheritance, might prove to be a new syndrome. Many subsequent reports have since appeared indicating that the condition may begin at any age from late infancy, early childhood or adolescence to early adult life. Proximal muscles of both the upper and lower limbs are usually affected first giving a clinical picture like that of muscular dystrophy, save for the presence of fasciculation in many cases; the electromyogram and muscle biopsy indicate denervation atrophy but serum creatine kinase activity may be slightly raised. The course of the condition is very variable from case to case but deterioration is usually slow and arrest frequently occurs. In a recent review of the literature and of 15 personal cases Gardner-Medwin, Hudgson, and Walton (1967) give reasons for suggesting that the condition is simply a benign variant of Werdnig-Hoffmann disease, as cases of this type have been observed within sibships in which previous children have died from classical infantile spinal muscular atrophy.

BENIGN CONGENITAL HYPOTONIA (AMYOTONIA CONGENITA)

SYMPTOMS

The condition is usually present at birth, though frequently it is not observed until the child is old enough to attempt to raise its head. The most striking feature of the disorder is the extreme hypotonicity of all the muscles, which renders it possible for the limbs to be placed in bizarre attitudes. The muscles, though somewhat weak, are not actually paralysed, but the child may be unable to maintain any posture against the force of gravity. It is, therefore, at first unable to raise its head and, later, to sit or to stand, though it is able to move its legs if it is supported beneath the axillae. The tendon reflexes are usually present but may be depressed. The intercostal muscles and diaphragm usually escape. Electromyography may show no abnormality and muscle biopsy shows no pathological change in muscle fibres though these may be smaller than normal.

DIAGNOSIS

The diagnosis is not easy, as many conditions are characterized by muscular hypotonia in infancy. Congenital laxity of the ligaments (as in families of contortionists) may result in excessive mobility at joints but the muscles are powerful.

In Werdnig-Hoffmann disease the weakness and hypotonia are more severe, the tendon reflexes are lost, and there may be indrawing of the lower ribs during inspiration as a result of intercostal weakness. Mental defect and mild flaccid diplegia may be difficult to distinguish in the early stages as may other causes of symptomatic hypotonia. Serum enzyme studies, electromyography, and muscle biopsy are of particular value in excluding spinal muscular atrophy, muscular dystrophy, and other myopathies, while motor nerve conduction velocity measurement and lumbar puncture may be necessary to exclude infantile polyneuropathy. Even so the diagnosis will occasionally remain in doubt and will only be clarified by repeated observation and examination of the child over a period of many months. Many rare and obscure benign congenital myopathies (Turner, 1949; Tizard, 1969) may be indistinguishable from benign congenital hypotonia in the early stages.

PROGNOSIS

The general tendency of the disorder is to improve, and, if the patient survives intercurrent infections, a considerable degree of recovery may occur. A few patients recover completely but others have small weak and hypotonic muscles throughout life and are then classified as cases of 'benign congenital myopathy'.

TREATMENT

Treatment must be directed to educating voluntary movement and to maintaining the nutrition of the muscles by active and passive movements.

REFERENCES

BATTEN, F. E., and HOLMES, G. (1912–13) Progressive spinal muscular atrophy of infants (Werdnig-Hoffmann type), *Brain*, **35**, 38.

DUBOWITZ, V. (1964) Infantile muscular atrophy. A prospective study with particular reference to a slowly progressive variety, *Brain*, **87**, 707.

GARDNER-MEDWIN, D., HUDGSON, P., and WALTON, J. N. (1967) Benign spinal muscular atrophy arising in childhood and adolescence, *J. neurol. Sci.*, **5**, 121.

GREENFIELD, J. G., CORNMAN, T., and SHY, G. M. (1958) The prognostic value of muscle biopsy in the 'floppy infant', *Brain*, **81**, 461.

GREENFIELD, J. G., and STERN, R. O. (1927). The anatomical identity of the Werdnig-Hoffmann and Oppenheim forms of infantile muscular atrophy, *Brain*, **50**, 652.

HOFFMANN, J. (1891) Weiterer Beitrag zur Lehre von der progressiven neurotischen Muskelatrophie, *Dtsch. Z. Nervenheilk.*, **1**, 95.

HOFFMANN, J. (1893) Über chronische spinale Muskelatrophie im Kindesalter, *Dtsch. Z. Nervenheilk.*, **3**, 427.

HOFFMANN, J. (1897) Weiterer Beitrag zur Lehre von der hereditären progressiven spinalen Muskelatrophie im Kindesalter, *Dtsch. Z. Nervenheilk.*, **10**, 292.

KUGELBERG, E., and WELANDER, L. (1956) Heredo-familial juvenile muscular atrophy simulating muscular dystrophy, *Arch. Neurol. Psychiat. (Chicago)*, **15**, 500.

OPPENHEIM, H. (1900) Über allgemeine und localisierte Atonie der Muskulatur (Myatonie) im frühen Kindesalter, *Mschr. Psychiat. Neurol.*, **8**, 232.

PAINE, R. S. (1963) The future of the 'floppy infant'. A follow-up study of 133 patients, *Develop. med. Child. Neurol.*, **5**, 115.

SPILLER, W. G. (1913) The relation of the myopathies, *Brain*, **36**, 75.

TIZARD, J. P. M. (1969) Neuromuscular disorders of infancy, in *Disorders of Voluntary Muscle*, 2nd ed., ed. WALTON, J. N., London.

TURNER, J. W. A. (1949) On amyotonia congenita, *Brain*, **72**, 25.

WALTON, J. N. (1956) Amyotonia congenita: a follow-up study, *Lancet*, i, 1023.

WALTON, J. N. (1957) The limp child, *J. Neurol. Psychiat.*, **20**, 144.

WERDNIG, G. (1890) Über einen Fall von Dystrophia musculorum mit positivem Rückenmarksbefunde, *Wien. med. Wschr.*, **40**, 1796.

WERDNIG, G. (1891) Zwei frühinfantile hereditäre Fälle von progressiver Muskelatrophie unter dem Bilde der Dystrophie, aber auf neurotischer Grundlage, *Arch. Psychiat*, **22**, 437.

FACIAL HEMIATROPHY

Synonym. Parry-Romberg syndrome.

Definition. A trophic disorder of uncertain aetiology, characterized by progressive wasting of some or all of the tissues of one side of the face and sometimes extending beyond these limits.

PATHOLOGY

Facial hemiatrophy, which was first described by Romberg in 1846, consists essentially of an atrophy which usually involves all the tissues of the face—the skin, the subcutaneous fat and connective tissue, the muscles, cartilage, and bone. The muscular atrophy is due to a disappearance, not of the muscle fibres, but of the fat and connective tissue of the muscle. The tongue and soft palate often suffer in addition. The cartilage of the nose frequently becomes atrophic: that of the ear, larynx, and tarsus is less often affected. In two cases the changes characteristic of interstitial neuritis have been observed in the trigeminal nerve on the affected side.

The cerebral hemisphere on the affected side may be atrophic. Stief (1933) described great vasodilatation of the ipsilateral hemisphere and round cell infiltration of the cervical sympathetic on the affected side.

AETIOLOGY

It is a disorder of early life, usually developing during the second decade, and is sometimes congenital. A number of cases, however, have been observed in which the onset has occurred in middle life or even old age. Among the predisposing causes local trauma to the head, face, or neck appears important. The disorder has sometimes been ascribed to local infections in the neighbourhood of the jaw and pharynx, for example alveolar abscess, and its onset has followed the extraction of teeth. General infections have been held responsible, but their importance is difficult to assess, except in the case of pulmonary tuberculosis, which has been described too frequently for its association with facial hemiatrophy to be a coincidence. Those who attribute the latter to a disorder of the cervical sympathetic believe that this may be involved in an apical pleurisy of tuberculous origin.

The immediate pathogenesis of facial hemiatrophy is unknown. Its association with scleroderma has been emphasized. Nevertheless, the two conditions appear to be distinct. Some workers have attributed it to a lesion of the trigeminal nerve. It is true that neuralgic pain is not uncommon in facial hemiatrophy, and facial anaesthesia has occasionally been observed. Lesions of the trigeminal nerve, however, are common, whereas facial hemiatrophy is rare, and it is unlikely that the former is the cause of the latter. Archambault and Fromm (1932) summarized the arguments in favour of attributing facial hemiatrophy to a disturbance of the sympathetic nervous system. The disorder has not uncommonly been observed in association with symptoms of paralysis of the cervical sympathetic, both of peripheral and of central origin, but either may occur without the other, and their relationship remains obscure.

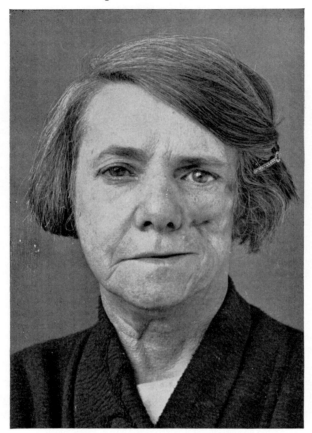

FIG. 91. Facial hemiatrophy associated with atrophy of the ipsilateral cerebral hemisphere. [See also FIG. 92.]

SYMPTOMS

Wasting may begin at any point of the face and may either remain limited to one region, so that it has been described as corresponding to one division of the trigeminal nerve, or may spread, either slowly or quickly, to the whole face, sometimes extending to the side of the neck and even, as in a case of Martin's, involving the breast on the same side. Some authors would accept that cases of progressive hemiatrophy of the whole body are closely related. When the disorder is well developed the patient's appearance is striking, the affected half of the face being sunken and wrinkled and presenting the appearance of old age, in marked contrast to the normal side [FIG. 91]. Very rarely both sides of the face are affected. The atrophy frequently involves the soft palate, tongue, and mucous membrane of the gums on the same side. Muscular weakness is absent. Falling of the hair of the face and scalp on the affected side is not uncommon. Pigmentary anomalies of the skin, such as vitiligo, frequently occur, and facial naevus has been described. Pains of a neuralgic character may develop and these are frequently associated with tender spots. True tic douloureux may occur. Sensory impairment is rare but cutaneous anaesthesia and analgesia have

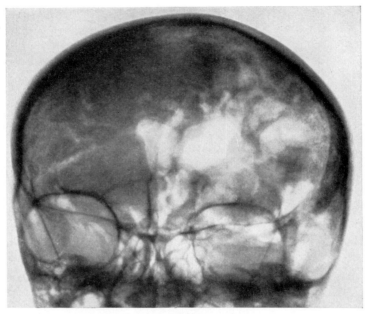

FIG. 92. Facial hemiatrophy with atrophy of the ipsilateral hemisphere resulting in dilatation of the ventricle on the same side and causing a local collection of air over the surface of the hemisphere in the region of the atrophy. Radiogram by Dr. Jupe. [Same patient as FIG. 91.]

been encountered. Sweating and lacrimal secretion may be either diminished or increased on the affected side. Ocular sympathetic paralysis—myosis, ptosis, and enophthalmos—has been encountered in a proportion of cases, and I have seen unilateral Argyll Robertson pupil. In other cases the pupil on the affected side has been larger than on the normal side.

Epileptiform convulsions, in some cases Jacksonian and in others generalized, have occurred in a small number of cases. I have seen one such case [FIG. 91] in which left facial hemiatrophy was associated with right-sided epilepsy, hemiplegia, hemianaesthesia, hemianopia, and aphasia, and atrophy of the left cerebral hemisphere was demonstrated by encephalography [FIG. 92]. Migraine is common. Facial hemiatrophy is sometimes associated with syringomyelia, and the presence of scleroderma elsewhere in the body has often been observed.

DIAGNOSIS

The clinical picture is so striking that it can hardly be confused with anything else.

PROGNOSIS

The wasting may become arrested before the whole of the face is involved, but there is no means of determining whether or not this will occur. The disorder causes no disability apart from its cosmetic effect.

TREATMENT

No known treatment will arrest the progress of the disease. For cosmetic purposes Gersuny introduced melted paraffin into the subcutaneous tissues but this treatment is dangerous and has now been discarded. X-ray irradiation is the most satisfactory method of relieving the neuralgic pains but the usual treatment of trigeminal neuralgia may be required.

REFERENCES

ARCHAMBAULT, L., and FROMM, N. K. (1932) Progressive facial hemiatrophy, *Arch, Neurol. Psychiat. (Chicago)*, **27**, 529.

STIEF, A. (1933) Über einen Fall von Hemiatrophie des Gesichtes mit Sektionsbefund, *Z. ges. Neurol. Psychiat.*, **147**, 573.

WARTENBERG, R. (1925) Zur Klinik und Pathogenese der Hemiatrophia faciei progressiva, *Arch. Psychiat. Nervenkr.*, **74**, 602.

WARTENBERG, R. (1945) Progressive facial hemiatrophy, *Arch. Neurol. Psychiat. (Chicago)*, **54**, 75.

14

DISORDERS OF THE SPINAL CORD
AND CAUDA EQUINA

ANATOMY OF THE SPINAL CORD
AND CAUDA EQUINA

THE spinal cord lies within the vertebral canal, extending from the foramen magnum, where it is continuous with the medulla oblongata, to the level of the first or second lumbar vertebra. It is oval in shape, being flattened from before backwards, and exhibits two enlargements, in the cervical and lumbar regions, corresponding to the outflow of nerves to the limbs. At its lower end the spinal cord terminates in the conus medullaris, from the end of which a delicate filament, the filum terminale, is prolonged downwards as far as the posterior surface of the coccyx.

The surface of the cord exhibits several longitudinal grooves, the deep anterior median fissure and the shallower posterior median sulcus, while on the lateral aspect are two sulci, the anterolateral and the posterolateral. From the last two a series of root filaments emerge on each side of the cord. At intervals several filaments from the posterolateral sulcus unite to form a dorsal root, upon which is situated a ganglion, the dorsal root ganglion, and similarly those from the anterolateral sulcus unite to form a ventral root. One ventral and the corresponding dorsal root on one side join together just distally to the dorsal root ganglion to form a spinal nerve. Thus from each side there arises a series of spinal nerves, and the spinal cord is regarded as divided into segments, one corresponding to each pair of spinal nerves. There are eight cervical, twelve dorsal or thoracic, five lumbar, five sacral segments, and one coccygeal. Since the spinal cord ends at the first or second lumbar vertebra, all the spinal nerves below the first lumbar descend to their respective foramina in a leash known as the cauda equina.

The spinal cord, like the brain, is surrounded by three meninges. The pia mater is a fibrous membrane, which forms the immediate covering of the cord, and from which fine septa penetrate into its substance. The arachnoid is a delicate, transparent membrane, which lies superficially to the pia mater, from which it is separated by the subarachnoid space; this contains the cerebrospinal fluid, and it is bridged by numerous trabeculae. The arachnoid extends as low as the second sacral vertebra. Outside the arachnoid lies the dura mater, which forms a lining to the vertebral canal, from which it is separated by the epidural space containing fatty tissue, and a thin-walled venous plexus. The dura mater extends a little lower than the arachnoid, to the second or third sacral vertebra. The spinal cord is suspended within its dural sheath by a series of ligamenta denticulata, which extend laterally from the sides of the cord to terminate in tooth-like attachments to the inner aspect of the dura.

On transverse section the substance of the cord is seen to be divided into the central grey and peripheral white matter. The grey matter is composed of ganglion cells and nerve fibres, and the white matter of fibres only. The grey matter forms an H-shaped mass composed of an anterior and a posterior horn on each side, united by the grey commissure, in the centre of which is situated the central canal. The anterior horns of grey matter contain the ganglion cells, the axons of which compose the anterior roots and which constitute the lower motor neurones. These cells are not uniformly scattered throughout the anterior horns, but are arranged in definite groups. In the cervical and lumbar enlargements it is possible to distinguish an anterolateral and a posterolateral, an anteromesial and a posteromesial, and a central group. According to Bing: 'It may be said that the centres for the spinal musculature are to be found in the dorsomesial group, those for the muscles of the proximal segments of the limbs in the ventromesial, while the two lateral groups govern the remaining segments of the extremities. The centres for the coarser movements of flexion and extension are in the neighbourhood of the periphery, while those for the finer movements (e.g. of toes and fingers) lie nearer the central groups.'

The white matter, which consists of the longitudinal bundles of nerve fibres, is regarded as being divided into three columns. The anterior column lies between the anterior fissure and the anterior horn of grey matter with its emerging roots. The lateral column is situated on the lateral side of the grey matter, between the ventral and dorsal roots, that is, between the anterolateral and posterolateral sulci. The posterior column lies between the posterior median septum and the posterior horn of grey matter and the dorsal root. The paths of the fibres entering the spinal cord by the posterior roots are described elsewhere [see p. 44]. The anatomical situation of the various fibre tracts of the spinal cord is best appreciated by reference to the diagram [FIG. 8, p. 44].

THE BLOOD SUPPLY OF THE SPINAL CORD

Arteries. The spinal cord is richly supplied with blood. There are two posterior spinal arteries, each derived from the corresponding vertebral or posterior inferior cerebellar artery and passing downwards upon the side of the medulla oblongata and throughout the whole length of the spinal cord, where they lie either in front of, or behind, the dorsal nerve roots. The single anterior spinal artery is formed by the union of a branch from each vertebral artery, and descends throughout the whole length of the spinal cord in the anterior median fissure. The spinal arteries are reinforced by segmental arteries, which enter the intervertebral foramina and are derived from the vertebral, intercostal, and lumbar arteries. The two most important of these are one in the lower cervical and one, the artery of Adamkiewicz, in the lower thoracic or upper lumbar region. The spinal cord is thus surrounded by a basocorona or arterial wreath, which unites the spinal arteries and which sends branches horizontally inwards to supply the white matter and the greater part of the posterior horns of grey matter. The anterior horns of grey matter are supplied by branches of the anterior spinal artery, and distributed to the anterior horn on each side alternately.

The direction of blood flow in the anterior spinal artery may not be the same throughout. Bolton (1939) suggested that the direction of blood flow is downwards in the anterior spinal artery, and in the posterior spinal artery down to the lower cervical region, but that in the rest of the posterior spinal artery blood flow is derived from the terminal portion of the anterior spinal artery and is directed upwards as far as the upper thoracic region. Within the cord the anterior spinal artery supplies all but the posterior portion of the posterior columns and posterior horns, which are supplied by the posterior spinal arteries. Descending branches from the spinal arteries also supply the roots of the cauda equina.

Veins. The spinal veins derived from the substance of the spinal cord terminate in a plexus in the pia mater, in which six longitudinal channels have been described. These pass upwards into the corresponding veins of the medulla oblongata and so drain into the intracranial venous sinuses. Segmental veins pass outwards along the nerve roots to join the internal vertebral venous plexus, in which also blood flows upwards to the intracranial venous sinuses. Venous drainage through the intervertebral foramina is relatively unimportant, but thrombophlebitis and neoplasms may reach the spinal veins by this route.

REFERENCES

BOLTON, B. (1939) The blood supply of the spinal cord, *J. Neurol. Psychiat.*, N.S. **2**, 137.
CORBIN, J. L. (1961) *Anatomie, pathologie artérielle de la moelle*, Paris.
HUGHES, J. T. (1966) *Pathology of the Spinal Cord*, London.

PARAPLEGIA

By paraplegia is meant paralysis confined to the lower limbs. This may be caused by a disorder of function at different levels. It may be psychogenic—in hysteria. It may occur as a result of a cerebral lesion, when it is so placed as to damage the corticospinal fibres from the leg areas of the motor cortex only. Cerebral paraplegia may thus be produced by a meningioma arising in the falx (a parasagittal meningioma), by thrombosis of the superior sagittal sinus, by congenital cerebral lesions (Little's disease), and in rare instances by thrombosis of an unpaired anterior cerebral artery. In such cases the lower limbs are usually spastic in extension. Paraplegia of flaccid type due to a lesion of the spinal cord is very much commoner and is the form usually encountered. Spinal paraplegia may be associated either with extension or with flexion of the lower limbs, paraplegia-in-extension or paraplegia-in-flexion. Paraplegia may also be caused by a lesion of the anterior horn cells of the lumbosacral region of the spinal cord, e.g. in poliomyelitis or, rarely, motor neurone disease, or by a lesion of the cauda equina, or of the peripheral nerves to the lower limbs, as in polyneuritis, or of the muscles, as in myopathy. We are here concerned mainly with paraplegia due to lesions of the spinal cord.

After a partial lesion of the cord two mutually antagonistic reflex activities emerge, extensor hypertonia and the flexor withdrawal reflex [see p. 55]. The former is recognized as physiologically equivalent to decerebrate rigidity in the animal, which, it will be remembered, is probably dependent upon the connexions of the reticular formation nuclei with the spinal cord. The flexor withdrawal reflex, on the other hand, utilizes short spinal reflex arcs. After a lesion which involves the corticospinal tracts only, both sets of reflexes are potentially active, but extensor hypertonia predominates as a persistent tonic activity, giving way only occasionally to the flexor withdrawal reflex when a noxious stimulus excites the latter. If, however, a spinal lesion involves a sufficient transverse extent of the cord to destroy not only the corticospinal fibres but also the descending tracts, upon which extensor hypertonia depends, the flexor reflex, freed from its antagonist, manifests greatly heightened activity and dominates the picture. Violent flexor spasms occur in the lower limbs, which in severe cases finally become fixed in an attitude of flexion, with the heels approximated to the buttocks. Paraplegia-in-flexion may be the outcome of a slowly progressive lesion of the cord, in which case it follows paraplegia-in-extension after an intermediate phase in which the balance swings between the two reflex systems. On the other hand, after a traumatic lesion, causing immediate and complete severance of the cord, because the reticulospinal tract is interrupted from the beginning, as soon as the stage of spinal shock has passed, paraplegia-in-flexion tends to develop unless prevented.

PARAPLEGIA-IN-FLEXION

In paraplegia-in-flexion three main reflex activities are demonstrable: (1) the flexor withdrawal reflex, (2) excretory, and (3) sexual reflexes. We must also consider (4) the 'mass reflex', and (5) the tendon reflexes.

1. *The flexor withdrawal reflex* has already been briefly described [see p. 56]. In paraplegia-in-flexion its activity is much enhanced. Its receptive field is enlarged and it may be elicitable by a noxious stimulus applied to any part of the lower limbs and abdominal wall, or even, with a high dorsal lesion, as high as the nipple. The motor response is extremely vigorous, and strong flexion of the lower limb occurs at all joints, with upward movement of the great toe and separation of the other toes. This is usually unilateral, but the opposite lower limb may also become flexed. The activity of the flexor reflex is depressed by spinal shock and by cutaneous or urinary infection. Both its receptive field and its motor response then shrink until it can be obtained only from the outer border of the sole, and yields only a contraction of the inner hamstring muscles.

2. *Excretory Reflexes.* When reflex activity of the divided spinal cord is well established, in traumatic cases about three weeks after transection, reflex evacuation of the bladder and rectum, and reflex sweating occur. The volume of fluid required to evoke reflex contraction of the bladder wall varies in different cases, but is usually about 150–200 ml. Reflex emptying of the bladder can be facilitated by deep breathing or by noxious stimuli applied to the skin of the lower limbs. Reflex evacuation of the rectum occurs in response to a volume of from 100–180 ml. Sweating occurs reflexly in response to cutaneous stimuli from the areas of skin supplied by the fibres of the sympathetic nervous system which leave the spinal cord below the level of the lesion.

3. *Sexual Reflexes.* In paraplegia-in-flexion the cremasteric, dartos, and bulbocavernosus reflexes are present, and reflex erection of the penis and seminal emission can be evoked by handling the organ. Spontaneous priapism may occur. These sexual reflexes may be associated with contractions of the abdominal recti, the leg flexors, and the adductors of the thigh.

4. *The Mass Reflex*. Reflex facilitation is probably responsible for the phenomenon named by Head and Riddoch (1917) the 'mass reflex', in which stimulation of the skin of the lower limbs and, when the lesion is high, of the lower
abdominal wall evokes reflex flexion of the lower trunk muscles and the lower
limbs, evacuation of the bladder and rectum, and sweating.

5. *The Tendon Reflexes*. The tone of the extensor muscles is minimal in
paraplegia-in-flexion, but the tendon reflexes can usually be elicited. Ankle
clonus, however, hardly ever occurs.

PARAPLEGIA-IN-EXTENSION

In paraplegia-in-extension tone predominates in the adductors of the hips
and the extensors of the hips, knees and ankles with a resulting posture of extension of the hip and knee and plantar-flexion of the ankles. The knee- and ankle-
jerks are exaggerated, and patellar and ankle clonus are frequently present. The
elicitation of the knee-jerk may evoke a sharp contraction of the adductors of the
opposite hip, the crossed adductor-jerk. Reflex extension of the limb can often be
obtained by applying a noxious stimulus, such as a scratch from a pin, to the skin
of the upper third of the thigh, and spontaneous extensor spasms may occur.

With this prevalence of extensor tone the flexor withdrawal reflex is relatively
inhibited. Its field of elicitation is small compared with that found in paraplegia-
in-flexion. After it has been evoked, the limb regains its primary posture of
extension by an active return of tone to the extensor muscles. Flexor withdrawal
of one limb is usually associated with increased extension of the other, the crossed
extensor reflex. The excretory reflexes which accompany paraplegia-in-flexion
are absent, and the motor concomitant of erection of the penis is extension
instead of flexion of the lower limbs.

REFERENCES

HEAD, H., and RIDDOCH, G. (1917) The automatic bladder, excessive sweating, and some
    other reflex conditions, in gross injuries of the spinal cord, *Brain*, **40,** 188.
MEDICAL RESEARCH COUNCIL (1924) Report of the Committee upon Injuries of the
    Nervous System, *Spec. Rep. Ser. med. Res. Coun. (Lond.)*, No. 88.
PEDERSEN, E., ed. (1962) Spasticity and neurological bladder disturbances, *Acta neurol.
    (Kbh.)*, **38,** Suppl. 3.
SCARFF, J. E. (1960) Injuries of the vertebral column and spinal cord, in *Injuries of the
    Brain and Spinal Cord*, 4th ed., ed. BROCK, S., p. 530, New York.
SIMPSON, J. A. (1963) Current neurological concepts of spinal cord injuries, in *Spinal
    Injuries: a Symposium of the Royal College of Surgeons*, ed. HARRIS, P., p. 10,
    Edinburgh.
WALSHE, F. M. R. (1914–15) The physiological significance of the reflex phenomena in
    spastic paralysis of the lower limbs, *Brain*, **37,** 269.
WALSHE, F. M. R. (1919) On the genesis and physiological significance of spasticity and
    other disorders of motor innervation: with a consideration of the functional relation-
    ships of the pyramidal system, *Brain*, **42,** 1.
WALSHE, F. M. R. (1923) On variations in the form of reflex movements, notably the
    Babinski plantar response, under different degrees of spacticity and under the
    influence of Magnus and de Kleijn's tonic neck reflex, *Brain*, **46,** 281.
WALSHE, F. M. R. (1923) The decerebrate rigidity of Sherrington in man, *Arch. Neurol
    Psychiat. (Chicago)*, **10,** 1.

THE INNERVATION OF THE BLADDER AND RECTUM

ANATOMY AND PHYSIOLOGY

The sympathetic fibres to the bladder are derived chiefly from the first and second lumbar ganglia, with contributions from the third and fourth. These fibres ultimately unite to form the presacral nerve or superior hypogastric plexus, which lies in front of the bifurcation of the aorta. From this plexus are derived the two hypogastric nerves, each of which ends in the vesical plexuses on the lateral aspect of the bladder. The parasympathetic nerve supply from the second and third sacral nerves also joins the vesical plexuses. It is doubtful if there is any separately innervated internal sphincter. When the parasympathetic is stimulated the longitudinal fibres of the detrusor pull the neck open and the circular fibres exert pressure on the contents. The physiology of micturition is discussed by Ruch (1960).

In infancy the evacuation of the bladder occurs reflexly, the reflex arc running through the sacral region of the cord. The development of control over bladder evacuation is associated with the growth of inhibition of the evacuation reflex, the path of the inhibitory impulses running in the sympathetic, which maintains closure of the sphincter and inhibition of the detrusor muscles. At the same time it becomes possible voluntarily to overcome this inhibition and so to initiate the act of micturition, which is then completed reflexly. Thus we can recognize three nervous mechanisms controlling bladder function—the sacral reflex arc for evacuation; the inhibitory influence of the sympathetic; and voluntary control overcoming the last-named and initiating micturition.

The paths in the central nervous system traversed by impulses concerned in sympathetic and voluntary bladder control are imperfectly known, but probably both afferent and efferent pathways lie in the posterior marginal part of the lateral columns of the spinal cord (McMichael, 1945). The voluntary initiation of micturition usually occurs in response to an awareness of distension of the bladder. The part of the postcentral gyrus lying at the vertex of the cerebral hemisphere is the cortical centre for sensations derived from the bladder, and the corresponding area of the precentral gyrus is probably the site of origin of motor impulses initiating the act of micturition. It is well recognized that parasagittal lesions which affect this area bilaterally may give rise to retention of urine or sometimes incontinence. Andrew and Nathan (1964) have shown that the area concerned is localized in the superior frontal gyrus and that unilateral or, more often, bilateral lesions in this region may give urgency and frequency of micturition and incontinence; the sensation giving rise to the desire to micturate is diminished or absent.

INVESTIGATION OF BLADDER FUNCTION

In order to diagnose the nature of a bladder disturbance and treat it appropriately it is necessary to test bladder function. *Cystometry* consists in measuring the rise of intravesical pressure induced by increasing volumes of fluid. Either the tidal drainage apparatus is used, or any device by which a funnel and manometer can be attached to the catheter. The intravesical pressure is recorded after the injection of each 50 ml. of fluid.

DISTURBANCES OF BLADDER FUNCTION

Lesions involving the Sacral Reflex Arc

Since the sacral reflex arc is concerned in evacuation of the bladder, its interruption usually causes retention of urine, which is produced by the unopposed action of the sympathetic. In tabes dorsalis the reflex is interrupted on its afferent side, owing to degeneration of the afferent neurones. Lesions of the conus medullaris of the spinal cord interrupt the central fibres of the reflex. Lesions of the cauda equina, if they destroy the second and third sacral roots, interrupt both the afferent and the efferent paths of the reflex and hence usually cause retention of urine. Even after severe lesions of the conus or cauda equina, however, 'reflex' evacuation of the bladder may occasionally develop, under the influence of a more peripheral autonomous nervous mechanism, probably the vesical plexus. However, in cauda equina lesions and in tabes the bladder is more usually atonic, that is, it accepts a very large volume of urine without reflexly contracting to raise the intravesical pressure.

Lesions of the Spinal Cord above the Conus Medullaris

Incomplete lesions of the spinal cord may affect principally either the inhibitory fibres destined for the sympathetic outflow or the fibres concerned in the voluntary initiation of micturition. In the former case, the patient complains of difficulty in holding urine, and micturition is precipitate. This is a common symptom in the early stages of multiple sclerosis. Moderately severe but still incomplete lesions of the spinal cord tend to impair voluntary control over micturition, so that retention of urine develops, owing to uninhibited action of the sympathetic. Retention of urine is thus produced by spinal compression in its later stages, by transverse myelitis, and in the more advanced stages of multiple sclerosis.

After complete interruption of conduction in the spinal cord, either by transection or by severe transverse lesions above the conus, there occurs an enhancement of reflex activity in the distal portion, and reflex evacuation of the bladder may then develop through the agency of the sacral reflex arc. It may be facilitated by stimuli applied to the sacral cutaneous areas. But after some massive lesions of the spinal cord the bladder may be atonic, presumably due to concurrent involvement of the cauda equina, perhaps as a result of ischaemia.

Cerebral Lesions

The fibres concerned in the voluntary initiation of micturition may be interrupted at levels of the nervous system above the spinal cord, and retention of urine may then develop, usually in association with severe bilateral corticospinal tract lesions. Lesions involving the vertical region of the precentral cortex on both sides may in the same way cause retention of urine, as Foerster has shown, and impairment of function of this part of the cerebral cortex or of its descending paths is probably responsible for difficulty in micturition and retention of urine, or for urgency and incontinence (Andrew and Nathan, 1964), which are not uncommon symptoms of intracranial tumour, anterior communicating artery aneurysms and of diffuse cerebral lesions such as presenile dementia or diffuse atherosclerosis.

Nocturnal enuresis in otherwise normal children probably arises in the first place as a result of delay in the development of inhibition of reflex bladder evacuation. Later, for psychological reasons, the child acquires abnormal conditioned reflexes whereby bladder evacuation continues to occur during sleep. Sometimes, however, enuresis in childhood is due to spinal cord or cauda equina lesions associated with spina bifida occulta.

TREATMENT OF BLADDER DISTURBANCES

In the treatment of disturbances of the bladder function the underlying physiological principles must be borne in mind. When retention of urine occurs, adequate bladder drainage, usually with the aid of an indwelling catheter, becomes necessary, and steps must be taken to combat the risk of infection of the urinary tract and to treat it, when it develops, with appropriate urinary antiseptics or antibiotics. (See p. 630 for the care of the bladder in paraplegia.)

In view of the fact that retention of urine is usually due to a relative preponderance of sympathetic influence, the action of the parasympathetic may be reinforced by drugs which stimulate its nerve endings. Injection of carbachol, B.P., 1 ml., may be given subcutaneously, or 1–3 mg. of carbachol orally, but if despite bladder contraction induced by this drug or by distigmine (*Ubretid*), 0·5 mg. by injection or 5 mg. by mouth, there is no evacuation, catheterization will be required. In chronic cases division of the internal sphincter (bladder neck resection) may help.

Interruption of the sympathetic supply to the bladder by resection of the presacral nerve has been carried out in a small number of cases and good results are claimed for this operation but its effect is rarely lasting. The same operation has been employed to interrupt pain impulses from the bladder in painful conditions such as inoperable carcinoma.

In cases of frequency of micturition or precipitate micturition due to predominant action of the parasympathetic, drugs which paralyse parasympathetic nerve endings are indicated, and belladonna or, preferably, propantheline, 15 mg. three or four times daily, is useful in such cases. At the same time ephedrine may be employed to stimulate the sympathetic. Propantheline owes what value it possesses in the treatment of nocturnal enuresis to its inhibitory effect upon the parasympathetic. Drug treatment alone, however, is rarely successful in this condition and requires to be combined with the education of reflex inhibition produced by suggestion, if necessary in the hypnotic state. Frequently, also, the child requires help to solve its psychological problems at school or in the home.

In patients with incontinence after spinal cord lesions every effort must be made to re-establish reflex bladder evacuation at regular intervals. Regular clamping and release of an indwelling catheter every 2–3 hours during the acute stage may help to initiate this process. The atonic bladder of cauda equina lesions can usually be evacuated by manual compression. Satisfactory incontinence apparatuses are available for the male but not, as yet, for the female patient.

THE INNERVATION OF THE RECTUM

The nerve supply of the rectum is identical with that of the bladder and micturition and defaecation are physiologically comparable except that in the rectum voluntary control is exerted over the external sphincter only and the rectum lacks voluntary inhibition.

After destruction of the sacral innervation of the rectum automatic activity, dependent upon a peripheral nervous plexus develops, the rectum contracting and the sphincter relaxing in response to a rise of tension within the rectum. This reflex activity is rendered more massive and complete when the sacral innervation is intact, e.g. after complete transverse division of the spinal cord above the sacral enlargement. Owing to the small force of the rectal contraction, however, it is at best not very efficient and since the tone of the external sphincter is unaffected by transverse spinal lesions the tendency is for all disturbances of rectal innervation to cause constipation, though after complete transverse division of the spinal cord reflex defaecation may occur and may be facilitated by cutaneous stimuli applied to the sacral cutaneous areas. In most patients with spinal cord or cauda equina lesions, satisfactory control of the bowels is eventually achieved by means of twice-weekly enemas or suppositories or by manual evacuation of the faeces.

REFERENCES

ANDREW, J., and NATHAN, P. W. (1964) Lesions of the anterior frontal lobes and disturbances of micturition and defaecation, *Brain*, **87,** 233.

BARRINGTON, F. J. F. (1931–2) Discussion on the innervation of the bladder, *Proc. roy. Soc. Med.,* **25,** 557.

DENNY-BROWN, D., and ROBERTSON, E. G. (1933) The state of the bladder and its sphincters in complete transverse lesions of the spinal cord and cauda equina, *Brain,* **56,** 397.

DENNY-BROWN, D., and ROBERTSON, E. G. (1935) An investigation of the nervous control of defaecation, *Brain,* **58,** 256.

HOLMES, G. (1933) Observations on the paralysed bladder, *Brain,* **56,** 383.

LANGWORTHY, O. R., KOLB, L. C., and LEWIS, L. G. (1940) *The Physiology of Micturition,* Baltimore.

LEARMONTH, J. R. (1931) A contribution to the neurophysiology of the urinary bladder in man, *Brain,* **54,** 147.

McLELLAN, F. C. (1939) *The Neurogenic Bladder,* Baltimore.

McMICHAEL, J. (1945) Spinal tracts subserving micturition in a case of Erb's spinal paralysis, *Brain,* **68,** 162.

PEDERSEN, E., ed. (1962) Spasticity and neurological bladder disturbances, *Acta neurol. (Kbh.),* **38,** Suppl. 3.

RUCH, T. C. (1960) Central control of the bladder, in *Handbook of Physiology,* ed. FIELD, J., Section I, Vol. ii, 1207.

VORIS, H. C., and LANDES, H. E. (1940) Cystometric studies in cases of neurologic disease, *Arch. Neurol. Psychiat. (Chicago),* **44,** 118.

THE CARE OF THE PARAPLEGIC PATIENT

The general management of a patient suffering from paraplegia requires much care and is of as much importance as the correct treatment of the cause of his disability, for his disorder renders him extremely susceptible to complications which may prove fatal, and, even when less serious, may considerably retard recovery.

DIET

The nutrition of the paraplegic patient is of the utmost importance: the loss of protein through pressure-sores and albuminuria may amount to 50 g. daily. The caloric requirements are 3,500, and the diet should include 125 g. of protein, a high vitamin intake, and 3,500–4,000 ml. of fluid. Milk should be given sparingly as the calcium increases the risk of urinary calculi. Anaemia may call for iron or even blood transfusion. When protein loss and wasting are severe, courses of treatment with anabolic steroid drugs may be of value.

CARE OF THE SKIN

In paraplegia the skin is extremely liable to injuries which are slow in healing, and readily become infected. The factors which lead to bed-sores are—shock in the early stages after injury, vasomotor paralysis, small traumata, and local anaemia caused by pressure. Bed-sores are most likely to develop over the bony prominences, especially the heels, the tuber ischii, the sacrum, and the great trochanter.

The paraplegic patient should be nursed if possible on a 'Ripple' bed. Care should be taken that the bed-clothes are warm and dry and free from rucks, and that a hot-water bottle is not placed in contact with the skin. The patient should be bathed daily, the skin being thoroughly cleansed with soap and water, and carefully dried. After this the back is well rubbed with methylated spirit or eau-de-Cologne, and dusted with a dusting powder. Areas of reddening of the skin or of loss of epidermis may heal quickly if protected by means of a waterproof spray of acrylic resin (*Nobecutane*) or by using a silicone barrier cream or plastic antiseptic spray (*Noxyflex, Octaflex*). The posture of the patient should be changed every two hours both by day and night. If he develops an acute infection the liability to bed-sores increases, and he should be moved every hour. The value of pads to protect pressure points is doubtful. The lower limbs should be kept extended and the calves should rest upon small pillows with the heels projecting beyond them. The weight of the bed-clothes is taken from the lower limbs by means of a cradle. If sweating is troublesome, atropine, 0·5 mg., or propantheline, 15 mg., may be given before the patient settles down for the night. Flexor spasms of the lower limbs are not likely to be severe if the skin and bladder are healthy. As far as possible, contact of the limbs with the bed-clothes should be reduced, and sedatives such as phenobarbitone or chlorpromazine may be given if necessary.

THE TREATMENT OF PRESSURE-SORES

If an ulcer has already developed, all necrotic tissue should first be removed to allow free drainage, and cultures should be made weekly. *Trypure Novo* dispersible powder (Evans Medical Ltd.) is helpful in removing sloughs. At first the bed-sores may be cleaned with hydrogen peroxide and a dressing of penicillin

(20,000 Units in 10 ml. of normal saline) applied for a few days. After that eusol or saline dressings or tulle gras should be used. The dressing should be well covered with adhesive plaster attached to skin some distance away from the pressure points and changed every day. Systemic chemotherapy may be required. Occasionally skin-grafting is necessary.

CARE OF THE BLADDER

When retention of urine occurs as a result of a lesion of the nervous system cystitis almost invariably develops, and if untreated leads to ascending pyelonephritis. Retention of urine must therefore be treated by some form of drainage of the bladder. The alternatives available are (1) catheterization every 8 hours, (2) the use of a self-retaining catheter, (3) suprapubic cystostomy. Tidal drainage is a form of bladder lavage which can be used with methods 2 and 3: it is likely to succeed only in the hands of assistants familiar with its use. Opinions still differ as to the best way to deal with the paralysed bladder. In general, repeated catheterization or a self-retaining catheter, with or without tidal drainage, is suitable for short periods, and in the absence of severe urinary infection. When urinary infection cannot be otherwise controlled, suprapubic cystostomy may have to be carried out but fortunately it is rarely needed. Manual control of catheter drainage can be obtained by a screw clip applied to the drainage tube, and operated by the patient. When the catheter has to be removed to be changed, it can be left out for several hours, during which time observations are made on the patient's ability to hold urine, which can be tested by abdominal straining or suprapubic manual pressure. In this way, and by estimations of residual urine, the bladder's recovery of activity can be assessed.

The greatest care must be taken that the catheter and all the vessels and apparatus employed are sterile, and the operator must be scrupulous in his observance of an aseptic technique. Balanitis is a potential source of infection and it may even be advisable that a male patient should be circumcised. The tidal drainage apparatus should be capable of being used as a cystometer. Suitable lavage solutions are $\frac{1}{2}$ per cent. acetic acid, 1 in 10,000 potassium permanganate, and solution 'M' of Suby and Albright. All solutions should be given at a temperature of 105° F.

If the urinary tract becomes infected the organisms must be cultured and the appropriate chemotherapy used. Unless a sulphonamide is being given the urine should be kept acid with sodium acid phosphate, ammonium chloride, or ammonium mandelate.

Cystoscopy and radiography of the urinary tract, including pyelography, may be necessary to exclude hydronephrosis and renal and vesical calculus; and estimation of renal function may be called for.

The object to be aimed at is an automatic bladder voiding sterile urine. Neither the grossly atonic bladder nor an organ much contracted owing to infection will become automatic. Division of the internal sphincter has been carried out when the detrusor muscle is reflexly active but the sphincter does not relax (Thompson, 1945). (For further details of care of the paralysed bladder see Guttmann, 1946; Petkoff, 1945; Joelson, 1945; Hamm, 1945; War Department Technical Bulletin, 1945; and Hardy, 1956.)

CARE OF THE RECTUM

The constipation which is usually a troublesome complication of paraplegia should be treated by the administration of an aperient at night, two or three times a week, and by washing out the rectum the next day with an enema. In paraplegia the bowel empties itself very slowly after an enema and 'leaking' may occur for an hour or more, a point which is important to bear in mind in order to avoid the bed becoming wet and soiled. If the rectum and large bowel are allowed to become distended, sloughing of the mucous membrane is liable to occur, and in any case abdominal distension causes the patient serious discomfort. Such distension should be treated by the administration of an enema, after which a rectal tube should be left in position. Often regular manual evacuation of faeces by the patient himself (rubber gloves must be supplied to prevent paronychia and other skin sepsis on the hands) is useful. A hypodermic injection of 1 ml. of *Pituitrin* is often useful for dispelling gas by increasing the tone of the intestinal muscle.

MUSCULAR SPASMS AND SPASTICITY

Involuntary spasmodic movements of the lower limbs are a troublesome and intractable symptom in many cases of paraplegia. Spasmodic extension may occur when extension is the predominant attitude of the lower limbs. Spasmodic flexion, which is encountered in paraplegia-in-flexion, is much commoner. Flexor movements are reflexly excited by moving contact of the lower limbs with the bed-clothes, a slight movement of the limb being sufficient in many cases to excite a violent flexor spasm. As far as possible, contact of the limbs with the bed-clothes should be reduced. Light massage, passive movements, and a warm bath at bed-time frequently have a sedative effect, and the spasms may be diminished in frequency and severity by the use of sedative drugs, of which the best are chlordiazepoxide (*Librium*), 10 mg. three or four times daily, and diazepam (*Valium*), 5 mg. three or four times a day. Mephenesin carbamate (*Tolseram*), 0·5–1·0 G. three or four times daily, and drugs such as chlorzoxazone and orphenadrine citrate are in general less effective.

In patients with no hope of recovery, flexor spasms have been treated by the intrathecal injection of phenol in *Myodil* or glycerin, and by anterior rhizotomy. In selected cases injection of 1 ml. of xylocaine, followed by 1–2 ml. of 45 per cent. alcohol into the motor points of selected muscles (e.g. hamstrings), after localization of the motor point or motor end-plate zone by electrical stimulation on the skin, is very helpful (Tardieu *et al.*, 1964). Anterior rhizotomy has the disadvantage of leading to muscular wasting and increasing the risk of pressure-sores. In irrecoverable cases division of the obturator nerves and appropriate tenotomies may be helpful. Regular mechanical traction applied to the flexed limbs, combined with appropriate tenotomies have been shown to be valuable by Platt, Russell, and Willison (1958). The use of intrathecal injections is described by Nathan (1959, 1965) and Kelly and Gautier-Smith (1959).

PHYSIOTHERAPY AND COMPENSATORY TRAINING

There are few paraplegic patients who will not be able to get about in a wheelchair, and many more than was once thought possible can be taught to walk.

Physiotherapy therefore aims at obtaining the maximum development of all those muscles in which voluntary power remains, and preventing flexor contractures of the lower limbs. Exercises are carried out with the help of slings as in the Guthrie-Smith apparatus, special attention being paid to the trunk muscles. Massage and passive movements are carried out in the lower limbs once or twice daily, and the muscles are stimulated with faradism or galvanism. As soon as possible the patient is allowed to sit up in a wheel-chair, the need for frequent changes of posture being still borne in mind. In suitable cases walking is later attempted, and may be achieved even when no voluntary power remains in the lower limbs apart from hip flexion or 'rocking' movements of the pelvis. Appropriate walking instruments or calipers will be necessary, locking at the knee and not carried high enough to exert pressure on the buttocks. A toe-raising spring can be incorporated. When the trunk muscles are paralysed a brace of the Taylor type will be necessary. The patient at first must be supported by parallel bars, later he uses elbow-crutches. When the lower limbs are completely paralysed, the pelvis must be rotated and tilted by the abdominal muscles; first one leg, and then the other is swung forward in this way. It may be possible for a patient to learn to 'walk' on crutches by swinging his trunk by means of the pectoralis, latissimus dorsi, serratus anterior, and trapezius muscles if these are over-developed and he has enough strength in his fingers to grasp the crutches, and can move them forward with his pectorals and deltoids. (For details see Deaver and Brown, 1945; Guttmann, 1946; and Lowman, 1947.)

PSYCHOTHERAPY

Not the least important part of the physician's task is to help the patient to adjust himself to a new mode of life—a life not of inactivity but of different activities. At first he will need to be convinced that an active and useful life is still possible. Occupational therapy should be begun early: games play an important part. In most cases the patient must be trained for a new occupation, and the co-operation of an employer sought. Family adjustments have also to be made. Coitus is not always impossible. An erection may be stimulated by handling the penis and, with the co-operation of an instructed wife, success may be achieved. Even when intercourse is impossible, in the case of a wife who is anxious to have a child, ejaculation may follow the intrathecal injection of small doses of neostigmine, following which artificial insemination may be possible.

INJURIES OF THE SPINAL CORD

AETIOLOGY

The spinal cord may be injured directly by penetrating wounds, for example, stabs or gun-shot wounds, in which case it may be penetrated by a missile or by fragments of bone. More frequently in civil life it suffers indirectly as a result of injuries of the vertebral column, either fractures, dislocations, or fracture-dislocations. The commonest sites of spinal injury in civil life are the lower cervical region and the thoracolumbar junction. The upper cervical region suffers next in frequency (Jefferson, 1928). Though the spinal column may be injured as the result of a blow leading to fracture at the site of the impact, more frequently it is injured by transmitted violence. Forcible extension of the neck may cause fracture of the dens or contusion of the cervical cord, but most spinal injuries are the result of forcible flexion. A blow on the head which does not expend its violence in fracturing the skull may, by forcibly flexing the cervical spine, cause dislocation in the lower cervical region or herniation of an intervertebral disc. Pre-existing cervical spondylosis which narrows the cervical canal greatly increases the risk of damage to the spinal cord by injuries which cause forcible extension of the neck. Blows upon the shoulders, such as are caused by heavy objects falling from a height, result in forcible flexion of the lower part of the spine, which usually yields at the thoracolumbar junction. This type of injury is produced chiefly by industrial accidents. Fracture-dislocation may similarly result from the patient's falling from a height on to the feet or buttocks. Lifting a heavy weight, falls, and strains may cause displacement of an intervertebral disc.

The spinal cord may be injured in the infant during birth as a result of violent traction. Such injuries may arise in three ways. Traction on the head may cause dislocation of the upper cervical spine, which is usually immediately fatal. Traction separating the head and shoulders, by exerting tension on the brachial plexus and cervical spinal roots, may injure the spinal cord as well as producing a brachial plexus palsy. In addition, violent traction, especially in a breech presentation, may cause fracture-dislocation in the thoracic or lumbar regions.

Spontaneous fracture-dislocation of the spine may occur when the vertebrae are diseased, for example, in tuberculous caries or in primary or secondary neoplasm of the vertebral column. The blast of a bomb or shell explosion may injure the spinal cord without damaging the spine.

PATHOLOGY

'*Concussion* of the spinal cord' is the term employed when the cord is injured by transmitted violence without fracture or dislocation of the vertebral column, e.g. by the passage of a bullet near the spine without penetration of the dura. The axis cylinders are broken up but the myelin sheaths remain intact. Spinal *contusion* is defined as bruising of the cord without rupture of the pia mater, resulting from compression. The contused cord is swollen and exhibits small haemorrhages. Holmes has described the formation of cylindrical cavities extending upwards or downwards for several segments, usually situated in the ventral part of the posterior columns or in the posterior horn of grey matter, and filled with brownish, gelatinous material. Microscopically, besides oedema and haemorrhages the contused cord exhibits swelling of the axis cylinders and disintegration of their myelin sheaths. In severe cases both completely disappear and the cord may be markedly softened. Ascending and descending degeneration of the long tracts follows the focal lesion. *Laceration* of the cord implies an injury of greater severity than contusion, leading to rupture of the pia mater and in the most severe cases the cord is completely transected. Barnett *et al.* (1966) have recently shown that a progressive myelopathy due to ascending cavitation of the cord above the level of the lesion may develop in some cases of traumatic paraplegia some years after the injury. When a wound penetrates the dura mater, meningitis is liable to occur as a complication of spinal injury. Rupture of the pia in such cases increases the risk of myelitis developing. Injuries of the vertebral column may damage the spinal roots as they pass through the intervertebral foramina.

SYMPTOMS

The symptoms of spinal injury depend upon the severity and situation of the lesion. Injury to the cord does not necessarily follow damage to the vertebral column; for example, dislocation of the cervical spine without injury to the cord is not rare. An injury to the cord in the upper cervical region is usually rapidly, if not immediately, fatal, since it causes paralysis both of the diaphragm and of the intercostal muscles.

Complete interruption of the spinal cord leads immediately to flaccid paralysis with loss of all sensation and most reflex activity below the site of the lesion, and paralysis of the bladder and rectum. Muscular paralysis and sensory loss are irrecoverable, but, as after from one to four weeks the stage of spinal shock passes off, reflex activity develops in the divided portion of the cord and the patient presents the picture of paraplegia-in-flexion [see p. 623]. For the motor symptoms of spinal interruption at different levels, see pages 650–2.

Lesions of the cord less severe than complete interruption, such as spinal contusion, may lead to an equally severe immediate disturbance of function, or symptoms may increase in severity for several days *pari passu* with the development of oedema in the cord. Slight spinal injuries cause motor symptoms of incomplete division [see p. 622] without complete sensory loss, or, if the injury is limited to one-half of the cord, a partial or complete Brown-Séquard syndrome [see p. 45]. Spinal concussion may cause temporary complete paraplegia with sensory loss mainly of the posterior column type.

Injuries of the Cauda Equina. Fracture-dislocation of the spine below the first lumbar vertebra damages only the roots of the cauda equina. In civil life unilateral injuries of the cauda are rare, though the severity and extent of the injury may differ on the two sides. Paralysis of the bladder, rectum, and sexual functions immediately follows the injury. The motor, sensory, and reflex disturbances are similar to those more gradually produced by slow compression of the cauda equina and are described on page 652.

DIAGNOSIS

The diagnosis is usually obvious, the only question being the nature of the injury to the cord. Myelography may be necessary to determine the presence and degree of cord compression.

PROGNOSIS

The prognosis of a severe injury of the spinal cord is always grave. If the respiratory muscles are not immediately paralysed and if the patient survives the stage of shock, death may occur from urinary or cutaneous infection, or, in the case of penetrating wounds, from meningitis or myelitis. Nevertheless, experience of the results of war injury of the spinal cord shows that it is possible for a patient with a completely divided cord to retain good general health in-definitely under careful supervision. When the cord has been incompletely divided, the prognosis is better, but, in the absence of infections of the bladder and skin, the limit of functional improvement will be reached when the shock has passed off, usually in from one to two months after the injury. After spinal concussion recovery is usually good, though some abnormal physical signs may remain. The prognosis of cauda equina injuries is better than that of injuries of the cord itself, since the roots of the cauda are capable of regeneration.

TREATMENT

The scope of surgery in the treatment of injuries of the spinal cord has been much discussed, and the modern tendency in this respect is conservative. It has to be recognized that in most cases the maximal injury has been produced at the time of the accident and the condition of the cord is both non-progressive and irreparable. Moreover, for several weeks after the injury spinal shock may render it impossible to decide whether interruption of the cord is complete. When there is reason to believe that the cord has been completely divided, surgery cannot accomplish anything, and open operation is contra-indicated by the presence of local sepsis, visceral complications, and secondary infective conditions. On the other hand, when there is radiographic evidence of gross bony deformity, disc protrusion or the presence of a foreign body in the spinal canal, and clinical examination indicates that the cord has not been completely divided, and when in such cases recovery of function has begun but has become arrested, surgical intervention offers the hope of relieving compression or cicatricial contraction, which may be retarding recovery. In such cases an exploratory laminectomy is indicated, and this may also be required to deal with severe persistent root pains, due to compression of dorsal nerve roots. The scope of manipulative reduc-tion of vertebral deformity in cases of spinal injury is not as yet defined, but this procedure may sometimes be indicated as an early treatment of cases of in-complete division following vertebral injury when the surgeon can feel sure that it entails no risk of increasing the severity of the damage. In cases of injury of the cauda equina the most that can be hoped from operation is the relief of pressure which may be retarding regeneration of the roots. The general manage-ment of cases of injury of the spinal cord and cauda equina is described on page 628.

REFERENCES

BALDWIN, R. S. (1934) Spinal concussion: a histologic study of two cases, *Arch. Neurol. Psychiat. (Chicago)*, **32,** 493.

BARNETT, H. J. M., BOTTERELL, E. H., JOUSSE, A. T., and WYNN-JONES, M. (1966) Progressive myelopathy as a sequel to traumatic paraplegia, *Brain*, **89,** 159.

BEDFORD, P. D., COSIN, L. Z., and McCARTHY, T. F. (1961) Bedsores, *Lancet*, ii, 76.

BROCK, S. (1960) *Injuries to the Brain and Spinal Cord and their Coverings*, 4th ed., London.

BYERS, R. K. (1930) Late effects of obstetrical injuries at various levels of the nervous system, *New Engl. J. Med.*, **203,** 507.

DEAVER, G. G., and BROWN, M. E. (1945) The challenge of crutches, *Arch. phys. Med.*, **26,** 397, 515, 573, 747.

ELSON, R. A. (1965) Anatomical aspects of pressure sores and their treatment, *Lancet*, i, 884.

FORD, F. R. (1925) Breech delivery in its possible relations to injury of the spinal cord, *Arch. Neurol. Psychiat. (Chicago)*, **14**, 742.

GUTTMANN, L. (1946) Rehabilitation after injuries to the spinal cord and cauda equina, *Brit. J. phys. Med.*, **9**, 162–71.

HAMM, F. C. (1945) War wounds of the spinal cord, *J. Amer. med. Ass.*, **129**, 158.

HARDY, A. G. (1956) The care of the bladder in traumatic paraplegia, *Postgrad. med. J.*, **32**, 328.

JEFFERSON, G. (1927–8). Discussion on spinal injuries, *Proc. roy. Soc. Med.*, **21**, 625.

JOELSON, J. J. (1945) War wounds of the spinal cord, *J. Amer. med. Ass.*, **129**, 157.

KELLY, R. E., and GAUTIER-SMITH, P. C. (1959) Intrathecal phenol in the treatment of reflex spasms and spasticity, *Lancet*, ii, 1102.

LOWMAN, E. W. (1947) Rehabilitation of the paraplegic patient, *Arch. Neurol. Psychiat. (Chicago)*, **58**, 610.

MEDICAL RESEARCH COUNCIL (1924) Report of the Committee on Injuries of the Nervous System, *Spec. Rep. Ser. med. Res. Coun. (Lond.)*, No. 88.

NATHAN, P. W. (1959) Intrathecal phenol to relieve spasticity in paraplegia, *Lancet*, ii, 1099.

NATHAN, P. W. (1965) Chemical rhizotomy for relief of spasticity in ambulant patients, *Brit. med. J.*, **1**, 1096.

PETKOFF, B. P. (1945) War wounds of the spinal cord, *J. Amer. med. Ass.*, **129**, 154.

PLATT, G., RUSSELL, W. R., and WILLISON, R. G. (1958) Flexion spasms and contractures in spinal-cord disease, *Lancet*, i, 757.

TARDIEU, G., HARIGA, J., TARDIEU, C., GAGNARD, L., and VELIN, J. (1964) Traitement de la spasticité par infiltration d'alcool dilué au point moteur ou par injection épidurale, *Rev. neurol.*, **110**, 563.

THOMPSON, G. S. (1945) Restoration of function by transurethral operation, *Nav. med. Bull. (Wash.)*, **45**, 207.

WALSHE, F. M. R., and ROSS, J. (1936) The clinical picture of minor cord lesions in association with injuries of the cervical spine: with special reference to the diagnostic and localising value of the tendon reflexes of the arm (inversion of the radial reflex), *Brain*, **59**, 277.

War Department. Technical Bulletin, T.B. Med. 162. (1945). Convalescent care and rehabilitation of patients with spinal cord injuries, *War Med. (Chicago)*, vii. 199.

HAEMATOMYELIA

Definition. The term 'haematomyelia' implies the occurrence of bleeding within the substance of the spinal cord. Haemorrhages occur within the cord in a variety of pathological states. Petechial haemorrhages are found in acute inflammatory conditions, such as poliomyelitis, in toxic states, in blood diseases, especially those accompanied by purpura, in asphyxia, and as a sequel of severe convulsions. Haemorrhages also occur as a result of injury, in spinal concussion and contusion, as well as laceration of the cord following fracture-dislocation of the spine and the penetration of the spinal canal by bullets. The term 'haematomyelia', however, is usually reserved for a focal extravasation of blood within the spinal cord occurring in the absence of any of the conditions already mentioned.

AETIOLOGY

Haematomyelia in the sense just defined may develop in the absence of any discoverable exciting factor. Not uncommonly, however, it follows an event which may be supposed to have exposed the spinal cord to transmitted violence, though this often seems slight in proportion to the severity of the resulting symptoms. Blows on the spine and falls are sometimes held responsible. There is evidence that a congenital abnormality, for example an intramedullary angioma, may be the commonest factor, and spontaneous haemorrhage into a syringomyelic cavity may occur. Haematomyelia usually occurs in early adult life, and males are more frequently affected than females. Recent evidence suggests that, particularly in cases attributable to trauma, a syndrome similar to that produced by haematomyelia may in fact be due to central softening within the spinal cord rather than haemorrhage, resulting often from contusion of the cord such as may occur particularly in the cervical region in patients suffering from previously symptomless cervical spondylosis, frequently after acute flexion or hyperextension of the neck.

PATHOLOGY

The cervical enlargement is the commonest site of haemorrhage, and haemorrhages elsewhere are rare. The bleeding occurs primarily in the central grey matter and tends to spread upwards and downwards, assuming a round or oval form, according to its longitudinal extent. It may extend into the white matter, but usually this suffers from compression rather than from direct invasion by the haemorrhage. At first red, the haemorrhage in the later stages becomes brown and may finally be represented by a cystic cavity containing yellow fluid. Surrounding regions of the cord exhibit an infiltration with compound granular cells, and glial reaction. There is destruction and disappearance of the ganglion cells of both anterior and posterior horns of grey matter at the site of the haemorrhage, and some degree of ascending and descending degeneration is usually found in the tracts of the white matter.

SYMPTOMS

The onset of symptoms is usually rapidly progressive, though after an injury there may be a sudden impairment of function of the spinal cord, followed later by a progressive increase in symptoms. Sometimes the onset is more gradual, and the symptoms may increase in severity over a period of several days. In cases of central softening after acute flexion or hyperextension injuries to the neck, neurological disability is usually maximal immediately after the injury and progressive improvement occurs during the subsequent weeks or months. Since the cervical enlargement is the commonest site of haemorrhage, symptoms of a lesion in this situation will alone be described in detail. In some cases the patient complains at the onset of severe pain in the neck radiating down one or both upper limbs. In other cases pain is absent, but there may be paraesthesiae, such as numbness and tingling. Muscular weakness rapidly develops. It is usually most marked in the upper limbs, one of which may suffer more than the other. In the upper limbs the paralysis is due to destruction of the anterior horn cells and hence is associated with muscular atrophy and diminution or loss of the tendon reflexes. It may be limited to the muscles innervated by the upper segments, cervical 5 and 6, or by the lower segments, cervical 8 and thoracic 1, of the cervical enlargement. Below the level of the haemorrhage the motor symptoms are those of spastic paralysis which may be slight or severe in the lower limbs and may affect the two sides unequally.

The most prominent sensory changes are due to destruction of the sensory fibres in the grey matter of the cord at the level of the haemorrhage. When this extends into the posterior horns and destroys the ganglion cells, all forms of sensibility will be impaired or lost over the whole or part of the upper limbs. When the destruction is limited to the region of the anterior white commissure there is no disturbance of appreciation of light touch, posture, or passive movement, but analgesia and thermo-anaesthesia occur over several segmental cutaneous areas below the upper level of the haemorrhage, which interrupts the fibres subserving these forms of sensibility at their decussation. The picture is thus similar to that of syringomyelia and a 'cape-like' distribution of the dissociated anaesthesia is frequently seen. It is not uncommon to find also some impairment of appreciation of pain, heat, and cold, over the trunk or lower limbs on one or both sides, owing to compression of the spinothalamic tract. Postural sensibility may be impaired in the lower limbs, but not as a rule to a severe extent, owing to compression of the posterior columns.

The tendon reflexes effected by muscles which are the site of atrophic paralysis are diminished or lost. Those of the lower limbs are usually exaggerated. The abdominal reflexes are diminished or lost and the plantar reflexes are extensor when the corticospinal tracts are damaged. Sphincter disturbances are usually proportional to the severity of the paraplegia.

Dorsal and lumbar haematomyelia are characterized by the rapid development of more or less complete paraplegia and sensory loss below the level of the lesion. Retention of urine is common.

The cerebrospinal fluid may be normal or may show an increase in its protein content, with or without xanthochromia.

DIAGNOSIS

Apart from traumatic lesions, there are few conditions in which a lesion of the spinal cord develops so rapidly as in haematomyelia. The onset of transverse myelitis is more often subacute rather than acute, and it is often preceded for days or even for weeks by pains in the spine. It is often associated with inflammatory changes in the cerebrospinal fluid and when, as in some cases, it is syphilitic in origin, the serological reactions in the fluid and probably also in the blood will be positive. Anterior poliomyelitis can be differentiated from haematomyelia by its more gradual, febrile onset, by the wide distribution of the atrophic paralysis, by the absence of sensory loss and of corticospinal lesions, and by the occurrence of a pleocytosis in the cerebrospinal fluid. Haemorrhage into a syringomyelic cavity constitutes a form of haematomyelia which it is important to recognize. However, this is a rare complication and haematomyelia is generally distinguishable from the syndrome of syringomyelia by virtue of its acute onset. The pre-existence of syringomyelia may be suggested by a history of cyanosis, painless injuries or trophic lesions of the fingers, and by the presence of bulbar symptoms and of associated abnormalities, such as scoliosis. The very rare condition of intramedullary abscess of the spinal cord can give a clinical picture very similar to that of haematomyelia but there is usually fever and leucocytosis and evidence of a focus of pyogenic infection elsewhere.

PROGNOSIS

The mortality rate is low, and most sufferers from haematomyelia survive. Death may occur from upward extension of the haemorrhage leading to paralysis of the diaphragm, through involvement of the spinal origin of the phrenic nerves, or from infection of the urinary tract or other complications of paraplegia. In patients who survive, considerable improvement may be expected and it is often particularly striking in traumatic cases with presumed central cord softening in which it may be concluded that much of the initial disability may have been due to transient disturbance of function as a result of concussion of the cord. Atrophic paralysis and sensory loss due to destruction of the grey matter are permanent, but even these diminish in extent, as recovery occurs in ganglion cells and fibres which have been compressed but not completely destroyed. A steady improvement may be expected in the power of the lower limbs and in many cases this may return to normal, though exaggeration of the tendon reflexes and extensor plantar responses may persist. When haemorrhage has occurred into a syringomyelic cavity, much less improvement in the immediate symptoms can be expected and the prognosis is that of syringomyelia.

TREATMENT

Complete rest is essential as long as the haemorrhage continues. It is doubtful if any special posture is of value. Sedative drugs should be given and analgesics when necessary. Vasoconstrictor drugs should be avoided, since they tend to raise the blood pressure. When paraplegia is present this will require appropriate treatment. Two weeks after the onset physiotherapy may safely be begun.

REFERENCES

BENDA, C. E. (1929) Zur Klinik der traumatischen Hämatomyelie. Zugleich ein Beitrag zur Differentialdiagnose zwischen Tumor Spinalis und Blutung, *Nervenarzt*, **1**, 28.

CHEVALLIER, P., and DESOILE, H. (1930) L'hématomyélie des jeunes sujets (importance des lésions vasculaires hérédo-syphilitiques), *Rev. Médecine*, **47**, 486.

DAVISON, C. (1960) General pathological considerations in injuries of the spinal cord, in *Injuries of the Brain and Spinal Cord*, 4th ed., ed. BROCK, S., New York.

DOERR, C. (1906; 1906–7) *Die spontane Rückenmarksblutung (Hämatomyelie)*, Zürich, and *Dtsch. Z. Nervenheilk.*, **32**, 1.

LÉPINE, J. (1900) *Étude sur les hématomyélies*, Thèse de Lyon.

RICHARDSON, J. C. (1938) Spontaneous haematomyelia: a short review and a report of cases illustrating intramedullary angioma and syphilis of the spinal cord as possible causes, *Brain*, **61**, 17.

COMPRESSION OF THE SPINAL CORD

AETIOLOGY AND PATHOLOGY

Compression of the spinal cord may be due to:

Disease of the Vertebral Column. The commonest of such diseases leading to spinal compression are tuberculous osteitis (Pott's disease), secondary carcinoma, and cervical spondylosis with protrusion of intervertebral discs [FIGS. 93 and 105]. Less frequent causes include primary neoplasms arising from vertebrae, such as sarcoma, myeloma, osteoma, haemangioma, and other forms of osteitis, such as staphylococcal osteitis, syphilitic osteitis and osteitis, deformans of Paget. Rarely, achondroplasia and severe kyphoscoliosis due to juvenile osteochondritis may have the same effect. The cord may occasionally be compressed by prolapse of an intervertebral disc elsewhere than at the cervical level (e.g. in the dorsal region) or as a result of erosion of vertebrae from without by sarcoma, or by aneurysm of the aorta. Compression due to vertebral injury is described on page 632.

Intravertebral Causes of Compression. These include extradural abscess due either to metastatic infection or vertebral osteitis, pachymeningitis due to syphilis, tuberculosis, or exceptionally to pyogenic organisms, infiltration of the meninges with reticulosis or leukaemic deposits, meningitis circumscripta serosa and other forms of arachnoiditis, parasitic cysts, such as the hydatid and cysticercus, and extramedullary and intramedullary spinal tumours.

Vertebral Disease

1. *Separation of the odontoid process* of the axis, occurring either as a congenital abnormality or as the result of trauma or rheumatoid arthritis may, by permitting abnormal movement of the atlas on the axis lead in time, sometimes after many years, to a delayed myelopathy resulting from compression of the spinal cord.

2. *Intervertebral disc protrusion* is commonest in the cervical region. An acute central prolapse of a disc may give symptoms and signs of acute or subacute cord compression and pain may not be prominent, whereas a lateral protrusion will give pain in the arm due to root compression (brachial neuralgia). Chronic protrusions are the result of degeneration of the discs: they may be single or multiple, and are usually encountered during or after middle age. Such a slow, progressive degenerative process (cervical spondylosis) gives the condition of so-called spondylotic myelopathy. Its effect upon the spinal cord is complex: in addition to directly compressing it, the protruding discs may interfere with its blood supply; while, owing to tethering of the cord by the ligamenta denticulata and of the spinal roots by narrowing of the intervertebral foramina, ordinary neck movements may produce cumulative trauma. The result is a condition of patchy degeneration—cervical myelopathy.

3. *Neoplasms of the Vertebral Column.* Secondary carcinoma is the commonest vertebral neoplasm. It is rare before the age of 35. The primary growth is most frequently situated within the breast, thyroid, prostate, or lung, less frequently in the uterus, stomach, kidney, or elsewhere. Although the vertebral metastasis may be blood-borne, the spine is not uncommonly involved at the same segmental level as the primary growth, which in such cases probably reaches it via the perineural lymphatics. The carcinomatous deposits erode the spongy portions of the vertebral bodies, which finally collapse. The spinal cord may be compressed as a result of the spinal deformity or by an intravertebral extension of the growth. Usually the spinal roots are compressed earlier than the cord

itself so that root pain may be present for some time before vertebral collapse gives acute cord compression.

Sarcoma may arise from a vertebra or invade the spinal column from the neighbouring tissues. Cavernous haemangioma is a rare vertebral tumour. Myeloma usually arises simultaneously in numerous vertebral bodies and frequently also in other bones, especially the ribs, but solitary myelomas of the spine giving cord compression are not uncommon. Erosion of vertebral bodies leads to collapse. Bence-Jones proteose is found in the urine. Osteomas are rare tumours which usually arise from the posterior part of a vertebral body and hence compress the cord anteriorly. So-called chondromas are usually intervertebral disc protrusions associated with spondylosis. Deposits of reticulosis and leukaemic metastases usually infiltrate the dura mater extensively on its outer surface but may occasionally invade the cord itself.

4. *Tuberculous spinal osteitis* usually occurs in children and young adults but no age is exempt. It is now much less common in the developed countries than it was twenty or thirty years ago as a result of pasteurization of milk, as most cases of skeletal tuberculosis used to be due to the bovine bacillus. The infective process generally begins in the body of the vertebra, and spreading to adjacent bodies leads to their collapse and so produces an angular deformity of the spine. It is rare for the deformity as such to be an important factor in compression of the spinal cord, which is more frequently due either to an extradural tuberculous abscess or to tuberculous pachymeningitis. In addition to actual compression of the cord, which may, however, be absent, interference with the vascular supply of subjacent segments, either by compression of radicular arteries or endarteritis, is an important factor in the production of paraplegia. Paraplegia occurs in about 11 per cent. of patients with Pott's disease, usually within two or three years of the onset, but in some cases after many years of apparent quiescence. The dorsal cord is commonly affected.

5. *Syphilitic spinal osteitis* is a rare cause of spinal compression and produces effects similar to those of tuberculous caries. In Paget's osteitis deformans, softening and collapse of vertebrae occur without abscess formation. Slowly progressive spastic weakness of the lower limbs due to spinal cord compression may also occur in some achondroplastic dwarfs and in patients with severe kyphoscoliosis and resultant acute angulation of the vertebral column.

6. *Spinal extradural* or *epidural abscess* is due as a rule to staphylococcal infection, arising either as a result of blood-borne invasion of the extradural space by the infecting organism or, more commonly, resulting from vertebral osteomyelitis. In the early stages the symptoms are those of pain in the back and/or root pains with fever, leucocytosis, and spinal tenderness. If untreated, sensorimotor symptoms in the limbs and sphincter disturbance may herald irreversible paraplegia or tetraplegia due to cord compression and interference with its blood supply. Surgical exploration and decompression of the spinal cord and treatment with the appropriate antibiotics must be carried out before this stage is reached; the condition is a neurosurgical emergency. Very rarely an intramedullary spinal abscess of metastatic origin develops and gives a clinical picture like that of intramedullary tumour of acute onset with pyrexia.

Spinal Tumour

Spinal tumours are conveniently divided into extradural and intradural growths, the latter being further subdivided into those arising outside the spinal cord—extramedullary tumours, and within the cord—intramedullary tumours. Excluding secondary carcinoma of the vertebrae Elsberg (1925) found that 10 per cent. of spinal tumours were extradural, 67 per cent. were extramedullary, and 14 per cent. were intramedullary.

The origin and nature of extradural tumours have been described in the previous section. The commonest extramedullary tumours are meningiomas and neurofibromas. According to Antoni the latter are twice as common as the former, while in Elsberg's series the former were two and a half times as frequent as the latter. Neurofibromas usually arise from spinal roots, the posterior more frequently than the anterior. They may be single or multiple and may or may not be associated with generalized neurofibromatosis. Exceptionally, an extramedullary neurofibroma may grow out through an intervertebral foramen, thus adopting a dumb-bell shape. The extraspinal portion may be palpable. Meningiomas may arise either from spinal roots or from the meninges. While neurofibromas may be seen at any level of the spinal canal and occur equally in the two sexes, meningiomas almost always occur in the dorsal region and much more often in females than in males. Sarcoma may be either localized or diffuse. Psammoma is probably a calcified endothelioma. Lipomas occasionally occur but are usually seen in relation to occult spina bifida and spinal dysraphism. Chordomas are rare, malignant tumours arising from a remnant of the notchocord. Spinal chordomas are almost invariably situated in the sacrococcygeal region. Dermoid cysts and other forms of teratomatous growth may also develop within the spinal canal.

Kernohan, Woltman, and Adson (1931), who investigated the histology of intramedullary spinal tumours, claimed to have recognized varieties corresponding to most of the cerebral gliomas. Forty-two per cent. of intramedullary tumours, according to these authors, are ependymomas, and the remainder includes spongioblastomas, astroblastomas, medulloblastomas, oligodendrogliomas, ganglioneuromas, very rare intramedullary metastases of carcinoma and haemangioblastomas. Angiomatous malformations occasionally occur and may have a considerable longitudinal extent. They may cause spinal subarachnoid haemorrhage as well as spinal cord compression; spinal subarachnoid bleeding is also occasionally seen in patients with neurofibromas, angioblastic meningiomas and particularly with ependymomas of the filum terminale. Leukaemic deposits may occur within the cord and gumma and tuberculoma are occasionally found. Spinal tumour may arise as a complication of syringomyelia. Cavitation, however, may occur within a spinal tumour or in the adjacent region of the cord.

Both sexes are equally liable to spinal tumour, which may develop at any age, but in over 80 per cent. of cases symptoms first appear between the ages of 20 and 60. The thoracic region of the cord is the commonest site of extradural and extramedullary tumours, the lower cervical of intramedullary tumours. Approximately two-thirds of extramedullary tumours are situated on the dorsal or dorsolateral aspects of the cord and approximately one-third on the ventral or ventrolateral aspects (Elsberg, 1925).

Meningeal Inflammation

Spinal compression may be due to pachymeningitis. This rare condition is sometimes syphilitic but may be metastatic from a pyogenic infection leading to extradural abscess. Tuberculous pachymeningitis occurs as a result of extension of infection from tuberculous osteitis. The condition known as meningitis circumscripta serosa or adhesive spinal arachnoiditis is not completely understood. Adhesions are found between the leptomeninges and may be circumscribed or extensive. Occasionally they enclose encysted collections of cerebrospinal fluid. Meningococcal infection, lymphocytic choriomeningitis, syphilis, and spinal trauma may play a part in aetiology. Tuberculous meningitis limited to the spinal cord is a cause of adhesive arachnoiditis in some tropical countries. Although adhesive arachnoiditis interferes with the functions of the cord and spinal roots, spinal compression probably plays comparatively little part in its ill effects and it may be that interference with its blood supply is more important.

Parasytic Cysts

Hydatid cysts are not uncommon causes of spinal compression in some countries. They are usually extradural. Cysticercus cysts are also occasionally encountered.

Effects of Compression upon the Cord

Spinal compression, however produced, affects the cord in several ways. Direct pressure interferes with conduction in the spinal roots and in the cord itself. Pressure upon the ascending longitudinal spinal veins leads to oedema of the cord below the site of compression. Compression of the longitudinal and radicular spinal arteries leads to ischaemia of the segments of the cord which they supply. These vascular disturbances cause local oedema of the cord with degeneration of the ganglion cells and of the white matter. Areas of softening may develop— so-called compression myelitis. In general, slow spinal compression affects the pyramidal (corticospinal) tracts first, the posterior columns next, and the spino-thalamic tracts last but there are many exceptions to this rule. It is suggested that this may be due to the fact that the pyramidal tracts are supplied by terminal branches of the anterior spinal artery which are thus most susceptible to compression ischaemia. Alternatively it has been suggested that the pyramidal tract lies closest to the attachments of the ligamentum denticulatum which is subjected to traction when the cord is compressed. Finally, obstruction of the subarachnoid space causes loculation of the cerebrospinal fluid below the point of compression and leads to characteristic changes in its composition.

SYMPTOMS

The symptoms of compression of the spinal cord differ to some extent according to whether the source of compression is extradural, extramedullary, or intramedullary and according to its segmental level. The frequency, however, with which it is impossible to determine the relationship of the site of compression to the cord before operation indicates the similarity of the symptoms produced by pressure arising in different situations. It will be convenient, therefore, first to describe the general symptoms of spinal compression, and then to discuss how they may differ according to the site and segmental level of the lesion.

Mode of Onset

The onset of symptoms is usually gradual, especially when they are due to a spinal tumour, but is often rapid in carcinoma of the vertebral column, in spinal extradural abscess and in acute compression due to other causes. In Pott's disease it is usually gradual but paraplegia may develop acutely. Approximately two-thirds of sufferers from spinal tumour come to operation between the first and second years after the onset of symptoms. Sometimes the interval is considerably longer. The first symptoms are usually sensory, the commonest being pain radiating in the distribution of one or more spinal roots. Root pains are usually severe in vertebral collapse from all causes, and in pachymeningitis. In the case of spinal tumours they are most frequently encountered when the tumour is extramedullary (particularly when it is a neurofibroma), and least in intramedullary tumours. The pains may be unilateral or bilateral, and are frequently described as burning or constricting and may be associated with soreness of the skin and tenderness of the deeper structures. They are often intensified by movements of the spine, and by coughing and sneezing, and they may be temporarily relieved by changes in posture. Pain in the back may occur, and is especially frequent in the case of tumours of the cauda equina, and malignant disease of the vertebral column. Compression of the spinothalamic tracts may cause pain of a peculiarly unpleasant character referred to distant parts. Thus pain in a lower limb may be a symptom of compression of the cervical cord. Paraesthesiae may also be produced by compression of the ascending sensory tracts, and take the form of numbness, coldness, or a sense of weight, swelling or tightness in the limbs. Compression of the posterior columns often gives sensations suggesting that the limb is enclosed in a tight bandage or stocking or that it is being constricted by a tight band or string.

Motor symptoms usually develop later than sensory. Weakness, stiffness, and unsteadiness of a limb may occur. When the cervical cord is compressed the order in which the limbs are affected is usually, as Elsberg points out, first one upper limb, then the lower limb on the same side, next the opposite lower limb, and finally the opposite upper limb, but cervical spondylosis may present with paraparesis. When the compression is situated below the cervical enlargement motor symptoms are confined to the lower limbs, one usually becoming weak before the other. Exceptionally, paraplegia develops rapidly. This is particularly likely to occur when an acute flexion or hyperextension injury of the neck is experienced by an individual with previously asymptomatic cervical spondylosis. Sphincter disturbances are usually late in appearing, even in the case of tumours of the conus medullaris and cauda equina.

The initial symptoms of a spinal angioma are extremely variable and may not appear till middle age. They are rarely those of focal spinal compression, but often indicate an insidiously progressive but rather patchy lesion in the thoracic or lumbar region. Exceptional modes of onset are subarachnoid haemorrhage or haematomyelia.

Motor Symptoms

Compression of ventral roots or of the anterior horns of grey matter leads to a progressive lower motor neurone lesion, characterized by weakness, wasting, and fasciculation of the muscles innervated by the affected segments. These symptoms are most conspicuous when the cervical or lumbosacral regions are compressed. Wasting of the intercostal muscles is similarly produced by a lesion of the thoracic cord but may be very difficult to detect.

Compression of the corticospinal tracts causes spastic weakness of the muscles below the level of the lesion. One side of the body is frequently involved before the other, but later spastic paraplegia-in-extension develops and as interruption of conduction in the cord becomes complete this may give place to paraplegia-in-flexion.

Objective Sensory Changes

Compression of dorsal spinal roots at the level of the lesion causes apparent hyperaesthesia and hyperalgesia (hyperpathia) in the corresponding cutaneous areas. Anaesthesia and analgesia may follow. Compression of the long ascending sensory tracts leads to impairment of sensibility in distant parts of the body. Several forms of dissociated sensory loss are encountered. Compression of the spinothalamic tract causes impairment of appreciation of pain, heat, and cold on the opposite side of the body, but owing to a lamination of the fibres of the tract certain cutaneous areas may escape. Thus it is common to find sensibility unimpaired over the areas supplied by the sacral segments of the cord ('sacral sparing'). Less frequently the sacral segments are affected early, but an area of normal cutaneous sensibility intervenes between them and an area of sensory loss at a higher level. The upper limit of the area of analgesia and thermo-anaesthesia is frequently several segments below the level of the lesion. This discrepancy occurs when the uppermost sensory fibres compressed in the cord are those which have decussated several segments below. It is exceptional to find that appreciation of pain, heat, and cold is affected to an equal extent. Not uncommonly cold is still felt over an area which is anaesthetic to heat, and sometimes a cold object, though not recognized as cold, evokes an unpleasant painful sensation. Cutaneous anaesthesia to light touch is frequently absent until the late stages, probably on account of the bilateral path of fibres subserving this form of sensibility. Appreciation of posture, passive movement, and vibration is impaired to a variable extent, and frequently more upon one side than upon the other. Although these forms of sensibility, which depend upon the integrity of the posterior columns, are likely to be affected early when the source of compression is posteriorly situated, they frequently also suffer when the cord is compressed from in front probably due to pressure against the infolded ligamentum subflavum.

Tenderness of the spine on pressure or percussion may arise in two ways. When vertebrae are diseased, inflamed or subjected to erosion by a tumour, their spinous processes are likely to be tender. When the vertebrae are normal, however, compression of the spinal cord or dorsal roots may lead to tenderness of the spines of the vertebrae innervated by the segments affected. In the latter case the tender vertebra is not necessarily the one overlying the lesion, but is often situated at a lower level, since the segments of the spinal cord do not correspond with the vertebrae in which they are situated (see below). When the cervical cord is compressed, flexing or extending the cervical spine frequently causes pain, numbness, or tingling, radiating into the regions innervated by the affected part of the cord. This symptom (so-called 'electric shock-like' sensations or Lhermitte's sign) may occur with both extramedullary and intramedullary tumours.

The Reflexes

Compression of the spinal cord at a given segmental level leads to diminution or loss of reflexes when the central portion of the reflex arc passes through the segment affected. When the corticospinal tract is simultaneously compressed, reflexes below the level of the lesion show the changes associated with cortico-spinal lesions, that is, the tendon reflexes are exaggerated, the cremasteric and abdominal reflexes are diminished or lost, and the plantar reflexes are extensor. The reflexes are, therefore, often of value in the localization of a spinal lesion, especially when a reflex mediated by one spinal segment is diminished and one transmitted by a slightly lower segment is exaggerated. For example, a lesion extending down to the fifth or even the sixth cervical segment but not involving the seventh cervical is likely to lead to diminution or loss of the biceps- and supinator-jerks, which depend upon the integrity of the former segments, while the triceps-jerk, of which the reflex arc passes through the seventh cervical segment, may be exaggerated. The segmental levels of the various spinal reflexes are given on page 54.

The Sphincters

The sphincters are not as a rule affected in the earliest stages of spinal compression, but later precipitancy or difficulty of micturition usually develops, and later still retention of urine is common, or the bladder may be emptied automatically. Constipation usually occurs, but when there is severe paraplegia there may be incontinence of faeces. Sphincter changes may occur at an earlier stage in the case of tumours involving the cauda equina and conus medullaris than when the compression is situated at a higher level.

Autonomic Symptoms

Autonomic symptoms may be of value in the localization of a spinal lesion. When there is considerable interruption of conduction in the spinal cord the control of higher centres over autonomic functions below the level of the lesion is impaired. In such cases excessive sweating frequently occurs over the parts of the body thus isolated from higher control. It is important to note that since the sympathetic outflow from the spinal cord is limited to the region between the first thoracic and the second lumbar segments, the upper level of the cutaneous distribution of autonomic disturbances does not as a rule correspond to that of the sensory symptoms of a lesion at a given level of the spinal cord [see p. 900]. Fay (1928) emphasized the value of vasomotor and pilomotor reactions in the determination of the upper level of a lesion of the cord. Oedema of the lower limbs is often seen in cases of severe spinal compression, as in paraplegia from other causes.

The Spine

The spine may exhibit angular deformity, local tenderness, and pain on movement when the vertebrae are diseased. In cervical spondylosis, however, both pain and limitation of movement are often very slight. A spinal bruit may be present when there is an angioma (Matthews, 1959).

The Cerebrospinal Fluid

Examination of the cerebrospinal fluid is of great diagnostic importance, since obstruction of the spinal subarachnoid space produces characteristic changes in its chemical composition, and its pressure below the block. Care is, however, necessary in cases of suspected extradural abscess and lumbar puncture should not be performed at or near the site of spinal pain or tenderness in view of the risk of introducing organisms into the subarachnoid space.

Chemical Changes. The essential chemical abnormality is a rise in the protein content of the fluid, which usually lies between 0·1 and 0·5 g. per 100 ml. but may be even higher if the block is complete. In addition the fluid is yellow in colour—xanthochromia—in about 40 per cent. of cases, and may coagulate spontaneously. An excess of mononuclear cells in the fluid may be present when the source of compression is inflammatory (e.g. spinal extradural abscess), and exceptionally in cases of tumour. A rise in the protein content of the fluid is most marked in cases of extramedullary spinal compression, and may be slight when the source of pressure is extradural or intramedullary. It is important to note that the protein may be normal or only slightly raised when the cord is compressed in the cervical region, whatever the cause of compression. A rise of the protein content has been observed in the fluid removed *above* a tumour of the cauda equina.

Manometry. Manometry is carried out by the method described on page 125. The pressure of the fluid is not infrequently subnormal below an obstruction of the spinal subarachnoid space, and variations in pressure corresponding to the pulse and respiration are often diminished or absent.

Queckenstedt's Test. This test affords valuable evidence of spinal subarachnoid block and should be carried out, as described on page 126, in every case in which this is suspected. If obstruction of the spinal subarachnoid space completely cuts off the lumbar sac from the cerebral subarachnoid space, jugular compression produces no alteration in the pressure of the fluid below the obstruction. If the obstruction be incomplete, both the rise and the fall of the pressure may be slower than normal. If a lesion in the cervical region is suspected it may be valuable to repeat the test with the head flexed, in the neutral position and in hyperextension as a total block may be present in only one of these positions. It must be remembered that holding the breath, coughing, sneezing, grunting, and abdominal compression may raise the pressure of the cerebrospinal fluid, even below an obstruction. If no rise of pressure in the spinal manometer follows jugular compression, this may be accepted as almost conclusive evidence of obstruction of the spinal subarachnoid space. A normal Queckenstedt's test, however, cannot with equal certainty be accepted as indicating that spinal compression is absent. Thus the test is not sufficiently accurate to exclude cord compression completely and when suspicion of such a lesion remains, opaque myelography is indicated. Indeed, many workers have now discarded this test in view of the fact that myelography may be difficult or impossible after a prior lumbar puncture carried out below a spinal block as the removal of the cerebrospinal fluid may have caused a shrinkage of the spinal subarachnoid space.

The presence of a tumour of the cauda equina may lead to a failure to obtain cerebrospinal fluid by lumbar puncture at the site of election below the fourth lumbar vertebra, if it completely fills the spinal canal at this point. Cisternal myelography will then be indicated.

Exacerbation of Symptoms following Lumbar Puncture. In cases of spinal subarachnoid block, especially when this is due to a spinal tumour, the withdrawal of cerebrospinal fluid below the level of the block by lumbar puncture may lead to a shift in the position of the tumour and a temporary or even permanent intensification of the symptoms, especially root pains, weakness, and retention of urine. Queckenstedt's test may evoke root pain. Thus hasty lumbar puncture is unwise in cases of suspected spinal tumour. On suspicion of such a diagnosis it is wiser to seek a neurosurgical opinion and to arrange myelography at a time when the neurosurgeon will be able to operate immediately, particularly if clinical deterioration follows the procedure.

Radiography

Radiography of the spine should be carried out in all cases of spinal compression. When this is due to disease of the vertebral column only X-ray examination may enable the cause of the compression to be discovered. It renders visible the vertebral destruction due to tuberculous caries, and other forms of osteitis, secondary carcinoma, primary vertebral neoplasm, and the changes associated with traumatic lesions. It should, however, be noted that a spinal extradural abscess due to acute vertebral osteitis may be present without visible radiological abnormalities in the early stages. Chronic disc protrusion is likely to be associated with narrowing of the corresponding disc space, and bony spurs from the bodies of adjacent vertebrae: its presence can be confirmed by myelography [FIG. 93]. Many patients, particularly manual workers, have severe degenerative changes in the discs of the cervical spine without symptoms so that when radiological findings of spondylosis are present in a patient with signs of spinal cord compression it cannot necessarily be assumed that spondylosis is the cause so that myelography will usually be necessary. A tumour arising within the vertebral canal may by erosion lead to its diffuse enlargement, in which case the distance between the pedicles will be increased, or it may pass outwards through the intervertebral foramen with local destruction of bone. Oblique views will then demonstrate enlargement of the intervertebral foramen and a soft-tissue shadow of a 'dumb-bell' tumour may also be seen.

Myelography

While some workers prefer to use air or oxygen injected intrathecally by lumbar puncture for the demonstration of lesions causing spinal cord compression, most radiologists prefer the use of an opaque oily contrast medium (*Myodil, Pantopaque*) of which 5–6 ml. is usually injected by lumbar puncture

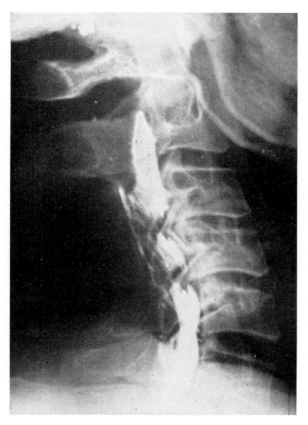

FIG. 93. Myelography in cervical spondylosis with intervertebral disc protrusion at C.3–4 and C.4–5, and compression of the spinal cord. Note that the osteophytes are limited to the posterior aspects of the bodies

with the patient in the sitting position. This preparation is generally non-irritant and few complications are known to result from its use although iodine sensitivity should be excluded before it is used. Occasionally low back pain and root pains in the legs and even retention of urine may follow myelography but these complications are as a rule transient; untoward long-lasting sequelae (due to adhesive arachnoiditis) are so rare that in Great Britain no attempt is made to remove the injected oil. In the United States, however, for medicolegal reasons, the lumbar puncture needle is generally left *in situ* and the oil is withdrawn when the radiological examination has been completed. Following injection the patient is examined on a tilting table under an X-ray screen and anteroposterior and lateral radiographs can be taken at appropriate spinal levels as the flow of contrast medium is observed. Usually the examination is carried out with the patient prone but supine myelography is also essential when a lesion at or near the foramen magnum is suspected. If the contrast medium is arrested below a compressive lesion or when a lesion in the cauda equina is suspected it may be necessary to inject the medium by cisternal rather than lumbar puncture in order to outline the upper extent of the lesion. In cases of cervical myelopathy radiographs should be taken in several positions of the head. When a complete block is present, re-screening after 24 hours may show that some contrast medium has passed the obstruction [FIGS. 93, 94].

Symptoms of Spinal Compression at different Levels

The symptoms of spinal compression at a given level consist of: (1) symptoms of a lower motor neurone lesion, that is, atrophic paralysis with diminution or loss of the tendon reflexes in the muscles innervated by the segments compressed; (2) symptoms of an upper motor neurone lesion, that is, spastic paralysis with exaggeration of the tendon reflexes, diminution or loss of the abdominal and cremasteric reflexes and an extensor plantar reflex on one or both sides below the level of the compression (in advanced cases paraplegia-in-extension in the lower limbs may give place to paraplegia-in-flexion); (3) symptoms of dorsal root irritation, pain and hyperalgesia, may be present, with a segmental distribution corresponding to the segments compressed; (4) various types of sensory loss already described, with an upper level at or somewhat below the segmental level of the site of compression; (5) autonomic changes, e.g. excessive sweating below the level of the lesion. The following are the principal motor and reflex disturbances resulting from compression of the spinal cord at different levels. The distribution of the sensory changes can best be ascertained from the figures on pages 42 and 43.

The Upper Cervical Region.

Spinal compression at this level or at the foramen magnum usually causes considerable pain in the neck and occiput, which is intensified by movements of the cervical spine. Pain, paraesthesiae, and weakness in the upper limbs are early symptoms and loss of proprioceptive sensation in the hands may be particularly prominent. Wasting may occur in both upper limbs although the cervical enlargement is not compressed. Compression of the phrenic nerves or of their nuclei may lead to diminution in the amplitude of the movements of the diaphragm. A tumour in this region may extend upwards through the foramen magnum and cause symptoms through compression of the medulla and of the lowest cranial nerves. Compression of the spinal tract and nucleus of the fifth nerve may cause relative analgesia and thermo-anaesthesia over the face, and the ninth, tenth, and eleventh cranial nerves may also suffer. Signs of corticospinal tract compression are present in both upper and lower limbs with exaggeration of *all* deep tendon reflexes. Postural sense and appreciation of vibration are usually impaired over one or both upper limbs.

The Fifth or Sixth Cervical Segments.

Atrophic paralysis is present in the

muscles innervated by these segments, namely, the rhomboids, deltoids, spinati, biceps, and brachioradialis. There is spastic paralysis of the remaining muscles of the upper limbs and of the trunk and lower limbs. The biceps- and supinator-

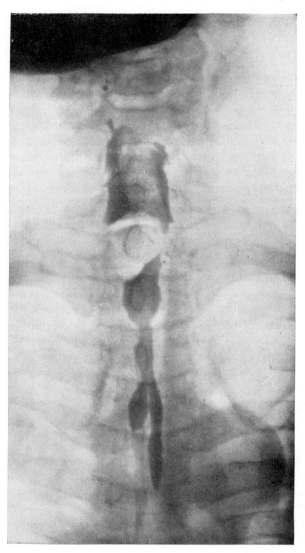

FIG. 94. Myelography in a case of spinal meningioma, a lobulated growth extending from the first to the fourth thoracic vertebra

jerks are diminished or lost, but a tap on the lower end of the radius may evoke exaggerated reflex flexion of the fingers (inversion of the radial reflex (Babinski)). The triceps-jerks are preserved and may be exaggerated while an attempt to elicit the biceps-jerk may actually give a triceps-jerk (inversion of the biceps reflex).

The Eighth Cervical and First Thoracic Segments. Atrophic paralysis involves the flexors of the wrist and fingers and the small muscles of the hands. Paralysis of the ocular sympathetic may be present. The tendon reflexes of the upper limbs are preserved. There is spastic paralysis of the trunk and lower limbs. Compression of the spinal cord at this level is virtually unknown in cervical spondylosis so that wasting of the small hand muscles does not occur due to this cause.

Mid-thoracic Region. Atrophic paralysis is confined to the intercostals innervated by the segments involved. Movements of the diaphragm are normal. There is spastic paralysis of the muscles of the abdomen and lower limbs.

Ninth and Tenth Thoracic Segments. The lower halves of the abdominal recti are paralysed; the upper halves are normal. Consequently the umbilicus is drawn upwards when the patient raises his head against resistance. The upper abdominal reflexes are preserved, while those of the lower segments are lost. There is spastic paralysis of the lower limbs.

Twelfth Thoracic and First Lumbar Segments. The abdominal recti are normal, but the lower fibres of obliquus internus and transversus abdominis are paralysed. The abdominal reflexes are preserved, but the cremasteric reflexes are diminished or lost. There is spastic paralysis of the lower limbs.

Third and Fourth Lumbar Segments. Flexion of the hip is preserved. There are atrophic paralysis of quadriceps and the adductors of the hips, with diminution or loss of the knee-jerks, and spastic paralysis of the remaining muscles of the lower limbs, with exaggeration of the ankle-jerks and extensor plantar responses.

First and Second Sacral Segments. Flexion of the hip, adduction of the thigh, extension of the knee, and dorsiflexion of the foot are preserved. There are atrophic paralysis of the intrinsic muscles of the foot and of the calf muscles, and weakness of flexion of the knee and of all muscles moving the hip-joint, except the flexors and adductors. The knee-jerks are preserved; the ankle-jerks and plantar reflexes are lost. The anal and bulbocavernosus reflexes are preserved.

Third and Fourth Sacral Segments. The large bowel and bladder are paralysed and retention of urine and faeces occurs, due to the uninhibited action of the internal sphincters. The external sphincters are paralysed and the anal and bulbocavernosus reflexes are lost. There is usually sensory loss in the perineum and buttocks in 'saddle' distribution. The motility and reflexes of the lower limbs are normal.

Compression of the Cauda Equina

Compression of the cauda equina is most frequently due to a neoplasm, but the nerve roots may be compressed by fat in cases of spina bifida occulta, by the constriction of a fibrous band (Léri, 1926), or by chronic arachnoiditis. An important source of compression of a single root, or even of multiple roots, occurring sometimes acutely is a displaced intervertebral disc [see p. 799]. Rarely, spondylolisthesis may have the same effect as may bony stenosis of the lumbar canal which more often gives the syndrome of recurrent ischaemia of the cauda equina on effort [see p. 682]. The clinical picture is a variable one, depending upon the site and extent of the source of compression. It may be virtually impossible clinically to distinguish between a neoplasm arising in the cauda equina itself and one arising in the conus medullaris but extending into the cauda. A small tumour may for a long time compress only one or two roots on one side. A large and massive growth may involve the whole of the cauda. For anatomical reasons the lower roots are more likely to be compressed than the upper, since they suffer alone when a growth is situated in the lowest part of the spinal canal, and they are also implicated, together with the upper roots, by tumours at a higher level.

In many cases of compression of the cauda equina by tumour, pain is the earliest symptom. It is usually located in the lumbar or sacral regions of the spine as a dull, aching pain which is liable to be exacerbated by jerky movements, coughing, and sneezing. Less frequently the pain is referred to one or both lower limbs in the distribution of certain of the lower spinal roots, and it may also be referred to the bladder or rectum.

Motor symptoms consist of atrophic paralysis, the distribution of which depends upon the roots affected. Most frequently there is paralysis of the muscles below the knee, though the tibialis anterior may escape, and of the hamstrings and glutei. In such cases the ankle-jerks are diminished or lost, and the plantar reflexes may also be unelicitable; but the knee-jerks are often preserved.

The distribution of the sensory loss also depends upon which spinal dorsal roots are involved. Compression of the lower sacral roots leads to a characteristic saddle-shaped area of anaesthesia and analgesia extending over the perineum, buttocks, and back of the thighs. Compression of the upper sacral and fifth lumbar roots produces an area of sensory loss over the foot and over the posterior and outer aspect of the leg. When the lowest sacral segments are involved, though the external genitals are anaesthetic, and the patient may be unaware of the passage of a catheter through the urethra, some sensibility usually remains in the bladder, so that the patient is aware of its distension, and cystitis may give rise to pain.

Disturbance of function of the bladder and bowel is usually a late development. Compression of the third and fourth ventral and dorsal sacral roots interrupts the reflex arc upon which evacuation of the bladder and rectum depends. The result is retention of urine and faeces due to the unopposed contraction of the internal sphincters, although the external sphincters are paralysed. Impotence occurs in the male. When the lowest sacral roots are compressed the anal and bulbocavernosus reflexes are lost, but these will be preserved as long as these roots escape.

Trophic symptoms may occur in the lower limbs, which are frequently cold and cyanosed, and tend to become oedematous if they are allowed to hang down. Slight injuries over the analgesic areas are apt to lead to sores which do not quickly heal and which leave permanent scars.

DIAGNOSIS

The diagnosis of spinal compression involves four stages: (1) Spinal compression must be distinguished from other lesions which may give rise to similar symptoms. (2) When the existence of spinal compression has been established, its segmental level must be determined. (3) An attempt should then be made to decide whether the compression is extradural, extramedullary, or intramedullary; and (4) what is its pathological nature.

Diagnosis from other Disorders

When the earliest symptom is pain spinal compression is liable to be confused with visceral disorders of which pain is a prominent symptom, for example, pleurisy, angina pectoris, cholecystitis, gastric and duodenal ulcer, and renal calculus. This error can only be avoided by a thorough examination of the nervous system, which will usually yield some indication of a lesion of the spinal cord, and also by the absence of physical signs of visceral disease. Spinal compression requires to be distinguished from spinal syphilis, multiple sclerosis, syringomyelia, and motor neurone disease, the last three of which may be simulated by cervical myelopathy due to spondylosis. On clinical grounds this distinction can usually be made with considerable confidence, but the diagnosis can only be clinched by examination of the cerebrospinal fluid and myelography.

Localization of Segmental Level

In the localization of the segmental level of spinal compression segmental symptoms, especially atrophic paralysis and root pains and hyperalgesia, are of the first importance. Next in value is the upper limit of the area of sensory loss, though this is not always easy to define. When it can be accurately determined. the segmental level of the upper limit of the area of analgesia may be taken as indicating the lowest segment compressed but it must be remembered that a sensory 'level' for pain sensation may suggest that the lesion is several segments lower than its actual site. Thus a level on the thoracic cage is not infrequently observed in patients with lesions of the cervical cord.

The clinical diagnosis of a tumour of the cauda equina from a tumour of the conus medullaris is often difficult, and may be impossible. If, however, in spite of paralysis of the bladder and rectum, the anal and bulbocavernosus reflexes are preserved and if sensory loss is of the dissociated type, that is, if sensibility to pain, heat, and cold is lost, while that to light touch is preserved, it is likely that the lesion involves the conus rather than the roots. The presence of an extensor plantar response on one or both sides indicates that the spinal cord is compressed at least as high as the fifth lumbar segment.

Relationship of Spinal Segments to Vertebrae. Since the spinal cord terminates at the level of the lower border of the first lumbar vertebra, spinal segments do not correspond numerically with the vertebral arches by which they are enclosed. Having localized a source of compression in terms of spinal segments, the surgeon requires to know beneath which laminal arch he may expect to find it. To ascertain which spinal segment is related to a given vertebra:

For the cervical vertebrae, add 1.
For thoracic 1–6, add 2.
For thoracic 7–9, add 3.
The tenth thoracic arch overlies lumbar 1 and 2 segments.

The eleventh thoracic arch overlies lumbar 3 and 4.
The twelfth thoracic arch overlies lumbar 5.
The first lumbar arch overlies the sacral and coccygeal segments.

It must be remembered that owing to the obliquity of the lower thoracic spinous processes a spinous process in this region is situated at the level of the body of the vertebra below. Despite these valuable clinical guides it is, except in very unusual or urgent circumstances, unwise to operate without confirmation of the level of the lesion by myelography.

The Relationship of the Source of Compression to the Cord

Angular deformity of the spine, and radiographic evidence of vertebral destruction indicate clearly that vertebral disease is responsible for the spinal compression. In the absence of such evidence the differentiation of extradural, extramedullary, and intramedullary sources of spinal compression is often difficult, and may be impossible. In extradural compression root pains not uncommonly occur early, and symptoms of spinal compression are usually bilateral and symmetrical in their development. Motor symptoms usually appear first, to be followed later by sphincter disturbances, and sensory changes are frequently late. The protein content of the cerebrospinal fluid is often not greatly increased and usually lies between 40 and 150 mg. per 100 ml. The distinction between extramedullary and intramedullary compression is often impossible before operation. The early onset of unilateral root pains and the development of symptoms indicating that compression is mainly exerted upon one-half of the cord favour an extramedullary source of compression. In such cases, moreover, blockage of the spinal subarachnoid space tends to occur early and the protein content of the spinal fluid is usually high. In cases of intramedullary compression root pains are less frequent and motor symptoms are usually bilateral. An area of dissociated sensory loss extending over a series of segments just below the level of the lesion is suggestive of an intramedullary growth. Subarachnoid blockage occurs later and the protein content of the fluid is usually lower in the case of intramedullary than in the case of extramedullary compression.

Diagnosis of the Cause

1. *Vertebral Disease*. When spinal compression is due to vertebral collapse there is usually considerable pain in, and rigidity of, the spine; angular deformity is common, and radiographic evidence of vertebral destruction will usually be found. *Tuberculous caries* is to be suspected when these symptoms are present in a young patient who shows evidence of infection, such as pyrexia, sweating, and a raised sedimentation rate, with possibly in addition signs of a tuberculous abscess or of a tuberculous focus elsewhere, but it may occur at any age and without general symptoms. *Secondary carcinoma* of the vertebral column is usually seen in middle-aged patients. The onset of the spinal symptoms is often rapid and attended by considerable pain. There is often a history of an operation for carcinoma and, in the absence of this, careful clinical and radiological examination usually enable the primary growth to be found. The diagnosis of other forms of vertebral disease, for example, myelomatosis and osteitis deformans of Paget,

can usually be established radiographically. When the former is suspected the appropriate tests should be carried out. The presence of *cervical spondylosis* can be demonstrated radiographically, but it must be remembered that this is very common after middle age, and is not always the cause of the patient's symptoms.

2. *Spinal Tumour.* Spinal tumour is to be suspected in cases in which there is a gradual onset and a slowly progressive development of symptoms of spinal compression, in the absence of evident disease of the vertebral column. It is usually impossible to anticipate the nature of the spinal tumour, but a careful search should be made for cutaneous pigmentation and other symptoms of neurofibromatosis, which may be associated with an intrathecal neurofibroma.

3. *Meningitis.* It is often impossible to diagnose either hypertrophic pachymeningitis or arachnoiditis before operation. The occurrence of multiple levels of segmental sensory disturbance, and a patchy or streaky arrest of contrast medium are in favour of arachnoiditis.

Such rare causes of spinal compression as reticulosis, leukaemic deposits, and parasitic cysts can be suspected only when clinical examination reveals evidence of the disease elsewhere.

PROGNOSIS

General Considerations

The prognosis of compression of the spinal cord depends upon (1) the nature of the source of compression and the extent to which it can be relieved, (2) the severity and duration of the disturbance of function when the patient comes under observation, and (3) the level of the cord compressed. The influence of the nature of the compressing agent upon prognosis is further considered below. The more severe the interruption of conduction in the cord, the less likely is recovery to be complete. Hence the development of paraplegia-in-flexion, which indicates a severe degree of interruption of the cord, is of bad prognostic import, and little functional improvement can be expected in such cases. The longer the history of symptoms of compression, the less complete is recovery likely to be, though even when such symptoms as spastic weakness of the lower limbs have been present for two years, a remarkable degree of recovery may occur if the cause can be removed. It cannot be stressed too strongly that rapidly-advancing spinal cord compression demands immediate investigation and treatment so that the latter can be carried out before the circulation to the cord is irreversibly embarrassed. The outlook is best when the site of compression is situated in the middle or lower thoracic regions although it should be remembered that surgical operations in this region, particularly when carried out for the relief of anteriorly-situated lesions, such as the rare dorsal disc protrusions, are hazardous, first because the spinal canal is very narrow in this region, and secondly because the blood supply of the cord is at its most precarious at this point. When the upper cervical cord is compressed the proximity of the spinal centres innervating the diaphragm adds to the risk both of the compression itself and of operations upon this region. Compression of the lumbosacral region and cauda equina is especially liable to lead to disturbance of function of the bladder and bowel, and hence there is a high incidence of infection of the urinary tract in such cases. In all cases of spinal compression the presence of infection of the urinary tract and of severe bed-sores adds to the gravity of the prognosis.

Tuberculous Spinal Osteitis

The mortality rate of tuberculous caries of the spine has been reduced by modern chemotherapy. Spinal compression naturally increases the risk of death, but about 70 per cent. of patients with paraplegia recover completely. Others are left with some spastic weakness of the lower limbs. The prognosis both as to life and as to recovery of function is better in children than in adults. The sudden development of paraplegia rapidly becoming complete is usually due to 'concertina' collapse of a vertebral body or to thrombosis of vessels supplying the cord, and in both conditions the outlook is poor. When long-standing paraplegia-in-flexion is present there is no hope of recovery.

Secondary Carcinoma of the Vertebrae

Few patients survive more than twelve months after the development of symptoms indicating the presence of metastatic carcinomatous deposits within the vertebral column, death occurring either as a direct result of disturbance of function caused by the primary growth, or from cachexia due to widespread metastases.

Spinal Tumour

The prognosis of spinal tumour depends primarily upon the extent to which the growth can be removed. Accordingly, the outlook is much better in the case of extramedullary tumours, a large proportion of which can be removed completely, than when the tumour is intramedullary. Few intramedullary tumours can be successfully removed without considerable damage to the spinal cord although some ependymomas are encapsulated and can be 'shelled out' with subsequent improvement. The mortality rate of operations for spinal tumours is under 5 per cent. in the best hands. A considerable functional improvement may be expected to follow the successful removal of a spinal tumour in all but the most advanced cases, even when symptoms of compression have been present for several years. Improvement, however, may be slow and may be expected to continue for a year or more after operation. Angiomas tend to be insidiously progressive in spite of all treatment but some can be removed successfully (Shephard, 1966).

Acute Intervertebral Disc Prolapse and Cervical Spondylosis

Acute central protrusion of a cervical intervertebral disc is usually best treated conservatively by means of immobilization of the neck in a plaster collar but if cord compression is severe laminectomy and decompression may be needed and if carried out sufficiently early the prognosis is good. Acute compression of the cauda equina, say by a central disc prolapse, demands immediate operation, especially if the sphincters are involved and here again the prognosis is good. Operative treatment is also indicated as a rule in cord compression due to prolapse of a dorsal intervertebral disc but the operation is risky, recovery is often incomplete, and irreversible paraplegia due to cord infarction is an all-too-frequent complication. In cervical myelopathy due to spondylosis the natural tendency of the disorder is to become arrested, but most patients are left with a varying degree of residual disability.

Arachnoiditis

The response to operation is often disappointing and only about 30 per cent. of cases recover, especially when a cyst can be removed.

TREATMENT

The treatment of compression of the spinal cord involves (1) the appropriate treatment of the source of the compression, and (2) when paraplegia is present, adequate care of the paralysed limbs, the skin, the urinary tract, and the bowels, along the lines laid down on page 628, for upon the careful treatment of the paraplegia may depend not only the patient's life but also the rate at which recovery of function occurs.

Tuberculous Spinal Osteitis

A patient suffering from tuberculous caries of the spine requires appropriate chemotherapy and orthopaedic treatment, usually immobilization in a plaster bed.

Laminectomy is rarely desirable, since most patients rapidly improve on the treatment described. An exploratory operation, however, may be carried out when paraplegia has continued unimproved after several months of treatment or when a sudden increase in its severity occurs.

Cervical Spondylosis

In some cases immobilization of the neck by means of a plaster or plastic collar is sufficient. In rapidly progressive cases, especially when the patient is relatively young, surgical decompression may be necessary. This is particularly likely to be indicated when myelography indicates that the cord is being compressed by significant disc protrusions at one or two levels. Surgery is probably contra-indicated if three or more discs are involved. The choice between posterior decompression by laminectomy and anterior removal of the discs with spinal fusion (the Cloward operation) is a matter for decision depending upon clinical and myelographic findings in the individual case.

Secondary Carcinoma of Vertebrae

Treatment of this condition can only be palliative as a rule, and morphine should be given in doses adequate for the relief of pain. In occasional cases of acute compression emergency laminectomy and decompression is indicated in order to relieve pressure and to obtain a surgical biopsy of the tumour as a preliminary to radiotherapy. The question as to whether the lesion should be irradiated depends upon the general condition of the patient and the situation and prognosis of the primary lesion being known. Many patients have relief of pain as a result and in some cord compression is relieved so that this treatment is usually indicated if the lesion is radiosensitive and unless the patient is *in extremis* as a result of the primary growth and/or multiple metastases elsewhere. Powerful analgesics and, in selected cases, surgical methods of pain relief (cordotomy, stereotaxic thalamotomy) may be required.

Spinal Tumour

Laminectomy should be performed, and when the tumour is extradural or extramedullary it should be removed as far as possible. For the treatment of intramedullary tumours Elsberg recommended incising the posterior aspect of the cord, slightly to one side of the median septum, and allowing the tumour to extrude itself, a second operation being performed a week later for the removal of the extruded portion. It is, however, sometimes possible to dissect out and remove an intramedullary tumour without serious damage to the cord. When a spinal tumour for any reason cannot be removed, the operation of laminectomy may lead to a temporary improvement by diminishing the pressure upon the cord. X-ray irradiation may be of value as an accessory method of treatment following operation, especially for intramedullary tumours. Angiomas are only rarely operable, and their response to radiotherapy is uncertain.

Meningitis

When spinal pachymeningitis is of long standing, it leads to softening of the spinal cord through interference with its vascular supply. In such cases little benefit can be expected to follow operation. At an earlier stage, however, when the symptoms are mainly due to constriction of the cord, improvement may follow laminectomy and removal of granulation tissue. When arachnoiditis is found at operation, an attempt should be made to free the cord from adhesions and to rupture or remove any localized cysts which may be present. Tuberculous spinal meningitis requires the appropriate chemotherapy.

The after-treatment of patients suffering from spinal compression and who have undergone laminectomy, should include massage and passive movements of the paretic limbs and re-educational exercises, in order to promote functional recovery [see p. 628].

REFERENCES

ABRAHAMSON, L., McCONNELL, A. A., and WILSON, G. R. (1934) Acute epidural spinal abscess, *Brit. med. J.*, **1**, 1114.

ADSON, A. W. (1938) Intraspinal tumors; surgical consideration. Collective review, *Surg. Gynec. Obstet.*, **67**, 225.

ALLEN, I. M. (1930) Tumours involving the cauda equina: a review of their clinical features and differential diagnosis, *J. Neurol. Psychopath.*, **11**, 111.

ANTONI, N. (1962) Spinal vascular malformations (angiomas) and myelomalacia, *Neurology (Minneap.)*, **12**, 795.

BLAKESLEE, G. A. (1928) Compression of the spinal cord in Hodgkin's disease, *Arch. Neurol. Psychiat. (Chicago)*, **20**, 130.

BRAIN, W. R. (1948) Rupture of the intervertebral disk in the cervical region, *Proc. roy. Soc. Med.*, **41**, 509.

BRAIN, W. R., NORTHFIELD, D. W. C., and WILKINSON, M. (1952) The neurological manifestations of cervical spondylosis, *Brain*, **75**, 187.

BRICE, J., and McKISSOCK, W. (1965) Surgical treatment of malignant extradural spinal tumours, *Brit. med. J.*, **1**, 1341.

BUCY, P. C., and OBERHILL, H. R. (1950) Intradural spinal granulomas, *J. Neurosurg.*, **7**, 1.

BULL, J. W. D. (1948) Rupture of the intervertebral disk in the cervical region, *Proc. roy. Soc. Med.*, **41**, 513.

BUTLER, R. W. (1934–5) Paraplegia in Pott's disease, with special reference to the pathology and aetiology, *Brit. J. Surg.*, **22**, 738.

CAIRNS, H., and RUSSELL, D. S. (1931) Intracranial and spinal metastases in gliomas of the brain, *Brain*, **54**, 377.

CAMPBELL, A. M. G., and PHILLIPS, D. G. (1960) Cervical disk lesions with neurological disorder, *Brit. med. J.*, **2**, 481.

CRITCHLEY, M., and GREENFIELD, J. G. (1930) Spinal symptoms in chloroma and leukaemia, *Brain*, **53**, 11.

ELKINGTON, J. ST. C. (1936) Meningitis serosa circumscripta spinalis, *Brain*, **59**, 181.

ELSBERG, C. A. (1925) *Tumors of the Spinal Cord*, New York.

ELSBERG, C. A. (1929) Tumors of the spinal cord, *Arch. Neurol. Psychiat. (Chicago)*, **22**, 949.

ELSBERG, C. A., and CONSTABLE, K. (1930) Tumors of the cauda equina, *Arch. Neurol. Psychiat. (Chicago)*, **23**, 79.

FAY, T. (1928) Vasomotor and pilomotor manifestations: their localizing value in tumors and lesions of the spinal cord, *Arch. Neurol. Psychiat. (Chicago)*, **19**, 31.

GLOBUS, J. H., and DOSHAY, L. J. (1929) Venous dilatations and other intraspinal vessel alterations, including true angiomata, with signs and symptoms of cord compression, *Surg. Gynec. Obstet.*, **48**, 345.

HASSIN, G. B. (1928) Circumscribed suppurative nontuberculous peripachy-meningitis, *Arch. Neurol. Psychiat. (Chicago)*, **20**, 110.

HAWK, W. A. (1936) Spinal compression caused by ecchondrosis of the inter-vertebral fibrocartilage: with a review of the recent literature, *Brain*, **59**, 204.

HIRSON, C. (1965) Spinal subdural abscess, *Lancet*, ii, 1215.

HOWELL, C. M. H. (1936–7) Arachnoiditis, *Proc. roy. Soc. Med.*, **30**, 33.

IRVINE, D. H., FOSTER, J. B., NEWELL, D. J., and KLUKVIN, B. N. (1965) Prevalence of cervical spondylosis in a general practice, *Lancet*, i, 1089.

KERNOHAN, J. W., WOLTMAN, H. W., and ADSON, A. W. (1931) Intramedullary tumors of the spinal cord, *Arch. Neurol. Psychiat. (Chicago)*, **25**, 679.

LÉRI, A. (1926) *Études sur les affections de la colonne vertébrale*, Paris.

LOVE, J. G., and WALSH, M. N. (1943) Protruded intervertebral disk, *Surg. Gynec. Obstet.*, **77**, 497.

MATTHEWS, W. B. (1959) The spinal bruit, *Lancet*, ii, 1117.

MONIZ, E. (1925) La pachyméningite spinale hypertrophique et les cavités médullaires, *Rev. neurol. (Paris)*, **32**, 433.

NASSAR, S. I., and CORRELL, J. W. (1968) Subarachnoid hemorrhage due to spinal cord tumors, *Neurology (Minneap.)*, **18**, 87.

PENNING, L. (1961) Atlanto-axial instability and functional X-ray examination, *Medicamundi*, **7**, 113.

ROSS, J. C., GIBBON, N. O. K., and DAMANSKI, M. (1964) Bladder dysfunction in non-traumatic paraplegia, *Lancet*, i, 779.

SEDDON, H. J. (1934–5) Pott's paraplegia: prognosis and treatment, *Brit. J. Surg.*, **22**, 769.

SHEPHARD, R. H. (1966) A reappraisal of spinal intradural angiomas with particular emphasis on treatment by excision, *Proc. roy. Soc. Med.* (film), **59**, 796.

STOOKEY, B. (1924) A study of extradural spinal tumors, *Arch. Neurol. Psychiat (Chicago)*, **12**, 663.

STOOKEY, B. (1927) Adhesive spinal arachnoiditis simulating spinal cord tumor, *Arch. Neurol. Psychiat. (Chicago)*, **17**, 151.

STOOKEY, B. (1928) Compression of the spinal cord due to ventral extradural cervical chondromas, *Arch. Neurol. Psychiat. (Chicago)*, **20**, 275.

SYMONDS, C. P., and MEADOWS, S. P. (1937) Compression of the spinal cord in the neighbourhood of the foramen magnum, *Brain*, **60**, 52.

TILNEY, F., and ELSBERG, C. A. (1926) Sensory disturbances in tumors of the cervical spinal cord, *Arch. Neurol. Psychiat. (Chicago)*, **15**, 444.

WEIL, A. (1931) Spinal cord changes in lymphogranulomatosis, *Arch. Neurol. Psychiat.* (*Chicago*), **26,** 1009.

WOLTMAN, H. W., KERNOHAN, J. W., ADSON, A. W., and CRAIG, W. McK. (1951) Intramedullary tumors of spinal cord and gliomas of intradural portion of filum terminale; fate of patients who have these tumors, *Arch. Neurol. Psychiat.* (*Chicago*), **65,** 378.

WYBURN-MASON, R. (1943) *Vascular Abnormalities and Tumours of the Spinal Cord,* London.

Discussion on vascular tumours of the brain and spinal cord, *Proc. roy. Soc. Med.,* 1930–1, **24,** 363.

SYRINGOMYELIA

Synonym. Status dysraphicus.

Definition. A chronic disease characterized pathologically by the presence of long cavities, surrounded by gliosis, which are situated in relation to the central canal of the spinal cord and frequently extend up into the medulla (syringobulbia). The principal clinical features are areas of cutaneous analgesia and thermo-anaesthesia, with preservation of appreciation of light touch and postural sensibility, muscular wasting, and trophic changes, especially in the upper limbs, and symptoms of corticospinal tract degeneration in the lower limbs. The term 'syringomyelia' was first used by Ollivier in 1824.

PATHOLOGY

The pathological changes characteristic of syringomyelia are most frequently situated in the lower cervical and upper thoracic regions of the spinal cord. Extension to the medulla is common, and the process may reach the pons or even as high as the internal capsule. A thoracicolumbar and lumbosacral incidence is rare and is usually due to a true hydromyelia associated with congenital anomalies of the lower spine, although ascending cavitation occurring after traumatic transverse lesions of the cord has been reported.

The affected region of the cord is enlarged, mainly in the transverse plane [FIG. 95]. In some cases the enlargement is sufficient to cause erosion of the bones of the spinal canal or at least widening of its anteroposterior diameter. Transverse section of the cord reveals a cavity surrounded by a zone of translucent gelatinous material. The cavity, which often possesses diverticula, contains clear or yellow fluid. The pathological process appears to originate most frequently at the base of one posterior horn of the grey matter of the spinal cord. Less frequently it begins in the midline in the grey matter, near the central canal. Exceptionally this canal itself appears dilated. In the medulla the region affected is the posterolateral part, in the neighbourhood of the spinal nucleus of the trigeminal nerve, and the nucleus ambiguus. Fissures may radiate from the fourth ventricle into this region. Microscopically, the gelatinous material lining the cavity contains glial cells and fibres.

The expansion of the cavity and surrounding gliosis lead to compression of the anterior horns of the grey matter, thus causing atrophy of the anterior horn cells, and degeneration of their axons in the ventral roots and peripheral nerves. Compression of the long ascending and descending tracts of the cord occurs somewhat later, and leads to secondary degeneration, which is most marked first in the corticospinal tracts, later in the spinothalamic tracts, and later still the posterior columns. Haemorrhage into a syringomyelic cavity constitutes one uncommon form of haematomyelia.

AETIOLOGY

There has been general agreement in the past that in most cases syringomyelia is based upon a congenital abnormality and is the outcome of abnormal closure

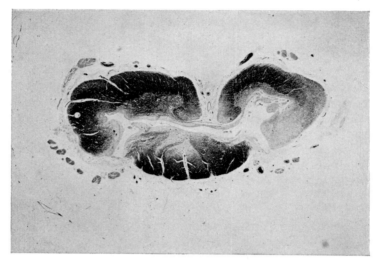

FIG. 95. Syringomyelia: spinal cord. Cavitation surrounded by gliosis

of the central canal of the spinal cord in the embryo. It has been suggested that incomplete closure leaves cavities around which a secondary gliosis develops, and alternatively that during closure spongioblasts are included in the region of the central canal and that these later form glial tissue which undergoes cavitation. Disturbances of the blood supply are probably of secondary importance in aetiology, and there is no good reason to suspect that infection plays any part in causation. Trauma has been held to be of aetiological importance. It has been suggested that intra-uterine haemorrhage within the cord may form the starting-point of syringomyelia, though there is no evidence of this. Occasionally also in adult life the symptoms of syringomyelia have been held to date from an accident. It is probable, however, that in such cases the trauma, if it possesses any significance, is not the primary cause of syringomyelia, but merely excites a latent abnormality into activity.

A familial, and even an hereditary, incidence of syringomyelia are well established, although exceptional. Multiple cases have been described in sibs, but the condition is usually sporadic. In this connexion it is interesting that congenital abnormalities have been observed in otherwise normal relatives of a patient suffering from syringomyelia. The occasional familial occurrence of syringomyelia relates it to myelodysplasia [see p. 671], and the common occurrence of spina bifida, both in patients with syringomyelia and in their relatives, affords support for the theory that syringomyelia is based upon defective closure of the central canal of the developing spinal cord. Recent work by Gardner (1965) and by Appleby *et al.* (1968) suggests that despite the occasional finding that a syringomyelic cavity may lie alongside an apparently intact central canal, in the great majority of cases the condition is due initially to a true hydromyelia (dilatation of the central canal) and that this may later develop diverticula which are no longer lined by ependyma but which dissect downwards in the centre of the cord. Such a dilatation appears to depend usually upon the presence of a Chiari type anomaly or of some other congenital abnormality (e.g. the Dandy–Walker syndrome of closure of the foramina of Magendie and Luschka) in the neighbourhood of the foramen magnum.

Although in most cases syringomyelia possesses the congenital pathological basis already described, cavitation may occur within the spinal cord as a result of intramedullary tumour, the cavity developing either within the tumour, or outside it due to hydromyelia. A spinal tumour may rarely develop in a patient already suffering from syringomyelia.

The age of onset of symptoms in syringomyelia ranges between 10 and 60. Usually it lies between 25 and 40. Males suffer more frequently than females in the proportion of about three to one.

SYMPTOMS

The symptoms of syringomyelia are readily interpreted as the outcome of the progressive lesion in the central region of the spinal cord.

Mode of Onset

The onset is usually insidious but rarely develops rapidly over the course of a few weeks. Wasting and weakness of the small muscles of the hands are the commonest early symptoms, but the patient may notice the loss of feeling in the hands or the resulting injuries. Less often pain or trophic lesions first attract attention.

Sensory Symptoms

At the earliest stage there is an elongated cavity surrounded by gliosis, situated in most cases at the base of one posterior horn of grey matter, and extending longitudinally through several segments, usually in the lower cervical and upper thoracic segments of the cord. The effect of such a lesion is to interrupt on one side the decussating sensory fibres derived from several consecutive dorsal roots. Since the fibres which decussate shortly after entering the cord are those which conduct impulses concerned in the appreciation of pain, heat, and cold, these forms of sensibility are impaired while other forms are preserved. This is the dissociated sensory loss described by Charcot, and is usually first observed along the ulnar border of the hand, forearm, and arm, and upper part of the chest and back on one side in a 'half-cape' distribution with a horizontal lower border across the chest wall and ending sharply at the midline. Sometimes, however, the impaired sensibility occupies the 'glove' area. When the lesion is centrally situated from the first, or has extended from one side of the cord to the other, the area of dissociated sensory loss is bilateral. As the lesion extends upwards and downwards in the cord, the area of sensory impairment extends to the radial sides of the upper limbs and the neck, and downwards over the thorax, exhibiting at this stage a distribution *en cuirasse*. The areas over which appreciation of pain, heat, and cold are first impaired, and later lost, are not always, nor even usually, co-terminous, but any one may be more extensive than the others. When the lesion reaches the upper cervical segments, it begins to involve the spinal tract and nucleus of the trigeminal nerve, which receives fibres conducting impulses concerned in the appreciation of pain, heat, and cold from the face. Progressive destruction of these fibres causes extension of the area of dissociated sensory loss in a concentric manner from behind forwards on the face, sensibility on the tip of the nose and upper lip sometimes being last affected. Exceptionally the disorder begins in the medulla, in which case sensibility is first impaired on the face.

The progressive extension of the spinal lesion later causes compression of the lateral spinothalamic tracts on one or both sides, leading to loss of appreciation of pain, heat, and cold over the lower parts of the body. There is sometimes an area of normal sensibility over the abdomen intervening between the area of thoracic anaesthesia due to interruption of the decussating fibres and the area of sensory loss on one or both lower limbs due to compression of the spinothalamic tracts. Sensation over the posterior aspects of the lower limbs is usually affected last. When the spinothalamic tract is compressed at the level of the medulla, appreciation of pain, heat, and cold is impaired or lost over the whole of the opposite half of the body. The posterior columns are usually the last of the sensory pathways to suffer, but in the late stages appreciation of posture, passive movement, and vibration is likely to be impaired, especially in the lower limbs, and there may be extensive anaesthesia to light touch.

Thermo-anaesthesia may be detected by the patient, owing to the fact that hot water no longer feels hot over the affected parts of the body, and his analgesia exposes him to injuries, especially burns of the fingers, which he does not notice at the time, because they are painless. Spontaneous pains, though usually absent, are sometimes troublesome, and the patient may describe burning, aching, or shooting pains which may in some respects resemble the lightning pains of tabes but more often the pain is continuous and may then cause considerable distress. Such pains in one side of the face or in the upper limb may be the first symptom. When the lesion begins in the thoracicolumbar or lumbosacral regions of the cord the dissociated loss has a corresponding distribution.

Optic atrophy is exceptional, but has occasionally been described presumably due to associated occult hydrocephalus.

Motor Symptoms

The earliest motor symptoms are usually muscular weakness and wasting, due to atrophy of the anterior horn cells produced by compression. Since the lesion usually begins in the cervicothoracic region of the cord, muscular wasting usually first appears in the small muscles of the hands. It may be bilateral from the beginning, or one hand may suffer before the other. As the lesion extends, the muscular wasting spreads to involve the forearms, and later the arms, shoulder girdles, and upper intercostals. It is often slight, and is never as severe as is seen in advanced cases of motor neurone disease. Fasciculation is usually absent. Contractures may develop, especially in the muscles of the hand and forearm. Extension of the lesion to the posterolateral part of the medulla often involves the nucleus ambiguus, causing paresis of the soft palate, pharynx, and vocal cord. The other motor functions in which the cranial nerves are concerned are less frequently affected, though I have seen paralysis of the mandibular muscles, lateral rectus, facial muscles, and soft palate on one side as a result of haemorrhage into a syringomyelic cavity in the pons and medulla. The tongue is occasionally involved. Nystagmus is commonly present in syringomyelia. It is usually rotary in character, and has been ascribed to involvement of the vestibular and cerebellar connexions within the brain stem. Paralysis of the ocular sympathetic on one or both sides may be present, and leads to small and often irregular pupils, with ptosis and slight enophthalmos. The reaction to light is preserved.

Compression of the corticospinal tracts in the spinal cord causes weakness, with slight spasticity and extensor plantar responses in the majority of cases in the later stages. The loss of power, however, is rarely severe. The tendon reflexes are exaggerated in the lower limbs, and usually diminished or lost in the upper limbs particularly on the side of the dissociated anaesthesia, presumably due to interruption of the reflex arc; only rarely are they exaggerated in the arms, depending upon the predominance of upper or lower motor neurone lesions. The sphincters are usually little affected.

Trophic Symptoms

Trophic symptoms are conspicuous. True hypertrophy involving all the tissues may be present in one limb or one-half of the body or even of the tongue. Loss of sweating or excessive sweating may occur, usually over the face and upper limbs. Excessive sweating may be spontaneous or may be excited reflexly when the patient takes hot or highly-seasoned food. Twenty per cent. of patients exhibit osteo-arthropathy—Charcot's joints. The shoulders, elbows, and cervical spine are most frequently affected, less often the joints of the hands, the temporomandibular joint, the sternoclavicular and acromioclavicular joints, and the joints of the lower limbs. Atrophy and decalcification of the bones in the region of the joints with erosion of joint surfaces are the usual radiographic findings, the hypertrophic varieties of arthropathy being unusual [FIG. 96]. The development of the joint changes is not usually associated with pain. The affected joint is often enlarged, and movement evokes loud crepitus but is generally painless. The long bones are frequently brittle. Trophic changes in the skin include cyanosis, probably due to a vasomotor paralysis, hyperkeratosis, and thickening of the subcutaneous tissues, leading to a swelling of the fingers described as 'la main succulente'. The analgesia, as already described, renders the patient exceptionally liable to minor injuries, and the poor nutrition of the hands delays healing. Ulceration, whitlows, and necrosis of bone are not uncommon. Gangrene rarely occurs. The scars of former injuries are usually evident upon the palmar surface of the fingers [FIG. 97].

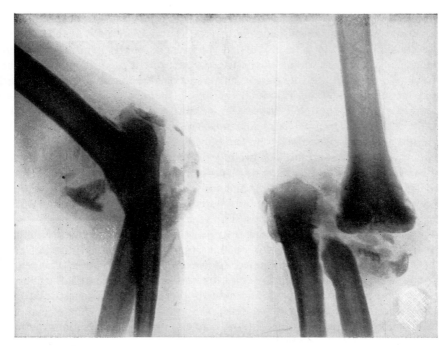

FIG. 96. Syringomyelia: Charcot elbow

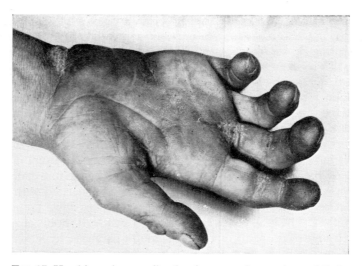

FIG. 97. Hand in syringomyelia, showing muscular wasting and fleshy
fingers with scars of burns

Syringobulbia

The medulla may be involved by upward extension from the spinal cord, or may be the initial site of the disorder. In the latter case the onset of symptoms may be sudden or gradual. Trigeminal pain, vertigo, facial, palatal, or laryngeal palsy, or wasting of the tongue may be the presenting symptom. The physical signs of syringobulbia have been described above.

Morvan's Disease

Morvan, in 1883, described the occurrence of painless whitlows upon the fingers of both hands [FIG. 98]. Similar lesions have also been described on the

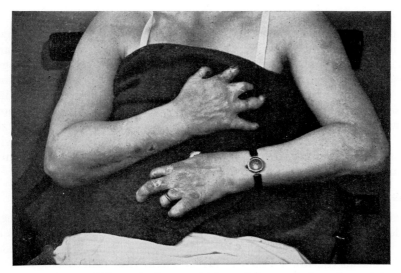

FIG. 98. A case of Morvan's disease, with loss of the terminal portions of the fingers

feet, and cutaneous ulceration may occur. Pain is not always absent. These trophic lesions are associated with muscular wasting of the hands and dissociated sensory loss over the upper extremities and sometimes over the feet. Perforating ulcers of the feet may occur. Morvan's disease is a rarity. Though it has been regarded as a form of syringomyelia in which trophic symptoms are unusually prominent, it is more probably the result in most cases of a progressive sensory neuropathy which may be inherited and which is due to degeneration of posterior root ganglion cells.

Associated Abnormalities

A large number of abnormalities have been described in association with syringomyelia, occurring either in affected individuals or in members of their families. Bremer (1926) drew attention to the following anomalies: deformities of the sternum, kyphoscoliosis, a difference in the size of the breasts, increase in the ratio between arm and body length, acrocyanosis of the hands, curved fingers, circumscribed sensory disturbances, enuresis, and so-called stigmas of degeneracy, such as anomalies of the hair and ears. Common abnormalities which may be added to Bremer's list include cervical rib, spina bifida, and pes cavus, while acromegaly is an occasional complication. Light brown pigmentation either in spots or diffuse sheets, often with a segmental distribution is common, especially on the shoulders.

The Cerebrospinal Fluid

The cerebrospinal fluid usually shows no abnormality unless the cavity has been large enough to cause a block when the protein content of the fluid may be raised.

Radiology

Straight radiographs of the cervical spine may show in some cases congenital anomalies (e.g. fusion of vertebral bodies) or may demonstrate that the antero-posterior diameter of the spinal canal is greater than normal. Prone myelography will usually confirm that the spinal cord itself is enlarged but supine examination of the region of the foramen magnum using injected air or contrast medium is necessary to show the descent of the cerebellar tonsils (Chiari type 1 anomaly) with which most cases are now known to be associated. When no such abnormality is demonstrated air encephalography or even ventriculography with air or contrast medium may be needed to show the closure of the exit foramina of the fourth ventricle which is present in some other cases.

DIAGNOSIS

There is little difficulty in making a diagnosis of syringomyelia when the disorder is advanced, since the association of wasting and trophic lesions of the hands with extensive dissociated sensory loss, and symptoms of corticospinal tract lesions in the lower limbs is highly distinctive. The diagnosis is much more difficult in the early stages and this is particularly important if treatment is to be effective. Intramedullary tumour of the spinal cord (especially ependymoma) may closely simulate syringomyelia. As a rule, however, it progresses more rapidly and blockage of the spinal subarachnoid space, with resulting changes in the cerebrospinal fluid, is likely to occur. The same is true of extramedullary spinal tumours with the addition that pain is usually a more prominent symptom of this lesion than of syringomyelia. Haematomyelia, though it may produce similar symptoms to syringomyelia, develops acutely. It must be remembered that haemorrhage into a syringomyelic cavity constitutes one form of haematomyelia. Cervical spondylosis, though it may cause wasting of proximal upper limb muscles and parasthesiae in the hands as well as spastic weakness of the lower limbs, does not cause dissociated sensory loss over the upper limbs. Cervical arthropathy may be hard to distinguish from spondylosis. Motor neurone disease may simulate syringomyelia when it begins with wasting of the small muscles of the hands, especially when the corticospinal fibres to the lower limbs are simultaneously involved. Sensory loss, however, is absent, and muscular wasting develops much more rapidly. In motor neurone disease muscular fasciculation is almost constantly present and is frequently widespread, whereas in syringomyelia it is less common. Cervical rib may cause symptoms which resemble those of the early stage of syringomyelia, and the distinction between the two is rendered difficult by the fact that they may coexist. Pain along the ulnar border of the hand and forearm is a common result of cervical rib, but rare in syringomyelia, and it is usual for the latter condition to come under observation at a stage at which sensory loss possesses an extent larger than can be attributed to a cervical rib. Peroneal muscular atrophy is distinguished from syringomyelia by the fact that muscular wasting of the lower limbs usually precedes that of the upper. The trophic symptoms of Raynaud's disease may simulate syringomyelia, but the dissociated sensory loss is absent in the former, while in the latter the attacks of blanching of the fingers observed in Raynaud's disease do not occur.

Syringobulbia presents little difficulty in diagnosis when the medullary lesion is an upward extension of cervical syringomyelia. When it occurs alone, however, it must be distinguished from other lesions of the medulla. Thrombosis of the posterior inferior cerebellar artery, which usually leads to sensory loss similar to that found in syringobulbia, is distinguished by its acute onset. Tumours of the medulla may closely simulate syringobulbia, especially as symptoms of increased intracranial pressure may be slight or absent, but the onset is more rapid, and extension to the pons, leading to paralysis of the lateral rectus or of conjugate ocular deviation and to facial paresis, is common in the case of medullary tumours and rare in syringobulbia. Progressive bulbar palsy is distinguished by the absence of sensory loss. The diagnosis of basilar impression, which may closely simulate syringomyelia, can be established only radiographically [see p. 917].

PROGNOSIS

The course of syringomyelia, if untreated, is progressive, though progress is frequently slow and remissions may occur, so that the patient's condition may remain unchanged for many years. A sudden intensification of symptoms may be produced by haemorrhage into a syringomyelic cavity, and occasionally distension of the spinal cord may become so marked as to produce a complete transverse lesion leading to paraplegia. Both of these events, however, are exceptional, and sufferers from syringomyelia frequently live many years, death occurring either from bulbar paralysis, leading to bronchopneumonia, or from some independent disease.

TREATMENT

In the past, apart from physiotherapeutic measures designed to reduce spasticity, delay contractures and improve movement in weakened limbs, treatment of this condition was largely symptomatic. The protection of analgesic areas and early treatment of cutaneous lesions in order to promote healing were also regarded as essential and remain obligatory today. In some cases continuous pain has required powerful analgesics and occasionally surgical methods for its relief, if intractable (medullary tractotomy or stereotaxic thalamotomy), have been required. Some surgeons have recommended laminectomy for decompression of the swollen spinal cord with aspiration or incision and drainage of the cavity but the results of the procedure have usually been disappointing. For many years radiotherapy, introduced first in 1905, had a considerable vogue and was believed to be particularly successful in relieving pain while some have suggested that sensory loss and muscular weakness and trophic changes were often reduced by this method. In recent years, however, its use has declined progressively.

The recent discovery that in most cases the condition is secondary to hydromyelia resulting from a developmental anomaly (Chiari malformation or Dandy-Walker syndrome) in the region of the foramen magnum (Gardner, 1965; Appleby et al., 1968) has prompted many surgeons to recommend that the upper cervical cord and lower medulla should be decompressed at the foramen magnum and that if the exit foramina of the fourth ventricle are occluded they should be opened up and the upper end of the central canal should then be occluded with muscle; aspiration of the central cavity may also be necessary. If carried out sufficiently early in the course of the disease, the results of these procedures seem encouraging in that dissociated sensory loss may gradually disappear and reflex changes may be reversed. Surgical treatment should thus be seriously considered in all cases seen within a few years of the onset but is unlikely to be helpful if the condition is long-established.

REFERENCES

APPLEBY, A., FOSTER, J. B., HANKINSON, J., and HUDGSON, P. (1968) The diagnosis and management of the Chiari anomalies in adult life, *Brain*, **91**, 131.

BREMER, F. W. (1926) Klinische Untersuchungen zur Ätiologie der Syringomyelie, der 'Status dysraphicus', *Dtsch. Z. Nervenheilk.*, **95**, 1.

CRUCHET, R., and DELMAS-MARSALET, P. (1939) Sur la maladie de Morvan, *Confin. neurol. (Basel)*, **2**, 32.

CURTIUS, F., and LORENZ, I. (1933) Über den Status dysraphicus, klinischerbbiologische und rassenhygienische Untersuchungen an 35 Fällen von Status dysraphicus und 17 Fällen von Syringomyelie, *Z. ges. Neurol. Psychiat.*, **149**, 1.

CZERNY, L. J., and HEINISMANN, J. I. (1930) Beiträge zur Pathologie und Röntgentherapieder Syringomyelie, *Z. ges. Neurol. Psychiat.*, **125**, 573.

GARDNER, W. J. (1965) Hydrodynamic mechanism of syringomyelia; its relationship to myelocele, *J. Neurol. Psychiat.*, **28**, 247.

JONESCO-SISESTI, N. (1929) *Tumeurs médullaires associées à un processus syringomyélique*, Paris.

JONESCO-SISESTI, N. (1932) *La syringobulbie*, Paris.

KIRCH, E. (1928) Über die pathogenetischen Beziehungen zwischen Rückenmarksgeschwülsten und Syringomyelie, *Z. ges. Neurol. Psychiat.*, **117**, 231.

LASSMAN, L. P., JAMES, C. C. M., and FOSTER, J. B. (1968) Hydromyelia, *J. neurol. Sci.*, **7**, 149.

PETRÉN, K., and LAURIN, E. (1925) Diagnosis of spinal tumors, with especial consideration of Röntgen-ray treatment of tumors and of syringomyelia, *Arch. Neurol. Psychiat. (Chicago)*, **14**, 1.

POUSSEPP, L. (1928) Traitement chirurgical de la syringomyélie, *Arch. franco-belges Chir.*, **30**, 293.

RILEY, H. A. (1930) Syringomyelia or myelodysplasia, *J. nerv. ment. Dis.*, **72**, 1.

SCHLESINGER, H. (1902) *Die Syringomyelie*, Leipzig.

MYELODYSPLASIA

Myelodysplasia is the term employed by Fuchs (1909) to describe a condition which he believes to be due to incomplete closure of the neural tube in the embryo. It is frequently familial and sometimes hereditary, and in some respects superficially resembles lumbar syringomyelia. Unlike the latter condition, however, it is non-progressive. The symptoms usually indicate a disturbance of function of the lumbosacral region of the spinal cord, though other parts may be affected. Myelodysplasia is closely related to spina bifida, with which it is usually associated. In the former, however, the spinal cord appears to be principally affected, in the latter the cauda equina.

Lumbosacral myelodysplasia has been held responsible for a variety of disturbances which are occasionally familial. The following are the principal symptoms: impairment of sphincter control, leading especially to enuresis; deformities of the feet, for example, pes cavus and syndactylism of the toes; wasting of the muscles below the knees, with impairment of the ankle-jerks; dissociated sensory loss of a syringomyelic character over one or both legs; and trophic disturbances of the feet, such as delayed healing of wounds, chronic ulceration, and gangrene. Spina bifida is almost always present but may only be apparent radiologically.

The commonest anatomical abnormality of the spinal cord is *diastematomyelia* (a bifid state of the lower cord). In many cases the two spinal cords are contained within a single dural tube but in others each of the two cords has its own dural sheath and the two are separated by a bony or fibrocartilaginous septum which may prevent the normal ascent of the cord as the vertebral column grows or else it may compress one or other spinal cord (James and Lassman, 1964). Either this anomaly itself or other associated lesions within the spinal cord which are commonly present in cases of 'spinal dysraphism' may demand surgical treatment which often produces considerable improvement. Rarely a similar anatomical anomaly in the cervical region may give a clinical picture resembling that of syringomyelia.

Myelodysplasia is distinguished from syringomyelia by the fact that it is frequently familial, by its non-progressive character, and by its predominant incidence upon the lower limbs. Other causes of muscular wasting and of trophic lesions of the feet must be excluded, especially peroneal muscular atrophy, familial polyneuritis, tabes, and gangrene of vascular origin.

The spinal defect upon which the symptoms depend is non-progressive, but there is a tendency for trophic lesions to occur and the patient may be progressively crippled by these.

X-ray irradiation of the affected region of the spinal cord has been tried, but has been largely discarded. It seems that in selected cases, particularly when the lesion is in the lumbar region, laminectomy with removal of bands which constrict or tether the spinal cord or its roots is sometimes beneficial.

REFERENCES

BIJE, L. (1956) *Status Dysrhaphicus*, Baarn.
BRUNS, F. (1903) Familiare symmetrischer Gangran und Arthropathie, *Neurol. Zbl.*, **22,** 599.

CURTIUS, F., and LORENZ, I. (1933) Über den Status dysraphicus, klinischerbbiologische und rassenhygienische Untersuchungen an 35 Fällen von Status dysraphicus und 17 Fällen von Syringomyelie, *Z. ges. Neurol. Psychiat.*, **149**, 1.

FUCHS, A. (1909) Über den klinischen Nachweis kongenitaler Defektbildungen in den unteren Rückenmarksabschnitten (Myelodysplasia), *Wien. med. Wschr.*, **59**, 2142, 2262.

JAMES, C. C. M., and LASSMAN, L. P. (1964) Diastematomyelia, *Arch. Dis. Childh.*, **39**, 125.

LICHTENSTEIN, B. W. (1940) Spinal dysraphism. Spina bifida and myelodysphasia, *Arch. Neurol. Psychiat. (Chicago)*, **44**, 792.

RILEY, H. A. (1930) Syringomyelia or myelodysplasia, *J. nerv. ment. Dis.*, **72**, 1.

THÉVENARD, A. (1942) L'arthropathie ulcéro-mutilante familiale, *Rev. neurol. (Paris)*, **74**, 193.

SPINA BIFIDA

Synonym. Rachischisis, spinal dysraphism.

Definition. Incomplete closure of the vertebral canal, which is usually associated with a similar anomaly of the spinal cord, or, when less severe, with other less striking intraspinal abnormalities.

AETIOLOGY AND PATHOLOGY

In the early embryo the nervous system is represented by the neural groove, the lateral folds of which unite dorsally to form the neural tube. An arrest in this process of development leads to defective closure of the neural tube, associated with a similar defect in the closure of the bony vertebral canal—spina bifida. A number of varieties of spina bifida are described, differing in respect of the nature and severity of the spinal defect. In the severe form a sac protrudes through the vertebral opening, which yields an impulse on crying and coughing, and compression of which in the infant increases the tension of the fontanelle. The sac may contain meninges only—meningocele; in more severe cases it contains both meninges and the flattened, opened or bifid spinal cord—myelocele or meningomyelocele. In such cases, when the cutaneous covering is incomplete, there may be a discharge of cerebrospinal fluid. Very rarely the central canal of the cord is closed but dilated—syringomyelocele. In the least severe cases there is no protrusion, but a defect in the laminae may be palpable as a depression, which is sometimes covered by a dimple or a tuft of hair (spina bifida occulta). There may, however, be no visible or palpable abnormality and the laminal defect may only then be detected radiologically. Spina bifida is sometimes hereditary.

The commonest site of spina bifida is the lumbosacral region. Occasionally it is found in the thoracic region, very rarely in the cervical. In lumbosacral spina bifida the spinal cord frequently retains its foetal length and extends as low as the sacrum. The flattened cord and nerve roots are often embedded in a pad of fat. Léri (1926) has described the occurrence in association with spina bifida of a fibrocartilaginous band compressing the cauda equina. James and Lassman (1967) have found in many cases of spina bifida occulta a variety of lesions including diastematomyelia, intramedullary dermoid, hydromyelia, cauda equina compression due to a fibrous band or to adhesions, ectopic dorsal nerve roots and subcutaneous lumbosacral lipoma communicating with a similar intraspinal lipoma. Spina bifida may be associated with other congenital abnormalities such as hydrocephalus due to atresia of the cerebral aqueduct or the Arnold-Chiari malformation of the medulla, occipital meningocele, cervical hydromyelia or syringomyelia, hare lip, and cleft palate. There may be general physical hypoplasia, with some degree of mental defect. Severe degrees of spina bifida may be incompatible with survival, the victim being stillborn or surviving birth only a short time. Paralysis of the lower limbs and of the sphincters is usually present in the latter case.

SYMPTOMS

Spina bifida occulta may give rise to no symptoms and may be an accidental discovery in the course of a routine examination. It is present in 17 per cent. of all spines X-rayed (Curtius and Lorenz, 1933). It is of considerable clinical importance, however, since it sometimes gives rise to symptoms, the cause of which is not immediately evident. In such cases a careful investigation of the history usually shows that symptoms were present at an early age, though improvement may have occurred, to be followed by a relapse in early adult life. However, in occasional cases, symptoms, say due to an intradural lipoma, may not appear until middle or late life. Such a relapse may be due to the effect of growth in causing tension upon the lower end of the cord and cauda equina, which are anchored at an abnormally low level, or to the compression of these structures by a lipoma, dermoid, or constricting band. The symptoms are those of a chronic lesion of the cauda equina, though frequently one function is more conspicuously affected than others.

Frequently it has been noted that the patient was slow in learning to walk and walked clumsily at first. Muscular wasting and weakness may be present in the muscles below the knees, with impairment or loss of the ankle-jerks and contracture of the calf muscles, leading to pes cavus. James and Lassman (1967) have drawn particular attention to a milder syndrome of progressive muscular imbalance and neurological deficit resulting in deformity of one or both feet in childhood with, in some cases, trophic ulceration and incontinence and point out that this syndrome resulting from minimal spinal dysraphism always demands investigation as early treatment may prevent progressive deformity. Sensation may be impaired over the cutaneous areas innervated by the lowest sacral segments, leading to the characteristic saddle-shaped area of analgesia over the buttocks and posterior surface of the thighs. Pain is usually inconspicuous. Sphincter disturbances are often prominent. Enuresis may be present, either constantly or intermittently, from infancy. The patient may have been late in gaining control over the bladder as a child, and this may never have become complete. Frequently nocturnal enuresis is associated with precipitate micturition by day. Less often retention of urine develops with secondary hydro-ureter and hydronephrosis and resulting impairment of renal function. Jancke (1916) described a sibship in which enuresis occurred in several generations and was associated with spina bifida in those members who were examined radiographically. The rectal sphincter is less often affected, though constipation or, less frequently, incontinence of faeces may occur. Impotence may be present in the male, either from the beginning of sexual life or after a period of normal potency. Trophic changes are conspicuous in some cases, and are rarely altogether lacking. In milder cases the feet are usually cold and cyanosed, and cutaneous injuries are slow in healing and tend to lead to ulceration, not only of the feet but also of the analgesic skin of the buttocks and thighs. Gangrene of the toes may occur and arthropathies have been described in the feet. Less common abnormalities include global atrophy of one lower limb, trophoedema of one lower limb (Léri), scleroderma, melanoleucoderma, and cutaneous naevi.

Cervical spina bifida occulta may be associated with hydromyelia or diastematomyelia causing symptoms resembling those of syringomyelia in the upper limbs, with wasting and trophic disturbances in the hands, and dissociated sensory loss.

The cerebrospinal fluid as a rule shows no abnormality, though lumbar puncture may be difficult or impossible at the usual level, owing to filling of the spinal canal with fat. Radiography shows defective fusion of the laminae in the affected region, usually the first sacral and fifth lumbar. Myelography is usually best performed by the cisternal route in such cases and is often successful in demonstrating diastematomyelia, an unusually low position of the conus medullaris, a typical filling defect due to a lipoma, or even a fibrous band constricting the cauda equina (Gryspeerdt, 1963).

DIAGNOSIS

The diagnosis of severe forms of spina bifida with a protruding sac is easy. Spina bifida occulta, however, may be missed, if it is not borne in mind as a possible cause of the symptoms of which the patient complains. All cases of enuresis for which no cause can be found, especially when precipitate micturition occurs by day, should be carefully investigated for the minor symptoms of spina bifida in the lower limbs, and radiographs of the lumbosacral spine should be taken. The more severe symptoms of spina bifida require to be differentiated from those of a tumour of the cauda equina, while, when trophic lesions are prominent, it is necessary to exclude Raynaud's disease and thrombo-angiitis obliterans. The fact that in spina bifida symptoms have often been present since birth is an important diagnostic point, and the rarity of pain and non-progressive character of the symptoms will help to exclude a tumour. The cerebrospinal fluid protein content is much more often raised when a tumour is present than in cases of dysraphism. The paroxysms of ischaemia characteristic of Raynaud's disease are absent in spina bifida and the arterial pulse is not reduced in volume, as is the case in thrombo-angiitis obliterans. X-ray examination of the spine and myelography afford confirmatory evidence.

PROGNOSIS

In the past, sufferers from the more severe degrees of spina bifida did not long survive. In the case of spina bifida occulta, although no improvement can be expected in the condition of the spinal cord and vertebral column, considerable functional improvement may follow appropriate treatment, especially in childhood. In selected cases benefit may follow operation. Spina bifida occulta does not usually shorten life, though occasionally death may occur as a result of infection of the urinary tract.

TREATMENT

Sharrard (1963) and others have shown that the survival rate of sufferers from meningomyelocele may be greatly increased and subsequent disability greatly reduced by operative closure of the sac within the first 48 hours of life. Subsequently neurosurgical treatment may be required for associated hydrocephalus and a variety of orthopaedic procedures may also be needed. Even if the lower limbs appear totally paralysed and anaesthetic, walking may eventually be possible with the aid of appropriate appliances if training is begun sufficiently early, usually towards the end of the second year of life. Incontinence of urine may be controlled in some cases by propantheline given in doses graded according to age, 15 mg. three times daily in the adult, while retention of urine may initially require catheterization followed later by bladder neck resection. Urinary infection will require appropriate antibiotics and incontinence of faeces is usually controlled eventually by the use of suppositories, regular enemas or even, in some cases, manual evacuation as the child grows older.

There is now good evidence that in cases of spina bifida occulta, operation carried out soon after symptoms first become apparent, to divide a constricting band, remove or decompress a lipoma or a dermoid cyst may produce considerable improvement and prevent progressive deformity. This is particularly important in childhood so that growth of an affected limb will not be impaired but operation may be equally successful if symptoms first develop in adult life.

REFERENCES

CURTIUS, F., and LORENZ, I. (1933) Über den Status dysraphicus, klinischerbäiologische und rassenhygienische Untersuchungen an 35 Fällen von Status dysraphicus und 17 Fällen von Syringomyelie, *Z. ges. Neurol. Psychiat.*, **149**, 1.

GOZZANO, M. (1926) A case of cervicodorsal spina bifida occulta, *Arch. Neurol. Psychiat. (Chicago)*, **15**, 702.

GRYSPEERDT, G. L. (1963) Myelographic assessment of occult forms of spinal dysraphism, *Acta radiol. (Stockh.)*, N.S., **1**, 702.

HASSIN, G. B. (1925) Spina bifida occulta cervicalis, *Arch. Neurol. Psychiat. (Chicago)*, **14**, 813.

JAMES, C. C. M., and LASSMAN, L. P. (1967) Results of treatment of progressive lesions in spina bifida occulta five to ten years after laminectomy, *Lancet*, ii, 1277.

JANCKE (1915–16) Über eine Bettnässerfamilie, zugleich ein Beitrag zur Erblichkeit der Spina bifida, *Dtsch. Z. Nervenheilk.*, **54**, 255; also, Röntgenbefunde bei Bettnässern, *Dtsch. Z. Nervenheilk.*, **55**, 334.

LASSMAN, L. P., and JAMES, C. C. M. (1967) Lumbosacral lipomas: critical survey of 26 cases admitted to laminectomy, *J. Neurol. Psychiat.*, **30**, 174.

LÉRI, A. (1926) *Études sur les affections de la colone vertébrale*, Paris.

LICHTENSTEIN, B. W. (1942) Distant neuro-anatomic complications of spina bifida (spinal dysraphism), *Arch. Neurol. Psychiat. (Chicago)*, **47**, 195.

ROBERTS, J. B. M. (1962) Spina bifida and the urinary tract, *Ann. roy. Coll. Surg. Engl.*, **31**, 69.

SHARRARD, W. J. W. (1963) Meningomyelocele: prognosis of immediate operative closure of the sac, *Proc. roy. Soc. Med.*, **56**, 510.

MYELITIS

Definition. Inflammation of the spinal cord, usually involving both the grey and the white matter, in a considerable part of its transverse extent. When the lesion is limited longitudinally to a few segments, it is described as transverse myelitis; when it spreads progressively upwards, as ascending myelitis.

AETIOLOGY

Myelitis may be a manifestation of meningovascular syphilis [see pp. 410–13]. It may be due to participation of the cord in acute or subacute encephalomyelitis due to a neurotropic virus or in acute disseminated encephalomyelitis, disseminated myelitis and optic neuritis, and acute disseminated encephalomyelitis complicating vaccination, smallpox, measles, chickenpox, or other specific fevers. An episode indistinguishable from an attack of transverse myelitis may be one presentation of multiple sclerosis.

Myelitis may be due to infections of the cord with pyogenic organisms, which may reach it through a penetrating wound, by extension from osteomyelitis of an adjacent vertebra, by inward spread from pyogenic meningitis, e.g. meningococcal meningitis, or through the blood stream from a focus of infection in any part of the body, the latter being the route of infection when myelitis complicates typhoid fever or brucellosis. Tuberculous myelitis may follow tuberculous caries of the spine.

PATHOLOGY

To the naked eye the spinal cord at the site of infection, which is usually the lower thoracic region, exhibits oedema and hyperaemia, and in severe cases actual softening—myelomalacia. Microscopically, the leptomeninges are congested and infiltrated with inflammatory cells. The substance of the cord exhibits congestion or thrombosis of the vessels with perivascular inflammatory infiltration, and oedema. There is degeneration of the ganglion cells of the grey matter, the myelin sheaths and axis cylinders of the white. The cord is diffusely infiltrated with inflammatory cells and with compound granular corpuscles. There is a hyperplasia of neuroglia. Ascending and descending degeneration can be traced in the long tracts. Abscess of the spinal cord is a very rare form of localized myelitis. The pus is to a variable extent encapsulated and, as it tends to spread longitudinally, the abscess usually assumes a spindle shape. When myelitis is due to pyogenic organisms, these may be demonstrable in films or on culture, and spirochaetes may be present in the syphilitic form, but in myelitis forming part of acute disseminated encephalomyelitis and in the form which occurs sporadically no infecting organism has yet been demonstrated and it seems likely that this is an acute demyelinating process due to hypersensitivity rather than infection.

SYMPTOMS

The onset of symptoms is acute or subacute, and there is often some pyrexia. There is usually considerable pain in the back at the level of the lesion. Flaccid paralysis, partial or complete, then develops more or less rapidly, being confined to part of the trunk and the lower limbs when the thoracic region of the cord is the part involved. Sensory loss, which may be complete or incomplete, is present and usually exhibits an upper level corresponding to the segmental site of the lesion. There may be a zone of hyperalgesia intervening between the area of sensory loss and that of normal sensibility above, and the spine may be tender in this region. There is an impairment of sphincter control, often amounting to complete paralysis of the bladder and rectum. The tendon reflexes are usually at first diminished or lost, and the abdominal reflexes are lost below the level of the lesion. The plantar reflexes may be absent for a few days after the onset and later become extensor. In the ascending form of myelitis there is a more or less rapid upward progression of the level of paralysis and sensory loss.

The cerebrospinal fluid usually contains a considerably increased protein content and an excess of cells, which are polymorphonuclear in cases of pyogenic myelitis, but usually exclusively or predominantly mononuclear in other forms. Queckenstedt's test usually indicates an absence of obstruction in the subarachnoid space, except in rare cases when meningeal adhesions develop. The V.D.R.L. and other serological reactions are negative, except in syphilitic cases.

DIAGNOSIS

The rapid onset of the symptoms of a transverse or ascending lesion of the spinal cord usually renders the diagnosis easy. Myelitis is distinguished from acute infective or post-infective polyneuritis (the Guillain-Barré syndrome) by the presence of extensor plantar reflexes, and of partial or complete sensory loss with a segmental upper level. Haematomyelia usually develops more rapidly than myelitis; it usually involves the cervical enlargement and causes greater damage to the grey than to the white matter of the cord. Syphilitic myelitis is distinguished by the history of infection and signs of cerebral syphilis, when these are present, and by positive serological reactions in the blood and cerebrospinal fluid. When myelitis forms part of an attack of acute disseminated encephalomyelitis, symptoms of cerebral lesions may be present, and in the cases following vaccination and the specific fevers the causal condition is usually readily discovered from the history. In disseminated myelitis and optic neuritis the diagnosis is clear when the latter precedes the former. Otherwise it must remain in doubt until optic neuritis develops. When myelitis complicates poliomyelitis, the patient exhibits in addition the typical atrophic paralysis. In zoster myelitis the diagnosis is established by the characteristic eruption. Though multiple sclerosis may be suspected as the cause of a transverse lesion of the spinal cord, especially in a young adult, this diagnosis can only be established if there is a history of previous and characteristic lesions of the nervous system, or if signs of this—for example, pallor of the optic discs or nystagmus—are present. Myelitis can be attributed to infection with pyogenic organisms only when a focus of such infection can be found or the organism grown.

PROGNOSIS

The prognosis depends upon the aetiology of the condition and its severity. Pyogenic myelitis is usually fatal, and so is the ascending form but occasional cases of intramedullary abscess have been treated successfully by means of antibiotics and surgical drainage and methods of mechanically-aided respiration have saved many patients who would previously have died of ascending myelitis. Any form of myelitis which is sufficiently severe to lead to a complete functional interruption of the cord is a very grave condition owing to the risk of death from urinary or cutaneous infection. However, even in such cases if complications are treated effectively, recovery is possible. In myelitis forming part of one of the various forms of acute disseminated encephalomyelitis the prognosis is often good, and if the patient survives the acute attack a large degree of functional recovery is the rule. In sporadic cases of myelitis a guarded prognosis should be given in view of the possibility that the cord lesion may be the first symptom of multiple sclerosis. For the prognosis of syphilitic myelitis see page 413, and for that of acute disseminated myelitis with optic neuritis see page 491.

TREATMENT

The general treatment of the patient must be carried out on the lines indicated for the treatment of paraplegia [see p. 628]. Any specific cause must receive appropriate treatment. For the treatment of syphilitic myelitis see page 413, and for that of acute disseminated myelitis with optic neuritis see page 493.

In those cases in which no cause for the condition can be demonstrated (these are the majority) there is now good evidence that treatment with ACTH, 80 Units intramuscularly daily, when given in the acute phase and continued for several weeks or months in diminishing dosage improves the outcome.

REFERENCES

BUZZARD, E. F., and GREENFIELD, J. G. (1921) *Pathology of the Nervous System*, London.
DAVISON, C., and KESCHNER, M. (1933) Myelitic and myelopathic lesions (a clinico-pathologic study). 1. Myelitis, *Arch. Neurol. Psychiat. (Chicago)*, **29**, 332.
HUGHES, J. T. (1966) *Pathology of the Spinal Cord*, London.

RADIATION MYELOPATHY

A syndrome of slowly progressive paraparesis, due to radiation injury to the spinal cord, may develop one to four years after a course of ionizing radiation given usually to the neck or mediastinum for the treatment of post-cricoid carcinoma or bronchial carcinoma with mediastinal spread. Weakness, spasticity, and sensory loss usually develop gradually and the condition often becomes arrested. The cerebrospinal fluid is usually normal and so, too, is myelography. The dose of radiation given has almost always exceeded 4,000 r and is usually of the order of 6,000–8,000 r. Pathologically, vacuolation and degeneration of the neurones and white-matter degeneration are seen while the spinal arterioles and capillaries are usually greatly thickened and show narrowing of their lumina.

REFERENCE

HUGHES, J. T. (1966) *Pathology of the Spinal Cord*, London.

SUBACUTE NECROTIC MYELITIS

This condition, first described by Foix and Alajouanine (1926) and subsequently by Greenfield and Turner (1939) and by Mair and Folkerts (1953) is commoner in men than in women and is commoner in the older age group, particularly in patients with chronic cor pulmonale. Clinically it is characterized by a slowly progressive and ascending weakness of the lower extremities with variable sensory loss and sphincter disturbance; there are signs of combined upper and lower motor neurone lesions and the clinical picture indicates a slowly progressive disorder of the cauda equina and lower spinal cord extending over several years. The protein content of the cerebrospinal fluid is usually raised and myelography, which is necessary to exclude a spinal tumour, is either negative or may demonstrate dilated blood vessels on the surface of the cord. Pathologically the cord is shown to be necrotic and there is widespread distension and often thrombosis of veins on the surface and within its substance. Some authors believe that the condition is due to a spinal thrombophlebitis (Blackwood, 1963), others that there is true venous angioma formation. No treatment is available though the condition is so rarely diagnosed in life that anticoagulants have not been given an adequate trial.

REFERENCES

BLACKWOOD, W. (1963) in *Greenfield's Neuropathology*, 2nd ed., ed. BLACKWOOD, W., McMENEMEY, W. H., MEYER, A., NORMAN, R. M., and RUSSELL, D. S., London.
FOIX, C., and ALAJOUANINE, T. (1926) La myélite nécrotique subaiguë, *Rev. neurol.*, **2**, 1.
GREENFIELD, J. G., and TURNER, J. W. A. (1939) Acute and subacute necrotic myelitis, *Brain*, **62**, 227.
MAIR, W. G. P., and FOLKERTS, J. F. (1953) Necrosis of the spinal cord due to thrombophlebitis (subacute necrotic myelitis), *Brain*, **76**, 563.

LANDRY'S PARALYSIS

In 1859 Landry first described a condition of acute ascending paralysis and subsequently the name 'Landry's paralysis' was commonly given to cases showing such a clinical presentation. It is now well recognized that this is a syndrome and not a single disease entity and the use of the term as a definitive diagnosis can no longer be justified. In very acute cases which present with sensory disturbance in the limbs followed by the rapid development of flaccid areflexic paralysis and a fatal outcome, usually within a few days, the condition can usually be classified pathologically as one of *acute necrotic myelopathy* (Hughes, 1966). *Transverse* or *ascending myelitis* as described above may also give rise to a clinical picture of ascending paralysis of variable severity, while *post-infective polyneuritis* or *polyradiculopathy* (the Guillain-Barré syndrome) is yet another cause. The episodes of ascending paralysis which may follow acute exanthemata or inoculation, particularly with rabies vaccine are plainly due to acute disseminated or ascending myelitis while during epidemics, occasional cases of poliomyelitis may present in this way, as may the acute polyneuropathy which complicates some cases of porphyria. A toxin produced by the bite of the Rocky Mountain wood tick has been known to produce similar symptoms which resolve when the tick is removed (Gibbes, 1938) while Symonds (1949) described such a syndrome associated with a high serum potassium due to renal failure. Thus the prognosis and management of cases so-called 'Landry's paralysis' are dependent upon the elucidation of the cause of the syndrome in every case.

REFERENCES

GIBBES, J. H. (1938) Tick paralysis in South Carolina, *J. Amer. med. Ass.*, **111,** 1008.
HUGHES, J. T. (1966) *Pathology of the Spinal Cord*, London.
LANDRY, O. (1859) Note sur la paralysie ascendante aiguë, *Gaz. hebd. Méd.*, **6,** 472.
SYMONDS, C. P. (1949) Reorientation in neurology, *Lancet*, i. 677.

INFARCTION AND ISCHAEMIA OF THE SPINAL CORD AND CAUDA EQUINA

The Blood Supply of the Spinal Cord and Cauda Equina

In the cervical and upper thoracic regions the major blood supply of the spinal cord is derived from the anterior spinal artery, which is formed by the union of the two anterior spinal branches which arise from the vertebral arteries within the cranial cavity. It runs in the anterior median fissure of the cord and receives small tributaries at different levels from the inferior thyroid arteries and from the costocervical trunk, each of which is derived from the corresponding subclavian artery. The anterior spinal artery supplies the anterior and lateral columns of the cord and the greater part of the spinal grey matter. The two small posterior spinal arteries also arise from the vertebrals intracranially and receive numerous small radicular tributaries entering the spinal cord along the posterior nerve roots; they supply the posterior columns of the cord. There are scanty circumferential vessels on the surface of the cord which form anastomoses between the anterior and posterior spinal vessels.

In the lower thoracic and lumbar regions the anterior and posterior spinal arteries receive large tributaries from the intercostal and lumbar branches of the aorta which contribute the major blood supply of the lower cord. One such vessel, the great anterior radicular artery of Adamkewicz (1882) which usually enters the spinal cord at about the T8 segment but may do so at any level from T8 to L4, appears to be of particular importance. The vessels in the lowest segments of the cord and the roots of the cauda equina receive tributaries from the iliolumbar and lateral sacral branches of the internal iliac arteries. Published work on the anatomy of the spinal cord arterial tree and upon its variable and inconstant but profuse venous drainage has been reviewed recently by Hughes (1966), Garland, Greenberg, and Harriman (1966), and by Henson and Parsons (1967).

Infarction of the Spinal Cord and Cauda Equina

Occlusion of the *anterior spinal artery* in the cervical region was shown by Spiller (1909) to produce infarction of the anterior and lateral columns of the cord from the fourth cervical to the third thoracic segments. Clinically the onset is abrupt, often with pain in the neck and back and paraesthesiae in the upper limbs followed by flaccid paralysis of both arms with loss of pain and temperature sensation below a variable level in the cervical region but with preservation of light touch and position and joint sense. Initially there is usually also flaccid paralysis of the lower limbs (spinal shock) but if the patient survives spastic weakness of the lower limbs develops with increased reflexes and extensor plantar responses. There is usually retention of urine and of faeces in the early stages but automatic bladder and bowel control may eventually be achieved. In severe cases paralysis remains complete and the prognosis is grave, but when infarction is less extensive the lower limbs may show a remarkable degree of recovery.

Anterior spinal artery occlusion in the dorsal region is commonly a complication of dissecting aneurysm of the aorta, though it may result from embolism as a result of disintegration of an atheromatous plaque in the aorta (Wolman and Bradshaw, 1967). When dissecting aneurysm is the cause and occasionally in other cases, there is severe pain in the back followed by total and permanent flaccid paralysis of the lower limbs, sphincter paralysis and loss of pain and temperature sensation up to a sensory 'level' at about the umbilicus (corresponding to the T10 segment of the cord), but with preservation of some light touch sensation and of position and joint sense.

While the clinical picture of anterior spinal artery occlusion has been recognized for many years, increasing attention has been paid more recently to the fact that infarction of the cord may sometimes be much more restricted, possibly due to occlusion of one posterior spinal artery or of one or more feeding or radicular arteries. In such cases weakness and sensory impairment may be restricted to one limb or may be asymmetrical in the two lower limbs and considerable or even complete recovery may take place after such a localized infarct. While rare by comparison with intermittent cerebral ischaemia, it also seems probable that transient episodes of weakness and of paraesthesiae in the lower extremities may well be due in many cases to *transient ischaemia of the spinal cord* or *cauda equina* (Wells, 1966; Garland, Greenberg, and Harriman, 1966; Henson and Parsons, 1967). Furthermore, there is now pathological evidence to suggest that repeated episodes of ischaemia or focal infarction may give rise to a slowly progressive spastic weakness of the lower limbs with variable sensory loss and signs of mixed upper and lower motor neurone involvement. In such cases of *atherosclerotic myelopathy*, a step-wise clinical course with episodes of deterioration alternating with periods of apparent arrest may suggest the nature of the disease, as may associated clinical evidence of atherosclerosis, but inflammatory, demyelinating, and neoplastic disorders must be excluded by means of radiology, cerebrospinal fluid examination, serological tests to exclude syphilis, and myelography. Rarely, collagen disease such as polyarteritis nodosa may give rise to episodes of spinal cord infarction.

Spinal cord embolism (Wolman and Bradshaw, 1967) due to the breakdown of an atheromatous plaque in the aorta so that fragments of cholesterol-containing debris are swept into the arteries of the cord, may give episodes of major infarction or chronic ischaemic myelopathy as described above. Similar episodes have been described in cases of subacute bacterial endocarditis; air and fat embolism of the cord appear to be very rare but decompression sickness (Caisson disease, p. 705) occurring during decompression in divers and compressed-air workers, in which bubbles of nitrogen appear in the circulating blood, commonly gives rise to transient episodes of spinal cord dysfunction and very occasionally to irreversible paraplegia (Haymaker, 1957).

Treatment, other than the usual nursing care of patients with paraplegia, is of little value in cases of spinal cord infarction. Vasodilator drugs may reasonably be given, but seem to be of little value and in cases of intermittent ischaemia or progressive myelopathy there are theoretical reasons for suggesting that anti-coagulant drugs may be worthy of a trial. Surgical treatment of an aortic dissecting aneurysm is of no value once cord infarction has occurred.

Intermittent Claudication or Ischaemia of the Spinal Cord or Cauda Equina

In 1906 Dejerine first suggested that transient weakness or numbness of one or both lower limbs occurring during exercise might be due to ischaemia of the spinal cord. It is now well recognized that in some patients the lower spinal cord or the roots of the cauda equina may suffer a degree of compression which is sufficient to restrict their arterial blood supply but is not sufficient to give rise to any symptoms or abnormal physical signs at rest. However, when the patient begins to walk he often develops first aching pain in one or both calves similar to that of true intermittent claudication, but the peripheral pulses in the legs and feet are found to be normal. If he continues to walk, paraesthesiae in one or both feet may then supervene and it is not uncommon for foot-drop to follow (in ischaemia of the cauda equina) or spastic weakness of one or both legs (in ischaemia of the cord). In suspected cases the symptoms may be precipitated by appropriate exercise under supervision; when the cauda equina is principally affected one or both ankle jerks may disappear, while if the lower cord is being compressed the plantar responses may become extensor.

The condition can usually be shown by radiography and myelography, which are obligatory investigations in such cases, to be due to either a central inter-vertebral disc protrusion (Blau and Logue, 1961) or, in cases involving the cauda equina, a bony stenosis of the lumbar canal resulting from an overgrowth (of unknown aetiology) of the bony laminae (Verbiest, 1954; Joffe, Appleby, and Arjona, 1966). In either event, laminectomy and decompression of the spinal canal usually produces complete relief of symptoms.

REFERENCES

BLAU, J. N., and LOGUE, V. (1961) Intermittent claudication of the cauda equina, *Lancet,* i, 1081.

DÉJERINE, J. (1906) Sur la claudication intermittente de la moelle épinière, *Rev. neurol.,* **33,** 1.

GARLAND, H., GREENBERG, J., and HARRIMAN, D. G. F. (1966) Infarction of the spinal cord, *Brain,* **89,** 645.

HAYMAKER, W. (1957) Decompression sickness, in *Handbuch der Speziellen Pathologischen Anatomie und Histologie,* vol. 13, ed. SCHOLZ, W., p. 1600, Berlin.

HENSON, R. A., and PARSONS, M. (1967) Ischaemic lesions of the spinal cord: an illustrated review, *Quart. J. Med.*, **36**, 205.

HUGHES, J. T. (1966) *Pathology of the Spinal Cord*, London.

JOFFE, R., APPLEBY, A., and ARJONA, V. (1966) 'Intermittent ischaemia' of the cauda equina due to stenosis of the lumbar canal, *J. Neurol. Neurosurg. Psychiat.*, **29**, 315.

SPILLER, W. G. (1909) Thrombosis of the cervical anterior median spinal artery: syphilitic acute anterior poliomyelitis, *J. nerv. ment. Dis.*, **36**, 601.

VERBIEST, H. (1954) A radicular syndrome from developmental narrowing of the lumbar vertebrae canal, *J. Bone Jt. Surg.*, **36B**, 230.

WELLS, C. E. C. (1966) Clinical aspects of spinovascular disease, *Proc. roy. Soc. Med.*, **59**, 790.

WOLMAN, L., and BRADSHAW, P. (1967) Spinal cord embolism, *J. Neurol. Neurosurg. Psychiat.*, **30**, 446.

15

INTOXICATIONS AND METABOLIC DISORDERS

ALCOHOL ADDICTION

AETIOLOGY

ALCOHOL addiction is a symptom of many different mental disorders and every case requires careful psychological investigation. It is more common in males than in females, is rare before the age of 20, and most frequently occurs in middle life. A parental incidence of alcoholism is frequently present, and there is a history of alcoholism in one or both parents of 30 per cent. of patients admitted to institutions for inebriates. Alcoholism may be a symptom of loss of self-control associated with the early stages of dementia, due, for example, to general paresis or cerebral arteriosclerosis. It may occur in schizophrenia or in manic-depressive psychosis. Though alcoholism is less common in females than males there appears to be a higher incidence of psychopathic personality in female than in male alcoholics. In some cases of dipsomania the periodicity of the outbreaks of alcoholism is due to a periodically recurrent depression in an individual with cyclothymia. Alcohol addicts who are not frankly psychotic are usually neurotic, and take alcohol as a means of escape from the difficulties of life. Business worries and domestic unhappiness are common secondary causes. The alcohol is often taken in the form of spirits; and the alcohol addict may also be a drug addict. Indeed there is some evidence that there are personality traits common to many of those who become addicted to any drug, of which alcohol is one.

INCIDENCE

It has been estimated that there are 4,390 alcoholics per 100,000 in the U.S.A. and at least 1,100 per 100,000 in England and Wales (Sim, 1968). There are important and complex differences in the incidence observed in various racial and ethnic groups (Jellinek, 1951; Williams and Glatt, 1965) but almost every country appears to have its 'skid-row' where down-and-out intractable drinkers and those who consume methyl alcohol tend to congregate (Bourne, Alford, and Bowcock, 1966; Edwards *et al.*, 1966; Olin, 1966).

PATHOLOGY

The prolonged consumption of alcohol produces degenerative changes in the central nervous system and in the peripheral nerves, which in their general features are similar to the effects of a large variety of other toxic agents. The brain is atrophied, and microscopically there is degeneration of the ganglion cells of the cerebral cortex. Degeneration of the middle layers of the corpus callosum is said to be characteristic (Marchiafava, 1933; Ironside, Bosanquet, and Mc-Menemey, 1961). There is an increase in the capillaries and a secondary glial hyperplasia. Haemorrhages are common. In cases of polyneuritis the peripheral nerves exhibit degeneration of their myelin sheaths and sometimes also of the axis cylinders. There is evidence that the neuritis, both central and peripheral, is not directly due to the alcohol, but is caused by deficiency of Vitamin B_1 [see p. 817]. This is also the cause of Wernicke's encephalopathy, which may complicate chronic alcoholism. Similarly alcoholic pellagra occurs. Victor and Adams (1961) conclude that whereas delirium tremens, alcoholic epilepsy, and alcoholic hallucinosis are due to habituation and alcohol withdrawal, and while Wernicke's disease, Korsakow's syndrome, polyneuropathy, retrobulbar neuropathy, and pellagra are due to nutritional deficiencies which are associated with alcoholism, the pathogenesis of alcoholic cerebellar degeneration, central pontine myelinolysis [see p. 507], of Marchiafava-Bignami disease and of alcoholic dementia is not yet fully understood and some of these disorders could prove to be due to a direct toxic effect of the long-continued ingestion of large quantities of alcohol. Cardiomyopathy and acute and chronic myopathic syndromes involving skeletal muscle have also been described in alcoholic patients (Perkoff, Hardy, and Velez-Garcia, 1966).

SYMPTOMS

Acute Alcoholic Intoxication

The action of alcohol upon the nervous system is paralytic, the highest functions being first affected. The earliest symptoms of intoxication, therefore, are those of altered behaviour, and the social value of alcohol in moderate doses rests upon its power of paralysing those inhibitions which manifest themselves as shyness, and of reducing, in the individual who takes it, his capacity for criticizing his own utterances, and those of others. In larger doses it produces irregularities in conduct, the nature of which depends upon the temperament of the individual, who may be excited, voluble, combative, depressed, or maudlin. There is impairment of memory, especially for recent events. The ability to carry out co-ordinated and complex motor acts is progressively impaired and since October 1967 in Great Britain it has been an offence in law to drive a motor vehicle when the blood alcohol exceeds 80 mg./100 ml. In the Scandinavian countries the legal limit is very much lower. Eventually articulation becomes impaired; the conjunctivae are congested; the pupils are usually dilated, but may be contracted, and there may be some impairment of the pupillary reaction to light; nystagmus is invariable and diplopia may occur. In still larger doses alcohol produces unconsciousness, and finally death, through extension of the paralysis to vital centres.

The relationship between the alcoholic content of the blood and the state of the nervous system is variable. A great deal depends upon the body weight of the drinker, upon whether the simultaneous or previous ingestion of food delays the absorption of the alcohol, and upon whether or not the individual in question is accustomed to taking alcoholic drinks. In general there are few if any signs of intoxication with a blood level of below 100 mg./100 ml. although between 50 and 100 mg./100 ml. some lack of inhibition and impairment of motor skills, with a slowing of reaction time, are generally apparent. Intoxication is usually clearly apparent in conversation with or on examining the individual with a blood level of 150 mg./100 ml. but he is usually still in reasonable control of his behaviour and faculties at about this level, whereas at 200 mg./100 ml. the signs of drunkenness are usually evident and consciousness is generally lost, except in habitual heavy drinkers or alcoholic subjects, at a level between 250 and 300 mg./100 ml. As a very rough guide, up to three single 'tots' of spirit or three half-pints of British beer will, in the average individual, give a blood level within an hour of between 50 and 75 mg./100 ml.

Methyl Alcohol

The consumption of methyl alcohol in the form of methylated spirits, industrial alcohol, anti-freeze, and filtered metal polish is mainly seen in the poor in countries where alcoholic drinks are expensive, or in exceptionally degenerate alcoholics. It may cause severe toxic confusional states, irreversible optic atrophy with bilateral central scotomata or even total blindness and sometimes rapid death.

Pathological Drunkenness

In certain individuals, especially those who have suffered from head injury or organic lesions of the brain, a comparatively small dose of alcohol may rapidly produce the symptoms of acute intoxication and this may also occur in individuals taking barbiturate drugs regularly, in whom alcohol has an additive effect.

Delirium Tremens

The precise cause of delirium tremens is still uncertain. It is most frequently seen as the result of a prolonged debauch in the chronic alcoholic, but may be precipitated in such an individual by acute infection, or operation, or an accident. The sudden deprivation of alcohol is undoubtedly the most important factor.

The onset may be acute, but there is often a prodromal period of nervousness, anorexia, and insomnia. The characteristic symptoms are tremor, and acute confusion, accompanied by hallucinations, which are principally visual. The tremor is coarse and generalized, and is most evident in the face, tongue, and hands. The patient is completely disorientated, and experiences visual hallucinations, which usually assume terrifying forms, especially animals. Auditory hallucinations may also be present, and cutaneous sensations may be interpreted as insects crawling under the skin. The emotional mood is usually one of terror, and the patient may attempt to escape from his surroundings, and attack with violence those around him. Convulsions may occur. In addition to these nervous disturbances, symptoms of a severe toxaemia are present. Hyperpyrexia is not uncommon, and there may be albuminuria. The tongue is furred, the pulse rapid, and cardiac dilatation may occur. Delirium tremens runs an acute course, and in most cases recovery occurs in three or four days. In cases which end fatally, death is due to heart failure in which dehydration plays an important part, or to intercurrent lobar pneumonia to which such individuals are peculiarly subject.

Acute Alcoholic Hallucinosis

This condition occurs in chronic alcoholics, either developing gradually or coming on suddenly after unusual excess. It is characterized by hallucinations which, unlike those in delirium tremens, are predominantly auditory and are often associated with delusions of persecution.

Dipsomania

In true dipsomania the patient has recurrent drinking-bouts ('the lost week-end'), the craving for alcohol suddenly developing after a period of abstinence. This condition is to be distinguished from pseudodipsomania, in which a chronic alcoholic exceeds his usual consumption of alcohol.

Korsakow's Psychosis

Korsakow's psychosis, though most frequently the result of chronic alcoholism with polyneuritis, may be due to other causes [see p. 982]. The characteristic feature of Korsakow's psychosis is a disturbance of attention and memory, which leads to the disorientation of the patient in space and time. His memory for recent events and his ability to retain new impressions are lost, and he fills the gap by confabulation, that is, the invention of a purely imaginary past. For example, one who has been bedridden for weeks describes with a wealth of detail a walk which he took on the previous day. Many clinical varieties of Korsakow's psychosis have been described, chiefly in terms of variations of the emotional mood, which is usually euphoric.

Alcoholic Cerebellar Degeneration

Victor, Adams, and Mancall (1959) described 50 cases of this condition which is characterized by ataxia of stance and gait and of leg movements with little or no involvement of the arms (apart from action tremor which is seen in a few cases); nystagmus and dysarthria are absent in most cases. The condition appeared to progress over a period of a few weeks or months and then to become arrested in most cases. Pathological observations in 11 cases revealed a degeneration of all neurocellular elements of the cerebellar cortex, particularly of the Purkinje cells and also degeneration of the olivary nuclei. In the cerebellum changes were most striking in the anterior and superior aspects of the vermis and of the hemispheres.

Marchiafava-Bignami Disease

This rare condition, originally described in Italian drinkers of crude red wine is now known to occur in other alcoholic patients. It is characterized clinically by disorders of emotional control and cognitive function followed by variable delirium, fits, tremor, rigidity, and paralysis and most patients eventually become comatose and die within a few months. Symmetrical demyelination with subsequent cavitation and destruction of axis cylinders is found in the corpus callosum and often, in varying degree, in the central white matter of the cerebral hemispheres, in the optic chiasm, and in the middle cerebellar peduncles (Victor and Adams, 1961).

Alcoholic Dementia

Prolonged addiction to alcohol leads in many cases to progressive mental deterioration. There is nothing distinctive in the nature of the resulting dementia, which is characterized, like other dementias, by impairment of memory and intellectual capacity, emotional instability, moral deterioration, and carelessness with regard to dress and person. Delusions may be present, a delusion of marital infidelity being particularly common.

Alcoholic dementia may be associated with dysarthria, tremor, sluggish pupillary reactions to light, and muscular weakness.

The full clinical picture of alcoholic polyneuritis may be present, but even in the absence of this the tendon reflexes are likely to be lost in the lower limbs.

Epilepsy

Epileptic attacks are not uncommon in chronic alcoholism, and are indistinguishable from the convulsions of idiopathic epilepsy. The convulsions of absinthe drinkers are due to the presence in the drink of the convulsant drug thujone. How other forms of alcohol cause epilepsy is not clearly understood. It would appear that fits may occur either at the height of a debauch ('rum fits' are then presumably due to the intoxication), or after withdrawal of alcohol when they may be compared with the attacks which occur on the withdrawal of other drugs such as barbiturates.

Polyneuritis

The symptoms of polyneuritis which may complicate any form of chronic alcoholism are described on page 818 and pellagra is described on page 731.

Central Pontine Myelinolysis

This rare complication of alcoholism is considered on page 507.

Alcoholic Myopathy

In 1962 Hed *et al.* described an acute muscular syndrome occurring in alcoholic patients after a debauch. Occasionally, muscle pain, tenderness and oedema were curiously localized in these cases but in others many skeletal muscles were involved. In severely affected individuals widespread muscle fibre necrosis, myoglobinuria, renal damage, and hyperkalaemia were found. Perkoff, Hardy, and Velez-Garcia (1966) described a similar reversible acute muscular syndrome occurring in chronic alcoholic patients; painful cramps and muscular tenderness were usually found, the serum creatine kinase activity was often raised and in most cases the serum lactate failed to rise after ischaemic work suggesting that glycogen utilization in the muscles was impaired. A subacute painless myopathy resolving after the withdrawal of alcohol has also been described by Ekbom *et al.* (1964).

Hepatic Encephalopathy

This syndrome which may complicate cirrhosis of the liver is not infrequently seen in alcoholic patients and is described on page 719.

DIAGNOSIS

The diagnosis of both acute and chronic alcoholic poisoning presents little difficulty if a reliable history is available. The early stages of acute alcoholic intoxication must be distinguished from the effects of acute lesions of the nervous system, especially those following head injury, and a smell of alcohol in the breath is not proof that the symptoms are due to intoxication. The diagnosis of alcoholic coma is described on page 975. The clinical picture in delirium tremens is highly distinctive, though I have seen it exactly simulated by cerebral thrombosis involving the frontal lobe and a similar picture follows withdrawal of barbiturates or amphetamines. The history, however, and careful examination of the nervous system will settle the matter. Korsakow's psychosis may be associated with focal cerebral lesions as well as with non-alcoholic forms of polyneuritis, and these must be distinguished from alcoholism by the history and clinical features. Alcoholic dementia must be distinguished from general paralysis. A history of alcoholic excess does not necessarily mean that this is the cause of the dementia, as alcoholism may complicate general paresis. In doubtful cases the cerebrospinal fluid and the blood serological reactions should be examined. In general paresis characteristic abnormalities are present in the fluid, and the serological reactions both in this and in the blood are positive. In arteriosclerotic dementia general arteriosclerosis is usually conspicuous, and there are frequently a history and signs of focal cerebral vascular lesions.

Alcoholic cerebellar degeneration must be distinguished from familial cerebellar ataxia and cerebellar degeneration secondary to carcinoma while the Marchiafava-Bignami syndrome may simulate a tumour of the corpus callosum and central pontine myelinolysis can produce symptoms and signs similar to those which occur in brain stem tumour, demyelination due to other causes or basilar artery thrombosis. Alcoholic myopathy must be distinguished from McArdle's syndrome of myophosphorylase deficiency and from other forms of endocrine and metabolic myopathy. In all of these conditions the history of excessive alcoholic intake is crucial.

PROGNOSIS

The prognosis of alcohol addiction depends upon the underlying cause, and the stage at which treatment is begun. When the habit is the expression of a psychotic or a seriously unbalanced personality, or when there is a strong hereditary tendency to alcoholism, the outlook is bad. A history of previous 'cures' and relapses also makes the outlook unsatisfactory. Voegtlin and his collaborators (1942) claim that nearly half the patients treated by 'conditioned reflex therapy' remain abstainers four years later. In the series of cases of delirium tremens reported by Tavel, Davidson, and Batterton (1961) the mortality rate was 11·8 per cent. The mortality rate of Korsakow's psychosis is from 30 to 50 per cent. In mild cases recovery may be complete. In more severe cases, and cases of long standing, there is likely to be some permanent mental enfeeblement.

The prognosis of chronic alcoholism in all its forms and the results of treatment are reviewed by McKinley and Moorhead (1967).

Alcoholic dementia runs a slow course in most cases, lasting for years. In the early stages withdrawal of alcohol leads to marked improvement, sometimes to complete recovery. In long-standing cases the brain has been permanently damaged, and recovery is incomplete. Exceptionally the course is much more rapid, and in a few weeks or months a rapidly progressive dementia terminates in coma and death, often preceded by a terminal hyperpyrexia. Central pontine myelinolysis and the Marchiafava-Bignami disease appear to be universally fatal within a few months of the onset. Alcoholic cerebellar degeneration usually becomes arrested after a period of deterioration and the various forms of myopathy slowly resolve when the alcohol is withdrawn.

TREATMENT

Alcohol Addiction

The successful treatment of alcohol addiction requires thorough supervision, so that the amount of alcohol taken can be completely controlled. If the patient is to be treated in his own home, reliable nurses will be required. Often treatment can only be carried out successfully in a nursing home or institution. Even so, many patients display remarkable cunning in obtaining access to supplies of alcohol and experience teaches that most alcoholics are accomplished and plausible liars. Complete and permanent abstinence from alcohol is the aim, but alcohol should never be suddenly withdrawn. The daily dose should be tapered, and in most cases the withdrawal can be accomplished within a week. Delirium tremens or other acute confusional states may follow sudden withdrawal. Chlorpromazine or other appropriate tranquillizers are generally necessary during the withdrawal period; drugs for the treatment of depression (amitriptyline, imipramine) are often necessary in addition. During the period of treatment a careful psychological investigation must be carried out to ascertain the presence of any underlying psychosis or neurosis, and in suitable cases the patient should receive psychotherapeutic treatment and/or appropriate drugs. The necessity for complete and permanent abstinence must be impressed upon the patient, as the slightest lapse in this respect may be followed by a relapse into the habit. Psychological help may be given by Alcoholics Anonymous (address in England, BM/AAL, London, W.C.1). It is a truism that chronic alcoholism is an incurable disease unless the patient really wishes to be cured when the association with others in a similar plight through A.A. may be invaluable. Unfortunately some patients may forswear alcohol and then become addicted to other drugs.

Voegtlin (1940) treats alcohol addiction by giving an injection of emetine and making the patient drink during the period of nausea, thus endeavouring to establish a conditioned reflex of aversion (for details see his papers). Apomorphine may similarly be used. The drug disulfiram (*Antabuse*) acts by sensitizing the patient to even a small dose of alcohol (Hald and Jacobsen, 1948; Martensen-Larsen, 1948). The usual dose is 0·5 G. daily; whenever a patient receiving this drug takes alcohol an unpleasant reaction with headache, intense flushing, and vomiting follows due to the release of acetaldehyde into the circulation. Unfortunately, some fatal reactions have been described and it is all too easy for the patient to discontinue the drug on leaving hospital unless very carefully supervised. Insulin may be used in various ways (Pullar-Strecker, 1945). Pullar-Strecker (1951) and Sim (1968) review the literature of these and other modes of treatment.

Delirium Tremens

The sufferer from delirium tremens should be treated as a patient with a severe toxaemia involving not only the nervous but also the cardiovascular system. Every effort must be made, therefore, to keep him in bed, and an adequate supply of experienced mental nurses is indispensable. It is unnecessary to give alcohol, but a high fluid intake is most important: Tavel *et al.* (1961) say that some severely ill patients may need up to 6 litres a day. Full doses of sedatives will be required: the most useful are the barbiturates and paraldehyde, although recent evidence suggests that chlordiazepoxide (*Librium*), 50 mg., may be marginally more effective (Sereny and Kalant, 1965). Phenothiazine derivatives are also valuable but are not without risk of inducing hypotension. Large doses of the B and C vitamins should be given by injection, say in the form of *Parentrovite*. The insulin-glucose-B$_1$ treatment (15 Units of insulin, 50 ml. of 50 per cent. glucose, and 50 mg. of vitamin B$_1$ intravenously) is often effective, and this dose can be repeated every four hours if required. Smith (1949) recommends ACTH and this drug is now generally given in a dosage of 20–40 Units 8-hourly for at least 48 hours. Antibiotic cover to prevent pneumonia and other infections is also necessary for four or five days.

Acute Alcoholic Hallucinosis

Hallucinosis should be treated on the same lines as delirium tremens.

Dipsomania

The sufferer from dipsomania should be urged to report to his doctor as soon as he experiences the slightest return of the craving, and treated as for alcohol addiction.

Alcoholic dementia and *Korsakow's psychosis* must be treated by the methods described for alcohol addiction and polyneuritis.

The treatment of *alcoholic polyneuritis* is described on page 819.

REFERENCES

BOURNE, P. G., ALFORD, J. A., and BOWCOCK, J. Z. (1966) Treatment of skid-row alcoholics, *Quart. J. Stud. Alcohol*, **27,** 242.

CARMICHAEL, E. A., and STERN, R. O. (1931) Korsakoff's syndrome: its histopathology, *Brain*, **54,** 189.

EDWARDS, G., HAWKER, A., WILLIAMSON, V., and HENSMAN, C. (1966) London's skid row, *Lancet*, i, 249.

EKBOM, K., HED, R., KIRSTEIN, L., and ASTROM, K. (1964) Muscular affections in chronic alcoholism, *Arch. Neurol. (Chicago)*, **10,** 449.

HALD, J., and JACOBSEN, E. (1948) A drug sensitizing the organism to ethyl alcohol, *Lancet*, ii, 1001.

HED, R., LUNDMARK, C., FAHLGREN, H., and ORELL, S. (1962) Acute muscular syndrome in chronic alcoholism, *New Engl. J. Med.*, **274,** 1277.

IRONSIDE, R., BOSANQUET, F. D., and McMENEMEY, W. H. (1961) Central demyelination of the corpus callosum (Marchiafava-Bignami disease), *Brain*, **84**, 212.

JELLINEK, E. M. (1951) W.H.O. Expert Committee on Mental Health. Subcommittee on Alcoholism. Report, *Wld Hlth Org., techn. Rep. Ser.* **42**, 20.

McKINLEY, R. A., and MOORHEAD, H. H. (1967) Alcoholism, in *Progress in Neurology and Psychiatry*, ed. SPIEGEL, E. A., Chap. 26, New York.

MARCHIAFAVA, E. (1932–3) The degeneration of the brain in chronic alcoholism, *Proc. roy. Soc. Med.*, **26**, 1151.

MARTENSEN-LARSEN, O. (1948) Treatment of alcoholism with a sensitizing drug, *Lancet*, ii, 1004.

OLIN, J. W. (1966) 'Skid-row' syndrome: a medical profile of the chronic drunkenness offender, *Canad. med. Ass. J.*, **95**, 205.

PERKOFF, G. T., HARDY, P., and VELEZ-GARCIA, E. (1966) Reversible acute muscular syndrome in chronic alcoholism, *New Engl. J. Med.*, **274**, 1277.

PULLAR-STRECKER, H. (1945) The use of insulin in the treatment of alcoholism and alcohol addiction, *Brit. J. Inebr.*, **43**, 14.

PULLAR-STRECKER, H. (1951) A review of the 1949/1950 literature of addiction, *Brit. J. Inebr.*, **48**, 3.

ROSENBAUM, M., and MERRITT, H. H. (1939) Korsakoff's syndrome. Clinical study of the alcoholic form, with special regard to prognosis, *Arch. Neurol. Psychiat. (Chicago)*, **41**, 978.

SERENY, G., and KALANT, H. (1965) Comparative clinical evaluation of chlordiazepoxide and promazine in treatment of alcohol-withdrawal syndrome, *Brit. med. J.*, **1**, 92.

SIM, M. (1968) *Guide to Psychiatry*, 2nd ed., Edinburgh.

SMITH, J. J. (1949) The treatment of acute alcoholic states with A.C.T.H. (adrenocorticotrophic) and A.C.E. (adrenocortical) hormones, *Quart. J. Stud. Alcohol*, **11**, 190.

TAVEL, M. E., DAVIDSON, W., and BATTERTON, T. D. (1961) A critical analysis of mortality associated with delirium tremens, *Amer. J. med. Sci.*, **242**, 18.

VICTOR, M., and ADAMS, R. D. (1961) On the etiology of the alcoholic neurologic diseases, *Amer. J. clin. Nutr.*, **9**, 379.

VICTOR, M., ADAMS, R. D., and MANCALL, E. L. (1959) A restricted form of cerebellar cortical degeneration occurring in alcoholic patients, *Arch. Neurol. (Chicago)*, **1**, 579.

VOEGTLIN, W. L. (1940) The treatment of alcoholism by establishing a conditioned reflex, *Amer. J. med. Sci.*, **199**, 802.

VOEGTLIN, W. L., LEMERE, F., BROZ, W. R., and O'HOLLAREN, P. (1942) Conditioned reflex therapy of alcoholic addiction: follow-up report of 1042 cases, *Amer. J. med. Sci.*, **203**, 525.

WILLIAMS, G. P., and GLATT, M. M. (1965) Unrecognized drinking, *Lancet*, ii, 1294.

DRUG ADDICTION

GENERAL CONSIDERATIONS

Drug addiction may be defined as the habitual use of a drug in order to modify the personality and diminish the strain of life. It is characterized by tolerance (increased doses are required to produce the desired effect), craving, and the development of severe symptoms on deprivation of the drug. Drugs of addiction include opium and its derivatives, morphine, heroin, eucodal, dilaudid, pethidine, and various synthetic drugs; and cocaine. Within recent years addiction to barbiturates, amphetamine and its derivatives and to lysergic acid diethylamide (LSD) and other hallucinogens has been recognized increasingly and more rarely, addiction to anaesthetic agents has been reported.

Drug habituation is a condition resulting from the repeated consumption of a drug in which there is a desire to continue taking the drug, but little or no tendency to increase the dose. The dependence is psychological and not physical, hence there are no physical symptoms of deprivation. Bromides, nicotine, and marihuana (cannabis) are drugs which may lead to habituation.

MORPHINE AND HEROIN ADDICTION
AETIOLOGY

The morphine and heroin addict often acquires his habit as a result of the legitimate administration of the drug for the relief of physical pain. As tolerance develops, increasing doses are required for this purpose. After a time he finds that he is unable to relinquish the drug without developing the symptoms of deprivation described below. Moreover, to avoid this, he requires increasing doses, so that he may need 1·0 G., or even more, a day. Morphine gives the addict no pleasurable sensations. As De Quincey wrote: 'Opium had long ceased to found its empire upon spells of pleasure; it was solely by the tortures connected with the attempt to abjure it that it kept its hold.' Very few, however, who receive narcotics for the relief of pain become addicts. The drug, besides relieving pain, blunts the edge of reality: to the psychologically unstable, therefore, it affords a way of escape from life's difficulties. Having experienced the sedative effects of morphine, they continue to take it for the relief of mental pain or distress, and are thus fettered to their habit by a double bond, psychological and physiological. Adams (1937) classified addicts into four groups:

1. Stabilized addicts who may lead useful lives on a fixed dose.
2. Accidental addicts, not necessarily psychopathic, who have often acquired addiction through treatment of a painful disease.
3. Natural addicts, essentially psychopathic.
4. Criminal addicts, who take to drugs for vicious purposes.

Doctors and nurses form a considerable proportion of addicts, since they have ready access to the drugs. Residence in a country where they are readily obtainable may also facilitate the acquisition of the habit. The number of drug addicts in the United States was officially said in 1955 to be 44,905, in Canada 3,295, and in Great Britain about 470, but numbers have greatly increased, particularly in Great Britain, within the last 10 years.

SYMPTOMS OF ADDICTION

The psychopathic addict undergoes a progressive mental deterioration, with loss of interest in his environment, intellectual efficiency, and self-respect. He becomes quite untrustworthy, and will commit almost any crime to obtain a supply of his drug, if he is faced by the prospect of deprivation. Physically he represents a picture of chronic toxaemia, including the specific symptoms attributable to the pharmacological action of the drug. He is wasted and shows trophic changes in the hair and nails. The pupils are usually contracted, and react sluggishly to light. The alimentary tract suffers severely; the appetite is poor and constipation is always present. There is severe fatigability, and muscular weakness, frequently with some ataxia. The pulse is of small volume, and the extremities are cold. Slight albuminuria may be present. Carelessness leads to infection of the skin at the site of the injections, and the resulting scars are usually to be found, while in some cases abscesses or ulcers may be present when the patient comes under observation.

SYMPTOMS OF DEPRIVATION

The addict who is suddenly deprived of his drug exhibits a highly characteristic train of symptoms. As the time for his usual injection passes he becomes restless and apprehensive, and yawning and sneezing develop, followed by the symptoms of an acute coryza. He feels cold, and contraction of the smooth muscles of the skin produces the appearance described as 'goose-flesh'. Later he complains of cramps in the abdomen, back, or lower limbs. His face is contracted in his distress; perspiration is excessive, and muscular spasms and twitching occur, most violently in the lower extremities. There is often a general tremor and the patient may be violent in his demands for the drug. Later, vomiting and diarrhoea occur, and lead to a stage of complete collapse, which may even terminate in death.

The pharmacology of drug addiction is fully discussed by Isbell and Fraser (1950) and by Sim (1968). Many explanations of the symptoms of deprivation have been proposed. The most plausible is a modification of Dixon's 'release' theory. Since morphine depresses many autonomic functions, tolerance must involve the balancing of increasing doses by a progressively higher 'gearing' of autonomic activity. When the morphine is suddenly withdrawn the autonomic nervous system 'races' like a motor-car engine when the clutch is suddenly thrown out. Nevertheless, psychological factors must also play a part, since it is said that in prisons, where abrupt withdrawal without medication is the rule, severe abstinence symptoms are rarely seen.

TREATMENT

Not every drug addict requires treatment. Stabilized addicts leading useful lives on a fixed dose, especially when past middle age, are often best left untreated. In Great Britain, the right of every doctor to prescribe opiates for addicts has now been proscribed by law and all addicts must now obtain their drugs from licensed doctors, usually working in psychiatric units or in centres for the treatment of drug addiction which are being established.

Treatment which should be carried out in an institution has been recently reviewed by Wolff (1945–6), Isbell and Fraser (1950), and by the British Interdepartmental Committee (1961). Abrupt withdrawal and slow withdrawal are both now regarded as unsatisfactory. Generally the drug is reduced over a period of 7 to 10 days. It is now regarded as unnecessary to cover the withdrawal by large doses of drugs of the atropine group. Adjuvant therapy includes the judicious use of sedatives and hypnotics, maintenance of fluid balance, hydrotherapy, and simple psychotherapy. Methadone and chlorpromazine in doses up to 100 mg. three times daily may be used to suppress the abstinence symptoms, and then withdrawn.

The after-treatment of the morphine addict is important, if a relapse is to be prevented. Convalescence under medical supervision should last for three months. Any painful condition which has necessitated morphine in the past should as far as possible be remedied. Psychotherapy may be required. It is desirable that the patient should abstain from alcohol, which predisposes to a relapse.

COCAINE ADDICTION

Coca leaves are chewed in South America for their sedative effects and their power of abolishing fatigue. Cocaine as a drug of addiction may be injected subcutaneously, drunk as coca wine, smoked, or taken as snuff. It acts to some extent as a sexual stimulant, and is stated to produce a sense of internal peace. Addicts suffer from mental deterioration, and, in severe cases, from confusional insanity. Hallucinations, especially of insects crawling under the skin, are common, and epilepsy may occur. Cocaine sniffing may lead to ulceration of the nasal septum. Addicts who are suddenly deprived of cocaine do not suffer, like morphine addicts, from severe deprivation symptoms. Treatment, therefore, is not required to counteract these, but is similar to the after-treatment of the morphine addict. Cocainism, however, is much more difficult to cure than morphine addiction.

REFERENCES

Adams, E. W. (1937) *Drug Addiction*, London.

Isbell, H., and Fraser, H. F. (1950) Addiction to analgesics and barbiturates, *Pharmacol. Rev.*, **2,** 355.

Light, A. B., Torrance, E. G., Karr, W. G., Fry, E. G., and Wolff, W. A. (1930) *Opium Addiction*, Chicago.

Maier, H. W. (1928) *La cocaïne*, Paris.

Sim, M. (1968) *Guide to Psychiatry*, 2nd ed., Edinburgh.

Vaillant, G. E. (1966) A 12-year follow-up of New York narcotic addicts, *Arch. gen. Psychiat.*, **15,** 599.

Wolff, P. O. (1945–6) The treatment of drug addicts, *Bull. Wld Hlth Org.*, No. 12.

Report of the Interdepartmental Committee on Drug Addiction (1961), London, H.M.S.O.

SEDATIVES AND HYPNOTICS

Barbitone, sodium barbitone, phenobarbitone, chloral, sulphonal, and allied drugs may be taken as drugs of habituation, either alone or with morphine, and addicts may become tolerant of enormous doses. All these drugs produce similar symptoms, both in cases of acute poisoning and in addicts, though some have in addition individual peculiarities.

Habituation to the Synthetic Hypnotics

When taken habitually (Glatt, 1966) these drugs lead to mental deterioration, dysarthria, nystagmus, muscular weakness, tremor, and incoordination. There is usually considerable emaciation. Veronal and sulphonal may lead to haematoporphyrinuria and polyneuritis. Chloral has a markedly toxic effect on the heart and on the skin, causing reddening of the face and a papular eruption. Treatment is carried out by means of gradual withdrawal: sudden withdrawal may cause convulsions. The artificial kidney may be used to eliminate the more soluble barbiturates. The general management is the same as that for morphine addiction.

Barbiturate Poisoning

In Great Britain the increasing use of barbiturates and of other sedative drugs for suicidal attempts has meant that this group of drugs now comes second to coal-gas poisoning as a method of attempted suicide (Cumming, 1961) and there are probably over 3,000 hospital admissions annually due to this cause.

In mild cases slurred speech, drowsiness, ataxia, and nystagmus are apparent but when the dose ingested is large the patients are stuporose or comatose and there is eventually total areflexia with hypotension and oliguria. Small blisters filled with serum may appear on the limbs in severe cases.

Management consists first in aspirating stomach contents, in identifying when possible the causative agent in stomach contents, blood or urine (or by searching the patient's belongings or questioning the relatives or family doctor concerning drugs which were in the patient's possession). Maintenance of an adequate airway, often by intubation, of the blood pressure by the use of appropriate drugs (e.g. methedrine), of the fluid and electrolyte intake by intravenous therapy and the administration of appropriate antibiotics with intensive nursing care to prevent pulmonary collapse and bed-sores are all essential. The use of analeptic drugs such as bemegride and amiphenazole has now been generally discarded in favour of the elimination of the offending drug by dialysis with the artificial kidney in severe cases. Catheterization is usually necessary and assisted respiration may be required for several days.

REFERENCES

CUMMING, G. (1961) *The Medical Management of Acute Poisoning*, London.
ESSIG, C. F. (1966) Non-narcotic addiction, *J. Amer. med. Ass.*, **196**, 714.
FLANDIN, C., BERNARD, J., and JOLY, F. (1934) *L'intoxication par les somnifères (intoxication barbiturique)*, Paris.
GLATT, M. M. (1966) Controlled trials of non-barbiturate hypnotics and tranquillisers, *Psychiat. Neurol.*, **152**, 28.
WRIGHT, J. T. (1955) The value of barbiturate estimations in the diagnosis and treatment of barbiturate intoxication, *Quart. J. Med.*, N.S. **24**, 95.

CHRONIC BROMIDE INTOXICATION

Chronic bromide intoxication may occur as a result of addiction, which is rare, or in consequence of the prolonged administration of bromide for therapeutic purposes. It used to be most often encountered in patients suffering from neurosis, hyperthyroidism, or epilepsy. Since the bromides are now much less frequently used, commoner sources of bromide intoxication are compounds of bromide with urea, such as carbromal and bromvaletone.

Bromide tends to replace the chlorides in the body, and a greater amount of bromide will be absorbed by a person with a low chloride intake than by one who is taking larger amounts of chloride. The blood bromide level is a rough index of the degree of intoxication, though individual susceptibility varies greatly. The normal level of bromide in the blood is under 3 mg. per 100 ml. According to Barbour, Pilkington, and Sargant (1936), levels of under 100 mg. per 100 ml. can usually be ignored; those between 100 and 200 mg. per 100 ml.

are likely to be associated with symptoms of intoxication in elderly patients or in those with impaired cardiovascular or renal efficiency, and levels of over 200 mg. per 100 ml. produce symptoms in most cases. There is evidence that bromide, like chloride, is excreted into the stomach and so may be reabsorbed.

In mild cases the symptoms are largely subjective, and consist of depression, fatigability, inability to concentrate, loss of memory, lack of appetite, and poor sleep. In more severe cases the mental state is usually one of confusion with some disorientation. The occurrence of terrifying hallucinations, especially at night, is rather characteristic. Physical symptoms are variable: when severe they consist of slurred speech, tremor and ataxia of the upper limbs, a staggering gait, and diminution or loss of the tendon reflexes. In more severe cases still the patient becomes stuporose. The rash usually regarded as characteristic of bromide intoxication is frequently absent.

The bromide must be immediately discontinued and the patient given increased sodium chloride and fluid by the mouth. Washing out the stomach helps to eliminate the drug. In severe cases the artificial kidney may be used. Restlessness is controlled if necessary by paraldehyde, by chlorpromazine, or by small doses of a barbiturate.

REFERENCES

BARBOUR, R. F., PILKINGTON, F., and SARGANT, W. (1936) Bromide intoxication, *Brit. med. J.*, **2**, 957.

MINSKI, L., and GILLEN, J. B. (1937) Blood bromide investigations in psychotic epileptics, *Brit. med. J.*, **2**, 850.

MARIHUANA (HASHISH, CANNABIS INDICA)

This drug which has been used by certain races in the Orient and in South America has recently been used more widely in Western countries, being often smoked in cigarettes. Its use is still illegal; it is a drug of habituation and not of addiction and in itself it is a minor nuisance rather than a serious social evil. It produces a transient sense of well-being and sometimes reversible hallucinations. Its danger is that for social reasons it may introduce its habituees to narcotics.

AMPHETAMINE ADDICTION

Amphetamines and their derivatives are commonly taken by young people in order to obtain temporary uplift, or mental alertness or to reduce desire for sleep. Addiction may also occur in young and middle-aged women who have received these drugs in therapeutic doses for the treatment of depression or fatigue or obesity. Connell (1958) has described acute psychotic states of a paranoid or hallucinatory nature while psychopathic and irresponsible behaviour is also common. Fits may occur as a result of intoxication or withdrawal. A common sign in addicts is continuous chewing, grinding of the teeth or licking of the lips, sometimes resulting in ulceration.

REFERENCE

CONNELL, P. H. (1958) *Amphetamine Psychosis*, Maudsley Monographs, No. 5, London.

HALLUCINOGENIC AGENTS

The use of hallucinogenic drugs such as LSD and mescaline is increasing and in some universities and other circles has developed almost into a cult. The danger of these drugs is that the induced hallucinations are sometimes terrifying and rarely pleasurable and the view that they produce increased perception is a dangerous delusion. Irreversible psychosis may result and addiction is increasing.

REFERENCE

SIM, M. (1968) *Guide to Psychiatry*, 2nd ed., Edinburgh.

LEAD POISONING

AETIOLOGY

The nervous symptoms of plumbism are usually due to chronic poisoning with lead. Industrial lead poisoning was at one time common, but has now been reduced by legislative restrictions. Lead poisoning still occurs, however, especially among plumbers and painters. In such cases the principal route of absorption of the lead is probably the digestive tract, though some may enter the body through the lungs. Water which has passed through lead pipes is an occasional source of poisoning, and beer and cider may be similarly contaminated. The first glass of these beverages, which has stayed in a lead pipe all night, is particularly poisonous. Lead nipple shields and sucking lead paint are the commonest cause of poisoning in children. Cosmetics containing lead are an occasional source of poisoning, which may also follow the use of lead obtained from diachylon plaster as a home-made abortifacient. Lead tetra-ethyl is a highly poisonous substance which has caused encephalopathy in the United States. It is used in small quantities in some forms of petrol. In chronic lead poisoning, as Aub and his fellow workers have shown, 95 per cent. of the lead is stored in the bones as insoluble phosphate. This lead storage is facilitated by a diet rich in calcium. In states of acidosis the stored lead is released into the blood stream, and its excretion in the faeces and urine is much increased. Hunter and Aub (1926–7) have shown that mobilization and excretion of lead can be similarly effected by parathyroid extract (parathormone). The undue mobilization of lead may precipitate an attack of encephalopathy. The researches of Aub seemed to throw new light upon the nature of so-called 'neuritis'. It has long been known that in this condition the muscles paralysed are usually those most used in the patient's occupation. Reznikoff and Aub (1927) produced experimentally selective muscular paralysis in animals with lead poisoning by fatiguing certain muscles. They believed that lactic acid liberated in the muscles by their contractions led to the local formation of lead acetate from the lead phosphate in the blood, and that from the lead acetate insoluble lead phosphate was precipitated in the muscle cells. However, recent pathological evidence suggests that there is no convincing evidence that lead damages the muscle fibres and indicates that muscular weakness is in fact due to peripheral neuropathy. Fullerton (1966) has shown that this heavy metal produces both axonal degeneration and demyelination in the peripheral nerves of guinea-pigs.

PATHOLOGY

There is much experimental evidence that lead poisoning produces a selective degeneration of the ganglion cells of the nervous system, and this is most marked in the spinal cord. Mott has described similar changes in chronic lead poisoning in man. Chronic cerebral symptoms and local and general progressive muscular atrophy in lead poisoning may, therefore, be due to degeneration of the ganglion cells of the cerebral cortex and of the anterior horns of the spinal cord respectively. In acute lead encephalopathy the brain is pale and oedematous, with an excess of fluid in the subarachnoid space. The symptoms of lead encephalopathy have been attributed to a spasm of the cerebral arteries, and the clinical picture has much in common with hypertensive encephalopathy, but there is evidence that the ganglion cells may be directly affected, that cerebral oedema is a prominent finding and that meningeal irritation may also occur (Smith et al., 1960). In guinea-pigs in which lead produced combined axonal degeneration and demyelination in peripheral nerves, epileptic seizures were also common and could be provoked by noise or movement (Fullerton, 1966).

SYMPTOMS

Acute Encephalopathy

This is an acute cerebral disturbance which is rare in adults but is commonly seen in children aged 1 or 2, and characterized by convulsions, delirium, and coma, often associated with papilloedema, and sometimes with cervical rigidity. The cerebrospinal fluid frequently shows abnormality; its pressure is increased, and there is an excess of globulin and of cells, which in adults are usually lymphocytes, though in children polymorphonuclear cells may be present. An increase in the sugar content of the fluid has also been described, and the presence of lead in it has been demonstrated. Between 20 and 30 per cent. of children who suffer from this condition suffer from recurring fits as a sequel (Coffin et al., 1966).

Chronic Encephalopathy

Mental changes and epileptiform convulsions have been observed as chronic manifestations of lead poisoning. Primary optic atrophy occasionally occurs. Laryngeal palsy is a rare symptom which has been described by Gowers and by Harris, who saw a case of bilateral abductor paralysis.

Lead Neuropathy

This condition usually affects the extensor muscles of the wrist and fingers, as a rule bilaterally, though the right side may suffer alone, especially in right-handed individuals. Wrist- and finger-drop occur, and the loss of synergic extension of the wrist causes weakness of flexion of the fingers. The brachioradialis muscle escapes and so, as a rule, does the abductor pollicis longus. In the upper-arm type of palsy the spinati, deltoid, biceps, brachialis, and brachioradialis muscles are affected. These are the abductor and external rotators of the shoulder and flexors of the forearm, and this distribution of paralysis may occur in workers employing these muscles chiefly, for example, in men grinding lead in a mortar. The lower limbs are occasionally affected, the muscles paralysed being those supplied by the lateral popliteal nerve, with the exception of the tibialis anterior, which usually escapes.

The paralysed muscles waste and demonstrate electrophysiological evidence of denervation with slowing of motor nerve conduction velocity, but fasciculation and sensory changes are absent.

Progressive Muscular Atrophy

Progressive muscular atrophy has been attributed to lead poisoning and is said to occur in a localized form involving the small muscles of the hand, when it is usually associated with the common paralysis of the extensors of the wrist and fingers. Fasciculation, which is absent from the muscles paralysed in lead neuropathy, is present in those degenerating through the action of lead on the anterior horn cells of the spinal cord. Rarely progressive muscular atrophy becomes generalized, and cases have been described in which it has been associated with signs of degeneration of the corticospinal tracts. Many workers are doubtful as to whether lead can be considered to be an aetiological agent in such cases and in the cases with localized atrophy it is still uncertain whether this is truly a disorder of the anterior horn cells or merely an unusual variant of motor neuropathy.

Other Symptoms

Other symptoms of lead poisoning are of diagnostic importance. The blue line should be sought on the gums. There may be a history of colic. There is often a secondary anaemia, with stippling of the red cells—punctate basophilia. Cardiovascular hypertrophy with high blood pressure may be present, or the symptoms of chronic nephritis. Gout is a rare complication today. In chronic lead poisoning in children X-rays may show a 'lead line', a band of increased density, at the diaphysial end of the growing bones. The normal content of lead in the blood is 10–60 μg. per litre. In lead encephalopathy there may be 100–200 μg. per ml. in the blood, and 100–1,000 μg. or more per litre of urine.

DIAGNOSIS

Acute lead encephalopathy must be distinguished from uraemia, in which there is always a high blood-urea content, and from hypertensive encephalopathy in which the blood pressure is usually higher. Meningitis may be simulated. Lead neuropathy is distinguished from a lesion of the radial nerve by the escape of the brachioradialis and by its gradual onset and by the involvement of muscles, perhaps on the opposite side or others not supplied by the radial nerve. In various other forms of polyneuropathy, foot-drop is usually associated with wrist-drop; pain in the limbs is often a prominent symptom; and there is usually sensory loss with a 'glove and stocking' distribution. Moreover, the blue line on the gums and other symptoms of lead poisoning are absent. The progressive muscular atrophy which may possibly be due to lead can only be distinguished from other forms of progressive muscular atrophy by the discovery of other symptoms of lead poisoning. In all doubtful cases the blood should be examined for evidence of anaemia and punctate basophilia, and lead should be sought in the urine and faeces.

Patients with lead poisoning excrete increased quantities of coproporphyrin III and of delta-amino-laevulinic acid in the urine so that a urinary screening test for porphyrin should be performed when the diagnosis is suspected.

PROGNOSIS

The outlook in acute encephalopathy is always serious, especially when convulsions occur, but with modern methods of treatment the prognosis has improved, and recovery, when it occurs, is often complete, but the patient may be left mentally subnormal, blind, or epileptic. Little improvement is to be expected in chronic encephalopathy. In lead neuropathy the prognosis is good, provided the patient abstains from contact with lead. Recovery, however, is usually slow, and may take one to two years. In progressive muscular atrophy believed to be due to lead no improvement is likely to occur, but the condition may become arrested.

TREATMENT

The patient with lead poisoning must be removed from contact with lead, and must never return to an occupation which exposes him to it. If he does so, relapse is certain. The first question to be settled is whether the patient requires active elimination of the lead or not. The treatment of lead poisoning has been revolutionized by the introduction of chelating agents. Disodium calcium ethylene-diamine-tetra-acetate (CaEDTA, *Versene*) forms with lead a chelate, which is a stable, water-soluble, and virtually non-ionized complex, which is excreted by the kidneys. Its successful use has been reported by Browne (1955) and Sidbury (1955), who treated nine patients. The drug can be given both orally and intravenously. The oral dose used by Sidbury was 30 mg. per kg. of body weight given before breakfast and supper with liberal amounts of water. Two methods have been used for the intravenous route: slow infusion of 1 G. on the first day and 2 G. a day thereafter for a total of five days in divided doses, twice daily in 250 ml. of 5 per cent. glucose in water; or 400 mg. was given once or twice a day in 5 or 10 ml. of saline. For children the dose is 60–75 mg. per kg. of body weight, given in the same ways. Both seemed equally satisfactory. There was marked improvement or complete disappearance of symptoms in all cases, including those of lead encephalopathy, on the third day of treatment, when blood and urine analyses showed that most of the readily available lead had been excreted. An alternative method of treatment is BAL in doses of 2–4 mg. per kg. of body weight given every 4 hours for up to 10 days. Since lead is deposited in the bones, patients who have been exposed to lead for long periods cannot eliminate the metal in a short time. They may therefore relapse and require further courses of treatment. Sidbury points out that this could be avoided if plumbism were recognized early. Wrist-drop and finger-drop may require to be treated by a splint. Lumbar puncture or the use of dexamethasone, 5 mg. three or four times daily to reduce cerebral oedema, may be helpful in the immediate treatment of encephalopathy.

REFERENCES

BROWNE, R. C. (1955) Metallic poisons and the nervous system, *Lancet*, i, 775.

COFFIN, R., PHILLIPS, J. L., STADLES, W. I., and SPECTOR, S. (1966) Treatment of lead encephalopathy in children, *J. Pediat.*, **69**, 198.

CUMINGS, J. N. (1959) *Heavy Metals and the Brain*, Oxford.

FULLERTON, P. M. (1966) Chronic peripheral neuropathy produced by lead-poisoning in the guinea-pig, *J. Neuropath. exp. Neurol.*, **25**, 214.

HUNTER, D. (1930) Goulstonian lectures. The significance to clinical medicine of studies in calcium and phosphorus metabolism, *Lancet*, i, 897, 947, 999.

HUNTER, D., and AUB, J. C. (1926–7) Lead studies. XV. The effect of the parathyroid hormone on the excretion of lead and of calcium in patients suffering from lead poisoning, *Quart. J. Med.*, **20**, 123.

McKHANN, C. F. (1932) Lead poisoning in children: the cerebral manifestations, *Arch. Neurol. Psychiat. (Chicago)*, **27**, 294.

MORRIS, C. E., HEYMAN, A., and POZEFSKY, T. (1964) Lead encephalopathy from whiskey, *Neurology (Minneap.)*, **14**, 493.

REZNIKOFF, P., and AUB, J. C. (1927) Lead studies. XIV. Experimental studies of lead palsy, *Arch. Neurol. Psychiat. (Chicago)*, **17**, 444.

SIDBURY, J. B., JR. (1955) Lead poisoning, *Amer. J. Med.*, **17**, 932.

SMITH, J. F., McLAURIN, R. L., NICHOLS, J. B., and ASBURY, A., (1960) Studies in cerebral oedema and cerebral swelling, *Brain*, **83**, 411.

Chelating Agents. Leader, *Lancet*, 1955, i, 754.

MANGANESE POISONING

This is an industrial disease due to the inhalation of manganese dust. The clinical features, which often appear within 6–9 months of exposure, are those of an extrapyramidal syndrome like Parkinsonism with slurred, monotonous speech, slowness and clumsiness of movement, facial masking and antero-pulsion or retropulsion. Personality change in the form of irritability and variable euphoria may be succeeded by intense fatigue, lethargy, and somno-lence. Little improvement usually follows removal of the patient from exposure to the dust but chelating agents or BAL may be of some value.

MERCURY POISONING

Acute mercurial poisoning may produce neurological symptoms and signs, but gastro-intestinal and renal damage dominate the clinical picture. Chronic mercurial poisoning in children may give 'pink disease' [p. 828] and one form in adults is Minamata disease [p. 716]. Chronic exposure to this metal in industry and even in police officers exposed to mercurial finger-print powder (which is no longer used) may give rise to a syndrome of tremor, variable limb weakness and ataxia and personality change often characterized by fatigability, insomnia, irritability, and erethism (childish over-emotionalism). BAL or chelating agents should be given in such cases.

REFERENCE

COHEN, M. M. (1955) Cerebral intoxication, in *Clinical Neurology*, ed. BAKER, A. B., Chap. 15, pp. 866–943, London.

CARBON MONOXIDE POISONING

AETIOLOGY

Carbon monoxide poisoning may occur as the result of the accidental or suicidal inhalation of coal-gas or of gas from a motor-car exhaust. Carbon monoxide may also be present in dangerous quantities in the air of coal-mines, especially after explosions. By combining with the haemoglobin of the blood to form carboxyhaemoglobin, carbon monoxide reduces the capacity of the blood to take up oxygen, and so leads to anoxaemia.

Absorption of the gas is cumulative, so that a concentration of 0·1 per cent. will saturate the blood up to 50 per cent. Effort increases absorption.

PATHOLOGY

In fatal cases the blood is cherry-red in colour and coagulates slowly. All the tissues are reddened. There is oedema of the lungs, and haemorrhages are found in the pleura and intestinal mucosa. Changes in the nervous system are of special importance and exhibit a predilection for the cerebral cortex, the hippocampus, cerebellum, and the corpus striatum. The changes are those of anoxia and similar appearances may be found to follow cardiac arrest or may complicate open-heart surgery. There is focal or laminar necrosis of the second and third cortical layers and often of the superficial white matter with striking degeneration in the Purkinje cells of the cerebellum and in Sommer's sector of Ammon's horn of the hippocampus. There may also be variable degrees of degeneration of the basal ganglia and occasional demyelination of the central white matter. When the patient survives for several days there is likely to be extensive ischaemic necrosis of the cerebral cortex and the lesions of the globus pallidus may progress to softening.

SYMPTOMS

McNally (1931) stated that the severity of the symptoms can be correlated with the degree of saturation of the blood with the gas. When this is less than 10 per cent. there are no symptoms. At between 10 and 20 per cent. the patient complains of slight headache and a tight sensation in the forehead, and there is a dilatation of the cutaneous vessels. At between 30 and 50 per cent. there is severe headache, weakness, giddiness, dimness of vision, nausea, vomiting, and collapse. At between 50 and 60 per cent. the patient becomes comatose and may convulse. Paralysis of the heart and respiration occurs, with tachycardia, tachypnoea, cyanosis, and, in some cases, glycosuria. Only a small proportion, even of patients who become comatose, end with permanent symptoms. Garland and Pearce (1967) have drawn particular attention to the striking variation in the clinical picture which may occur in such cases, including such features as major seizures, cortical blindness, dysphasia, apraxia and various forms of agnosia with mental changes ranging from retardation to frank psychotic behaviour. Some patients leave hospital apparently recovered only to relapse into coma in from one to three weeks, or into a state of akinetic stupor, or confusion and visual agnosia with catatonic postures.

No explanation has yet been advanced for this syndrome of so-called post-anoxic encephalopathy whilst there is some evidence that its incidence is reduced if activity is greatly limited in the early stages after poisoning (Plum, Posner, and Hain, 1962). A mild Parkinsonism may make its appearance within six weeks of recovery from the initial coma.

PROGNOSIS

In mild cases there is usually complete recovery, but in severe cases the patient may remain comatose for days or even for weeks, and on recovery may exhibit symptoms of permanent damage to the brain, including dementia, aphasia, apraxia, choreo-athetoid movements, and Parkinsonism. Polyneuropathy may occur. However, even a confusional state lasting for as long as two months does not necessarily mean that the patient may not recover completely (Garland and Pearce, 1967).

TREATMENT

The patient should at once be moved from exposure to the gas, preferably to the open air, care being taken to protect the body from loss of heat. Inhalations of oxygen should be given and these may with advantage contain 5 per cent. of carbon dioxide to increase the pulmonary ventilation, the object being as rapidly as possible to replace carboxyhaemoglobin by oxyhaemoglobin. If the patient is unconscious, artificial respiration should be carried out by administering the mixture of oxygen and carbon dioxide with a respirator. Smith *et al.* (1962) recommend treatment with oxygen at two atmospheres pressure; this is especially valuable when carbon monoxide poisoning is complicated by barbiturate poisoning or a cerebrovascular accident. Suitable treatment for heart failure may be required. In the later stages treatment is symptomatic.

REFERENCES

DENNY-BROWN, D. (1960) Diseases of the basal ganglia, *Lancet*, ii, 1104.
DRINKER, C. K. (1938) *Carbon Monoxide Asphyxia*, New York.
GARLAND, H., and PEARCE, J. (1967) Neurological complications of carbon monoxide poisoning, *Quart. J. Med.*, **36**, 445.
HILLER, F. (1924) Ueber die krankhaften Veränderungen im Zentralnervensystem nach Kohlenoxydvergiftung, *Z. ges. Neurol. Psychiat.*, **93**, 594.
KANT, F. (1926) Katatone Motilitätspsychose nach CO-Vergiftung, *Arch. Psychiat. Neurol.*, **78**, 365.
McNALLY, W. D. (1931) Carbon monoxide poisoning, *Illinois med. J.*, **59**, 383.
MEYER, A. (1958) in *Neuropathology*, GREENFIELD, J. G., BLACKWOOD, W., McMENEMEY, W. H., MEYER, A., and NORMAN, R. M., p. 234, London.
MEDICAL RESEARCH COUNCIL. Carbon monoxide poisoning. Use of carbon dioxide–oxygen mixture, *Brit. med. J.* (1958) **2**, 1408.
PLUM, F., POSNER, J. B., and HAIN, R. F. (1962) Post-anoxic encephalopathy, *Arch. intern. Med.*, **110**, 18.
SMITH, G., LEDINGHAM, I. McA., SHARP, G. R., NORMAN, J. N., and BATES, E. H. (1962) Treatment of coal-gas poisoning with oxygen at 2 atmospheres pressure, *Lancet*, i, 816.
STRECKER, E. A., TAFT, A. E., and WILLEY, G. F. (1927) Mental sequelae of carbon monoxide poisoning, with reports of autopsy in two cases, *Arch. Neurol. Psychiat. (Chicago)*, **17**, 552.
WILSON, G., and WINKLEMAN, N. W. (1924) Multiple neuritis following carbon monoxide poisoning: a clinicopathologic study, *J. Amer. med. Ass.*, **82**, 1407.

CAISSON DISEASE

AETIOLOGY AND PATHOLOGY

Caisson disease, also known as compressed-air sickness, diver's paralysis, and 'the bends', first made its appearance with the introduction of high-pressure caissons for submarine work. It also occurs in tunnel workers and others who work in compressed air. Divers may work in caissons which are open at the bottom and in which the air must be maintained at a high pressure, usually 30 to 35 lb. to the square inch, to balance the pressure of the water, which increases in proportion to the depth. As a result of the increased air pressure in the caisson, the tissues of those working in it absorb the gases of the air. If such individuals are suddenly transferred to normal atmospheric pressure, these gases, especially the nitrogen, are liberated in the tissues in the form of small bubbles, in a manner exactly comparable to the liberation of bubbles of carbon dioxide in a bottle of soda water when the cork is removed. The nitrogen is especially soluble in the body fats, and is thus liberated in large amounts in the nervous system. For this reason also fat men are more liable to caisson disease than those of spare build. The liberation of bubbles of gas causes not only disruption of the nerve tissue but also interference with its blood supply through blockage of small vessels.

SYMPTOMS

The first symptom is usually pain situated in the limbs, trunk, and epigastrium, and sometimes associated with vomiting. The pain usually begins in the knees and hips. Headache and vertigo may occur and in severe cases the patient may rapidly become comatose. Hemiplegia or paraplegia with sensory loss may occur.

PROGNOSIS

In severe cases the condition is fatal. In less severe cases recovery usually occurs, sometimes in a few hours, but disability may persist for days, weeks, or months.

TREATMENT

Prophylaxis consists in the slow decompression of workers exposed to high pressures. When symptoms have developed, immediate recompression is necessary, the patient being placed in an air lock for this purpose, and restoration to normal pressure must be extremely slow. Otherwise treatment is symptomatic.

REFERENCES

BEHNKE, A. R. (1966) Disorders due to alterations in barometric pressure, in *Principles of Internal Medicine*, 5th ed., ed. HARRISON, T. R., ADAMS, R. D., BENNETT, I. L., RESNIK, W. H., THORN, G. W., and WINTROBE, M. M., Chap. 25, New York.

DU BOIS, E. F. (1929) Physiology of respiration in relationship to the problems of naval medicine: part vi, Deep diving, *Nav. med. Bull. (Wash.)*, **27**, 311.

HILL, L. E. (1912) *Caisson Sickness and the Physiology of Work in Compressed Air*, London.

PATON, W. D. M., and WALDER, D. N. (1954) Compressed air illness, M.R.C. Special Report Series, No. 281, London, H.M.S.O.

ELECTRIC SHOCK

PATHOLOGY

The pathological changes produced in the nervous system by electric shock are highly characteristic. They consist of chromatolysis of the ganglion cells, wide dilatation of the perivascular spaces, holes or spaces in the brain itself due to fissures, vascular lesions ranging from focal petechial haemorrhages to actual disruption of large vessels, changes in the peripheral nerves such as fragmentation of the axons and neurilemma, and a peculiar spiral-like appearance of the muscle fibres. These changes may be associated with electrical burns of the skin.

AETIOLOGY

There has been much discussion as to the precise way in which electric shock injures the nervous system. The heating effect of the current may sometimes be sufficient to cause severe damage, as in legal electrocution or lightning stroke. The importance of the electrolytic effect of the current and of its mechanical effect has been stressed by some writers, but Pritchard (1934) pointed out that neither of these agencies could produce the pathological changes observed, and suggests that in the case of lightning stroke electrostatic charges on the surface of the body may be responsible for the disruptive changes found in the nervous system.

Changes in the central nervous system are most likely to occur when the current has been applied directly to the skull. The extreme variability of conditions is no doubt responsible for the unpredictability of the results of exposure to electric currents. Eleven thousand volts may cause only slight injury (Critchley, 1934). On the other hand, forty volts has been known to prove fatal. Death from electric shock, however, is rare, especially considering the risks of exposure in civilized life.

SYMPTOMS

A severe electric shock causes immediate loss of consciousness from syncope or concussion. If the patient does not lose consciousness there is usually severe pain associated with bizarre sensory disturbances, especially visual hallucinations. A typical immediate sequel of the shock is a transitory flaccid paraplegia with objective sensory disturbance, both disappearing after about twelve hours. Critchley classified the neurological sequelae of electric shock as follows: (1) cerebral, (2) spinal, (3) mixed cerebrospinal affection, (4) peripheral nerve lesions, isolated or multiple, and (5) psychological disorders, hysteria being particularly common. Symptoms of an isolated cerebral lesion are rare, but spinal atrophic paralyses leading to a clinical picture not unlike motor neurone disease are not uncommon. Brachial neuritis may follow a shock to the upper limbs and Critchley described a lasting polyneuritic syndrome following lightning stroke.

PROGNOSIS

Generalizations about prognosis are impossible on account of the varied character of the clinical picture.

TREATMENT

The first essential is immediate artificial respiration and, if necessary, external cardiac massage since by these methods it may be possible to revive a victim even though the heart has apparently ceased to beat. It is difficult to know how long artificial respiration should be carried on in the absence of any response, but there is some evidence that resuscitation has been effective even after a period of three hours. During artificial respiration the general treatment of shock should be carried out, and the after-treatment will depend upon the nature of the sequelae.

REFERENCES

CRITCHLEY, M. (1934) Neurological effects of lightning and of electricity, *Lancet*, i, 68.
JELLINEK, S. (1932) *Elektrische Verletzungen*, Leipzig.
MORRISON, L. R., WEEKS, A., and COBB, S. (1930) Histopathology of different types of electric shock on mammalian brains, *J. industr. Hyg.*, **12,** 324.
PRITCHARD, E. A. B. (1934) Changes in the central nervous system due to electrocution, *Lancet*, i, 1163.

TETANUS

Definition. Tetanus is an intoxication of the nervous system with the exotoxin of the tetanus bacillus. It is characterized by the progressive development of muscular rigidity which is subject to paroxysmal exacerbations.

AETIOLOGY

Tetanus is due to infection with the *Clostridium tetani*, a Gram-positive, anaerobic organism which bears spores. The spore is oval or rounded, and develops at one end of the bacillus, which then presents the appearance of a drumstick. The *Cl. tetani* is actively motile, its movement being due to flagella. Fildes (1929) has shown by immunological methods that a number of types exist, not all of which are toxic.

The *Cl. tetani* is widely distributed in the soil, and is found in the faeces of many animals, especially horses, and of a small proportion of normal human beings. The disease arises in man through contamination of wounds with the spores of the organism, especially as a result of accidents in which road dust or soil is introduced into the wound. Other, less common, sources of tetanus infection include vaccination, infection of wounds by contaminated dressings or catgut, and the injection of infected gelatine and drugs. Tetanus neonatorum, due to infection of the stump of the umbilical cord in newly born infants, and puerperal tetanus are common in some tropical countries.

The mere introduction of tetanus spores into a wound is not sufficient to cause the disease. It appears to be necessary that other organisms should also be present. There is frequently a foreign body, such as a splinter. The *Cl. tetani* do not spread beyond the wound, but they produce an exotoxin, by which the nervous system is poisoned. Animal experiments have suggested that the toxin reaches the nervous system by ascending the axis cylinders of the peripheral nerves. It has been shown that the dorsal root ganglia act as a filter which prevents the toxin entering the spinal cord by the dorsal roots. Its portal of entry is thus confined to the ventral roots. There is, however, some recent evidence to suggest that the toxin may also spread by the blood stream; thus Zacks and Sheff (1966) have found that the toxin could be isolated from brain, spinal cord, skeletal muscle, and spleen after injecting it into mice. Zacks *et al.* (1966) have also shown vesicles and dense intra-mitochondrial inclusions in the skeletal muscle of such animals. Having reached the brain stem and spinal cord, the toxin produces its characteristic effects by disturbing the normal regulation of the reflex arc. Afferent stimuli not only produce an exaggerated effect, but also reciprocal innervation is abolished and both prime movers and antagonists contract. Hence arises the characteristic muscular spasm.

When a small amount of toxin is slowly absorbed it reaches the anterior horn cells by the route already described. In such cases the first symptom is local spasm of the muscles in the neighbourhood of the wound. When a slightly larger amount of toxin is produced it enters the circulation by way of the lymphatics and reaches the nervous system diffusely by ascending all the peripheral motor nerves. The larger the volume of toxin, the more remains unabsorbed by the anterior horn cells and available to poison distant synapses and ultimately the vital centres. There is then no local tetanus; trismus is usually the first symptom and the spasm subsequently spreads rapidly, to involve the arms, trunk, and legs.

PATHOLOGY

Tetanus is essentially a disorder of function of the nervous system and no constant structural changes have been observed, though hyperaemia may occur in the spinal cord and brain, especially in the anterior horns of grey matter and there may be rupture of fibres and haemorrhages in the muscles which have been subjected to violent spasms.

SYMPTOMS

Incubation Period

The incubation period varies, but is usually 7 or 8 days. In patients who have had a prophylactic inoculation of antitoxin it may extend to several weeks. Exceptionally it is as short as one or two days or, conversely, it may seem, on occasion, to be as long as two or three weeks, when the clinical syndrome may be milder than in the average case, or the spasms may even be curiously localized in one or more limbs (local tetanus). Such a prolonged incubation period is commonest in those who have previously been immunized.

Descending Form

A prodromal phase of restlessness and irritability has been described. The first motor symptom is usually trismus, which is rapidly followed, or may be preceded, by stiffness of the neck. At this stage the patient is likely to attribute his symptoms to a chill. Within a few hours, however, the spasm extends to other muscles and dysphagia is often an early complaint. Spasm of the facial muscles may lead either to pursing of the lips or to retraction of the angles of the mouth—

the risus sardonicus. The eyes may be partly closed through contraction of the orbicularis oculi, or the eyebrows may be elevated by spasm of the frontalis. Examination reveals the presence of rigidity of the musculature of the limbs and trunk. There may be slight opisthotonos. The muscles of the abdominal wall are rigid, and the lower limbs, which are usually affected more than the upper, are fixed in a position of extension. As the disease progresses, this persisting general rigidity undergoes paroxysmal exacerbations which are attended by severe cramp-like pains. Opisthotonic spasm usually occurs in these attacks, but in some cases the spine is bent in other directions, for example, forwards or laterally. Spasm of the larynx and respiratory muscles leads to dyspnoea, and profuse sweating occurs. These convulsive paroxysms may be excited by external stimuli, for example, by attempting to feed the patient. Between the paroxysms the general muscular rigidity persists. The tendon reflexes are exaggerated, but, with the exceptions described below, there are no signs of organic lesions of the nervous system. Consciousness is retained to the end.

Death may occur in a convulsive attack from asphyxia, or, when severe spasms recur frequently, from heart failure. The disease may be apyrexial, but some fever is not uncommon, and hyperpyrexia is an important and serious complication in severe cases, the temperature even continuing to rise after death. Other risks include a negative nitrogen balance leading to uraemia, hypotension, and gastric dilatation, all most liable to occur between the 7th and 14th days, and motor paresis. Laryngeal spasm, apnoea, and pneumonia are also risks. In favourable cases the severity and frequency of the spasms gradually diminish, but the general rigidity frequently persists for several weeks, trismus being often the last abnormality to disappear.

Ascending or Local Form

In this form of tetanus the first symptom is local spasm of the muscles in the neighbourhood of the wound, whence persistent or intermittent spasm spreads to neighbouring muscles and in severe cases to the other limbs, head, and trunk. After recovery from this form of the disease the original local spasm may persist for days or weeks. In one reported case severe rigidity was present in one upper limb only (though trismus was also present in the early stages) for over five months, and in the first two or three months any attempt to use the affected limb produced severe spasms localized to it—'recruitment spasm' (Struppler, Struppler, and Adams, 1963).

Cephalic Tetanus

Cephalic tetanus is a rare variety of the ascending form and follows wounds of the head, face, and neck. Muscular paralysis is frequently present, usually involving the facial muscles on one side and may be associated with facial spasm on the opposite side. Trismus and pharyngeal spasm usually develop. When the wound has involved the orbit, ptosis, external ophthalmoplegia, and iridoplegia have been observed on one or both sides. Cephalic tetanus may remain localized or become generalized. It is usually fatal, but, when recovery occurs, facial paralysis and spasm may persist for weeks.

Splanchnic Tetanus

This term has been applied to a form of tetanus which follows abdominal wounds and in which the bulbar and respiratory muscles are early and severely affected.

Modified Tetanus

The symptoms of tetanus may be considerably modified by a previous immunization or prophylactic inoculation of antitoxin. The incubation period in such cases is usually longer than normal. There is a tendency for the spasm to remain localized to the muscles in the neighbourhood of the wound, and often, when generalized tetanus ensues, convulsions are absent, and if they occur are likely to be slight.

DIAGNOSIS

Conditions causing trismus may be confused with tetanus. Trismus is sometimes produced by painful lesions in the neighbourhood of the jaw such as dental abscess, or it may follow mandibular block with local anaesthetics. The presence of the causative lesion and the localized character of the spasm enable these cases to be distinguished from tetanus. Trismus may also occur in encephalitis, and in some cases, post-vaccinal encephalitis in which trismus was a prominent symptom was at first regarded as tetanus. Symptoms of organic lesions of the brain and spinal cord are always present in such cases and distinguish them from tetanus. The convulsions of strychnine poisoning superficially resemble those of tetanus, but develop more rapidly. Moreover, the fact that they follow reflex excitation is apparent from the beginning, whereas this is a late feature in tetanus. Strychnine poisoning also differs from tetanus in that muscular relaxation is complete between the paroxysms, and the upper limbs are more severely affected. A history of poisoning can usually be obtained. Rabies may also be confused with tetanus, but in this condition trismus is absent and dysphagia is the most conspicuous symptom. Further, muscular relaxation occurs between the paroxysms and there is almost always a history of a bite by a rabid animal. Tetany is distinguished from tetanus by the fact that the muscular spasm always begins in the periphery of the limbs and leads to the characteristic attitude of the hands. Trismus occurs only in the most severe attacks. Hysteria may cause either trismus or generalized rigidity associated with opisthotonos. Hysterical trismus, however, is not associated with rigidity elsewhere, while hysterical opisthotonos usually forms part of a hysterical convulsion which develops suddenly without pre-existing rigidity, is attended by impairment of consciousness, and is frequently associated with other signs of hysteria.

PROGNOSIS

The prognosis of tetanus unmodified by immunization or prophylactic inoculation of antitoxin is always extremely grave, though the outlook was somewhat improved by treatment with antitoxic serum. In one series of cases the mortality before the introduction of treatment with serum was 79 per cent. and afterwards 57·7 per cent. Corresponding figures for the London Hospital quoted by

Fildes (1929) were 81·7 per cent. and 71·8 per cent. In general, the shorter the incubation period the worse is the prognosis, and few patients with an incubation period of less than six days used to recover. Cole (1937–8) stressed the prognostic importance of the interval between the first symptom and the first generalized reflex spasms, which he calls 'the period of onset'. Nevertheless, the new methods of treatment recently introduced offer the hope of saving life even when the incubation period is short, and the mortality rate is now 30 per cent. or less. There may be some persistent motor weakness for many months after recovery.

TREATMENT

The patient should be nursed in isolation and kept as quiet as possible. The curative value of antitoxin is limited by the fact that the nervous system is largely impenetrable by immune bodies. Nevertheless, antitoxin can neutralize toxin in process of absorption and so reduce the dose, perhaps to one the tissues can neutralize. A massive dose—Cole uses 200,000 Units—should be given intravenously.

The modern treatment of tetanus is based upon the elimination of muscle spasm by tubocurarine chloride in doses of 15 mg. repeated as necessary up to a daily total of 150–650 mg., while artificial respiration is carried out with intermittent positive-pressure equipment through a tracheostomy tube, and naso-oesophageal feeding is employed.

Chlorpromazine is highly effective in the control of spasms and can be given instead in a dosage of 100 to 150 mg. four- or six-hourly intramuscularly or, in neonates, 25 mg. four- or six-hourly. It can be combined with barbiturates, e.g. amylobarbitone or pentobarbitone; or phenobarbitone intramuscularly. Antibiotics are given to prevent pulmonary infection. The continuous supervision of an anaesthetist and laryngologist is required. Nutrition and fluid and electrolyte balance must be watched, and many nursing difficulties need to be overcome (Shackleton, 1954; Forbes and Auld, 1955; Adams, 1958; Smith, 1958; Adams et al., 1959).

REFERENCES

ABEL, J. J., and others. Researches on tetanus, *Bull. Johns Hopk. Hosp.*, II, 1935, **56**, 84; III, 1935, **56**, 317; IV, 1935, **57**, 343; V, 1936, **59**, 307; VI, 1938, **62**, 91; VII, 1938, **62**, 522; VIII, 1938, **62**, 610.

ADAMS, E. B. (1958) Clinical trials in tetanus, *Proc. roy. Soc. Med.*, **51**, 1002.

ADAMS, E. B., WRIGHT, R., BERMAN, E., and LAURENCE, D. R. (1959) Treatment of tetanus with chlorpromazine and barbiturates, *Lancet*, i, 755.

COLE, L. (1937–8) The treatment and prognosis of tetanus, *Proc. roy. Soc. Med.*, **31**, 1205.

FILDES, P. (1929) Bacillus tetani, in *A System of Bacteriology*, Vol. 3, p. 298, London.

FORBES, G. R., and AULD, M. (1955) Management of tetanus, *Amer. J. Med.*, **18**, 947.

SHACKLETON, P. (1954) The treatment of tetanus, *Lancet*, ii, 155.

SHERRINGTON, C. S. (1917) Observations with antitetanus serum in the monkey, *Lancet*, ii, 964.

SMITH, A. C. (1958) The treatment of severe tetanus by paralysing drugs and intermittent pressure respiration, *Proc. roy. Soc. Med.*, **51**, 1006.

STRUPPLER, A., STRUPPLER, E., and ADAMS, R. D. (1963) Local tetanus in man, *Arch. Neurol.* (*Chicago*), **8**, 162.

ZACKS, S. I., HALL, J. A. S., and SHEFF, M. F. (1966) Studies in tetanus. IV. Intra-mitochondrial dense granules in skeletal muscles from human cases of tetanus intoxication, *Amer. J. Path.*, **48,** 811.

ZACKS, S. I., and SHEFF, M. F. (1966) Studies on tetanus. V. *In vivo* localization of purified tetanus neurotoxin in mice with fluorescein-labelled tetanus antitoxin, *J. Neuropath. exp. Neurol.*, **25,** 422.

BOTULISM

Definition. A form of food poisoning due to intoxication with the exotoxin of the *Clostridium botulinum* derived from infected foodstuffs, especially those preserved in tins, and characterized by extreme weakness and fatigability of both striated and unstriated muscle.

AETIOLOGY

The *Cl. botulinum* is a large, Gram-positive, anaerobic, spore-bearing organism, which is an inhabitant of the soil in certain regions and may contaminate food. It finds a most congenial environment in food preserved in tins, especially vegetables and fruit, and both bought and home-preserved foodstuffs may be contaminated with it. The commonest type is so-called Type E, and Type E spores have been shown to be plentiful in North American soil and littoral waters (Meyer, 1956). It produces a powerful exotoxin, to which the toxic effects are due. Tinned food infected with the bacillus may often be detected as tainted. Production of gas in the tin may abolish the normal vacuum, and the food often has a peculiar rancid odour and taste. This, however, may be disguised by sauces and dressings. There are many examples of severe and fatal poisoning occurring in a person who had only tasted the food to see if it was tainted. Cooking at boiling temperature for a few minutes destroys the toxin. There have been outbreaks of botulism in many countries, especially in Germany, where it was first attributed to eating infected sausages—hence the name, derived from 'botulus', a sausage—and in the United States. An outbreak leading to a number of deaths occurred at Loch Maree in Scotland in 1922. Botulism has frequently been observed in domestic animals which have eaten the remains of tainted food, and fowls which have been thus intoxicated may die before symptoms appear in human beings, who have eaten the same food. Contamination of fish by Type E may occur before they are caught and Whittaker, Gilbertson, and Garrett (1964) reported eight simultaneous cases due to eating white chubb fish from the Great Lakes area, fish which was contaminated with Type E spores.

Botulinus toxin acts presynaptically, by abolishing the release of acetylcholine at cholinergic nerve endings (Burgen, Dickens, and Zatman, 1949; Zacks, 1964).

PATHOLOGY

The changes in the nervous system consist of great congestion of both the brain and meninges, leading to oedema and perivascular haemorrhages.

SYMPTOMS

In man, symptoms usually develop between 18 and 36 hours after the ingestion of the tainted food, less frequently as early as 12 hours or as late as 48 hours or longer afterwards. In about one-third of all cases an acute gastro-intestinal disturbance, characterized by nausea, vomiting, and diarrhoea, occurs, but in most cases this is absent, constipation, probably due to paresis of the smooth muscle of the intestines, occurring early and persisting throughout the illness.

The earliest symptoms of muscular weakness are usually visual. Dimness of vision occurs as a result of paresis of accommodation; the pupils become dilated, and lose their reaction to light, and ptosis usually develops early. Paresis of the external ocular muscles leads to diplopia, and nystagmus may be present. In some cases complete ocular immobility occurs. Vertigo is not uncommon. Owing to weakness of the muscles concerned, swallowing and talking become difficult; attempts to swallow lead to choking and regurgitation of food through the nose; and there may be complete aphonia. Weakness of the jaw muscles renders mastication difficult or impossible, and the muscles of the trunk and limbs also become extremely weak. The muscular disturbance appears to be an extreme degree of fatigability, rather than an actual paralysis, since the patient may be able to carry out a movement moderately well on one occasion but be then unable to repeat it. The tendon reflexes are preserved and the plantar reflexes are flexor. There is usually no sensory disturbance. In most cases consciousness remains unimpaired up to the end, though occasionally there is a terminal coma, and terminal convulsions have been described.

The cerebrospinal fluid is usually normal. The temperature remains normal, unless a complicating infection, such as bronchopneumonia, develops. The pulse is usually rapid. Death occurs either from paralysis of the respiratory muscles or from bronchopneumonia.

DIAGNOSIS

The most useful diagnostic features are: (1) a previously healthy patient; (2) absence of fever; (3) abdominal symptoms; (4) weakness, malaise, and fatigability; (5) cranial nerve signs; and (6) a likely food source.

In cases in which an acute gastro-intestinal disturbance occurs the diagnosis from other forms of acute gastro-enteritis cannot usually be made before the onset of muscular weakness, unless domestic animals have already shown signs of poisoning. The dilated pupils may suggest belladonna poisoning, but the unclouded mental condition enables this to be excluded. When the diagnosis is doubtful it may be confirmed by the demonstration of the *Cl. botulinum* or of its toxins in the remains of food which has been consumed.

PROGNOSIS

The mortality varies in different outbreaks, ranging between 16 and 65 per cent. Death usually occurs between the fourth and eighth day. Convalescence is very slow in patients who recover.

TREATMENT

Prophylaxis consists in the careful scrutiny of all tinned foods, and the rejection, without tasting it, of any which appears to be tainted. The cooking of tinned products for ten minutes before use abolishes all risk of botulism. Antitoxin appears to possess greater prophylactic than curative value, but it can seldom be used before the onset of muscular symptoms. Fifty thousand Units of a polyvalent serum should be employed. The stomach should be washed out and a purge administered to remove as far as possible any toxin which may not have yet been absorbed. Antibiotics should also be given orally and parenterally, penicillin being the drug of choice in order to destroy surviving organisms in the gastro-intestinal tract which may still be producing exotoxin. Complete rest is of great importance to protect the muscles from all avoidable fatigue, and sedatives should be given if necessary. Nasal feeding and artificial respiration may be required. In view of the action of the toxin on the nerve endings neostigmine should be tried.

REFERENCES

AITKEN, R. S., BARLING, B., and MILES, A. A. (1936) A case of botulism, *Lancet*, ii, 780.
BURGEN, A. S. V., DICKENS, F., and ZATMAN, L. J. (1949) Action of botulinum toxin on the neuro-muscular junction, *J. Physiol. (Lond.)*, **109**, 10.
DICKSON, E. C. (1921) Botulism, in *Oxford Loose Leaf Medicine*, Vol. 5, ch. xi, p. 231, New York.
MEYER, K. F. (1956) The status of botulism as a world health problem, *Bull. Wld Hlth Org.*, **15**, 28.
MONRO, T. K., and KNOX, W. W. N. (1923) Remarks on botulism as seen in Scotland in 1922, *Brit. med. J.*, **1**, 279.
PETTY, C. J. (1965) Botulism; the disease and the toxin, *Amer. J. med. Sci.*, **249**, 345.
WHITTAKER, R. L., GILBERTSON, R. B., and GARRETT, A. S. (1964) Botulism, Type E. Report of 8 simultaneous cases, *Ann. intern. Med.*, **61**, 448.
ZACKS, S. I. (1964) *The Motor End-plate*, Philadelphia.

SAXITOXIN POISONING

Saxitoxin, a powerful neurotoxic agent, may produce symptoms in human subjects eating mussels or other shellfish which have been contaminated by dinoflagellates of the genus *Gonyaulax* which only occur in the sea at certain times of the year and in certain weather conditions. Epidemics have been reported from the Pacific Coast of the U.S.A. and from many places in Europe. A recent outbreak in Northumberland affecting 78 individuals has been described by McCollum *et al.* (1968); while the condition has been fatal all patients in this series recovered. Symptoms, which usually developed within 30 minutes to 12 hours after eating mussels, included paraesthesiae in the limbs and circumoral distribution, muscular weakness, ataxia, headache, vomiting, and choking sensations. Recovery was usually complete within 24–72 hours.

REFERENCE

McCOLLUM, J. P. K., PEARSON, R. C. M., INGHAM, H. R., WOOD, P. C., and DEWAR, H. A. (1968) An epidemic of mussel poisoning in North-East England, *Lancet*, ii, 767.

ERGOTISM

'Ergotism' is the term applied to poisoning with the toxins produced by the fungus *Claviceps purpurea* of rye. Two forms occur, one characterized by gangrene—the gangrenous form—the other by nervous phenomena, especially muscular spasms and generalized convulsions—the convulsive form.

Poisoning with ergot is usually due to the consumption of bread made from contaminated flour. The gangrenous form is occasionally produced by the administration of ergot in the attempt to procure abortion, or therapeutically. Very rarely it may result from the excessive use of ergotamine tartrate given as a treatment for migraine or of the closely-related drug dimethysergide (*Deseril*) given as a prophylactic in this condition, though retroperitoneal fibrosis is a more important complication of treatment with the latter remedy. Many patients who take abnormally large amounts of these drugs may complain of pains in the limbs and of paraesthesiae, blanching of digits and coldness in the extremities but the fully-developed syndrome of ergotism is rare in patients using these remedies. Ergotism is rare in England, but is commoner on the continent of Europe, where it was especially prevalent during the Middle Ages. Epidemics have occurred in France, Germany, Sweden, Norway, Finland, Russia, and elsewhere, and in the last-named country ergotism is apparently still endemic. The gangrenous and convulsive forms differ in their geographical distribution, the former occurring to the west, and the latter to the east, of the Rhine, though mixed epidemics have sometimes been observed where these regions meet. There is reason to believe that the gangrenous form is due to poisoning with ergotoxin or ergotamine, but the convulsive form appears to depend upon the coexistence of two factors, consumption of an unknown constituent of ergot, which is not the alkaloid, together with a deficiency of vitamin A in the diet (Mellanby, 1931; Barger, 1931).

Convulsive ergotism is associated with degeneration of the spinal cord, especially of the dorsal columns, and also of the peripheral nerves. Thickening of the media and hyaline degeneration of the intima of the arteries, sometimes associated with thrombosis, are the changes found in the gangrenous form.

The onset of gangrenous ergotism may be insidious or rapid. Gangrene is usually preceded by severe burning pains, hence the name St. Anthony's fire. Gangrene may involve only the nails, or the fingers or toes or whole limbs, the gangrenous part separating spontaneously without pain or the loss of blood. Convulsive ergotism begins with muscular fasciculation, followed by clonic and tonic muscular spasms, leading to abnormal postures and finally, in severe cases, generalized convulsions. Anaesthesia of the limbs, hemiplegia, and paraplegia may occur.

REFERENCES

BARGER, G. (1931) *Ergot and Ergotism*, London.
MELLANBY, E. (1931) The experimental production and prevention of degeneration in the spinal cord, *Brain*, **54**, 247.
VON STORCH, T. J. C. (1938) Complications following the use of ergotamine tartrate. Their relation to the treatment of migraine headache, *J. Amer. med. Ass.*, **111**, 293,

MINAMATA DISEASE

Between 1953 and 1956 a disorder characterized by symptoms and signs of peripheral neuropathy, cerebellar ataxia, visual and hearing loss and inconstant pyramidal tract involvement, and sometimes by the development of a progressive encephalopathy, was noted in villagers living near Minamata Bay in Kyushu Island, Japan. In fatal cases widespread neuronal damage was found in the granular layer of the cerebellum and in the cerebral cortex. The condition usually followed the ingestion of fish and circumstantial evidence suggested that it was due to the toxic action of a mercurial compound contained in the effluent which flowed into Minamata Bay from a fertilizer factory.

REFERENCE

MCALPINE, D., and ARAKI, S. (1958) Minamata disease, *Lancet*, ii, 629.

THE NEUROLOGICAL MANIFESTATIONS OF ACUTE PORPHYRIA

There are two distinct disorders of porphyrin metabolism. One is the very rare congenital or erythropoietic type, in which light sensitivity is present from birth and neurological manifestations do not occur, and the other, as Dean and Barnes (1955) have shown, includes acute intermittent porphyria, porphyria cutanea tarda, and symptomless porphyrinuria. Porphyria cutanea tarda is characterized by the development of light sensitivity in adult life, while symptomless porphyria, which Dean and Barnes (1958) have called hyperporphyrinism is not genetically determined, is of no serious pathological significance, and can be distinguished from inherited porphyria by biochemical tests. As it is in cases of acute porphyria that neurological manifestations occur, this alone will be considered further.

Macalpine, Hunter, and Rimington (1968) have suggested that King George III of England suffered from a psychotic illness due to porphyria and gave reasons for suggesting that the disorder was present in many members of the Royal Houses of Stuart, Hanover, and Prussia.

AETIOLOGY AND PATHOLOGY

Acute intermittent porphyria is inherited as a Mendelian dominant. There are two principal types, namely the Swedish type, which is commonest in Europe (Waldenstrom, 1957), which is seen most often in females between 16 and 50 years, in which acute attacks are often precipitated by drugs, especially barbiturates, light sensitivity does not occur and there is a high excretion of porphobilinogen G and of δ-amino-laevulinic acid during the acute attacks and for a long time afterwards. In the South African type (Dean and Barnes, 1958) the age and sex incidence is similar, acute attacks are always precipitated by drugs and are often fatal; light sensitivity is found in some affected individuals, particularly males, and there is a high excretion of porphobilinogen in the acute attack but this returns to normal as soon as the patient recovers. The fundamental fault appears to lie in the liver, where it is believed that porphyrin metabolism is abnormal. The pathological changes in the nervous system have been studied by Hierons (1957), who found changes in the anterior horn cells of the spinal cord at all levels, and considerable loss of myelin in the peripheral nerves. Demyelination of the spinal cord was present in only one case. He thought it unlikely that these changes were secondary to vascular abnormalities. The cerebral changes are more difficult to interpret on account of the frequent presence of hypertension, possibly associated with vascular spasm, and anoxia resulting from respiratory paralysis. It is possible, however, that the mental disturbances which may occur in acute porphyria are due to a direct, and possibly reversible, metabolic effect of the disease.

Goldberg (1959) suggests that related to the metabolic disturbance of the liver there is a disorder of the metabolism of the nervous system of which demyelination is the pathological expression. The exact nature of this association is not yet clear. Rimington (1961) discusses theories of the biochemical disorder in acute porphyria, and suggests that the biochemical lesion interferes with the production of acetylcholine. Dagg et al. (1965) drew attention to the similarity of lead poisoning to acute porphyria. In both conditions there is a considerable increase in the excretion of δ-amino-laevulinic acid. They suggest that the abdominal, cardiovascular, and neurological manifestations may be explained on a neurogenic basis with focal demyelination of peripheral and autonomic nerves and in the central nervous system. However, Cavanagh and Mellick (1965) found no evidence of demyelination in the peripheral nerves of four fatal cases and suggested that the lesion lay distally in the axon.

SYMPTOMATOLOGY

The syndrome of acute intermittent porphyria may present with the acute clinical picture, or with cutaneous lesions alone, or with a combination of the two. The biochemical lesion may exist without producing any symptoms, particularly in the sibs of affected patients.

The onset of symptoms usually occurs in adolescence or early adult life, and the acute manifestations are frequently precipitated by the administration of barbiturates, Sedormid, drugs of the sulpha group, or over-indulgence in alcohol.

Early symptoms of involvement of the nervous system include restlessness, emotional instability and mood disorder, sometimes going on to a confusional state. Epileptic attacks are common, and are sometimes the presenting feature. Severe involvement of the cerebral hemispheres may lead to stupor or coma, or status epilepticus.

The other characteristic clinical picture is a polyneuropathy, usually predominantly motor, and leading to muscular weakness, initially chiefly proximal in the limbs, but becoming generalized and sometimes involving the respiratory and bulbar muscles. Though subjective sensory symptoms are common, objective sensory loss is rare.

General symptoms often usher in the attacks, especially acute abdominal pain with nausea, vomiting, and constipation. As already mentioned, hypertension may occur, and there may be impairment of renal function. The skin may exhibit scars, erosions or bullae, and a bronze pigmentation and hirsutism are common.

During the acute attack, the urine contains large amounts of the porphyrin precursors, δ-amino-laevulinic acid and porphobilinogen. In the Swedish type, there is very little increase in urinary and faecal porphyrin excretion except in the acute attack, while in the South African type urinary and faecal porphyrins show a much greater increase, again particularly during an attack. The urine from patients with acute intermittent porphyria is not necessarily abnormally coloured, even during the attack, though in many cases the patient will have noted darkening, and the typical 'port-wine' colour which darkens on standing, at the outset.

DIAGNOSIS

As far as the neurological symptoms are concerned, it is necessary to bear in mind the possibility of porphyria as a cause of otherwise unexplained confusional states, coma, epilepsy, or polyneuropathy occurring particularly in early adult life, and especially if the symptoms have been precipitated by the administration of any of the drugs known to be apt to precipitate acute porphyria.

PROGNOSIS

Acute porphyria is always a serious disease, and the mortality rate may be as high as 50 per cent. In Berman's (1961) series of 81 cases, there were 22 deaths, only 12 of which were attributed solely to the porphyric illness. In 10 cases the cause of death was cardio-respiratory failure, and in 2 cardiac arrest—a mortality rate of 15·6 per cent. All those patients had severe paralysis. However, even though the patient may be gravely ill, complete recovery may occur.

TREATMENT

Prophylaxis obviously includes the avoidance of the drugs known to precipitate attacks in the case of known sufferers, and the investigation of sibs for evidence of asymptomatic metabolic disorder. Treatment is primarily symptomatic, and the usual treatment of bulbar and respiratory paralysis may be called for. Otherwise, chlorpromazine seems to be of particular value for relief of pain and other symptoms. It may be given in a dose of 25 mg. three or four times a day, and a single dose of 100 mg. is reported to have been followed by a complete remission (Welby, Street, and Watson, 1956). Gajdos and Gajdos-Torok (1961) have suggested that the intramuscular injection of adenosine-5-monophosphoric acid may produce prompt improvement.

REFERENCES

BERMAN, S. (1961) Neurologic disorders in porphyria. A brief clinical survey of 81 cases. Reports at the VII International Congress in Neurology, Rome, p. 33.

CAVANAGH, J. B., and MELLICK, R. S. (1965) On the nature of the peripheral nerve lesions associated with acute intermittent porphyria, *J. Neurol. Psychiat.*, **28**, 320.

DAGG, J. H., GOLDBERG, A., LOCHHEAD, A., and SMITH, J. A. (1965) The relationship of lead poisoning to acute intermittent porphyria, *Quart. J. Med.*, **34**, 163.

DEAN, G., and BARNES, H. D. (1955) The inheritance of porphyria acuta, cutanea tarda, and symptomless porphyrinuria, *Brit. med. J.*, **2**, 89.

DEAN, G., and BARNES, H. D. (1958) Porphyria. A South African screening experiment, *Brit. med. J.*, **1**, 298.

DOBRINER, K., and RHOADS, C. P. (1940) The porphyrins in health and disease, *Physiol. Rev.*, **20**, 416.

EALES, L. (1960) Cutaneous porphyria, *S. Afr. J. Lab. clin. Med.*, **6**, 63.

EALES, L. (1961) Porphyrins and the porphyrias, in *Annual Reviews of Medicine*, Palo Alto, Calif.

GAJDOS, A., and GAJDOS-TOROK, M. (1961) Adenosine therapy for porphyria, *Lancet*, ii, 175.

GOLDBERG, A. (1959) Acute intermittent porphyria, *Quart. J. Med.*, **28**, 183.

HAEGER, B. (1958) Urinary δ-aminolaevulinic acid and porphobilinogen in different types of porphyria, *Lancet*, ii, 606.

HIERONS, R. (1957) Changes in the nervous system in acute porphyria, *Brain*, **80**, 176.

MACALPINE, I., HUNTER, R., and RIMINGTON, C. (1968) Porphyria in the Royal Houses of Stuart, Hanover and Prussia, *Brit. med. J.*, **1**, 7.

MASON, V. R., COURVILLE, C., and LISKIND, E. (1933) The porphyrins in human disease, *Medicine (Baltimore)*, **12**, 355.

RIMINGTON, C. (1961) Neurological disorders in porphyria. Reports at the VII International Congress in Neurology, Rome, p. 21.

WALDENSTROM, J. (1957) The porphyrias as inborn errors of metabolism, *Amer. J. Med.*, **22**, 758.

WELBY, J. C., STREET, J. P., and WATSON, C. J. (1956) Chlorpromazine in the treatment of porphyria, *J. Amer. med. Ass.*, **162**, 174.

THE NEUROLOGICAL SYMPTOMS OF HEPATIC FAILURE

Neurological symptoms may appear as the result of hepatic failure from any cause, e.g. of acute virus hepatitis, eclampsia, portal cirrhosis, Wilson's disease, haemochromatosis, acute chemical poisoning, or the terminal stages of biliary cirrhosis. They may arise spontaneously or be precipitated in patients with chronic liver disease by gastro-intestinal haemorrhage, acute alcoholic intoxication, the administration of morphine or barbiturates, paracentesis, diuretics, or surgery. They may also follow the operation of portacaval anastomosis (Sherlock, 1963).

The causes of the disturbances of central nervous function are complex and not fully understood, and are discussed by Sherlock (1963). The essential factor appears to be that as a result of abnormal anastomoses between the portal and systemic arterial systems, either arising naturally or produced by surgery, nitrogenous material intended for the liver enters the systemic circulation. Measurement of the blood ammonia gives a rough index of the severity of the condition which has more recently been called porto-systemic encephalopathy.

One of the most constant pathological features in the brain is the presence in the cortex and in the basal ganglia of Alzheimer type 2 cells which are believed to be glial in origin, and show no cytoplasm with ordinary staining methods (Adams and Foley, 1953). These cells are also present in Wilson's disease.

Neurological symptoms in chronic hepatic disease may be intermittent, and sometimes predominantly psychiatric for long periods. In other cases, and in acute hepatic failure, they develop rapidly and progressively. Psychiatric symptoms consist of changes in the personality, abnormalities of mood and behaviour, and drowsiness deepening into stupor and coma. Speech is likely to be slurred, and there may be aphasia. A 'flapping' tremor is rather characteristic when the arms are outstretched, but may occur in other toxic states also. Neurological signs suggestive of focal cerebral damage or dysfunction are occasionally seen (Pearce, 1963). Extrapyramidal rigidity and tremor may be present with or without signs of corticospinal lesions or cerebellar deficiency. Muscle twitching may occur. More recently myelopathy with spasticity and increased limb reflexes but with flexor plantar responses has been described (Liversedge and Rawson, 1966) and in some cases a syndrome of chronic choreo-athetosis has been observed (Toghill, Johnston, and Smith, 1967).

In severe cases delta waves which may be triphasic will be present in the EEG. In milder cases there is a slowing of the dominant frequency. The EEG can be used as a sensitive indicator of the response to treatment as well as for diagnosis (Laidlaw and Read, 1961). The cerebrospinal fluid is usually normal.

The clinical and biochemical signs of the causal hepatic disorder will be present. Jaundice may be slight or absent in chronic hepatic failure due to cirrhosis.

Treatment consists first in reducing the absorption of nitrogenous substance from the bowel. Hence a protein intake of less than 20 g. daily is necessary and neomycin, 1–2·5 G. daily, may be given in an attempt to sterilize the bowel and to reduce absorption. *Lactobacillus acidophilus* has been used for the same purpose (Macbeth, Kass, and McDermott, 1965) while surgical exclusion of the colon has also been successful (Walker *et al.*, 1965).

REFERENCES

ADAMS, R. D., and FOLEY, J. M. (1953) The neurological disorder associated with liver disease, in *Metabolic Disorders of the Nervous System*, A.R.N.M.D., Baltimore.
BROWN, I. A. (1957) *Liver-brain Relationships*, Springfield, Ill.
LAIDLAW, J., and READ, A. E. (1961) The EEG diagnosis of manifest and latent delirium, *J. Neurol. Psychiat.*, **24**, 58.
LIVERSEDGE, L. A., and RAWSON, M. D. (1966) Myelopathy in hepatic disease and portacaval anastomosis, *Lancet*, i, 277.
MACBETH, W. A. A. G., KASS, E. H., and McDERMOTT, W. V. (1965) Treatment of hepatic encephalopathy by alteration of intestinal flora with *Lactobacillus acidophillus*, *Lancet*, i, 399.
PEARCE, J. M. S. (1963) Focal neurological syndromes in hepatic failure, *Postgrad. med. J.*, **39**, 653.
READ, A. E., LAIDLAW, J., and SHERLOCK, S. (1961) Neuropsychiatric complications of portacaval anastomosis, *Lancet*, i, 961.
SHERLOCK, S. (1963) *Diseases of the Liver and Biliary System*, 3rd ed., Oxford.
TOGHILL, P. J., JOHNSTON, A. W., and SMITH, J. F. (1967) Choreoathetosis in porto-systemic encephalopathy, *J. Neurol. Psychiat.*, **30**, 358.
WALKER, J. G., EMLYN-WILLIAMS, A., CRAIGIE, A., ROSENOER, V. M., AGNEW, J., and SHERLOCK, S. (1965) Treatment of chronic portal-systematic encephalopathy by surgical exclusion of the colon, *Lancet*, ii, 861.

BIOCHEMICAL DISORDERS ASSOCIATED WITH MENTAL RETARDATION

An increasing number of biochemical disorders has been discovered during recent years to be associated with retardation of mental development. Some of these are considered elsewhere in this book, for example Wilson's disease [see p. 534], erythroblastosis foetalis [see p. 566], lead poisoning [see p. 698], and the lipidoses and leucodystrophies [see p. 567]. Some conditions remain to be considered, which have in common their liability to produce mental subnormality, though it will be noticed that in some cases the same or allied disorders may be detected in adult life. The subject has recently been reviewed by Moncrieff (1960) and by Crome and Stern (1967).

AMINO ACID DISORDERS

Crome and Stern (1967) have tabulated no fewer than 47 metabolic disorders, many involving amino acid metabolism, which may be associated with mental retardation. Many of these can only be recognized by means of highly specialized chromatographic techniques applied to the examination of infants' urine. Ideally, were it not for the many difficulties, such screening tests should be carried out in all new-born infants. Only some of the commoner and more important conditions will be considered here.

PHENYLKETONURIA

Phenylketonuria, also known as phenylpyruvic oligophrenia or amentia, is a hereditary (recessive) metabolic disorder first described by Fölling in 1934. It is characterized by a defect in the hydroxylation of phenylalanine to tyrosine, which leads to the urinary excretion of phenylpyruvic acid. Unless the condition is detected and treated during the first few weeks of life, amentia generally results though it is now clear that occasionally mildly-affected individuals may first be recognized in adult life and may show only minor degrees of subnormality. It has been estimated (Brimblecombe et al., 1961) that there are about 40 new cases in the United Kingdom every year. The importance of recognizing such cases is that they may transmit the disease in its more severe form to their children.

The child usually appears normal at birth, but subsequently fails to develop and may suffer from convulsions. Most such children have blonde hair and a fair complexion, and skin changes have been described, which may be the result of diminished skin pigmentation. The degree of mental deficiency is usually severe, and is associated with a non-specific clumsiness of gait and movement, and often with stereotyped repetitive movements. The EEG shows 'a marked generalized abnormality with poverty of rhythmic activity, excess of large irregular slow waves, and large discharges with variable focal distribution' (Pampiglione, 1961).

The presence of phenylpyruvic acid in the urine is demonstrated by adding to the acidified urine a few drops of fresh 5 per cent. ferric chloride solution, which produces a deep bluish-green colour. A simple and more reliable paper-strip test is now available (Brimblecombe et al., 1961).

Treatment consists in putting the child as early as possible on a diet containing a restricted amount of phenylalanine. This is discussed in detail by Brimble-combe *et al.* (1961). They state that of all the ten cases that they have been able to discover in which treatment was begun by the age of 6 weeks, and in which the dietary control of phenylalanine was satisfactory, there was no example of mental deficiency. They also draw attention to the dangers of excessive phenyl-alanine restriction.

HARTNUP DISEASE

Baron *et al.* (1956) first described this hereditary metabolic disorder. Milne *et al.* (1960) collected from the literature 11 patients who were members of 7 unrelated families. The disease appears to be inherited as an autosomal recessive factor. It is characterized by renal amino-aciduria and an excessive excretion of indican and indolic acids. Milne *et al.*, as a result of their investigations, suggest that there may be defective transport of tryptophan across the cells of the jejunum and of the proximal renal tubules.

A curious feature of the disorder is the episodic character of the symptoms. The main clinical features are a photosensitive rash typical of pellagra, mental deterioration, and attacks of cerebellar ataxia. The disease occurs in childhood and tends to improve with increasing age, and in some patients the clinical manifestations have been very mild. The rash may respond to nicotinamide therapy and the attacks of ataxia recover spontaneously. It is suggested that the cerebellar ataxia may be due to intoxication by retained indolic acids, in which case alkalinization of the urine by sodium bicarbonate will increase the excretion of indolic acids and provide an easy method of therapy.

OTHER SYNDROMES ASSOCIATED WITH AMINO ACID DIS-ORDERS

A number of other syndromes, mostly rather rare, have been found to be associated with disorders of the metabolism of amino acids. The term *oculo-cerebral dystrophy* includes several syndromes characterized by eye changes, such as cataract, enophthalmos and corneal opacities, mental retardation, and amino-aciduria. In another syndrome, mental retardation, convulsions, and ataxia are associated with excretion of large quantities of arginin-succinic acid in the urine. There are also two syndromes in which mental retardation is associated with amino acids in the urine which give it a characteristic smell, leading to the terms oast-house syndrome and maple-syrup syndrome. Finally, amino-aciduria is a characteristic of Wilson's disease. These conditions, among others discovered recently, are reviewed by Holt and Milner (1964) and tabulated by Crome and Stern (1967).

DISORDERS OF CARBOHYDRATE METABOLISM

GALACTOSAEMIA

Mental retardation can be associated with an abnormal metabolism of lactose, due to a defect of the enzyme galactose-1-phosphate uridyl transferase, which is inherited as an autosomal recessive factor. The mental defect occurs with varying degrees of severity, and in severe cases enlargement of the liver is associated with jaundice, and the child later develops cataracts. A reducing substance will be found in the urine, and the diagnosis is established by incubating red blood cells obtained from the umbilical cord with galactose. In affected babies an accumulation of galactose-1-phosphate can be demonstrated. In such cases a lactose-free diet appears to give good results.

FRUCTOSURIA

Two metabolic disorders are associated with fructosuria. The first is essential fructosuria, which is symptomless, and may be confused with diabetes mellitus on account of the positive result of testing the urine with Benedict's solution. The other syndrome is known as fructose intolerance, a hereditary disorder in which the absorption of fructose leads to an abnormally high blood fructose associated with hypoglycaemia. This condition may be, but is not always, associated with mental retardation. Dormandy and Porter (1961) have recently reported a case of familial fructose and galactose intolerance.

HYPOGLYCAEMIA

According to Moncrieff (1960) there are various forms of hypoglycaemia in childhood, and as a result of repeated or prolonged hypoglycaemic attacks severe cerebral damage may occur, with mental deterioration. The pathological changes in such cases are similar to those of anoxia [see p. 703] but the Purkinje cells of the cerebellum are peculiarly sensitive to hypoglycaemia so that surviving children are often ataxic. Ingram, Stark, and Blackburn (1967) have reviewed 26 children who suffered from hypoglycaemic coma between the ages of 10 weeks and 11 years. Twelve were diabetic, 1 had islet cell adenomatosis, and in 13 the cause of the hypoglycaemia was unknown. Nine of the 23 children seen at follow-up were mentally retarded, 4 were epileptic, and 10 showed signs of ataxia or ataxic diplegia. In addition to an idiopathic type, and hypoglycaemia in diabetes and islet cell adenomatosis, as just pointed out, episodes of hypoglycaemia may occur in association with a raised blood fructose, and the same thing may happen in galactosaemia.

WATER AND ELECTROLYTE DISTURBANCES

Nephrogenic diabetes insipidus is a congenital defect of water metabolism, frequently but not always associated with mental retardation. It has been attributed to an abnormality of the renal tubules, and appears to be transmitted as a sex-linked recessive disorder, only males being affected. It is unknown whether the mental disorder is the result of the dehydration as such, or the associated raised level of blood sodium. Moncrieff says that very early detection, followed by frequent administration of water, holds out hope of a normal development, and that this is the only condition in which a baby who may be a potential ament can be endowed with a mind by giving a great deal of water.

Both an abnormally high and an abnormally low blood sodium level have been found to be associated with persistent cerebral damage.

REFERENCES

BARON, D. N., DENT, C. E., HARRIS, H., HART, E. W., and JEPSON, J. B. (1956) Hereditary pellagra-like skin rash with temporary cerebellar ataxia, constant renal amino-
aciduria and other bizarre biochemical features, *Lancet*, ii, 421.

BRIMBLECOMBE, F. S. W., BLAINEY, J. D., STONEMAN, M. E. R., and WOOD, B. S. B. (1961)
Dietary and biochemical control of phenylketonuria, *Brit. med. J.*, 2, 793.

CROME, L. C., and STERN, J. (1967) *Pathology of Mental Retardation*, London.

DORMANDY, T. L., and PORTER, R. J. (1961) Familial fructose and galactose intolerance,
Lancet, i, 1189.

HOLT, K. S., and MILNER, J. (eds.) (1964) *Neurometabolic Disorders in Childhood*, Edinburgh.

INGRAM, T. T. S., STARK, G. D., and BLACKBURN, I. (1967) Ataxia and other neurological disorders as sequels of severe hypoglycaemia in childhood, *Brain*, 90, 851.

MILNE, M. D., CRAWFORD, M. A., GIRAO, C. B., and LOUGHRIDGE, L. W. (1960) The
metabolic disorder in Hartnup disease, *Quart. J. Med.*, 29, 407.

MONCRIEFF, A. (1960) Biochemistry of mental defect, *Lancet*, ii, 273.

PAMPIGLIONE, E. (1961) EEG in inborn errors of metabolism. Reports at the VII International Congress in Neurology, Rome, p. 15.

CARBON DIOXIDE INTOXICATION

In patients with chronic respiratory disease, especially chronic bronchitis
and emphysema, it has become increasingly apparent that neurological manifestations may result from the fact that the respiratory centre appears to become
insensitive to carbon dioxide which is retained in the circulation as bicarbonate
as a result of chronic alveolar hypoventilation. In some such cases a chronic
syndrome characterized by headache, lethargy, drowsiness, and fluctuating confusion persists over a period of many weeks or months. In some cases, however,
an acute syndrome characterized by severe headache and vomiting, convulsions,
papilloedema, and rapid impairment of consciousness has been described, due
to increasing cerebral oedema and may be precipitated by the administration of
oxygen. In many such patients it is necessary to give steroid drugs and diuretics
to reduce brain swelling but intermittent positive pressure respiration, monitored
by measurements of the blood pO_2 and pCO_2 is the most effective treatment,
in order to remove the accumulated CO_2 and, in time, to restore the sensitivity
of the respiratory centre.

REFERENCES

FISHMAN, A. P., TURINO, G. M., and BERGOFOLLY, E. H. (1957) The syndrome of
alveolar hypoventilation, *Amer. J. Med.*, 23, 333.

MANFREDI, F., SIEKER, H. O., SPOTO, A. P., and SALTZMAN, H. A. (1960) Severe carbon
dioxide intoxication, *J. Amer. med. Ass.*, 173, 999.

STUART-HARRIS, C. H., and HANLEY, T. (1957) *Chronic Bronchitis, Emphysema and Cor
Pulmonale*, Bristol.

16

DEFICIENCY DISORDERS

THE isolation of the vitamins and the study of their physiological properties and of the effects of their lack upon animals in experimental conditions led to the hope that vitamin deficiency in man would be recognizable in a similarly clear-cut manner, but greater clinical experience of nutritional disorders during the Second World War has produced a more critical approach to a problem which is now seen to be more complex than was thought at first. The sick man suffering from nutritional deficiency has usually been partially starved for a long time. His disorder is often chronic; different vitamins are likely to have been lacking in varying proportions in different circumstances; other dietary elements will probably have been inadequate also; finally dysentery and other acute and chronic infections are complicating factors acting both by their toxins and also by interfering with the absorption of food. We are thus presented with varying and partially overlapping clinical pictures which we are often unable to correlate with particular forms of deficiency. It seems best, therefore, first to review the physiology of those vitamins whose lack is believed to cause nervous disorders and then to describe the chief syndromes which appear to be caused by nutritional deficiency.

The B Group of Vitamins

Experimental work has led to the isolation of a number of factors in the vitamin B complex, four of which need especially to be considered in relation to nervous disease: these are vitamin B_1 (aneurine or thiamine), nicotinic acid, riboflavine, and pyridoxine. The B group of vitamins are present in greatest amount in brewers' yeast, in the germ and aleurone layer of ripe wheat, and also in egg yolk and mammalian liver, and in smaller amounts in milk, green vegetables, potatoes, and meat.

Vitamin B_1 (Aneurine or Thiamine)

This vitamin plays an important part in the metabolism of carbohydrates. It forms a compound with pyrophosphoric acid which acts as co-enzyme to the enzyme which breaks down pyruvic acid, one of the intermediate products in the breakdown of glucose. A deficiency of aneurine, by interfering with the breakdown of pyruvic acid, leads to an accumulation of pyruvate in the blood, which can be detected chemically. Experimental workers have described the signs of acute and chronic aneurine deficiency in pigeons. Acute deficiency causes opisthotonos, chronic deficiency 'locomotor ataxia', weakness of the legs, and cardiac failure. Histologically there is a degeneration of the peripheral nerves, and haemorrhages are found in the brain.

The minimum requirement of aneurine in the day's food is not more than $1\frac{1}{2}$ to

2 mg. Aneurine deficiency may be detected by a subnormal blood level (less than 3 μg. per 100 ml.), diminished urinary excretion after a test dose, or a raised level of pyruvate in the blood.

Nicotinic Acid

Nicotinic acid or niacin acts as a co-enzyme in intracellular oxidation processes. The daily requirements of an adult are probably about 20 mg. A saturation test has been used to detect nicotinic acid deficiency in man. Deficiency of nicotinic acid produces in dogs a condition known as 'black-tongue', which is very similar to human pellagra.

Riboflavine

Riboflavine also acts as a co-enzyme in the breakdown of carbohydrate. The daily minimal requirement in man is probably 2–3 mg. Riboflavine deficiency causes angular stomatitis, glossitis, injection of the limbus of the cornea, and in some cases abnormal vascularization of the cornea: its possible role in causing nervous symptoms is discussed below [see p. 734].

Pyridoxine

Pyridoxine (vitamin B_6) aids the conversion of tryptophan to N-methyl nicotinamide. In infants reared on a pyridoxine-deficient diet, convulsions and anaemia were noted. In adults living on a diet deficient in this vitamin or in those receiving desoxypyridoxine, or more often, isoniazid given for the treatment of tuberculosis (both of these substances are pyridoxine antagonists), symmetrical polyneuropathy, optic atrophy and/or microcytic anaemia may develop and each can be corrected by administration of this vitamin.

REFERENCES

BEAUPRE, E. M., and GROUNEY, P. M. (1963) Pyridoxine-responsive anaemia with neuropathy, *Ann. intern. Med.*, **59, 724**

BICKNELL, F., and PRESCOTT, F. (1953) *The Vitamins in Medicine*, 3rd ed., London.

SPILLANE, J. D. (1964) Drug-induced neurological disorders, *Proc. roy. Soc. Med.*, **57,** 135.

STANNUS, H. S. (1944) Some problems in riboflavin and allied deficiencies, *Brit. med. J.*, **2**, 103, 140.

SWANK, R. L. (1940) Avian thiamin deficiency. A correlation of pathology and clinical behaviour, *J. exp. Med.*, **71**, 683.

SWANK, R. L., and PRADOS, M. (1942) Avian thiamine deficiency, *Arch. Neurol. Psychiat. (Chicago)*, **47,** 97.

VILTER, R. W., MUELLER, J. E., GLAZER, H. S., JARROLD, A. J., THOMPSON, C., and HAWKINS, V. R. (1963) The effect of vitamin B_6 deficiency produced by desoxypyridoxine in human beings, *J. Lab. clin. Med.*, **42, 335**.

BERIBERI

AETIOLOGY

The discovery that beriberi was due to dietary deficiency and that one substance lacking in the diet of natives suffering from this disorder was the water-soluble vitamin now known as vitamin B_1, aneurine, or thiamine, which was contained in the germinal layer discarded from polished rice, was of the greatest value in the prevention and treatment of the disease. The designation of this vitamin, the antineuritic vitamin, however, tended to obscure the problems in the aetiology of beriberi which still remain unsolved. It is clear that aneurine is not an antineuritic vitamin in the sense that its absence from the diet necessarily causes neuritis, for this does not occur in animals unless they are given carbo-hydrates, and in man a fall in the ratio of aneurine to carbohydrate and protein in the diet is also a causal factor, beriberi occurring when the ratio of mg. of aneurine per 1,000 non-fat calories falls below 0·3. Since we now know that aneurine is necessary for the normal metabolism of carbohydrates, these observa-tions seem to show that the nervous system and heart suffer in beriberi either from an inability to metabolize carbohydrates normally or, as Walshe has suggested, from poisoning with pyruvate or some other product of incomplete carbohydrate breakdown. Other causal factors are chronic diarrhoea which inter-feres with the absorption of aneurine, liver disease which probably impairs its storage, and physical exertion which increases the need of the tissues for it. Some believe that a lack of other vitamins of the B group contributes to the causation of beriberi.

Any or all of these factors may combine with dietary deficiency to cause beri-beri among prisoners of war or ill-nourished natives. There is no doubt that beriberi can occur also in patients whose diet is not deficient in aneurine but who suffer from a disorder of the alimentary canal which renders its absorption defective. Such lesions include pyloric stenosis, gastro-enterostomy, ulcerative colitis, dysentery, and steatorrhoea. In addition to impairing absorption these disorders may lead to the adoption of a deficient diet. Chronic alcoholism may cause beriberi by leading to a defective intake and absorption of aneurine. At the same time the high calorie value of the alcohol increases the need for aneurine and hence the relative deficiency. Pregnancy also increases the demand for the vitamin. Vitamin B deficiency is also seen, even in highly-developed countries, in elderly people living alone on inadequate diets and it may even result from the anorexia which sometimes accompanies chronic endogenous depression.

PATHOLOGY

The changes in the nervous system are those of degenerative or parenchy-matous neuritis [see p. 810], involving both the somatic peripheral nerves and the autonomic nerves. This is the so-called 'dry' form. The affected neurones exhibit degenerative changes, especially at the periphery, and chromatolysis is found in the ganglion cells of the anterior horns and dorsal root ganglia of the spinal cord, and of the motor nuclei of the cranial nerves. The changes in the muscles are those characteristic of degeneration of the lower motor neurones. In the 'wet' form of beriberi there are myocardial degeneration, with enlargement of the right side of the heart, chronic venous congestion of the liver and spleen, effusions in the pleural cavities and pericardium, ascites, and oedema of the skin and subcutaneous tissues. Patients dying in the acute stage of the disease exhibit congestion and haemorrhagic injection of the pyloric end of the stomach and the duodenum.

SYMPTOMS

The onset in some cases is very rapid, especially in infants—'the acute pernicious' type of Wright. In others it is more gradual, and mild or larval forms occur. In the most acute cases nervous symptoms typical of polyneuritis develop within twenty-four or forty-eight hours. These consist of paraesthesiae and tenderness of the limbs, sensory loss, and progressive atrophic paralysis, with loss of reflexes. The paralysis may rapidly spread to involve all the muscles of both upper and lower limbs and finally the laryngeal muscles, intercostals, and diaphragm. Symptoms of cardiac involvement include dyspnoea and palpitations, tachycardia, cardiac dilatation, and signs of heart failure. Oedema may be slight or extreme. Disturbance of function of the alimentary canal leads to flatulence, and constipation or diarrhoea.

In chronic cases the clinical picture is that of a more or less severe polyneuritis with or without cardiac failure. The presence or absence of oedema is the basis of the distinction between the so-called 'wet' and 'dry' forms of the disease.

The pyruvic acid in the blood is often raised in beriberi above the normal content of 0·4–1·0 mg. per 100 ml. The pyruvate content of the cerebrospinal fluid is similarly raised. In doubtful cases a pyruvate tolerance test may be helpful (Joiner, McArdle, and Thompson, 1950).

DIAGNOSIS

The diagnosis of polyneuritis in general is discussed on page 812. In the wet form of beriberi the combination of polyneuritis and cardiac failure is unique. The dry form requires to be distinguished from polyneuritis due to other causes. Tenderness of the calves and excessive sensitivity of the skin on the soles of the feet are often more striking in B_1-deficiency neuropathy than in any other. Beriberi should be suspected when the diet has been deficient for any reason or a disorder of the alimentary canal has interfered with absorption. Confirmation is afforded by a raised level of pyruvate in the blood or by a pyruvate tolerance test. It should be remembered that many heavy metals produce polyneuropathy by acting as competitive inhibitors of co-enzyme A or by combining with SH groups which are necessary in this reaction so that the possibility of occult heavy metal poisoning should be borne in mind. If such a metal is responsible then an abnormal pyruvate tolerance test may not be corrected by the administration of thiamine.

PROGNOSIS

In untreated fulminating cases death may occur within a few days from heart failure. Patients who survive the acute stage without treatment are likely to be left with the symptoms of a chronic polyneuritis with or without heart failure. Most patients who receive early and thorough treatment during the acute stage make a complete recovery, and remain well as long as they continue to take an adequate diet. Treatment may bring about some improvement in patients who have reached the chronic stage, but these are not likely to make a complete recovery.

TREATMENT

The heart failure must be treated by absolute rest in bed. The diet should consist of frequent small feeds with a minimum of carbohydrates and fluid. Aneurine should be injected intravenously. As much as 50 mg. may be given in this way if necessary on the first day and smaller doses on subsequent days as required. There is usually an immediate response, but diuretics and digoxin may also be needed. Oral treatment with 50 mg. thiamine three times daily should be continued for some days, the dose later being reduced to a maintenance level of 5–10 mg. daily. The usual therapeutic treatment of polyneuritis should be carried out, a diet rich in aneurine should be given, and the possibility that the patient is also suffering from the lack of other vitamins should be borne in mind. Indeed, it is wise to give nicotinic acid, riboflavine and pyridoxine as well and to be sure that there is no evidence of associated vitamin B_{12} deficiency. Chronic alcoholics should be treated for alcohol addiction. Patients in whom aneurine deficiency is secondary to disease of the stomach, duodenum, or intestine or to endogenous depression will need appropriate treatment.

REFERENCES

BICKNELL, F., and PRESCOTT, F. (1953) *The Vitamins in Medicine*, 3rd ed., London.

COWGILL, G. R. (1938) The physiology of vitamin B_1, *J. Amer. med. Ass.*, **110,** 805.

GOODHART, R. S., and SINCLAIR, H. M. (1940) Deficiency of vitamin B_1 in man as determined by the blood cocarboxylase, *J. biol. Chem.*, **132,** 11.

JOINER, C. L., MCARDLE, B., and THOMPSON, R. H. S. (1950) Blood pyruvate estimations in the diagnosis and treatment of polyneuritis, *Brain*, **73,** 431.

VICTOR, M., and ADAMS, R. D. (1961) On the etiology of the alcoholic neurological diseases, *Amer. J. clin. Nutr.*, **9,** 379.

WALSHE, F. M. R. (1918–19) On the 'deficiency theory' of the origin of beri-beri in the light of clinical and experimental observations on the disease with an account of a series of 40 cases, *Quart. J. Med.*, **12,** 320.

WILLIAMS, R. R. (1938) The chemistry of thiamin, *J. Amer. med. Ass.*, **110,** 727.

WILLIAMS, R. R. (1961) *Toward the Conquest of Beriberi*, Cambridge, Mass.

WRIGHT, H. (1903) On the classification and pathology of beri-beri, *Stud. Inst. med. Res. Kuala Lumpur*, No. 3.

WERNICKE'S ENCEPHALOPATHY

Synonym. Polio-encephalitis haemorrhagica superior.

Definition. An acute or subacute disorder affecting chiefly the midbrain and hypothalamus, caused by vitamin deficiency, chiefly if not exclusively of aneurine, and characterized pathologically by congestion, capillary proliferation, and petechial haemorrhages, and clinically by disorders of memory and consciousness, ophthalmoplegia, and ataxia.

AETIOLOGY

Experimental work shows that a pathological condition which appears to be identical with Wernicke's encephalopathy can be produced in animals by putting them on a diet deficient in aneurine. In man the fasting level of pyruvate in the blood has been found to be invariably elevated, and to return to normal after the administration of aneurine parallel with the clinical improvement of the patient. It has been suggested, however, that the Wernicke syndrome may not represent a simple aneurine deficiency, being complicated in some cases by lack of other nutritional factors.

The aneurine deficiency may be due to various causes. An inadequate diet was the cause of Wernicke's encephalopathy occurring in prisoners of war, and in civil life the causes are the same as those which produce beriberi, namely, inadequate diet, chronic alcoholism, gastro-intestinal disorders, especially carcinoma of the stomach, and persistent vomiting of pregnancy. The condition has also been recorded as occurring after gastectomy.

The rare condition of subacute necrotizing encephalopathy [p. 578] which occurs in acidotic infants in which raised blood levels of lactate and pyruvate are found is believed to be a closely related disorder, resulting, however, from an inborn error of metabolism and not from primary aneurine deficiency (Procopis, Turner, and Selby, 1967).

PATHOLOGY

Recent observations have confirmed Wernicke's original description of the pathology of this disorder, the essential lesion consisting of foci of marked congestion with many small petechial haemorrhages affecting particularly the hypothalamus and the grey matter of the upper part of the brain stem. The corpora mammillaria are constantly involved, and frequently there is also a zone of congestion with petechiae in the grey matter immediately surrounding the third ventricle, i.e. throughout the hypothalamus and medial part of the thalamus on each side. Foci are also frequently seen in the posterior colliculi of the midbrain, and less frequently in the grey matter of the floor of the fourth ventricle and other regions. They have also been described in the optic nerves. Histologically the essential lesion appears to be the vascular disorder, namely, great dilatation and proliferation of capillaries with small perivascular haemorrhages. Damage to the nerve cells is usually surprisingly slight.

SYMPTOMS

The onset is usually insidious. Vomiting and nystagmus are early symptoms. The patient may experience a sense of unreality; he has difficulty in concentrating and sleeps badly. This condition passes into a confusional state which ends in stupor and coma. In less severe and acute cases the mental changes are usually those of Korsakow's syndrome with defects of recent memory and confabulation. The ophthalmoplegia usually begins with weakness of the lateral recti and may become complete. There is usually some degree of ataxia of the limbs. Retinal haemorrhages may be present. In many cases Wernicke's encephalopathy is accompanied by polyneuritis, but this is not always so.

DIAGNOSIS

The diagnosis should be suggested by the occurrence of cerebral symptoms in a patient in whom one of the predisposing causes already mentioned is present, and may be confirmed by finding a raised pyruvate level in the blood. Wernicke's encephalopathy is most likely to be confused with some form of acute encephalitis in which, however, fever is likely to be present, and there will probably be a pleocytosis in the cerebrospinal fluid. Associated features of the Korsakow syndrome and polyneuropathy will clinch the diagnosis.

PROGNOSIS

Wernicke's encephalopathy if untreated is likely to prove fatal. In prisoner-of-war camps the condition when diagnosed early and treated with the inadequate supplies of aneurine usually available had a mortality rate of 50 per cent. Intensive early treatment, however, leads to rapid and complete recovery, except that in some cases the Korsakow psychosis may persist for many months or occasionally for years after recovery from the acute stage. The latter syndrome does not respond to aneurine as completely and promptly as Wernicke's encephalopathy and recovery from it may be incomplete [see p. 689].

TREATMENT

The treatment is that of beriberi [see p. 729]. In view of the possibility that other deficiencies besides that of aneurine may be present it is advisable to give nicotinic acid as for pellagra and 5 mg. of riboflavine daily in addition.

REFERENCES

CAMPBELL, A. C. P., and BIGGART, J. H. (1939) Wernicke's encephalopathy (polio-encephalitis haemorrhagica superior): its alcoholic and non-alcoholic incidence, *J. Path. Bact.*, **48**, 245.

CAMPBELL, A. C. P., and RUSSELL, W. R. (1941) Wernicke's encephalopathy: the clinical features and their probable relationship to vitamin B deficiency, *Quart. J. Med.*, N.S. **10**, 41.

JOLLIFFE, N., WORTIS, H., and FEIN, H. D. (1941) The Wernicke syndrome, *Arch. Neurol. Psychiat. (Chicago)*, **46**, 569.

MEYER, A. (1944) The Wernicke syndrome, *J. Neurol. Psychiat.*, N.S. **7**, 66.

PRADOS, M., and SWANK, R. L. (1942) Vascular and interstitial cell changes in thiamine-deficient animals, *Arch. Neurol. Psychiat. (Chicago)*, **47**, 626.

PROCOPIS, P. G., TURNER, B., and SELBY, G. (1967) Subacute necrotizing encephalopathy in an acidotic child, *J. Neurol. Neurosurg. Psychiat.*, **30**, 349.

VICTOR, M., and ADAMS, R. D. (1961) On the etiology of the alcoholic neurological diseases, *Amer. J. clin. Nutr.*, **9**, 379.

WORTIS, H., BUEDING, E., STEIN, M. H., and JOLLIFFE, N. (1942) Pyruvic acid studies in the Wernicke syndrome, *Arch. Neurol. Psychiat. (Chicago)*, **47**, 215.

PELLAGRA

Definition. A disease which appears to be caused chiefly by deficiency of an element in the vitamin B_2 complex, nicotinic acid, though lack of other essential food factors may also be important. It is characterized by cutaneous lesions, mental changes, glossitis, diarrhoea, and degeneration of the brain, spinal cord, and peripheral nerves.

AETIOLOGY

Pellagra is endemic in the poorer strata of the population in many South European countries, in Africa, and especially in the Southern States of the U.S.A. It is rare in Great Britain, where it has been found most often in patients in mental hospitals and in alcoholics. It may occur at any age, and both sexes are affected with equal frequency. It is commonly, but not exclusively, found among white maize-eaters. Its aetiology was until recently obscure. It has been attributed to a diet deficient in proteins, to the ingestion of toxic substances contained in the maize and to other hypothetical toxins, but recent evidence shows that the main cause is a deficiency of an element in the vitamin B complex, nicotinic acid. This is also known as the pellagra-preventing (P.P.) factor. More recently still it has been demonstrated that the amino acid, tryptophan, is a nicotinic acid precursor and dietary deficiency of tryptophan or nicotinic acid or both may produce the syndrome. The administration of nicotinic acid produces immediate improvement in patients suffering from pellagra, and will prevent the development of pellagra if added to a diet which otherwise produces it. Endemic pellagra is attributed to a deficiency of nicotinic acid in the diet. As in the case of other deficiency diseases, however, defective absorption of nicotinic acid from the alimentary canal is sometimes the cause of 'secondary' pellagra which may occur though there is an ample supply of the essential substance in the diet. 'Secondary' pellagra may thus occur after dysentery or long-continued diarrhoea, after operation or cancer involving the stomach or small intestine, and in alcohol addicts. The combination of alcoholism and a deficient diet is an important cause of pellagra in some countries. Pellagra-like skin lesions may be seen in Hartnup disease, due to an inborn error of metabolism in which cerebellar ataxia, amino-aciduria, and an excretion of excess indole-acetic acid in the urine are observed. Rarely, similar skin lesions also appear in patients treated with isoniazid, a vitamin B_6 inhibitor. Finally, in patients with the carcinoid syndrome (malignant argentaffinoma), the circulating serotonin may cause tryptophan deficiency and a pellagra-like syndrome. The disease of dogs, canine black tongue, like human pellagra, can be prevented and cured by nicotinic acid. Maize is said to contain an antivitamin to nicotinic acid, and tryptophan in some way counterbalances lack of nicotinic acid.

PATHOLOGY

The meninges are thickened and the brain may be oedematous or atrophic. Chromatolysis and pigmentation are found in the ganglion cells throughout the central nervous system and in the autonomic ganglia. The spinal cord exhibits demyelination of many of the long tracts. This is most marked in the posterior columns in the upper thoracic and cervical regions, but the corticospinal and spinocerebellar tracts also suffer. Changes in the peripheral nerves are less conspicuous, and consist mainly of degeneration of the myelin sheaths. Pigmentation and hyaline degeneration have been described in the cerebral arterioles and capillaries.

The principal lesions outside the nervous system are atrophy of the stomach and intestine, and ulceration of the large bowel.

SYMPTOMS

The disease may run a protracted course lasting for many years. The first attack and subsequent exacerbations tend to occur in the spring. The early attacks are characterized by gastro-intestinal disturbances, especially diarrhoea, associated with the development of the cutaneous lesions. The latter begin as an erythema involving the parts of the body exposed to light, while later the deeper layers of the skin are involved, leading to desquamations, thickening, and finally atrophy. Exceptionally the cutaneous lesions may be absent. The tongue exhibits glossitis, with loss of the epithelium, and similar changes occur in the pharynx. Gastric achylia is the rule and porphyrinuria is sometimes present. Nervous changes develop later. Many abnormal mental states occur, depending no doubt partly on the psychological constitution of the patient. Mania and melancholia may develop, the latter sometimes leading to suicide. Often the terminal state is a dementia. Visual impairment and diplopia may occur. Dysarthria and dysphagia may develop in the later stages, together with tremor and ataxia, especially in the lower limbs. The tendon jerks may be increased at first, but later tend to be lost. The plantar reflexes may be extensor. Sensory symptoms consist of pain in the limbs with tenderness of the muscles and superficial anaesthesia and analgesia. There may be loss of appreciation of passive movements of the toes.

Nicotinic acid deficiency has also been regarded as the cause of an encephalopathy leading to stupor or coma occurring alone or associated with pellagra, polyneuritis, ophthalmoplegia, or scurvy. Urinary excretion tests may be of value in diagnosis.

DIAGNOSIS

The clinical picture is unique, and can hardly be confused with anything else, but in the absence of the cutaneous lesions the nervous condition may resemble subacute combined degeneration.

PROGNOSIS

The prognosis in the past was poor, most patients after many years ending their days in mental hospitals. Early treatment on modern lines, however, may be expected to bring about a cure in many cases.

TREATMENT

Treatment is primarily dietetic. Nicotinic acid should be given. Spies (1938) recommended 0·5 G. per day given in five doses of 100 mg. each for oral administration. If it is necessary to give the substance parenterally 10 to 20 mg. may be injected in sterile saline four times a day. Parenteral administration may be necessary where there is reason to think that absorption from the alimentary canal is defective. In encephalopathy 100 mg. of nicotinamide should be given intravenously and the same dose intramuscularly daily, together with 1,000 mg. divided between five doses orally. In the present state of knowledge, it is unwise to rely entirely upon nicotinic acid. Sebrell (1938) advised a high calorie diet, 3,000 to 4,000 Calories, including at least one quart of milk daily, together with other vitamin supplements.

REFERENCES

Aetiology of pellagra and the nutritive value of maize, *Lancet*, 1938, i. 282.

BICKNELL, F., and PRESCOTT, F. (1953) *The Vitamins in Medicine*, 3rd ed., London.

ELLINGER, P., BENESCH, R., and HARDWICK, S. W. (1945) Nicotinamide methochloride elimination tests on normal and nicotinamide-deficient persons, *Lancet*, ii, 197.

GRANT, J. M., ZSCHIESCHE, E., and SPIES, T. D. (1938) The effect of nicotinic acid on pellagrins maintained on a pellagra-producing diet, *Lancet*, i, 939.

GREENFIELD, J. G., and HOLMES, J. M. (1939) A case of pellagra. The pathological changes in the spinal cord, *Brit. med. J.*, **1**, 815.

JOLLIFFE, N., BOWMAN, K. M., ROSENBLUM, L. A., and FEIN, H. D. (1940) Nicotinic acid and deficiency encephalopathy, *J. Amer. med. Ass.*, **114**, 307.

LANGWORTHY, O. R. (1931) Lesions of the central nervous system characteristic of pellagra, *Brain*, **54**, 291.

SEBRELL, W. H. (1938) Vitamins in relation to the prevention and treatment of pellagra, *J. Amer. med. Ass.*, **110**, 1665.

SPIES, T. D. (1938) The response of pellagrins to nicotinic acid, *Lancet*, i, 252.

SPILLANE, J. D. (1947) *Nutritional Disorders of the Nervous System*, Edinburgh.

SYDENSTRICKER, V. P. (1958) The history of pellagra, its recognition as a disorder of nutrition and its conquest, *Amer. J. clin. Nutr.*, **6**, 409.

SYDENSTRICKER, V. P., and CLECKLEY, H. M. (1941) Effects of nicotinic acid in stupor, lethargy and various other psychiatric disorders, *Amer. J. Psychiat.*, **98**, 83.

NUTRITIONAL NEUROPATHIES OF OBSCURE ORIGIN

For many years doctors practising in the tropics have been familiar with clinical pictures which have been found to occur either alone or in association with beriberi, pellagra, or ariboflavinosis. Fresh attention was directed to these syndromes during the Spanish Civil War and the Second World War. They appear to be due to defective nutrition though some may be due to toxic substances in food; various views are held about their causation. Treatment with riboflavine, aneurine, and nicotinic acid has not afforded conclusive evidence that any of these alone is the deficient factor and it seems probable that in many cases there are multiple deficiencies as well as some imbalance between various constituents of the diet.

Painful Feet. There are burning sensations in the soles, especially severe at night and accompanied by hyperalgesia and sweating, and later by a changeable and patchy hyperaesthesia. Other nervous abnormalities are usually absent. This syndrome has been attributed to deficiency of nicotinic acid, but deficiency of pantothenic acid now seems more likely to be the cause.

Spinal Ataxia. This begins with dysaesthesiae in the feet, gradually followed by unsteadiness of gait. Sensory loss is prominent. Appreciation of vibration is lost first in the lower limbs, then awareness of passive movement, first in the toes, then more proximally. Cutaneous sensory loss appears later and spreads up to the knees or even the waist. The knee- and ankle-jerks are usually exaggerated but the plantar reflexes are flexor. The condition has been the subject of extensive reports from West Africa (Money, 1961; Monekosso, 1964), from Tanganyika (Haddock, Ebrahim, and Kapur, 1962) and from Senegal (Collomb *et al.*, 1967). In many cases the clinical picture is purely one of sensory ataxia, often of remarkably sudden onset, but amblyopia and optic atrophy and pyramidal tract involvement have been found to be associated in some cases.

Osuntokun (1968) has recently reported 84 cases seen in Western Nigeria and has found plasma and urinary thiocyanate levels to be raised in such patients. He gives reasons for suggesting that the condition is due to chronic exposure to dietary cyanide, obtained from culinary derivatives of cassava, the tuber of manioc.

Cranial Nerve Disorders. The commonest of these is acute or subacute retrobulbar neuritis. Nerve-deafness, laryngeal palsy, anosmia, and trigeminal anaesthesia may also occur, with or without spinal ataxia. In Moore's cases (1937) retrobulbar neuritis was associated with soreness of the tongue and mouth and scrotal dermatitis while Monekosso and Ashby (1963) found an association of nutritional amblyopia and spinal ataxia in occasional cases.

Spastic Paraplegia. This was the rarest of these disorders among prisoners of war. Mental changes may occur at the onset. Spillane (1947) points out its resemblance to lathyrism. Cruickshank, Montgomery, and Spillane (1961) have reported cases of paraplegia of gradual or sudden onset in Jamaica associated with loss of posterior column sensibility, retrobulbar neuritis, nerve-deafness, and occasionally distal wasting of the limb muscles. Montgomery *et al.* (1964) have analysed the clinical findings in 206 cases and the pathological findings in 10. There were 25 cases with ataxia, optic atrophy, and nerve-deafness resembling the other tropical neuropathies described above, and almost certainly due to malnutrition. In 181 cases, however, the picture was one of a spastic paraparesis; most patients showed positive blood tests for syphilis, but these were negative in the spinal fluid. They consider the possibility that toxic food substances (bush tea) or nutritional deficiencies could in some way modify the clinical and pathological picture of neurosyphilis and so produce this syndrome. Mani *et al.* have recently described 35 cases from Southern India which seem identical to those observed in Jamaica. They found no evidence of cyanide intoxication in their cases and nothing to indicate that syphilis was responsible. While unidentified dietary toxins may account for the condition they raise the possibility that it could be due to a slow virus infection.

Treatment

The treatment of these tropical neuropathies must include the provision of a full balanced diet with vitamin supplements, particularly of the B group. If given before irreversible pathological changes have occurred there is often an encouraging response except in cases of West Indian or South Indian spastic paraplegia in which the usual treatment for syphilis should also be given but improvement, if any, is usually slight.

Lathyrism

The consumption of lathyrus peas, which are often eaten in India, may produce a slowly-progressive spastic paraplegia, especially when the peas are contaminated with seeds of the weed akta (*vicia sativa*) which contain certain alkaloids and a cyanogenetic glycoside. The toxic principle has been identified as β-amino-proprionitrile (Sinclair and Jelliffe, 1961).

REFERENCES

BRAIN, W. R. (1947) Malnutrition of the nervous system, *Brit. med. J.*, **2**, 763.

COLLOMB, H., QUERE, M. A., CROS, J., and GIORDANO, G. (1967) Les neuropathies dites nutritionnelles au Sénégal, *J. neurol. Sci.*, **5**, 159.

CRUICKSHANK, E. K., MONTGOMERY, R. D., and SPILLANE, J. D. (1961) Obscure neurologic disorders in Jamaica, *Wld Neurol.*, **2**, 99.

DENNY-BROWN, D. (1947) Neurological conditions resulting from prolonged and severe dietary restriction, *Medicine (Baltimore)*, **26**, 41.

HADDOCK, D. R. W., EBRAHIM, G. J., and KAPUR, B. B. (1962) Ataxic neurological syndrome found in Tanganyika, *Brit. med. J.*, **2**, 1442.

MANI, K., MANI, A., and MONTGOMERY, R. D. (1969) A spastic paraplegic syndrome in South India, *J. neurol. Sci.*, in the press.

MONEKOSSO, G. L. (1964) Clinical survey of a Yoruba village, *W. Afr. med. J.*, **13**, 47.

MONEKOSSO, G. L., and ASHBY, P. H. (1963) The natural history of an amblyopia syndrome in Western Nigeria, *W. Afr. med. J.*, **12**, 226.

MONEY, G. L. (1961) Etiology of funicular myelopathies in Tropical Africa, *Wld Neurol.*, **2**, 526.

MONTGOMERY, R. D., CRUICKSHANK, E. K., ROBERTSON, W. B., and McMENEMEY, W. H. (1964) Clinical and pathological observations on Jamaican neuropathies— a report on 206 cases, *Brain*, **87**, 425.

MOORE, D. F. (1937) Nutritional retrobulbar neuritis followed by partial optic atrophy, *Lancet*, i, 1225.

OSUNTOKUN, B. O. (1968) An ataxic neuropathy in Nigeria. A clinical, biochemical and electrophysiological study, *Brain*, **91**, 215.

SINCLAIR, H. M., and JELLIFFE, D. B. (1961) *Tropical Nutrition and Dietetics*, London.

SPILLANE, J. D. (1947) *Nutritional Disorders of the Nervous System*, Edinburgh.

SPILLANE, J. D., and SCOTT, G. I. (1945) Obscure neuropathy in the Middle East, *Lancet*, ii, 262.

VITAMIN B₁₂ NEUROPATHY (SUBACUTE COMBINED DEGENERATION OF THE SPINAL CORD)

Synonyms. Posterolateral sclerosis; combined system disease.

Definition. A deficiency disease, usually associated with pernicious anaemia, and characterized pathologically by degeneration of the white matter of the spinal cord, which is most evident in the posterior and lateral columns, and of the peripheral nerves and brain, and clinically by paraesthesiae, sensory loss, especially impairment of deep sensibility, ataxia, and paraplegia. Subacute combined degeneration was described as progressive pernicious anaemia in tabetic patients by Leichtenstern in 1884, and the spinal cord changes were associated with the anaemia by Lichtheim in 1887. The first complete clinical and pathological account was given by Russell, Batten, and Collier in 1900. The therapeutic value of liver was the discovery of Minot and Murphy in 1926 and led to the recognition of extrinsic and intrinsic factors by Castle and his collaborators. Lester Smith in England and Rickes and his colleagues in America isolated the essential factor, cyanocobalamin, vitamin B₁₂, from the liver in 1948.

Richmond and Davidson (1958) for various reasons suggest that vitamin B$_{12}$ neuropathy is a better name than subacute combined degeneration.

PATHOLOGY

Macroscopical changes in the nervous system are slight. Slight cerebral atrophy has been described, and on section of the cord demyelination is evident in the greyish appearance of the white matter. Microscopically, two types of lesion are found in the spinal cord, necrotic foci and degeneration of the long tracts. It has been suggested that the latter may be secondary to the former.

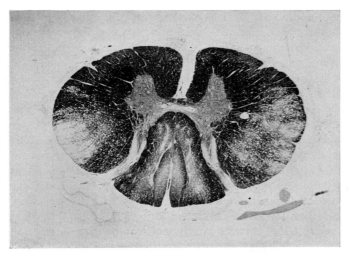

Fig. 99. Vitamin B$_{12}$ neuropathy. Spinal cord; C. 3

The necrotic foci, which first appear in the lower cervical and upper thoracic regions of the spinal cord, are irregular patches of demyelination situated in the white matter, near the surface, and are possibly related to the entering blood vessels. They are most marked in the posterior columns, and the corticospinal and ascending cerebellar tracts. Degeneration of the long tracts is most evident in the upper part of the cord in the ascending tracts, and in the lower part in the descending tracts. Both types of lesion are characterized by demyelination, and in the most severely affected regions both the myelin sheaths and the axis cylinders disappear, leaving vacuolated spaces separated by a fine glial meshwork [Fig. 99]. Similar focal areas of degeneration have been described in the white matter of the brain, together with more diffuse degenerative changes in the cerebral association fibres (Adams and Kubik, 1944). Degeneration is often present in the peripheral nerves, and the muscles are usually smaller than normal and exhibit a simple atrophy.

In the majority of cases the pathological changes of pernicious anaemia are found in patients dying of vitamin B$_{12}$ neuropathy. These include glossitis, anaemia, hyperplasia of the red marrow in the long bones, slight or moderate enlargement of the spleen, and the presence of iron in the reticulo-endothelial system. Magnus and Ungley (1938) have described in pernicious anaemia a profound atrophy of all coats of the stomach wall, localized to the body and sparing the pyloroduodenal region. The sera of about 60 per cent. of patients with pernicious anaemia contain antibodies which are capable of interfering with the ability of intrinsic factor to promote normal physiological handling of vitamin B_{12}. Immunofluorescent techniques have revealed that the antigen involved is a constituent of gastric parietal cells (*British Medical Journal*, 1966).

AETIOLOGY

Vitamin B_{12} neuropathy is a disease of middle life, the average age of onset being about 50. It may, however, begin as early as 26 or as late as 70. Both sexes are equally affected. Its familial occurrence is rare, but is well authenticated, and families have been described in which multiple cases of vitamin B_{12} neuropathy and pernicious anaemia have occurred in the same family, sometimes in more than one generation.

In almost all cases vitamin B_{12} neuropathy is associated with megalocytic anaemia, but the relationship between the two disorders is a complicated one. At first it was believed that the degeneration of the spinal cord was secondary to the anaemia, but that this view is incorrect is shown by the fact that the anaemia may be slight or even, exceptionally, absent, when the spinal degeneration is severe, while only 10 per cent. of patients with Addisonian anaemia suffer from vitamin B_{12} neuropathy (see Waters and Mollin, 1961). It must also be noted that psychiatric syndromes of confusion, depression and dementia have been observed as a result of avitaminosis B_{12} with normal findings in the peripheral blood and marrow (Strachan and Henderson, 1965). There is also evidence to suggest that tobacco amblyopia may be due to traces of cyanide in tobacco smoke which interfere with the utilization of vitamin B_{12} and that the condition may be corrected by the administration of hydroxocobalamin but not by cyanocobalamin (*vide infra*) (Chisholm, Bronte-Stewart, and Foulds, 1967).

It is now known that the importance of gastric achylia lies not in the absence of the gastric acidity but in the lack of an intrinsic factor, secreted by the normal stomach, which facilitates the absorption of an extrinsic factor, contained in the food. This is cyanocobalamin, a cobalt-containing complex isolated in a red crystalline form from the liver by Smith (1948) and Rickes *et al.* (1948) and called by the latter vitamin B_{12}. Recent work suggests that the only function of the intrinsic factor is to render possible the absorption of the extrinsic factor, which occurs in the terminal portion of the ileum, and which is necessary for normal haemopoiesis and the maintenance of the nutrition of the nervous system. While failure to secrete the intrinsic factor is the usual fault, impaired absorption may cause vitamin B_{12} neuropathy; so, too, may inadequate intake as in vegans, a sect of strict vegetarians, who refuse to eat any animal products (Smith, 1962).

Although vitamin B_{12} neuropathy is usually associated with pernicious anaemia, the blood count may be normal. Vitamin B_{12} neuropathy may also occur after the operations of partial or total gastrectomy, and intestinal disease, such as idiopathic steatorrhoea, regional ileitis, tropical sprue, and resections, diverticulosis and fistulae of the small intestine. In such cases a megalocytic anaemia may be due to either folic acid or vitamin B_{12} deficiency, and folic acid given for the anaemia may aggravate the neurological symptoms of B$_{12}$ deficiency.

SYMPTOMS

Nervous Symptoms

The clinical picture is usually a mixture of posterior column, corticospinal tract, and peripheral nerve degeneration.

The onset of symptoms is usually gradual, but is sometimes rapid. The first symptoms are generally paraesthesiae, and consist of tingling sensations, first felt in the tips of the toes, and later in the fingers. Less frequently both upper and lower extremities are thus involved simultaneously, or both the hands may be first affected. Other paraesthesiae of which patients complain include sensations of numbness, coldness, and tightness, while pains of a burning or stabbing character, sometimes resembling the lightning pains of tabes, may occur in the limbs and back. The paraesthesiae, which usually begin in the periphery of the lower limbs, tend to spread slowly towards and up the trunk, and a sense of constriction around the chest or abdomen is common. Motor symptoms consisting of weakness and ataxia develop at a variable interval after the paraesthesiae, and begin in the lower limbs. The patient may first notice that he easily becomes tired when walking, or that he walks unsteadily and tends to stumble.

Objective sensory changes are almost constantly present, and the forms of sensibility mediated by the posterior columns are always affected. Postural sensibility and appreciation of passive movement and of vibration are impaired first in the lower, and later in the upper limbs. Cutaneous sensibility to light touch, pin-prick, heat, and cold is impaired at first over the periphery of the extremities, leading to the characteristic 'glove and stocking' distribution of superficial sensory loss. The calves may be tender on pressure. The proximal border of the anaesthetic areas moves gradually towards the trunk, and on the trunk itself moves slowly upwards.

In some cases weakness and spasticity, in others ataxia, predominate in the lower limbs, but both weakness and ataxia are usually present in all four limbs, and are more severe in the lower. Incoordination in the lower limbs, which is mainly the outcome of defective postural sensibility, is evident in the ataxic gait and the presence of Romberg's sign. Moderate muscular wasting is usually present in the later stages in the extremities, especially in the peripheral muscles.

The reflexes vary considerably. In more than 50 per cent. of cases the ankle-jerks are absent when the patient comes under observation; the knee-jerks are lost rather less frequently; in other cases both are exaggerated. The plantar reflexes are flexor at first in about 50 per cent. of cases, but later become extensor in all but a small proportion. In a few cases, in which the degeneration is confined to the posterior columns, ataxia is the predominant symptom throughout and signs of corticospinal defect are lacking. Conversely, spastic paraplegia may alone be present.

Sphincter disturbances consist, in the early stages, of difficult or precipitate micturition, and later of retention of urine or incontinence. Impotence occurs early.

Bilateral primary optic atrophy with some visual impairment is observed in about 5 per cent. of cases and may even be the presenting feature, when central scotomata may be found (Freeman and Heaton, 1961) [see p. 150]; nystagmus may be present. The pupils may be small, but react normally. Otherwise the cranial nerves are usually normal, though dysarthria may occur.

Mental changes sometimes occur and their importance has been stressed by McAlpine (1929), Holmes (1956), Fraser (1960), and Strachan and Henderson (1965). They may be present in the absence of anaemia and of signs of spinal cord disease. There may be a mild dementia, with impaired memory and intellectual capacity, or a confusional psychosis with disorientation and paranoid tendencies, or Korsakow's psychosis; or the mental disorder may be predominantly affective, and manifest itself in irritability or depression with a suicidal tendency. The cerebrospinal fluid is normal. In cases of pernicious anaemia, with or without symptoms and signs of involvement of the brain and spinal cord, the EEG may show diffuse slow activity and returns to normal after appropriate treatment (Walton *et al.*, 1954).

Associated Symptoms

Gastric achlorhydria is constantly present in Addisonian anaemia, but free acid may be present in the gastric juice when the neuropathy is due to nutritional deficiency or malnutrition. There is usually anaemia, commonly of the Addisonian or macrocytic variety, characterized by a high colour index and mean cell volume, the presence of megalocytes or even megaloblasts in the circulating blood, poikilocytosis, anisocytosis, polychromatophilia, and leucopenia, with a relative lymphocytosis. Even when the blood count is apparently normal it may be possible to demonstrate an excessive number of the large red cells characteristic of pernicious anaemia or an abnormal marrow on sternal puncture. Glossitis is common, but appears to be more closely related to the anaemia than to the neurological symptoms. It may be slight or absent when the anaemia is not severe. Other symptoms may be present if the anaemia is severe. These include dyspnoea, the characteristic lemon tint of the skin, cardiac dilatation, haemic murmurs, and oedema, which is most marked in the lower limbs. The spleen is palpable in only a small proportion of cases. Gastro-intestinal symptoms are common, especially anorexia, flatulence, and diarrhoea particularly when the neuropathy is secondary to intestinal disease. Bodily nutrition is well maintained at first, but general wasting is usually marked in the later stages.

DIAGNOSIS

The neurological picture must be distinguished from tabes, multiple sclerosis, spinal compression, and polyneuritis. Tabes is distinguished by the absence of extensor plantar responses, except when it happens to be associated with meningovascular syphilis. Reflex iridoplegia is usually present in tabes, and in most cases the V.D.R.L. reaction is positive in either the blood or the cerebrospinal fluid, if not in both.

In multiple sclerosis there is usually evidence of the disseminated character of the lesions, and especially of cerebral involvement, with pallor of the optic discs and nystagmus. The ankle-jerks are usually exaggerated in multiple sclerosis and very rarely diminished. Difficulty in diagnosis is most likely to arise in the form of multiple sclerosis characterized by progressive spastic paraplegia which is not uncommon in middle-aged patients. This, however, usually runs a much more chronic course than subacute combined degeneration, and anaemia and gastric achlorhydria are absent.

Spinal compression may lead to an ataxic paraplegia of gradual onset. Careful investigation of the physical signs, however, often indicates a well-defined level at the upper limit of the motor disability and sensory loss, and characteristic changes will usually be found in the cerebrospinal fluid and on myelography. Cervical spondylosis may cause a myelopathy closely resembling the spinal lesions of vitamin B$_{12}$ neuropathy, but in addition cervical spondylosis and the neuropathy may coexist, in which case the most careful investigation of both will be required to assess their relative importance.

Polyneuritis may simulate subacute combined degeneration, when paraesthesiae, occurring in the extremities, are associated with ataxia of the lower limbs, loss of the tendon reflexes, and sensory loss of the 'glove and stocking' distribution. It is not surprising that there should be a close resemblance between the two conditions, since it is certain that some of the symptoms of vitamin B$_{12}$ neuropathy are in fact due to degeneration of the peripheral nerves. Furthermore there is evidence from investigations of pyruvate metabolism that vitamin B$_{12}$ and B$_1$ deficiency may coexist (Hornabrook and Marks, 1960). In 'pure' polyneuritis, however, there is never any evidence of involvement of the corticospinal tracts. Pain and tenderness of the muscles and muscular weakness in the distal segments of the limbs are more severe as a rule than in vitamin B$_{12}$ neuropathy.

When vitamin B$_{12}$ neuropathy is suspected on neurological grounds a blood count should be made and the gastric acidity investigated. The presence of anaemia and of gastric achlorhydria affords strong support for the diagnosis, since, apart from their accidental occurrence, these symptoms are not constantly associated with any condition with which vitamin B$_{12}$ neuropathy is likely to be confused. If there is no anaemia sternal marrow puncture may still show the characteristic abnormality of red cell formation, but this too may be normal. In untreated cases an assay of the serum vitamin B$_{12}$ is diagnostic. The normal range using the *Euglena gracilis* test is from 100 to 960 $\mu\mu$g. per ml. In vitamin B$_{12}$ neuropathy the serum vitamin B$_{12}$ is usually below 80 $\mu\mu$g. per. ml. It should be noted that chlorpromazine and other drugs may interfere with estimation of the serum B$_{12}$, giving falsely low levels (Herbert, Gottlieb, and Altschule, 1965). Another useful test is the investigation of vitamin B$_{12}$ absorption using radioactive B$_{12}$ (Berlyne, Liversedge, and Emery, 1957). In pernicious anaemia the absorption is almost nil, but if the intrinsic factor is given as well it becomes normal. In untreated patients the response to treatment is also a helpful test (Mollin, 1957–8, 1959). When doubt remains as to whether a low serum B$_{12}$ is due to Addisonian pernicious anaemia or to some other cause the Schilling test and a search for gastric parietal-cell antibodies in the serum may be valuable.

PROGNOSIS

The average duration of the illness of pernicious anaemia before the introduction of the modern treatment was about two years. Now it is possible by means of cyanocobalamin or hydroxocobalamin to restore the blood to normal and maintain the patient in good health indefinitely. Such patients need never develop vitamin B_{12} neuropathy. When this has already developed, it can always be arrested, but the degree of recovery depends upon the stage which the disease has reached. The peripheral nerves are capable of regeneration, but this is not possible in the spinal cord, though doubtless here already damaged fibres may be restored to normal. A striking improvement therefore may be expected in the polyneuritic symptoms with disappearance of paraesthesiae and pains in the limbs, sensory loss of the 'glove and stocking' distribution, and muscular wasting, and with return of the tendon reflexes and improvement in co-ordination. Extensor plantar reflexes and spastic weakness and gross loss of postural sensibility, however, usually persist unchanged. Even in patients in whom the disease has been arrested by treatment the development of an infection, especially localized suppuration, may lead to a severe exacerbation.

TREATMENT

The essential factor which is lacking in vitamin B_{12} neuropathy must be administered to the patient intramuscularly in the form of vitamin B_{12}. The intramuscular route is usually the most convenient, but recent work suggests that oral treatment with vitamin B_{12}-peptide may be equally effective (Mooney and Heathcote, 1963). The state of the blood is no guide to the dosage required for the nervous symptoms (Ungley, 1949), which is usually much larger than that needed to combat the anaemia.

Treatment should be begun with 1,000 μg. of vitamin B_{12} given every 2 or 3 days for 5 doses to restore the tissue stores. After this 100 μg. should be given weekly for 6 months, after which 100 μg. a month is usually sufficient but may need to be increased if infection or renal insufficiency develops. The oral B_{12}-peptide is given in a dosage of 100–300 μg. (equivalent) daily. Vitamin B_{12} must be given for the rest of the patient's life. Folic acid is not only useless for the treatment of vitamin B_{12} neuropathy but may be deleterious as the administration of folate load produces a secondary B_{12} deficiency.

Bed rest may be required at first. The diet should be ample and well supplied with vitamins. If there is any suspicion of B_1 deficiency, aneurine should be given. Re-educational exercises are of great value. Analgesics and sedatives may be required at first and in advanced cases, which are now fortunately rare, the usual care of the skin, bladder, rectum, and paralysed muscles necessitated by paraplegia will be required.

REFERENCES

ADAMS, R. D., and KUBIK, C. S. (1944) Subacute combined degeneration of the brain, *New Engl. J. Med.*, **231**, 1.

BERK, L., DENNY-BROWN, D., FINDLAND, M., and CASTLE, W. B., (1948) Effectiveness of vitamin B_{12} in combined system disease, *New Engl. J. Med.*, **239**, 328.

BERLYNE, G. M., LIVERSEDGE, L. A., and EMERY, E. W. (1957) Radioactive vitamin B_{12} in the diagnosis of neurological disorders, *Lancet*, i, 294.

BRITISH MEDICAL JOURNAL (1966) Parietal-cell antibody and gastritis, Leading Article, *Brit. med. J.*, **1**, 643.

CHISHOLM, I. A., BRONTE-STEWART, J., and FOULDS, W. S. (1967) Hydroxocobalamin versus cyanocobalamin in the treatment of tobacco amblyopia, *Lancet*, ii, 450.

DAVISON, C. (1931) Changes in the spinal cord in subacute combined degeneration following liver therapy, *Arch. Neurol. Psychiat. (Chicago)*, **25**, 1394.

FRASER, T. N. (1960) Cerebral manifestations of Addisonian pernicious anaemia, *Lancet*, ii, 458.

FREEMAN, A. G., and HEATON, J. M. (1961) The aetiology of retrobulbar neuritis in Addisonian pernicious anaemia, *Lancet*, i, 908.

GILDEA, E. F., KATTWINKEL, E. E., and CASTLE, W. B. (1930) Experimental combined system disease, *New Engl. J. Med.*, **202**, 523.

GREENFIELD, J. G., and CARMICHAEL, E. A. (1935) The peripheral nerves in cases of subacute combined degeneration of the cord, *Brain*, **58**, 483.

HERBERT, V., GOTTLIEB, C. W., and ALTSCHULE, M. D. (1965) Apparent low serum-vitamin-B$_{12}$ levels associated with chlorpromazine, *Lancet*, ii, 1652.

HOLMES, J. M. (1956) Cerebral manifestations of vitamin B$_{12}$ deficiency, *Brit. med. J.*, **2**, 1394.

HORNABROOK, R. W., and MARKS, V. (1960) The effect of vitamin B$_1$ therapy on blood-pyruvate levels in subacute combined degeneration of the cord, *Lancet*, ii, 893.

MAGNUS, H. A., and UNGLEY, C. C. (1938) The gastric lesion in pernicious anaemia, *Lancet*, i, 420.

McALPINE, D. (1929) Nervous and mental aspects of pernicious anaemia, *Lancet*, ii, 643.

MOLLIN, D. L. (1957–8) The megaloblastic anaemias, in *Lectures on the Scientific Basis of Medicine*, Vol. 7, p. 94, London.

MOLLIN, D. L. (1959) Radioactive B$_{12}$ in the study of blood diseases, *Brit. med. Bull.*, **15**, 8.

MOONEY, F. S., and HEATHCOTE, J. G. (1963) Oral treatment of subacute combined degeneration of spinal cord, *Brit. med. J.*, **1**, 1585.

RICHMOND, J., and DAVIDSON, S. (1958) Subacute combined degeneration of the spinal cord in non-Addisonian anaemia, *Quart. J. Med.*, **27**, 517.

RICKES, E. L., BRINK, N. G., KONIUSZY, F. R., WOOD, T. R., and FOLKERS, K. (1948) Crystalline vitamin B$_{12}$, *Science*, **107**, 396.

RUSSELL, J. S. R., BATTEN, F. E., and COLLIER, J. (1900) Subacute combined degeneration of the spinal cord, *Brain*, **23**, 39.

SMITH, A. D. M. (1962) Veganism: a clinical survey with observations on vitamin B$_{12}$ metabolism, *Brit. med. J.*, **1**, 1655.

SMITH, E. L. (1948) Purification of anti-pernicious anaemia factors from liver, *Nature (Lond.)*, **161**, 638.

STRACHAN, R. W., and HENDERSON, J. G. (1965) Psychiatric syndromes due to avitaminosis B$_{12}$ with normal blood and marrow, *Quart. J. Med.*, **34**, 303.

STRAUSS, M. B., and CASTLE, W. B. (1932) The extrinsic (deficiency) factor in pernicious and related anaemias, *Lancet*, ii, 111.

UNGLEY, C. C. (1949) Subacute combined degeneration of the cord, *Brain*, **72**, 382.

UNGLEY, C. C., and SUZMAN, M. M. (1929) Subacute combined degeneration of the cord: symptomatology and effects of liver therapy, *Brain*, **52**, 271.

WALTON, J. N., KILOH, L. G., OSSELTON, J. W., and FARRALL, J. (1954) The electroencephalogram in pernicious anaemia and subacute combined degeneration of the cord, *Electroenceph. clin. Neurophysiol.*, **6**, 45.

WATERS, A. H., and MOLLIN, D. L. (1961) Studies on the folic acid activity of human serum, *J. clin. Path.*, **14**, 335.

FOLATE DEFICIENCY

Folate deficiency produced by malabsorption (as in steatorrhoea and intestinal 'blind-loop' syndromes) or by the use of anticonvulsant drugs, causes haematological abnormalities identical with those of pernicious anaemia, but until recently was not considered to cause neurological symptoms and signs. However,

it has recently been shown that some patients with polyneuropathy and myelopathy (Grant, Hoffbrand, and Wells, 1965) and others with mental illness,
including dementia (Carney, 1967) may be shown to be folate-deficient, with
serum values of less than 2 μg./ml. In some such cases improvement follows
the administration of folic acid, 5 mg. three times daily. While the exact role of
folate in the aetiology of these neurological disorders remains to be determined
it would appear that estimation of the serum folate should be carried out in cases
of unexplained polyneuropathy, myelopathy, and dementia.

REFERENCES

CARNEY, M. W. P. (1967) Serum folate values in 423 psychiatric patients, *Brit. med. J.*,
    2, 512.
GRANT, H. C., HOFFBRAND, A. V., and WELLS, D. G. (1965) Folate deficiency and
    neurological disease, *Lancet*, ii, 763.
HERBERT, V. (1964) Studies of folate deficiency in man, *Proc. roy. Soc. Med.*, **57**, 377.

17

THE NEUROLOGICAL MANIFESTATIONS OF NEOPLASMS ARISING OUTSIDE THE NERVOUS SYSTEM

THE presence of a neoplasm in the body may affect the nervous system in a number of different ways. The most familiar is by the spread of metastases to the nervous system itself, or the structures by which it is contained. During recent years, however, a number of other effects, the pathogenesis of which is quite obscure, have been noted.

Cerebral Metastatic Neoplasms

The commonest sites of a primary carcinoma, likely to give rise to cerebral metastases, are the bronchus, breast, kidney, stomach, prostate, and thyroid. It sometimes happens that it is the symptoms of a cerebral metastasis which first bring the patient under medical observation. This is particularly common in the case of carcinoma of the bronchus. Indeed the primary growth may be so small as not to be evident on plain X-rays of the lung. At the other extreme there may be a latent interval of many years between the removal of the primary growth and the development of a cerebral metastasis, e.g. in the case of a breast carcinoma.

The clinical features of secondary carcinoma of the brain are described elsewhere [p. 260]. Two diagnostic points are of importance: it may be possible to demonstrate the presence of neoplastic cells in the cerebrospinal fluid; and electroencephalography or isotope scanning may show abnormalities suggestive of multiple metastases when only one may be causing clinical symptoms (Strang and Ajmone-Marsan, 1961).

The likelihood that a cerebral metastasis is solitary is of obvious importance in relation to treatment. Russell and Rubinstein (1959) noted that in a series of 117 cases of cerebral metastasis from bronchial carcinoma a solitary secondary was found in the brain in 30 per cent., but in only 2 of these cases were solitary metastases the only secondary growth found in the body, though in 6 others the extracranial deposits were restricted to the hilar glands.

Direct Invasion of the Nervous System by Tumour

The commoner tumours which arise outside the nervous system, but within the skull or spinal canal, are considered in the sections dealing with intracranial and spinal tumours. Other tumours arising from structures in the neighbourhood of the nervous system, and directly invading it, are comparatively rare. They include chordomas, osteomas, chondromas and sarcomas of bone, glomus jugulare tumours, malignant tumours arising in the orbit, nasal sinuses, and nasopharynx. Myeloma is considered below.

Carcinomatous Meningitis

Exceptionally metastatic carcinoma of the nervous system may present with the clinical features of meningitis as the result of spread of a metastatic growth to the basal leptomeninges. The identification of tumour cells in the cerebro-spinal fluid is a valuable aid to diagnosis.

Cranial Metastases

The main clinical importance of metastatic growths in the cranial bones is that such tumours readily spread to the dura and may then lead to a subdural haematoma.

Spinal Metastases

Metastatic carcinoma of the spine is discussed elsewhere [see pp. 640 and 655].

Direct Invasion of Plexuses and Peripheral Nerves

Nerve plexuses or peripheral nerves are sometimes invaded by either a primary tumour or by metastatic growths in neighbouring lymph nodes. This is particularly likely to occur in the case of tumours of the apex of the lung, the thyroid, breast, uterus, and rectum. Involvement of peripheral nerves by haematogenous metastases is rare except in lymphoma.

Myeloma (Plasmacytoma)

Myelomas may arise within the bones of the skull, or the spine (Clarke, 1954), and may then invade the nervous system secondarily.

Polyneuropathy has been described in association with myeloma by Victor, Banker, and Adams (1958) and is not the result of compression of nervous structures by tumour tissue. The pathological change in the peripheral nerves is degenerative, and the lower limbs may be affected alone, or with the upper as well. Thickened carpal ligaments may lead to the carpal tunnel syndrome. The condition is unrelated to amyloid disease, and in some cases clinical, radio-logical, and even biochemical evidence of myeloma may be lacking.

NEUROLOGICAL COMPLICATIONS OF THE RETICULOSES

Macroglobulinaemia (Waldenström's Syndrome)

Some 25 per cent. of patients with macroglobulinaemia suffer from neuro-logical complications, most of which appear to be due to increased serum viscosity and macroglobulin levels. The subject has recently been reviewed by Solomon (1965). The principal abnormalities are retinopathy, with papilloe-dema and haemorrhages in some cases, various manifestations of encephalopathy, including strokes, and headache, auditory symptoms, such as tinnitus, deafness, and vertigo, and postural hypotension. Peripheral neuropathy occurs but it is doubtful whether this is a symptom of increased serum viscosity. Those symp-toms which are can usually be relieved by plasmaphoresis.

Progressive Multifocal Leuco-encephalopathy

Progressive multifocal leuco-encephalopathy was originally described by Åström, Mancall, and Richardson (1958) and by Cavanagh *et al.* (1959). The subject has recently been reviewed by Richardson (1965) who has had access to 44 cases.

It is characterized by foci of demyelination in the white matter of the cerebral hemispheres, sometimes also involving the brain stem and cerebellum and, sparsely, the spinal cord. These areas range in size from some just visible to the naked eye to large confluent areas. Usually the myelin sheaths disappear with preservation of the axis cylinders. Inflammatory infiltration is often absent but there is a characteristic change in most cases in the astrocytes, which are enlarged with bizarre nuclei, often showing mitotic changes, and in all cases, the nuclei of the oligodendrocytes are paler than normal and contain inclusion bodies.

Progressive multifocal leuco-encephalopathy is a rare disorder occurring as a terminal event, usually in patients suffering from disorders of the reticulo-endothelial or blood-forming systems, i.e. the reticuloses and myelocytic leukaemias. It has also been observed in sarcoidosis, tuberculosis, and in a small number of cases of carcinomatosis and other disorders. It was speculatively thought to be due to the invasion of the nervous system by a virus in patients who, owing to their primary disorder, had lost the normal immune reactions, and this view now appears to have been confirmed by the observations of Zu Rhein and Chou (1965), Silverman and Rubinstein (1965) and Howatson, Nagai, and Zu Rhein (1965), who have, with the electron microscope, identified in the oligodendrocytes particles which appear to be forms of the polyoma virus. The demyelination is attributed to destruction of the oligodendrocytes by the virus and the changes in the nuclei of the astrocytes to viral invasion.

The disorder usually terminates fatally from three to six months from the onset, and is characterized by the symptoms of massive destruction of the white matter in the cerebral hemispheres and/or cerebellum, i.e. hemiplegia, quadriplegia, aphasia, visual field defects or blindness, dysarthria, and ataxia. Convulsions are rare. The patient dies in coma. The cerebrospinal fluid is usually normal.

Subacute 'Poliomyelitis'

Recently, Walton, Tomlinson, and Pearce (1968) have reported a patient with Hodgkin's disease who developed subacute muscular weakness and wasting and in whom pathological examination revealed inflammatory changes like those of poliomyelitis in the anterior horns of the spinal cord; electron microscopy showed viral-like particles in these lesions.

NEUROPATHY AND MYOPATHY ASSOCIATED WITH CARCINOMA

During recent years abnormalities in various parts of the nervous system and in the muscles have been noticed to occur with increasing frequency in association with neoplasms of the viscera, but unrelated to the presence of metastases. Denny-Brown(1948) under the heading 'Primary Sensory Neuropathy with Muscular Changes associated with Carcinoma' described 2 cases of bronchial carcinoma in patients whose predominant neurological symptoms were gross loss of sensibility and an associated ataxia. Lennox and Prichard (1950) reported 5 cases of peripheral neuritis among 299 cases of carcinoma of the bronchus. Brain, Daniel, and Greenfield (1951) reported 4 cases of subacute cortical cerebellar degeneration associated with carcinoma of the bronchus in 2 and the ovary in 1.

There have been many recent additions to the literature and the subject has recently been reviewed in *The Remote Effects of Cancer on the Nervous System* (Brain and Norris, 1965). Brain and Adams (1965) provide the following classification of these disorders in terms of the anatomical level involved.

CLASSIFICATION OF NON-METASTATIC CARCINOMATOUS NEUROLOGICAL DISEASES

I. ENCEPHALOPATHY
    1. Multifocal leuco-encephalopathy
    2. Diffuse polio-encephalopathy
        (*a*) With mental symptoms
        (*b*) Subacute cerebellar degeneration
        (*c*) Brain stem lesions
    3. Encephalopathy due to disordered metabolic or endocrine functions or nutritional deficiency, especially
        (*a*) Hypercalcaemia with or without bone metastases
        (*b*) Hyperadrenalism
        (*c*) Hypoglycaemia
        (*d*) Hyponatraemia and water intoxication
        (*e*) Hyperviscosity states especially in macroglobulinaemia

II. MYELOPATHY
    1. Chronic myelopathy
        (*a*) Long tract degeneration
        (*b*) Long tract and neuronal degeneration
        (*c*) including cases simulating motor neurone disease
    2. Subacute necrotic myelopathy
    3. Nutritional myelopathy

III. NEUROPATHY
    1. Sensory neuropathy with dorsal column degeneration
    2. Peripheral sensorimotor neuropathy (polyneuropathy or neuritis)
    3. Metabolic, endocrine, and nutritional neuropathies

IV. MUSCULAR DISORDERS
    1. Polymyopathy
    2. Disorders of neuromuscular transmission
        (*a*) Myasthenic myopathy with paradoxical potentiation
        (*b*) Myasthenia gravis

3. Polymyositis and dermatomyositis
4. Metabolic myopathies secondary to disordered endocrine function, especially
   (a) Hyperadrenalism
   (b) Hypercalcaemia
   (c) Hyperthyroidism

THE INCIDENCE OF CARCINOMATOUS NEUROMYOPATHY

Croft and Wilkinson (1965) have published a survey of the incidence of carcinomatous neuromyopathy in a large number of men and women with carcinoma at various sites. Their figures show that in a consecutive series of 1,476 cases of cancer at various sites, there was an over-all incidence of neuromyopathy of 6·6 per cent., the highest figures being 16·4 per cent. for carcinoma of the ovary, 14·2 per cent. for carcinoma of the lung, 9 per cent. for carcinoma of the stomach, compared with 4·4 per cent. for carcinoma of the breast. The following table shows the incidence of different types of carcinomatous neuromyopathy encountered in the unselected series of 1,476 patients with cancer and in 44 cases specifically referred to them as suffering from neuromyopathy (the selected group).

Type of Neuromyopathy

	Cerebellar degeneration	Motor neurone type	Sensory neuropathy	Mixed peripheral neuropathy	Myasthenic	Neuro-muscular	Other	Total
Unselected series	3 (2·9%)	3 (2·9%)	—	15 (14·6%)	2 (1·9%)	72 (70%)	8 (7·7%)	103
Selected group	6 (13·6%)	3 (6·8%)	6 (13·6%)	14 (31·8%)	—	10 (22·8%)	5 (11·4%)	44
All patients	9 (6·1%)	6 (4·1%)	6 (4·1%)	29 (19·7%)	2 (1·4%)	82 (55·8%)	13 (8·8%)	147

Croft and Wilkinson used the term 'neuromuscular' here to cover a considerable group of cases of muscular wasting in which it was impossible to be sure on clinical grounds whether the condition was primarily myopathic or neuropathic, or both combined.

Thus Croft and Wilkinson's figures show that lung carcinoma is responsible for over 50 per cent. of all cases of neuromyopathy associated with carcinoma and that evidence of neuromyopathy is to be found in 14·2 per cent. of all patients with lung carcinoma routinely examined, and in 4·4 per cent. of all patients with breast carcinoma. The neuromuscular type of disturbance accounted for approximately 50 per cent. of the types of neuromyopathy encountered irrespective of the site of the primary growth.

PATHOLOGY

Neuropathology

The rare progressive multifocal leuco-encephalopathy has already been dealt with [p. 747]. Apart from this, when the central nervous system is involved as a remote effect of carcinoma and in the absence of metastases, the pathological picture may be described as a polio-encephalomyelopathy, that is, it is characterized by neuronal destruction and inflammatory infiltration, both diffuse and perivascular, the neuronal degeneration and inflammatory infiltration varying independently of one another. These changes are always to some extent diffuse, but when the damage falls predominantly upon one particular part of the nervous system, this determines the clinical picture, and this relative selectivity in many cases is responsible for the recognizable syndromes. In the brain the inflammatory changes may affect predominantly the limbic lobe, the brain stem, or the cerebellum, when loss of Purkinje cells is always a striking feature, and in some cases none can be found. In the spinal cord the anterior horn cells may be destroyed at varying levels, and there may be ascending and descending tract degeneration. In some cases the cells of the posterior root ganglia are widely destroyed, and this results in Wallerian degeneration in the posterior columns and peripheral nerves.

The peripheral nerves may be attacked, leading to a peripheral sensorimotor neuropathy, recently studied by Croft, Urich, and Wilkinson (1967). The peripheral nerves showed a variable degree of loss of axons, and of loss of myelin sheaths, usually in excess of the damage to the axons. Sparse lymphocytic infiltration was sometimes seen.

The Pathology of the Muscles

The pathological changes in the muscles are often slight in proportion to the degree of muscular weakness. Shy and Silverstein (1965) report changes suggestive of a myopathic lesion, i.e. loss of cross-striations, floccular, cloudy and granular changes, and internally-placed nuclei with an increase of endomysial connective tissue. Many cases showed basophilic fibres with large vesicular nuclei, and prominent nucleoli characteristic of regeneration of muscle. Inflammatory changes were inconstant and not usually marked. Some authors regard carcinomatous myopathy as a variant of polymyositis (Rose and Walton, 1966).

CLINICAL FEATURES

Encephalitic Form

When the brain is chiefly involved, symptoms will depend upon the region chiefly affected. The onset of symptoms is often insidious and may cover a wide range of psychiatric disorders, such as dementia, deterioration of memory, or disorder of mood, such as depression, anxiety, or agitation. When the brain stem is chiefly affected, the symptoms will depend upon the distribution of the lesions, ranging from ophthalmoplegia to bulbar palsy, often with nystagmus, ataxia, sometimes involuntary movements, and evidence of bilateral pyramidal tract damage.

Subacute Cerebellar Degeneration

This syndrome has recently been reviewed by Brain and Wilkinson (1965). The onset is usually subacute with rapidly progressive loss of cerebellar function, leading to ataxia in both upper and lower limbs and dysarthria. Nystagmus, however, is absent in half the cases. The tendon reflexes may be diminished or lost, and the plantar reflexes extensor.

Myelopathy

The symptoms are those of motor neurone disease, or amyotrophic lateral sclerosis. The patient may present with symptoms of bulbar palsy, weakness of one or both upper limbs or of the lower limbs, or of generalized weakness and lassitude. Wasting and fasciculation are found in the affected muscles. The tendon reflexes may be exaggerated or diminished and the plantar reflexes may be flexor or extensor. Brain, Croft, and Wilkinson (1965) in a recent review of this syndrome note that it not infrequently runs a more benign course than classical motor neurone disease.

Sensory Neuropathy

This is the clinical condition associated with degeneration of the posterior root ganglion cells. The patient develops, usually subacutely, sensory impairment, which tends to involve all forms of sensation in both upper and lower limbs, and is often accompanied by distressing paraesthesiae. There is sensory ataxia, and the tendon reflexes are likely to be diminished or lost. Muscular wasting and weakness may also be present.

Peripheral Sensorimotor Neuropathy (Polyneuropathy)

Croft, Urich, and Wilkinson (1967) divide their patients into three groups. These are (1) a mild and often terminal peripheral neuropathy occurring in the course of known malignant disease. (2) Subacute or acute severe peripheral neuropathy, often occurring before any evidence of malignant disease is present, and (3) patients similar to those in the second group but in whom the neuropathy follows a remitting, or sometimes relapsing, course.

The symptoms are the classical ones of a polyneuropathy with distal weakness and wasting and sensory loss, symmetrical in the upper and lower limbs with diminution or loss of tendon reflexes.

Electrodiagnostic tests in some cases yielded evidence of a sensorimotor neuropathy, in others, motor conduction velocities were markedly reduced, and in two of the cases studied by Croft, Urich, and Wilkinson, there was also electrical evidence of a myopathy.

Cerebrospinal Fluid

Both in patients with involvement of the central nervous system and in those with polyneuropathy the cerebrospinal fluid may be normal. The cell count usually is normal. There may be a moderate rise in protein. Changes in the colloidal gold curve are common, especially a tendency to a paretic curve.

Symptoms of Neuromyopathy

The carcinomatous neuromyopathies are by far the commonest of the remote effects of malignant disease. Symptoms of muscular weakness may, and often do, ante-date the symptoms of malignancy, sometimes by several years. The predominant complaints of all patients are difficulty in standing, in rising from a sitting position, and in climbing stairs. The muscles most frequently involved are the proximal ones. Involvement of the bulbar muscles may occur. The tendon reflexes in the affected muscles are diminished or lost and occasionally fasciculation is seen. The symptoms of a neuromyopathy may be associated with those of one of the characteristic central nervous system syndromes.

Electrodiagnostic tests give results characteristic of a myopathy. There is a short mean action potential duration and a marked increase in the number of short polyphasic potentials. Some patients may show electrical evidence of neuropathic involvement as well.

The Myasthenic Syndrome

One of the rarer manifestations of malignancy is the myasthenic syndrome, usually associated with bronchogenic carcinoma (see Lambert and Rooke, 1965). The initial symptom is weakness and easy fatigability of the legs, less frequently the arms; some patients may have blurring of vision or ptosis. There is an appreciable delay in the development of strength and the onset of maximal voluntary contraction, but with prolonged exertion weakness develops more rapidly than in normal persons. The fatigability may not respond at all to anticholinesterase drugs or to a lesser extent than in myasthenia gravis; it is, however, corrected by guanidine.

There are characteristic electrical reactions. The action potential and the twitch evoked in a muscle by a single supramaximal stimulus are greatly reduced in amplitude even though the strength of voluntary contraction may be normal or nearly so. Repetitive stimulation of the nerve at a slow rate produces a further decrease in amplitude but stimulation at fast rates leads to a progressive increase in response (paradoxical potentiation).

SUBACUTE NECROTIC MYELOPATHY

This rare disorder is characterized clinically by a subacute onset of the symptoms of an ascending lesion of the spinal cord, partial or complete, and usually terminating fatally in days or weeks. The patient develops paraplegia with some impairment of sensibility and loss of sphincter control. The cerebrospinal fluid may be normal but more frequently there is a rise of protein and there may be an excess of cells, either mononuclear or polymorphs. Pathologically there is a massive and symmetrical necrosis which may extend to the whole spinal cord or involve principally the thoracic region. The blood vessels show adventitial thickening and fibrosis, and necrosis.

Mancall and Rosales (1964) found 9 cases in the literature and added 2 more of their own. In 10 out of the 11 cases the myelopathy was associated with a carcinoma. In the 11th case there was a sarcoma, and I have seen a clinically identical condition associated with a reticulum-cell sarcoma.

NEUROMETABOLIC DISORDERS ASSOCIATED
WITH NEOPLASMS

It has recently been observed that tumours of various kinds may disturb metabolism, and so lead to neurological symptoms which may bring the patient under observation. The most important of such symptoms are mental disturbances and muscular weakness. The principal syndromes of this kind are reviewed in *The Remote Effects of Cancer on the Nervous System* (Brain and Norris, 1965) and summarized by Brain and Adams (1965).

Hypercalcaemia

The production of hypercalcaemia by a tumour of the parathyroid gland has long been recognized. However, there are at least two other ways in which tumours arising elsewhere may produce hypercalcaemia. It is thought that a tumour arising in some organ other than the parathyroid gland may produce a parathormone-like substance which leads to hypercalcaemia. Sarcoidosis may also produce hypercalcaemia in a manner not fully understood. When a tumour metastasizes widely to bones the resulting bone destruction may liberate calcium into the blood stream faster than it can be excreted, and so cause a hypercalcaemia. Myelomatosis may also produce this effect. Hypercalcaemia, however produced, may lead to cerebral symptoms, such as drowsiness, confusion or stupor, or to muscular weakness (Lemann and Donatelli, 1964; Watson, 1963; Dent and Watson, 1964).

Adrenal Hypercorticism

A tumour, usually a bronchogenic carcinoma, may produce corticotrophin-like material and so lead to adrenal hypercorticism. This does not usually in the early stages lead to the typical symptoms of Cushing's syndrome, but is likely to present as a result of hypokalaemic alkalosis, the symptoms of Cushing's syndrome developing only later. Clinically this syndrome may present with symptoms of a confusional psychosis or dementia, or those of a myopathy (O'Riordan *et al.*, 1966; Friedman, Marshall-Jones, and Ross, 1966).

Hypoglycaemia

Some tumours other than those arising in the pancreas may produce hypoglycaemia. These have usually been of mesenchymal origin. It is thought that in some cases the tumour elaborates a material with insulin-like activity which nevertheless differs in structure from insulin, while in other cases some other explanation is necessary to understand the mode of production of the hypoglycaemia. The presenting symptoms are likely to be those familiar as a result of hypoglycaemia, namely, an encephalopathy characterized by stupor, coma, and convulsions.

Hyponatraemia

Hyponatraemia is most likely to occur in association with a bronchogenic carcinoma which is assumed to be secreting a substance with the effects of antidiuretic hormone (inappropriate ADH secretion). The result is hyponatraemia, hypotonicity of extracellular fluid, and a hypertonic urine with sodium wasting. The patient may present with a so-called water-intoxication-type of periodic paralysis, or encephalopathy characterized by coma, convulsions, and a raised pressure of cerebrospinal fluid.

REFERENCES

ADAMS, R. D., DENNY-BROWN, D., and PEARSON, C. M. (1953) *Diseases of Muscle*, London.

ÅSTRÖM, K.-E., MANCALL, E. L., and RICHARDSON, E. P. (1958) Progressive multifocal leuko-encephalopathy, *Brain*, **81**, 93.

BRAIN, W. R., and ADAMS, R. D. (1965) A guide to the classification and investigation of neurological disorders associated with neoplasms, Chapter 21, in *The Remote Effects of Cancer on the Nervous System*, ed. BRAIN, W. R., and NORRIS, F., New York.

BRAIN, W. R., CROFT, P. B., and WILKINSON, M. (1965) Motor neurone disease as a manifestation of neoplasm (with a note on the course of classical motor neurone disease), *Brain*, **88**, 479.

BRAIN, W. R., DANIEL, P. M., and GREENFIELD, J. G. (1951) Subacute cerebellar degeneration and its relation to carcinoma, *J. Neurol. Neurosurg. Psychiat.*, **14**, 59.

BRAIN, W. R., and HENSON, R. A. (1958) Neurological syndromes associated with carcinoma, *Lancet*, ii, 971.

BRAIN, W. R., and NORRIS, F. (1965) *The Remote Effects of Cancer on the Nervous System*, New York.

BRAIN, W. R., and WILKINSON, M. (1965) Subacute cerebellar degeneration in patients with carcinoma, Chapter 3, in *The Remote Effects of Cancer on the Nervous System*, ed. BRAIN, W. R., and NORRIS, F., New York.

CAVANAGH, J. B., GREENBAUM, D., MARSHALL, A. H. E., and RUBINSTEIN, L. J. (1959) Cerebral demyelination associated with disorders of the reticuloendothelial system, *Lancet*, ii, 524.

CLARKE, E. (1954) Cranial and intracranial myelomas, *Brain*, **71**, 61.

CROFT, P. B., URICH, H., and WILKINSON, M. (1967) Peripheral neuropathy of sensori-motor type associated with malignant disease, *Brain*, **90**, 31.

CROFT, P. B., and WILKINSON, M. (1965) The incidence of carcinomatous neuromyo-pathy with special reference to carcinoma of the lung and the breast, Chapter 6, in *The Remote Effects of Cancer on the Nervous System*, ed. BRAIN, W. R., and NORRIS, F., New York.

DENNY-BROWN, D. (1948) Primary sensory neuropathy with muscular changes associated with carcinoma, *J. Neurol. Neurosurg. Psychiat.*, **11**, 73.

DENT, C. E., and WATSON, L. C. A. (1964) Hyperparathyroidism and cancer, *Brit. med. J.*, **2**, 218.

FRIEDMAN, M., MARSHALL-JONES, P., and ROSS, E. J. (1966) Cushing's syndrome: adrenocortical hyperactivity secondary to neoplasms arising outside the pituitary-adrenal system, *Quart. J. Med.*, **35**, 193.

HEATHFIELD, K. W. G., and WILLIAMS, J. R. B. (1954) Peripheral neuropathy and myopathy associated with bronchogenic carcinoma, *Brain*, **77**, 122.

HENSON, R. A., RUSSELL, D. S., and WILKINSON, M. (1954) Carcinomatous neuropathy and myopathy, *Brain*, **77**, 82.

HOWATSON, A. F., NAGAI, M., and ZU RHEIN, G. (1965) Polyoma-like virions in human demyelinating brain disease, *Canad. Med. Ass. J.*, **93**, 379.

HUTCHINSON, E. C., LEONARD, B. J., MAWDSLEY, C., and YATES, P. O. (1958) Neurological complications of the reticuloses, *Brain*, **81**, 75.

LAMBERT, E. H., and ROOKE, E. D. (1965) Myasthenic state and lung cancer, Chapter 8, in *The Remote Effects of Cancer on the Nervous System*, ed. BRAIN, W. R., and NORRIS, F., New York.

LAMBERT, E. H., ROOKE, E. D., EATON, L. M., and HODGSON, C. H. (1961) Myasthenic syndrome occasionally associated with bronchial neoplasm. Neurophysiologic studies, in *Myasthenia Gravis*, ed. VIETS, H. R., p. 362, Springfield, Ill.

LEMANN, J., and DONATELLI, A. A. (1964) Calcium intoxication due to primary hyperparathyroidism: a medical and surgical emergency, *Ann. intern. Med.*, **60**, 447.

LENNOX, B., and PRICHARD, S. (1950) The association of bronchial carcinoma and peripheral neuritis, *Quart. J. Med.*, N.S. **19**, 97.

LLOYD, O. C., and URICH, H. (1959) Acute disseminated demyelination of the brain associated with lymphosarcoma, *Lancet*, ii, 529.

MANCALL, E. L., and ROSALES, R. K. (1964) Necrotizing myelopathy associated with visceral carcinoma, *Brain*, **87**, 639.

O'RIORDAN, J. L., BLANSHARD, G. P., MOXHAM, A., and NABARRO, S. (1966) Corticotrophin-secreting carcinomas, *Quart. J. Med.*, **35**, 137.

RICHARDSON, E. P. (1965) Progressive multifocal leukoencephalopathy, Chapter 2, in *The Remote Effects of Cancer on the Nervous System*, ed. BRAIN, W. R., and NORRIS, F., New York.

ROSE, A. L., and WALTON, J. N. (1966) Polymyositis: a survey of 89 cases with particular reference to treatment and prognosis, *Brain*, **89**, 747.

RUSSELL, D. S., and RUBINSTEIN, L. J. (1959) *Pathology of Tumours of the Nervous System*, p. 213, London.

SHY, G. M., and SILVERSTEIN, I. (1965) A study of the effects upon the motor unit by remote malignancy, *Brain*, **88**, 515.

SILVERMAN, L., and RUBINSTEIN, L. J. (1965) Electron microscopic observations on a case of progressive multifocal leukoencephalopathy, *Acta neuropath. (Berl.)*, **5**, 215.

SOLOMON, A. (1965) Neurological manifestations of macroglobulinemia, Chapter 12, in *The Remote Effects of Cancer on the Nervous System*, ed. BRAIN, W. R., and NORRIS, F., New York.

STRANG, R., and AJMONE-MARSAN, C. (1961) Brain metastases, *Arch. Neurol. (Chicago)*, **4**, 8.

VICTOR, M., BANKER, B. Q., and ADAMS, R. D. (1958) The neuropathy of multiple myeloma, *J. Neurol. Neurosurg. Psychiat.*, **21**, 73.

WALTON, J. N., TOMLINSON, B., and PEARCE, G. W. (1968) Subacute 'poliomyelitis' and Hodgkin's disease, *J. neurol. Sci.*, **6**, 435.

WATSON, L. C. A. (1963) Hypercalcaemia and cancer, *Postgrad. med. J.*, **39**, 646.

ZU RHEIN, G., and CHOU, S. M. (1965) Particles resembling papova viruses in human cerebral demyelinating disease, *Science*, **148**, 1477.

18

DISORDERS OF PERIPHERAL NERVES

TUMOURS OF NERVES

THE connective tissue of a peripheral nerve may be the site of a tumour, either benign—a fibroma, or malignant—a sarcoma. Such tumours do not differ from similar tumours elsewhere. Tumours peculiar to peripheral nerves consist of tumours arising from the nerve elements and those arising from the nerve sheaths. Primary tumours of the nerve elements are extremely rare, but a neuroepithelioma has occasionally been described on a peripheral nerve. The perineurial fibroblastoma is a tumour arising from the nerve sheath. It is seen in several syndromes, variants of neurofibroblastomatosis, of which von Reckling-hausen's disease is the best known [see p. 581]. Peripheral nerves may, of course, be compressed or invaded by primary or secondary tumours arising in other tissues.

TRAUMATIC AND ALLIED LESIONS OF PERIPHERAL NERVES

Work carried out by Seddon and his collaborators has done much to elucidate the nature of the different degrees of nerve injury. Seddon (1944 b) describes three well-defined types of nerve injury. *Neurotmesis* is complete anatomical division. *Axonotmesis* is a 'lesion in continuity' in which more or less of the supporting structure of the nerve is preserved but there is nevertheless such disturbance of the nerve fibres that true Wallerian degeneration occurs peripherally. *Neuropraxia* is the term applied to a 'transient block', a minimal lesion producing paralysis which is usually incomplete, is unaccompanied by peripheral degeneration, and recovers rapidly and completely. The subject is exhaustively reviewed in the light of experience gained in the Second World War in *Medical Research Council Special Report Series*, No. 282, 1954.

Ischaemic Lesions. Ischaemic lesions may involve motor and sensory nerves and also the muscles. They may occur as a result of arterial injury or occlusion, of which tourniquet paralysis is one form; or closed fractures, resulting in ischaemic paralysis. The anterior tibial syndrome is a form of ischaemic paralysis of the muscles in which the anterior tibial muscles after being subjected to unaccustomed effort, swell within their tight fascial compartment and may undergo partial or complete infarction. Richards (1954) discusses neurovascular lesions.

Pressure Neuropathy. Repeated or prolonged pressure upon a nerve leads to ischaemia, the response to which is oedema extending both above and below the source of pressure. The initial disturbance of function is neuropraxial but this may be followed by axonotmesis, and if the pressure is not relieved fibrosis develops and prevents recovery. This is the lesion underlying the neuropathy caused by herniated intervertebral disc, narrowed intervertebral foramen, cervical rib, median nerve compression in the carpal tunnel, ulnar nerve compression at the elbow, meralgia paraesthetica, and Morton's metatarsalgia.

NEUROTMESIS

Neurotmesis occurs as a result of open wounds, direct blunt injuries, traction upon the nerve, and some forms of local chemical poisoning, e.g. with sulphonamides. Retrograde degeneration occurs in the central stump for 2 or 3 cm. and the peripheral stump undergoes Wallerian degeneration. The axons of the central end soon sprout, and form a neuroma composed of nerve fibres and scar tissue on the central stump.

SYMPTOMS OF COMPLETE DIVISION

Complete division of a mixed peripheral nerve causes motor, sensory, vasomotor, sudomotor, and trophic symptoms corresponding in anatomical distribution to the region in which these functions are supplied by the divided nerve.

Motor Symptoms

Interruption of the motor fibres of the nerve leads to a lower motor neurone paralysis of the muscles which it innervates. The muscles innervated exhibit a flaccid paralysis, and rapidly waste. The reflexes in which they participate are diminished or lost, and reaction of degeneration develops. Investigation of the motor functions of a nerve involves testing the patient's power to contract the muscles both as prime movers and also as synergists. The observer must be on his guard to detect trick movements, for it is often possible for a movement which is normally effected by a paralysed muscle to be carried out by another muscle when the segment of the limb is first placed in an appropriate position. The electrical reactions of the muscles must also be tested, and in the case of the small muscles of the hand electrical testing often gives more reliable information as to the extent of the paralysis than does voluntary movement. Electromyography is particularly valuable in this connexion, while if the nerve which has been divided is one in which conduction can be measured electrically, soon after the injury has occurred conduction in the segment distal to the lesion quickly becomes greatly slowed and is later lost.

Sensation

The methods of carrying out tests of sensibility are described elsewhere [see p. 37]. Division of a sensory nerve causes complete loss of cutaneous sensibility only over the area exclusively supplied by the nerve, the *autonomous zone*. This is surrounded by an *intermediate zone*, which is the area of the nerve's territory overlapped by the supply of adjacent nerves. The autonomous and intermediate zones together constitute the *maximal zone* which is the full extent of the nerve's distribution. The cutaneous area over which appreciation of light touch is lost is usually considerably greater than the area characterized by a loss of appreciation of pin-prick. In investigating the former the area of skin to be tested should always be shaved. The area over which appreciation of pin-prick is lost is often ill defined and merges gradually into the intermediate zone in which this form of sensibility is present, though grossly impaired. In some cases, even of complete division of a nerve, the completely analgesic area is surrounded by a zone in which, although a stronger stimulus than normal is necessary to evoke pain, the painful sensation is more than usually disagreeable ('hyper-pathia'). The term 'deep sensibility' is used to include the appreciation and localization of pressure, and the pain induced by deep pressure, and the recognition of posture and passive movements of the joints. Impairment of deep sensibility, when present as a result of nerve division, is confined to a peripheral area which is less extensive than the area anaesthetic to light touch.

Vasomotor, Sudomotor, and Trophic Functions

Vasomotor and trophic disturbances which follow destruction of a motor or a mixed nerve are probably due, at least in part, to the interruption of efferent sympathetic fibres concerned in vasoconstriction. These disturbances are most marked after injuries of the median, ulnar, and sciatic nerves. After complete division of a nerve the analgesic area of skin becomes dry and inelastic, and ceases to sweat. The surface becomes scaly owing to retardation of desquamation; the affected area is blue and colder than normal, especially in cold weather; and the limb becomes oedematous when it is allowed to hang down. The analgesic area is exceptionally liable to injury, and when injured heals slowly, so that ulcers may develop. The growth of the nails is retarded. Adhesions between tendons and their sheaths, and fibrous changes in the muscles and joints are to be regarded as complications rather than as direct results of the nerve injury, since they can be prevented by repeated passive movements of the joints.

AXONOTMESIS

This type of lesion is best illustrated by the experimental crushing of a peripheral nerve with forceps, after which all the nerve fibres are broken but the connective tissue of the nerve survives to some extent. It may be associated with open wounds or follow direct blunt injuries, such as fractures and dislocations, traction or compression, as well as local action by physical and chemical agents. Peripheral to the injury degeneration is complete, but in acute cases regeneration always occurs, and functional recovery is always more rapid and more complete than after complete division and suture. At first, however, the symptoms are the same as after neurotmesis.

NEUROPRAXIA

In neuropraxia, although the functions of the nerve are temporarily impaired or even apparently completely lost, recovery occurs so quickly that it is impossible that it could be caused by regeneration. Lesions of this type may be produced by any of the causes of axonotmesis, provided the nerve is not actually severed. Pressure is the commonest cause. In neuropraxia according to Seddon (*a*) the loss of function is predominantly motor; (*b*) there is little wasting, and the electrical reactions of the muscles persist unchanged; (*c*) subjective sensory disturbances—numbness, tingling, and burning—are common; (*d*) objective sensory disturbances are generally partial, and often minimal as far as touch, pain, heat, and cold are concerned; (*e*) loss of postural sensibility and vibration sense are common; and (*f*) loss of sweating is unusual. The lesion is usually therefore a dissociated one, the motor and proprioceptive fibres suffering most, probably because the largest fibres are the most vulnerable, but in occasional cases all motor and sensory function is temporarily lost. Recovery is fairly rapid, beginning usually after two to three weeks, and becoming complete within six or eight weeks, though, occasionally, complete restoration of function may be delayed until the fourth month. Recovery progresses irregularly and follows no anatomical order, but is always complete.

DIAGNOSIS OF THE NATURE OF A NERVE LESION

The appropriate treatment of a peripheral nerve lesion depends upon an accurate diagnosis of its nature and severity. The symptoms of neurotmesis and axonotmesis are for a long time indistinguishable. It is possible to wait until sufficient time has elapsed for regeneration to occur and, if it does not, to conclude that the nerve has been completely divided, but if suture is delayed more than five or six months the prospects of recovery are impaired. Moreover, the whole of a nerve may not be equally severely injured and combinations of neurotmesis, axonotmesis, and neuropraxia occur. It is always necessary to take into account the nature of the injury since experience is often a guide to the type of nerve injury to be expected. It is often possible to recognize neuropraxia by the features described above. Electrical tests may be useful (Bowden, 1954 *a*). In other cases if there is any doubt as to the nature of the lesion the nerve should always be explored within two or three months of the injury: exploration is often an essential part of diagnosis.

SPECIAL METHODS IN THE DIAGNOSIS OF NERVE LESIONS

In most cases clinical examination and the ordinary electrical tests will suffice to diagnose lesions of peripheral nerves and follow their progress towards recovery but methods of measuring both motor and sensory conduction velocity have greatly increased diagnostic precision. Other methods are occasionally helpful. Gilliatt and Wilson (1954) drew attention to the increase in sensory symptoms produced by temporary ischaemia obtained by applying a pneumatic tourniquet to the limb. *Sweating* responses after exposure to heat may be used to demarcate a denervated area (Guttmann, 1940), see page 899. This may be particularly useful in distinguishing between a lesion of a spinal root, plexus and peripheral nerve, e.g. cervical rib and ulnar neuropathy, and in demonstrating a peripheral nerve lesion coexisting with a lesion of the spinal cord, e.g. a lateral popliteal nerve lesion in a patient anaesthetic from a spinal injury. *Procaine nerve-block* (Highet, 1942 *b*) may be applied either to an injured nerve or to neighbouring nerves when the diagnosis is complicated by anomalous muscle movements or when it is uncertain to which nerve a sensory area belongs.

Electromyography (Weddell, Feinstein, and Pattle, 1943; Bowden, 1954 *a*; Buchthal, 1962; Norris, 1963; Barwick and Richardson, 1969) is a delicate method of electrical analysis of nervous and muscular activity which is of value in the diagnosis of the degree of nerve injury and regeneration. Electrical methods have been greatly developed during recent years, in the study of sensory and motor neurone conduction in peripheral nerve lesions (Simpson, 1956; Gilliatt and Sears, 1958; Buchthal and Rosenfalck, 1966; Downie, 1969). (See also under lesions of the median nerve, p. 781, and ulnar nerve, p. 784.) Finally, axon responses may be used to diagnose the site of the lesion (Bonney, 1954).

Electromyography

Electromyography may be used in various ways in the diagnosis of lesions of the lower motor neurone and muscles. The electrical muscle potentials are measured by inserting a needle electrode into the muscle. Recordings are then made with the muscle at rest, with slight voluntary contraction, and with maximal voluntary contraction. The potentials are amplified and made visible by means of cathode ray oscilloscopy, and they are also rendered audible through a loud-speaker (see Bowden, 1954 *a*; Gilliatt, 1957; Kugelberg, 1947, 1949; Norris, 1963; Barwick and Richardson, 1969).

Normal Muscle. When a normal muscle is tested at rest there is no evidence of electrical activity. On slight voluntary contraction motor-unit potentials of 500 to 1,000 microvolts in amplitude, and 4 to 8 milliseconds in duration, are recorded. These may be monophasic, biphasic, or triphasic in shape. On vigorous voluntary contraction of the muscle an interference pattern develops. Since the patient recruits as many motor units as possible, and they fire asynchronously, each one interferes with the ones which precede and follow it [FIG. 100 *a*].

The Completely Denervated Muscle. After complete transection of a nerve, and when sufficient time—about two weeks—has elapsed to allow the distal segment to degenerate, fibrillation or fasciculation potentials are evident in the resting muscle. A fibrillation potential which arises from the spontaneous discharge of a single muscle fibre is usually 50 to 100 microvolts in amplitude, 1 to 2 milliseconds in duration, and monophasic or biphasic in shape. No change in the muscle is produced by voluntary contraction. Fasciculation will be found only when the lesion is in or near the spinal cord, for it represents a spontaneous discharge of all the muscle fibres innervated by a single nerve fibre. Fasciculation potentials are similar to motor unit potentials and are therefore 500 to 1,000 microvolts in amplitude, 4 to 8 milliseconds in duration, and may be monophasic, biphasic, or triphasic in shape. The only difference between these and normal motor unit potentials is that fasciculation potentials occur spontaneously in a resting muscle, while normal motor unit potentials occur only on voluntary contraction [FIG. 100 *b*].

The Partially Denervated Muscle. The electromyogram in the partially denervated muscle is what might be expected from a combination of degeneration of some lower motor neurones with preservation of others. If the inserted needle is in the region of denervated muscle, fibrillation or fasciculation potentials will be observed. On slight voluntary contraction intact motor units will fire, and

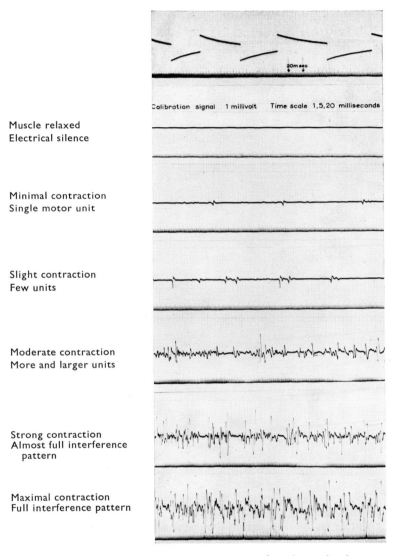

Muscle relaxed
Electrical silence

Minimal contraction
Single motor unit

Slight contraction
Few units

Moderate contraction
More and larger units

Strong contraction
Almost full interference
pattern

Maximal contraction
Full interference pattern

Calibration signal 1 millivolt Time scale 1,5,20 milliseconds

FIG. 100 *a*. Normal electromyograms. (FIGS. 100 *a*, *b*, and *c* are by the courtesy of Dr. H. R. A. Townsend.)

the size, shape, and duration of their motor unit potentials will be normal, but vigorous muscular contraction will not bring into action a sufficient number of additional units to produce a normal interference pattern [FIG. 100 *c*]. Thus the interference pattern is reduced.

The Myopathic Muscle. In myopathy we have to deal with a disorder of function which is not based on the pattern of innervation. As a rule no fibrillation or fasciculation is seen at rest but in occasional cases of myopathy (and

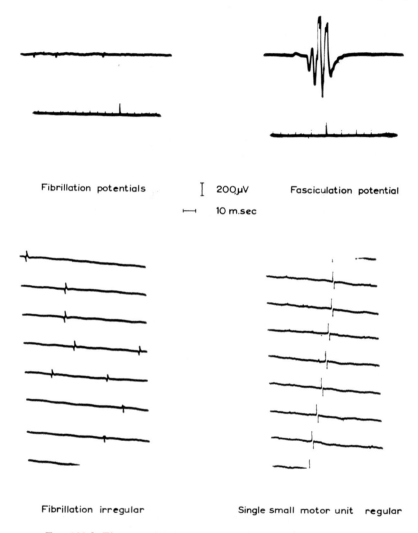

Fibrillation potentials I 200μV   Fasciculation potential

⊢—⊣ 10 m.sec

Fibrillation irregular   Single small motor unit   regular

FIG. 100 *b*. Electromyograms showing fibrillation and fasciculation

especially in polymyositis) the disease process may affect intramuscular nerve endings or alternatively focal necrosis of part of a muscle fibre may separate the remainder of the fibre from its motor end-plate so that fibrillation potentials may then be seen. On slight voluntary contraction there may be some normal muscle fibres which respond, but these will be fewer than usual. Consequently the population of muscle fibres within the individual motor units is reduced so that the duration and amplitude of the motor unit potentials is diminished and many are broken-up or polyphasic. On maximal contraction more motor units may fire, but as these will have diseased muscle fibres in them there will be a low-voltage and complex interference pattern made up of many short-duration and polyphasic potentials [FIG. 100 c].

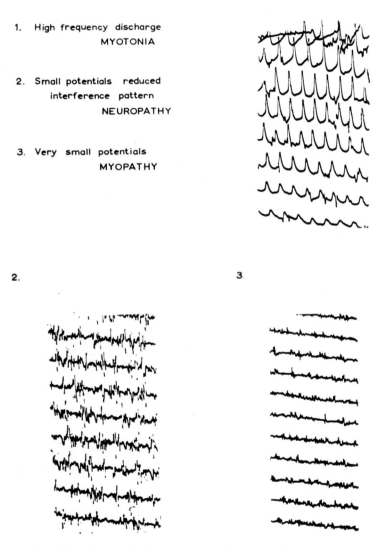

1. High frequency discharge
MYOTONIA

2. Small potentials reduced
interference pattern
NEUROPATHY

3. Very small potentials
MYOPATHY

FIG. 100 c. Abnormal electromyograms: compare with FIG. 100 a

Myotonia is associated with characteristic chains of oscillations of high frequency [FIG. 100 c] which are evoked by movement of the exploring needle within the muscle and which give rise to a characteristic recurring 'dive-bomber' sound in the loud-speaker.

Conduction Time. When the lower motor neurones are abnormal in the peripheral nerves, tests of conduction time are of value. The nerve is stimulated directly, and the time taken for the resulting impulse to evoke a response in the muscle measured. For instance, the ulnar nerve may be stimulated at the elbow and also at the wrist and the evoked muscle potential in the hypothenar eminence is recorded. It is then possible to measure the conduction velocity from elbow to wrist and from wrist to muscle (terminal latency). The median, radial, and lateral popliteal nerves are commonly examined in this way. The normal motor conduction velocity at a temperature of 20–25° C. in the adult is 50–60 m./sec. in the median and ulnar nerves and 45–50 m./sec. in the lateral popliteal, and the normal maximum terminal latency from wrist to thenar eminence in the median nerve is 4·5–5·0 m./sec. (Norris, 1963). A slowing of conduction time is observed both in diffuse conditions, such as polyneuritis, and when there is local pressure on the nerve at some point. In general, demyelinating lesions slow conduction in nerve trunks whereas axonal lesions do not as surviving axons conduct at normal rates. Sensory conduction time can be measured similarly, for instance by applying a ring electrode to a finger and then recording the sensory volley ascending the appropriate nerve.

SYMPTOMS OF RECOVERY

Recovery of function after complete division of a nerve occurs by means of a down-growth of the nerve fibres from the central end, and can therefore take place only when the divided ends lie in apposition or have been brought together by suture. The time required for recovery depends principally upon the distance which the regenerating fibres have to travel from the site of injury to their normal destinations and also upon the integrity of the peripheral sheaths of Schwann cells into which the regenerating axons must grow. After complete division and suture many axons are misdirected so that recovery is often incomplete. The average rate of motor nerve recovery in man is 1·5 mm. per day. There has been much theoretical discussion concerning the interpretation of sensory changes which characterize returning function, but there is considerable agreement as to the facts. The first indication that nerve fibres have passed into the distal part of the nerve may be a peculiar sensitivity of the nerve trunk below the site of the union. Mechanical stimulation readily evokes a tingling sensation which is referred by the patient into the cutaneous territory of the nerve (Tinel's sign). Before other objective signs of recovery appear, the patient may say that the part feels more life-like or is less numb. The first objective sign of returning function is a diminution in the area of impairment of deep sensibility. Painful sensibility returns next, but for a long time exhibits characteristics which distinguish it from normal painful feeling. During this stage of recovery, a stronger stimulus than normal may be required to evoke pain, but the response is of a peculiarly unpleasant quality, and is a diffuse and badly localized sensation ('hyperpathia' or the stage of 'protopathic sensation' according to Head). Somewhat later the affected area becomes sensitive to the extremes of heat and cold. The appreciation of light touch, and its accurate localization and tactile discrimination—Head's 'epicritic sensation'—do not recover until many months after the return of painful sensibility, and frequently never recover completely. When recovery of appreciation of light touch occurs it is associated with the disappearance of the uncomfortable and irradiating character of painful sensibility.

With the return of painful sensibility, vasomotor changes become less conspicuous and the skin heals more readily. There is frequently considerable sensory recovery before there is any return of motor power. The response of the paralysed muscles to faradic stimulation may return before voluntary muscular contraction, but this is not always the case. In testing voluntary power the limb should always be placed in such a position that the movement to be carried out is not opposed by the force of gravity. Further, when a muscle can act both as a prime mover and as a synergist it should be tested in both these capacities, as return of power may be demonstrable in one before the other.

The above description of recovery applies only to a nerve which has been completely divided and sutured. After axonotmesis recovery is somewhat more rapid and much more often complete; after neuropraxia, as already stated, it is more rapid still, and always complete.

The following scheme is recommended by the Medical Research Council to assess recovery, which is divided into motor (voluntary power) and sensory:

I. MOTOR RECOVERY

Stage 0. No contraction.

Stage 1. Return of perceptible contraction in the proximal muscles.

Stage 2. Return of perceptible contraction in both proximal and distal muscles.

Stage 3. Return of function in both proximal and distal muscles of such an extent that all *important* muscles are of sufficient power to act against resistance.

Stage 4. Return of function as in Stage 3 with the addition that *all* synergic and isolated movements are possible.

Stage 5. Complete recovery.

II. SENSORY RECOVERY

Stage 0. Absence of sensibility in the autonomous zone.

Stage 1. Recovery of deep cutaneous pain sensibility within the autonomous zone.

Stage 2. Return of some degree of superficial cutaneous pain and touch sensibility within the autonomous zone.

Stage 3. Return of superficial cutaneous pain and touch sensibility throughout the autonomous zone with disappearance of any over-response.

Stage 4. Return of sensibility as in stage 3 with the addition that there is recovery of 2-point discrimination within the autonomous zone.

TREATMENT

NON-OPERATIVE TREATMENT

Treatment is directed to maintaining the nutrition of the paralysed muscles, preventing contractures in their antagonists, and keeping the joints mobile, so that when regeneration of the nerve fibres occurs the limb may be in the best possible condition to profit by the return of nervous function. Even if operation on the nerve should be required, the treatment of the limb is the same before and after operation. A splint is sometimes necessary to obtain relaxation of the paralysed muscles, in order to avoid their being stretched by the force of gravity or by their non-paralysed antagonists. The appropriate splints are described in the sections dealing with the individual nerves, and see Bowden (1954 b). Passive movements of the various joints must be carried out daily in order to maintain their mobility. Various agencies are available for improving the nutrition of the paralysed muscles. The limb must always be kept warm, and extra stockings or long woollen gloves should be worn in cold weather. Heat may be used to stimulate the circulation and can be most simply applied by soaking the limb in a bath of hot water. Radiant heat and diathermy can also be used. Electricity may be employed to stimulate the paralysed muscles. The limb should first be warmed, and the minimal current, whether galvanic or faradic, which will cause a contraction of the muscle, should be employed, the two terminals being placed over the muscle to be stimulated. Recent work has shown the value of galvanism in promoting recovery after complete denervation. As soon as voluntary power begins to return, the patient may be encouraged to assist recovery by active exercises, in which at first the movement is assisted by the physiotherapist. Later re-education in skilled movements forms an important part of the treatment, and the patient must be prevented from carrying out 'trick movements'.

OPERATIVE TREATMENT

The technique of the surgery of the peripheral nerves does not come within the scope of this book, but it is desirable to discuss the indications for surgical treatment, which have been considerably clarified by experience during the Second World War. On the whole, recovery is more complete after secondary suture than after primary suture. In all cases of open wounds, therefore, when there is a risk of infection, primary suture should never be performed. If the nerve is seen, its condition should be noted, and, if it has been divided, steps taken to prevent retraction of the stumps. Secondary suture can then be performed two or three months later. An exception to this rule has been made in the case of small penetrating wounds of warfare and clean glass cuts which almost invariably heal well after suture, but Seddon prefers secondary suture for these injuries also. When the patient presents himself with a healed wound and the past treatment of the nerve injury is unknown, the nerve should be explored, unless the clinical condition and electrophysiological tests suggest that the lesion is neuropraxial. After closed injuries with fractures medical treatment should be carried out for long enough to permit regenerating nerve fibres to reach the most proximal muscle supplied by the nerve, calculating the rate of regeneration at 1 mm. a day and allowing a slight margin. If there is then no recovery of function in that muscle, the nerve should be explored. Severe traction injuries, e.g. of the brachial plexus, should be treated medically.

The prognosis of nerve suture, and factors influencing recovery have been reviewed by Davis (1949), Seddon (1949, 1954 b), and Zachary (1954).

CAUSALGIA
SYMPTOMS

Causalgia is a distressing symptom, usually associated with incomplete lesions of a peripheral nerve. Though it may occur as a result of a lesion of any nerve, it is most frequently met with when the inner cord of the brachial plexus or the median or the sciatic nerve is damaged. It consists of intense and persistent burning pain, which is subject to paroxysmal exacerbations, which may be excited not only by actual contact with the limb but also by any event which excites an emotional reaction in the patient. The pain usually begins a week or two after the injury. The appearance of the affected limb is characteristic. In a case of median nerve causalgia the hand is pink and sweating; the skin is tight and glossy; the nails are curved, grow rapidly, and are tender; the finger pads are wasted, so that the nail-beds protrude; the joints are stiff and swollen, and the bones rarefied and brittle. Tenderness may be evoked either by superficial or by deep stimulation or both, in a small proportion of cases only by the latter. Superficial tenderness usually extends over the whole cutaneous area innervated by the nerve, and thus is more extensive than the area of anaesthesia produced by nerve section, which corresponds to the area exclusively supplied by the nerve. The affected nerve may be tender throughout the whole length of the limb, even as high as the brachial plexus. There may be little or no associated muscular paralysis. Owing to the extreme tenderness of the affected part the patient makes every effort to protect the limb from all forms of external stimulation. Similar symptoms may be referred to the stump following amputation.

The most plausible explanation of causalgia is that the pain is due to the liberation of an irritant substance at the nerve endings, but an artificial synapse between the efferent sympathetic and afferent somatic fibres at the site of the injury probably plays a part. The subject has been reviewed by Rasmussen and Freedman (1946), Mayfield (1951), and by Barnes (1954).

TREATMENT

The most effective treatment appears to be sympathetic block, with or without excision of the damaged area of the nerve, and resuturing. If the patient is seen early, medical treatment should be given a trial and this may be combined with procaine block of the sympathetic. Medical treatment consists of moist local applications at the temperature which the patient finds most comforting, sedatives and analgesics. The limb should not be immobilized, and active and passive movements should be carried out as far as they can be tolerated.

Surgical treatment should not be too long delayed, since in long-standing cases even extensive interruption of pain fibres in the dorsal roots or spino-thalamic tract may be ineffective. If procaine block of the sympathetic relieves the pain, sympathectomy should be carried out. It is not necessary to remove the stellate ganglion to relieve the pain in the upper extremity. Some surgeons also excise the damaged area of nerve, but if sympathectomy relieves the pain the peripheral nerve can be dealt with on the principles which determine the treatment of nerve injuries.

Causalgic symptoms in amputation stumps in the absence of active infection are usually due to painful neuromas. These can be dealt with by dividing the nerve as high above the bulb as possible, crushing and ligaturing the end, and injecting the nerve with absolute alcohol, but recent evidence suggests that repeated percussion of the neuroma in the amputation stump with an appropriate instrument may be more effective in the long run.

SYMPTOMS AND TREATMENT OF INDIVIDUAL NERVE LESIONS

THE PHRENIC NERVE

The phrenic nerve is derived from the anterior primary divisions of the third, fourth, and fifth cervical spinal nerves, the main contribution coming from the fourth. It is the motor nerve to the diaphragm. Irritation of the phrenic nerve causes a dry, unproductive, 'barking' cough: rarely it may cause hiccup. Paralysis of the nerve causes loss of movement of the diaphragm on the affected side. The effects of this are most evident when the lesion is bilateral. The diaphragm fails to descend on inspiration and may actually be drawn upwards. There is increased eversion of the costal margins with indrawing of the upper abdominal wall on inspiration. Diaphragmatic paralysis causes no symptoms as long as the patient is at rest, but dyspnoea may occur on exertion. The resulting diminution in expansion of the bases of the lungs renders the patient liable to develop a basal bronchopneumonia.

Diaphragmatic paralysis is most frequently produced by lesions involving the anterior horn cells of the spinal cord in the third, fourth, and fifth cervical segments, for example, direct trauma, poliomyelitis, transverse myelitis, and tumours of the spinal cord. The phrenic nerve may be intentionally divided for therapeutic purposes or injured during operations on the neck, and may be compressed by aneurysm of the aorta or by intrathoracic neoplasms or enlargement of the mediastinal glands. It may undergo degeneration in polyneuritis due to alcohol, diphtheria, lead, or other toxins or may be involved in post-infective polyneuropathy (the Guillain-Barré syndrome).

THE NERVES OF THE UPPER LIMB
THE BRACHIAL PLEXUS

The brachial plexus [FIG. 101] is formed from the anterior primary divisions of the fifth, sixth, seventh, and eighth cervical and the first thoracic spinal nerves. It sometimes receives a contribution from the second thoracic nerve. Variations in the position of the brachial plexus are not uncommon. In the so-called 'prefixed' type there is a contribution from the fourth cervical nerve; the fifth cervical branch is large and there may be no branch from the second thoracic. In the 'post-fixed' type there may be no branch from the fourth cervical, and that from the fifth is comparatively small, whereas the second thoracic branch is quite distinct. The spinal segmental representation of muscles may be slightly higher or slightly lower than normal, according to whether the plexus is pre-fixed or post-fixed.

The contributions to the plexus from the anterior primary divisions soon divide into anterior and posterior trunks, and from these are formed the three cords of the plexus. The lateral cord is formed by a union of anterior trunks of the fifth, sixth, and seventh nerves. From it arise the lateral anterior thoracic and musculocutaneous nerves and the lateral head of the median nerve. The medial or inner cord is formed by a combination of the anterior trunk of the eighth cervical with the contribution of the first thoracic nerve to the plexus. It

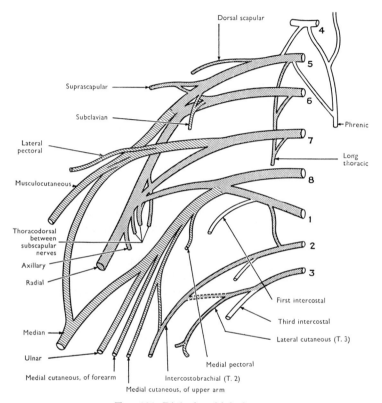

FIG. 101. Right brachial plexus

gives origin to the medial head of the median nerve, the ulnar nerve, the medial cutaneous nerves of the arm and forearm, and the medial anterior thoracic nerve. The posterior cord is formed by the union of the posterior trunks from the fifth, sixth, seventh, and eighth cervical and sometimes the first thoracic nerves. It gives rise to the axillary and radial nerves, the two subscapular nerves, and the nerve to the teres major.

Certain muscles are innervated by nerves which leave the brachial plexus proximal to the formation of the three cords. The most important of these are: the dorsal scapular nerve, from the fifth cervical, which supplies the levator scapulae and the rhomboid muscles; the long or posterior thoracic nerve, from the fifth, sixth, and seventh cervical nerves, which supplies the serratus anterior; and the suprascapular nerve, from the fifth and sixth cervical nerves, which supplies the supraspinatus and the infraspinatus.

LESIONS OF THE BRACHIAL PLEXUS

If we consider with the brachial plexus the spinal nerves from which it is derived we find that it is liable to damage at many points and from many causes. One or more of the spinal nerves may be involved by a lesion of the cervical spine, including congenital abnormality such as fusion of vertebrae—Klippel-Feil syndrome—fracture-dislocation, herniated intervertebral disc, spondylosis occurring alone or with any of the foregoing, and, rarely, tuberculous or syphilitic caries or malignant deposits. The plexus itself is liable to be damaged by stabs and gun-shot wounds, by fracture of the clavicle, and by dislocation of the upper end of the humerus. Its component parts may be torn by forcible separation of the head and shoulder or by abduction of the arm, or compressed by abnormalities of the thoracic inlet. The plexus is occasionally involved in neoplastic deposits in cervical lymph nodes or invaded by apical pulmonary neoplasm, and it may be compressed by a neurofibroma. The character of the motor and sensory disturbances resulting from lesions of the brachial plexus depends upon the situation of the lesion and the part of the plexus involved.

Total Plexus Paralysis

This is a rare occurrence. When the lesion is close to the vertebral column all the muscles supplied by the plexus will be paralysed and the cervical sympathetic may also be involved. When the plexus is involved at the level of the cords, the spinati, rhomboids, serratus anterior, pectorals, and cervical sympathetic may escape. Appreciation of light touch, pain, and temperature is lost over the fore-arm and hand and over the outer surface of the arm in its lower two-thirds. Postural sensibility and appreciation of passive movement are lost in the fingers. All the tendon reflexes in the upper limb are lost.

Upper Plexus Paralysis (Erb–Duchenne type)

This is due to a lesion of the branch from the fifth cervical nerve to the brachial plexus. Occasionally the sixth cervical contribution may be involved, but this is exceptional. Upper plexus paralysis is usually the result of indirect violence, the nerve being torn by undue separation of the head and shoulder. It is a common form of birth injury resulting from traction on the head when there is difficulty in delivering one shoulder. It may occur in adults as a result of a fall on the shoulder forcing the head to one side, and occasionally follows an anaesthetic in patients in whom, during the operation, the arm has been held abducted and externally rotated. The muscles paralysed as a result of interruption of the fifth cervical branch are the biceps, deltoid, brachialis, brachioradialis, supraspinatus, infraspinatus, and the rhomboids. When the sixth cervical branch is involved in addition, there may be weakness, but not as a rule complete paralysis, of the serratus anterior, latissimus dorsi, triceps, pectoralis major, and extensor carpi radialis.

The position of the limb resulting from upper plexus paralysis is characteristic. It hangs at the side internally rotated at the shoulder, with the elbow extended and the forearm pronated. There is wasting of the paralysed muscles. Paralysis of the deltoid renders abduction at the shoulder impossible. The elbow cannot be flexed on account of paralysis of the flexors. External rotation at the shoulder is lost owing to paralysis of the spinati. Movements of the wrist and fingers are unaffected. The biceps and supinator jerks are lost. Sensory loss may be absent, but there is sometimes a small area of anaesthesia and analgesia overlying the deltoid.

The results of operative treatment of upper plexus paralysis are disappointing, and surgical intervention is inadvisable, except in those rare instances in which the upper part of the plexus has been divided by a stab or gun-shot wound. It is contra-indicated if tests show the lesion to be proximal to the dorsal root ganglia (Bonney, 1954). The 'flare' response which follows local scratching of the skin is an axon reflex which is lost in lesions occurring distal to the ganglia. Thus if the 'flare' response is present, and particularly if myelography demonstrates a pattern of root-sleeve filling which indicates that the fifth root or spinal nerve has been torn from its origin from the spinal cord, the prognosis is very poor. The arm should be put up in an adjustable abduction splint with a movable joint at the elbow, and the usual after-treatment of peripheral nerve lesions should be carried out. When the lesion is distal to the ganglia, however, the prognosis is on the whole better as actual division or tearing of the nerve is much less common, especially when the cause of the paralysis is birth injury. Complete recovery occurs in at least 50 per cent. of cases. In infants recovery is often rapid and may be complete in from three to six months. In adults it may take as long as two years. Zachary recommends transplantation of latissimus dorsi and teres major to the outer side of the humerus to restore external rotation of the arm in those cases where recovery is incomplete.

Lower Plexus Paralysis (Dejerine–Klumpke type)

The contribution of the first thoracic nerve to the brachial plexus may be torn as a result of traction on the arm when it is in an abducted position. Lower plexus paralysis is sometimes encountered as a result of birth injury, or may be produced by a fall during which the patient endeavours to save himself by clutching something with the hand. The first thoracic nerve is usually affected alone, but the eighth cervical may also be involved. The resulting paralysis and wasting involves all the small muscles of the hand, a claw-hand resulting from the unopposed action of the long flexors and extensors of the fingers. When the eighth cervical nerve is also involved there may be wasting and weakness of the ulnar flexors of the wrist and fingers. Cutaneous anaesthesia and analgesia are present in a narrow zone along the ulnar border of the hand and for a variable distance up the forearm. There is frequently an associated paralysis of the cervical sympathetic.

LESIONS OF THE CORDS OF THE PLEXUS

The effects of lesions of the cords of the plexus can readily be deduced from a knowledge of their respective contributions to the nerves of the upper limb which have already been described.

The Lateral Cord. The lateral cord is occasionally injured in dislocations of the humerus. Its interruption causes paralysis of the biceps, coracobrachialis, and of all the muscles supplied by the median nerve, except the intrinsic muscles of the hand. Sensation is affected to a variable extent on the radial aspect of the forearm.

The Posterior Cord. This is rarely damaged. A lesion of the posterior cord causes paralysis of the muscles supplied by the axillary and radial nerves, and loss of sensibility over the areas of their cutaneous supply.

Middle Plexus Paralysis. This is also rare and is equivalent to interruption of the posterior cord with the addition of paralysis of the latissimus dorsi as a result of involvement of the thoracodorsal nerve.

The Medial Cord. Injury to the medial cord of the plexus is most commonly produced by subcoracoid dislocation of the humerus. It causes paralysis of the muscles supplied by the ulnar nerve, together with those intrinsic muscles of the hand which are supplied by the median. Sensory loss occurs along the ulnar border of the hand and forearm. Treatment is that appropriate to the individual nerves involved.

Diagnosis of the Site of the Lesion

It is important in relation to both prognosis and treatment to decide the precise site of the lesion. Axon responses to histamine and reflex vasodilatation to cold may decide this, being absent when the lesion is distal to the dorsal root ganglion and present when it is proximal (Bonney, 1954).

COSTOCLAVICULAR SYNDROMES INCLUDING CERVICAL RIB

AETIOLOGY AND PATHOLOGY

The adoption by man of an upright posture and the release of his upper limb as an organ of prehension has imposed certain stresses upon the nervous and vascular supply of the limb, and rendered the bony structure of the upper thoracic outlet liable to congenital abnormalities which may interfere with nerves and blood vessels. There may be a rudimentary rib derived from the seventh cervical vertebra—cervical rib, which may be associated with a prefixed brachial plexus. The first true rib may be congenitally abnormal. The brachial plexus may be post-fixed, and the contribution from the first thoracic nerve may be unusually large with an addition from the second thoracic segment.

The production of symptoms by these factors is complex and not fully understood. The eighth cervical and first thoracic contributions to the plexus may rest upon, and be compressed by, a cervical rib, or an enlarged seventh cervical transverse process, or a fibrous band uniting such a structure to the first rib or by the scalenus anterior muscle. Or it may be compressed by an abnormal or even a normal first rib. The subclavian artery in such cases often arises at a higher level than normal, and may be compressed by a bony abnormality, by the scalenus anterior muscle, or, on abducting the arm, by the clavicle, as it lies between the clavicle and the first rib.

As already mentioned, the scalenus anterior muscle may play a part in the production of symptoms but there seems to be no justification for isolating a 'scalenus anterior syndrome'. The mutual relations of the various structures of the upper thoracic outlet are constantly being altered by the respiratory movements and by movements of the upper limb, which contribute a cumulative traumatic factor, which may in time lead to the production of fibrous tissue— an additional element in compression. The third part of the subclavian artery may become the site of an aneurysmal dilatation, in which thrombosis may be a source of embolism in the upper limb or even in the vertebral artery giving brain stem ischaemia, or the artery itself may become thrombosed. Finally, loss of tone in the shoulder girdle, or the traction due to carrying heavy weights, or dropping of the shoulder-girdle after thoracoplasty, may precipitate symptoms in middle life though the bony abnormalities are congenital, or may cause symptoms though the bony structures are normal. These factors probably explain why in right-handed persons symptoms usually occur on the right side, though cervical ribs are generally bilateral, and why women are more prone than men to develop symptoms in middle life.

Symptoms may be either nervous or vascular, or both, and the vascular symptoms can probably be explained as the result of intermittent or persistent vascular occlusion without invoking disturbances of sympathetic innervation. The occasional coexistence of Horner's syndrome is difficult to explain except as a result of traction upon the cervicothoracic ganglion. It must be remembered that cervical ribs are a fairly common abnormality, and are frequently present without causing symptoms: in fact it has been estimated that symptoms occur in only 5 to 10 per cent. of cases. Moreover, they may be associated with other abnormalities which may give rise to symptoms, notably syringomyelia.

Symptoms rarely arise in childhood, but occur with increasing frequency between the third and fifth decades of life.

SYMPTOMS

With Structural Abnormalities. The onset is usually gradual, and the symptoms of which the patient complains may be mainly sensory, motor, or vascular, or a combination of these may be present. The commonest sensory symptom is pain, which is referred to the ulnar border of the hand and distal half of the forearm and may be associated with numbness, tingling, or other paraesthesiae. Typically the pain is relieved by raising the hand above the head, which diminishes the pressure of the nerve upon the rib. Careful sensory investigation frequently reveals either hyperalgesia or relative analgesia in a narrow zone corresponding to the cutaneous distribution of the eighth cervical or first thoracic segment along the ulnar border of the hand and of the distal part of the forearm or occasionally on the medial aspect of the upper arm. Exceptionally, pain in the neck at the site of the rib may be the only symptom of which complaint is made. Motor symptoms consist of weakness and wasting, the distribution of which depends in part upon the position of the plexus. It is usually confined to the small muscles of the hand, and may begin either in those supplied by the median or in those supplied by the ulnar nerve. Less frequently the muscles of the ulnar side of the forearm are affected, and this is most likely to occur when the plexus is post-fixed. Horner's syndrome may be present.

Vascular symptoms are due to compression of the subclavian artery. Attacks of blanching or cyanosis of the fingers occur, and sometimes even gangrene. The radial pulses are frequently unequal, that upon the affected side possessing a smaller volume than its fellow, and sometimes becoming obliterated when the shoulder is retracted. The course of the subclavian arteries is frequently abnormal when cervical ribs are present, and the artery can be felt passing obliquely across the posterior triangle of the neck from a point ½ to 1 inch above the lower border of the sternomastoid to a point behind the middle of the clavicle. Thrombosis or stenosis of the subclavian artery may occur as a result of the pressure of the rib, and there is often a systolic bruit or palpable thrill over the vessel. Symonds has reported a case in which the thrombus extended from the subclavian artery on the right side into the right common carotid, and a portion, becoming detached, was carried as an embolus into the right internal carotid; vertebral artery embolism is probably more common (Gunning *et al.*, 1964). There may be an aneurysm of the third part of the subclavian, and embolism may occur peripherally.

The cervical rib may be visible or palpable as a bony swelling in the neck, pressure over which may cause pain or tingling referred to the ulnar border of the hand and forearm, or obliteration of the radial pulse. The presence of cervical ribs can be demonstrated radiographically, but it must be remembered that the symptoms may be due to a fibrous band, which will not be seen in radiograms, or to a normal first rib. The whole cervical and upper thoracic spine should be included in the X-rays.

Without Structural Abnormalities. Though the symptoms may be as severe as in the former group they tend to be less so, and to be sensory rather than motor, and subjective rather than objective. Pain and paraesthesiae are referred along the ulnar border of the forearm and hand. Symptoms may be entirely nocturnal, developing only when the patient has been lying down for some time.

DIAGNOSIS

A cervical rib is distinguished from motor neurone disease by the presence of pain and analgesia, and by the absence of muscular fasciculation. In syringomyelia, wasting of the small muscles of the hands is associated with analgesia and thermo-anaesthesia, but the sensory loss is usually much more extensive than that associated with a cervical rib, and signs of corticospinal degeneration are likely to be present. Cervical rib is a congenital abnormality which may be present in cases of syringomyelia. The radiographic demonstration of the presence of a rib must not, therefore, be taken as proof that the rib is the cause of the patient's symptoms. Tumour of the apex of the lung will be visible radiographically. Lesions of the median or ulnar nerve, especially when they arise from occupational pressure in the palm, may be confused with cervical rib, but the diagnosis is established by the characteristic distribution of the motor and sensory symptoms of lesions of these nerves. For other causes of wasting in the hands see page 785.

TREATMENT

Only surgical treatment affords permanent relief from a structural abnormality, and to obtain the best results it should be undertaken early. The precise operation required depends upon the nature of the abnormality present but the characteristic clinical syndrome described above, even in the absence of any radiological abnormality, demands exploration of the root of the neck. It may be necessary simply to divide a constricting fibrous band or to remove a cervical rib or a large seventh cervical transverse process, or a portion of the first rib, if that is the offender. It may be sufficient to divide the scalenus anterior muscle, thus allowing the first rib to drop. Following operation there is rapid relief of the sensory symptoms, and considerable improvement in muscular power may be expected. If there is severe muscular atrophy before operation, it is unlikely that full recovery will occur: hence the importance of operating early. The usual treatment of peripheral nerve lesions must be carried out. When symptoms occur without bony abnormality in middle life, rest in bed may give relief, and in suitable cases exercises designed to strengthen the muscles which lift the shoulder girdle are helpful. Experience will dictate the arrangement of pillows and the posture most suitable for nocturnal brachialgia.

THE LONG THORACIC NERVE

The long thoracic nerve is derived by three roots from the fifth, sixth, and seventh cervical nerves. The upper two roots pass through the scalenus medius muscle. The nerve, which supplies the serratus anterior, is injured alone most frequently as a result of pressure upon the shoulder, either from a sudden blow or from the prolonged pressure of carrying weights on the shoulder. Occasionally it is a site of neuritis, of the 'shoulder-girdle' type [see p. 808], and it may be involved in inflammation secondarily to apical pleurisy. When the lesion is a neuritis, there may be considerable pain at the onset. Isolated lesions of this nerve are comparatively rare but 'winging' of the scapula, presumably due to this cause is occasionally seen as a sequel of pneumonia or of other infective illnesses or may rarely arise spontaneously for no obvious cause.

The serratus anterior fixes the scapula to the chest wall when forward pressure is exerted with the upper limb. It brings the scapula forward when the upper limb is thrust forward, as in a fencing lunge, and it assists in elevating the limb above the head by rotating the scapula. Paralysis of the serratus anterior causes no deformity of the scapula when the limb is at rest. If, however, the patient is asked to push the limb forward against resistance, the inner border of the scapula becomes winged, especially in its lower two-thirds [FIG. 102]. He is unable to raise the limb above the head in front of him. The usual treatment of the paralysed muscle is carried out, but recovery does not always occur. In such cases Sherren (1908) recommended transplanting the sternocostal portion of the pectoralis major from the arm to the inferior angle of the scapula.

THE AXILLARY (CIRCUMFLEX) NERVE

The axillary nerve arises from the posterior cord of the brachial plexus. It innervates the teres minor and deltoid muscles, and supplies cutaneous sensibility to an oval area, the long axis of which extends from the acromion process to half-way down the outer aspect of the arm [Fig. 7, pp. 42, 43]. Injury to the axillary nerve, therefore, causes wasting and paralysis of the deltoid muscle, with paralysis of abduction of the arm and anaesthesia and analgesia corresponding to its cutaneous supply. The axillary nerve may be injured as

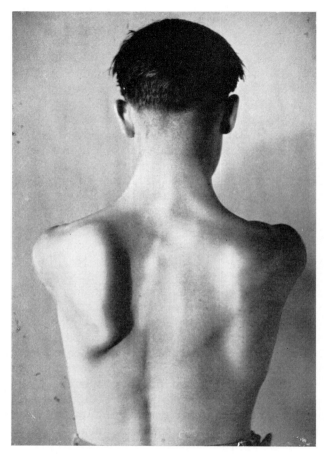

Fig. 102. Winging of the scapula due to paralysis of the left
serratus anterior

a result of surgical lesions in the region of the neck of the humerus and is some-times affected by shoulder girdle neuritis ('neuralgic amyotrophy') in which case there is usually severe and persistent pain in the shoulder region for several hours or even for one or two days before the paralysis is noted. The arm should be splinted in a position of abduction at the shoulder, and the usual treatment for peripheral nerve lesions applied.

THE RADIAL OR MUSCULOSPIRAL NERVE

The radial nerve constitutes the termination of the posterior cord of the brachial plexus and is derived from the fifth, sixth, seventh, and eighth cervical spinal nerves. It innervates the following muscles in the order given: triceps, anconeus, brachioradialis, extensor carpi radialis longus, and, through the posterior interosseous nerve, extensor carpi radialis brevis, supinator, extensor digitorum, extensor digiti minimi, extensor carpi ulnaris, the three extensors of the thumb, and extensor indicis. It supplies sensibility to the lower half of the radial aspect of the arm and the middle of the posterior aspect of the forearm. It also carries sensation from a variable area on the dorsum of the hand extending from the wrist distally as far as the interphalangeal joint of the thumb and the metacarpophalangeal joints of the index and middle fingers, and bounded laterally by the radial border of the thumb, and medially by the axis of the middle metacarpal [FIGS. 7 a and 7 b].

Complete interruption of the radial nerve in or above the axilla causes paralysis and wasting of all the muscles it supplies. Paralysis of the triceps leads to inability to extend the elbow. Paralysis of the brachioradialis is detected through failure of this muscle to contract when the patient flexes the elbow with the forearm midway between pronation and supination, the brachioradialis acting as a flexor of the elbow and not as a supinator. Paralysis of the supinator leads to loss of supination. Paralysis of the extensors of the wrist and fingers causes wrist-drop and finger-drop. Not only is the patient unable to extend the wrist as a primary movement, but synergic extension of the wrist fails to occur in association with flexion of the fingers, with a resulting impairment of the power of this movement. In investigating extension of the thumb special attention must be paid to extension at the carpometacarpal and metacarpophalangeal joints, since extension at the terminal joint may be carried out by some of the intrinsic muscles of the hand. The long extensors of the fingers produce extension only at the metacarpophalangeal joints, extension at the other joints being brought about by the interossei and lumbricals. In a case of radial paralysis, when the patient attempts to extend the fingers, the last-named muscles contract synergically and produce flexion at the metacarpophalangeal and extension at the interphalangeal joints. Following a pressure palsy of the radial nerve sensory loss is variable and may be absent but if present is found usually on the dorsum of the hand between the thumb and index finger. Radial nerve conduction studies may be helpful in determining the site of the lesion (Downie and Scott, 1967).

When the nerve is injured, as most frequently happens, in the lower third of the arm, the triceps usually escapes paralysis, and the branch to the brachioradialis, and less frequently that to the extensor carpi radialis longus, may also escape, the distribution of the paralysis coinciding with that following a lesion of the posterior interosseous nerve. The radial nerve is frequently injured where it winds round the humerus as a result of fractures of that bone. It is also liable to compression in the axilla through the use of a crutch, and when the arm of an anaesthetized patient is allowed to hang over the edge of the operating table, and during sleep, especially when the patient is intoxicated. In such cases pressure may be due to the arm hanging over the back of a chair ('Saturday-night paralysis'), and I have known radial palsy occur in a man who went to sleep on Hampstead Heath on a Bank Holiday with a girl lying on his arm. As Kopell and Thompson (1963) point out, the deep branch of the radial nerve can be compressed by the fibrous edge of the extensor carpi radialis brevis, or as it passes through a slit in the supinator muscle, and this can give a radial nerve palsy without sensory symptoms or signs, the picture being virtually indistinguishable from that due to a posterior interosseous nerve lesion. This may follow trauma and is not infrequently associated with a 'tennis elbow' syndrome.

Splinting is of great importance in the treatment of radial paralysis. A splint must be used to maintain extension of the wrist, but although extension at the metacarpophalangeal joints must be ensured, these joints must not be rigidly fixed. A system of elastic extension should, therefore, be used for the fingers. The thumb and finger-tips are covered with the fingers of a leather or plastic glove, to which elastic tapes are attached. These are carried back over the dorsum of the hand to be attached to a bracelet, which is fixed to the splint beneath the wrist. The usual treatment of a peripheral nerve lesion is carried out.

The prognosis of lesions of the radial nerve is good as most are due to simple pressure and are thus neuropraxial. Even after complete division and suture, signs of returning muscular function are usually evident in from four to eight months, according to the level of the lesion. When the deep branch of the radial posterior interosseous nerve is involved and electrical tests indicate a complete lesion the nerve should be explored.

THE MUSCULOCUTANEOUS NERVE

The musculocutaneous nerve is a branch of the lateral cord of the brachial plexus, its fibres being derived from the fifth and sixth cervical spinal nerves. It supplies the biceps and part of the brachialis, the principal flexors of the elbow, and its sensory distribution is to the radial border of the forearm as low as the carpometacarpal joint of the thumb [FIGS. 7 a and 7 b].

Division of the musculocutaneous nerve, therefore, causes weakness of flexion of the elbow-joint, though some power of flexion can still be carried out by the brachioradialis and the part of the brachialis which is innervated by the radial nerve. Sensation is impaired over the cutaneous distribution of the nerve. The musculocutaneous nerve is rarely injured alone, but may be damaged by dislocation of the head of the humerus or by penetrating wounds. Very rarely it may, like the radial nerve, be affected by simple pressure and transient paralysis of the biceps has been known to occur in a man falling asleep with his wife's head lying across his upper arm.

The forearm should be supported in a sling and the usual treatment of a peripheral nerve lesion carried out.

THE MEDIAN NERVE

The fibres of the median nerve are derived from the sixth, seventh, and eighth cervical and first thoracic spinal segments. It is formed by the union of two heads from the inner and outer cords of the brachial plexus. In the forearm it supplies the following muscles, to which branches are given in the order named: pronator teres, flexor carpi radialis, palmaris longus, flexor digitorum superficialis, flexor pollicis longus, flexor digitorum profundus, pronator quadratus. In the hand it usually supplies the two radial lumbricals, opponens pollicis, abductor pollicis brevis, and the outer head of the flexor pollicis brevis. Sometimes it supplies the first dorsal interosseous. Seddon (1954 *a*) describes anomalies in the nerve supply of the muscles of the hand.

Traumatic Lesions. After a complete lesion of the median nerve above its highest muscular branch there is, therefore, paralysis of pronation of the forearm. Occasionally this may result from compression of one or both heads which form the nerve as a result of sclerosis in the wall of the axillary artery to which they are closely related in the axilla. More often the nerve can be trapped or compressed as it passes through the pronator teres muscle at the elbow (the pronator

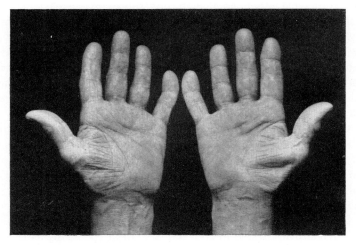

FIG. 103. Partial thenar atrophy due to compression of both median nerves in the carpal tunnel

syndrome) or kinked against the fibrous edge of the flexor digitorum superficialis (Kopell and Thompson, 1963). The radial flexor of the wrist is paralysed, so that when the wrist is flexed against resistance the hand deviates to the ulnar side. There is inability to flex the terminal phalanx of the thumb and the phalanges of the index finger. There is weakness of flexion of the phalanges of the remaining fingers, especially the middle finger, but not complete paralysis, since the ulnar half of the flexor digitorum profundus is supplied by the ulnar nerve. Flexion at the metacarpophalangeal joints is carried out by the interossei and lumbricals, of which only the two outer lumbricals are innervated by the median nerve. Paralysis of the muscles of the thenar eminence supplied by the median nerve leads to weakness of abduction of the thumb, a movement which must be tested in a plane at right angles to the palm, and opposition of the thumb is lost. Wasting is present in the paralysed muscles and is especially conspicuous in the thenar eminence, where wasting of the abductor pollicis brevis renders the first metacarpal unduly prominent [FIG. 103]. A lesion of the median nerve or of the anterior interosseous nerve in the middle of the forearm may paralyse the superficial flexor of the index finger, while allowing those of the other three fingers, the branches to which leave the nerve at a higher level, to escape. When the nerve is injured at the wrist, paralysis is confined to the hand. When investigating muscular power after a median nerve lesion it must be remembered that the abductor pollicis longus may be used in a trick movement as a radial flexor of the wrist, and that opposition of the thumb may be simulated by the combined action of the adductors and the abductor pollicis longus.

Sensory loss following a lesion of the median nerve is somewhat variable, especially in regard to the appreciation of pin-prick [FIGS. 7 a and 7 b]. Loss of this form of sensibility may be confined to the terminal phalanges of the index and middle fingers, the affected area being somewhat more extensive on their palmar than on their dorsal aspect. Appreciation of pin-prick is, however, more often lost over a somewhat larger area, including the palmar aspect of the terminal phalanx of the thumb. Loss of appreciation of light touch is more constant in its outline, which runs along the radial border of the thumb to the base of the thenar eminence, thence across the palm to the cleft between the middle and ring fingers, and includes approximately half of the palmar aspect of the ring finger on the radial side. On the dorsum it includes the radial aspect of the terminal two-thirds of the ring finger and the dorsal aspect of the middle and index fingers as far proximally as the middle of the proximal phalanges. From the radial side of the index finger the border passes along the fold of the first interosseous space and up the inner border of the thumb as far as the ulnar edge of the nail. Deep sensibility is usually lost in the terminal phalanges of the index and middle fingers. The median nerve is the commonest site of causalgia, which only occurs, however, when the lesion is incomplete.

The median nerve may be injured at any point of its course by stab or gun-shot wounds. It is occasionally damaged in dislocation of the shoulder. The commonest acute traumatic lesion in civil life is a cut at the wrist, usually the result of the hand having been put through a window pane. In such cases the ulnar nerve may also be damaged.

TREATMENT

To prevent stretching of the paralysed muscles the thumb is held in a position of palmar abduction and opposition by means of a splint consisting of a leather or plastic cuff at the wrist to which are attached two strips of elastic which run to a moulded cylinder fitted over the metacarpophalangeal joint and made from a plaster cast of the thumb (Highet, 1942 a). The usual treatment for the paralysed muscles is carried out. Causalgia requires special treatment, see page 767. Signs of returning sensibility usually precede motor recovery. After suture of the nerve the latter occurs in from three months to a year, depending upon the situation of the lesion and the distance of individual muscles below it. Voluntary power usually reappears first in pronator teres and in flexor carpi radialis. Sensory recovery is frequently incomplete, especially in respect of appreciation of light touch upon the index finger, but the proportion of useful motor and sensory recoveries is high—88 and 79 per cent. respectively (Seddon, 1949).

THE CARPAL TUNNEL SYNDROME

Compression of the median nerve in the carpal tunnel (Brain, Wright, and Wilkinson, 1947) occurs spontaneously, chiefly in middle-aged women, and in pregnancy. It may also occur after fractures and arthritis involving the wrist-joint, in acromegaly, myxoedema and amyloidosis, and in pyogenic infections of the hand. It results either from lesions which reduce the size of the carpal tunnel, from tenosynovitis with swelling of flexor tendon sheaths due to over-use, or from soft tissue swelling due to fluid retention (as in pregnancy or myxoedema). Pain and tingling are felt in the cutaneous distribution of the nerve to the digits, often awakening the patient at night, and constituting one form of acroparaesthesiae. Cutaneous sensory loss over the digits renders the manipulation of small objects difficult, and is sometimes accompanied by wasting and weakness of abductor brevis and opponens pollicis, causing conspicuous hollowing of the outer thenar eminence [FIG. 103]. Often, however, pain and paraesthesiae may be the only symptoms for many months and years and are often accentuated by using the hand or by warmth, and the only abnormal physical signs may be some blunting of sensation in the thumb and fingers supplied by the median nerve and/or tingling in the appropriate distribution produced by a sharp tap over the carpal ligament. The application of a tourniquet to the upper arm above arterial blood pressure may quickly produce ischaemic paraesthesiae in the affected fingers (Gilliatt and Wilson, 1954; Fullerton, 1963). The demonstration of slowed conduction and increased terminal latency in electromyography is of diagnostic value in doubtful cases (Simpson, 1956; Fullerton, 1963; Preswick, 1963; McLeod, 1966).

The carpal tunnel syndrome in pregnancy may be expected to recover after labour (Wilkinson, 1960). Diuretics and local injections of hydrocortisone (Foster, 1960) may produce temporary improvement, but in most long-standing cases only surgical division of the transverse carpal ligament is likely to be effective.

THE ULNAR NERVE

The ulnar nerve is derived from the eighth cervical and first thoracic spinal nerves. It gives off no branches above the elbow, where it lies behind the medial condyle of the humerus. It supplies branches to the following muscles in the forearm in the order stated: flexor carpi ulnaris, and the inner half of flexor digitorum profundus. In the hand it usually supplies the palmaris brevis, the muscles of the hypothenar eminence, the two inner lumbricals, the palmar and dorsal interossei, the transverse and oblique heads of the adductor pollicis, and the inner head of the flexor pollicis brevis. The first dorsal interosseous muscle is sometimes supplied by the median. Seddon (1954 a) describes the anomalies of the nerve supply of the muscles of the hand.

Interruption of the ulnar nerve at or above the level of the elbow causes paralysis of these muscles. As a result of paralysis of the flexor carpi ulnaris the hand deviates to the radial side on flexion of the wrist against resistance. Another method of demonstrating weakness of this muscle is as follows: the patient closes his hand and the examiner adducts it, placing his finger on the tendon of the flexor carpi ulnaris. When the patient extends his fingers this tendon can normally be felt to tighten. Paralysis of the ulnar half of the flexor digitorum profundus abolishes flexion of the little finger at the interphalangeal joints, and weakens flexion of the ring finger at these joints. Paralysis of the muscles of the hypothenar eminence abolishes abduction of the little finger, and impairs flexion of this finger at the metacarpophalangeal joint. Paralysis of the interossei abolishes abduction and adduction of the fingers. In examining this movement it is important that the hand should be kept with the palm pressed against a flat surface, as the long extensors and flexors of the fingers act to some extent as abductors and adductors. Further, the fingers cannot be held with the meta-carpophalangeal joints flexed and the interphalangeal joints extended. Paralysis of the transverse and oblique heads of the adductor pollicis weakens adduction of the thumb, and this is most evident when the patient attempts to press the thumb firmly against the index finger.

Wasting of the paralysed muscles is evident on the ulnar side of the flexor aspect of the forearm, the hypothenar eminence, the interosseous spaces, and the ulnar half of the thenar eminence [FIG. 104]. Paralysis of the small muscles of the hand causes 'claw-hand', this posture being produced by the unopposed action of their antagonists. Since the interossei cause flexion of the fingers at the metacarpophalangeal joints and extension at the interphalangeal joints, when these muscles are paralysed the opposite posture is maintained by the long flexors and extensors, namely, hyperextension at the metacarpophalangeal joints and flexion at the interphalangeal joints. This is usually most marked in the ring and little fingers, since the two radial lumbricals, which are supplied by the median nerve, to some extent compensate for loss of action of the interossei on the index and middle fingers.

After a lesion of the ulnar nerve at or above the elbow loss of deep sensibility is usually limited to the little finger. The area of analgesia to pin-prick is variable, but usually covers the little finger, the ulnar border of the palm, and often the ulnar half of the ring finger. The area of anaesthesia to light touch includes the little finger and the ulnar half of the ring finger, together with the ulnar border of the hand, both on the dorsum and the palmar aspects as far as the wrist, the area being bounded on the radial side by a line continuous with the axis of the ring finger [FIGS. 7 a and 7 b].

When the ulnar nerve is divided at the wrist, the flexor carpi ulnaris and the ulnar half of the flexor digitorum profundus escape paralysis, which is confined to the small muscles of the hand supplied by the nerve. When the lesion is below the point at which the dorsal branch is given off, the area of sensory loss is less than that described above. On the palmar aspect of the hand the area over which sensibility is lost is the same as when the nerve is divided above the wrist, but on the dorsal aspect appreciation of light touch is lost over the terminal two phalanges of the little finger, and the ulnar half of these phalanges of the ring finger, and loss of appreciation of pin-prick is usually confined to the terminal phalanx of the little finger. In such cases all the muscles supplied by the ulnar nerve in the hand are likely to be affected. When the deep palmar branch alone is involved there is no sensory loss and the hypothenar muscles escape.

Ulnar Nerve Lesions

Lesions of the ulnar nerve above the elbow are rare, but it may be involved in a penetrating wound. At the elbow it may suffer as a result of fractures and dislocations involving the lower end of the humerus, and the elbow-joint. In

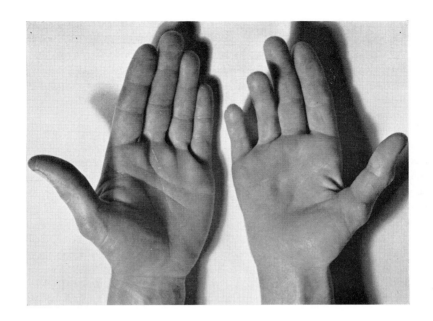

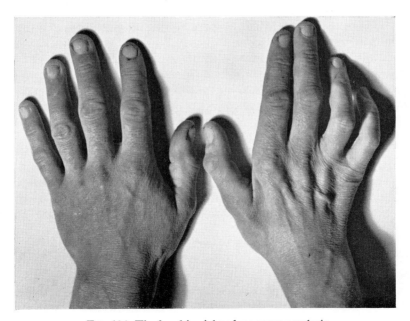

FIG. 104. The hand in right ulnar nerve paralysis

such cases the injury to the nerve may be immediate. Occasionally, however, it is involved years after an injury which has led to cubitus valgus. Similarly the nerve may be damaged by osteophytic outgrowths following arthritis of the elbow-joint, or by a ganglion. I have known it compressed by a Charcot elbow. However, the commonest site of chronic irritation or compression of the nerve in this situation is as it passes between the humeral and ulnar heads of the flexor carpi ulnaris (the cubital tunnel) (Kopell and Thompson, 1963).

In individuals possessing a shallow groove for the nerve behind the internal condyle of the humerus or an unusual degree of physiological cubitus valgus, the nerve may suffer from undue mobility, tending to slip forwards over the internal condyle when the elbow is flexed. Occupations involving repeated flexion of the elbow occasionally cause symptoms through the long-continued minor trauma involved. In all these cases of chronic injury of the nerve at the elbow-joint the lesion is a localized pressure neuropathy associated with fibrous thickening of the nerve at the site of trauma, where a spindle-shaped swelling can often be felt. The earliest symptoms are pain and paraesthesiae referred to the cutaneous distribution of the nerve. These symptoms may at first be apparent only when the patient awakens in the morning after sleeping with the elbow flexed. In long-standing cases there are usually weakness and wasting of the muscles innervated by the nerve in addition. Pressure on the nerve behind the elbow, or where it enters the cubital tunnel, may then reproduce the patient's paraesthesiae. Ulnar paralysis is occasionally met with as a result of pressure on the nerve at the elbow during sleep. At the wrist the ulnar nerve may be injured by cuts, and the median nerve may be simultaneously involved. The entire palmar branch of the nerve, including its superficial sensory component is occasionally compressed or injured on the anterior aspect of the wrist. A pressure neuropathy of the deep palmar branch of the ulnar nerve sometimes occurs in individuals whose occupation involves prolonged or recurrent pressure upon the outer part of the palm. In such cases the muscles of the hypothenar eminence usually escape damage and there is no sensory loss. Both at the wrist and in the palm the cause of compression may be a ganglion.

Motor nerve conduction time may be valuable in localizing the lesion, estimating its severity, and assessing recovery (Ebeling, Gilliatt, and Thomas, 1960). When the lesion is at the elbow, motor conduction is markedly slowed in the segment of the nerve around the elbow, while in lesions of the deep palmar branch of the nerve, conduction in the forearm is normal but terminal latency is increased.

TREATMENT

The treatment of lesions of the ulnar nerve is conducted on the same general lines as for other peripheral nerve lesions. Highet's 'knuckle-duster' splint is designed to maintain the hand in a posture of flexion at the metacarpophalangeal and extension at the interphalangeal joints (Highet, 1942 *a*). It has been modified in order to restore the metacarpal arch (Bowden, 1954 *b*). When the nerve is the site of pressure neuropathy as a result of abnormalities of the elbow-joint or wrist, an appropriate operation will be required to free it from pressure. When the nerve suffers from chronic irritation, it must be brought to lie in front of the internal condyle of the humerus. In such cases operation rapidly relieves sensory symptoms, but recovery of voluntary power is necessarily slower. In lesions of the deep palmar branch of the nerve, exploration is usually indicated, as it may be possible to remove a ganglion which is compressing the nerve. After suture of the nerve, sensibility usually begins to recover before voluntary power. Motor recovery, which occurs to a useful extent in about 80 per cent. of cases (Seddon, 1949), usually begins in the flexor carpi ulnaris and flexor digitorum profundus, and is most complete in these muscles and in the abductor digiti minimi. It may take two years after suture at the elbow.

DIGITAL NERVE NEUROPATHY

As Kopell and Thompson (1963) point out, one or more digital nerves in the hand may suffer compression in the intermetacarpal tunnel. This gives rise to burning pain and sensory impairment on the contiguous halves of two adjacent digits. Repeated digital nerve blocks with local anaesthetic agents may relieve the discomfort but not the sensory impairment.

DIAGNOSIS OF WASTING OF THE MUSCLES OF THE HAND

Lesions of the median and ulnar nerves require to be diagnosed from other causes of wasting of muscles of the hand. These muscles are innervated by the anterior horn cells of the eighth cervical and first thoracic segments of the spinal cord, mainly the latter. The causes of their wasting, therefore, include lesions of their lower motor neurones at any point between this spinal segment and the muscles, together with certain other conditions in which primary muscular degeneration or reflex muscular wasting occurs.

Lesions of Acute Onset Involving the Anterior Horns

The commonest of such acute lesions is *poliomyelitis*. This is usually easily distinguished by the acute onset, commonly in childhood, the non-progressive character of the wasting, the presence of muscular wasting with a patchy and asymmetrical distribution elsewhere in the body, the cyanosis of the affected extremity, and the absence of sensory loss. *Vascular lesions of the spinal cord* are rare. Thrombosis of a branch of the anterior spinal artery may cause destruction of the anterior horn cells. In such cases the spinothalamic tract is usually damaged simultaneously. *Haematomyelia* or cord contusion following acute hyperextension injuries of the neck may destroy the anterior horn cells of the cervical enlargement. Wasting is usually not confined to muscles innervated by the first thoracic segment and is usually associated with extensive sensory loss over the upper limbs and often with involvement of the long ascending and descending tracts of the cord.

Lesions of Slow Onset Involving the Anterior Horns

The commonest chronic lesion is *motor neurone disease*, which frequently begins with wasting of the small muscles of one or both hands. This condition is distinguished by its progressive course, the presence of muscular fasciculation and, sooner or later, wasting of other muscle groups, the frequent coexistence of corticospinal degeneration, and the absence of sensory loss. In *syringomyelia* wasting of the hand muscles is often an early symptom. Fasciculation is usually absent. The diagnosis depends upon the characteristic associated analgesia and thermo-anaesthesia, trophic lesions, and the frequent involvement of the cortico-spinal tracts. In *tumour of the spinal cord* the signs of a progressive focal lesion at the cervical enlargement are usually accompanied by pain and are sooner or later associated with those of spinal subarachnoid block.

Lesions of the Ventral Roots

The ventral roots are occasionally involved in the localized *leptomeningitis of syphilitic origin*, in which the substance of the cord usually also suffers. The ventral root lesion can be distinguished from a lesion of the anterior horn cells only when the dorsal roots are also involved, leading to root pains, often with some impairment of sensibility over the segmental cutaneous areas.

Lesions of the Spinal Nerve

The spinal nerve consists of a fusion of the ventral and the dorsal root, and a lesion of the first thoracic nerve, therefore, causes root-pain and frequently some sensory loss along the ulnar border of the hand and forearm, in addition to muscular wasting of the small muscles of the hand. The spinal nerve may be the site of neuropathy, though this is rare in the case of the first thoracic nerve and this nerve is rarely affected by intervertebral disc disease or spondylosis, in which conditions, contrary to widespread misconceptions, wasting of small hand muscles is excessively rare. It may, however, be compressed as a result of collapse or hyperostosis of the vertebral column. A traumatic lesion of the first thoracic spinal nerve is responsible for the *Dejerine-Klumpke type of birth palsy*. Lesions involving the first dorsal segment of the spinal cord, its ventral roots and spinal nerve, usually cause paralysis of the cervical sympathetic, the pre-ganglionic fibres of which leave the cord at this level.

Lesions of the Medial Cord of the Brachial Plexus

Lesions of the medial cord of the plexus, for example the pressure of a *cervical rib*, cause wasting of some or all the muscles supplied by the ulnar nerve, including those in the forearm together with the small muscles of the hand supplied by the median. The distribution of pain and sensory loss involves the eighth cervical and first thoracic segmental areas, that is, roughly, the supply of the ulnar nerve, together with the distal half or two-thirds of the ulnar border of the forearm.

Lesions of the Median and Ulnar Nerves

All lesions situated between the anterior horn cells of the first thoracic segment and the medial cord of the brachial plexus, inclusive, cause wasting of the small muscles of the hand. Distally to the medial cord of the plexus the innervation of these muscles is divided between the ulnar and median nerves. Lesions of these nerves, as has already been described, are distinguished by the characteristic distribution of the muscular wasting and sensory loss. Apart from localized lesions of these nerves, wasting of the small muscles of the hand may occur in various forms of *polyneuropathy* in which sensory loss of peripheral distribution and tenderness of the muscles are usually present, and the same symptoms frequently occur in the lower limbs. In *peroneal muscular atrophy* wasting of the hands usually follows that of the feet. The onset of the wasting in early life, its gradual ascent of the limbs stopping short at the elbows and knees, and the associated peripheral sensory impairment are distinguishing features.

Muscular Dystrophy

Wasting of the small muscles of the hand is found in some forms of *muscular dystrophy*, especially the so-called *distal* type of *myopathy*, and much less frequently in *dystrophia myotonica* in which forearm muscles are wasted but not so much those of the hands. The diagnosis depends upon the age of onset, the symmetrical character, distribution, and progressive course of the wasting, the absence of muscular fasciculation, sensory loss and signs of involvement of the central nervous system, and the familial or hereditary nature of the disorder.

Trophic Disorders

Reflex muscular wasting secondary to *arthritis* of the joints of the hand must not be overlooked. It is easily recognized on account of pain, swelling, and bony changes in the joints. In the so-called *shoulder-hand syndrome*, pericapsulitis of the shoulder-joint is often associated initially with painful swelling of the hand but subsequently there may be atrophy of the small hand muscles and even of the bones (Sudeck's atrophy). *Ischaemia* due to arteriosclerosis or thrombo-angiitis is a rare cause of muscular wasting, more frequently seen in the lower than in the upper limb. *Ischaemic myositis* (ischaemic contracture) caused by the pressure of a splint too tightly applied to the forearm leads to paralysis, wasting, and contracture of the muscles of the forearm and hand, with or without sensory loss, due to compression and degeneration of the nerves.

THE NERVES OF THE LOWER LIMB

THE LUMBOSACRAL PLEXUS

The lumbar plexus is formed by contributions from the twelfth thoracic and the first, second, third, and fourth lumbar spinal nerves; the sacral plexus, from the fourth and fifth lumbar and the first, second, and third sacral nerves. The principal nerves derived from the lumbar plexus are the femoral and the obturator, and from the sacral plexus the sciatic and the superior and inferior gluteal nerves. The lumbosacral plexus may be compressed by neoplastic metastases or one of its roots by a protruded intervertebral disc. The symptoms of this are described in the sections dealing with individual nerves. The plexus may be injured by the pressure of the foetal head or obstetric forceps during delivery and it is occasionally affected by pelvic deposits of endometriosis; either the obturator or the sciatic nerves may thus be damaged on one or both sides. The lumbosacral cord is most frequently affected, leading to unilateral or bilateral paralysis of the anterior tibial and peroneal muscles. (See also under the sciatic nerve, p. 789.)

THE LATERAL CUTANEOUS NERVE OF THE THIGH

The lateral cutaneous nerve of the thigh is derived from the dorsal parts of the second and third lumbar nerves. Passing through the psoas major muscle it enters the thigh beneath the lateral end of the inguinal ligament, and, piercing the fascia lata of the thigh about 4 inches distal to the anterior superior iliac spine, it divides into an anterior and a posterior branch which supply sensibility to the lateral aspect of the thigh and the lateral part of its anterior aspect from the buttock almost as low as the knee [FIGS. 7 a and 7 b]. Either where the nerve emerges from the pelvis or where it passes through or beneath the inguinal ligament or through the fascia lata it may become constricted by fibrous tissue with the production of pain, numbness, and paraesthesiae referred to the cutaneous distribution of the nerve, especially of its anterior branch. This condition, which is known as 'meralgia paraesthetica' usually afflicts middle-aged men but also occurs in women, particularly when overweight. It may follow the application of a plaster corset. The pain and numbness are often brought on by walking or standing, which may suggest arterial disease. The site of the pain, which is usually associated with relative anaesthesia and analgesia of the skin of the outer aspect of the thigh, is distinctive. The disorder is usually benign, has little more than a nuisance value, and may remit spontaneously. When pain is more troublesome repeated infiltration of local anaesthetic around the lateral half of the inguinal ligament may relieve symptoms, but if this is unsuccessful, operative decompression or division of the nerve may be indicated. For a review see Stevens (1957).

THE OBTURATOR NERVE

The obturator nerve is derived from the second, third, and fourth lumbar nerves by roots which are situated anteriorly to those of the femoral nerve. The union of these roots occurs in the psoas muscle and the nerve emerges from the pelvis by the obturator foramen. It gives a branch to the hip-joint and supplies the following muscles: adductor longus and gracilis, adductor brevis usually, and sometimes pectineus, obturator externus, and adductor magnus. Its cutaneous supply is variable and is distributed to the skin of the distal two-thirds of the medial aspect of the thigh [FIGS. 7 a and 7 b]. It also supplies a branch to the knee-joint.

Injury to the obturator nerve causes paralysis of the adductors of the thigh, except for the flexor fibres of the adductor magnus, which are innervated by the sciatic. Sensory loss is usually absent. The nerve is most frequently injured in the course of a difficult labour, occasionally as a result of dislocation of the hip or obturator hernia. No splint is required. The usual treatment of lower motor neurone paralysis is applied to the paralysed muscles.

The nerve may occasionally be compressed in the obturator canal by an obturator hernia or as a result of osteitis pubis following genito-urinary surgery. Pain down the medial aspect of the thigh is the most prominent symptom and may demand intrapelvic section of the nerve at the expense of permanent adductor paralysis (Kopell and Thompson, 1963).

THE FEMORAL NERVE

The femoral nerve is derived from the lumbar plexus, arising from the dorsal parts of the second, third, and fourth lumbar nerves, posterior to the obturator nerve. The nerve is formed in the psoas major muscle, and after passing through the pelvis enters the thigh beneath the inguinal ligament, lateral to the femoral sheath and femoral vessels. In the abdomen it sends a branch to the iliacus muscle and in the femoral triangle it breaks up into terminal branches which supply the pectineus, sartorius, and quadriceps. It gives articular branches to the hip- and knee-joints. Its intermediate and medial cutaneous branches supply the medial and internal aspects of the thigh in its lower two-thirds, and by the saphenous nerve it supplies sensibility to the inner aspect of the leg and foot as far distally as midway between the medial malleolus and the base of the great toe [FIGS. 7 a and 7 b].

After a lesion of the femoral nerve there may be slight weakness of flexion of the hip owing to paralysis of the iliacus, but the principal motor disturbance is weakness of extension of the knee owing to paralysis of the quadriceps, which is wasted. As a result of this the leg gives way in walking and cannot be used to raise the body on stairs. The knee-jerk is lost, and sensibility is lost over the cutaneous area innervated by the nerve. Causalgia may occur in the distribution of the saphenous nerve after partial lesions of the nerve.

The femoral nerve may be involved in psoas abscess or in new growths within the pelvis, or injured as a result of fractures of the pelvis or of the femur, or by dislocation of the hip. Lesions of this nerve are rarely seen as a result of gun-shot wounds of the thigh, as the proximity of the femoral artery renders the majority of such injuries rapidly fatal. The commonest lesion is a neuropathy which is sometimes secondary to diabetes ('diabetic amyotrophy'), or to lumbar spondylosis, sometimes due to the pressure of a herniated intervertebral disc upon one of the roots, and in some cases of unknown aetiology. In a series of 23 cases, Thage (1965) found that seven were due to diabetes, two were traumatic, one was due to neurinoma, five to lumbar disc lesions, and eight were idiopathic.

No splint is required in the treatment of lesions of the femoral nerve. Support to the leg may be given by means of a strong elastic band running from a belt over the front of the thigh to be attached to a gaiter round the calf. The usual treatment of lower motor neurone paralysis should be applied to the quadriceps. For the diagnosis, symptoms, and treatment of femoral neuropathy see page 809.

THE SCIATIC NERVE

The sciatic nerve is derived from the sacral plexus, which is formed by a fusion of the ventral primary divisions of the fourth and fifth lumbar and of the first, second, and third sacral spinal nerves. The nerve is composed of two divisions which are destined to form the tibial (medial popliteal) and common peroneal (lateral popliteal) nerves. These two divisions, though bound together by connective tissue, are separable up to the sacral plexus from which they are separately derived, the tibial coming from the ventral divisions of the fourth and fifth lumbar and first, second and third sacral nerves, while the common peroneal comes from the dorsal divisions of the fourth and fifth lumbar and first and second sacral nerves. The sciatic nerve, in addition to its two principal components, contains nerves to the hamstrings and a nerve to the short head of the biceps muscle. It leaves the pelvis by passing through the great sciatic notch below the piriformis muscle into the buttock and then descends in the back of the thigh, lying between the great trochanter of the femur and the tuberosity of the ischium. It terminates at a variable point between the sciatic notch and the proximal part of the popliteal fossa by dividing into the common peroneal and tibial nerves.

In addition to supplying motor nerves to the semitendinosus, semimembranosus, the long head of the biceps, the short head of the biceps, and adductor magnus, the sciatic is the motor nerve to all the muscles below the knee. The superficial peroneal branch of the common peroneal nerve supplies the peronei longus and brevis; the deep peroneal nerve supplies the tibialis anterior, extensor digitorum longus, extensor hallucis longus, peroneus tertius, and extensor digitorum brevis. The tibial nerve supplies muscular branches in the following order: gastrocnemius, popliteus, plantaris, and soleus, and by the terminal part innervates the popliteus, the deep part of the soleus, tibialis posterior, flexor digitorum longus, and flexor hallucis longus. The medial and lateral plantar nerves supply the small muscles of the feet.

After complete interruption of the sciatic nerve there is paralysis of flexion of the knee, which is carried out by the hamstrings, and of all the muscles below the knee. Foot-drop occurs as a result of paralysis of the anterior tibial group of muscles and of the peronei. The patient is able to stand and to walk, but drags the toes of the affected foot and is unable to stand on his toes on the paralysed side.

The sensory distribution of the sciatic nerve lies entirely below the knee [FIGS. 7 a and 7 b]. After complete division of the nerve, light touch is the form of sensibility which is most extensively lost. Anaesthesia to cotton wool extends over the whole of the foot, with the exception of a zone about $1\frac{1}{2}$ inches wide along the inner aspect, extending about 2 inches distal to the internal malleolus, this area being supplied by the saphenous nerve. On the leg the area of anaesthesia to light touch includes the outer aspect, roughly from the midline in front to the midline behind as far up as 2 inches below the upper end of the fibula. Analgesia to pin-prick is less extensive than anaesthesia to light touch. Below, the two areas approximately coincide, but above, the area of analgesia is less extensive than that of anaesthesia by 2 or 3 inches. Appreciation of pressure and of vibration is lost over the whole of the foot, with the exception of the proximal two-thirds of the inner aspect, and postural sensibility and appreciation of passive movement are lost in the toes.

The knee-jerk is unaffected, but the ankle-jerk is lost and so also is the plantar reflex. Vasomotor and trophic changes are usually conspicuous after complete division of the sciatic. The leg is congested and swollen, especially when it is allowed to hang down. The skin is dry, and sweating is lost over the foot, except along the inner border, where it is supplied by the saphenous nerve. Perforating ulcers may develop on the sole.

The sciatic nerve may be damaged as a result of fractures of the pelvis and femur, and gun-shot wounds of the buttock and thigh. In civil life one of the commonest causes of a sciatic nerve lesion is a misplaced injection given too far medially in the buttock, while there is evidence that rarely the nerve may undergo entrapment or compression as it traverses the sciatic notch. It may be compressed within the pelvis by neoplasms, or by the foetal head during delivery. The common peroneal division is much more susceptible to injury than the tibial. Complete division of the whole nerve is rare.

The differential diagnosis of lesions of the sciatic nerve is discussed in the section dealing with sciatica.

THE COMMON PERONEAL (LATERAL POPLITEAL) NERVE

After division of the common peroneal nerve there is paralysis with wasting of the peronei and of the anterior tibial group of muscles. The power of dorsiflexion of the foot and toes and of eversion of the foot is lost, and foot-drop results. Inversion is lost when the foot is dorsiflexed, but a weak movement of inversion is possible in association with plantar flexion. When the nerve is divided above the point of origin of its lateral cutaneous branch, sensation is impaired over the dorsum of the foot, including the first phalanges of the toes, and over the antero-external aspect of the leg in its lower half or two-thirds, the area of anaesthesia to light touch being somewhat more extensive than the area of anaesthesia to pin-prick [FIGS. 7 a and 7 b]. When the lesion is situated below the origin of the lateral cutaneous branch, sensation is impaired over the dorsum of the foot only, and the anaesthetic area is usually bounded by a line passing upwards from the space between the fourth and fifth toes parallel with the outer border of the foot. Deep sensibility is unimpaired.

The common peroneal nerve may be injured as a result of penetrating wounds in the neighbourhood of the knee-joint, and of fractures involving the upper end of the fibula. It is sometimes entrapped or compressed or irritated by fibrous constricting bands as it winds round the neck of the fibula and may suffer from compression by a tight bandage applied to the knee, or by pressure during sleep. In certain occupations, as in slaters working on roofs, the nerve may be compressed if the individual habitually works with one leg flexed and lying under the other with its outer aspect against the roof surface. In the case of neuritis and compression of the nerve, the muscles which it innervates do not always suffer equally. The peronei are usually more gravely affected than the anterior tibial group, and the area of sensory loss is often less than that found after complete division.

A common peroneal nerve palsy, of which the most striking symptom is foot-drop, may result from the causes mentioned and often recovers in two or three months but rarely surgical exploration of the nerve at the fibular neck is required. The diagnosis can be confirmed by measurements of nerve conduction velocity in the nerve.

THE TIBIAL (MEDIAL POPLITEAL) NERVE

After division of the tibial nerve the calf muscles and the muscles of the sole are paralysed and wasted and the foot assumes the position of talipes calcaneo-valgus. The ankle-jerk is lost, and the plantar reflex may also be unelicitable.

There is as a rule no loss of deep sensibility. There is anaesthesia to light touch over the skin of the sole, including the plantar aspect of the toes and the dorsal aspect of their terminal phalanges. The area of analgesia to prick is less extensive and does not include the toes [FIGS. 7 a and 7 b].

POSTERIOR TIBIAL NERVE

Rarely the posterior tibial nerve may be compressed behind and below the medial malleolus giving rise to sensory loss over almost the entire sole of the foot (the tarsal tunnel syndrome).

PLANTAR AND INTERDIGITAL NERVES

Plantar nerves may occasionally be compressed as they enter the medial aspect of the sole of the foot giving a picture of sensory loss slightly less extensive than that of posterior tibial nerve compression (Kopell and Thompson, 1963). Neuropathies of plantar interdigital nerves giving rise to pain and analgesia in the adjacent halves of two contiguous toes have also been described and may rarely be associated with neuroma formation.

TREATMENT

After lesions of the sciatic nerve and of the common peroneal nerve it is important to prevent dropping of the foot. The patient should, therefore, wear a night-splint, and during the day the foot-drop must be overcome by wearing a shoe with a toe-raising spring. (For suitable designs, see Bowden, 1954 b.) The usual treatment of peripheral nerve lesions should be carried out, including exercises and electricity. Recovery is always slow after complete division of the nerve. When the sciatic nerve trunk has been divided return of voluntary power cannot be expected for from a year to eighteen months, and may take much longer. It may be necessary to carry out treatment for three years. In the case of division of the common peroneal nerve return of power may be expected to be demonstrable in from nine months to a year, but it is likely to be at least two years before the maximum degree of recovery is attained. Useful motor recovery occurs in about 50 per cent. of cases after suture. In the case of the tibial nerve motor recovery is better than sensory. In the rare cases of posterior tibial or plantar nerve compression, surgical decompression is indicated in intractable cases, while in certain cases of interdigital neuropathy, excision of a neuroma or division of the affected nerves may be necessary to relieve persistent pain.

REFERENCES

BARNES, R. (1954) Peripheral nerve injuries, *Spec. Rep. Ser. med. Res. Coun. (Lond.)*, **282**, 156.

BARWICK, D. D., and RICHARDSON, A. T. (1969) Clinical electromyography, in *Disorders of Voluntary Muscle*, 2nd ed., ed. WALTON, J. N., London.

BONNEY, G. (1954) The value of axon responses in determining the site of lesion in traction injuries of the brachial plexus, *Brain*, **77**, 588.

BOWDEN, R. E. M. (1954 a) Peripheral nerve injuries, *Spec. Rep. Ser. med. Res. Coun. (Lond.)*, **282**, 263.

BOWDEN, R. E. M. (1954 b) Peripheral nerve injuries, *Spec. Rep. Ser. med. Res. Coun. (Lond.)*, **282**, 298.

BRAIN, W. R., WRIGHT, A. D., and WILKINSON, M. (1947) Spontaneous compression of both median nerves in the carpal tunnel, *Lancet*, i, 277.

BUCHTHAL, F. (1957) *An Introduction to Electromyography*, Copenhagen.

BUCHTHAL, F. (1962) The electromyogram, *Wld Neurol.*, **3**, 16.

BUCHTHAL, F., and ROSENFALCK, A. (1966) Evoked action potentials and conduction velocity in human sensory nerves, *Brain Research*, **3**, special issue.

DAVIS, D. R. (1949) Some factors affecting the results of treatment of peripheral nerve injuries, *Lancet*, i, 877.

DOWNIE, A. W. (1969) Studies in nerve conduction, in *Disorders of Voluntary Muscle*, 2nd ed., ed. WALTON, J. N., London.

DOWNIE, A. W., and SCOTT, T. R. (1967) An improved technique for radial nerve conduction studies, *J. Neurol. Neurosurg. Psychiat.*, **30**, 332.

EBELING, P., GILLIATT, R. W., and THOMAS, P. K. (1960) A clinical and electrical study of ulnar nerve lesions in the hand, *J. Neurol. Neurosurg. Psychiat.*, **23**, 1.

FOERSTER, O. (1929) in LEWANDOWSKY's *Handbuch der Neurologie*, Ergänzungsband, 2. Teil, 1. Abschnitt. Spezielle Anatomie und Physiologie der peripheren Nerven, Berlin.

FOERSTER, O. (1929) in LEWANDOWSKY's *Handbuch der Neurologie*, Ergänzungsband, 2. Abschnitt. Die Symptomatologie der Schussverletzungen der peripheren Nerven, Berlin.

FOERSTER, O. (1929) in LEWANDOWSKY's *Handbuch der Neurologie*, Ergänzungsband, 2. Teil, 3. Abschnitt. Die Therapie der Schussverletzungen der peripheren Nerven, Berlin.

FOSTER, J. B. (1960) Hydrocortisone and the carpal-tunnel syndrome, *Lancet*, i, 454.

FULLERTON, P. M. (1963) The effect of ischaemia on nerve conduction in the carpal tunnel syndrome, *J. Neurol. Neurosurg. Psychiat.*, **26**, 385.

GILLIATT, R. W. (1957) Clinical electromyography, in *Modern Trends in Neurology*, ed. WILLIAMS, W., p. 65, London.

GILLIATT, R. W., and SEARS, T. A., (1958) Sensory nerve action potentials in patients with peripheral nerve lesions, *J. Neurol. Neurosurg. Psychiat.*, **21**, 109.

GILLIATT, R. W., and WILSON, T. G. (1954) Ischaemic sensory loss in patients with peripheral nerve lesions, *J. Neurol. Neurosurg. Psychiat.*, **17**, 104.

GUNNING, A. J., PICKERING, G. W., ROBB-SMITH, A. H. T., and ROSS RUSSELL, R. (1964) Mural thrombosis of the subclavian artery and subsequent embolism in cervical rib, *Quart. J. Med.*, **33**, 133.

GUTTMANN, L. (1940) Topographic studies of disturbances of sweat secretion after complete lesions of peripheral nerves, *J. Neurol. Psychiat.*, N.S. **3**, 197.

HARRIS, W. (1930) Discussion on injuries to the brachial plexus, *Proc. roy. Soc. Med.*, (Sect. Neurol.) **23**, 1281.

HIGHET, W. B. (1942 *a*) Splintage of peripheral nerve injuries, *Lancet*, i, 555.

HIGHET, W. B. (1942 *b*) Procaine nerve block in the investigation of peripheral nerve injuries, *J. Neurol. Psychiat.*, N.S. **5**, 101.

KOPELL, H. P., and THOMPSON, W. A. L. (1963) *Peripheral Entrapment Neuropathies*, Baltimore.

KUGELBERG, E. (1947) Electromyograms in muscular disorders, *J. Neurol. Neurosurg. Psychiat.*, **10**, 122.

KUGELBERG, E. (1949) Electromyography in muscular dystrophies, *J. Neurol. Neurosurg. Psychiat.*, **12**, 129.

McLEOD, J. G. (1966) Digital nerve conduction in the carpal tunnel syndrome after mechanical stimulation of the finger, *J. Neurol. Neurosurg. Psychiat.*, **29**, 12.

MAYFIELD, F. H. (1951) *Causalgia*, Springfield, Ill.

NORRIS, F. H. (1963) *The EMG*, New York.

POLLOCK, L. J., and DAVIES, L. (1931–2) Peripheral nerve injuries, *Amer. J. Surg.*, **15** 179, 390, 573; **16**, 141, 353; **17**, 139, 301, 462.

PRESWICK, G. (1963) The effect of stimulus intensity on motor latency in the carpal tunnel syndrome, *J. Neurol. Neurosurg. Psychiat.*, **26**, 398.

RASMUSSEN, T. B., and FREEDMAN, H. (1946) Treatment of causalgia; analysis of 100 cases, *J. Neurosurg.*, **3**, 165.

RICHARDS, R. L. (1954) Peripheral nerve injuries, *Spec. Rep. Ser. med. Res. Coun.* (*Lond.*), **282**, 186.

ROSENTHAL, A. M. (1961) Electrodiagnostic testing in neuromuscular diseases, *J. Amer. med. Ass.*, **177**, 829.

SEDDON, H. J. (1944 *a*) The early management of peripheral nerve injuries, *Practitioner*, **152**, 101.

SEDDON, H. J. (1944 *b*) Three types of nerve injury, *Brain*, **66**, 237.

SEDDON, H. J. (1949) The practical value of peripheral nerve repair, *Proc. roy. Soc. Med.*, **42**, 427.

SEDDON, H. J. (1954 *a*) Peripheral nerve injuries, *Spec. Rep. Ser. med. Res. Coun.* (*Lond.*), **282**, 1.

SEDDON, H. J. (1954 *b*) Peripheral nerve injuries, *Spec. Rep. Ser. med. Res. Coun.* (*Lond.*), **282**, 389.

SEDDON, H. J., MEDAWAR, P. B., and SMITH, H. (1943) Rate of regeneration of peripheral nerves in man, *J. Physiol.* (*Lond.*), **102**, 191.

SHERREN, J. (1908) *Injuries of Nerves and Their Treatment*, London.

SIMPSON, J. A. (1956) Electrical signs in the diagnosis of carpal tunnel and related syndromes, *J. Neurol. Neurosurg. Psychiat.*, **19**, 275.

SPEIGEL, I. J., and MILOWSKY, J. L. (1945) Causalgia: a preliminary report, *Arch. Neurol. Psychiat.* (*Chicago*), **53**, 448.

STEVENS, H. (1957) Meralgia paraesthetica, *Arch. Neurol. Psychiat.* (*Chicago*), **77**, 557.

STOPFORD, J. S. B. (1927) Disturbances of sensation following section and suture of a peripheral nerve, *Brain*, **50**, 391.

SUNDERLAND, S. (1968) *Nerves and Nerve Injuries*, Edinburgh.

TELFORD, E. D., and MOTTERSHEAD, S. (1947) The 'costoclavicular syndrome', *Brit. med. J.*, **1**, 325.

THAGE, O. (1965) The 'quadriceps syndrome', *Acta neurol. scand.*, **41**, Suppl. 13, 245.

WALSHE, F. M. R. (1942) The anatomy and physiology of cutaneous sensibility: a critical review, *Brain*, **65**, 48.

WALSHE, F. M. R., JACKSON, H., and WYBURN-MASON, R. (1944). On some pressure effects associated with cervical and with rudimentary and 'normal' first ribs, and the factors entering into their causation, *Brain*, **67**, 141.

WEDDELL, G., FEINSTEIN, B., and PATTLE, R. E. (1943) The clinical application of electromyography, *Lancet*, i, 236.

WILKINSON, M. (1960) The carpal-tunnel syndrome in pregnancy, *Lancet*, i, 453.

ZACHARY, R. B. (1945) Thenar palsy due to compression of the median nerve in the carpal tunnel, *Surg. Gynec. Obstet.*, **81**, 213.

ZACHARY, R. B. (1954) Peripheral nerve injuries, *Spec. Rep. Ser. med. Res. Coun.* (*Lond.*), **282**, 354.

SPINAL RADICULITIS AND RADICULOPATHY

In the cervical region the ventral and dorsal spinal roots of each segment lie close together within the intervertebral foramen to form the radicular nerve. The dorsal root ganglion lies just peripherally in the gutter of the transverse process. Beyond that the two roots fuse to form the spinal nerve. In the lumbar region the ganglia lie in the foramina. Each radicular nerve has an investment of dura mater and the leptomeninges. The term radiculitis is sometimes applied indiscriminately to inflammatory lesions of the spinal roots proper and of the spinal nerve, though the latter should be termed spinal neuritis.

Lesions of dorsal roots are commoner than those of ventral roots. Either or both may be involved in syphilitic spinal leptomeningitis, spinal arachnoiditis, or pyogenic leptomeningitis or pachymeningitis. The dorsal roots are the site of degeneration in tabes dorsalis, and of inflammation in herpes zoster, and occasionally in various forms of encephalomyelitis. They may be compressed by extramedullary spinal tumour, or irritated by abnormal constituents of the cerebrospinal fluid, such as blood after subarachnoid haemorrhage, or substances introduced for diagnostic or therapeutic purposes. A radiculitis limited to the cauda equina has been described.

Diseases of the vertebral column may damage either spinal roots or spinal nerves. A growth which invades the spinal theca or a herniated intervertebral disc may compress spinal roots, but when there is vertebral collapse, due to primary or secondary neoplasm, tuberculous or other infection, Paget's osteitis, or traumatic fracture-dislocation, it is usually the radicular nerves which are compressed in the intervertebral foramina. The radicular nerves occasionally undergo compression in severe scoliosis and in spondylosis, and are sometimes the site of neuritis after serotherapy. The cause is sometimes obscure.

An irritative lesion of a single dorsal root causes pain of a lancinating or burning character, which is often precipitated or intensified by coughing or sneezing and sometimes by movements of the spine, and is associated with hyperaesthesia and hyperalgesia over the full segmental distribution of the root. According to Foerster, no detectable sensory loss is produced by surgical division of a single dorsal root, owing to the overlapping of adjacent root areas. When more than one adjacent root is interrupted, the area of sensory loss is that area which is exclusively supplied by the combined roots involved, and the area of analgesia is larger than that of anaesthesia to light touch. A lesion of a ventral root causes atrophic paralysis of any muscle exclusively supplied by that root, and a partial lower motor neurone lesion of any muscle to whose innervation it contributes. Fasciculation may occur in affected muscles. A lesion of a radicular nerve produces the same symptoms as a lesion of the corresponding ventral and dorsal root combined.

The diagnosis of radiculitis depends first upon the recognition of the segmental character of the sensory and motor symptoms. The nature of the lesion can be ascertained only by taking into account the whole clinical picture, the presence of associated symptoms of a lesion of the spinal cord and vertebral column and the results of examination of the cerebrospinal fluid and X-rays of the spine, especially the intervertebral foramina. Broadly speaking, an acute onset of root symptoms alone suggests an inflammatory lesion or acute disc protrusion, an insidious onset of root symptoms with or without symptoms of a lesion of the spinal cord at the same level suggests compression, and the coexistence of pain in the back, limitation of movements of the spine, and local spinal tenderness or deformity at the same level points to disease of the spine as the cause.

SENSORY NEUROPATHY DUE TO DEGENERATION OF THE DORSAL ROOT GANGLIA

This is an unusual but striking syndrome characterized clinically by the subacute onset of a severe sensory ataxia with gross sensory loss, particularly of posterior column sensibility, but often of all forms, with loss of reflexes. The causes are various including carcinoma [see p. 751], syphilis, diabetes, and unknown factors. Pathologically there is a selective loss of dorsal root ganglion cells and their fibres in dorsal roots, posterior columns of the spinal cord, and peripheral nerves (McAlpine and Page, 1951; Bosanquet and Henson, 1957).

Hereditary sensory neuropathy is a disorder usually included in the hereditary ataxia group in which there is usually progressive peripheral impairment of all forms of sensibility, beginning early in life and in which degeneration of dorsal root ganglia is the primary lesion; it is inherited by an autosomal recessive mechanism. Insensitivity to pain may be so extensive in the trunk and extremities that a diagnosis of congenital insensitivity to pain may be made erroneously; painless perforating ulcers of the feet commonly result, with painless fracture or resorption of bones in the feet and even in the phalanges (Morvan's syndrome).

SPINAL RADICULOPATHY DUE TO INTERVERTEBRAL DISC DISEASE

Disorders of the spinal column associated with lesions of the intervertebral discs are by far the commonest cause of painful root compression. Such lesions are situated chiefly in the cervical and lumbar regions of the spine, though they occur occasionally in the thoracic region. The principal cause is undoubtedly the tendency of the intervertebral discs to degenerate with increasing age and this no doubt explains the occurrence of degeneration of both cervical and lumbar intervertebral discs in the same patient. Other factors, especially trauma, may play a part.

The intervertebral disc consists of a central portion, the nucleus pulposus, which obeys the laws of fluids and is surrounded by the annulus fibrosus, a strong but somewhat fibro-cartilaginous and elastic membrane binding the bodies of the vertebrae together. When force is exerted upon the disc it is distributed laterally in all directions, and if the force is too strong for the resistance of the annulus fibrosus the nucleus pulposus will herniate through it. Such protrusions may occur either in the midline or posterolaterally into the spinal canal, or more laterally into the intervertebral foramen [FIG. 105]. This is described as a nuclear herniation. There is, however, another type of disc protrusion, the annular protrusion, which is produced in a different way. A degenerated intervertebral disc tends to collapse, in which case the annulus bulges in all directions. The protruded material becomes vascularized and its fibrous elements are increased. A nuclear herniation is originally soft, but in time undergoes a similar transformation into fibrocartilage, so that the end result of both a nuclear and an annular protrusion may be a hard calcified boss. For anatomical reasons the effects of cervical and lumbar protrusions are somewhat different and must be considered separately.

CERVICAL DISC LESIONS AND BRACHIAL RADICULOPATHY

Cervical intervertebral discs are bounded on their lateral margins by an articulation known as the uncovertebral joint which lies on the anteromedial side of the intervertebral foramen, the posterior boundary of which is formed by the articulation between the pedicles of the two adjacent vertebrae. The cervical spinal roots may therefore be compressed, either by posterolateral protrusions of the intervertebral disc into the spinal canal or, as the radicular

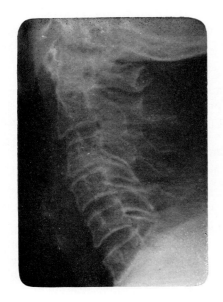

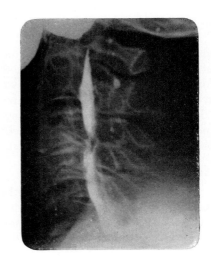

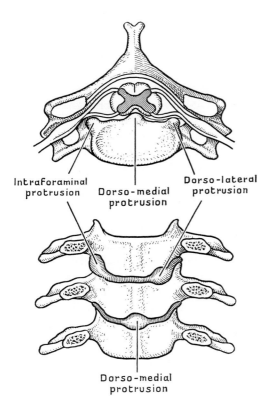

Intraforaminal
protrusion   Dorso-medial   Dorso-lateral
protrusion   protrusion

Dorso-medial
protrusion

FIG. 105. Cervical spondylosis

Above: Gross narrowing of C.3–4 intervertebral disc with posterior osteophyte
causing narrowing of spinal canal shown
in myelogram (on right)

Left: Sites of intervertebral disc protrusion

nerve, within the intervertebral foramen, either by an acute disc protrusion or as the result of narrowing of the foramen by osteophytes, especially those arising from uncovertebral joints. Such pressure, as Frykholm (1951) has shown, leads to fibrosis of the root sheaths.

The pathological changes of the chronic syndrome of cervical spondylosis may involve one pair of intervertebral joints or more than one and are more often related to single or multiple annular protrusions with eventual bony boss formation, though this process may occur in patients who have suffered previous acute protrusions; when the joint lesions are multiple the joints affected may be adjacent to one another or they may not. Since age is the chief factor in causing the degeneration of the intervertebral discs most patients are middle-aged or older, but acute cervical disc protrusion may occur at an earlier age.

Acute Protrusions

Acute protrusions may occur either spontaneously or as the result of trauma. A patient suffering from an acute protrusion usually gives a history of recurrent attacks of pain in the neck often diagnosed as 'fibrositis'. Suddenly a pain more severe and lasting than the previous ones occurs. The neck may feel as though it is fixed, and both active and passive movements cause an intensification of the pain, which may be very severe. Anteroposterior movements of the head (which occur mainly at the atlanto-occipital joints) and rotation (which occurs largely at the atlanto-axial joint) are restricted only by protective muscle spasm. It is lateral movements which are particularly painful, especially towards the side of the lesion (Spurling's sign). The pain is also referred within the distribution of the spinal nerve which is compressed. On examination the neck is usually held rigidly, and sometimes slightly flexed towards the side of the lesion. The muscles innervated by the spinal nerve compressed are usually somewhat wasted and hypotonic, but severe muscular weakness or wasting is unusual. The tendon reflexes which they mediate are diminished, and sometimes lost. It may be possible to demonstrate some hyperalgesia and hyperaesthesia within the corresponding dermatome, or some diminution of cutaneous sensibility. Plain X-rays usually show little abnormality, though there may be slight narrowing of the affected intervertebral disc. Myelography may show an obliteration of the corresponding root sheath.

The treatment of spontaneous acute protrusion of an intervertebral disc involving one spinal nerve in the neck is a combination of traction on the head, to relieve pressure upon the protruding disc, and/or immobilization. In the acute phase a soft 'Gamgee' tissue collar or one made of newspaper may be helpful and powerful analgesics are usually required. After the acute phase has passed, immobilization may be continued by means of a plastic collar. If these methods fail surgical exploration may be required but this is rarely necessary in acute cervical disc lesions.

CERVICAL SPONDYLOSIS

The duration and the history of symptoms of cervical spondylosis are extremely variable and radicular symptoms may be acute, subacute, or insidious in their onset. They are, in fact, often absent in cases of cervical cord compression (myelopathy). Acute involvement of one spinal nerve leads to symptoms resembling those of a spontaneous acute protrusion of a single intervertebral disc into the intervertebral foramen, as described above. Pain, however, is not always limited to one dermatome, but may extend down the upper limb to involve to a greater or lesser extent all the digits, in which case a clinical picture resembling the classical one of 'brachial neuritis or neuralgia' is produced. An insidious onset is characterized by dysaesthesiae consisting of a burning and tingling sensation, sometimes accompanied by pain, radiating down the upper limb into one or more digits and tending to be particularly troublesome at night. Motor symptoms are usually slight or absent and only exceptionally is there a complaint of weakness, but occasionally wasting accompanied by fasciculation may be severe enough to simulate motor neurone disease.

On examination of the patient there is commonly some diminution of the appreciation of light touch and pin-prick within the distribution of the dermatomes corresponding to the affected radicular nerves. There may also be localized areas of tenderness in the corresponding muscles. Appreciation of posture and passive movement is usually unimpaired. There is likely to be slight muscular wasting accompanied by hypotonia in the muscles innervated by the affected spinal nerves, but muscular weakness is usually slight. The tendon reflexes innervated from the affected segments are likely to be diminished or lost. Active and passive movements of the neck are somewhat limited in extent, but relatively painless. There may be some local tenderness on pressure.

Plain X-rays usually show narrowing of intervertebral discs with posterior osteophytes, and, in the oblique views, of the intervertebral foramina owing to the projection of osteophytes from the uncovertebral joints.

TREATMENT

In most cases there is a satisfactory response to immobilization in a plaster or plastic collar which is usually required for two or three months. Both traction and manipulation have their advocates, but the latter is probably not free from risk. Surgical decompression of the intervertebral foramina has been carried out, but is rarely likely to be required. Various forms of physiotherapy are useful adjuvants to treatment. In the acute stage analgesic drugs and rest in bed are necessary with the arm supported on a pillow, and when the patient gets up, in a sling, but care must be taken that immobilization does not lead to a 'frozen shoulder'.

LUMBAR DISC LESIONS AND SCIATICA

The term sciatica has come to be applied to a benign syndrome characterized especially by pain beginning in the lumbar region and spreading down the back of one lower limb to the ankle, usually intensified by coughing or sneezing, and associated with little weakness or sensory loss but sometimes with diminution or loss of the ankle-jerk. In most cases spontaneous recovery occurs rather slowly with some liability to recurrence. During recent years it has been established that sciatica thus defined is usually due to herniation of one or more of the lumbar intervertebral discs. It seems best, therefore, to discuss sciatica under this heading and to consider other causes of sciatic pain in relation to diagnosis.

AETIOLOGY

Lumbar disc protrusion is often the result of trauma, a history of which is obtainable in at least half of all cases. The commonest type of stress is that produced by lifting a heavy object in a bent-forward position or by a fall in a similar posture. Since 75 per cent. of patients are in or beyond the fourth decade it would appear that degenerative changes which begin in the prime of life predispose towards herniation but the syndrome is not uncommon in young adults and may even occur in children. The changes in the lumbar spine associated with pregnancy may also cause it. Thickening of the ligamentum flavum has often been noted in addition.

The age-incidence shows a peak with 35 per cent. of cases in the fourth decade, and between 75 and 80 per cent. of patients are males. Almost all lumbar herniations occur between the fourth and fifth lumbar or fifth lumbar and first sacral bodies, with a relative frequency of two to three. A disc protrusion compresses the spinal nerve which is running to the foramen one segment below, the fourth lumbar disc the fifth lumbar nerve, and the fifth lumbar disc the first sacral nerve. Sometimes protrusions occur from two or more discs. The compressed nerve becomes swollen and tense. Occasionally an acute lumbar disc protrusion results in the sequestration of a portion of the disc which acts as a major space-occupying lesion in the lumbar canal, involving multiple spinal nerves in the cauda equina.

SYMPTOMS

In most cases the onset is subacute, and sciatica is frequently preceded by lumbar pain, which may have occurred intermittently for years. The pain may immediately follow an injury such as a strain or a fall, or there may be a latent interval of days or even weeks. After two or three days of pain in the lumbar spine the pain radiates down the back of one leg from the buttock to the ankle. It is often possible to distinguish three elements in the pain: (1) pain in the back, aching in character and intensified by spinal movements; (2) pain deep in the buttock and thigh, also aching or gnawing in character and influenced by the posture of the limb; and (3) pain radiating to the leg and foot, momentarily increased by coughing and sneezing. When the first sacral root is compressed the pain radiates to the outer border of the foot. When the pressure is upon the fifth lumbar root it spreads from the outer aspect of the leg to the dorsum or the inner border of the foot. In general the pain is intensified by stooping, sitting, and walking. The patient is usually most comfortable lying in bed on the sound side with the affected leg slightly flexed at the hip and knee. The pain interferes with sleep and when it is very severe he may be able to obtain relief only by getting up and walking about. There is often a feeling of numbness, heaviness, or deadness in the leg, especially along the outer side of the foot.

There are muscular hypotonia and slight wasting, not only of the muscles supplied by the sciatic nerve, but usually also of the glutei and sometimes of all the muscles of the lower limb. Compression of the first sacral root causes weakness of the small muscles of the foot and the calf muscles and the ankle-jerk is diminished or lost. Compression of the fifth lumbar root causes weakness of the peronei—occasionally complete foot-drop—and the ankle-jerk is preserved. The knee-jerk may be slightly exaggerated, partly as a reflex result of the pain and partly owing to hypotonia of the hamstrings, the antagonists of the quadriceps, but if the fourth lumbar root is involved it may be diminished. The plantar reflex is flexor. There is tenderness on pressure in the buttock and thigh, straight-leg-raising is limited by pain, and stretching the sciatic nerve by extending the knee with the hip flexed causes severe pain—Lasègue's sign. There is rarely much sensory loss, though often there is some blunting of light touch and pin-prick over the outer half of the foot and three outer toes and lower part of the outer aspect of the leg when the first sacral root is involved. The fourth and fifth lumbar cutaneous areas are shown in FIGURES 7a and 7b. Scoliosis is often associated with sciatica, the lumbar spine being flexed, usually towards the affected side, less frequently towards the opposite side. Some rigidity of the lumbar spine is usually present, and there may be a tender spot at the level of the fifth lumbar transverse process. In the case of large central disc protrusions in the lumbar region pain is sometimes bilateral though often more severe on one side, muscular weakness is more widespread, several tendon reflexes may be lost (e.g. one knee-jerk and both ankle-jerks), sensory loss is more extensive, indicating involvement of motor roots, and sphincter control may be impaired. This condition should be regarded as a neurosurgical emergency. An excess of protein, up to 70 or 80 mg. per 100 ml., is present in the cerebrospinal fluid in about 80 per cent. of cases, but the cell count is normal.

X-ray examination should be carried out in all cases of sciatica, since many causes of sciatic pain are associated with bony changes visible in radiograms. Straight X-rays are not of great value in the diagnosis of herniated disc. The lumbosacral disc is often normally narrower than the other lumbar discs, so little stress can be laid upon narrowing of this disc. Narrowing of the fourth lumbar disc is more likely to be significant especially if associated with sclerosis of adjacent vertebral bodies or local arthritis. Myelography after the injection of an opaque fluid or air may demonstrate a filling defect, but is only indicated if the picture is unusually severe and if surgical treatment is contemplated; a herniated disc may be present in spite of a negative myelogram.

DIAGNOSIS

Sciatica due to a lumbar disc protrusion must be distinguished from: (1) compression of the nerve roots by a tumour within the spinal canal; (2) inflammatory, degenerative, and neoplastic lesions of the spine and pelvis involving the roots; and (3) neoplasms of the pelvic viscera. The principal points of distinction are that in herniated disc the onset of symptoms is fairly rapid, the buttock and posterior aspect of the thigh are tender on pressure, muscular wasting is slight, sensory loss is slight, and the course of the disorder during the first months after the onset is stationary or tends to improvement. In sciatic compression the onset is usually gradual, the nerve is not tender on pressure, muscular wasting is conspicuous, and sensory loss is more pronounced. Further, both of these symptoms are progressive.

In such cases the abdomen and pelvis must be thoroughly examined for sources of compression, and the lumbar spine and pelvis should be X-rayed.

Attention must also be paid to the general condition of the patient, and inquiry made for symptoms suggestive of a pelvic neoplasm and as to recent loss of weight. Rectal examination should never be omitted; and in women vaginal examination is advisable also. A complete examination of the nervous system is required to exclude tumours within the spinal canal and syphilis as a cause of sciatic pain, and if these are suspected the cerebrospinal fluid should also be examined, and if necessary a myelogram carried out.

Whether true sciatic neuritis occurs is now very doubtful: if it occurs at all it is certainly very rare, and the diagnosis should be accepted with reserve even when investigations appear to exclude all other causes.

The distinction of sciatica from femoral neuropathy has been described in the section dealing with the latter.

Herniated disc requires to be distinguished from arthritis of the hip-joint, with which sciatica may be associated. In herniated disc movements of the hip-joint are painless, provided the sciatic nerve is not stretched. The lower limb can be rotated and abducted without pain, whereas these movements are painful and often limited in arthritis of the hip. In the latter condition the ankle-jerk is preserved. X-rays will confirm the diagnosis.

Congenital abnormalities of the lumbosacral junction, such as spondylolis-thesis and sacralization of the fifth lumbar vertebra, may cause low back pain but only occasionally true sciatica, unless the fifth lumbar root is compressed. This abnormality will be apparent on the X-ray film.

Fibrositis of the glutei may cause pain referred down the leg and on extending the knee with the hip flexed, but no sensory loss or diminution of the ankle-jerk is present and both local and referred pain are abolished by the infiltration with procaine of tender spots in the buttock.

Vascular lesions within the distribution of the femoral artery, such as atheroma and thrombo-angiitis obliterans, are occasional causes of pain in the leg in middle age and later in life: intermittent claudication is not always present in these cases. The diagnosis is readily established by diminution in the volume of the femoral, dorsalis pedis, or posterior tibial pulses. The syndrome of intermittent ischaemia of the cauda equina with pain, paraesthesiae or weakness of the leg occurring only on exertion and relieved by rest can usually be distinguished from sciatica, due to a single lateral disc protrusion, by myelography [see p. 682].

PROGNOSIS

In mild cases the stage of severe pain lasts only two or three weeks and the patient recovers in a month or two, except that he may from time to time experience aching in the course of the nerve and stooping may still excite some pain in the affected leg. In more severe cases there may be slight improvement after several weeks, but the condition then becomes stationary and the patient continues to suffer from considerable pain for a number of months. Recovery, however, ultimately occurs, except for the residual disabilities just mentioned. Recovery from symptoms may occur though the disc protrusion remains. For this reason, perhaps, relapses are common. In some cases they occur at frequent intervals, so that the patient is hardly free from pain over a period of several years. In other cases the second attack may be delayed until ten or more years after the first. Operation gives good results in 90 per cent. of cases operated upon, with a mortality rate of 1 per cent. or less, but even after operation a relapse may occur.

TREATMENT

Most patients with lumbar intervertebral disc protrusion recover completely if treated conservatively. Operation should therefore be reserved for patients with large central disc protrusions involving multiple roots (in whom it is obligatory, especially if the sphincters are involved) and for those with marked motor weakness (e.g. foot-drop) present from the outset. It is probably indicated also in those whose symptoms do not respond to other measures and become chronic, those who relapse, and those with gross and persistent symptoms of root compression, sufficiently severe to cause disability. Probably not more than 10 per cent. will require operation, but the percentage will be higher among manual workers, in whom inability to do the necessary physical work may itself constitute an indication for surgery.

Conservative treatment consists of rest in bed and analgesics, to which may be added various measures designed to immobilize the lower part of the spine and the affected lower limb. When rest in bed for two or three weeks has been tried and failed, immediate relief is sometimes given by the application of a plaster jacket which fixes the lumbar spine in slight extension. The patient, who is allowed to walk about, should wear the plaster for three months. Alternatively many patients are relieved by the application of continuous lumbar traction for two or three weeks followed by the provision of a light lumbar support or corset which is worn for three months or longer. Manipulation also has its advocates and is remarkably successful in some patients with intractable pain. An 'overlay' of depression and anxiety commonly occurs in patients with lumbar disc disease and as a result of tension in the lumbar muscles accentuates and perpetuates pain. Antidepressive remedies and tranquillizing drugs such as amitriptyline and diazepam are particularly valuable in some patients. About 70 per cent. of patients respond satisfactorily to conservative treatment (Pearce and Moll, 1967) but in those who continue to have pain, provided there is no evidence of a severe 'functional overlay', surgical treatment is probably indicated.

Sacral Epidural Injection

In some cases benefit may be derived from stretching the nerve roots by epidural injection at the sacral hiatus. This can readily be palpated at the lower end of the sacrum, where it is covered by the dorsal sacrococcygeal ligament. The foramen is bounded above by the concave lower border of the sacrum in the midline and at the sides by the two lateral tubercles. The patient either lies on one side or assumes the knee-elbow position. The site of the injection is painted with iodine and anaesthetized with procaine, and a fine lumbar-puncture needle is passed through the ligament upwards and slightly forwards. Twenty ml. of 1 per cent. procaine solution are first injected, and this is followed by an injection of normal saline, of which 80 ml. or more can usually be injected, the solution being at body temperature. The object of the injection being to stretch the nerve roots, a sufficient volume of saline must be injected to raise the tension in the epidural space. It is necessary, therefore, to continue injecting saline until a considerable resistance is encountered, provided always that it does not cause severe pain. Epidural injection yields relief of pain in about 50 per cent. of cases. Sometimes the result is dramatic, the patient being completely and permanently relieved. A second injection may be given after an interval of two or three days if necessary. Various other solutions have been used for this injection, but they do not appear to possess any advantage over saline, which has the additional recommendation of being perfectly safe.

Physical therapy in its various forms is merely palliative but graduated exercises are of value when the pain has gone.

RADICULITIS OF THE CAUDA EQUINA

Rarely the cauda equina is the site of a neuritis of obscure origin, of subacute or insidious onset. The symptoms and signs are those of a cauda equina lesion [see p. 652], and its inflammatory nature is indicated by a pleocytosis, usually mononuclear, in the cerebrospinal fluid with some rise of protein. This syndrome has been described in ankylosing spondylitis (Matthews, 1968) but in most instances, repeated investigation or eventual pathological observations in such cases has demonstrated that the condition is due either to tumour (e.g. ependymoma of the filum terminale), to mechanical compression of roots, or to ischaemia resulting from atherosclerosis or stenosis of the lumbar canal.

REFERENCES

BOSANQUET, F. D., and HENSON, R. A. (1957) Sensory neuropathy in diabetes mellitus, *Folia psychiat. neerl.*, **60,** 107.

BRADFORD, F. K., and SPURLING, R. G. (1941) *The Intervertebral Disk*, Springfield, Ill.

DANDY, W. E. (1943) Recent advances in the treatment of ruptured (lumbar) intervertebral disks, *Ann. Surg.*, **118,** 639.

DANDY, W. E. (1944) Newer aspects of ruptured intervertebral disks, *Ann. Surg.*, **119,** 481.

FALCONER, M. A., GLASGOW, G. L., and COLE, D. S. (1947) Sensory disturbances occurring in sciatica due to intervertebral disc protrusions, *J. Neurol. Neurosurg. Psychiat.*, **10,** 72.

FALCONER, M. A., McGEORGE, M., and BEGG, A. C. (1948 *a*) Surgery of lumbar intervertebral disk protrusion, *Brit. J. Surg.*, **35,** 225.

FALCONER, M. A., McGEORGE, M., and BEGG, A. C. (1948 *b*) Cause and mechanism of symptom-production in sciatica and low-back pain, *J. Neurol. Neurosurg. Psychiat.*, **11,** 13.

FRYKHOLM, R. (1951) Cervical nerve root compression resulting from disc degeneration and root-sleeve fibrosis, *Acta chir. scand.*, Supp. 160.

LOVE, J. G., and SCHORN, V. G. (1965) Thoracic disk protrusions, *J. Amer. med. Ass.*, **191,** 627.

LOVE, J. G., and WALSH, M. N. (1940) Intraspinal protrusion of intervertebral disks, *Arch. Surg. (Chicago)*, **40,** 454.

McALPINE, D., and PAGE, F. (1951) Sensory neuropathy due to posterior root ganglion degeneration, *Arch. Mddx Hosp.*, **1,** 250.

MACEY, H. B. (1940) Clinical aspects of protruded intervertebral disks, *Arch. Surg. (Chicago)*, **40,** 433.

MATTHEWS, W. B. (1968) The neurological complications of ankylosing spondylitis, *J. neurol. Sci.*, **6,** 561.

O'CONNELL, J. E. A. (1944) Maternal obstetrical paralysis, *Surg. Gynec. Obstet.*, **29**, 374.

O'CONNELL, J. E. A. (1950) The indications for and results of the excision of lumbar intervertebral disk protrusions, a review of 500 cases, *Ann. roy. Coll. Surg. Engl.*, **6**, 403.

PEARCE, J., and MOLL, J. M. H. (1967) Conservative treatment and natural history of
acute lumbar disc lesions, *J. Neurol. Neurosurg. Psychiat.*, **30**, 13.

PENNYBACKER, J. (1940) Sciatica and the intervertebral disk, *Lancet*, ii, 532.

SHINNERS, B. M., and HAMBY, W. B. (1949) Protruded lumbar intervertebral discs,
J. Neurosurg., **6**, 450.

SPURLING, R. G., and GRANTHAM, E. G. (1940) Neurologic picture of herniations of the
nucleus pulposus in the lower part of the lumbar region, *Arch. Surg. (Chicago)*, **40**,
375.

WILKINSON, M. (1960) The morbid anatomy of cervical spondylosis and myelopathy,
Brain, **83**, 589.

'INTERSTITIAL NEURITIS'

While 'interstitial neuritis' was a diagnosis commonly made in the past to
explain a lesion of a single peripheral nerve for which no obvious cause could
be demonstrated there is growing evidence to indicate that such an inflammatory
process does not exist as a specific pathological entity. In most cases so diagnosed in the past it is now well recognized that the condition almost certainly
resulted from mechanical compression of the nerve in question or of its component roots, or from ischaemia, due either to peripheral vascular disease
(Richards, 1951; Gairns, Garven, and Smith, 1960) or to a diffuse inflammatory
disorder of arteries such as polyarteritis nodosa (Lovshin and Kernohan, 1948)
in which an arteritis of the vasa nervorum may occur resulting in a 'mononeuritis multiplex'. It is also well recognized that some individuals have
a peculiar liability to develop peripheral nerve lesions (of the lateral popliteal,
ulnar, or median nerves and less frequently of other mixed nerves) as a result of
transient and minimal trauma; these patients may develop recurrent palsies
of the affected nerve or nerves and this liability often appears to be inherited
(Earl *et al.*, 1964).

REFERENCES

EARL, C. J., FULLERTON, P. M., WAKEFIELD, G. S., and SCHUTTA, H. S. (1964) Hereditary neuropathy with liability to pressure palsies, *Quart. J. Med.*, **33**, 481.

GAIRNS, F. W., GARVEN, H. S. D., and SMITH, G. (1960) The digital nerves and the
nerve endings in progressive obliterative vascular disease, *Scot. med. J.*, **5**, 382.

LOVSHIN, L. L., and KERNOHAN, J. W. (1948) Peripheral neuritis in periarteritis nodosa,
Arch. intern. Med., **82**, 321.

RICHARDS, R. L. (1951) Ischaemic lesions of peripheral nerves: a review, *J. Neurol.
Psychiat.*, **14**, 76.

'NEURITIS' OF THE FACE AND SCALP

Pain is commonly experienced in the distribution of one or more of the
cutaneous nerves of the face and scalp and has been attributed to 'neuritis',
but the nature of the pathological process in such cases is speculative. In some
cases there may well be mechanical compression or irritation of the affected
nerve, in others emotional tension is almost certainly a factor. The term 'neuritis'
may reasonably be used to identify cases in which the aetiology cannot be

identified with certainty provided it is not taken to imply the presence of a specific pathological process. Occasionally all the branches of one trigeminal nerve are involved. More frequently the affection is limited to one branch, usually the supra-orbital or auriculotemporal, less often the infra-orbital. The great occipital nerve is also a common site of neuritis.

SYMPTOMS

The onset is usually acute, and pain in the face and scalp may follow a cold, tonsillitis, or an attack of influenza. The patient complains of pain situated within the distribution of the affected nerve. The pain usually occurs in paroxysms lasting for several hours, most frequently towards the close of the day, when he is fatigued. An attack of pain is also readily precipitated by exposure to cold. When the pain is severe it interferes with sleep. It is of a dull, aching character, intensified by exacerbations in which it is described as shooting along the course of the nerve. There is often hyperpathia in the area of skin supplied by the nerve, and when this includes the scalp it is noticed on combing and brushing the hair. The nerve trunk is tender on pressure, which causes irradiation of pain throughout the nerve. The cutaneous hypersensitivity is readily demonstrated by pricking with a pin.

DIAGNOSIS

There are numerous causes of paroxysmal pain in the face and scalp, and careful investigation is required to exclude other conditions before falling back on a diagnosis of 'neuritis.'

Infection of the nasal air sinuses is a common cause of such pain, frontal sinusitis being associated with supra-orbital neuralgia, and infection of the maxillary antrum with pain in the distribution of the infra-orbital nerve. In ethmoiditis the pain is chiefly at the root of the nose, and in infection of the sphenoidal sinus is usually referred to the forehead or occiput. In acute cases of sinus infection there is usually a history of influenza or a cold in the head with or without a purulent nasal discharge. There may be visible oedema over the frontal sinus or antrum. Transillumination and examination of the nose will usually reveal the site of infection, and in doubtful cases the sinuses should be X-rayed.

The tympanic membranes should always be examined to exclude a latent otitis media.

The teeth are a common cause of facial pain. Search should be made for carious teeth, and the possibility that there is an unerupted tooth must always be considered. This may be present, as may also a buried root, in an apparently edentulous patient, and can be detected only by X-ray examination of the jaws. Pain of dental origin is often accentuated by chewing or by the ingestion of hot or cold foods.

A careful examination of the pharynx should be made for a growth, which may occasionally cause pain referred to the ear and neck.

The eye is occasionally the source of referred neuralgic pain, the commonest ocular cause being glaucoma, which may be missed unless this possibility is borne in mind. Pain may also be referred to the face in disease of the heart and lungs.

Intractable neuralgia may follow herpes zoster involving the first division of the trigeminal nerve. The history of the eruption and the residual scars render the diagnosis easy.

Trigeminal neuralgia, tic douloureux, is distinguished by the brevity of the attacks of pain and the characteristic precipitating factors.

In migraine the paroxysms of headache occur at comparatively long intervals and are often associated with vomiting and preceded by the characteristic prodromal symptoms. There is usually a long history.

Periodic migrainous neuralgia gives attacks of severe pain in and around the eye, lasting for up to two hours and occurring daily or twice daily in bouts lasting for several weeks or months.

Temporal or cranial arteritis occurs in the elderly and often gives rise to pain and tenderness in the scalp, particularly in the temporal and occipital regions; the temporal arteries are usually tortuous and tender and the erythrocyte sedimentation rate is raised.

Tabes is an occasional cause of paroxysmal pain in the face or scalp, but is readily recognized by its other clinical features.

The various intracranial causes of pain in the face and head must be borne in mind, especially lesions of the trigeminal fibres in the brain stem such as syringo-bulbia, and thrombosis of the posterior inferior cerebellar artery, in both of which pain is usually associated with analgesia and thermo-anaesthesia.

Occipital pain may be due to lesions of the cervical region of the spinal cord or of the vertebral column at this level, especially cervical spondylosis, and is sometimes the result of fibrositis of the cervical muscles.

Psychogenic pain is distinguished from neuritis by its lack of relation to a nerve trunk, its failure to respond to analgesic drugs, and by the patient's exaggerated emotional reaction to the pain. However, it must be stressed that chronic tension of the muscles attached to the scalp, occurring in association with anxiety and/or depression, may give rise to pain of exactly the type described, and this is not infrequently unilateral. This is particularly true of the so-called 'atypical facial pain' which usually occurs in the upper jaw in young or middle-aged women and which is often attributed erroneously to 'neuritis' but which in the great majority of cases is of purely psychogenic origin.

PROGNOSIS

In most cases the prognosis of neuritis of the face and scalp is good and there is a rapid response to treatment. Occasionally, however, especially in individuals of a neurotic temperament, the pain proves intractable.

TREATMENT

The first essential is to exclude the organic causes of facial pain referred to above by means of appropriate investigations. Simple analgesic drugs are often effective but the fact that many cases respond even more satisfactorily to a combination of antidepressive and tranquillizing remedies is sufficient to indicate that in a high proportion of such cases there is no organic cause for the pain.

If a pain persists despite the measures outlined it is occasionally necessary to inject the nerve trunk with 2 per cent. procaine solution, the supra-orbital nerve being injected at the supra-orbital notch, the infra-orbital at its foramen, by the methods described in the section on trigeminal neuralgia. The great occipital nerve can be similarly injected, and when occipital pain is due to fibrositis of the cervical muscles relief may sometimes be obtained from procaine injection of any tender spots in the muscles. However, these measures are rarely necessary.

BRACHIAL NEURITIS

The term 'brachial neuritis' was formerly used to describe the symptoms which are now known to be usually caused by radiculitis due to cervical spondylosis. No distinctive clinical picture of true brachial neuritis exists and like 'sciatic neuritis' the term has ceased to serve a useful purpose.

SHOULDER-GIRDLE NEURITIS (NEURALGIC AMYOTROPHY)

Localized neuritis of one or more nerves innervating the shoulder-girdle muscles was well recognized before the Second World War and was also observed during the war, especially in the Near East. The patients were often in hospital for an operation or acute infection. Pain is usually the initial symptom; it may be intense for several days and is followed by muscular wasting and weakness. The muscles most often affected are the serratus anterior, spinati, deltoid, and trapezius in that order. When the deltoid is involved there may be sensory loss over the distribution of the axillary (circumflex) nerve. The lesions may be bilateral. In mild cases there is a slow recovery; in more severe cases the muscular atrophy is permanent. The cause is unknown but an identical syndrome may follow 7–10 days after the injection of foreign serum ('serum neuropathy'). Treatment is symptomatic.

INTERCOSTAL NEURITIS

Intercostal neuritis is a rare disorder which is diagnosed much more frequently than it occurs. It is characterized by paroxysmal pain throughout the distribution of an intercostal nerve, associated frequently with cutaneous tenderness in the area supplied by the nerve, especially at the point of emergence of its lateral cutaneous branch. Before diagnosing intercostal neuritis the utmost care must be taken to exclude the many other disorders which may be associated with pain of this character. Such pain may be due to inflammation of spinal dorsal roots, especially in syphilis, or their compression by a neoplasm of the spinal cord. It may precede or follow an attack of herpes zoster. The spinal nerve may be compressed as a result of localized collapse of the vertebral column, most commonly due to tuberculous caries, secondary carcinoma, or traumatic lesions. Spondylitis is often associated with root pains, and these may also be produced by scoliosis. Pleurisy, both tuberculous and neoplastic, is sometimes mistakenly diagnosed as intercostal neuralgia, and the thorax is a common site of referred pain in visceral disease, especially in mitral stenosis and diseases of the upper abdominal viscera. Pain in the distribution of an intercostal nerve is also seen in some patients after thoracotomy and may be intractable.

TREATMENT

Intercostal neuritis should be treated with analgesics and counter-irritants. Local anaesthetic injections may give temporary relief and if all else fails the nerve may be injected with alcohol or phenol, care being taken that the needle does not penetrate the pleura. In occasional cases, surgical division of two or three intercostal nerves close to the spine may be needed but even after this operation pain may recur after a few months.

FEMORAL NEURITIS

The term 'femoral neuritis' dates from the time when sciatica was attributed to sciatic neuritis and a similar clinical picture within the distribution of the femoral nerve was thought to be due to an inflammation of its roots. It is now recognized, however, that this syndrome is usually due to an intervertebral disc protrusion in the upper lumbar spine, pain being referred into the third or fourth lumbar dermatome and accompanied by wasting and weakness of the quadriceps and diminution or loss of the knee-jerk. It may also be due to diabetes ('diabetic amyotrophy') or to involvement of the nerve in inflammatory or neoplastic processes in the pelvis. Treatment depends upon the nature of the lesion.

SCIATIC NEURITIS

As in the case of brachial and femoral neuritis it is now doubtful whether true sciatic neuritis ever occurs except as part of a more diffuse inflammatory or toxic process involving many nerves. Isolated sciatic nerve lesions invariably prove to be due to trauma or to compression of the nerve or of its component roots.

REFERENCES

HARRIS, W. (1926) *Neuritis and Neuralgia*, London.

PARSONAGE, M. J., and TURNER, J. W. A. (1948) Neuralgic amyotrophy. The shoulder-girdle syndrome, *Lancet*, i, 973.

SPILLANE, J. D. (1943) Localized neuritis of the shoulder girdle, *Lancet*, ii, 532.

TAYLOR, R. A. (1960) Heredofamilial mononeuritis multiplex with brachial predilection, *Brain*, **83**, 113.

POLYNEURITIS (POLYNEUROPATHY)

Synonyms. Multiple symmetrical peripheral neuritis; multiple neuritis; parenchymatous neuritis.

Definition. Polyneuritis is a clinical picture, the essential feature of which is an impairment of function of many peripheral nerves simultaneously, resulting in a symmetrical distribution of flaccid muscular weakness, and usually also of sensory disturbances, affecting as a rule the distal more than the proximal segments of the limbs, and sometimes also involving the cranial nerves. A simultaneous disorder of the highest cerebral functions, leading to mental disturbances is sometimes associated. Polyneuritis thus defined may be caused by a very large number of agencies, which may operate in several different ways and even at different points of the peripheral nerves. Among such agencies are numerous endogenous and exogenous toxins, acute infections which directly attack the nerves, and vitamin deficiency.

Peripheral neuritis of this kind was recorded by Lettsom in 1789 and an epidemic in Paris was described by Robert Graves in 1828. Todd first conceived that the terminal branches of the peripheral nerves might undergo degeneration, and this was demonstrated pathologically by Dumenil in 1864. Joffroy in 1879 contributed to the classification of polyneuritis and Grainger Stewart gave it the name multiple symmetrical peripheral neuritis in 1881. Korsakow described the mental changes not uncommonly associated with polyneuritis in 1889.

As Simpson (1962) pointed out in a valuable review, except in the case of leprosy, true inflammation in peripheral nerves is rare and most such disorders are more correctly termed 'neuropathy'. Recent pathological studies have demonstrated that most polyneuropathies are demyelinating (the myelin sheath and/or Schwann cell are attacked by the disease) but some are due to axonal degeneration. In demyelinating neuropathies nerve conduction is usually markedly delayed while in axonal degenerations there may be no conduction at all, or, if denervation is partial, the surviving axons conduct at a normal rate.

While many forms of polyneuropathy affect both sensory and motor fibres, some appear to involve motor fibres selectively while in predominantly sensory neuropathies the process may involve more severely the rapidly-conducting, heavily-myelinated 'A' fibres which mainly carry touch and tactile discrimination, or alternatively the slowly-conducting, finely-myelinated 'C' fibres which mainly carry pain. Factors determining such selective involvement are still unknown.

AETIOLOGY

The following classification includes the most important causes (see also *Classification of the Neuromuscular Diseases—Research Group on Neuromuscular Diseases of the World Federation of Neurology*, 1968):

1. TOXIC SUBSTANCES:

   Metals: Arsenic, antimony, mercury (pink disease, Minimata disease), copper, phosphorus, bismuth, lead, thallium.

   Organic substances: Acrylamide, 'bush tea', carbon monoxide, carbon bisulphide, chloroquine, vincristine sulphate, thalidomide, dinitrobenzol, sulphonal, chloral, chloretone, organic chlorine compounds used as insecticides, tetrachlorethane, aniline, triorthocresylphosphate (ginger paralysis and apiol paralysis), sulphanilamide and its compounds, streptomycin, isoniazid, nitrofurantoin, immune sera.

2. DEFICIENCY AND METABOLIC DISORDERS:

   Beriberi, chronic alcoholism, pregnancy, and chronic diseases of and operations on the gastro-intestinal tract, hunger oedema, pellagra, vitamin B_{12} neuropathy, folic acid deficiency.

   Diabetes, myxoedema, uraemia, acromegaly, porphyria.

   Amyloid disease.

   Neuropathy in A-α and β-lipoproteinaemia and in dysglobulinaemia.

3. INFECTIVE CONDITIONS:

   (a) *Local infection of nerves*:
   Leprosy, very rarely syphilis, brucellosis, and leptospirosis.

   (b) *Polyneuritis complicating acute or chronic infections*:
   Septicaemia, puerperal sepsis, typhoid, paratyphoid, scarlet fever, dysentery, influenza, tuberculosis, syphilis, gonorrhoea, mumps, typhus, malaria, meningitis, measles, smallpox, focal infection.

   (c) *Infections with organisms whose toxins have an affinity for the peripheral nerves*:
   Diphtheria, tetanus, dysentery.

4. POST-INFECTIVE (?ALLERGIC) POLYNEUROPATHY:

   Acute post-infective polyradiculoneuropathy (the Guillain-Barré syndrome).
   Some cases of subacute and chronic polyneuropathy.
   ? Recurrent polyneuropathy.

5. COLLAGEN AND ALLIED DISORDERS:

   Disseminated lupus erythematosus, polyarteritis nodosa, giant-cell arteritis, rheumatoid polyneuritis, sarcoidosis, systemic sclerosis.

6. GENETICALLY-DETERMINED POLYNEUROPATHY:

   Progressive hypertrophic polyneuritis of Dejerine and Sottas, Refsum's syndrome, familial polyneuritis, neuropathy in metachromatic leucodystrophy, in the Krabbe form of diffuse sclerosis, in primary amyloidosis, in porphyria and in A-α and β- lipoproteinaemia.

7. POLYNEURITIS OF OBSCURE ORIGIN:

   Recurrent polyneuritis. Chronic progressive polyneuritis. Carcinomatous neuropathy, myelomatosis.

In some cases the toxin is introduced into the body from without. In others it is formed within the body as a result of bacterial action or of metabolic disturbances. Yet again the source may be undiscoverable. Sometimes the toxin appears to possess a specific affinity for the peripheral nerves, and it has been suggested that it may combine with the phospholipids of the myelin sheaths. Such toxins probably ascend the peripheral nerves. We thus encounter both a local neuritis involving the nerves supplying the region in which the toxin originates, for example, palatal paralysis in diphtheria, and also generalized polyneuritis, in which the toxin is disseminated in the blood stream and so reaches the peripheral nerves throughout the body, subsequently ascending them from their terminations.

The role of avitaminosis in the causation of polyneuritis is more complex than used to be thought and is discussed on page 725. Deficiency of other factors may also be important.

PATHOLOGY

There have been important recent advances in knowledge concerning the pathology of peripheral neuropathy (polyneuritis) of various types. These have come partly from post-mortem studies but have been based more particularly on experimental studies in animals and upon nerve biopsy studies, utilizing techniques for the examination of single teased nerve fibres stained with osmic acid. Methods involving osmic acid staining of transverse sections of nerves in which fibres can be counted and their diameters measured have also made valuable contributions, as has electron microscopy. The sural nerve is the one most conveniently biopsied but has the occasional disadvantage that, being wholly sensory, it is not invariably diseased in neuropathies which are predominantly motor in type. Such studies have demonstrated that in many forms of neuropathy (in diabetes, the Guillain-Barré syndrome, carcinomatous neuropathy, familial hypertrophic neuropathy, and metachromatic leucodystrophy) the disease process affects predominantly the Schwann cells and results in segmental demyelination of peripheral nerves, with a progressive shrinkage of the myelin away from the nodes of Ranvier and the eventual denuding of axons which frequently remain intact. In this phase, conduction in the affected nerves is markedly slowed. Recovery is accompanied by re-myelination but the newly-formed myelin is often thinner than normal and the internodal distances are less than normal; however, nerve conduction velocity may recover eventually to normal. In other forms of neuropathy (Gilliatt, 1966) including those due to alcoholism, porphyria, triorthocresylphosphate, isoniazid, vincristine, and thalidomide, the process appears to be one of axonal degeneration and segmental demyelination is slight or absent so that nerve conduction velocity is reduced comparatively little. Recent work suggests that in the neuropathies due to lead and acrylamide (Fullerton, 1966; Fullerton and Barnes, 1966) both the axons and their myelin sheaths may be affected simultaneously.

SYMPTOMS AND PROGNOSIS

The symptoms and prognosis and further details of the pathology of the commoner and more important forms of polyneuritis are described under their respective headings.

DIAGNOSIS

As a rule the diagnosis of polyneuritis is easy, owing to the characteristic symmetrical and peripheral distribution of the muscular weakness and wasting, pain, tenderness, and sensory impairment. Electrical measurements of nerve conduction may be useful in establishing the peripheral nerves as the site of the lesion. The association of pain, ataxia, and loss of tendon reflexes in the lower limbs may simulate tabes. The pain of polyneuritis, however, when present, is of a persistent, burning, and tearing character and is quite different from the lightning pains of tabes, and is associated with tenderness of the deep tissues on pressure, whereas in tabes these are insensitive. Although the pupillary reaction to light may be sluggish in polyneuritis, especially in the alcoholic form, a true Argyll Robertson pupil is never found, and the V.D.R.L. reaction is negative, except in patients who happen to suffer both from syphilis and from polyneuritis. As stated elsewhere, some of the symptoms of subacute combined degeneration are due to an associated polyneuritis. The true cause of these symptoms, however, is usually easily established by the presence of extensor plantar responses, impairment of appreciation of vibration over the trunk as well as the limbs, and the presence of anaemia, glossitis, and gastric achylia, though the last may be present in patients suffering from polyneuritis due to other causes. When a diagnosis of polyneuritis has been made, the diagnosis of the cause is based upon distinctive features of the history and symptoms peculiar to the different varieties, and upon investigative findings which are described under their respective headings.

TREATMENT

The first step in treatment is the removal of the patient from exposure to the causal toxin, and its elimination from the body, or the correction of abnormal metabolic states or vitamin deficiency. The steps necessary for this are described in the sections dealing with the various forms of polyneuritis.

Rest in bed is essential only when the severity of the muscular weakness is such that the patient cannot walk or in those forms of polyneuritis (such as beriberi) in which the heart is also involved. In the more usual cases, continuing activity is important.

Local treatment consists of the prevention of muscular contractures, the maintenance of the nutrition of the muscles, and the promotion of the recovery of voluntary power. Wrist-drop and foot-drop must be prevented by the use of appropriate splints. As long as muscular tenderness is severe, splints cannot be borne, and the feet must then be supported by means of a sandbag placed beneath the soles, the weight of the bed-clothes being taken by a cradle. Later, aluminium or plastic night-shoes may be used to support the feet at a right angle. When contractures have already developed they must be overcome by the use of an extension apparatus, and tenotomy of the tendo calcaneus may be required. Daily active and passive movements should be instituted as soon as the patient is able to bear them. Analgesic drugs will be required when the pain is severe.

REFERENCES

FULLERTON, P. M. (1966) Chronic peripheral neuropathy produced by lead poisoning in guinea-pigs, *J. Neuropath. exp. Neurol.*, **25**, 214.

FULLERTON, P. M. and BARNES, J. M. (1966) Peripheral neuropathy in rats produced by acrylamide, *Brit. J. industr. Med.*, **23**, 210.

GILLIATT, R. W. (1966) Nerve conduction in human and experimental neuropathies, *Proc. roy. Soc. Med.*, **59**, 989.

MILLER, H. G. (1966) Polyneuritis, *Brit. med. J.*, **2**, 1219.

RESEARCH COMMITTEE ON NEUROMUSCULAR DISEASES (1968) Classification of the neuro-muscular disorders, *J. neurol. Sci.*, **6**, 165.

SIMPSON, J. A. (1962) The neuropathies, in *Modern Trends in Neurology*, 3rd series, ed. WILLIAMS, D., London.

SIMPSON, J. A. (1964) Biology and disease of peripheral nerves, *Brit. med. J.*, **2**, 709.

THAGE, O., TROJABORG, W., and BUCHTHAL, F. (1963) Electromyographic findings in polyneuropathy, *Neurology (Minneap.)*, **13**, 273.

ACUTE POST-INFECTIVE POLYNEURITIS

Synonyms. Acute toxic polyneuritis; febrile polyneuritis; syndrome of Guillain and Barré; polyradiculoneuropathy.

Definition. An acute diffuse post-infective disease of the nervous system involving the spinal roots and peripheral nerves, and occasionally the cranial nerves.

AETIOLOGY

Acute post-infective polyneuritis or polyradiculoneuropathy is now probably the commonest form of polyneuritis in Great Britain. A number of cases were observed among troops during the 1914–18 war (Guillain, Barré, and Strohl, 1916; Holmes, 1917; Bradford, Bashford, and Wilson, 1918). Most of the reported cases have occurred in males between the ages of 20 and 50 years but the condition may occur in either sex at any age. Although this syndrome is clearly defined it is by no means certain that all cases are of uniform aetiology. In the past it was known as acute infective polyneuritis but no infecting organism has ever been isolated from such cases though it has been known to follow a variety of specific and non-specific infective illnesses, but may arise apparently spontaneously. The current view is that it is an inflammatory disorder due to allergy or hypersensitivity, perhaps as a result of a variety of unidentified allergens, but the possibility still exists that some cases could be due to an as yet unidentified virus infection. It may also follow surgical operations (Arnason and Asbury, 1968). Waksman and Adams (1955) have produced a similar condition in animals by injecting an emulsion of peripheral nerve to which they have been sensitized, suggesting a possible allergic basis. A similar disorder has been observed in dogs following the bite of a racoon, so-called 'coonhound paralysis' (Cummings and Haas, 1967).

PATHOLOGY

Naked-eye abnormalities are slight and consist of variable congestion of the meninges, and in fatal cases there may be petechial haemorrhages in the substance of the spinal cord. Microscopically the spinal cord exhibits chromatolysis of the ganglion cells, both of the anterior horns and of the dorsal roots, with slight perivascular infiltration with small, round cells. The spinal roots and peripheral nerves, especially those containing motor fibres, show marked degenerative changes in their myelin sheaths, with proliferation of the cells of the neurilemma, and in some cases swelling and fragmentation of the axis cylinders. There is an inflammatory exudate with round cells and haemorrhages. In long-standing cases denervation atrophy is found in the muscles. Perivascular inflammatory infiltration has been observed in the brain, and infiltration with round cells may be present in the liver, kidneys, and lungs, the kidneys sometimes showing areas of acute nephritis.

Since there is evidence of inflammatory and degenerative changes throughout the whole course of the lower motor neurone, the condition may be better described as a polyneuronitis than as a polyneuritis.

SYMPTOMS

There is often an initial febrile illness in which no nervous symptoms appear, followed by a period of latency, which may last from a few days to several weeks, at the end of which paralysis develops. More frequently the patient first comes under observation in the paralytic stage, symptoms of the initial stage being slight or absent. There is now increasing evidence to indicate that some cases of subacute or chronic polyneuropathy are aetiologically similar.

The first symptoms may be headache, vomiting, slight pyrexia, and pains in the back and limbs, which may be associated with a feeling of stiffness in the neck. More often the paralytic symptoms, which are often the first manifestations but sometimes develop after the prodromal symptoms described, usually come on suddenly accompanied sometimes by headache and a recurrence of the pyrexia. Less frequently the onset of the paralytic symptoms is gradual. The paralysis may affect all four limbs simultaneously or may begin in the lower limbs and spread to the upper. In contrast with other forms of polyneuritis all the muscles of a limb are usually affected, those of the proximal segments suffering as much as, or even more severely than, those of the distal segments. Occasionally weakness is even limited to proximal limb muscles and may be asymmetrical. In severe cases the muscles of the neck and trunk are also involved, and there is often paralysis of the facial muscles on both sides, though this is occasionally unilateral. Dysphagia may occur as a result of pharyngeal paralysis, but the palate usually escapes. External ophthalmoplegia is occasionally seen. In occasional cases the affection is confined to the cranial nerves (cranial polyneuritis or polyneuritis cranialis). The paralysed muscles are flaccid, but a severe degree of wasting is exceptional. Superficial and deep reflexes are usually diminished or lost, but may be retained in spite of weakness of voluntary movement in the muscles concerned. The sensory symptoms characteristic of polyneuritis are usually but not invariably present, and in the early stages the patient complains of pain, numbness, and tingling in the limbs. All forms of sensibility may be impaired over the peripheral segments of the limbs and the muscles may be tender but even in the presence of typical paraesthesiae sensory abnormalities on examination are often conspicuous by their absence. Bilateral optic neuritis leading to visual impairment is rare but papilloedema is seen occasionally: bilateral deafness is even rarer. The sphincters are rarely involved and never to a severe extent, though there may at times be slight retention of urine necessitating catheterization. Cerebral symptoms are usually absent and consciousness is unclouded throughout, but a confusional or Korsakow's psychosis rarely develops.

General symptoms of toxaemia may be present, including tachycardia and slight cardiac dilatation, and albuminuria and an erythematous rash. The blood may show a moderate polymorphonuclear leucocytosis. The characteristic change in the cerebrospinal fluid is a great excess of protein (occasionally up to 1 g. per 100 ml.) with either a normal cell count, or at most only a moderate excess of mononuclear cells. This is the 'dissociation albumino-cytologique' stressed by Guillain, Barré, and Strohl (1916). The fluid may be yellow or brown and clot spontaneously. The high protein may persist for many weeks even after recovery. Nevertheless the same clinical picture may coexist with a spinal fluid that is virtually normal, particularly in the early stages.

DIAGNOSIS

Acute post-infective polyneuritis is readily distinguished from other forms of polyneuritis by the acute onset, the rapid development of the paralysis, and the severe involvement of the proximal limb muscles. It is distinguished from poliomyelitis by the symmetrical character of the paralysis, the presence of sensory loss, and by the slightness or absence of muscular wasting in the later stages. Electrical nerve-conduction tests which almost invariably demonstrate slowing of motor conduction in affected limbs localize the lesion to the peripheral nerves. In subacute or chronic cases there may be difficulty in distinguishing the condition from other forms of polyneuritis, particularly since in occasional cases, peripheral nerves may become enlarged. Many acute cases have been diagnosed in the past as examples of Landry's paralysis but for reasons given previously [p. 679] this disorder is a syndrome of multiple aetiology and this diagnostic label should no longer be used. Acute myelitis, especially the ascending form, may also cause widespread flaccid paralysis, but in this condition the plantar reflexes are usually extensor, sensory loss is more extensive and involves the whole body below the level of the lesion, and sphincter disturbances are present.

PROGNOSIS

The mortality rate of the disease was high in the past in some epidemics, death usually occurring from paralysis of the respiratory muscles, with or without terminal bronchopneumonia. Slight remissions were not infrequent, but were often followed by severe relapses. In sporadic cases, however, the outlook is usually good, but improvement is slow and the paralysis, having reached its height, tends to remain stationary for some weeks. Sometimes recovery is incomplete. In the most favourable cases the patient is not likely to be convalescent in less than from three to six months and in occasional cases the condition may smoulder on for one or two years but may nevertheless recover completely.

TREATMENT

In the past, no effective treatment for the condition was known but, among others, Graveson (1957) and Jackson, Miller, and Schapira (1957) suggested that the condition could be effectively controlled by cortisone or corticotrophin (ACTH). While many workers employ these drugs in all cases and there is a general impression that ACTH (80 Units daily intramuscularly at first, reducing gradually but continuing maintenance dosage for several months or even up to one or two years) is more effective than cortisone, others are equally adamant that such treatment does not modify the natural history of the illness. Undoubtedly some cases appear to respond dramatically, relapse after withdrawal and respond again, but some appear totally steroid-resistant and the use of immunosuppressive agents has not been strikingly successful. The usual treatment of polyneuritis must be carried out [see p. 813]. Much depends upon good nursing. Bulbar and respiratory paralysis should be treated with intermittent positive pressure respiration as in poliomyelitis [see p. 459].

Complications including respiratory infections will demand appropriate antibiotics. Hypernatraemia with water retention which occurs in occasional cases may demand diuretics (Posner *et al.*, 1967).

REFERENCES

ARNASON, B., and ASBURY, A. K. (1968) Idiopathic polyneuritis after surgery, *Arch. Neurol. (Chicago)*, **18**, 487.

BRADFORD, J. R., BASHFORD, E. F., and WILSON, J. A. (1918–19) Acute infective polyneuritis, *Quart. J. Med.*, **12**, 88.

CLARKE, E. S., BAYLISS, R. I. S., and COOPER, R. (1954) Cardiovascular manifestations of the Guillain-Barré syndrome, *Brit. med. J.*, **2**, 1504.

CUMMINGS, J. F., and HAAS, D. C. (1967) Coonhound paralysis. An acute idiopathic polyradiculoneuritis in dogs resembling the Landry–Guillain–Barré syndrome, *J. neurol. Sci.*, **4**, 51.

GILPIN, S. F., MOERSCH, F. P., and KERNOHAN, J. W. (1936) Polyneuritis, *Arch. Neurol. Psychiat. (Chicago)*, **35**, 937.

GRAVESON, G. S. (1957) Acute polyneuritis treated with cortisone, *Lancet*, i, 340.

GUILLAIN, G., BARRÉ, J. A., and STROHL, A. (1916) Sur un syndrome de radiculo-névrite avec hyperalbuminose du liquide céphalo-rachidien sans réaction cellulaire. Remarques sur les caractères cliniques et graphiques des réflexes tendineux, *Bull. Soc. méd. Hôp. Paris*, **40**, 1462.

GUILLAIN, G., and others (1938) *Les polyradiculonévrites avec dissociation albumino-cytologique et à évolution favorable*, Brussels.

HAYMAKER, W., and KERNOHAN, J. W. (1949) The Landry–Guillain–Barré syndrome, *Medicine (Baltimore)*, **28**, 59.

HOLMES, G. (1917) Acute febrile polyneuritis, *Brit. med. J.*, **2**, 37.

JACKSON, R. H., MILLER, H., and SCHAPIRA, K. (1957) Polyradiculitis (Landry–Guillain–Barré syndrome). Treatment with cortisone and corticotrophin, *Brit. med. J.*, **1**, 480.

JANEWAY, R., and KELLY, D. (1966) Papillodema and hydrocephalus associated with recurrent polyneuritis, *Arch. Neurol. (Chic.)*, **15**, 507.

POSNER, J., ERTEL, N. H., KOSSMANN, R. J., and SCHEINBERG, L. C. (1967) Hyponatremia in acute polyneuropathy, *Arch. Neurol. (Chic.)*, **17**, 530.

WAKSMAN, B. H., and ADAMS, R. W. (1955) Allergic neuritis, an experimental disease of rabbits induced by the injection of peripheral nerve tissue and adjuvants, *J. exp. Med.*, **102**, 213.

ALCOHOLIC POLYNEURITIS
AETIOLOGY

The cause of alcoholic polyneuritis is not fully understood. It has been thought to be a form of beriberi, the deficiency of aneurine being due to a combination of defective diet, impaired absorption owing to a catarrhal condition of the alimentary canal, and increased need caused by the high calorie value of the alcohol. It has been stated that if the deficiency of aneurine is repaired the patient may continue to improve though permitted to take alcohol. On the other hand, Brown (1941) found that the administration of aneurine did not hasten recovery from alcoholic polyneuritis. This, however, does not necessarily mean, as has been supposed, that the polyneuritis is not initially due to aneurine deficiency, for chronic beriberi polyneuritis responds poorly to aneurine. Alcoholic beriberi with heart failure and oedema undoubtedly occurs: whether 'dry' alcoholic polyneuritis is similarly caused is at present unsettled. Alcoholic polyneuritis is more frequently the result of the consumption of spirits than of other forms of alcoholic drink. The sex and age incidence are those of alcoholic addiction, most patients being middle-aged, and males being affected more often than females. At present it is impossible to be sure that deficiency of other vitamins or dietary factors may not play a part.

PATHOLOGY

The changes in the nervous system are those of degenerative or parenchy-matous neuritis [see p. 811], involving both the somatic peripheral nerves and the autonomic nerves. Although there is some slowing of conduction in peripheral nerves (Mawdsley and Mayer, 1965) this is rarely severe and pathological evidence suggests that the lesion is predominantly axonal, with little segmental demyelination (Gilliatt, 1966). The affected neurones exhibit degenerative changes especially at the periphery, and chromatolysis is found in the ganglion cells of the anterior horns and dorsal root ganglia of the spinal cord, and of the motor nuclei of the cranial nerves. The changes in the muscles are those characteristic of degeneration of the lower motor neurones.

SYMPTOMS

Sensory disturbances usually play a prominent part in the clinical picture. In the early stages the patient complains of numbness, tingling, and paraesthesiae in the hands and feet, and especially pain in the extremities. The pain may be very severe and is described as burning or 'like tearing flesh off the bones'. Cramp-like pains occur in the calves and are especially severe at night. Following the early sensory disturbances the limbs become weak, the lower limbs usually being more severely affected than the upper.

As is the rule in polyneuritis, both motor and sensory symptoms affect predominantly the periphery of the limbs and in a symmetrical manner. In severe cases both wrist-drop and foot-drop are present, the latter causing a 'steppage' gait, and there is some wasting of the peripheral muscles of all four limbs. Weakness is most marked in the peripheral segments. If the patient can move his limbs, sensory ataxia can usually be demonstrated, and in one form of disorder—the so-called pseudotabetic variety—ataxia is conspicuous in the lower limbs and is due to loss of postural sensibility. There is a blunting of all forms of sensibility in the periphery of the limbs, cutaneous anaesthesia, and analgesia usually extending up to the elbows and knees. Postural sensibility and appreciation of passive movements are impaired in the fingers and toes. At the same time pressure upon the muscles, especially those of the calves, is usually intensely painful, and scratching the sole may also evoke severe pain. In both cases pain may be delayed. Exceptionally pain and tenderness are slight or absent.

The tendon reflexes are diminished or lost, the ankle-jerks disappearing before the knee-jerks. The plantar reflexes may also be lost, but if present are flexor. The skin of the extremities is often oedematous and sweating. Muscular contractures readily develop, especially in the flexors of the fingers, the hamstrings, and the calf muscles, and fibrous adhesions readily occur in the tendon sheaths and around the joints. The sphincters are usually unaffected.

Abnormalities in the cranial nerves are inconstant. The pupils tend to be contracted and may react sluggishly to light. Nystagmus is common. Neuritis of the cranial nerves may be present, the vagus being most frequently involved, with a resulting tachycardia, and the facial next in frequency. Korsakow's psychosis, Wernicke's encephalopathy [see p. 729], or alcoholic dementia may complicate the picture. The cerebrospinal fluid may be normal, or its protein content may be considerably increased. A blood pyruvate estimation will be helpful in assessing aneurine deficiency. The symptoms of alcoholic poisoning of other organs besides the nervous system may be present. Gastritis is common and the liver may be enlarged. Myocardial failure may also occur, and pulmonary tuberculosis is a not uncommon complication. Patients are often obese and florid but are occasionally wasted due to malnutrition.

DIAGNOSIS

The diagnosis of polyneuritis has been described on page 812.

PROGNOSIS

The prognosis of alcoholic polyneuritis depends upon how early treatment is begun, and how far it is possible to remove or prevent the recurrence of the causal factor. When treatment can be begun early the prognosis is good, and in mild cases the symptoms disappear in a few weeks. In more severe cases recovery takes several months, and in long-standing cases recovery may be incomplete, especially in respect of return of power to the peripheral muscles. In some cases, in spite of early treatment and the withdrawal of alcohol, the disorder runs a rapidly progressive course with increasing mental confusion, terminating either by death in coma or heart failure or from an intercurrent pneumonia.

TREATMENT

Vitamin B_1 (aneurine or thiamine) should certainly be given and may usefully be combined with other vitamins in an intramuscular injection of *Parentrovite* or of some similar multi-vitamin preparation. Subsequently a vitamin-rich diet is necessary but should for some time be supplemented by giving thiamine, 50 mg. daily. The treatment of alcohol addiction must be combined with that of the polyneuritis [see p. 690]. The coincident catarrhal condition of the alimentary canal should receive attention.

REFERENCES

Brown, M. R. (1941) Alcoholic polyneuritis, *J. Amer. med. Ass.*, **116**, 1615.
Gilliatt, R. (1966) Nerve conduction in human and experimental neuropathies, *Proc. roy. Soc. Med.*, **59**, 989.
Jolliffe, N. (1938) The role of vitamin B_1 deficiency in the production of polyneuritis in the alcohol addict, *Brit. J. Inebr.*, **36**, 7.
Mawdsley, C., and Mayer, R. F. (1965) Nerve conduction in alcoholic polyneuropathy, *Brain*, **88**, 335.
Strauss, M. B. (1938) The therapeutic use of vitamin B_1 in polyneuritis and cardiovascular conditions, *J. Amer. med. Ass.*, **110**, 953.
Victor, M., and Adams, R. D. (1953) The effect of alcohol on the nervous system, *Res. Publ. Ass. nerv. ment. Dis.*, **32**, 526.

ISONIAZID NEUROPATHY

A sensorimotor neuropathy has been described in patients receiving isoniazid, usually in doses of 300 mg. daily or more, for the treatment of tuberculosis, and may be accompanied by mental symptoms and skin changes similar to those of pellagra. It is believed to be due to a conditioned pyridoxine deficiency and can be prevented as a rule by the administration of pyridoxine, 25–50 mg. daily. It has been shown that the neuropathy occurs in individuals who detoxicate isoniazid slowly and that the ability to detoxicate the drug slowly or rapidly is genetically determined.

REFERENCES

CARLSON, H. B., ANTHONY, E. M., RUSSELL, W. F., and MIDDLEBROOK, G. (1956) Prophylaxis of isoniazid neuropathy with pyridoxine, *New Engl. J. Med.*, **255,** 118.
CLARKE, C. A., PRICE EVANS, D. A., HARRIS, R., McCONNELL, R. B., and WOODROW, J. C. (1968) Genetics in medicine. A review. Part II. Pharmacogenetics, *Quart. J. Med.*, **37,** 183.
McCONNELL, R. B., and CHEETHAM, H. D. (1952) Acute pellagra during isoniazid therapy, *Lancet*, ii, 959.

ARSENICAL POLYNEURITIS
AETIOLOGY

Polyneuritis may follow either acute or chronic arsenical poisoning, more usually the latter. The arsenic may have been administered with intent to murder or in an attempt at suicide. It may have been taken accidentally or medicinally. For murderous purposes white arsenic or sodium arsenite, which is contained in certain rat-poisons and weed-killers, has usually been employed. Arsenic has also been obtained from fly-papers for this purpose. Accidental arsenical poisoning may occur in occupations involving handling arsenic, though this is rare, or as a result of taking food contaminated with arsenic, as in the Manchester epidemic in 1900, when poisoning was produced by the consumption of beer brewed with glucose containing arsenic. Poisoning has also been produced by the inhalation of arsenic from wallpapers, in which it has been used as a dye. Medicinal arsenical poisoning is rare today, but was more frequent in the past, when Fowler's solution was administered for long periods in the treatment of chorea, multiple sclerosis, and pernicious anaemia. Polyneuritis is rare after treatment with arsenobenzene derivatives.

The observation that arsenical poisoning causes an accumulation of pyruvate in the blood suggests that arsenic, like other heavy metals, may act by reacting with a thiol group which is an essential component of an enzyme concerned with pyruvate metabolism, and may provide a link between arsenical polyneuritis and polyneuritis due to vitamin deficiency (Peters, Stocken, and Thompson, 1945).

A sensorimotor polyneuropathy virtually identical with that due to arsenic may be produced on occasion by other heavy metals including gold, mercury, zinc, bismuth, antimony, and thallium and the mechanism is believed to be similar. Thallium, which has been used commercially as a rat poison and as an insecticide or as a depilatory, has been responsible for a number of such cases.

PATHOLOGY

See page 811.

SYMPTOMS

The symptoms of arsenical polyneuritis resemble those of the alcoholic variety. As in the latter, sensory symptoms are conspicuous, and pain is usually severe. Muscular weakness is usually more conspicuous in the lower than in the upper limbs. Korsakow's psychosis or a confusional state may be present. In the diagnosis of arsenical polyneuritis the presence of abnormalities outside the nervous system assumes great importance. In chronic arsenical poisoning gastro-intestinal symptoms may be absent. Excessive salivation is not uncommon, and there is often a secondary anaemia. Cutaneous symptoms are usually present. These may consist of erythema or even of exfoliative dermatitis. In long-standing cases there is often cutaneous pigmentation. This is absent from the exposed parts and consists of a fine mottling of the skin, with patches of a light chocolate colour, the intervening areas being white. Hyperkeratosis of the palms and soles is often found, the thickened skin presenting a smooth, somewhat waxy appearance. Herpes zoster is a common complication. The blood pyruvate is raised and even when the resting level is normal, a pyruvate tolerance curve demonstrates that the serum pyruvate rises well above the normal upper limit of 1·3 mg. per 100 ml. after a loading dose of glucose.

DIAGNOSIS

The diagnosis of polyneuritis is described on page 812. The diagnosis of arsenical from other forms of polyneuritis depends upon the presence of the abnormalities just described, especially the cutaneous symptoms of arsenical poisoning, and upon the demonstration by appropriate toxicological tests of arsenic in the hair, nails, urine, or faeces.

PROGNOSIS

The prognosis of arsenical polyneuritis is good, provided the general symptoms of arsenical poisoning are not too far advanced when the patient comes under treatment. Recovery of voluntary power, however, is slow and may take one or two years.

TREATMENT

Dimercaprol was the first drug to be of value; calcium versenate, another chelating agent, is also effective in promoting the excretion of arsenic but both may well be supplanted by penicillamine (Simpson, 1962). In addition the general treatment of polyneuritis should be carried out [see p. 813].

REFERENCES

HASSIN, G. B. (1930) Symptomatology of arsenical polyneuritis, *J. nerv. ment. Dis.*, **72,** 628.
PETERS, R. A., STOCKEN, L. A., and THOMPSON, R. H. S. (1945) British Anti-Lewisite (BAL), *Nature (Lond.)*, **156,** 616.
SIMPSON, J. A. (1962) The neuropathies, in *Modern Trends in Neurology*, 3rd series, ed. WILLIAMS, D., London.

ORGANIC CHLORINE COMPOUNDS USED AS INSECTICIDES

Campbell (1952) has reported 5 cases of polyneuritis and 3 of retrobulbar neuritis following the use of an insecticide containing ortho- and para-dichloro-benzene, DDT, and pentachlorophenol. He suggested that the last might be the toxic factor.

REFERENCE

CAMPBELL, A. M. G. (1952) Neurological complications associated with insecticides and fungicides, *Brit. med. J.*, **2**, 415.

LEAD NEUROPATHY

Lead poisoning has been considered in detail on page 698. Lead may produce a predominantly motor type of polyneuropathy, often affecting predominantly those muscles in common use in the individual's occupation (e.g. wrist-drop in battery-makers). In experimental studies in the guinea-pig, Fullerton (1966) found that lead produced a combination of segmental demyelination and axonal degeneration.

REFERENCE

FULLERTON, P. M. (1966) Chronic peripheral neuropathy produced by lead poisoning in guinea-pigs, *J. Neuropath. exp. Neurol.*, **25**, 214.

THALIDOMIDE NEUROPATHY

Thalidomide, used some years ago as a hypnotic in Britain and in Europe was withdrawn from the market when it was found to produce phocomelia in the foetus if taken by the mother during the early months of pregnancy. After regular administration of the drug for several months many patients were found to develop a predominantly sensory neuropathy giving rise to unpleasant burning dysaesthesiae in the hands and feet accompanied by peripheral impairment of pain sensation often restricted to the digits (Fullerton and Kremer, 1961). While in milder cases slow recovery often occurred following withdrawal of the drug, in a number of severe cases painful paraesthesiae and sensory loss have persisted for many years.

REFERENCE

FULLERTON, P. M., and KREMER, M. (1961) Neuropathy after intake of thalidomide (Distaval), *Brit. med. J.*, **2**, 855.

POLYNEURITIS DUE TO TRIORTHOCRESYLPHOSPHATE

During the spring of 1930 thousands of cases of polyneuritis, some of them fatal, occurred in the United States, owing to the consumption of fluid extract of ginger adulterated with triorthocresylphosphate. The condition became known as 'ginger paralysis'. Recent outbreaks of polyneuritis in South Africa, Germany, Morocco, and the Merseyside area have been traced to cresyl esters in cooking-oil. The same toxic substance has been proved responsible for causing poly-neuritis in women who have taken apiol as an abortifacient. Triorthocresylphos-phate irreversibly inhibits pseudocholinesterase but since not all inhibitors of pseudocholinesterase produce degeneration of peripheral nerves some other factor would seem to be at work.

Both in man and in experimental animals triorthocresylphosphate produces a chromatolysis of the anterior horn cells of the spinal cord and of the ganglion cells of the motor nuclei of the pons and medulla, degeneration of the fasciculus gracilis and the corticospinal tracts in the spinal cord, and destruction of the myelin sheaths and axis cylinders of the peripheral nerves. Cavanagh (1953, 1964) has shown that changes occur initially in those nerve fibres which are longest and of the greatest diameter, both in the peripheral and central nervous system and suggests that the primary pathological process is one of 'dying-back' of the axon. Symptoms of polyneuritis have developed from ten to twenty days after the consumption of adulterated ginger, and consisted of bilateral wrist-drop and foot-drop, with wasting of the distal muscles of the limbs. Pain in the limbs was common, but sensory loss was inconstant. In many cases the paralysis has proved to be permanent. Acute retrobulbar neuritis has been described in apiol poisoning. For treatment see page 813.

REFERENCES

ARING, C. D. (1942) The systemic nervous affinity of triorthocresylphosphate (Jamaica ginger palsy), *Brain*, **65**, 34.

CAVANAGH, J. B. (1954) The toxic effects of tri-ortho-cresyl phosphate on the nervous system, *J. Neurol. Neurosurg. Psychiat.*, **17**, 163.

CAVANAGH, J. B. (1953) Organo-phosphorus neurotoxicity: a model 'dying back' process comparable to certain human neurological disorders, *Guy's Hosp. Rep.*, **112**, 303.

CAVANAGH, J. B. (1964) Peripheral nerve changes in ortho-cresyl phosphate poisoning in the cat, *J. Path. Bact.*, **87**, 365.

HOTSTON, R. D. (1946) Outbreak of polyneuritis due to orthotricresyl phosphate poisoning, *Lancet*, i, 207.

SMITH, M. I., ELVOLVE, E., and FRAZIER, W. H. (1930) Pharmacological action of certain phenol esters, with special reference to the etiology of so-called ginger paralysis, *Publ. Hlth Rep. (Wash.)*, **45**, 2509.

WEBER, M. L. (1936–7) Follow-up study of thirty-five cases of paralysis caused by adulterated Jamaica ginger extract, *Med. Bull. Veterans' Adm. (Wash.)*, **13**, 228.

NITROFURANTOIN NEUROPATHY

Nitrofurantoin (*Furadantin*) is a drug now widely used in the treatment of urinary infection. Cases have been reported in which a symmetrical sensori-motor peripheral neuropathy developed during treatment with this drug and was shown to occur only in those with severe impairment of renal function (Ellis, 1962; Loughridge, 1962). It is now clear that this drug should be used with great caution if the blood urea (or non-protein nitrogen) is above normal or if there are other indications of substantially impaired renal function.

REFERENCES

ELLIS, F. G. (1962) Acute polyneuritis after nitrofurantoin therapy, *Lancet*, ii, 1136.

LOUGHRIDGE, L. W. (1962) Peripheral neuropathy due to nitrofurantoin, *Lancet*, ii, 1133.

URAEMIC POLYNEUROPATHY

Since the original report of Asbury, Victor, and Adams (1962) it has become abundantly clear that a mixed sensorimotor polyneuropathy may occur frequently in patients who are uraemic as a result of chronic renal failure. In many cases improvement follows treatment of the renal disease, as by intermittent dialysis, but this is not invariable. Demyelination appears to be the primary pathological process.

REFERENCE

ASBURY, A. K., VICTOR, M., and ADAMS, R. D. (1962) Uremic polyneuropathy, *Trans. Amer. neurol. Ass.*, **87**, 100.

CHLOROQUINE NEUROMYOPATHY

A motor polyneuropathy, unaccompanied by symptoms or signs of sensory dysfunction, may develop in patients receiving treatment with chloroquine, usually in doses of 500 mg. daily or more for one year or longer. Histological studies indicate that the muscle fibres are also affected as they commonly show striking vacuolation which appears to be due to the accumulation of glycogen.

REFERENCE

WHISNANT, J. P., ESPINOSA, R. E., KIERLAND, R. R., and LAMBERT, E. H. (1963) Chloroquine neuromyopathy, *Proc. Mayo Clin.*, **38**, 501.

VINCRISTINE NEUROMYOPATHY

Vincristine sulphate, used increasingly of late for the treatment of medulloblastoma in childhood and of intracranial gliomas in adult life, has been found to produce in many cases a sensorimotor polyneuropathy. Pathological and electrophysiological studies suggest that the damage is primarily axonal but focal necrosis of muscle fibres is also found (Bradley *et al.*, 1969).

REFERENCE

BRADLEY, W. G., LASSMAN, L. P., PEARCE, G. W., and WALTON, J. N. (1969) The neuromyopathy of vincristine in man, *J. neurol. Sci.* (in the press).

NEURITIS COMPLICATING SEROTHERAPY

Neuritis is a rare sequel of serotherapy. It has been described after the administration of serum in the treatment of tetanus, diphtheria, and scarlet fever. Nervous symptoms usually occur two or three days after the onset of typical symptoms of serum sickness. The commonest lesion is a spinal neuritis, the fifth cervical spinal nerve being most commonly affected on one or both sides, with pain in the corresponding segmental distribution and paralysis of the muscles innervated, especially the deltoid. This syndrome is almost identical with that of 'shoulder-girdle neuritis' (neuralgic amyotrophy) [see p. 808]. Less frequently the whole brachial plexus may be involved, leading to brachial neuritis, or polyneuritis may occur. Cerebral symptoms, probably resulting from cerebral oedema, rarely occur. Optic neuritis has been described. Complete recovery usually occurs in from one to eighteen months, though occasionally muscular weakness persists. Treatment appropriate to the situation of the lesion must be carried out.

REFERENCES

ALLEN, I. M. (1931) The neurological complications of serum therapy, with report of a case, *Lancet*, ii, 1128.

BARON, J. H. (1958) A.T.S. cervical polyradiculitis treated by cortisone, *Brit. med. J.*, **2**, 678.

POLYNEURITIS IN PREGNANCY

It is better to speak of polyneuritis in pregnancy than polyneuritis of pregnancy since any form of polyneuritis may occur in pregnancy. Some writers stress the importance of nutritional factors. Persistent vomiting, unsuitable diet, and increased requirements due to the needs of the foetus may all contribute to nutritional deficiency in pregnancy, though whether of one or more factors is uncertain. Where beriberi is endemic, pregnancy appears to predispose to it. Bilateral retrobulbar neuritis resembling that ascribed by Moore to vitamin deficiency has been observed by Ballantyne (1941) in hyperemesis gravidarum. Ungley (1933) has described recurrent neuritis in pregnancy and the puerperium in three members of the same family.

When there is reason to suspect nutritional deficiency vitamin supplements should be given.

REFERENCES

BALLANTYNE, A. J. (1941) Ocular complications in hyperemesis gravidarum, *J. Obstet. Gynec.*, **48**, 206.

STRAUSS, M. B., and McDONALD, W. J. (1933) Polyneuritis of pregnancy, *J. Amer. med. Ass.*, **100**, 1320.

UNGLEY, C. C. (1933) Recurrent polyneuritis, *J. Neurol. Psychiat.*, **14**, 15.

UNGLEY, C. C. (1938) On some deficiencies of nutrition and their relation to disease, *Lancet*, i, 925.

DIABETIC POLYNEURITIS

AETIOLOGY

It is improbable that hyperglycaemia alone is the cause of the neuritis which sometimes complicates diabetes. Age plays a part in causation, since neuritis is seen almost exclusively in the middle-aged and elderly. It is probable that atheroma of the vasa nervorum is a predisposing factor in some cases. However, in young and middle-aged patients it is now generally agreed that the neuropathy is of metabolic origin, being associated as a rule with uncontrolled diabetes. The exact metabolic defect has not yet been identified, although a disorder of pantothenic acid metabolism has been postulated (Bosanquet and Henson, 1957).

PATHOLOGY

See page 811. Nerve conduction studies (Gilliatt and Willison, 1962) and the pathological examination of teased nerve fibres (Thomas and Lascelles, 1965) indicate that the neuropathy is demyelinating. When isolated peripheral nerve lesions occur, however (mononeuropathy), pathological evidence has indicated that ischaemia with localized infarction of nerve trunks is the cause (Raff, Sangalang, and Asbury, 1968).

SYMPTOMS

Loss of tendon reflexes and of vibration sense in the lower limbs is very common in diabetes in the absence of other signs of neuritis. Severe polyneuritis is exceptional. In such cases sensory symptoms usually predominate over motor, and the lower limbs are more affected than the upper. Pure sensory neuropathy may occur [see p. 795]. Pain in the calves may be considerable, and loss of postural sensibility is often marked in the lower limbs, leading to severe ataxia. 'Diabetic amyotrophy' (Garland, 1957), characterized by pain, tenderness, and weakness of muscles, usually limited to the anterior aspect of one or both thighs, is probably a form of diabetic neuritis and may well be due in most cases to a femoral nerve neuropathy. Arthropathy may occur. Isolated lesions of other peripheral nerves, particularly the lateral popliteal, also occur. Ocular palsies occurring in diabetes have been ascribed to neuritis of the oculomotor nerves, but are more probably due to vascular lesions involving the nerve trunks or mid-brain [see p. 155]. In elderly diabetics the pupils are often contracted and may react sluggishly to light ('diabetic pseudotabes'). Absent circulatory reflexes, and particularly an abnormal response to the Valsalva manoeuvre (Sharpey-Schafer and Taylor, 1960), are found in some cases and are due to disease in the afferent pathway. Primary optic atrophy may occur. In some cases, chronic diarrhoea, often nocturnal, and even steatorrhoea may occur and have been attributed to a neuropathy of autonomic visceral nerves (see Simpson, 1962). Other complications of diabetes may be present, including impaired peripheral circulation, owing to arterial atheroma, which may lead to gangrene of the extremities or perforating ulcer.

DIAGNOSIS

The diagnosis of polyneuritis is described on page 812. The origin of the diabetic form is settled by the discovery of glycosuria and hyperglycaemia. The symptoms of metabolic neuritis must be distinguished from those of vascular occlusion with resultant ischaemic neuropathy. Confusion is not likely to arise if the arterial pulse is carefully examined both in the proximal and peripheral parts of the limbs.

PROGNOSIS

The prognosis of diabetic neuritis is good, provided that the patient responds satisfactorily to treatment for diabetes, that vascular degeneration is not severe, and that trophic lesions, such as gangrene and perforating ulcers, are absent.

TREATMENT

The usual treatment of diabetes must be carried out.

Vitamins appear to be of no value but measures appropriate to the usual management of polyneuritis may be indicated [p. 813].

REFERENCES

BOSANQUET, F. D., and HENSON, R. A. (1957) Sensory neuropathy in diabetes mellitus, *Psychiat. Neurol. Neurochirurg.*, **60,** 107.

GARLAND, H. (1957) Diabetic amyotrophy, in *Modern Trends in Neurology* (2nd series), ed. WILLIAMS, D., p. 229, London.

GILLIATT, R. W., and WILLISON, R. G. (1962) Peripheral nerve conduction in diabetic neuropathy, *J. Neurol. Neurosurg. Psychiat.*, **25,** 11.

GOODMAN, J. I., BAUMOEL, S., FRANKEL, L., MARCUS, L. J., and WASSERMANN, S. (1953) *The Diabetic Neuropathies*, Springfield, Ill.

JORDAN, W. R. (1936) Neuritic manifestations in diabetes mellitus, *Arch. intern. Med.*, **57,** 307.

RAFF, M. C., SANGALANG, V., and ASBURY, A. K. (1968) Ischaemic mononeuropathy multiplex associated with diabetes mellitus, *Arch. Neurol. (Chic.)*, **18,** 487.

RUNDLES, R. W. (1945) Diabetic neuropathy, *Medicine (Baltimore)*, **24,** 111.

SHARPEY-SCHAFER, E. P., and TAYLOR, P. J. (1960) Absent circulatory reflexes in diabetic neuritis, *Lancet*, i, 559.

SIMPSON, J. A. (1962) The neuropathies, in *Modern Trends in Neurology*, 3rd series, ed. WILLIAMS, D., London.

THOMAS, P. K., and LASCELLES, R. G. (1965) Schwann-cell abnormalities in diabetic neuropathy, *Lancet*, i, 1355.

WOLTMAN, H. W., and WILDER, R. M. (1929) Diabetes mellitus. Pathologic changes in the spinal cord and peripheral nerves, *Arch. intern. Med.*, **44,** 576.

HYPOGLYCAEMIC NEUROPATHY

In patients with an insulin-secreting pancreatic islet-cell adenoma, motor weakness may occur and can occasionally be accompanied by peripheral paraesthesiae. It has been suggested that this syndrome is due to a peripheral neuropathy (Lambert, Mulder, and Bastron, 1960) but Tom and Richardson (1951) suggested that hyperinsulinism may damage the anterior horn cells of the spinal cord rather than the peripheral nerves.

REFERENCES

LAMBERT, E. H., MULDER, D. W., and BASTRON, D. W. (1960) Regeneration of peripheral nerves with hyperinsulinism neuropathy. Report of a case, *Neurology (Minneap.)*, **11,** 125.

TOM, M. I., RICHARDSON, J. C. (1951) Hypoglycaemia from islet-cell tumour of pancreas with amyotrophy and cerebrospinal nerve cell changes; a case report, *J. Neuropath.*, **10,** 57.

MYXOEDEMA NEUROPATHY

Bilateral compression of the median nerves in the carpal tunnels is a common complication of myxoedema (Murray and Simpson, 1958) but it has also been suggested that a symmetrical, predominantly sensory, neuropathy involving all four limbs may occur in such cases and responds to treatment with L-thyroxine (Nickel *et al.*, 1961).

REFERENCES

MURRAY, I. P. C., and SIMPSON, J. A. (1958) Acroparaesthesiae in myxoedema, *Lancet*, i, 1360.

NICKEL, S. N., FRAME, B., BEBIN, J., TOURTELOTTE, W. W., PARKER, J. A., and HUGHES, B. R. (1961) Myxoedema neuropathy and myopathy. A clinical and pathological study, *Neurology (Minneap.)*, **11,** 125.

AMYLOID NEUROPATHY

Amyloidosis is commonly divided into primary and secondary forms. Secondary amyloidosis is associated with chronic suppuration, and other chronic infective conditions and occasionally with malignant disease, particularly plasmacytoma. Primary amyloidosis occurs in the absence of any of these predisposing causes and is usually familial. So far as the amyloidosis is concerned it is doubtful whether the two forms differ, but in secondary amyloidosis the conspicuous features are usually those of diffuse visceral involvement by the amyloid disease, while primary amyloidosis is likely to present more selectively, and not uncommonly with symptoms resulting from involvement of the peripheral nerves.

The first symptoms are usually sensory, and consist of painful dysaesthesiae of the distal parts of the upper or lower limbs. The physical signs are those of a polyneuropathy with distal sensory loss, muscular wasting and weakness, and diminution or loss of the tendon reflexes. Hyperpathia is sometimes prominent. On the other hand, painless ulcers may occur. The peripheral nerves are characteristically thickened, and tougher than normal.

There may be an increase of protein or of the number of cells in the cerebrospinal fluid.

Other symptoms of amyloid disease, notably macroglossia, myocardial involvement, and impairment of renal function may be present. Involvement of autonomic nerves commonly gives rise to gastro-intestinal symptoms, orthostatic hypotension, and impotence (Munsat and Poussaint, 1962).

The serum protein may be low, with increased globulin and an abnormal protein found on electrophoresis. The Congo-red test may or may not be positive. Biopsy is the best method of confirming the diagnosis and may be carried out on the skin, gum, rectum or, most suitably in neurological cases, on a palpably thickened cutaneous nerve running from an area of abnormal sensation.

The diagnosis has to be made from other forms of peripheral neuropathy, especially those associated with thickening of the peripheral nerves, i.e. leprosy, chronic hypertrophic polyneuritis, and some forms of recurrent polyneuritis.

Death usually occurs in from one to five years from cardiac failure. Treatment is symptomatic.

REFERENCES

ANDRADE, C. (1952) Peculiar form of peripheral neuropathy; familial atypical generalized amyloidosis with special involvement of peripheral nerves, *Brain*, **75**, 408.

CHAMBERS, R. A., MEDD, W. E., and SPENCER, H. (1958) Primary amyloidosis, *Quart. J. Med.*, **27**, 207.

MUNSAT, T. L., and POUSSAINT, A. F. (1962) Clinical manifestations and diagnosis of amyloid polyneuropathy, *Neurology (Minneap.)*, **12**, 413.

PINK DISEASE

Synonyms. Erythroedema polyneuritis; trophodermatoneurosis; vegetative neurosis; acrodynia.

Definition. A disease affecting young children, characterized by irritability, photophobia, a red discoloration, with slight swelling of the hands and feet, and symptoms of polyneuritis.

PATHOLOGY

The pathology of pink disease was investigated by Paterson and Greenfield (1924), and by Wyllie and Stern (1931). The changes in the nervous system consisted of degeneration, especially of myelin, in the peripheral nerves. In the spinal cord there was chromatolysis of the anterior horn cells. Histologically the cutaneous lesions consisted of hyperkeratosis, hypertrophy of the sweat glands, and lymphocytic infiltration of the corium, with oedema.

AETIOLOGY

The victims of the disease are young children between the ages of 4 months and 7 years, the onset usually occurring between the ages of 9 and 18 months. Males are affected slightly more often than females. The disease used to be widely prevalent, but was especially common in Australia and in North America. Small local epidemics were characteristic. Most cases occurred between the autumn and early spring. Some workers regarded it as infective, others as a deficiency disease. A somewhat similar condition has been produced in rats by feeding them on a restricted diet, and pink disease in some respects resembles pellagra. There is no evidence, however, that it is due to a deficiency of any known vitamin. The prominence in the clinical picture of symptoms of autonomic disturbance has led to its being regarded as a disorder of the vegetative nervous system. Warkany and Hubbard (1948) suggested that mercury administered in teething powders or ointments was the causal agent. This now seems to be established (see mercury poisoning, p. 702) and since the withdrawal of these powders and of calomel from the market, the disease has virtually disappeared.

SYMPTOMS

The earliest symptoms were usually those of a mild infection of the upper respiratory tract or of the alimentary canal. Shortly afterwards the child became miserable and irritable, and suffered from insomnia and loss of appetite. At the same time the hands and feet became bluish-red, slightly swollen, and cold. In addition there was often an erythematous rash over the face, trunk, and extremities. There was always excessive sweating, and desquamation occurred on the hands and feet. The rash was extremely irritating, and the child frequently adopted a characteristic posture, crouching in bed with its knees drawn up and its face buried in the pillow, to shield it from the light.

In severe cases trophic disturbances were present, including ulceration of the mouth, falling-out of teeth, nails and hair.

There was no true paralysis, but the muscles became extremely hypotonic, and in chronic cases the tendon reflexes were lost and analgesia of peripheral distribution was sometimes demonstrable.

Pyrexia was absent after the prodromal stage. The pulse was rapid and the blood pressure was often slightly raised. The urine often contained a trace of albumin and detectable amounts of mercury but the cerebrospinal fluid was normal.

DIAGNOSIS

The combination of symptoms and their occurrence in early childhood were unique, and the condition was, therefore, unlikely to be confused with any other.

PROGNOSIS

The mortality was low, approximately 5 per cent., death being due to cardiac failure, or more usually to an intercurrent infection, such as bronchopneumonia. The disease ran a chronic course and usually lasted from three months to a year.

TREATMENT

Treatment was mainly symptomatic. Bower (1954) found that ganglion-blocking drugs were worth a trial when autonomic symptoms predominated. Feeding often proved to be difficult on account of anorexia and irritability and sedatives were generally required. Slow improvement was shown to follow the withdrawal of drugs containing mercury and chelating agents were rarely required.

REFERENCES

BOWER, B. D. (1954) Pink disease: the autonomic disorder and its treatment with ganglion-blocking agents. *Quart. J. Med.*, N.S. **23**, 215.

PATERSON, D., and GREENFIELD, J. G. (1923–4) Erythroedema polyneuritis, *Quart. J. Med.*, **17**, 6 (contains 17 refs.).

WARKANY, J., and HUBBARD, D. M. (1948) Mercury in the urine of children with acrodynia, *Lancet*, i, 829.

WYLLIE, W. G., and STERN, R. O. (1931) Pink disease: its morbid anatomy, with a note on treatment, *Arch. Dis. Childh.*, **6**, 137.

DIPHTHERIA

AETIOLOGY

Neuritis is the commonest and most important of the nervous complications of diphtheria, the exotoxin of *Corynebacterium diphtheriae* having an affinity for the peripheral nerves. It is most frequently observed during childhood and is rare in adult life. According to Rolleston (1929), in spite of the general belief to the contrary, the occurrence of paralysis bears a definite relationship to the severity of the local infection, which is usually faucial but may be extrafaucial. The introduction of antitoxin has greatly reduced the incidence of paralysis, which is almost unknown in patients who have received antitoxin on the first day of their illness, and becomes progressively more frequent the longer the administration of this remedy is delayed.

Palatal paralysis is usually attributed to the ascent of the toxin from the common faucial site of infection to the medulla. A local ascent of the nerves by the toxin is responsible for the local development of paralysis following a cutaneous infection, the muscles paralysed being those supplied by the spinal segment from which the infected region is innervated (Walshe, 1918–19). Paralysis of accommodation and generalized polyneuritis are due to the dissemination of the toxin by the blood stream to the ciliary muscle, and the peripheral nerves.

PATHOLOGY

The pathology of the neuritis is that of a segmental demyelination (Fisher and Adams, 1956; Morgan-Hughes, 1965) which is accompanied by characteristic slowing of motor nerve conduction, a finding which may persist for some time after clinical recovery. The neuropathic effects of the toxin have been shown experimentally to be dose-dependent; the toxin becomes unavailable for inactivation by antitoxin within one hour and small diameter nerve fibres are more severely affected (Cavanagh and Jacobs, 1964). Hemiplegia, a rare complication of diphtheria, appears usually to be due to a vascular lesion, either embolism or thrombosis of a cerebral artery, or to an area of so-called acute haemorrhagic encephalitis.

SYMPTOMS

Paralysis of the palate, which is usually the earliest nervous symptom, may occur within a few days of the onset of the infection. Usually, however, it develops during the second or third week. It is generally bilateral but may be unilateral. Maher (1948) distinguishes defective elevation and deviation of the uvula. It causes the voice to acquire a nasal character and leads to regurgitation of fluids through the nose on swallowing. The palatal reflex is usually lost.

Paralysis of accommodation develops as a rule during the third or fourth week and leads to dimness of vision for near objects. It is usually bilateral, very rarely unilateral, and may pass unnoticed in myopic subjects who do not require to accommodate for near vision. The pupillary reactions to light and on convergence are unimpaired. Paresis of external ocular muscles is not very rare, the lateral rectus being most often affected.

The symptoms of generalized polyneuritis, which are not always preceded by paralysis of the palate and of accommodation, do not develop until between the fifth and seventh week after infection. At this stage paralysis of the constrictors of the pharynx, of the intrinsic muscles of the larynx, associated with laryngeal anaesthesia, and paralysis of the diaphragm are the most serious complications, on account of the dysphagia and dyspnoea to which they lead. The adductors of the vocal cords are more often paralysed than the abductors. Paralysis of the neck muscles may occur.

The lower limbs are usually more severely affected than the upper, and movements of peripheral segments suffer more than those of proximal. Sensory loss is common, cutaneous anaesthesia and analgesia of the 'glove and stocking' distribution being associated with tenderness of the muscles on pressure. Postural sensibility is often grossly impaired, leading to marked ataxia, especially in the lower limbs, the so-called 'pseudotabetic form' of diphtheritic paralysis.

The tendon reflexes are lost early and may remain absent for months or even for years. Loss of the tendon reflexes may occur in the absence of other symptoms of the polyneuritis and, with or without palatal palsy, may constitute the only nervous symptoms of diphtheria. The plantar reflexes may be unobtainable but are usually flexor, though Rolleston has drawn attention to the occurrence of extensor plantar responses, an indication that the corticospinal tracts may rarely be involved in the intoxication. The sphincters are usually unaffected, but impotence has frequently been described. The 'cardiac paralysis' of the early stages is probably due to the effect of the toxin on the myocardium, but at any stage tachycardia may occur as a result of vagal paralysis. The cerebrospinal fluid may be normal or its protein content may be increased.

Diphtheritic hemiplegia is fortunately rare. The symptoms are similar to those of other acquired forms of infantile hemiplegia [see p. 562]. Meningism is not very uncommon in the acute stage of diphtheria. Cervical rigidity or opistho-tonos may be associated with rigidity of the limbs, so-called 'spasmodic diph-theria'. The cerebrospinal fluid in such cases, though its pressure may be increased, is normal in composition. Permanent bulbar palsy is a rare sequel of diphtheria.

DIAGNOSIS

For the diagnosis of polyneuritis see page 812. The diphtheritic form is usually easily recognized on account of the age of the patient and the occurrence of such characteristic features as palatal paralysis and paralysis of accommodation. The diphtheria bacillus should always be sought at the site of infection, but may be absent. In doubtful cases the Schick test may be of diagnostic value, since a positive reaction indicates that the patient probably has not had diphtheria. A negative reaction, however, is of little significance.

PROGNOSIS

The prognosis of the paralysis is usually good if the child survives. Paralysis of the palate and of accommodation disappears in from three to six weeks, and recovery from the paralysis of the limbs is usually complete, though this may take several months. Paralysis of the pharynx, larynx, and diaphragm, though equally recoverable, is of serious import owing to the risk of bronchopneumonia which it involves. Permanent paralysis of the limbs is fortunately very rare. Hemiplegia is a serious complication, as not only may it prove fatal, but in patients who survive recovery is usually incomplete, and epilepsy and mental defect may occur as sequels.

TREATMENT

The routine treatment of diphtheria includes injection of adequate doses of antitoxin as early as possible. If this has been carried out, the administration of further doses when paralysis develops is of doubtful value. Paralysis of the limbs should be treated on the lines laid down for the treatment of polyneuritis [see p. 813]. Paralysis of the pharynx and larynx necessitates special care in feed-ing. Food should be soft and semi-fluid, and if, in spite of this, coughing occurs, it will be necessary to employ nasal feeding. Bulbar and respiratory paralysis should be treated as in poliomyelitis [see p. 459].

REFERENCES

CAVANAGH, J. B., and JACOBS, J. M. (1964) Some quantitative aspects of diphtheritic neuropathy, *Brit. J. exp. Path.*, **45**, 309.

FISHER, C. M., and ADAMS, R. D. (1956) Diphtheritic polyneuritis: a pathological study, *J. Neuropath. exp. Neurol.*, **15**, 243.

MAHER, R. M. (1948) Significance of palatal movements in diphtheria, *Lancet*, i, 57.

MORGAN-HUGHES, J. A. (1965) Changes in motor nerve conduction velocity in diph-theritic polyneuritis, *Rev. Pat. nerv. ment.*, **86**, 253.

ROLLESTON, J. D. (1913) Diphtheritic hemiplegia, *Clin. J.*, **42**, 12.

ROLLESTON, J. D. (1929) *Acute Infectious Diseases*, 2nd ed., London.

WALSHE, F. M. R. (1917–18) On the pathogenesis of diphtheritic paralysis, Part I, *Quart. J. Med.*, **11**, 191.

WALSHE, F. M. R. (1918–19) On the pathogenesis of diphtheritic paralysis, Part II, *Quart. J. Med.*, **12**, 14.

POLYNEURITIS IN COLLAGEN DISORDERS

The occurrence of polyneuropathy in association with sarcoidosis, disseminated lupus erythematosus, scleroderma, and rheumatoid arthritis raises problems of pathogenesis which are not yet completely solved (Hart and Golding, 1960; Kibler and Rose, 1960; Steinberg, 1960). In polyarteritis nodosa it is due to vascular lesions of the peripheral nerves, a mononeuritis multiplex. It seems probable that involvement of the vasa nervorum is a pathological process common to all of the disorders in this group. In disseminated lupus, systemic sclerosis, and polyarteritis nodosa the neuropathy may show some improvement with steroid drugs. In rheumatoid arthritis, Pallis and Scott (1965) identify five different types of peripheral neuropathy. Isolated lesions of major peripheral nerves in either the upper or lower limbs, digital neuropathy in the upper limbs and distal sensory neuropathy in the lower limbs are in their view relatively benign and often recover. However, the syndrome of distal sensorimotor polyneuropathy involving all four limbs carries a uniformly poor prognosis. It seems to arise more commonly in patients who have been treated with steroid drugs, given for their rheumatoid disease and most affected individuals die of a diffuse vasculitis.

REFERENCES

HART, F. D., and GOLDING, J. R. (1960) Rheumatoid neuropathy, *Brit. med. J.*, **1**, 1594.
KIBLER, R. F., and ROSE, F. C. (1960) Peripheral neuropathy in collagen diseases, *Brit. med. J.*, **1**, 1781.
PALLIS, C. A., and SCOTT, J. T. (1965) Peripheral neuropathy in rheumatoid arthritis, *Brit. med. J.*, **1**, 1141.
STEINBERG, V. L. (1960) Neuropathy in rheumatoid diseases, *Brit. med. J.*, **1**, 1600.

LEPROUS NEURITIS

AETIOLOGY

Leprosy is due to infection with the *Mycobacterium leprae* of Hansen, an acid-fast bacillus, staining like the tubercle bacillus by Ziehl-Neelsen's method. The mode of infection is uncertain, but the disease is probably contagious. The organism has a predilection for the mucous membranes and peripheral nerves. Macular, infiltrative, and polyneuritic forms are described (Cochrane, 1954).

PATHOLOGY

The characteristic lesion is a granuloma, the leprous nodule, composed of large connective-tissue cells, the lepra-cells, containing the lepra bacilli and surrounded by epithelioid and plasma cells and fibroblasts. Khanolkar (1951) points out that through healthy or slightly altered skin the bacilli spread in or along nerve fibres. The peripheral nerves are invaded by the nodules, the infection usually beginning at the periphery and gradually ascending the nerve, leading to marked irregular thickening. The axis cylinders and later the myelin sheaths degenerate. The dorsal root ganglia, the trigeminal ganglia, the sympathetic ganglia, and the anterior horns of the spinal cord may be invaded, and within the cord fibres derived from the dorsal root ganglia undergo degeneration. The pathology has been reviewed in detail by Dastur (1967).

SYMPTOMS

In the maculo-anaesthetic form anaesthesia is related to the cutaneous lesions. a polyneuritic form without skin lesions also occurs.

The onset of symptoms is gradual. Prodromal symptoms of a toxaemic nature may be present. These are followed by pains referred to the distribution of the peripheral nerves in the limbs and often by a sense of numbness of the extremities. Symptoms tend to be symmetrical, anaesthesia of the 'glove and stocking' distribution developing, together with atrophic paralysis of the muscles of the peripheral segments of the limbs. Facial anaesthesia and paralysis due to involvement of the fifth and seventh cranial nerves are often seen. Trophic changes are conspicuous in the limbs. Bullae, ulceration, and necrosis of the phalanges occur, and the fingers may all be lost. Thickening of the peripheral nerves is usually, but not invariably, palpable.

DIAGNOSIS

Leprous neuritis must be distinguished from other forms of polyneuritis, especially from progressive hypertrophic polyneuritis, in which also palpable thickening of the peripheral nerves may occur, from syringomyelia, and from Raynaud's disease. Bacteriological examination and biopsy may be necessary.

PROGNOSIS

Modern chemotherapy with sulphone drugs has much improved the prognosis. Recovery is usually complete in a few years apart from residual nerve damage.

TREATMENT

For the treatment of leprosy the reader is referred to textbooks of tropical medicine. Cochrane (1954) gives a useful review.

REFERENCES

COCHRANE, R. G. (1954) in *Modern Trends in Dermatology*, ed. MACKENNA, R. M. B., p. 153, London.

DASTUR, D. K. (1967) The peripheral neuropathology of leprosy, in *Symposium on Leprosy*, ed. ANTIA, N. H., and DASTUR, D. K., Bombay.

JULIÃO, O. F. (1945) *Contribuïção para o estudo do diagnóstico clínico da lepra nervosa*, São Paulo.

KHANOLKAR, V. R. (1951) Studies in the histology of early lesions of leprosy, *Indian Council of Med. Res. Spec. Rep. Series*, 19.

PROGRESSIVE HYPERTROPHIC POLYNEURITIS

Definition. A rare disease, frequently familial, characterized by conspicuous enlargement of the peripheral nerves, associated with the symptoms of slowly progressive polyneuritis, and sometimes other abnormalities. The disease was first described in 1889 by Gombault and Mallet, but is usually associated with the names of Dejerine and Sottas, who reported two cases in 1893. Refsum (1946) described a familial disorder, which has been shown to be associated with hypertrophic polyneuritis, and which he named heredopathia atactica polyneuritiformis but in the latter condition a specific biochemical substrate of the disorder has now been identified [see p. 576].

PATHOLOGY

There is a great increase in the volume of the peripheral nerves, though some may be affected more than others. The sciatic nerve in a case reported by Harris and Newcomb (1929) measured $1\frac{1}{2}$ in. in diameter. In addition to the nerves of the limbs the cranial nerves may be involved, and similar changes have been described in the sympathetic nerves, the cauda equina, and the spinal roots. The thickening is principally due to hypertrophy and proliferation of the cells of the neurilemma, which may coalesce into masses penetrated by nerve fibres or may be flattened into layers resembling an onion. The remarkable proliferation of the Schwann cells has been studied with the electron microscope by Weller (1967) and by Thomas and Lascelles (1967). The interfibrillar connective tissue of the nerve sheaths also undergoes hypertrophy, though to a lesser extent. The myelin sheaths of the nerves degenerate, especially peripherally. Degeneration of the axis cylinders is variable. Plasmatic swellings of spinal ganglia have been described. Within the spinal cord degeneration of the posterior columns is frequently, but not invariably, present, and is probably secondary to the changes in the nerves. It is most marked in the lumbosacral region and in the cervical cord is confined to the fasciculus gracilis. Compression of the spinal cord giving rise to 'long tract signs' has been rarely reported in such cases and appears to be a mechanical effect produced by hypertrophied spinal roots. The muscles exhibit a simple atrophy. The pathological changes in Refsum's syndrome are similar, and a cardiomyopathy has been described in the latter disease by Cammermeyer (1956) and Gordon and Hudson (1959). It should also be noted that hypertrophy of peripheral nerves does not only occur in these two conditions. It has been observed in chronic diabetic neuritis and in recurrent post-infective polyneuropathy (*vide infra*).

AETIOLOGY

Although sporadic cases occur, the classical disease is invariably inherited. Russell and Garland (1930) have described fully developed or abortive cases in four generations of the same family. Croft and Wadia (1957) have followed up Russell and Garland's family, and consider that the inheritance of Dejerine and Sottas' malady is a Mendelian dominant. Although it is described as polyneuritis, it is unlikely that it is inflammatory in nature. In many ways, apart from the peripheral nerve enlargement, the condition closely resembles peroneal muscular atrophy clinically, but it seems that it could also be related to neurofibromatosis. The onset of symptoms usually occurs in childhood, but exceptionally is deferred until adult life. Refsum's disease, by contrast, like many other inherited metabolic disorders, is a condition of autosomal recessive inheritance.

SYMPTOMS

Symptoms may begin in childhood or adult life. Sensory symptoms are usually prominent in the early stages, and patients frequently complain of shooting pains in the limbs, which may be associated with a sense of numbness in the hands and feet. Difficulty in walking is often an early complaint. Muscular weakness and wasting develop as in polyneuritis symmetrically in the peripheral muscles of the limbs. Either the hands or the feet may be first affected, or both may suffer simultaneously. The wasting rarely extends above the knees or the elbows. Coarse fasciculation is frequently present in the affected muscles, which exhibit the reaction of degeneration. Claw-hand and claw-foot may follow the muscular atrophy, but pes cavus may be present as a congenital abnormality.

Cutaneous sensory loss of the 'glove and stocking' distribution is found, and postural sensibility is also impaired.

Argyll Robertson pupils have been described in a small proportion of cases, and the pupils, though reacting normally, may be small, probably on account of oculosympathetic paralysis. Nystagmus is frequently present. The deep reflexes are diminished or lost in the affected muscles; the plantar reflexes may be lost; exceptionally extensor plantar reflexes have been described but this is probably due to mechanical compression of the spinal cord (*vide supra*) (Symonds and Blackwood, 1962). Kyphoscoliosis is sometimes present, and arthropathic changes have been observed in the joints of the limbs. Palpable thickening of the peripheral nerves is a valuable diagnostic sign but is not invariably present. The cerebrospinal fluid protein may be raised.

DIAGNOSIS

There is little difficulty in making a correct diagnosis in a patient presenting the symptoms of a slowly progressive polyneuritis and in whom the peripheral nerves are thickened. The only common condition in which comparable thickening of the nerves occurs is neurofibromatosis, and in this disease it is rare to find palpable thickening of the deep nerves, such as the ulnar, and polyneuritic symptoms are absent. Leprosy, amyloidosis, and sarcoidosis are unlikely to cause confusion. The inherited disorder must also be distinguished from the other forms of metabolic or post-infective polyneuritis (e.g. diabetic and amyloid neuropathy and recurrent or post-infective polyneuritis) in which enlargement of nerves may occur. From these it can be differentiated by its familial incidence, and slow progressive course, and by the absence of the common causes of polyneuritis. Unless thickening of the nerves can be felt, it may be difficult or impossible to distinguish it from peroneal muscular atrophy. In this condition, as in other forms of demyelinating neuropathy, nerve conduction is markedly slowed. Biopsy of a superficial cutaneous nerve may help to settle the diagnosis.

PROGNOSIS

The course of the disease is extremely slow and is usually steadily progressive, though remissions may occur. When the onset is in childhood patients usually survive to adult life, becoming increasingly crippled, and finally bedridden. Death occurs from some intercurrent disease.

TREATMENT

No treatment is known to influence the course of the disease, but treatment on the lines indicated for polyneuritis will help to maintain the power of the limbs as long as possible.

REFERENCES

CAMMERMEYER, J. (1956) Neuropathological changes in hereditary neuropathies: manifestations of the syndrome heredopathia atactica polyneuritiformis in the presence of interstitial hypertrophic polyneuritis, *J. Neuropath. exp. Neurol.*, **15**, 340.

CROFT, P. B., and WADIA, N. H. (1957) Familial hypertrophic polyneuritis, *Neurology*, (*Minneap.*) **7**, 356.

DE BRUYN, R. S., and STERN, R. O. (1929) A case of the progressive hypertrophic polyneuritis of Dejerine and Sottas, with pathological examination, *Brain*, **52**, 84.

DEJERINE, J., and SOTTAS, J. (1893) Sur la névrite interstitielle hypertrophique et progressive de l'enfance, *C.R. Soc. Biol. (Paris)*, **50**, 63.

GORDON, N., and HUDSON, R. E. B. (1959) Refsum's syndrome—heredopathia atactica polyneuritiformis, *Brain*, **82**, 41.

HARRIS, W., and NEWCOMB, W. D. (1929) A case of relapsing interstitial hypertrophic polyneuritis, *Brain*, **52**, 108.

REFSUM, S. (1946) Heredopathia atactica polyneuritiformis, *Acta psychiat. scand.*, Suppl. 38.

RUSSELL, W. R., and GARLAND, H. G. (1930) Progressive hypertrophic polyneuritis, with case reports, *Brain*, **53**, 376.

SYMONDS, C. P., and BLACKWOOD, W. (1962) Spinal cord compression in hypertrophic neuritis, *Brain*, **85**, 251.

THOMAS, P. K., and LASCELLES, R. G. (1967) Hypertrophic neuritis, *Quart. J. Med.*, **36**, 223.

WELLER, R. O. (1967) An electron microscopic study of hypertrophic neuropathy of Dejerine and Sottas, *J. Neurol. Neurosurg. Psychiat.*, **30**, 111.

CHRONIC PROGRESSIVE POLYNEURITIS

The term 'chronic progressive polyneuritis' or 'slow chronic polyneuritis' (Harris, 1935) has been applied to rare cases of polyneuritis which cannot be attributed to any of the common toxic causes and which run a slowly progressive course. Nothing is known about the causation of this condition which may well be one of multiple aetiology. The pathological changes in the nervous system consist of widespread degeneration of the peripheral nerves, especially of their motor fibres. There is progressive weakness of the limbs, associated with some wasting, especially of the peripheral segments, and sensory loss of the type characteristic of polyneuritis. Pain is often less severe than in the more rapidly developing forms. The cranial nerves may be involved in the later stages, leading to dysarthria and dysphagia. Increase in the severity of the symptoms continues for a number of months and the disease may terminate fatally, as in one patient which was reported by Hyland and Russell (1930). Complete recovery, however, may occur or the disorder may become arrested, leaving the patient with some permanent muscular weakness, associated with contractures.

The number of cases so classified has gradually decreased over the years as modern methods of investigation have been employed. Many are probably related aetiologically to the post-infective variety and in such cases in which no cause for the neuritis can be demonstrated, a trial of corticosteroid drugs is always justifiable. Even so, there remain a small number of patients with poly-neuritis whose disease defies classification and whose condition fails to show a response to any form of treatment.

REFERENCES

HARRIS, W. (1935) Chronic progressive (endotoxic) polyneuritis, *Brain*, **58**, 368.
HYLAND, H. H., and RUSSELL, W. R. (1930) Chronic progressive polyneuritis, with report of a fatal case, *Brain*, **53**, 278.

RECURRENT POLYNEURITIS

Recurrent or relapsing polyneuritis is a rare form of polyneuritis, in which repeated attacks occur, usually separated by intervals of several years. Only a small number of such cases have been reported. Ungley (1933) reviewed the literature and reported three members of the same family who suffered from recurrent polyneuritis in pregnancy and the puerperium. Austin (1958) collected 30 cases from the literature and added two more. One of my patients was a boy of 15, whom I saw in his fourth attack, the first having occurred when he was 4 years of age, each attack being followed by complete recovery. In a middle-aged woman, who was seen in her third attack, there was some permanent muscular wasting and weakness. No cause could be found. In one-third of the cases col-lected by Austin there was thickening of the peripheral nerves. The cerebrospinal fluid protein may be raised. The recurrent form appears to be closely related to the chronic progressive and post-infective varieties and should receive the same treatment. Corticosteroids may give symptomatic relief.

REFERENCES

AUSTIN, J. H. (1958) Recurrent polyneuropathies and their corticosteroid treatment, *Brain*, **81**, 157.
UNGLEY, C. C. (1933) Recurrent polyneuritis, *J. Neurol. Psychopath*, **14**, 15.

POLYNEURITIS CRANIALIS

The term 'polyneuritis cranialis' has been used in two senses.

1. Certain of the cranial nerves may be involved in polyneuritis in association with the nerves of the limbs. The cranial nerves are commonly attacked in acute post-infective polyneuritis, but there is probably no form of polyneuritis in which cranial nerves may not suffer. They are usually symmetrically affected. The facial nerve is most frequently involved, leading to facial paralysis, which is usually bilateral, and next in frequency the bulbar nerves, leading to dysphagia, and the trigeminal. The oculomotor nerves are less frequently affected, and the optic nerves usually escape, though I have seen bilateral optic neuritis associated with severe polyneuritis. Exceptionally the cranial nerves may be alone affected in polyneuritis or there may be only slight involvement of the nerves of the limbs, indicated by paraesthesiae or diminution in the tendon reflexes.

2. The term 'polyneuritis cranialis' has also been applied to an inflammatory lesion of multiple cranial nerves within the skull. This usually follows osteomye-litis of the bones of the base of the skull or basal pachymeningitis secondary to

nasal sinusitis or chronic otitis media. The lesion may involve the anterior group, third, fourth, fifth, and sixth on one or both sides, or the posterior group, seventh to twelfth usually on one side only, but in some cases almost all the nerves may suffer. This condition must be distinguished from compression of multiple cranial nerves by neoplastic infiltration of the meninges. It must also be distinguished from the syndrome of multiple cranial nerve involvement, often beginning unilaterally, which may be seen in patients with nasopharyngeal carcinoma, in sarcoidosis or in other granulomatous meningitides including syphilis and torulosis. Unilateral or bilateral facial nerve palsy has been described as a complication of acute leukaemia and recurrent (often familial) unilateral or bilateral facial palsy, often associated with a congenitally fissured tongue, is often referred to as Melkersson's syndrome (Stevens, 1965).

REFERENCES

FISHER, M. (1956) An unusual variant of acute idiopathic polyneuritis (syndrome of ophthalmoplegia, ataxia and areflexia), *New Engl. J. Med.*, **255**, 57.

FORSTER, F. M., BROWN, M., and MERRITT, H. H. (1941) Polyneuritis with facial diplegia, *New Engl. J. Med.*, **225**, 51.

STEVENS, H. (1965) Melkersson's syndrome, *Neurology (Minneap.)*, **15**, 263.

TAYLOR, E. W., and McDONALD, C. A. (1932) The syndrome of polyneuritis with facial diplegia, *Arch. Neurol. Psychiat. (Chicago)*, **27**, 79.

VIETS, H. R. (1927) Acute polyneuritis with facial diplegia, *Arch. Neurol. Psychiat. (Chicago)*, **17**, 794.

YUDELSON, A. B. (1927) Facial diplegia in multiple neuritis, *J. nerv. ment. Dis.*, **65**, 30.

19

DISORDERS OF MUSCLE

THE ANATOMY AND PHYSIOLOGY OF MUSCLE

A VOLUNTARY muscle is composed of muscle fibres, each of which is a multi-nucleate cell, consisting of myofibrils, sarcoplasm, and a number of discrete intracellular organelles including mitochondria, ribosomes, and the sarcotubular system. Each fibre is enclosed within a sarcolemmal sheath, deep to which the muscle nuclei are situated and each has a motor end-plate in which the nerve fibre terminates. Under normal conditions muscle fibres never contract singly, but the functional unit of muscle activity is known as the motor unit, being that group of muscle fibres supplied by a single anterior horn cell and its motor nerve axon. Discharge of such a single anterior horn cell results in the simultaneous contraction of all of the muscle fibres which it innervates. Anatomical and physiological evidence (see Sissons, 1969) suggests that sometimes all of the muscle fibres of a motor unit may be localized within a single bundle of fibres or fasciculus, but more often several fasciculi, which may be widely separated within the muscle, may be innervated by a single anterior horn cell so that the components of the motor unit may be anatomically separated within the individual muscle. Contraction of the muscle fibres which make up a motor unit is preceded by electrical excitation of the fibre membranes. The appearance of this electrical activity in the electromyogram depends on physical factors such as the dimensions of the electrode used, as well as on the muscle chosen for examination. For example, in the biceps brachii of a healthy young adult, the electrical activity of a single motor unit usually appears as a di- or triphasic wave with a duration of 5–10 msec. and an amplitude of less than 250 μV; however, the variation in form, amplitude, and duration is considerable (see Buchthal, 1957). Recent evidence suggests that these so-called motor unit action potentials may on occasions be produced not by the electrical activity of the entire motor unit, but simply by the electrical activity of one of its component fasciculi which may be referred to as a sub-unit.

An important advance in our knowledge of the physiology of muscular contraction was the discovery of a humoral element in the transmission of the nerve impulse at the myoneural junction. It was Dale (1934) who first demonstrated that acetylcholine played an important part in this process. There is now good evidence to indicate that the synaptic vesicles in the motor nerve terminal are actually packets of acetylcholine. Single packets of acetylcholine are continually being released spontaneously and give rise to small depolarizations (miniature end-plate potentials) which can be recorded electrically with a micro-electrode in the region of the end-plate. The arrival of a nerve impulse at the motor end-plate results in the synchronous release of many packets of acetylcholine which produces a localized depolarization of the muscle fibre membrane in the region of the end-plate; this is the end-plate potential. When the end-plate potential reaches a certain critical size it triggers off an excitatory wave, the action potential, which then travels away from the end-plate along the surface membrane of the fibre (see Buller, 1969; Zaimis, 1969). At rest the inside of the fibre membrane is some 80 millivolts negative with respect to the outside, but during the action potential the polarization of the membrane momentarily reverses, so that for about one millisecond the inside of the fibre becomes positive. This reversal of electrical polarity is caused by increased sodium permeability of the fibre membrane. There is evidence that the wave of excitation spreads inwards into the substance of the muscle fibre along the transverse system of tubules, the 'T' system (see Huxley, 1964) and that the consequent mobilization of calcium ions in the sarcoplasmic reticulum initiates contraction of the myofibrils.

Ultrastructural investigations of skeletal muscle have demonstrated that the unit of structure of the individual myofibril is the sarcomere, extending from one Z-line (situated in the midst of the 'I'-band) to the next. Attached to each Z-line are a series of thin filaments of the protein actin. There is also a second type of filament which is rather thicker and is composed of myosin; these filaments correspond to the dark (birefringent) A-bands of the myofibrils. Each filament of myosin is surrounded by a hexagonal array of actin filaments; in addition, molecular cross-bridges reach out from the myosin to the actin filaments. It is thought that, during contraction, the cross-bridges repeatedly disengage and re-engage at successive sites on the actin filaments. The propulsion imparted to the actin filaments causes them to slide over the myosin filaments so as to inter-digitate more fully with the latter; in this way the whole myofibril, and conse-quently its parent fibre, shortens. The biochemical changes which accompany muscle contraction are extremely complicated (for recent reviews see Peachey, 1968, and Gergely, 1969) but it is plain that among the many biochemical reactions which occur, creatine phosphate is broken down in the presence of calcium to creatine and phosphate, and adenosine triphosphate (ATP) is broken down to adenosine diphosphate (ADP). The release of high-energy phosphate bonds provides much of the energy required for muscular contraction.

It is also important to recognize that skeletal muscles are not homogeneous in that in man they contain at least two main types of muscle fibre which are morphologically and histochemically distinct. One type of fibre, the so-called Type I fibre, tends to be somewhat smaller than the second type; it contains myofibrils which are generally somewhat slender and a high concentration of mitochondria. Histochemical stains demonstrate that this type of fibre contains a high concentration of enzymes such as succinic dehydrogenase which are con-cerned with aerobic metabolism. In the larger Type II fibre, whose myofibrils are generally more coarse and more widely dispersed, there are fewer mito-chondria and histochemical studies indicate that these fibres contain a higher concentration of glycogen and of enzymes such as phosphorylase and myofibrillar adenosine triphosphatase which are concerned with anaerobic metabolism. In man, all skeletal muscles contain an admixture of Type I and Type II fibres, so that in transverse sections stained histochemically, a characteristic checker-board pattern is observed (see Dubowitz, 1968). Physiological experiments also indicate that these fibres are functionally different. Thus in the animal kingdom it is known that there are certain muscles such as soleus which are made up predominantly of Type I fibres (so-called red muscle). These muscles are considered to be concerned largely with the maintenance of posture and, upon stimulation, are found to contract and relax relatively slowly. By contrast, other muscles concerned more directly with motor activity, such as the flexor digitorum longus, are made up predominantly of Type II fibres (white muscle) and are more rapidly contracting (fast 'twitch' muscles). Recent experiments (see Dubowitz, 1968) demonstrate that in some unknown manner the motor nerve appears to control not only the physiological behaviour, but also the histochemical structure, of the muscle fibres in that transposition of its motor nerve supply from a fast muscle to a slow muscle, and vice versa, may completely alter the physiological and histochemical characteristics of the muscle fibres.

Finally, before commenting upon individual diseases of muscle, it is important to mention briefly a number of drugs which may act upon the neuromuscular junction. Acetylcholine, when released at the neuromuscular junction, is broken down by cholinesterase which is normally present in the subneural apparatus and can be demonstrated histochemically. The drug curare acts on the post-junctional membrane, where it reduces or prevents the depolarizing effect of the transmitter excited by the nerve impulse (Hunt and Kuffler, 1950; Riker, 1953). Drugs such as physostigmine and neostigmine destroy cholinesterase and allow acetylcholine liberated at the myoneural junction to accumulate. Initially the accumulation of acetylcholine produces muscular contraction as a result of depolarization of the muscle fibre membrane, but if this substance accumulates in excess, the depolarization persists and may result in blockage of the muscle action potential (depolarization block). Whereas drugs such as tubocurarine and gallamine compete with acetylcholine for the end-plate chemical receptors and are thus known as competitive inhibitors, drugs such as decamethonium and suxamethonium produce muscle paralysis as a result of depolarization block (see Zaimis, 1969).

REFERENCES

BUCHTHAL, F. (1957) *An Introduction to Electromyography*, Copenhagen.
BULLER, A. J. (1969) Physiology of the motor unit, in *Disorders of Voluntary Muscle*, ed. WALTON, J. N., 2nd ed., London.
DALE, H. (1934) Chemical transmission of the effects of nerve impulses, *Brit. med. J.*, **2**, 835.
DUBOWITZ, V. (1968) *Developing and Diseased Muscle*, London.
GERGELY, J. (1969) Biochemical aspects of muscular structure and function, in *Disorders of Voluntary Muscle*, ed. WALTON, J. N., 2nd ed., London.
HUNT, C. C., and KUFFLER, S. W. (1950) Pharmacology of the neuromuscular junction, *Pharmacol. Rev.*, **2**, 96.
HUXLEY, A. F. (1964) Muscle, *Ann. Rev. Physiol.*, **26**, 131.
PEACHEY, L. D. (1968) Muscle, *Ann. Rev. Physiol.*, **30**, 401.
RIKER, W. F. (1953) Excitatory and anti-curare properties of acetyl choline and related quaternary ammonium compounds at the neuromuscular junction, *Pharmacol. Rev.*, **5**, 1.
SISSONS, H. A. (1969) Anatomy of the motor unit, in *Disorders of Voluntary Muscle*, ed. WALTON, J. N., 2nd ed., London.
ZAIMIS, E. (1969) The chemistry of neuromuscular transmission, in *Disorders of Voluntary Muscle*, ed. WALTON, J. N., 2nd ed., London.

GENERAL COMMENTS ON DISORDERS OF MUSCLE

The past 15 or 20 years have seen increasing world-wide interest in diseases of muscle. A comprehensive classification of the neuromuscular disorders has recently been produced by the Research Group on Neuromuscular Diseases of the World Federation of Neurology (1968). It includes, however, many disorders which affect muscle through disease of spinal cord, anterior horn cells, and peripheral nerves which have been dealt with in other parts of this volume (see CHAPTERS 13, 14, and 18). This chapter will therefore be concerned with those disorders which primarily affect voluntary muscle and the myoneural junction. The term 'myopathy' may reasonably be used (Walton, 1966) to define any disease or syndrome in which the patient's symptoms and/or physical signs can be attributed to pathological, biochemical, or electrophysiological changes which are occurring in the muscle fibres or in the interstitial tissues of the voluntary musculature and in which there is no evidence that the symptoms related to the muscular system are in any way secondary to disordered function of the central or peripheral nervous system. Within this group, therefore, are to be included many degenerative disorders which appear to be genetically determined, as well as others of a primary biochemical character and yet others in which the disease process appears to be essentially one of inflammation. The construction of this chapter will be different from many of the others in this book in that the clinical and genetic aspects of the various conditions to be considered are first described in turn, and the chapter concludes with commentaries upon differential diagnosis by means of clinical and investigative methods.

REFERENCES

RESEARCH GROUP ON NEUROMUSCULAR DISEASES (1968) Classification of the neuromuscular disorders, *J. neurol. Sci.*, **6**, 165.

WALTON, J. N. (1966) Diseases of muscle, *Abstr. Wld Med.*, **40**, 1, 81.

PROGRESSIVE MUSCULAR DYSTROPHY

Muscular dystrophy can be defined as genetically-determined primary degenerative myopathy (Walton, 1966; Walton and Gardner-Medwin, 1969), but this definition can no longer be regarded as being entirely satisfactory as there are a number of myopathies, to which reference will be made in this chapter, which are genetically determined but which are not normally regarded as being muscular dystrophies in the accepted sense of the term. However, this definition may reasonably be retained, despite its defects, as the condition appears to be due to some factor or factors present in the individual's genetic constitution from birth; pathological and other evidence indicates that the disease is primarily one of the muscle cell and the process is at present classified as being degenerative as there is no evidence available to indicate its fundamental nature, though it is widely presumed that it may in the end prove to be the result of the absence of one or more enzymes within the muscle cell.

CLASSIFICATION

Classification of the muscular dystrophies is by no means an academic matter as it is the only safe guide to prognosis and genetic counselling. The traditional clinico-anatomical classification of this group of diseases into the pseudohypertrophic, pelvic girdle atrophic, facioscapulohumeral, juvenile scapulohumeral, distal, ocular, late-life, and congenital forms has proved to be unsatisfactory both clinically and genetically, since if, for instance, one classifies all cases showing pseudohypertrophy into one group, this is then shown to be heterogeneous with several different forms of inheritance and little clinical uniformity. Important contributions to this problem have been made recently by Tyler and Wintrobe (1950), Stevenson (1953), Becker (1953, 1957), Walton and Nattrass (1954), Morton and Chung (1959), Dubowitz (1960), and Emery and Walton (1967). The most satisfactory clinico-genetic classification based upon current knowledge would appear to be that proposed by Walton and Gardner-Medwin (1969):

The 'pure' muscular dystrophies
  (*a*) X-linked muscular dystrophy
      Severe (Duchenne type)
      Benign (Becker type)
  (*b*) Autosomal recessive muscular dystrophy
      Limb-girdle types
      Childhood muscular dystrophy (except Duchenne)
      Congenital muscular dystrophies
  (*c*) Facioscapulohumeral muscular dystrophy
  (*d*) Distal muscular dystrophy
  (*e*) Ocular muscular dystrophy
  (*f*) Oculopharyngeal muscular dystrophy

Although this classification would seem to be the most satisfactory that can be devised based upon present knowledge, there are still a number of cases which are seen from time to time which are difficult to fit into any of the groups described. Many more detailed family studies will be required, using rigid clinical and genetic criteria, before a final and definitive classification can be achieved. Though the nature of the pathological process causing muscular weakness and wasting in these cases is similar in character, though different in tempo, in the various groups, there are other features such as differences in the pattern of muscular involvement and in the degree to which enzymes such as creatine kinase leak into the serum in the different varieties, which strongly suggest that they may in the end prove to be different diseases from the aetiological standpoint.

It will now be convenient to consider the general clinical features of the muscular dystrophies, before describing the distinctive clinical characteristics of the various sub-varieties.

CLINICAL FEATURES OF THE MUSCULAR DYSTROPHIES

These depend upon which muscles are first involved by the disease process and upon the rate of progress of the disease. Weakness in the muscles around the pelvic girdle characteristically gives rise to slowness in walking, inability to run, frequent falling, difficulty in climbing stairs or in rising from the floor and eventually the patients develop accentuation of the lumbar lordosis and a characteristic waddling gait. Climbing up the legs on rising from the floor (Gowers' sign) is a characteristic feature of the condition [FIG. 106] but is by no means specific for muscular dystrophy, as it occurs in any condition in which pelvic

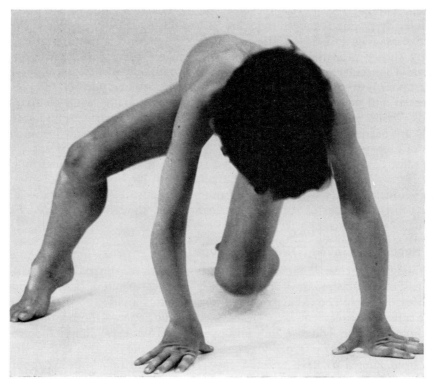

FIG. 106. A boy suffering from the Duchenne type muscular dystrophy rising from the floor

girdle muscles are weakened and thus may be seen in various benign forms of spinal muscular atrophy, congenital myopathy, and polymyositis. Weakness in the shoulder girdles gives an unusually sloping appearance of the shoulders with a tendency for the scapulae to rise prominently when the patient attempts to abduct the arms. Many patients utilize trick movements by placing one hand beneath the other elbow in an attempt to lift the hand to the face or head. Facial weakness in its characteristic form, as seen in the facioscapulohumeral variety, causes inability to whistle and to pout the lips or to close the eyes, while distal weakness (as seen in the distal variety) gives rise to weakness of grip and of fine finger movements and foot-drop. Contractures are a common feature of all forms of muscular dystrophy in the late stages, but are seen particularly in the severe Duchenne type. They may result from weakness developing in a group of muscles whose antagonists remain comparatively powerful (this explains the partial foot-drop with turning in of the feet and toes which is seen in advancing cases of the Duchenne type and which typically causes the children to walk on their toes; it results from progressive weakness of the anterior tibial group at a time when the calf muscles remain powerful). Contractures may also be due to postural changes which develop in a patient confined to a wheelchair; in such a situation the biceps and hamstrings show a particular tendency to shorten. One of the most important clinical characteristics of all forms of muscular dystrophy is that muscles are picked out by the disease in a curiously selective manner and this is also one of the most difficult features to explain on any theory of pathogenesis. Though there are certain differences in the pattern of muscular involvement seen in the various sub-varieties, it is common in the upper limbs, for instance, to find that the serrati and pectoral muscles are weakened and atrophic, as are biceps and brachioradialis, while deltoid and triceps remain relatively powerful. In the lower limbs quadriceps and anterior tibials are particularly weakened and the calf muscles are spared, but in some cases of limb-girdle muscular dystrophy the hamstrings and quadriceps appear to be affected to an equal degree. Such a selective pattern of muscular involvement is very strongly suggestive of muscular dystrophy, but a similar affection of individual muscles with sparing of others may also be seen in some of the more benign varieties of spinal muscular atrophy, though it is rarely as consistent.

The Severe X-Linked (Duchenne) Type

Although it is clear that this condition is due to a sex-linked recessive gene, over half of the affected boys appear to be isolated cases and in these individuals the disease is presumed to have resulted from genetic mutation occurring perhaps in the cells of one segment of the ovary in either the patient's mother or maternal grandmother. The evidence indicating sex-linked recessive inheritance comes first from the inspection of pedigrees, secondly from the fact that several women have been known to have affected children by more than one male, thirdly from the finding of families in which there is crossing-over with red-green colour blindness, and fourthly from the fact that two cases of the disease have now been reported in patients of female morphology suffering from Turner's syndrome (ovarian agenesis) with an XO chromosome constitution (Walton, 1956a; Ferrier, Bamatter, and Klein, 1965; Emery and Walton, 1967).

The condition usually first becomes clinically apparent towards the end of the third year of life with difficulty in walking, frequent falling, and difficulty in climbing stairs. The pelvic-girdle muscles are thus first affected, but involvement of the shoulder girdles soon follows. Enlargement of the calf muscles and sometimes of quadriceps, deltoids, and other muscles as well, occurs in about 90 per cent. of cases at some stage but later disappears as the disease advances. This enlargement has often been referred to as pseudohypertrophy in view of the fact that muscle biopsy may demonstrate, in some such muscles, a marked infiltration of fat, but there is good histological evidence now to suggest that in many cases this initial enlargement can be due to a true muscular hypertrophy with enlargement of individual muscle fibres. Most patients show slow progressive deterioration so that the majority are unable to walk by the time they are 10 years old. False or apparent clinical improvement may occur between the ages of 5 and 8 years, when the rate of deterioration due to the disease is apparently outstripped by the processes of normal physical development. Once the child is confined to a wheelchair, progressive deformity with muscular contractures and skeletal distortion and atrophy occur, and death usually results from inanition, respiratory infection, or cardiac failure towards the end of the second decade. Some of the children waste progressively, but some become excessively obese and no explanation for this discrepancy is forthcoming. Macroglossia is not infrequent and occasionally certain incisor teeth are absent. The intelligence quotient in these cases is 10 per cent. or more lower than in a group of control children of comparable age and sex (Dubowitz, 1965; Murphy, Thompson, Corey, and Conen, 1965). Marked skeletal atrophy and deformity occur and the shafts of long bones may become pencil-thin and fracture on minimal trauma (Walton and Warrick, 1954). Cardiac involvement is probably invariable in such cases, though it may not be detectable in the early stages. Persistent tachycardia is common and of particular importance is the characteristic electrocardiogram which shows tall R waves in the right precordial leads and deep Q waves in the limb leads and left precordial leads (Skyring and McKusick, 1961).

While as yet no effective treatment for this tragic progressive disorder has been discovered, and methods of management will be discussed later, an important recent advance has been the discovery that the female carriers of the gene can usually be detected by means of serum creatine kinase estimation, quantitative electromyography, and possibly muscle biopsy. This fact is of particular importance to the sisters of dystrophic boys, who have a 50-50 chance of being carriers. A carrier female, who may rarely show clinical evidence of minor degrees of muscle weakness and possibly enlargement of the calves, is likely to pass the disease on to half of her sons, and half her daughters will themselves be carriers; it is not, therefore, surprising that most young women who are found to be carriers decide not to have children. If all carriers can be detected and if most do not reproduce, then undoubtedly the incidence of the disease will fall in the future, though some cases will continue to arise as a result of genetic mutation. The principles of carrier detection and the recent literature on this topic have been reviewed recently by Gardner-Medwin (1968) and by Walton and Gardner-Medwin (1969).

The Benign X-Linked (Becker) Type of Muscular Dystrophy

The existence of a distinct benign X-linked recessive form of muscular dystrophy was first suggested by Becker and Kiener (1955) and subsequent reports have made it clear that the benign cases are distinct and not simply part of a spectrum of severity related to the Duchenne type. This disorder differs from the severe Duchenne variety in that the onset of the disease is usually between the fifth and twenty-fifth year, the disorder may be transmitted by affected males through carrier daughters to their grandsons, there is gradually progressive weakness and wasting of the pelvic and later of the pectoral muscles, and most patients become unable to walk 25 years or more after the onset.

Cardiac involvement is absent in most families, contractures and skeletal deformity occur late, if at all, and some such patients, though severely disabled, survive to a normal age.

Limb-Girdle Muscular Dystrophy

This form of the disease occurs equally in the two sexes and usually begins in the second or third decade of life, but occasionally first appears in middle life.

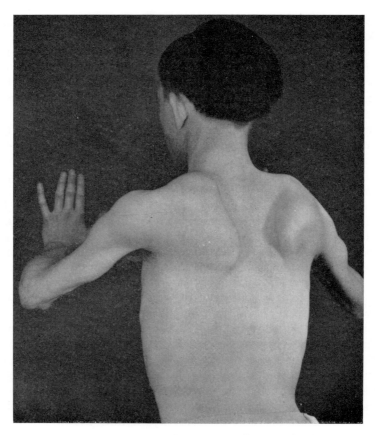

FIG. 107. A patient suffering from limb-girdle muscular dystrophy, demonstrating bilateral winging of the scapulae.

Though genetic evidence plainly indicates that in most families the condition is inherited by an autosomal recessive mechanism and that its incidence is therefore considerably increased by consanguinity, many cases are sporadic and it has been suggested that some may be due to manifestation in the heterozygote (Morton and Chung, 1959; Chung and Morton, 1959). In about half the cases, muscle weakness begins in the shoulder-girdle muscles [FIG. 107] and may then remain limited to these for many years before eventually spreading to involve the pelvic girdle. In the other half, by contrast, the pelvic-girdle muscles are first involved and as a rule the weakness spreads to the shoulders in about

10 years. Enlargement of calf muscles is not uncommon in these cases. The severity of the disease varies a good deal from case to case and from family to family. Often muscular weakness and wasting are asymmetrical initially, and sometimes the disease process appears temporarily to arrest, but in most patients the degree of disability is severe within 20 years of the onset. There is some evidence to suggest that in the patients in whom weakness begins in the upper limbs the disease runs a more benign course than in those in whom the pelvic-girdle muscles are first involved. There may be considerable difficulty in distinguishing cases beginning in the pelvic girdle on purely clinical grounds from cases of benign spinal muscular atrophy and from other forms of myopathy of metabolic origin; electromyography and muscle biopsy are of particular value in making the distinction. Contractures and skeletal deformity occur late in the course of this disease by comparison with the Duchenne type, but progress much more rapidly when the patient is unable to walk. Most sufferers are severely disabled in middle life and many die before the normal age.

Childhood Muscular Dystrophy with Autosomal Recessive Inheritance

This is one of the most difficult categories of muscular dystrophy to characterize. Proof of autosomal recessive inheritance is rarely possible and the arguments for the very existence of this condition have depended upon the occasional occurrence of muscular dystrophy in young girls and in a few families in which consanguinity of the parents has made autosomal recessive inheritance likely. It seems possible, indeed likely, that in some of the earlier cases which were reported, the condition may, in fact, have been one of benign spinal muscular atrophy which often affects girls and may mimic muscular dystrophy very closely. However, cases reported by Kloepfer and Talley (1958), Jackson and Carey (1961), and some of those described by Johnston (1964) seem convincing. This form of the disease is similar to the Duchenne type but rather more benign. The onset may be in the second year or as late as the fourteenth, but is most often in the second half of the first decade. Progression is comparatively slow and patients usually become unable to walk in their early twenties, but sometimes as early as 15 years or as late as 43 years. The pattern of weakness is very similar to that observed in the typical severe X-linked Duchenne type (Walton and Gardner-Medwin, 1969).

Congenital Muscular Dystrophy

It was Batten who in 1909 suggested that the syndrome of amyotonia congenita, as first described by Oppenheim (1900), might be due to a simple atrophic myopathy of congenital origin. However, he may well have been describing the condition which has been variously entitled benign congenital myopathy (Turner, 1940, 1949; Turner and Lees, 1962) or benign congenital hypotonia with incomplete recovery (Walton, 1956 b), a disorder which differs from the muscular dystrophies in its relatively non-progressive course and in the absence of specific histological abnormalities in the muscle fibres. However, Banker, Victor, and Adams (1957), Pearson and Fowler (1963), Gubbay, Walton, and Pearce (1966), and Zellweger, Afifi, McCormick, and Mergner (1967) describe cases with congenital hypotonia and severe, but relatively non-progressive, muscular weakness in which the muscle histology was typical of muscular dystrophy. In several of these children there were widespread contractures suggesting arthrogryposis multiplex congenita. The proper nosological status of these non-progressive muscle disorders remains uncertain, but in a few cases congenital muscular dystrophy is rapidly progressive and terminates fatally within the first year of life (Wharton, 1965). Patients with congenital dystrophy intermediate in severity between the static and rapidly progressive groups make it unlikely that sub-division on the grounds of severity alone is justifiable.

The essential features of this disorder are severe hypotonia present from birth with the subsequent development of more or less progressive muscular wasting and weakness. The diagnosis from spinal muscular atrophy of infancy can only be made with confidence by means of electromyography, serum enzyme studies, and muscle biopsy. Sibs are not infrequently affected, but more definite evidence of autosomal recessive inheritance of this disorder is lacking.

Facioscapulohumeral Muscular Dystrophy

This form, which is inherited by an autosomal dominant mechanism (Tyler and Wintrobe, 1950; Stevenson, 1953), occurs equally in the two sexes and can begin at any age from childhood until adult life, though it is usually recognized first in adolescence. A possible autosomal recessive mode of inheritance has been suggested in certain families, but if this does occur it is very uncommon. Facial involvement is apparent at an early stage and is generally accompanied by weakness of shoulder-girdle muscles, which is often remarkably selective with bilateral winging of the scapulae and involvement of the pectoral muscles but with sparing of others. Biceps and brachioradiales are often selectively involved and there is difficulty in raising the arms above the head. Muscular hypertrophy or pseudo-hypertrophy is uncommon but may occasionally be seen in the calves and deltoids. In the lower extremities many such patients show selective involvement of the anterior tibial muscles with bilateral foot-drop and some few, showing unusually rapid progress, demonstrate a particularly severe accentuation of the lumbar lordosis at a comparatively early stage of the disease. The condition which has been referred to as scapuloperoneal muscular dystrophy may be no more than a variant of this form, but on the other hand most cases of scapuloperoneal muscular atrophy have been shown to be due to neuropathic, as distinct from myopathic, changes. In most patients with facioscapulohumeral dystrophy the condition is benign, runs a prolonged course with periods of apparent arrest, and muscular contractures and skeletal deformity are late in developing. There are some patients in whom the disease process is apparently abortive and after certain muscles are selectively involved, the spread of weakness appears to cease spontaneously. The patients tend to show a very characteristic pouting appearance of the lips with a typical transverse smile; most affected individuals survive and remain active until a normal age. Cardiac involvement is rare and the range of intelligence is normal.

Distal Muscular Dystrophy

This form of the disease is rare in Britain and in the United States, but Welander (1951, 1957) has reported her experience of over 250 cases. In her experience the condition is inherited as an autosomal dominant character, begins usually between the ages of 40 and 60 years and affects both sexes, though it seems to be commoner in men than in women. Weakness begins in the small muscles of the hands and in the anterior tibial muscles and calves, but eventually spreads proximally, in contradistinction to the weakness observed in peroneal muscular atrophy (Charcot-Marie-Tooth disease) with which this disorder is most often confused. The condition in Sweden is comparatively benign and slowly progressive, but sporadic cases seen in other countries of the world tend to show a rather more rapid course and more severe disability (see Walton and Gardner-Medwin, 1969).

Ocular Myopathy

This disorder usually begins with progressive bilateral ptosis (Hutchinson, 1879; Fuchs, 1890; Kiloh and Nevin, 1951). It used to be generally referred to in the literature as progressive nuclear ophthalmoplegia, but it has been clearly demonstrated that the condition is due to a true myopathy of the external ocular muscles even when this occurs in patients also suffering from heredo-familial disease of the nervous system, some of whom also demonstrate pig-mentary retinal degeneration (Walsh, 1957). Diplopia is rare and in most cases bilateral external ophthalmoplegia develops slowly and progressively over a period of many years. Usually there is also some weakness of the upper facial muscles and often the neck and shoulder-girdle muscles are affected to some extent. The facial weakness is particularly severe in the orbicularis oculi, but is not as intense as that seen in facioscapulohumeral muscular dystrophy.

Oculopharyngeal Muscular Dystrophy

Victor, Hayes, and Adams (1962) separated those cases of ocular myopathy with dysphagia as a group to which they gave the name oculopharyngeal myopathy. Bray, Kaarsoo, and Ross (1965) supported this sub-division and defined the other distinguishing clinical features, of which the most valuable is the age of onset (mean 23 years for the ocular cases and 40 for the oculopharyn-geal). Many of the reported cases have been of French-Canadian stock (see Barbeau, 1966) and occasional cases, often sporadic, have occurred elsewhere. The inheritance in familial cases is dominant. The disorder bears some slight resemblances to dystrophia myotonica, not only in some of its clinical and genetic features, but in the probable involvement of smooth muscle (Lewis, 1966) and reports of abnormalities of immunoglobulins (Russe, Busey, and Barbeau, 1969) in some families.

MYOTONIC DISORDERS

Myotonia, which occurs not only in man but also in certain goats (Brown and Harvey, 1939), is the continued active contraction of a muscle which persists after the cessation of voluntary effort or stimulation; an electrical after-discharge in the electromyogram (EMG) can be seen to accompany the phenomenon. Clinically, it is best demonstrated as a slowness in relaxation of the grip or by a persistent dimpling after a sharp blow on a muscle belly (e.g. in the thenar eminence or tongue). It appears to be due to an abnormality of the muscle fibre itself as it persists after section or blocking of the motor nerve and after curarization (Denny-Brown and Nevin, 1941). Three hereditary syndromes, all with autosomal dominant inheritance, have been described, namely myotonia congenita, dystrophia myotonica, and paramyotonia congenita. Only in one of these, namely dystrophia myotonica, are dystrophic changes observed within some of the affected muscles. Transitional cases may be seen suggesting a close relationship between the three disorders, and Maas and Paterson (1950) suggested that these syndromes may be merely different manifestations of the same disorder. However, the difference between the course and prognosis of typical cases of dystrophia myotonica on the one hand and of myotonia congenita on the other, and the fact that in the vast majority of families the conditions breed true, suggest that for the present they should be regarded as different diseases. The evidence on this question has been reviewed by Caughey and Myrianthopoulos (1963). Further nosological problems arise over the close relationship between paramyotonia and the periodic paralyses. It seems clear that all of these disorders are more closely related to each other than they are to the pure muscular dystrophies.

In a rare and little-understood syndrome, a clinically similar but probably distinct phenomenon is associated with myokymia (benign coarse fasciculation), cramps, hyperhidrosis, and sometimes muscle wasting (Gamstorp and Wohlfart, 1959; Greenhouse et al., 1967). The cases of continuous muscle fibre activity described by Isaacs (1967) and Mertens and Zschocke (1965) seem to be similar. Although the failure of relaxation in these cases is similar to myotonia, no dimple is induced by percussion and electromyography shows that the after-discharge is different in form.

MYOTONIA CONGENITA

Myotonia congenita (Thomsen, 1876; Nissen, 1923; Thomasen, 1948) usually begins at birth but symptoms may be delayed until the end of the first or even into the second decade. Myotonia is usually generalized, giving painless stiffness which is accentuated by rest and cold and gradually relieved by exercise. It is particularly easy to demonstrate this phenomenon by asking the patient to grip firmly and then to relax, when difficulty in opening the hand will be experienced. The phenomenon can also be demonstrated by percussion of affected muscles and is often well seen in the thenar eminence and tongue; percussion in either situation results in the formation of a dimple in the muscle which only slowly disappears. Diffuse hypertrophy of muscles usually persists throughout life in these cases, though the myotonia tends to improve. Rarely myotonia may increase during exertion (myotonia paradoxa) when it must be distinguished from the cramping stiffness of McArdle's disease. Hypertrophia musculorum vera (Friedreich, 1863; Spiller, 1913) may well be a variant of this condition.

DYSTROPHIA MYOTONICA

Dystrophia myotonica (myotonia atrophica) was described by Steinert (1909) and Batten and Gibb (1909) and has been reviewed by Thomasen (1948) and

Caughey and Myrianthopoulos (1963). It is a diffuse systemic disorder in which myotonia and distal muscular atrophy are accompanied by cataracts, frontal baldness in the male [FIG. 108], gonadal atrophy, cardiomyopathy, impaired pulmonary ventilation, mild endocrine anomalies, bone changes, mental defect or dementia and abnormalities of the serum immunoglobulins. The affected families show progressive social decline in successive generations, diminished fertility, and an increased infantile mortality rate. The presenting symptom of the condition is usually weakness in the hands, difficulty in walking and frequent falling and myotonia is only rarely obtrusive. Poor vision, loss of weight,

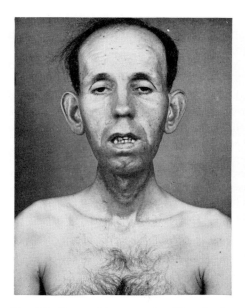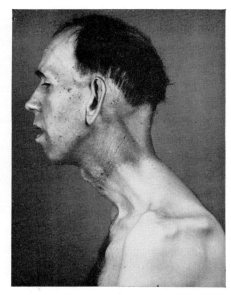

FIG. 108. Dystrophia myotonica. Note the frontal alopecia, myopathic facies and wasting of the sternocleidomastoids

impotence or loss of libido, ptosis and increased sweating are common. The condition is usually observed to begin between the ages of 20 and 50 but clinical features of the disorder may be recognized in offspring of affected individuals in the second decade. Recently it has become apparent that the condition may present in infancy and childhood with severe muscular weakness and hypotonia and delay in walking and these children may erroneously be regarded as examples of benign congenital hypotonia unless the existence of myotonic dystrophy in other members of the family is recognized (Pruzanski, 1966).

The facial appearance is characteristic [FIG. 108]; ptosis and involvement of other external ocular muscles may be seen. Wasting of the masseters, temporal muscles, and sternomastoids is almost invariable and in the extremities there is distal weakness and wasting involving mainly forearm muscles, the anterior tibial group and the calves and peronei. Slit-lamp examination reveals cataracts in about 90 per cent. of cases. Cardiac involvement is very common and the pulmonary vital capacity and maximum expiratory pressure are often impaired (Kilburn, Eagan, Sieker, and Heyman, 1959; Kaufman, 1965); as a result, many patients tolerate barbiturate anaesthesia poorly. Disordered oesophageal contraction can often be demonstrated by contrast radiography or manometry. The testes are usually small and histologically the changes in these organs resemble those of Klinefelter's syndrome though the nuclear sex is male. Irregular menstruation and infertility and prolonged parturition are common in affected females. Pituitary function is usually normal but there may be a selective failure of adrenal androgenic function and occasionally thyroid activity and glucose utilization are impaired (Marshall, 1959; Caughey and Myrianthopoulos, 1963). Hyperostosis of the skull vault, localized or diffuse, and a small sella turcica are frequent radiological findings (Jequier, 1950; Walton and Warrick, 1954). Both mental defect and progressive dementia occur. Rosman and Kakulas (1966) have described neuronal heterotopias in the brain at autopsy in 4 cases and investigation in life may reveal a high incidence of abnormality in the electro-encephalogram (Barwick, Osselton, and Walton, 1965) or progressive cerebral ventricular enlargement (Refsum, Lounum, Sjaastad, and Engeset, 1967). Excessive catabolism of immunoglobulin-G has been demonstrated in these patients by Wochner, Drews, Strober, and Waldmann (1966).

Most patients show progressive deterioration and become severely disabled and unable to walk within 15 to 20 years of the onset. Death from respiratory infection or cardiac failure usually occurs well before the normal age.

PARAMYOTONIA CONGENITA

This condition, first described by Eulenburg (1886), is characterized by myotonia which is apparent only on exposure to cold, and in addition the patients experience attacks of unexplained generalized muscular weakness similar to those of familial periodic paralysis. The condition is closely related to hyper-kalaemic periodic paralysis or adynamia episodica hereditaria (Gamstorp, 1956). Resnick and Engel (1967) have, however, described patients with myotonia who suffered attacks of periodic paralysis of the hypokalaemic variety. Thus although the nosological status of paramyotonia congenita remains confused (Pratt, 1967) it remains a useful diagnostic category for patients in whom myotonia and weakness are induced by cold, so long as it is recognized that the particular precipitants and any associated electrolyte changes in each family must be worked out if useful advice and treatment are to be given.

TREATMENT

Muscular Dystrophy

Regrettably there is no evidence that any form of drug treatment has any influence upon the course of muscular dystrophy. Many remedies have been tried in the past and have been found wanting and none is to be recommended for routine administration, though complications such as respiratory infection may demand appropriate antibiotics. There is good evidence to suggest that physical exercise is of value in delaying the march of the weakness and the onset of contractures and it is advisable to institute a regular programme of exercise, which may be started under the supervision of a skilled physiotherapist and subsequently continued at home by the patients, who, like their parents and other relatives, should be given appropriate instructions. Passive stretching of those tendons, such as the tendons of Achilles, which show a tendency to shorten, should also be carried out regularly, particularly in Duchenne type cases. In certain selected cases the wearing of light spinal supports is helpful in delaying skeletal deformity and occasionally calipers and night-splints are successful in helping affected individuals to walk for longer periods than they would otherwise be able to do. Recent evidence suggests that surgical division of the Achilles tendons in selected cases, a procedure which has long been regarded as being contra-indicated, may be beneficial, provided this is followed by immediate mobilization of the patient in walking plasters or calipers. Immobilization of patients with muscular dystrophy is in general to be avoided as far as ever possible as this frequently causes deterioration. Not least in importance is the psychological management of these patients which may demand considerable reserves of patience and understanding on the part of parents, doctors, nurses, and social workers. Optimism and encouragement, however unjustifiable in the face of continuing deterioration, are greatly needed.

Myotonia

In dystrophia myotonica, no treatment is known which will influence the progressive muscular wasting and weakness which eventually develops. In paramyotonia, the treatment of the attacks of periodic paralysis is similar to that required in patients with familial periodic paralysis and depends upon whether the paralysis is shown to be hypo- or hyperkalaemic in type. Myotonia itself may, however, be substantially relieved by means of appropriate drugs. These are particularly valuable in patients with myotonia congenita, but are also helpful in some with myotonic dystrophy in whom the myotonia is severe. Of drugs used in the past, including quinine, prednisone, and procainamide, the latter is probably the most successful in a dosage of 250–500 mg. three or four times daily, depending upon tolerance (Leyburn and Walton, 1959). Recently it has been shown (Munsat, 1967) that, if anything, hydantoin sodium (*Epanutin* or *Dilantin*) is even more successful in a dosage of 100 mg. three times daily.

REFERENCES

BANKER, B. O., VICTOR, M., and ADAMS, R. D. (1957) Arthrogryposis multiplex due to congenital muscular dystrophy, *Brain*, **80**, 319.

BARBEAU, A. (1966) The syndrome of hereditary late onset ptosis and dysphagia in French Canada, in *Progressive Muskeldystrophie, Myotonie, Myasthenie*, ed. KUHN, E., New York.

BARWICK, D. D., OSSELTON, J. W., and WALTON, J. N. (1965) Electroencephalographic studies in hereditary myopathy, *J. Neurol. Neurosurg. Psychiat.*, **28**, 109.

BATTEN, F. E. (1909) The myopathies or muscular dystrophies; critical review, *Quart. J. Med.*, **3**, 313.

BATTEN, F. E., and GIBB, H. P. (1909) Myotonia atrophica, *Brain*, **32**, 187.

BECKER, P. E. (1953) *Dystrophia Musculorum Progressiva*, Stuttgart.

BECKER, P. E. (1957) Neue Ergebnisse der Genetik der Muskeldystrophien, *Acta Genet. med. (Roma)*, **7**, 303.

BECKER, P. E., and KIENER, F. (1955) Eine neue x-chromosomale Muskeldystrophie, *Arch. Psychiat. Nervenkr.*, **193**, 427.

BRAY, G. M., KAARSOO, M., and ROSS, R. T. (1965) Ocular myopathy with dysphagia, *Neurology (Minneap.)*, **15**, 678.

BROWN, G. L., and HARVEY, A. M. (1939) Congenital myotonia in the goat, *Brain*, **62**, 341.

CAUGHEY, J. E., and MYRIANTHOPOULOS, N. C. (1963) *Dystrophia Myotonica and Related Disorders*, Springfield, Ill.

CHUNG, C. S., and MORTON, N. E. (1959) Discrimination of genetic entities in muscular dystrophy, *Amer. J. hum. Genet.*, **11**, 339.

DENNY-BROWN, D., and NEVIN, S. (1941) The phenomenon of myotonia, *Brain*, **64**, 1.

DUBOWITZ, V. (1960) Progressive muscular dystrophy of the Duchenne type in females and its mode of inheritance, *Brain*, **83**, 432.

DUBOWITZ, V. (1965) Intellectual impairment in muscular dystrophy, *Arch. Dis. Childh.*, **40**, 296.

EMERY, A. E. H., and WALTON, J. N. (1967) The genetics of muscular dystrophy, in *Progress in Medical Genetics*, ed. STEINBERG, A. G., and BEARN, A. G., Vol. V, New York.

EULENBURG, A. (1886) Ueber eine familiäre, durch sechs Generationen verfolgbare Form congenitaler Paramyotonie, *Neurol. Zbl.*, **5**, 265.

FERRIER, P., BAMATTER, F., and KLEIN, D. (1965) Muscular dystrophy (Duchenne) in a girl with Turner's syndrome, *J. med. Genet.*, **2**, 38.

FRIEDREICH, N. (1863) Ueber congenitale halbseitige Kopfhypertrophie, *Virchows Arch. path. Anat.*, **38**, 474.

FUCHS, E. (1890) Ueber isolierte doppelseitige Ptosia, *Arch. Ophthal. (Chicago)*, **36**, 234.

GAMSTORP, I. (1956) Adynamia episodica hereditaria, *Acta paediat. (Uppsala)*, Suppl. 108.

GAMSTORP, I., and WOHLFART, G. (1959) A syndrome characterised by myokymia, myotonia, muscular wasting and increased perspiration, *Acta psychiat. scand.*, **34**, 181.

GARDNER-MEDWIN, D. (1968) Studies of the carrier state in the Duchenne type of muscular dystrophy. 2. Quantitative electromyography as a method of carrier detection, *J. Neurol. Neurosurg. Psychiat.*, **31**, 124.

GREENHOUSE, A. H., BICKNELL, J. M., PESCH, R. N., and SEELINGER, D. F. (1967) Myotonia, myokymia, hyperhidrosis and wasting of muscle, *Neurology (Minneap.)*, **17**, 263.

GUBBAY, S. S., WALTON, J. N., and PEARCE, G. W. (1966) Clinical and pathological study of a case of congenital muscular dystrophy, *J. Neurol. Neurosurg. Psychiat.*, **29**, 500.

HUTCHINSON, J. (1879) An ophthalmoplegia externa or symmetrical immobility (partial) of the eye with ptosis, *Trans. med.-chir. Soc. Edinb.*, **62**, 307.

ISAACS, H. (1967) Continuous muscle fibre activity in an Indian male with additional evidence of terminal motor fibre abnormality, *J. Neurol. Neurosurg. Psychiat.*, **30**, 126.

JACKSON, C. E., and CAREY, J. H. (1961) Progressive muscular dystrophy: autosomal recessive type, *Pediatrics*, **28**, 77.

JEQUIER, M. (1950) Dystrophie myotonique et hyperostose cranienne, *Schweiz. med. Wschr.*, **80**, 593.

JOHNSTON, H. A. (1964) Severe muscular dystrophy in girls, *J. med. Genet.*, **1**, 79.

KAUFMAN, L. (1965) Respiratory function in muscular dystrophy, in *Research in Muscular Dystrophy*, 2nd series, London.

KILBURN, K. H., EAGAN, J. T., SIEKER, H. O., and HEYMAN, A. (1959) Cardiopulmonary insufficiency in myotonic and progressive muscular dystrophy, *New Engl. J. Med.*, **261**, 1089.

KILOH, L. G., and NEVIN, S. (1951) Progressive dystrophy of external ocular muscles (ocular myopathy), *Brain*, **74**, 115.

KLOEPFER, H. W., and TALLEY, C. (1958) Autosomal recessive inheritance of Duchenne type muscular dystrophy, *Ann. hum. Genet.*, **22**, 138.

LEWIS, I. (1966) Late-onset muscular dystrophy: oculopharyng-oesophageal variety, *Canad. med. Ass. J.*, **95**, 146.

LEYBURN, P., and WALTON, J. N. (1959) The treatment of myotonia: a controlled trial, *Brain*, **82**, 81.

MAAS, O., and PATERSON, A. S. (1950) The identity of myotonia congenita, dystrophia myotonica and paramyotonia, *Brain*, **73**, 318.

MARSHALL, J. (1959) Observations on endocrine function in dystrophia myotonica, *Brain*, **82**, 221.

MERTENS, H. G., and ZSCHOCKE, S. (1965) Neuromyotonie, *Klin. Wschr.*, **43**, 917.

MORTON, N. E., and CHUNG, C. S. (1959) Formal genetics of muscular dystrophy, *Amer. J. hum. Genet.*, **11**, 360.

MUNSAT, T. L. (1967) Therapy of myotonia: a double-blind evaluation of diphenyl-hydantoin, procainamide and placebo, *Neurology (Minneap.)*, **17**, 359.

MURPHY, E. G., THOMPSON, M. W., COREY, P. N. J., and CONEN, P. E. (1965) Varying manifestations of Duchenne muscular dystrophy in a family with affected females, in *Muscle*, ed. PAUL, W. M., DANIEL, E. E., KAY, C. M., and MONCKTON, G., New York.

NISSEN, K. (1923) Beiträge zur Kenntnis der Thomsen'schen Krankheit (myotonia congenita) mit besonderer Berücksichtigung des hereditären Momentes und seiner Beziehungen zu den Mendelschen Vererbungsregeln, *Z. klin. Med.*, **96**, 58.

OPPENHEIM, H. (1900) Ueber allgemeine und localisierte Atonie der Muskulatur (mya-tonie) in frühen Kindesalter, *Mschr. Psychiat. Neurol.*, **8**, 232.

PEARSON, C. M., and FOWLER, W. G. (1963) Hereditary non-progressive muscular dystrophy inducing arthrogryposis syndrome, *Brain*, **86**, 75.

PRATT, R. T. C. (1967) *The Genetics of Neurological Disorders*, London.

PRUZANSKI, W. (1966) Variants of myotonic dystrophy in pre-adolescent life (the syndrome of myotonic dysembryoplasia), *Brain*, **89**, 563.

REFSUM, S., LOUNUM, A., SJAASTAD, O., and ENGESET, A. (1967) Dystrophia myotonica: repeated pneumoencephalographic studies in ten patients, *Neurology (Minneap.)*, **17**, 345.

RESNICK, J. S., and ENGEL, W. K. (1967) Myotonic lid lag in hypokalaemic periodic paralysis, *J. Neurol. Neurosurg. Psychiat.*, **30**, 47.

ROSMAN, N. P., and KAKULAS, B. A. (1966) Mental deficiency associated with muscular dystrophy. A neuropathological study, *Brain*, **89**, 769.

RUSSE, H., BUSEY, H., and BARBEAU, A. (1969) Immunoglobulin changes in oculopharyngeal muscular dystrophy, *Proc. 2nd Internat. Congr. Neurogenetics*, Montreal.

SKYRING, A., and McKUSICK, V. A. (1961) Clinical, genetic and electrocardiographic studies in childhood muscular dystrophy, *Amer. J. med. Sci.*, **242**, 534.

SPILLER, W. G. (1913) The relation of the myopathies, *Brain*, **36**, 75.

STEINERT, H. (1909) Myopathologische Beiträge: I. Ueber das klinische und anatomische Bild des Muskelschwunds der Myotoniker, *Dtsch. Z. Nervenheilk.*, **37**, 58.

STEVENSON, A. C. (1953) Muscular dystrophy in Northern Ireland, *Ann. Eugen. (Lond.)*, **18**, 50.

THOMASEN, E. (1948) *Thomsen's Disease, Paramyotonia, Dystrophia Myotonica*, Aarhus.

THOMSEN, J. (1876) Tonische Krämpfe in willkürlich beweglichen Muskeln in Folge von ererbter psychischer Disposition (ataxia muscularis?), *Arch. Psychiat. Nervenkr.*, **6**, 706.

TURNER, J. W. A. (1940) The relationship between amyotonia congenita and congenital myopathy, *Brain*, **63**, 163.

TURNER, J. W. A. (1949) On amyotonia congenita, *Brain*, **72**, 25.

TURNER, J. W. A., and LEES, F. (1962) Congenital myopathy—a fifty year follow-up, *Brain*, **85**, 733.

TYLER, F. H., and WINTROBE, M. M. (1950) Studies in disorders of muscle. I. The problem of progressive muscular dystrophy, *Ann. intern. Med.*, **32**, 72.

VICTOR, M., HAYES, R., and ADAMS, R. D. (1962) Oculopharyngeal muscular dystrophy. A familial disease of late life characterised by dysphagia and progressive ptosis of the eyelids, *New Engl. J. Med.*, **267**, 1267.

WALSH, F. B. (1957) *Clinical Neuro-ophthalmology*, 2nd ed., London.

WALTON, J. N. (1956 *a*) The inheritance of muscular dystrophy: further observations, *Ann. hum. Genet.*, **21**, 40.

WALTON, J. N. (1956 *b*) Amyotonia congenita: a follow-up study, *Lancet*, i, 1023.

WALTON, J. N. (1966) Diseases of muscle, *Abstr. Wld Med.*, **40**, 1, 81.

WALTON, J. N., and GARDNER-MEDWIN, D. (1969) Progressive muscular dystrophy, in *Disorders of Voluntary Muscle*, ed. WALTON, J. N., 2nd ed., London.

WALTON, J. N., and NATTRASS, F. J. (1954) On the classification, natural history and treatment of the myopathies, *Brain*, **77**, 169.

WALTON, J. N., and WARRICK, C. K. (1954) Osseous changes in myopathy, *Brit. J. Radiol.*, **27**, 1.

WELANDER, L. (1951) Myopathia distalis tarda hereditaria, *Acta med. scand.*, Suppl. 264, 1.

WELANDER, L. (1957) Homozygous appearance of distal myopathy, *Acta Genet. med. (Roma)*, **7**, 321.

WHARTON, B. A. (1965) An unusual variety of muscular dystrophy, *Lancet*, i, 603.

WOCHNER, R. D., DREWS, G., STROBER, W., and WALDMANN, T. A. (1966) Accelerated breakdown of immunoglobulin G (IgG) in myotonic dystrophy: a hereditary error of immunoglobulin catabolism, *J. clin. Invest.*, **45**, 321.

ZELLWEGER, H., AFIFI, A., McCORMICK, W. F., and MERGNER, W. (1967) Severe congenital muscular dystrophy, *Amer. J. Dis. Child.*, **114**, 591.

INFLAMMATORY DISORDERS OF MUSCLE

SPECIFIC INFECTIONS

Voluntary muscle may be involved as a secondary effect of suppuration arising in skin, bone, or connective tissue and widespread necrosis frequently occurs following trauma as a result of infection with the anaerobic organism of gas gangrene. Some viral infections may give rise to an acute myositis and this is particularly common in infection with certain viruses of the Coxsackie type. Thus in the syndrome often called Bornholm disease, pain in the muscles of the trunk and diaphragmatic involvement, giving pain on deep breathing and coughing, are frequently seen but the disorder is self-limiting and usually recovers within a few days. Muscle is only rarely involved in parasitic infestations, but muscular pain and weakness may occur in South American trypanosomiasis and in trichinosis, which usually develops after the ingestion of infested pork. Fleeting muscle pain and tenderness may be accompanied by peri-orbital oedema and *Trichinella spiralis* may be detected on muscle biopsy.

MUSCULAR INVOLVEMENT IN COLLAGEN OR CONNECTIVE TISSUE DISEASES

In cases of rheumatoid arthritis, pathological examination of muscle biopsy sections often demonstrates foci of inflammatory cell infiltration, but this focal nodular myositis is rarely accompanied by any specific muscular wasting and weakness save for that resulting secondarily from joint disease. In sarcoidosis, however, muscular involvement may be so widespread that occasional patients with this affliction present with a subacute weakness and wasting of proximal muscles and typical sarcoid granules may be observed on muscle biopsy (see Pearson, 1969). In polyarteritis nodosa, severe localized muscle pain, subcutaneous oedema, and tenderness may occur as a result of muscle infarction. Focal nodular myositis may occur in disseminated lupus erythematosus, but in occasional cases muscular involvement is more severe and diffuse and this syndrome may reasonably then be identified as one of polymyositis, although in occasional such cases histological investigation reveals a vacuolar myopathy (Pearson and Yamazaki, 1958).

POLYMYOSITIS

The classification and nosological status of polymyositis remains somewhat controversial. This name is usually given to identify a group of cases in which muscular wasting and weakness occurs and is sometimes associated with local muscle pain, tenderness and wasting or with evidence of some form of connective tissue or collagen disease. Muscle biopsy generally demonstrates areas of muscle fibre necrosis accompanied by interstitial or perivascular cellular infiltrates or both, though these are not invariable. The term is commonly used to include cases with florid skin change, which are more properly called dermatomyositis; it is usually taken to indicate the so-called idiopathic syndrome and excludes disorders such as polymyalgia rheumatica (*vide infra*) and also acute myositis resulting from infections with micro-organisms and viruses. The relationship of the myopathies seen in sarcoidosis, Sjogren's disease, and bronchogenic carcinoma to polymyositis is still somewhat obscure (Pearson, 1969), though with the exception of the specific myasthenic-myopathic syndrome (*vide infra*) which has been observed in patients with lung cancer, it seems probable that most cases of so-called carcinomatous myopathy in reality belong with the syndrome of polymyositis (Rose and Walton, 1966). Denny-Brown (1960) and Shy (1962) have suggested that such polymyopathies should be identified according to their aetiology and pathological characteristics. However, Walton and Adams (1958), Barwick and Walton (1963), and Rose and Walton (1966) concluded that the term 'polymyositis' should be retained as in many cases the aetiology of the condition remains obscure despite full investigation. Furthermore, a response to steroid therapy, suggesting a relationship to diseases of the connective tissue group, occurs in some patients in whom muscle biopsy findings are very non-specific. There is evidence to suggest that in occasional cases of polymyositis, involvement of distal branches of peripheral nerves occurs, possibly within the muscle, and these cases may reasonably be described as examples of neuromyositis (McEntee and Mancall, 1965).

AETIOLOGY

The recent work of Dawkins (1965) and Kakulas (1966) demonstrating that polymyositis may be produced in animals by the injection of muscle homogenates with Freund's adjuvant supports the view that this syndrome in the human may well be the result of hypersensitivity or of auto-immune processes. It is thus possible to suggest that polymyositis in which there is no clinical evidence to suggest that any tissue other than muscle is involved may be an organ-specific auto-immune disease, while in cases showing involvement of skin or joints it may be regarded as being a feature of a non-organ-specific auto-immune disease. The clear-cut relationship between polymyositis and dermatomyositis on the one hand, and malignant disease on the other, also suggests that the condition may sometimes be the result of a conditioned auto-immune response in patients suffering from cancer. However, attempts to demonstrate antimuscle antibodies in the serum of patients with polymyositis have to date failed to confirm the presumed auto-immune character of the disease (Stern, Rose, and Jacobs, 1967). The close relationship of the condition to other disorders of the connective tissue group can, however, be underlined by the occurrence of certain cases which may successively present manifestations of polymyositis, disseminated lupus erythematosus, and/or scleroderma or systemic sclerosis.

CLASSIFICATION

The original clinical classification proposed by Walton and Adams (1958), as modified by Rose and Walton (1966), seems to be reasonably satisfactory for clinical assessment and is given below:

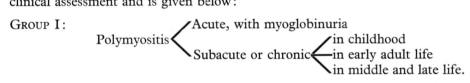

GROUP I:
Polymyositis — Acute, with myoglobinuria — Subacute or chronic — in childhood — in early adult life — in middle and late life.

GROUP II: Polymyositis with dominant muscular weakness but with some evidence of an associated collagen disease or dermatomyositis with severe muscular disability and with minimal or transient skin changes.

GROUP III: Polymyositis complicating severe collagen disease, e.g. rheumatoid arthritis, or dermatomyositis with florid skin changes and minor muscle weakness.

GROUP IV: Polymyositis complicating malignant disease (including 'carcinomatous myopathy' and dermatomyositis occurring in patients with malignant disease).

It must be accepted that some of the cases classified arbitrarily in these groups, and particularly some with myoglobinuria, as well as progressive cases of late onset, may be due to metabolic abnormalities unrelated aetiologically to the group of collagen or connective tissue disorders in which most cases of polymyositis rightfully belong.

INCIDENCE

Polymyositis is world-wide, occurs in many races and appears to be commoner in men. It is more common in adult life than muscular dystrophy, but is less common than the latter in childhood. About 15 per cent. of cases occur under the age of 15, another 15 per cent. between the ages of 16 and 30, about a quarter between 31 and 45, and a third between the ages of 46 and 60. The condition usually occurs spontaneously, but may follow a variety of febrile illnesses and has been known to develop after the administration of various drugs, including sulphonamides or following exposure to sunlight.

CLINICAL MANIFESTATIONS

Detailed analyses of the clinical manifestations of polymyositis have been given by many authors (Eaton, 1954; Garcin, Lapresle, Gruner, and Scherrer, 1955; Pearson and Rose, 1960; Barwick and Walton, 1963; Pearson, 1964). Muscle pain and tenderness occur in approximately 50 per cent. of cases, as does dysphagia. Cutaneous manifestations are seen in about two-thirds of all patients and may take the form of widespread erythema with desquamation seen particularly on the face and on other exposed areas of the trunk, but occasionally involving almost the whole body. A particularly characteristic heliotrope erythema around the eyes, together with periorbital oedema, is seen in some patients, as is congestion of the nail beds. In some cases the skin changes are slight and may take the form of no more than a faint butterfly-type rash on the face, while in others, particularly in childhood, there may be ulceration over bony prominences with subcutaneous calcification; the latter on occasion can be very extensive (calcinosis universalis). Raynaud's syndrome is a common association and many younger patients develop thickening and loss of elasticity of the skin over the fingers, face and anterior chest wall resembling those of generalized scleroderma or acrosclerosis.

In about a quarter of the patients joint pain and stiffness may be observed. Proximal limb muscles are almost invariably involved and it is characteristic that the neck muscles are weak in about two-thirds of all cases so that patients may have difficulty in holding up the head. Specific involvement of distal limb muscles, without proximal weakness, is uncommon, but weakness may be generalized in about a third of all cases, and in under a third contractures eventually develop. Facial weakness and involvement of external ocular muscles occur rarely. Occasionally myasthenic fatigability is striking and is partially responsive to edrophonium or neostigmine, but treatment with these and related drugs usually produces only temporary improvement. The deep tendon reflexes may be depressed in the affected muscles but are often surprisingly brisk despite the severity of the muscular weakness.

PROGNOSIS

Even without treatment the course of the illness is variable. Sometimes it runs a fluctuating course with spontaneous exacerbations and remissions; progressive deterioration with a fatal termination within a few weeks or months of the onset is seen particularly in acute dermatomyositis, but in some patients spontaneous arrest has been seen. However, before the introduction of steroid drugs, the over-all mortality of the disease was about 50 per cent. Slow insidious progression is seen, particularly in middle age, but spontaneous recovery may occur in childhood (Nattrass, 1954).

In a recent review of 89 cases observed and studied in north-east England, Rose and Walton (1966) found that 16 per cent. of their patients had associated malignant disease. Seventy-five patients in their series had received adequate steroid therapy and in the great majority the treatment was followed by subjective and objective clinical improvement accompanied by a progressive reduction in serum enzyme activity. Withdrawal of treatment during the first two years after the onset sometimes resulted in relapse. Most patients required treatment for at least three years and no deaths occurred under the age of 30. Most of the children and young adults recovered completely, but after the age of 30 a number of patients went on to develop evidence of diffuse connective tissue disease unresponsive to treatment, while after the age of 50 malignant disease which was present in a high proportion of cases adversely affected the prognosis.

TREATMENT

The condition should usually be treated with 60 mg. of prednisone daily, given for 4 or 5 days, thereafter reducing the dose to 40 mg. daily when clinical improvement appears and subsequently regulating the maintenance dose according to the level of serum creatine kinase activity and the clinical response. Occasionally even higher doses of prednisone may be required for short periods, and in resistant cases ACTH, 80 Units daily, is worth trying as an alternative and has the advantage in childhood of having less effect in the suppression of growth. Maintenance therapy may have to be continued for many years before the drug can be withdrawn. Respiratory and urinary infection should be treated with appropriate antibiotics and in occasional severe cases intermittent positive pressure respiration is necessary. Following the acute stage, active and passive movements carried out under the supervision of a skilled physiotherapist are valuable.

POLYMYALGIA RHEUMATICA

Polymyalgia rheumatica (Bagratuni, 1953; Gordon, 1960; Todd, 1961) occurs almost always in elderly patients whose principal complaint is one of widespread muscular pain, often with local tenderness, minor constitutional upset, and sometimes general malaise. Muscle weakness is not present as a rule, though pain may be so severe that movement is restricted and many patients are wrongly diagnosed as suffering from polymyositis. Difficulty in getting out of a bath or out of a low chair without help is characteristic. Muscle biopsy usually reveals normal muscle. Some patients go on to develop rheumatoid arthritis and Paulley and Hughes (1960) and others have suggested that there is a close relationship between this condition and cranial arteritis, which may develop in others. In all patients the erythrocyte sedimentation rate is substantially raised, but the electromyogram, serum enzyme studies, and muscle biopsy are usually negative. The response to steroid therapy is usually immediate and dramatic. The condition may well prove to be a disorder of intramuscular connective tissue rather than of muscle itself.

REFERENCES

BAGRATUNI, L. (1953) Polymyalgia rheumatica, *Ann. rheum. Dis.*, **12**, 98.
BARWICK, D. D., and WALTON, J. N. (1963) Polymyositis, *Amer. J. Med.*, **35**, 646.
DAWKINS, R. L. (1965) Experimental myositis associated with hypersensitivity to muscle, *J. Path. Bact.*, **90**, 619.
DENNY-BROWN, D. (1960) The nature of polymyositis and related muscular diseases, *Trans. Coll. Phycns Philad.*, **28**, 14.

EATON, L. M. (1954) The perspective of neurology in regard to polymyositis; study of 41 cases, *Neurology (Minneap.)*, **4**, 245.

GARCIN, R., LAPRESLE, J., GRUNER, J., and SCHERRER, J. (1955) Les polymyosites, *Rev. neurol.*, **92**, 465.

GORDON, I. (1960) Polymyalgia rheumatica, *Quart. J. Med.*, **116**, 473.

KAKULAS, B. A. (1966) Destruction of differentiated muscle cultures by sensitized cells, *J. Path. Bact.*, **91**, 495.

McENTEE, W. J., and MANCALL, E. L. (1965) Neuromyositis: a reappraisal, *Neurology (Minneap.)*, **15**, 69.

NATTRASS, F. J. (1954) Recovery from muscular dystrophy, *Brain*, **77**, 549.

PAULLEY, J. W., and HUGHES, J. P. (1960) Giant-cell arteritis, or arteritis of the aged, *Brit. med. J.*, **2**, 1562.

PEARSON, C. M. (1964) Polymyositis and related disorders, in *Disorders of Voluntary Muscle*, ed. WALTON, J. N., London.

PEARSON, C. M. (1969) Polymyositis and related disorders, in *Disorders of Voluntary Muscle*, ed. WALTON, J. N., 2nd ed., London.

PEARSON, C. M., and ROSE, A. S. (1960) Myositis, the inflammatory disorders of muscle, *Res. Publ. Ass. nerv. ment. Dis.*, **38**, 422.

PEARSON, C. M., and YAMAZAKI, J. N. (1958) Vacuolar myopathy in systemic lupus erythematosus, *Amer. J. clin. Path.*, **29**, 455.

ROSE, A. L., and WALTON, J. N. (1966) Polymyositis: a survey of 89 cases with particular reference to treatment and prognosis, *Brain*, **89**, 747.

SHY, G. M. (1962) The late onset myopathy, *Wld Neurol.*, **3**, 149.

STERN, G. M., ROSE, A. L., and JACOBS, K. (1967) Circulating antibodies in polymyositis, *J. neurol. Sci.*, **5**, 181.

TODD, J. W. (1961) Polymyalgia rheumatica, *Lancet*, ii, 1111.

WALTON, J. N., and ADAMS, R. D. (1958) *Polymyositis*, Edinburgh.

MYASTHENIA GRAVIS

Definition. A chronic disease with a tendency to remit and to relapse, characterized by abnormal muscular fatigability which may for a long time be confined to, or predominant in, an isolated group of muscles and is later associated in many cases with permanent weakness of some muscles. The fatigability is due to a disorder of conduction at the myoneural junction which can be temporarily relieved by neostigmine and similar drugs, and in some cases permanently benefited by removal of the thymus gland. Early descriptions were given by Wilks (1877) and Erb (1879), while the present name was coined by Jolly (1895). Walker (1934) was the first to describe the beneficial effect of physostigmine, and the first successful thymectomy was performed by Blalock in 1936.

CLASSIFICATION

As Simpson (1969) has pointed out, the symptom of myasthenia is not peculiar to one disease. Similar fatigability can be observed in muscles affected by polymyositis, systemic lupus, dermatomyositis, and one type of carcinomatous myopathy (*vide infra*). However, a therapeutic response to anticholinesterase drugs is necessary for the definition of true myasthenia gravis, and although some response may be found in the symptomatic myasthenias, it is rarely dramatic and often fails within a few weeks. Myasthenia gravis is therefore a clearly-recognizable disease in which the response to appropriate drugs is dramatic and sustained and it is one which has an individual natural history and pathology.

INCIDENCE AND NATURAL HISTORY

Myasthenia occurs in all races and affects both sexes, but is seen in women twice as often as in men (Osserman, 1958). Only occasionally is it seen in more than one member of the same family. The mean age of onset is about 26 years in women and 30 years in men, but the condition may sometimes arise for the first time in childhood and occasionally as late as 80 years. It often arises without apparent cause, but occasionally follows emotional upset, physical stress, febrile illness, or pregnancy. Most remissions occur within the first 5 years of the disease process, and most deaths also occur within this period. After the disease has been in progress for 10 years, death from myasthenia itself is rare and in many instances the disease is apparently burnt out by this stage (Simpson, 1969).

There is a close relationship between myasthenia gravis and thyrotoxicosis and the two diseases occur in combination in the same individual far more often than can be accounted for by chance. The condition which has been called acute thyrotoxic bulbar palsy is almost certainly due in most cases to myasthenia affecting bulbar muscles in a thyrotoxic individual.

Neonatal myasthenia is seen in about one in seven of the children born to myasthenic mothers, but in those who survive it usually recovers in between a week and three months after birth and does not recur.

SYMPTOMS AND SIGNS

The muscles most often affected by the disease are the external ocular, bulbar, neck and shoulder-girdle muscles in this descending order, but it is not uncommon to find that those of respiration and the proximal muscles of the lower extremities are also involved. The onset is usually gradual and ptosis of one or both upper lids is often the first symptom and is soon associated with diplopia due to paralysis of one or more of the external ocular muscles. These symptoms typically appear in the evening when the patient is tired and disappear after a night's rest. When the bulbar muscles are first involved, difficulty in swallowing and/or in chewing is described, again most evident in the course of a meal, and speech may become indistinct when the patient is tired.

On examination unilateral or bilateral ptosis is often found and is intensified by asking the patient to gaze upwards. Weakness of the external ocular muscles is usually asymmetrical and may progress to complete external ophthalmoplegia of one or both eyes. Occasionally conjugate ocular movements appear to be affected, but more often there is no functional relationship between the muscles involved in the two eyes. Paresis of accommodation has been described and the pupillary reflexes are usually normal but may be sluggish or exhibit fatigability.

The facial muscles are almost always seen to be affected. Weakness of the orbicularis oculi is a relatively constant sign; in the lower face the retractors of the angles of the mouth tend to suffer more than the elevators, so that a characteristic myasthenic snarling appearance on smiling is seen [FIG. 109]. Weakness of the jaw muscles leads to difficulty in chewing and weakness of the muscles of the soft palate, pharynx, tongue, and larynx to difficulty in swallowing and in articulation. The characteristic fatigability of speech may be demonstrated by asking the patient to count up to 50, during which time speech becomes

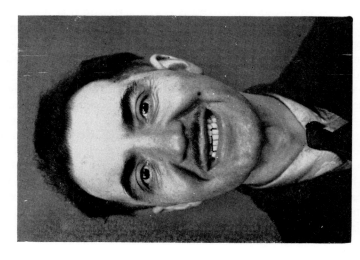

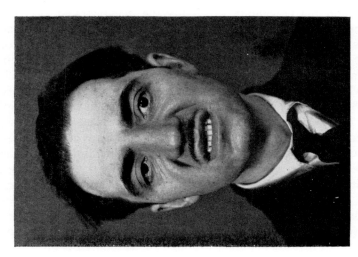

FIG. 109. Myasthenia gravis: facial movements before and after an injection of neostigmine. Note also the disappearance of ptosis and strabismus

progressively less distinct and palatal weakness may give a nasal character to the voice and occasional regurgitation of fluids through the nose on swallowing. Typically, weakness of the neck muscles tends to cause the head to fall forward, a sign seen most often in myasthenia gravis but also observed in some cases of polymyositis. In severe cases the weakness of the upper limbs is such that the hands cannot be lifted to the mouth and it is characteristic that muscle power may initially be reasonably satisfactory, but after testing a particular movement on several occasions, the strength rapidly declines. Breathlessness is always a sinister symptom in patients with myasthenia, as respiratory weakness may develop rapidly and may even cause sudden death.

Muscular wasting is not usually observed in the early stages, but in long-standing cases of myasthenia it is common to find permanent weakness and wasting, irreversible by drugs, in the external ocular muscles and in certain limb muscles, particularly the triceps brachii. While in the majority of cases muscular weakness eventually becomes widespread throughout the muscles of the head and neck, trunk and limbs, Grob (1953) and Ferguson, Hutchinson, and Liversedge (1955) have shown that in some cases the disease appears to remain limited to the external ocular muscles and never spreads to those of the bulb or limbs.

It is a notable feature of myasthenia gravis that the tendon reflexes almost always remain brisk, even in the presence of severe weakness.

DIAGNOSIS

The diagnosis of myasthenia depends not only upon the characteristic clinical picture and upon the fatigability which may be demonstrated electrically by means of repetitive supramaximal stimulation of a nerve such as the ulnar, with simultaneous recording of the evoked muscle potential from the hypothenar muscles, but also upon the clinical response to an injection of neostigmine or edrophonium hydrochloride. The quick-acting edrophonium hydrochloride (*Tensilon*), which is given initially in a dosage of 2 mg., followed immediately by a further 8 mg. intravenously if there is no severe reaction, has now supplanted neostigmine for diagnostic purposes (Osserman and Kaplan, 1953). Provocative tests designed to increase myasthenia, utilizing such drugs as curare and quinine, are dangerous and are rarely required. Churchill-Davidson and Richardson (1952) showed that myasthenic patients are abnormally resistant to the action of depolarizing neuromuscular blocking drugs such as decamethonium and that tolerance is particularly marked in clinically-unaffected muscles. However, depolarization block, if it occurs at all, is brief and soon changes to a longer competitive (curare-like) type of block. This dual response in the child or adult is characteristic of myasthenia gravis, though the response obtained in normal neonates is similar (Churchill-Davidson and Wise, 1963). This particular provocative test is rarely necessary for diagnosis.

AETIOLOGY

Simpson (1960) drew attention to the interrelationship between myasthenia gravis and a number of other diseases, including thyroid disorders, diabetes, rheumatoid arthritis, systemic lupus, and sarcoidosis. He suggested that myasthenia was probably an auto-immune disorder and that the thymus might produce an antibody against muscle end-plate protein. Strauss, Seegal, Hsu, Burkholder, Nastuk, and Osserman (1960) demonstrated a muscle-binding globulin in myasthenic serum and Marshall and White (1961) showed that direct injection of bacterial antigen into the guinea-pig thymus produced a histological reaction similar to that of myasthenia. Desmedt (1957) suggested that the lesion is presynaptic as the disorder of function is closely simulated by the administration of hemicholinium which impairs acetylcholine synthesis, while Dahlbäck, Elmqvist, Johns, Radner, and Thesleff (1961) demonstrated in their studies of isolated intercostal muscles removed from myasthenic and control patients, that there appeared to be a disturbance of transmitter formation or release. These and many other observations suggest that some kind of auto-immune response may prevent the proper release or formation of acetylcholine at the motor end-plate. The presence of morphological abnormalities in terminal nerve endings in myasthenic muscle (Coërs and Desmedt, 1959; Bickerstaff and Woolf, 1960) is as yet unexplained. Despite the suggestion that neonatal myasthenia must be due to a circulating toxin, possibly released from the thymus (Wilson, Obrist, and Wilson, 1953) no such substance has been demonstrated, but the existence of such a toxin, even if established, would not controvert the auto-immune theory.

TREATMENT

The standard treatment for myasthenia gravis is still neostigmine or the closely-related drug pyridostigmine (*Mestinon*). The usual dosage of neostigmine is to begin by giving a 15 mg. tablet three or four times a day, and almost always it is necessary to give in addition atropine, 0·6 mg. twice daily, to overcome the muscarinic side-effects of the drug. Recent evidence suggests that the long-acting *Mestinon*, which has been used by many workers in the past in combination with neostigmine which has seemed to act more quickly, is probably preferable as the standard medication and the initial dosage is 60 mg. three or four times daily, again with atropine or propantheline. The dosage is then steadily increased until maximum benefit is obtained. Some patients find that it is best to take the tablets every two hours, while some require them three-hourly. Other drugs which have been utilized in recent years include ambenonium hydrochloride (*Mytelase*) of which the usual dosage is 10–25 mg. three or four times daily. ACTH, immunosuppressive drugs, aldosterone inhibitors, and potassium chloride have all had their advocates (see Simpson, 1969) but none of these seem superior to the standard medication. Ephedrine sulphate is often used as an adjuvant in a dosage of 25 mg. three times daily.

The differential diagnosis between myasthenic and cholinergic crises, in which rapidly increasing muscular weakness occurs and in which serious respiratory weakness may threaten life, can be a matter of considerable difficulty. The most useful single test is to give an intravenous injection of edrophonium. If this increases muscle power, then it is likely that the weakness is myasthenic and requires more treatment, while if it reduces muscle power it is likely that the weakness is cholinergic and that treatment must be reduced. Any hint of impending respiratory insufficiency may be an indication for withdrawal of all drugs and for assisted respiration with positive pressure apparatus and tracheostomy. Unfortunately some patients show a differential sensitivity of different muscles to various drugs. It is not unknown to find that a sufficient dose of pyridostigmine which improves power in the limb muscles may be sufficient to cause cholinergic paralysis of the diaphragm.

The place of thymectomy is still in some doubt. Simpson (1958, 1969) has reviewed the problem in detail and has pointed out that thymectomy benefits both sexes but that the extent of improvement is greatest in women, who would otherwise have a worse prognosis than men. Benefit following the operation may occur at any time, but the results are best in young women with a short history suffering from severe myasthenia. However, it would appear that any patient who is deteriorating despite optimum medication has nothing to lose in the hands of an experienced surgeon and may improve. The prognosis for life seems to be worse if a thymoma is present and radiotherapy is generally recommended to the thymus in these cases before operation. Even after thymectomy, two out of three patients with a thymoma die within five years, but the survivors may benefit to the same extent as those without a tumour.

THE MYASTHENIC-MYOPATHIC SYNDROME

This syndrome is generally associated with oat-cell carcinoma of the bronchus, though it has been occasionally described in patients with carcinoma in other sites. The clinical picture is usually one of subacute muscular fatigability with weakness and wasting affecting the proximal parts of the limbs and trunk, but occasionally the external ocular and bulbar muscles are involved (Rooke, Eaton, Lambert, and Hodgson, 1960). The weakness is often myasthenic in the sense that the patient complains of increased enfeeblement after exertion, but it has been observed in many such cases that muscle power may in fact increase after brief exercise, a reversed myasthenic effect. In contrast to true myasthenia gravis, the condition is only slightly improved by treatment with neostigmine or pyridostigmine, though there may be definite improvement in strength after an injection of edrophonium hydrochloride. However, the tendon reflexes in this condition, unlike those in true myasthenia, are almost always depressed or absent. In contrast to the findings in true myasthenia gravis, repetitive stimulation of motor nerves at tetanic rates may cause an increase in the amplitude of the evoked potentials in the hypothenar muscles and these patients are excessively sensitive to decamethonium. Not only is the progressive potentiation in muscular strength which follows an initial period of fatigue after exercise a distinguishing feature of this condition, but it has recently been shown (McQuillen and Johns, 1966) that the muscular weakness and fatigability may be greatly improved by the administration of guanidine, which has no convincing effect in true myasthenia gravis. Guanidine hydrochloride is given orally in a dose of 20–50 mg./kg. body weight (Lambert, 1966).

REFERENCES

Bickerstaff, E. R., and Woolf, A. L. (1960) The intramuscular nerve endings in myasthenia gravis, *Brain*, **83**, 10.

Churchill-Davidson, H. C., and Richardson, A. T. (1952) The action of decamethonium iodide (C.10) in myasthenia gravis, *J. Neurol. Neurosurg. Psychiat.*, **15**, 129.

CHURCHILL-DAVIDSON, H. C., and WISE, R. P. (1963) Neuromuscular transmission in the newborn infant, *Anaesthesiology*, **24**, 271.

COËRS, C., and DESMEDT, J. E. (1959) Mise en évidence d'une malformation caractéristique de la jonction neuromusculaire dans la myasthénie, *Acta neurol. belg.*, **59**, 539.

DAHLBÄCK, O., ELMQVIST, D., JOHNS, T. R., RADNER, S., and THESLEFF, S. (1961) An electrophysiologic study of the neuromuscular junction in myasthenia gravis, *J. Physiol. (Lond.)*, **156**, 336.

DESMEDT, J. E. (1957) Bases physiopathologiques du diagnostic de la myasthénie par le test de Jolly, *Rev. neurol.*, **96**, 505.

ERB, W. H. (1879) Ueber einen eigenthümlichen bulbaren (?) Symptomcomplex, *Arch. Psychiat. Nervenkr.*, **60**, 172.

FERGUSON, F. R., HUTCHINSON, E. C., and LIVERSEDGE, L. A. (1955) Myasthenia gravis. Results of medical management, *Lancet*, ii, 636.

GROB, D. (1953) Course and management of myasthenia gravis, *J. Amer. med. Ass.*, **153**, 529.

JOLLY, F. (1895) Ueber Myasthenia Gravis Pseudoparalytica, *Klin. Wschr.*, **32**, 1.

LAMBERT, E. H. (1966) Defects of neuromuscular transmission in syndromes other than myasthenia gravis, *Ann. N.Y. Acad. Sci.*, **135**, 367.

McQUILLEN, M. P., and JOHNS, R. J. (1966) The nature of the defect in the Eaton-Lambert syndrome, *Neurology (Minneap.)*, **17**, 527.

MARSHALL, A. H. E., and WHITE, R. G. (1961) Experimental thymic lesions resembling those of myasthenia gravis, *Lancet*, i, 1030.

OSSERMAN, K. E. (1958) *Myasthenia Gravis*, New York.

OSSERMAN, K. E., and KAPLAN, L. I. (1953) Studies in myasthenia gravis. Use of edrophonium chloride (Tensilon) in differentiating myasthenic from cholinergic weakness, *Arch. Neurol. Psychiat. (Chicago)*, **70**, 385.

ROOKE, E. D., EATON, L. M., LAMBERT, E. H., and HODGSON, C. H. (1960) Myasthenia and malignant intrathoracic tumor, *Med. Clin. N. Amer.*, **44**, 977.

SIMPSON, J. A. (1958) An evaluation of thymectomy in myasthenia gravis, *Brain*, **81**, 112.

SIMPSON, J. A. (1960) Myasthenia gravis: a new hypothesis, *Scot. med. J.*, **5**, 419.

SIMPSON, J. A. (1969) Myasthenia gravis and myasthenic syndromes, in *Disorders of Voluntary Muscle*, ed. WALTON, J. N., 2nd ed., London.

STRAUSS, A. J. L., SEEGAL, B. C., HSU, K. C., BURKHOLDER, P. M., NASTUK, W. L., and OSSERMAN, K. E. (1960) Immunofluorescence demonstration of a muscle binding, complement-fixing serum globulin fraction in myasthenia gravis, *Proc. Soc. exp. Biol. (N.Y.).*, **105**, 184.

WALKER, M. B. (1934) Treatment of myasthenia gravis with physostigmine, *Lancet*, i, 1200.

WILKS, S. (1877) Bulbar paralysis; fatal; no disease found, *Guy's Hosp. Rep.*, **37**, 54.

WILSON, A., OBRIST, A. R., and WILSON, H. (1953) Some effects of extracts of thymus glands removed from patients with myasthenia gravis, *Lancet*, ii, 368.

ENDOCRINE AND METABOLIC MYOPATHIES

ENDOCRINE MYOPATHIES

DISORDERS OF THE THYROID GLAND

Thyrotoxic Myopathy

Chronic thyrotoxic myopathy was first described by Bathurst in 1895 and it is well recognized that in severe cases of thyrotoxicosis weakness and wasting of proximal limb muscles, particularly in the upper extremities, may occur and may resolve when the thyroid disease is effectively treated. Ramsay (1965) described clinical and electromyographic studies carried out on 54 consecutive unselected patients with proven thyrotoxicosis and demonstrated that while few complained of muscular weakness, clinical examination showed demonstrable weakness in over 80 per cent. and the electromyogram showed a reduced mean action potential duration and a higher percentage of polyphasic potentials in more than 90 per cent. of cases. Four months after treatment of the thyrotoxicosis the EMG had returned to normal in most patients. These findings suggest that in thyrotoxicosis there is almost always a reversible abnormality of muscle function and that electromyography, using an objective technique, is probably the most sensitive indicator of this change.

Exophthalmic Ophthalmoplegia

Exophthalmic ophthalmoplegia, or endocrine exophthalmos, must be mentioned as the principal effect of this disorder is upon the external ocular muscles, which are greatly increased in bulk, as are the orbital contents as a whole. The subject was reviewed in detail by Brain (1959). The main symptoms are exophthalmos and diplopia and the degree of ophthalmoplegia is usually proportional to the severity of the exophthalmos. Sometimes the latter is so great [FIG. 110] that the eyelids cannot be closed and corneal ulceration ensues. Papilloedema may occur and, if not relieved, may progress to optic atrophy and blindness. In severe cases surgical decompression of the orbit is required and sometimes must be carried out as an emergency. Medical and hormonal treatment have been in general disappointing, but radiotherapy to the orbit or pituitary gland, or both, is sometimes of value.

Thyrotoxicosis and Myasthenia Gravis

About 5 per cent. of myasthenic patients have, or later develop, thyrotoxicosis (McArdle, 1969). Engel (1961) noted that myasthenia may become worse when hyperthyroidism increases. Both conditions must be treated in the usual manner, but it should be noted that the risks of thyroidectomy are greatly increased in patients suffering from myasthenia gravis.

Thyrotoxic Periodic Paralysis

An association between thyrotoxicosis and periodic paralysis has been observed, particularly among the Japanese. Okinaka and his colleagues (1957), in a study of 6,333 cases of hyperthyroidism, found that 8·9 per cent. of the males and 0·4 per cent. of the females had had attacks of periodic paralysis which were of hypokalaemic type. Adequate treatment of the hyperthyroidism results in the disappearance of the periodic attacks of weakness or in a marked decrease in their number and severity (Norris, Panner, and Stormont, 1968).

Myopathy in Hypothyroidism

Muscular hypertrophy with weakness and slowness of muscular contraction and relaxation has been described in children suffering from sporadic cretinism (Debré and Semelaigne, 1935). When a similar condition occurs in adults it is known as Hoffman's syndrome (Hoffman, 1896) and Wilson and Walton (1959) described cases in which the clinical evidence of hypothyroidism was relatively unobtrusive and the muscular symptoms predominated. This syndrome may superficially resemble myotonia and has then been called pseudomyotonia (Crispell and Parson, 1954) but it has also been shown that sometimes hypothyroidism may be superimposed upon a pre-existing and virtually symptomless myotonia congenita (Jarcho and Tyler, 1958). Recently, Astrom, Kugelberg, and

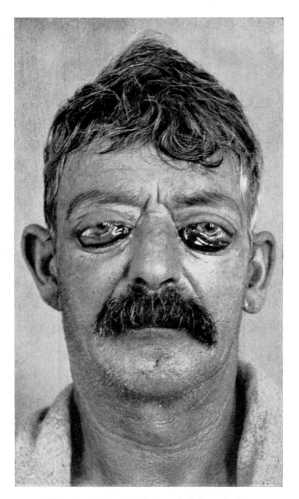

FIG. 110. Exophthalmic ophthalmoplegia

Müller (1961) have suggested that myxoedema may occasionally be associated with a true girdle myopathy causing mild proximal weakness and wasting similar to that seen in chronic thyrotoxic myopathy. In their cases improvement was observed on treatment with thyroxine.

DISORDERS OF THE PITUITARY AND ADRENAL GLANDS

In acromegaly and pituitary gigantism, generalized muscular weakness may be observed but is rarely an outstanding feature (Adams, Denny-Brown, and

Pearson, 1962). Similarly, widespread weakness with some atrophy has been described in hypopituitarism (Walton, 1960), but the exact nature of the myopathic change in such cases remains to be elucidated (Shy, 1960). General weakness is also seen in some cases of Addison's disease and is probably the result of the changes in plasma and muscle water and electrolytes. Treatment of the condition leads to a rapid improvement in muscular strength and no permanent muscle changes have been described in this disorder, though Witts, Lakin, and Thompson (1938) and Thorn (1949) noted contractures at the elbows and knees occurring in occasional cases of Addison's disease and suggested that these were due to changes of unknown nature occurring in the fasciae and tendons.

Cushing's Syndrome and Steroid Myopathy

In 1959 Müller and Kugelberg (1959) described six patients with Cushing's syndrome of whom five had weakness of the muscles of the pelvic girdle and thighs. Electromyography demonstrated myopathic changes in the affected muscles, and in the same year Perkoff et al. (1959) reported cases of muscle weakness and wasting occurring in patients under treatment with steroids. Since then both the naturally-occurring myopathy and the iatrogenic disorder have been frequently reported (Shy, 1960), and it seems that the latter is most often caused by steroids such as triamcinolone which have a fluorine atom in the 9α position (Harman, 1959). A similar syndrome has been described in patients receiving dexamethasone and betamethasone (Golding, Murray, Pearce, and Thompson, 1961); usually in such cases weakness resolves when prednisone is substituted, though occasional cases have been reported (Perkoff, Silber, Tyler, Cartwright, and Wintrobe, 1959) in which the latter drug has itself been responsible. Coomes (1965) has examined electromyographically 50 patients receiving corticosteroid drugs and has compared his findings with those obtained in a series of control individuals. He found that the mean action potential duration of motor action potentials obtained from one deltoid muscle was markedly reduced in patients showing striking side-effects of steroid therapy. He concluded that corticosteroid myopathy is commonest in those patients who show most side-effects of the treatment and that measurement of the mean action potential duration in the EMG recorded from an appropriate muscle appears to be a reliable method of detecting early myopathic change. Current evidence suggests that the myopathy quickly resolves once the steroid treatment is withdrawn.

ACTH Myopathy

Prineas et al. (1968) have reported the development of proximal muscle weakness and wasting in a series of pigmented patients who had undergone adrenalectomy for the treatment of Cushing's disease. Investigation clearly demonstrated that these patients were suffering from a myopathy and muscle biopsy sections showed a striking accumulation of fat within individual muscle fibres. It was concluded that this myopathy was the result of an excessive amount of circulating ACTH.

METABOLIC MYOPATHIES

Myopathy in Metabolic Bone Disease

Prineas, Mason, and Henson (1965) described two patients with chronic muscular weakness, one of whom had a parathyroid adenoma with osteomalacia and the other was found to be suffering from osteomalacia and idiopathic steatorrhoea. The main clinical features were proximal muscular wasting and weakness, pain and discomfort on movement, with hypotonia and brisk tendon reflexes. They suggested that in these cases a disturbance of vitamin D metabolism could interfere with the excitation-contraction coupling involving the entry of calcium into the muscle fibre during contraction. Similar cases have been described by Smith and Stern (1967).

Glycogen Storage Disease of Muscle

In 1951 McArdle described the case of a man of 30 who had generalized muscular pain and stiffness which increased during slight exertion. He showed that the blood lactate and pyruvate levels failed to rise after exercise and suggested that the disorder was due to a defect of glucose utilization. In 1959 two additional cases were reported (Schmid and Mahler, 1959; Mommaerts, Illingworth, Pearson, Guillory, and Seraydarian, 1959) and one of these also showed myoglobinuria. In both cases the muscle glycogen content was increased and myophosphorylase activity was absent. Mellick, Mahler, and Hughes (1962) described another case of myophosphorylase deficiency in which there was permanent muscular weakness in the girdle muscles, and Schmid and Hammaker (1961) described three cases in a single family in which the pattern of inheritance suggested an autosomal recessive mechanism; recently Adamson, Salter, and Pearce (1967) have also described 3 cases of variable severity in a single family. Engel, Eyerman, and Williams (1963) described 2 patients, one of whom had severe muscular weakness and wasting without cramps developing in late life, while a second, also in middle age, developed cramps after exercise without weakness and wasting and both patients showed a partial defect of muscle phosphorylase activity with a normal total glycogen content in the muscle.

It has become increasingly apparent in recent years that other forms of muscle glycogenosis, though rare, are more common than was at one time realized. In a child of 4 with a diffuse myopathy, Thomson, MacLaurin, and Prineas (1963) demonstrated a defect of phosphoglucomutase, and more recently Tarui et al. (1965) have also described a myopathic disorder resembling McArdle's disease which was demonstrated to be the result of phosphofructokinase deficiency. It has been well recognized that the condition now called limit dextrinosis (Illingworth, Cori, and Cori, 1956) gives glycogen storage in liver, skeletal muscle, and in heart and is due to a deficiency of debranching enzyme (amylo-1,6-glucosidase). This condition, however, like Pompe's disease which gives rise to glycogen storage in the heart, skeletal muscles, and central nervous system and which is due to amylo-1,4-glucosidase (acid maltase) deficiency, is usually incompatible with survival beyond the first few years of life. However, it has become apparent quite recently that acid maltase deficiency may be much less grave in its prognosis and several cases are now on record in which the patients presented with an apparently progressive myopathy of girdle muscles in late childhood or in adult life (Zellweger *et al.*, 1965; Courtecuisse *et al.*, 1965; Hudgson *et al.*, 1968). Thus the possible diagnosis of glycogen storage disease of muscle must now be considered in all cases of suspected limb-girdle muscular dystrophy arising in middle life, and muscle biopsy may be diagnostic as striking vacuolation of muscle fibres is usually thereby revealed and the vacuoles contain large quantities of glycogen. It seems more than probable that in the years to come, many more specific myopathic disorders related to individual enzyme defects may well be defined. Unfortunately none of these conditions yet appears to be amenable to any form of effective treatment.

It should also be mentioned that myopathy resulting from severe and prolonged hypoglycaemia has been described in patients suffering from islet cell adenoma of the pancreas (Mulder, Bastron, and Lambert, 1956).

PERIODIC PARALYSIS SYNDROMES

Hypokalaemic Periodic Paralysis

The classical hypokalaemic variety of periodic paralysis has been well recognized for many years and recently has been reviewed by McArdle (1969). This condition gives rise to attacks of flaccid weakness of the voluntary muscles but those of speech, swallowing, and respiration are usually spared. Attacks most often begin in the second decade and are most frequent in early adult life. Commonly they last for several hours and often start early in the morning on waking, after a period of rest following exertion, or after a heavy carbohydrate meal. During attacks the plasma potassium level is usually found to be low (less than 3 mEq./l.); there is positive balance of potassium and some or all of the retained potassium seems to pass into the muscle cell (Grob, Liljestrand, and Johns, 1957; Zierler and Andres, 1957). Shy *et al.* (1961) have shown that the resting membrane potential is normal during an attack of paralysis, and these authors and Pearce (1964) have demonstrated that electron microscopy of muscle biopsy specimens taken during an attack shows vacuoles resulting from dilatation of the sarcoplasmic reticulum. Conn and Streeten (1960) suggested that this form of periodic paralysis might be due to intermittent aldosteronism as it is well recognized that patients with primary aldosteronism due to tumours of the adrenal (Conn, 1955) do have attacks of muscular weakness. However, aldosteronism can be distinguished from periodic paralysis by the associated hypertension, alkalosis, and hypernatraemia and by the persistence of the hypokalaemia between the attacks; furthermore, in familial periodic paralysis increased aldosterone excretion is not usually found. Administration of potassium chloride, 4–6 G. daily, is the treatment of choice for attacks of the hypokalaemic type but rarely seems to shorten the episodes of weakness. Spironolactone, 25 mg. four times daily, and other aldosterone antagonists have been found, however, to reduce greatly the frequency and severity of the attacks (Poskanzer and Kerr, 1961 *a*). Occasionally in these cases muscular weakness is curiously localized to one or more muscle groups and sometimes after frequent episodes of weakness permanent atrophy of muscles develops, but on the whole the patients tend to improve spontaneously as they grow older.

Hyperkalaemic Periodic Paralysis (Adynamia Episodica Hereditaria)

In 1951 Tyler, Stephens, Gunn, and Perkoff described a group of cases in which the serum potassium level did not fall during the attacks and the patients were made worse by potassium chloride. Helweg-Larsen, Hauge, and Sagild (1955) described a similar condition and Gamstorp (1956) described two families containing such cases and entitled the condition adynamia episodica hereditaria (hyperkalaemic periodic paralysis is probably a more satisfactory title (Klein, Egan, and Usher, 1960)). This condition is closely related to paramyotonia for some of the patients show definite myotonia (Drager, Hammill, and Shy, 1958; Van der Meulen, Gilbert, and Kane, 1961) though in others the myotonia seems curiously limited to the muscles around the eye and can be evoked by placing ice-bags on the eyelids, a manoeuvre which tends to give a remarkable degree of lid-lag. Van't Hoff (1962) has referred to such cases as examples of myotonic periodic paralysis. In affected individuals the attacks are usually much shorter in duration than in the hypokalaemic variety, lasting on an average 30–40 minutes, and they may be precipitated immediately by exercise. Commonly there is a rise in the serum potassium level, though some patients have severe weakness when the level is no higher than 4 mEq./l., whereas in normal people a level of 8 mEq./l. is needed as a rule before weakness develops. Abbott et al. (1962) have shown that the muscle fibre membrane potential is lowered during the attacks in such cases. The attacks may be cut short by the intravenous administration of calcium gluconate, while acetazolamide, 250 mg. two or three times daily, hydrochlorothiazide, 25 mg. two or three times daily, and dichlorphenamide have all been used successfully for prophylaxis.

Sodium-responsive Normokalaemic Periodic Paralysis

The third type of periodic paralysis, entitled provisionally the so-called sodium-responsive normokalaemic variety (Poskanzer and Kerr, 1961 b) is probably a variant of the hyperkalaemic type, except for the fact that in these cases the attacks have been seen occasionally to last for days or weeks and have often developed at night. Nevertheless in these patients paralysis is always increased by the administration of potassium and improved by large doses of sodium chloride. It is in cases of this type that Shy, Gonatas, and Perez (1966) have described the appearance of very much increased numbers of mitochondria in muscle biopsy sections examined with the electron microscope and have referred to this change as pleoconial myopathy. Poskanzer and Kerr (1961 b) found that acetazolamide combined with 9-α-fluorohydrocortisone, 0·1 mg. daily, prevented the attacks.

This recent work has clearly indicated that careful investigation of every case of periodic paralysis is necessary in order to establish the nature of the patient's illness. Attempts to demonstrate a primary enzyme defect or a specific disorder of carbohydrate metabolism in such cases have so far been unsuccessful, but empirical treatment, both given prophylactically or in order to cut short the attacks, has proved to be successful once the character of the patient's attacks has been carefully defined by investigation.

MYOGLOBINURIA

Myoglobin may appear in the urine as a result of acute crush injury of muscle (Bywaters and Stead, 1945) and in localized ischaemic muscular necrosis, while, as already mentioned, it can occur in certain acute forms of polymyositis.

A specific syndrome of paroxysmal myoglobinuria of unknown aetiology has also been described; this is characterized by acute attacks of severe cramp-like muscle pain and tenderness associated with weakness or paralysis which are accompanied, within a few hours, by myoglobinuria. The condition usually clears up within two to three days with rest, but occasional cases show such severe and widespread muscle damage that death ensues. Korein, Coddon, and Mowrey (1959) have distinguished two types, of which Type I occurs predominantly in males in late adolescence or early adult life; the pain and myoglobinuria follow exercise, which must be curtailed as the recurrent attacks may eventually cause permanent weakness and wasting. In cases of Type II, which are seen particularly in childhood, an acute infection often precedes the muscle pain and myoglobinuria; the attacks are severe, with fever and leucocytosis, but tend to occur at progressively longer intervals and usually clear up with the passage of time.

REFERENCES

ABBOTT, B. C., CREUTZFELDT, O., FOWLER, B., and PEARSON, C. M. (1962) Membrane potentials in human muscle, *Fed. Proc.*, **21**, 318.

ADAMS, R. D., DENNY-BROWN, D., and PEARSON, C. M. (1962) *Diseases of Muscle: A Study in Pathology*, 2nd ed., New York.

ADAMSON, D. G., SALTER, R. H., and PEARCE, G. W. (1967) McArdle's syndrome (myophosphorylase deficiency), *Quart. J. Med.*, **36**, 565.

ASTROM, K. E., KUGELBERG, E., and MÜLLER, R. (1961) Hypothyroid myopathy, *Arch. Neurol. (Chic.)*, **5**, 472.

BATHURST, L. W. (1895) A case of Graves' disease associated with idiopathic muscular atrophy, *Lancet*, ii, 529.

BRAIN, W. R. (1959) Pathogenesis and treatment of endocrine exophthalmos, *Lancet*, i, 109.

BYWATERS, E. G. L., and STEAD, J. K. (1945) Thrombosis of the femoral artery with myoglobinuria and low serum potassium concentration, *Clin. Sci.*, **5**, 195.

CONN, J. W. (1955) Primary aldosteronism, a new clinical syndrome, *J. lab. clin. Med.*, **45**, 661.

CONN, J. W., and STREETEN, D. H. P. (1960) in *The Metabolic Basis of Inherited Disease*, ed. STANBURY, J. B., WYNGAARDEN, J. B., and FREDRICKSON, D. S., New York.

COOMES, E. N. (1965) Corticosteroid myopathy, *Ann. rheum. Dis.*, **24**, 465.

COURTECUISSE, V., ROYER, P., HABIB, R., MONNIER, C., and DEMOS, J. (1965) Glyco-genose musculaire par déficit d'alpha-1,4-glucosidase simulant une dystrophie musculaire progressive, *Arch. franç. Pédiat.*, **22**, 1153.

CRISPELL, K. R., and PARSON, W. (1954) Occurrence of myotonia in 2 patients following thyroidectomy for hyperthyroidism, *Trans. Amer. Goiter Ass.*, 399.

DEBRÉ, R., and SEMELAIGNE, G. (1935) Syndrome of diffuse muscular hypertrophy in infants causing athletic appearance: its connection with congenital myxedema, *Amer. J. Dis. Child.*, **50**, 1351.

DRAGER, G. A., HAMMILL, J. F., and SHY, G. M. (1958) Paramyotonia congenita, *Arch. Neurol. Psychiat. (Chicago)*, **80**, 1.

ENGEL, A. G. (1961) Thyroid function and myasthenia gravis, *Arch. Neurol. (Chic.)*, **4**, 663.

ENGEL, W. K., EYERMAN, E. L., and WILLIAMS, H. E. (1963) Late onset type of skeletal muscle phosphorylase deficiency. A new familial variety with completely and partially affected subjects, *New Engl. J. Med.*, **268**, 135.

GAMSTORP, I. (1956) Adynamia episodica hereditaria, *Acta paediat. (Uppsala)*, (Suppl.), **108**, 1.

GOLDING, D. N., MURRAY, S., PEARCE, G. W., and THOMPSON, M. (1961) Corticosteroid myopathy, *Ann. phys. Med.*, **6**, 171.

GROB, D., LILJESTRAND, A., and JOHNS, R. J. (1957) Potassium movement in patients with familial periodic paralysis, *Amer. J. Med.*, **23**, 356.

HARMAN, J. B. (1959) Muscular wasting and corticosteroid therapy, *Lancet*, i, 887.

HELWEG-LARSEN, H. F., HAUGE, M., and SAGILD, U. (1955) Hereditary transient muscular paralysis in Denmark; genetic aspects of family periodic paralysis and family periodic adynamia, *Acta genet. (Basel)*, **5**, 263.

HOFFMAN, J. (1896) Ein Fall von Thomsen'scher Krankheit, compliciert durch Neuritis multiplex, *Dtsch Z. Nervenheilk.*, **9**, 272.

HUDGSON, P., GARDNER-MEDWIN, D., WORSFOLD, M., PENNINGTON, R. J. T., and WALTON, J. N. (1968) Adult myopathy in glycogen storage disease due to acid maltase deficiency, *Brain*, **91**, 435.

ILLINGWORTH, B., CORI, G. T., and CORI, C. F. (1956) Amylo-1,6-glucosidase in muscle tissue in generalized glycogen storage disease, *J. biol. Chem.*, **218**, 123.

JARCHO, L. W., and TYLER, F. H. (1958) Myxoedema, pseudomyotonia and myotonia congenita, *Arch. intern. Med.*, **102**, 357.

KLEIN, R., EGAN, T., and USHER, P. (1960) Changes in sodium, potassium and water in hyperkalaemic periodic paralysis, *Metabolism*, **9**, 1005.

KOREIN, J., CODDON, D. R., and MOWREY, F. H. (1959) The clinical syndrome of paroxysmal paralytic myoglobinuria, *Neurology (Minneap.)*, **9**, 767.

MCARDLE, B. (1951) Myopathy due to a defect in muscle glycogen breakdown, *Clin. Sci.*, **10**, 13.

MCARDLE, B. (1969) Metabolic and endocrine myopathies, in *Disorders of Voluntary Muscle*, ed. WALTON, J. N., 2nd ed., London.

MELLICK, R. S., MAHLER, R. F., and HUGHES, B. P. (1962) McArdle's syndrome: phosphorylase-deficient myopathy, *Lancet*, i, 1045.

MOMMAERTS, W. F. H. M., ILLINGWORTH, B., PEARSON, C. M., GUILLORY, R. J., and SERAYDARIAN, K. (1959) A functional disorder of muscle associated with the absence of phosphorylase, *Proc. nat. Acad. Sci. (Wash.)*, **46**, 791.

MULDER, D. W., BASTRON, J. A., and LAMBERT, E. H. (1956) Hyperinsulin neuronopathy, *Neurology (Minneap.)*, **6**, 627.

MÜLLER, R., and KUGELBERG, E. (1959) Myopathy in Cushing's syndrome, *J. Neurol. Neurosurg. Psychiat.*, **22**, 314.

NORRIS, F. H., PANNER, B. J., and STORMONT, B. M. (1968) Thyrotoxic periodic paralysis, *Arch. Neurol. (Chic.)*, **19**, 88.

OKINAKA, S., SHIZUME, K., IINO, S., WATANABE, A., IRIE, M., NOGUCHI, A., KUMA, S., KUMA, K., and ITO, T. (1957) The association of periodic paralysis and hyperthyroidism in Japan, *J. clin. Endocr.*, **17**, 1454.

PEARCE, G. W. (1964) Tissue culture and electron microscopy, in *Disorders of Voluntary Muscle*, ed. WALTON, J. N., 1st ed., London.

PERKOFF, G. T., SILBER, R., TYLER, F. H., CARTWRIGHT, G. E., and WINTROBE, M. M. (1959) Studies in disorders of muscle. XII. Myopathy due to the administration of therapeutic amounts of 17-hydroxycortico-steroids, *Amer. J. Med.*, **26**, 891.

POSKANZER, D. C., and KERR, D. N. S. (1961 a) Periodic paralysis with response to spironolactone, *Lancet*, ii, 511.

POSKANZER, D. C., and KERR, D. N. S. (1961 b) A third type of periodic paralysis with normokalaemia and favourable response to sodium chloride, *Amer. J. Med.*, **31**, 328.

PRINEAS, J. W., HALL, R., BARWICK, D. D., and WATSON, A. J. (1968) Myopathy associated with pigmentation following adrenalectomy for Cushing's syndrome, *Quart. J. Med.*, **37**, 63.

PRINEAS, J. W., MASON, A. S., and HENSON, R. A. (1965) Myopathy in metabolic bone disease, *Brit. med. J.*, **1**, 1034.

RAMSAY, I. D. (1965) Electromyography in thyrotoxicosis, *Quart. J. Med.*, **34**, 255.

SCHMID, R., and HAMMAKER, L. (1961) Hereditary absence of muscle phosphorylase (McArdle's syndrome), *New Engl. J. Med.*, **264**, 223.

SCHMID, R., and MAHLER, R. (1959) Chronic progressive myopathy with myoglobinuria; demonstration of a glycogenolytic defect in the muscle, *J. clin. Invest.*, **38**, 1044.

SHY, G. M. (1960) Some metabolic and endocrinological aspects of disorders of striated muscle, *Res. Publ. Ass. nerv. ment. Dis.*, **38**, 274.

SHY, G. M., GONATAS, N. K., and PEREZ, M. C. (1966) Two childhood myopathies with abnormal mitochondria—1. Megaconial myopathy, 2. Pleoconial myopathy, *Brain*, **89**, 133.

SHY, G. M., WANKO, T., ROWLEY, P. T., and ENGEL, A. G. (1961) Studies in familial periodic paralysis, *Exp. Neurol.*, **3**, 53.

SMITH, R., and STERN, G. M. (1967) Myopathy, osteomalacia and hyperparathyroidism, *Brain*, **90**, 593.

TARUI, S., OKUNA, G., IKURA, Y., TANAKA, T., SUDA, M., and NISHIKAWA, M. (1965) Phosphofructokinase deficiency in skeletal muscle. A new type of glycogenosis, *Biochem. biophys. Res. Commun.*, **19**, 517.

THOMSON, W. H. S., MACLAURIN, J. C., and PRINEAS, J. W. (1963) Skeletal muscle glycogenosis; an investigation of two dissimilar cases, *J. Neurol. Neurosurg. Psychiat.*, **26**, 60.

THORN, G. W. (1949) *The Diagnosis and Treatment of Adrenal Insufficiency*, p. 144, Springfield, Ill.

TYLER, F. H., STEPHENS, F. E., GUNN, F. D., and PERKOFF, G. T. (1951) Studies on disorders of muscle. VII. Clinical manifestations and inheritance of a type of periodic paralysis without hypopotassaemia, *J. clin. Invest.*, **30**, 492.

VAN DER MEULEN, J. P., GILBERT, G. J., and KANE, C. A. (1961) Familial hyperkalaemic paralysis with myotonia, *New Engl. J. Med.*, **264**, 1.

VAN'T HOFF, W. (1962) Familial myotonic periodic paralysis, *Quart. J. Med.*, **31**, 385.

WALTON, J. N. (1960) Muscular dystrophy and its relation to the other myopathies, *Res. Publ. Ass. nerv. ment. Dis.*, **38**, 378.

WILSON, J., and WALTON, J. N. (1959) Some muscular manifestations of hypothyroidism, *J. Neurol. Neurosurg. Psychiat.*, **22**, 320.

WITTS, L. J., LAKIN, C. E., and THOMPSON, A. P. (1938) Discussion on Addison's disease at the Association of Physicians, *Quart. J. Med.*, **7**, 590.

ZELLWEGER, H., BROWN, B. I., McCORMICK, W., and TU, J. B. (1965) A mild form of muscular glycogenosis in two brothers with alpha-1,4-glucosidase deficiency, *Ann. paediat.*, **205**, 413.

ZIERLER, K. L., and ANDRES, R. (1957) Movement of potassium into skeletal muscle during spontaneous attack in family periodic paralysis, *J. clin. Invest.*, **36**, 730.

THE FLOPPY INFANT SYNDROME

It is well recognized that generalized muscular hypotonia in infancy can be due to a variety of causes. In a survey of 111 floppy infants, Paine (1963) found that 48 were suffering from various forms of cerebral palsy, 28 from mental retardation, 3 from cerebral degenerative disease, and 1 from brain tumour. There were 4 cases of spinal muscular atrophy and 4 of myopathy, while 18 were found to have a condition which could only be entitled 'benign congenital hypotonia' (Walton, 1956, 1957). Congenital muscular dystrophy as a cause of such a syndrome has already been considered [see p. 849]. The term 'benign congenital hypotonia' can still reasonably be reserved for those floppy infants in whom hypotonia is not demonstrated to be the result of any specific metabolic disorder or to be secondary to mental defect or central nervous disease and in which full investigation, including electromyography and muscle biopsy, fails to demonstrate any specific abnormality of the muscle fibres other than, in some cases, an over-all decrease in their diameter. While recent work has clearly indicated a remarkable variability in the clinical course of spinal muscular atrophy in infancy and childhood (Byers and Banker, 1961; Dubowitz, 1964; Gardner-Medwin, Hudgson, and Walton, 1967) it has recently become apparent that some floppy infants may be suffering from certain apparently specific though benign disorders of muscle which are relatively non-progressive. There remain, however, a substantial number of hypotonic infants who show gradual improvement and in whom no other diagnostic label than one of benign congenital hypotonia can yet be applied, since modern methods of investigation fail to demonstrate any cause for the widespread muscular hypotonia which they manifest. It must, however, be appreciated that this condition is no more than a syndrome which may eventually prove to be one of multiple aetiology. A number of the more specific forms of benign and relatively non-progressive myopathy which have been described in recent years will now be mentioned.

CENTRAL CORE DISEASE

In 1956 Shy and Magee described a family of children in which the affected individuals did not walk until about the age of 4 years. The patients showed profound and widespread muscular hypotonia and muscle biopsy revealed large muscle fibres, most of which showed one or sometimes two central cores which had different staining properties from other fibrils. Further cases have been described by Bethlem and Meyjes (1960) and by Engel et al. (1961). Dubowitz and Pearse (1960) found the central core to be devoid of oxidative enzymes and of phosphorylase activity and suggested that it was non-functioning. The condition is plainly benign and genetically determined, being probably the result of an autosomal recessive gene, but as in the several other conditions described below, its pathogenesis remains obscure.

NEMALINE MYOPATHY

In 1963 Shy et al. described another congenital non-progressive myopathy in which curious collections of rod-shaped bodies were found within the muscle fibres. It is now apparent that in many such cases the clinical diagnosis can be suspected as these patients usually show not only evidence of a diffuse myopathy, but also facial weakness, a high arched palate, prognathism of the lower jaw, and skeletal changes resembling those of arachnodactyly, though none of the other stigmata of Marfan's syndrome are present (Ford, 1960; Conen, Murphy, and Donohue, 1963; Engel, Wanko, and Fenichel, 1964). Examination of muscle from such cases with the electron microscope (Price et al., 1965; Hudgson et al., 1967) has shown that the subsarcolemmal rods appear to be due to a selective swelling and degeneration of Z-bands with consequent destruction of myofilaments in the adjacent part of the muscle fibre.

MITOCHONDRIAL MYOPATHIES

In children showing a similar clinical presentation to those of central core disease, yet another form of apparently specific pathological change in muscle has been observed by Shy and Gonatas (1964) and has been called 'megaconial myopathy' by Shy, Gonatas, and Perez (1966). One patient, an 8-year-old white female suffering from a slowly progressive weakness beginning at about the age of 3, showed marked involvement of all shoulder and pelvic-girdle muscles. Routine examination of the muscle biopsy with the light microscope did not reveal any significant abnormality, but ultrastructural investigations demonstrated enormously enlarged mitochondria measuring up to 5 μ in length in the subsarcolemmal region as well as throughout the fibre. Some of these mitochondria contained unusual rectangular crystalline-like inclusions of high density. Similarly abnormal mitochondria have, however, been described recently in a variety of different forms of muscle disease and the existence of this condition as an independent diagnostic entity is somewhat in doubt. It may prove that this megaconial change is a non-specific reaction occurring within muscle which is diseased due to a variety of causes (see Hudgson and Pearce, 1969).

Subsequently Shy and his colleagues (Shy, Gonatas, and Perez, 1966) reported another curious mitochondrial abnormality which they have provisionally entitled 'pleoconial myopathy'. In these cases enormous numbers of rounded mitochondria were seen within muscle fibres. The patients in whom this abnormality was found showed clinical features similar to those described by Poskanzer and Kerr (1961) in patients with so-called normokalaemic periodic paralysis. The specificity of this mitochondrial change is also now in doubt as abnormal numbers of mitochondria within skeletal muscle fibres have now been described in other forms of metabolic myopathy showing different clinical characteristics (see McArdle, 1969; Hudgson and Pearce, 1969).

MYOTUBULAR MYOPATHY

In a 9-year-old child with a form of Möbius disease characterized by facial diplegia, external ocular palsies, a decrease in muscle mass, moderate symmetrical muscle weakness, and poor development of all somatic muscles, Spiro, Shy, and Gonatas (1966) found changes which may represent the first example of cellular arrest in the human. The great majority of the muscle fibres contained central nuclei, often lying in chains, and the appearances in the muscle were very similar to those of the so-called myotubes seen in the normal foetus in the early months of intra-uterine life. Subsequent reports, recently reviewed by Campbell, Rebeiz, and Walton (1969), have, however, shown many differences between these structures and foetal myotubes, so that although this condition appears to be a clinical and morphological entity, its pathogenesis is still a matter of speculation.

It may nevertheless be concluded that although it is too early to be certain that all of the syndromes mentioned represent separate specific disorders of muscle, within this field of benign congenital myopathy new advances are taking place with great rapidity and many interesting histological abnormalities of the muscle fibre are being demonstrated by histochemical, biochemical, and ultrastructural techniques.

REFERENCES

BETHLEM, J., and MEYJES, F. E. P. (1960) Congenital non-progressive central core disease of Shy and Magee, *Psychiat. Neurol. Neurochir. (Amst.)*, **63**, 246.

BYERS, R. K., and BANKER, B. Q. (1961) Infantile muscular atrophy, *Arch. Neurol. (Chicago)*, **5**, 140.

CAMPBELL, M. J., REBEIZ, J. J., and WALTON, J. N. (1969) Myotubular, centronuclear or pericentronuclear myopathy, *J. neurol. Sci.*, 8, 425.

CONEN, P. E., MURPHY, E. G., and DONOHUE, W. L. (1963) Light and electron microscopic studies on 'myogranules' in a child with hypotonia and muscle weakness, *Canad. med. Ass. J.*, **89**, 983.

DUBOWITZ, V. (1964) Infantile muscular atrophy. A prospective study with particular reference to a slowly progressive variety, *Brain*, **87**, 707.

DUBOWITZ, V., and PEARSE, A. G. E. (1960) Oxidative enzymes and phosphorylase in central-core disease of muscle, *Lancet*, ii, 23.

ENGEL, W. K., FOSTER, J. B., HUGHES, B. P., HUXLEY, H. E., and MAHLER, R. (1961) Central core disease—an investigation of a rare muscle cell abnormality, *Brain*, **84**, 167.

ENGEL, W. K., WANKO, T., and FENICHEL, G. M. (1964) Nemaline myopathy: a second case, *Arch. Neurol. (Chic.)*, **11**, 22.

FORD, F. R. (1960) Congenital universal muscle hypoplasia, in *Diseases of the Nervous System in Infancy, Childhood and Adolescence*, Oxford.

GARDNER-MEDWIN, D., HUDGSON, P., and WALTON, J. N. (1967) Benign spinal muscular atrophy arising in childhood and adolescence, *J. neurol. Sci.*, **5**, 121.

HUDGSON, P., GARDNER-MEDWIN, D., FULTHORPE, J. J., and WALTON, J. N. (1967) Nemaline myopathy, *Neurology (Minneap.)*, **17**, 1125.

HUDGSON, P., and PEARCE, G. W. (1969) Ultramicroscopic studies of diseased muscle, in *Disorders of Voluntary Muscle*, ed. WALTON, J. N., 2nd ed., London.

McARDLE, B. (1969) Endocrine and metabolic myopathies, in *Disorders of Voluntary Muscle*, ed. WALTON, J. N., 2nd ed., London.

PAINE, R. S. (1963) The future of the 'floppy infant', *Develop. Med. Child Neurol.*, **5**, 115.

POSKANZER, D. C., and KERR, D. N. S. (1961) A third type of periodic paralysis with normokalaemia and favourable response to sodium chloride, *Amer. J. Med.*, **31**, 328.

PRICE, H. M., GORDON, G. B., PEARSON, C. M., MUNSAT, T. L., and BLUMBERG, J. M. (1956) New evidence for excessive accumulation of Z-band material in nemaline myopathy, *Proc. nat. Acad. Sci. (Wash.)*, **54**, 1398.

SHY, G. M., ENGEL, W. K., SOMERS, J. E., and WANKO, T. (1963) Nemaline myopathy, a new congenital myopathy, *Brain*, **86**, 793.

SHY, G. M., and GONATAS, N. K. (1964) Human myopathy with giant abnormal mitochondria, *Science*, **145**, 493.

SHY, G. M., GONATAS, N. K., and PEREZ, M. C. (1966) Two childhood myopathies with abnormal mitochondria—1. Megaconial myopathy, 2. Pleoconial myopathy, *Brain*, **89**, 133.

SHY, G. M., and MAGEE, K. R. (1956) A new congenital non-progressive myopathy, *Brain*, **79**, 610.

SPIRO, A. J., SHY, G. M., and GONATAS, N. K. (1966) Myotubular myopathy, *Arch. Neurol. (Chic.)*, **14**, 1.

WALTON, J. N. (1956) Amyotonia congenita—a follow-up study, *Lancet*, i, 1023.

WALTON, J. N. (1957) The limp child, *J. Neurol. Neurosurg. Psychiat.*, **20**, 144.

SOME MISCELLANEOUS DISORDERS OF MUSCLE

RESTLESS LEGS

The aetiology of this condition, which has been reviewed in detail by Ekbom (1960), is unknown. There is no evidence that it is a primary muscular disorder, but it gives rise to unpleasant aching in the muscles of the lower limbs when the patient rests in a chair and the symptoms are often particularly troublesome in bed. They may be associated with muscular cramps so that they interfere with sleep and after a period of restless shuffling the patient may be compelled to get up and to walk the floor to obtain relief. There are no abnormal physical signs on examination and no lesions within the muscles or peripheral nerves have been discovered. The aetiology of this troublesome syndrome is totally unexplained, but some patients are greatly helped by treatment with chlorpromazine given in a dosage of 50–100 mg. at night, and perhaps 25 mg. three times a day as well. Diazepam and hydantoinates are sometimes helpful in relieving the associated muscle cramps which occur in some cases.

TIBIALIS ANTERIOR SYNDROME

Severe boring pain in the tibialis anterior muscle may occur, particularly in male adults undertaking unaccustomed exercise. The condition is probably due to ischaemia followed by swelling of the tibialis anterior and its associated muscles lying within a tight fascial compartment. In very rare cases the pain may be intense, and widespread necrosis of the anterior tibial muscles may occur, and can even be fatal as a result of myoglobinuria. In mild chronic cases recurrent pain in the appropriate distribution occurs whenever the patient exerts himself. Relief may then be obtained by means of surgical decompression of the anterior crural compartment (Sirbou, Murphy, and White, 1944).

PROGRESSIVE MYOSITIS OSSIFICANS

Although localized myositis ossificans may occur as a result of the ossification of certain muscles as a result of their repeated involvement in the trauma of certain exercises or occupations and may occasionally occur in muscles in the region of the hip joint (particularly the adductors) following paraplegia or paraparesis, as after partial recovery from transverse myelitis, there is a genetically-determined progressive disorder in which widespread ossification of muscles occurs. Most of these patients are children who often have associated anomalies of their great toes or other digits and it seems that the ossification in muscle is preceded by sclerosis of intramuscular connective tissue (McKusick, 1956). This rare disorder, which is probably transmitted by a dominant gene which often shows incomplete penetrance (see Foster, 1969), often begins by giving rise to swelling or swellings in the neck which mimic congenital torticollis and eventually in most cases the muscles of the back, shoulder, and pelvic girdles become ossified. The overlying skin may ulcerate and in the terminal stages aspiration pneumonia and/or asphyxia may occur.

THE STIFF-MAN SYNDROME

In 1956 Moersch and Woltman reported on 14 patients who had suffered a progressive fluctuating muscular rigidity and spasm and used the term 'stiff-man syndrome' to describe this condition. The condition predominantly affects male adults who, after a prodromal phase of aching and tightness of the axial muscles, go on to develop a symmetrical continuous stiffness of the skeletal muscles upon which painful muscular spasms are superimposed; these may be precipitated by movement. The cause of the condition is unknown but there is evidence to suggest that it may be a disorder of spinal cord origin. Diazepam (Howard, 1963) may be remarkably successful in controlling the symptoms.

REFERENCES

EKBOM, K. A. (1960) Restless legs syndrome, *Neurology (Minneap.)*, **10**, 868.

FOSTER, J. B. (1969) The clinical features of some miscellaneous neuromuscular disorders, in *Disorders of Voluntary Muscle*, ed. WALTON, J. N., 2nd ed., London.

HOWARD, F. M. (1963) A new and effective drug in the treatment of stiff-man syndrome, *Proc. Mayo Clin.*, **38**, 203.

McKUSICK, V. (1956) *Heritable Disorders of Connective Tissue*, p. 184, St. Louis, Mo.

MOERSCH, F. P., and WOLTMAN, H. W. (1956) Progressive fluctuating muscular rigidity and spasm (stiff-man syndrome), *Proc. Mayo Clin.*, **31**, 421.

SIRBOU, A. B., MURPHY, M. J., and WHITE, A. S. (1944) Soft tissue complications of fractures of the leg, *Calif. west Med.*, **60**, 53.

DIFFERENTIAL DIAGNOSIS

The differential diagnosis of muscle disease depends first upon the clinical history and examination, secondly upon electromyographic and other neurophysiological evidence, thirdly upon the biochemical findings, and fourthly upon pathological changes in muscle as revealed by biopsy.

CLINICAL DIAGNOSIS

In the characteristic case of muscular dystrophy showing the usual slowly progressive pattern of increasing muscular weakness and selective atrophy of the proximal limb muscles, diagnosis is rarely in doubt. On the other hand, in an infant or child showing a picture of relatively diffuse non-progressive atrophy and weakness, it may be apparent that the condition belongs to one of the group of so-called benign congenital myopathies. There are, however, some cases in which differential diagnosis between a congenital non-progressive myopathy and progressive muscular dystrophy of early onset may be an extremely difficult matter on purely clinical grounds and may then depend upon ancillary investigations.

If the pattern of muscular weakness and wasting is obscured by subcutaneous fat or when muscular involvement is predominantly distal, as in myotonic dystrophy and distal myopathy, it may not always be easy to distinguish muscular dystrophy from neuropathic disorders such as progressive muscular atrophy, polyneuropathy, and peroneal muscular atrophy. Usually, however, the associated neurological signs, including fasciculation, and the sensory abnormalities which generally occur in polyneuropathy and peroneal muscular atrophy are sufficient to clarify the position. In early life, fasciculation is a useful sign, both in the tongue and in limb muscles, which may help to identify benign or pseudo-myopathic forms of spinal muscular atrophy, and electromyography is of particular value in distinguishing the latter disorder from muscular dystrophy, as the classical features of central denervation atrophy are almost always found.

Usually, therefore, it is comparatively easy to distinguish myopathy from neuropathy on clinical grounds alone, but it may be much more difficult to separate cases of sporadic muscular dystrophy from other forms of myopathy. The possibility of an endocrine cause for the muscular weakness must always be considered, and associated signs of endocrine disease and/or of metabolic bone disease should be sought carefully. It must also be noted that in untreated myasthenia gravis fatigability of muscles may not always be immediately apparent, and in any patient with proximal muscular weakness of comparatively recent onset, even when there is no involvement of ocular and bulbar muscles, a diagnostic injection of edrophonium chloride is indicated. Equivocal improvement following such an injection is sometimes seen in polymyositis and a more striking response may be observed in the myasthenic-myopathic syndrome complicating bronchial carcinoma, in which, however, the tendon reflexes are usually absent, whereas in true myasthenia they are brisk, and electrophysiological tests will usually be helpful in making the distinction. It should also be noted that in cases of periodic paralysis and of myoglobinuria, permanent muscular atrophy may eventually supervene, though in such cases there is invariably a clear-cut history of episodic attacks of weakness or of muscle pain and the diagnosis will then be elucidated by clinical methods.

The differential diagnosis between muscular dystrophy and subacute or chronic polymyositis may be an extremely difficult matter. Among the criteria of value in differential diagnosis are first, the rapidity of onset and occasional remissions which occur in polymyositis; secondly, the global weakness and wasting which occur in this disease, unlike the selective pattern which is more characteristic of dystrophy; thirdly, a positive family history, if present, clearly indicates a genetically-determined disorder of muscle; fourthly, the almost constant involvement of neck muscles and the frequent occurrence of dysphagia strongly favour polymyositis, while these features are rare in muscular dystrophy except in the oculopharyngeal variety (it should also be recalled that myasthenia may selectively involve the neck muscles in occasional cases); finally, associated phenomena such as skin changes and the Raynaud phenomenon are found to be present in many cases of polymyositis.

Even with the help of these and other clinical guides, there are nevertheless cases in which diagnosis remains in doubt and must then depend upon investigative findings.

ELECTROMYOGRAPHY

In neuropathic disorders, spontaneous fibrillation potentials may be recorded from a muscle undergoing an active process of denervation, while the pattern of motor unit activity on volition, though reduced from normal, clearly indicates that the surviving motor unit action potentials are either normal or increased in size. In myopathic disorders, by contrast, spontaneous activity in the form of fibrillation potentials is uncommon, though fibrillation has been found in some cases and is more frequently seen in polymyositis than in muscular dystrophy (Walton and Adams, 1958). In the myotonic disorders a characteristic discharge taking the form of chains of oscillations of high frequency, is seen, and similar spontaneous discharges evoked by movement of the exploring electrode, which, however, do not show the classical waxing and waning of the myotonic discharge but which continue at a standard frequency and then cease spontaneously, may be recorded in various forms of non-myotonic myopathy including polymyositis and have been called pseudomyotonic discharges. Volitional activity in the myopathic disorders, and particularly in muscular dystrophy and polymyositis, demonstrates a break-down of the motor unit action potentials corresponding to patchy degeneration of muscle fibres and as a result there is an increase in the proportion of short-duration and polyphasic motor unit action potentials (Kugelberg, 1947; Walton, 1952). Buchthal, Rosenfalck, and Erminio (1960) have shown that a decrease in mean action potential amplitude and duration, together with a reduced motor unit territory and fibre density, is seen particularly often in the Duchenne type of muscular dystrophy. In myotonic dystrophy and polymyositis they found that motor unit territory and the mean duration of the motor unit potentials were similarly reduced, but normal amplitudes were maintained. In polymyositis Buchthal and Pinelli (1953) found that the mean duration of the motor unit action potential was decreased by up to 60 per cent. and the incidence of polyphasic potentials was increased three times. In the more benign forms of muscular dystrophy (the limb-girdle and facio-scapulohumeral types) similar but less conclusive quantitative changes may be observed (Buchthal, 1962). Changes in the motor unit action potentials similar to those observed in muscular dystrophy are found in thyrotoxic myopathy (Havard et al., 1963), in steroid myopathy (Müller and Kugelberg, 1959), and in the myopathies of Addison's disease and sarcoidosis (Buchthal, 1962). Farmer, Buchthal, and Rosenfalck (1959) found that the absolute refractory period of voluntary muscle was reduced in cases of muscular dystrophy.

In myasthenia gravis the electromyogram may be entirely normal, except that a myopathic pattern, as described above, may be obtained from fatigued muscle. A progressive diminution in the amplitude of the action potentials in myasthenic muscle obtained in response to supramaximal stimulation of its motor nerve at rates of 3 per second and detected by surface electrodes (Harvey and Masland, 1941) is a useful diagnostic sign of myasthenia, but only occurs as a rule in muscles which are clinically affected by the disease (Botelho et al., 1952). At tetanic rates of stimulation (50 per second) the amplitude of the evoked muscle action potential may actually increase in cases of the myasthenic-myopathic syndrome complicating lung cancer (Lambert, Eaton, and Rooke, 1956) but a similar, though less striking, increment (Simpson, 1969) is occasionally seen in myasthenia gravis. No specific electromyographic appearances have been described in cases of familial periodic paralysis, but in patients with various forms of benign congenital myopathy the electromyogram may again reveal a myopathic pattern without any specific features (see Richardson and Barwick, 1969).

BIOCHEMICAL DIAGNOSIS

Many biochemical tests can be employed in differentiating the various forms of myopathy. Thus in the endocrine myopathies many tests apposite to the diagnosis of the individual endocrine deficiencies may well be required in certain cases. In the periodic paralysis syndromes, in addition to serial estimations of the serum potassium level and measures designed to precipitate attacks for diagnostic purposes, there are certain cases in which measurement of sodium and potassium output in the urine, and even of sodium and potassium balance, may be needed. In cases of severe generalized muscle pain and weakness, a search for myoglobin in the urine is essential, while in those patients who develop muscle pain after effort it is usually necessary to exclude certain forms of glycogen storage disease by the measurement of lactate and pyruvate in venous blood distal to a tourniquet following a period of ischaemic work; estimation of phosphorylase and of other glycolytic enzymes by histochemical and chemical methods applied to muscle biopsy samples, as well as the estimation of the total glycogen content of muscle, may also be needed.

In polymyositis the erythrocyte sedimentation rate is raised in about half the cases and there may be an elevation of the serum gamma-globulin level which can be demonstrated by electrophoresis (Barwick and Walton, 1963). Tests for circulating antibodies in the serum of such patients have been disappointing (Caspary, Gubbay, and Stern, 1964). Antimyosin antibody is found not only in some cases of polymyositis and in myasthenia gravis, but also in some patients with muscular dystrophy and neurogenic atrophy and in a proportion of normal individuals. Antinuclear factor is present, however, in a higher proportion of cases of polymyositis than of controls. Positive LE-cell preparations are occasionally seen in such cases (Pearson, 1969) but such examinations as the latex fixation and Rose-Waaler tests are of little diagnostic value.

Many other relatively non-specific biochemical findings have been described in cases of myopathy and have been reviewed by Pennington (1969). Thus an excessive output of creatine and a diminished creatininuria have been observed in many forms of myopathy but have little diagnostic significance. Aminoaciduria is also seen in a proportion of cases, while changes observed in serum lipid and protein levels lack specificity. Of the greatest diagnostic value, however, have been changes in serum enzyme activities. Sibley and Lehninger (1949) first demonstrated that the serum aldolase level was raised in patients with various muscle diseases including progressive muscular dystrophy. Subsequently many authors have used the assay of this enzyme in the diagnosis of muscular dystrophy and it has been found that the activity of this enzyme in the serum is raised to about ten times the normal upper limit in early cases of Duchenne type muscular dystrophy, while less striking increases are observed in the more benign varieties. Pearson (1957) showed that similar though less striking increases occurred in the serum activity of the transaminases (aminotransferases) and pointed out that a substantial rise in enzyme activity might occur long before overt clinical signs of Duchenne type dystrophy appeared— that is, in the preclinical phase of the disease. In 1959 Ebashi *et al.* reported a pronounced increase in creatine kinase activity in the serum of patients with muscular dystrophy and demonstrated that in early cases of the Duchenne type this increase might even be three hundredfold. It is now apparent that estimation of this enzyme in the serum is much the most sensitive early diagnostic test for this form of muscular dystrophy, and Pearce, Pennington, and Walton (1964) among others have confirmed that it is increased in preclinical cases. It is well recognized that the activity of this and other enzymes (see Pennington, 1969) which leak out of the diseased muscle into the serum is at its highest in the early stages of all forms of muscle disease and tends to decline as the disease advances. In the Duchenne type dystrophy, activity is probably highest at about the second or third year of life and declines progressively after the age of 10. Similar reductions are seen during the course of limb-girdle and facio-scapulohumeral dystrophy and in myotonic dystrophy, although in these three disorders the initial increases are very much less striking. In polymyositis the activity is highest in acute cases before treatment, but a rapid decline occurs following treatment, particularly if it is effective. Estimation of serum creatine kinase activity has recently been shown to be the most useful single test for the identification of the carrier state in female relatives of patients suffering from X-linked muscular dystrophy.

HISTOLOGICAL DIAGNOSIS

Traditionally, muscle biopsy has been one of the standard methods employed in the differential diagnosis of the various myopathies (Adams, Denny-Brown, and Pearson, 1962). Many pathological changes have been described in muscle and detailed reviews have been given recently by Pearson (1965), Pearce (1965), and Adams (1969). Increasing knowledge has led to decreasing confidence concerning the specificity of pathological changes seen in muscle biopsy specimens in so far as the differential diagnosis of myopathy is concerned. Although techniques such as intravital staining of the motor end-plates, histochemistry, tissue culture, and electron microscopy have been of considerable interest from the research standpoint, they have not as yet added great precision to the histological diagnosis of the myopathies except in such conditions as central core disease and nemaline or megaconial myopathy.

Among the most characteristic histological features observed in cases of muscular dystrophy of all types (Adams, Denny-Brown, and Pearson, 1962; Pearce and Walton, 1962; Pearson, 1965) are such changes as marked variations in fibre size, fibre splitting, the central migration of sarcolemmal nuclei [FIG. 111], areas of fibre atrophy, the formation of nuclear chains, areas of necrosis with phagocytosis of necrotic sarcoplasm [FIG. 112], and basophilia of sarcoplasm with an enlargement of sarcolemmal nuclei [FIG. 113] which show prominent nucleoli (changes construed as being due to abortive regeneration); infiltration with fat cells and connective tissue is also observed. When changes of the type described are uniformly distributed throughout the muscle sections, it is not usually difficult to accept that the diagnosis is one of muscular dystrophy. On the other hand, similar changes may be seen in polymyositis (Walton and Adams, 1958; Pearson, 1969; Adams, 1969), in which condition, however, signs of muscle fibre destruction and repair (necrosis, phagocytosis, and regenerative activity) are usually more striking and widespread, though they may be surprisingly slight even in acute cases. Most important in the diagnosis of polymyositis, but often scanty and only very rarely observed in muscular dystrophy, are interstitial or perivascular infiltrations of inflammatory cells such as lymphocytes and plasma cells [FIG. 114].

If, therefore, in a muscle section there is gross variation in fibre size with fibre-splitting, infiltration with fat and connective tissue and little phagocytosis

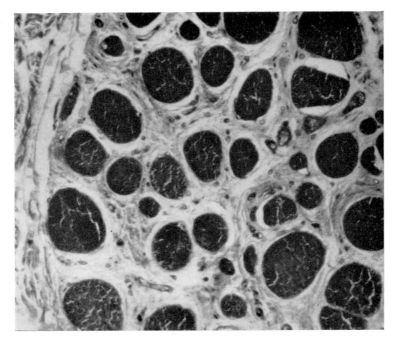

FIG. 111. Transverse section of biceps brachii biopsy from a case of advanced limb-girdle dystrophy showing rounding of fibres, random variation in size, central nuclei, fibre-splitting, and infiltration with connective tissue. H and E, ×240.

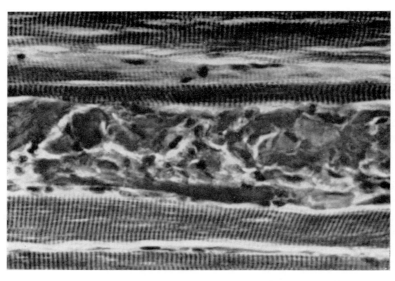

FIG. 112. Longitudinal section of quadriceps biopsy from a case of Duchenne type muscular dystrophy demonstrating focal necrosis and phagocytosis of a segment of muscle fibre. Picro-Mallory, ×640.

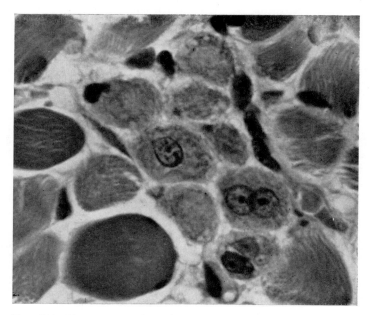

FIG. 113. Transverse section of a quadriceps biopsy from a case of preclinical Duchenne type dystrophy. H and E, ×640. Note the group of central fibres with sparse myofibrils and large vesicular nuclei with prominent nucleoli, demonstrating regenerative activity.

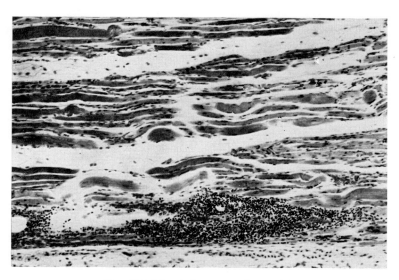

FIG. 114. Muscle in acute polymyositis

or regenerative activity, one may reasonably assume that the process is probably, but not certainly, dystrophic. If, by contrast, there is widespread necrosis and phagocytosis of muscle fibres with some, though not excessive, variation in fibre size, with profuse regenerative activity and massive infiltration of inflammatory cells between fibres and around blood vessels, it is not difficult to decide that one is probably dealing with a case of polymyositis. In between these two extremes, however, there is a considerable overlapping of the types of change

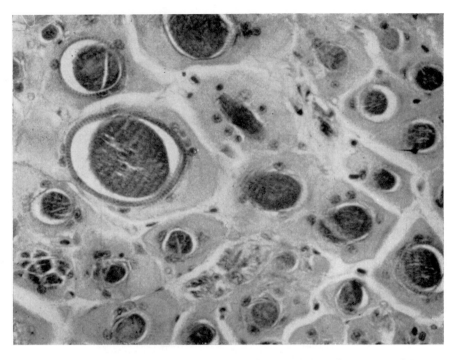

FIG. 115. Transverse section of quadriceps, obtained at autopsy from a case of dystrophia myotonica, PTAH ×480, demonstrating ringbinden and/or sarcoplasmic masses surrounding the transversely-sectioned central myofibrils of virtually every muscle fibre. (By kind permission of Dr. G. W. Pearce.)

which may be seen in dystrophy on the one hand and polymyositis on the other. Furthermore, in some cases of myasthenia gravis (Russell, 1953) degenerative changes are observed within muscle fibres, and lymphorrhages (collections of lymphocytes) may be seen around blood vessels or occasionally between fibres. Changes are often less striking in cases of the myasthenic-myopathic syndrome complicating bronchial carcinoma (Croft and Wilkinson, 1965), and although the pathological changes in muscle in cases of thyrotoxic and other endocrine myopathies may certainly be construed as being myopathic in the broadest sense, they are often slight and difficult to define.

The finding of striated annulets or so-called ringbinden (Wohlfart, 1951; Greenfield, Shy, Alvord, and Berg, 1957) in which striated myofibrils are seen

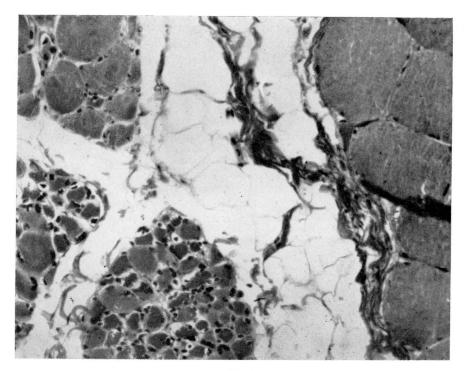

Fig. 116 (*a*).

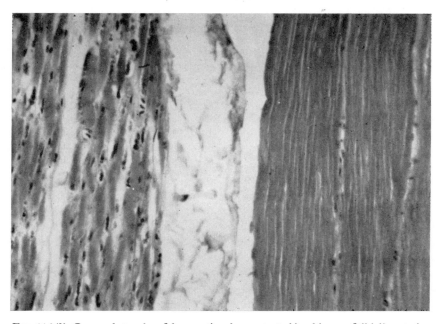

Fig. 116 (*b*). Grouped atrophy of denervation demonstrated in a biopsy of tibialis anterior from a patient with peroneal muscular atrophy. (*a*) Transverse section, H and E, ×640. (*b*) Longitudinal section, H and E, ×640.

to be encircling muscle fibres cut in transverse section, is often regarded as
being diagnostic of myotonic dystrophy [FIG. 115], though this is not absolutely
so as these abnormalities may occasionally be seen in other muscle diseases and
are probably due to the fracture of peripherally-situated myofibrils which then
wind around the intact portion of the fibre. In myotonic dystrophy, chains of
nuclei within muscle fibres are particularly striking and the nuclei are often
small and pyknotic, unlike the large vesicular nuclei occurring in chains which
are seen in some cases of Duchenne type dystrophy and of polymyositis and

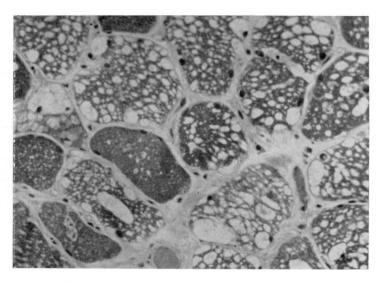

FIG. 117. Vacuolar myopathy in glycogen storage disease of muscle due
to acid maltase deficiency. Transverse section of quadriceps biopsy.
H and E, ×640.

which probably indicate abortive regenerative activity. Peripheral masses of
palely-staining homogeneous sarcoplasm lying in the periphery of muscle fibres
(so-called sarcoplasmic masses) are also characteristically seen in myotonic cases
[FIG. 115]. The 'myopathic' changes described can, in the great majority of
cases, be readily distinguished from those of denervation atrophy in which
groups of uniformly atrophic fibres can usually be seen lying alongside others
which are normal or larger than normal in size [FIG. 116 (a) and (b)].

Vacuolar change within muscle fibres is another pathological change of some
interest. Massive vacuoles within the substance of muscle fibres and often lying
in a subsarcolemmal position, and shown by alcoholic PAS staining to contain
glycogen, are characteristic of the various forms of glycogen storage disease of
muscle [FIG. 117] including Pompe's disease (Hudgson et al., 1968) and
McArdle's syndrome (Salter, Adamson, and Pearce, 1968). Widespread but less
striking vacuolar change can also be seen with the light microscope within the
muscle fibres of patients with periodic paralysis during attacks, and electron
microscopy (Shy et al., 1961) has confirmed that these vacuoles are due to

dilatation of the endoplasmic reticulum. Pearson and Yamazaki (1958) have also suggested that vacuolar change in muscle may be characteristic of disseminated lupus erythematosus, and similar histological abnormalities may be seen in the myopathy which may result from the long-continued administration of chloroquine (see Kakulas, 1969). While in certain muscular diseases such as McArdle's disease the histochemical demonstration that phosphorylase is absent

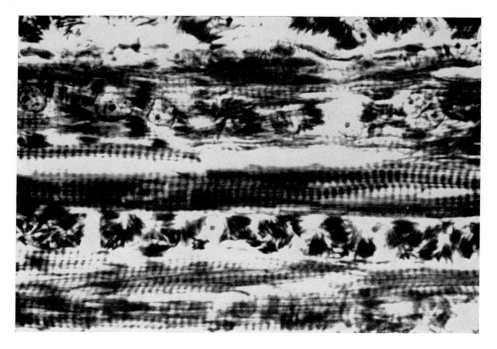

FIG. 118. Nemaline myopathy; longitudinal section of biopsy from biceps brachii, PTAH ×960. Note the collections of rods lying between the fibres. (From Hudgson, P., Gardner-Medwin, D., Fulthorpe, J. J., and Walton, J. N. (1967) *Neurology (Minneap.)*, **17**, 1125. By kind permission of the Editor.)

or reduced in quantity may be valuable diagnostically, the constellation of histochemical changes involving many different enzymes which have been described in some detail by Dubowitz and Pearse (1964), Engel (1965), Jasmin (1965), and many others, appear as yet to lack absolute specificity in so far as the diagnosis of muscle disease is concerned and there is still disagreement between various authors concerning interpretation. It should finally be mentioned that in cases of so-called benign congenital myopathy or hypotonia in which myopathic changes have been observed in the electromyogram, examination of muscle biopsy specimens under the light microscope has been singularly disappointing (Walton, 1957), and it is only since particular attention has been paid to these cases, using histochemical stains and electron microscopy, that entities such as central core disease, nemaline myopathy [FIGS. 118 and 119], and myotubular myopathy [FIG. 120] have been recognized. It is more than

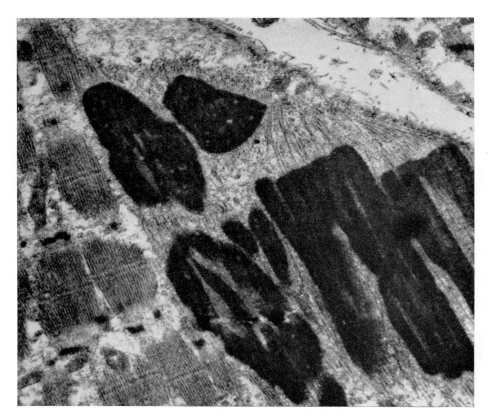

FIG. 119. Electron micrograph of longitudinal section of biceps brachii biopsy, ×25,000, demonstrating electron-dense nemaline rods, lying in the sub-sarcolemmal portion of a muscle fibre. (From Hudgson, P., Gardner-Medwin, D., Fulthorpe, J. J., and Walton, J. N. (1967) *Neurology* (*Minneap.*), **17**, 1125. By kind permission of the Editor.)

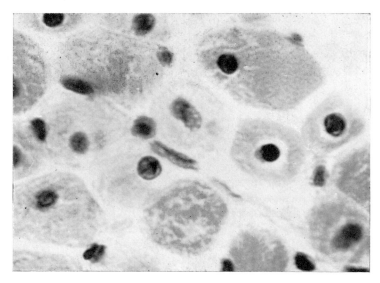

FIG. 120. Myotubular or centronuclear myopathy, transverse section of quadriceps biopsy. H and E, ×960. Note the central nuclei surrounded by clear 'halos' in several muscle fibres.

likely that the use of these highly-specialized techniques will in the future identify many more specific syndromes within this relatively difficult and little-understood group.

REFERENCES

ADAMS, R. D. (1969) Pathological reactions of the skeletal muscle fibre in man, in *Disorders of Voluntary Muscle*, ed. WALTON, J. N., 2nd ed., London.

ADAMS, R. D., DENNY-BROWN, D., and PEARSON, C. M. (1962) *Diseases of Muscle, A Study in Pathology*, 2nd ed., New York.

BARWICK, D. D., and WALTON, J. N. (1963) Polymyositis, *Amer. J. Med.*, **35**, 646.

BOTELHO, S. Y., DEATERLY, C. F., AUSTIN, S., and COMROE, J. H. (1952) Evaluation of the electromyogram of patients with myasthenia gravis, *Arch. Neurol. Psychiat. (Chicago)*, **67**, 441.

BUCHTHAL, F. (1962) The electromyogram, *Wld Neurol.*, **3**, 16.

BUCHTHAL, F., and PINELLI, P. (1953) Muscle action potentials in polymyositis, *Neurology (Minneap.)*, **3**, 424.

BUCHTHAL, F., ROSENFALCK, P., and ERMINIO, F. (1960) Motor unit territory and fibre density in myopathies, *Neurology (Minneap.)*, **10**, 398.

CASPARY, E. A., GUBBAY, S. S., and STERN, G. M. (1964) Circulating antibodies in polymyositis and other muscle-wasting disorders, *Lancet*, ii, 941.

CROFT, P. B., and WILKINSON, M. (1965) The incidence of carcinomatous neuromyopathy in patients with various types of carcinoma, *Brain*, **88**, 427.

DUBOWITZ, V., and PEARSE, A. G. E. (1964) Histochemical aspects of muscle diseases, in *Disorders of Voluntary Muscle*, ed. WALTON, J. N., 1st ed., London.

EBASHI, S., TOYOKURA, Y., MOMOI, H., and SUGITA, H. (1959) High creatine phosphokinase activity of sera of progressive muscular dystrophy, *J. Biochem. (Tokyo)*, **46**, 103.

ENGEL, W. K. (1965) Muscle biopsy, in *Clinical Orthopaedics and Related Research*, ed. DE PALMA, A. F., London.

FARMER, T. W., BUCHTHAL, F., and ROSENFALCK, P. (1959) Refractory and irresponsive periods of muscle in progressive muscular dystrophy and paresis due to lower motor neuron involvement, *Neurology (Minneap.)*, **9**, 747.

GREENFIELD, J. G., SHY, G. M., ALVORD, E. C., and BERG, L. (1957) *An Atlas of Muscle Pathology in Neuromuscular Diseases*, Edinburgh.

HARVEY, A. M., and MASLAND, R. L. (1941) A method for the study of neuromuscular transmission in human subjects, *Bull. Johns Hopk. Hosp.*, **69**, 1.

HAVARD, C. W. H., CAMPBELL, E. D. R., ROSS, H. B., and SPENCE, A. W. (1963) Electromyographic and histological findings in the muscles of patients with thyrotoxicosis, *Quart. J. Med.*, **32**, 145.

HUDGSON, P., GARDNER-MEDWIN, D., WORSFOLD, M., PENNINGTON, R. J. T., and WALTON, J. N. (1968) Adult myopathy in glycogen storage disease due to acid maltase deficiency, *Brain*, **91**, 435.

JASMIN, G. (1965) In *Muscle*, ed. PAUL, W. M., DANIEL, E. E., KAY, C. M., and MONCKTON, G., p. 569, Oxford.

KAKULAS, B. A. (1969) Experimental myopathies, in *Disorders of Voluntary Muscle*, ed. WALTON, J. N., 2nd ed., London.

KUGELBERG, E. (1947) Electromyogram in muscular dystrophy, *J. Neurol. Neurosurg. Psychiat.*, **10**, 122.

LAMBERT, E. H., EATON, L. M., and ROOKE, E. D. (1956) Defect of neuromuscular conduction associated with malignant neoplasms, *Amer. J. Physiol.*, **187**, 612.

MÜLLER, R., and KUGELBERG, E. (1959) Myopathy in Cushing's syndrome, *J. Neurol. Neurosurg. Psychiat.*, **22**, 314.

PEARCE, G. W. (1965) Histopathology of voluntary muscle, *Postgrad. med. J.*, **41**, 294.

PEARCE, G. W., and WALTON, J. N. (1962) Progressive muscular dystrophy: the histopathological changes in skeletal muscle obtained by biopsy, *J. Path. Bact.*, **83**, 535.

PEARCE, J. M. S., PENNINGTON, R. J. T., and WALTON, J. N. (1964) Serum enzyme studies in muscle disease—Part II: Serum creatine kinase activity in muscular dystrophy and in other myopathic and neuropathic disorders, *J. Neurol. Neurosurg. Psychiat.*, **27**, 96.

PEARSON, C. M. (1957) Serum enzymes in muscular dystrophy and certain other muscular and neuromuscular diseases. I. Serum glutamic oxalacetic transaminase, *New Engl. J. Med.*, **256**, 1069.

PEARSON, C. M. (1965) in *Muscle*, ed. PAUL, W. M., DANIEL, E. E., KAY, C. M., and MONCKTON, G., p. 423, Oxford.

PEARSON, C. M. (1969) Polymyositis and related disorders, in *Disorders of Voluntary Muscle*, ed. WALTON, J. N., 2nd ed., London.

PEARSON, C. M., and YAMAZAKI, J. N. (1958) Vacuolar myopathy in systematic lupus erythematosus, *Amer. J. clin. Path.*, **29**, 455.

PENNINGTON, R. J. T. (1969) Biochemical aspects of muscle disease, in *Disorders of Voluntary Muscle*, ed. WALTON, J. N., 2nd ed., London.

RICHARDSON, A. T., and BARWICK, D. D. (1969) Clinical electromyography, in *Disorders of Voluntary Muscle*, ed. WALTON, J. N., 2nd ed., London.

RUSSELL, D. S. (1953) Histological changes in the striped muscles in myasthenia gravis, *J. Path. Bact.*, **65**, 279.

SALTER, R. H., ADAMSON, D. G., and PEARCE, G. W. (1968) McArdle's syndrome (myophosphorylase deficiency), *Quart. J. Med.*, **36**, 565.

SHY, G. M., WANKO, T., ROWLEY, P. T., and ENGEL, A. G. (1961) Studies in familial periodic paralysis, *Exp. Neurol.*, **3**, 53.

SIBLEY, J. A., and LEHNINGER, A. L. (1949) Aldolase in the serum and tissues of tumour-bearing animals, *J. nat. Cancer Inst.*, **9**, 303.

SIMPSON, J. A. (1969) Myasthenia gravis and myasthenic syndromes, in *Disorders of Voluntary Muscle*, ed. WALTON, J. N., 2nd ed., London.

WALTON, J. N. (1952) The electromyogram in myopathy: analysis with the audio-frequency spectrometer, *J. Neurol. Neurosurg. Psychiat.*, **15**, 219.

WALTON, J. N. (1957) The limp child, *J. Neurol. Neurosurg. Psychiat.*, **20**, 144.

WALTON, J. N., and ADAMS, R. D. (1958) *Polymyositis*, Edinburgh.

WOHLFART, G. (1951) Dystrophia myotonica and myotonia congenita. Histopathological studies with special reference to changes in muscles, *J. Neuropath. exp. Neurol.*, **10**, 109.

20

DISORDERS OF THE AUTONOMIC NERVOUS SYSTEM

THE AUTONOMIC NERVOUS SYSTEM

THE 'autonomic' or 'vegetative' nervous system is the term applied to that part of the nervous system which is concerned in the innervation of unstriated muscle and many of the secretory glands. Physiologically it is divisible into two parts—the sympathetic and the parasympathetic, which to a large extent are mutually antagonistic in function, and employ anatomically separate pathways.

ANATOMY OF THE AUTONOMIC PERIPHERAL NERVES

In the case of both the sympathetic and the parasympathetic nerves two neurones intervene between the central nervous system and the innervated viscus, the efferent path being interrupted at a ganglion. The first neurone, which runs between the nervous system and the ganglion, is termed *preganglionic*. The second neurone, which runs from the ganglion to the viscus, is termed *postganglionic*.

SYMPATHETIC FIBRES
Efferent Paths

The sympathetic outflow from the central nervous system is limited to the region of the spinal cord lying between the first thoracic and the first lumbar segments inclusive.

Preganglionic Fibres. The preganglionic neurones are ganglion cells situated in the lateral horn of the grey matter of the spinal cord between these levels. The axons of these ganglion cells leave the spinal cord by the corresponding ventral roots and spinal nerves, from which they pass to the corresponding ganglia of the sympathetic chain. The preganglionic fibres are medullated, and the root by which they pass from the ventral root to the sympathetic ganglion is known as a white ramus. Arrived at the sympathetic ganglion, some preganglionic fibres terminate in the ganglion corresponding to the segment at which they leave the cord. Others pass upwards or downwards in the sympathetic chain, to terminate in ganglia above or below. Others again, passing through the ganglia of the sympathetic chain, emerge by special nerves, to terminate in more peripheral ganglia, the collateral sympathetic ganglia, or sympathetic plexuses, which are usually situated in close relationship with the blood vessels supplying the principal viscera. The most important of such nerves are the splanchnic nerves. The greater splanchnic nerve is derived from the ganglia of the sympathetic chain, from the fifth to the ninth or tenth thoracic segments, and runs to the coeliac plexus; the lesser splanchnic nerve, from the tenth and eleventh thoracic ganglia, goes to the aorticorenal plexus, and the lowest splanchnic nerve, from the eleventh thoracic ganglion, to the renal plexus.

The Sympathetic Chain. The sympathetic chain, which lies close to the vertebral column on either side, consists of a series of sympathetic ganglia possessing for the most part a segmental arrangement, linked together by sympathetic fibres. There are three cervical ganglia—superior, middle, and inferior—eleven thoracic, four lumbar, and four sacral ganglia, all paired, together with one unpaired coccygeal ganglion. Although all the preganglionic fibres emerge from the thoracic and first lumbar segments of the cord, by means of the sympathetic chain they are brought into relationship with spinal nerves through-out the whole length of the vertebral column.

Postganglionic Fibres. The postganglionic sympathetic fibres are non-medullated. Some arise from ganglion cells in each of the ganglia of the sympathetic chain and pass to the corresponding spinal nerve by a grey ramus, to be distributed to the tissues innervated by this nerve. Other postganglionic fibres take origin in collateral ganglia and pass to the various viscera.

Afferent Paths

Afferent sympathetic fibres, both medullated and non-medullated, enter the nervous system by the dorsal roots at all levels, having their ganglion cells in the thoracic root ganglia.

PARASYMPATHETIC FIBRES

The parasympathetic is also known as the craniosacral autonomic nervous system because its outflow is situated in the cranial and sacral regions. Unlike the sympathetic system, the ganglia of the parasympathetic are situated in the immediate neighbourhood of the innervated viscera. Thus the preganglionic fibres are long, and the postganglionic short. The principal preganglionic fibres of the cranial parasympathetic pass through the third nerve to the ciliary ganglion, through the seventh to the geniculate, pterygopalatine, submaxillary, and otic ganglia, through the ninth to the otic ganglion, and through the vagus to the ganglia of the thoracic and abdominal viscera supplied by this nerve. The vagus is the most important parasympathetic nerve. Its dorsal motor nucleus is the site of origin of the fibres which innervate the viscera it supplies. The sacral autonomic outflow is derived from the second and third sacral segments, and passes to the vesical plexus by the pelvic splanchnic nerves. The principal afferent fibres of the parasympathetic reach the central nervous system through the vagus nerve, having their ganglion cells in the inferior ganglion of that nerve.

PHYSIOLOGY

The physiology of the autonomic nervous system in respect of various organs is considered below. Certain generalizations which have been made concerning the functions of the sympathetic and the parasympathetic, and their mutual antagonism, must be mentioned.

The sympathetic dilates the pupil, widens the palpebral fissure, and in animals causes proptosis; it increases the rate of the heart and the conductivity of the atrioventricular bundle; it constricts most blood vessels, especially those of the skin and the splanchnic viscera, but dilates the coronary arteries and causes contraction of the spleen; it thus causes a rise of blood pressure and an increased blood flow, especially through the heart, lungs, brain, and muscles; it inhibits peristalsis in the alimentary canal, and promotes contraction of some at least of the sphincters; it is inhibitory to the detrusor muscle of the bladder; it causes erection of the hairs of the skin, and sweating; it excites the secretion of adrenaline, which, by stimulating the sympathetic nerve endings, in turn reinforces sympathetic action, and also raises the blood sugar by liberating sugar from the liver.

The parasympathetic, on the other hand, constricts the pupil, retards the heart and diminishes conductivity in the atrioventricular bundle, dilates the blood vessels, at least in certain situations, constricts the bronchioles, excites the secretion of tears and saliva, promotes peristalsis and inhibits the action of some at least of the alimentary sphincters, promotes contraction of the bladder, through the pelvic splanchnic nerves plays the principal part in sexual activity, and excites secretion of insulin, which lowers the blood sugar.

Whereas most sympathetic nerves are adrenergic (i.e. they act through the release of adrenaline at their nerve endings) and most parasympathetic nerves are cholinergic (acting through the release of acetylcholine) it seems that sudomotor sympathetic nerves (which cause sweating) are cholinergic.

The antagonism between the sympathetic and the parasympathetic has been stressed especially by Cannon, who points out that the changes produced by sympathetic stimulation are an appropriate preparation for violent activity. The sympathetic has thus been described as an activator for flight or fight, while the parasympathetic presides over anabolic, excretory, and reproductive activities. This is a suggestive generalization, though in some respects it oversimplifies the facts.

Degeneration of nerve cells in the lateral horn of grey matter of the dorsal cord may give rise to severe orthostatic hypotension and syncopal attacks [see p. 286], presumed to be due to sympathetic denervation and 'autonomic failure' (Bannister, Ardill, and Fentem, 1967).

SYMPATHETIC DENERVATION OF THE SKIN

The sympathetic nerve supply to the skin may be interrupted by lesions or surgical division of the outflow from the spinal cord in the white rami or ganglia, or of the peripheral nerves. In either case the area of skin denervated shows loss of (1) pilomotor, (2) vasomotor, and (3) sudomotor activity. (1) The pilomotor reflex consists of the appearance of gooseflesh by the application of cold or the scratch of a pin. (2) Vasomotor paralysis causes flushing, as a result of which the temperature of the denervated area becomes higher than that of the corresponding area on the normal side. This difference may be palpable or may require special methods of thermometry for its determination. (3) Loss of sweating may also be palpable, but is best investigated by applying to the skin a colour-indicator such as chinizarin 2–6-disulphonic acid. The patient is given 300–600 mg. of acetylsalicylic acid with one or two cups of hot tea and put under a radiant heat cradle. Where sweating occurs the skin becomes violet, the dry areas remaining light. (For details of this test see Guttmann, 1940.) Alternatively the skin may be painted with the following solution: chemically pure iodine, 1·5 to 2 g., castor oil, 10 ml., and absolute alcohol to 100 ml., after which fine rice starch powder is dusted on and the test continued as above.

HYPERHIDROSIS

Excessive sweating, e.g. from the palms, may be a congenital abnormality. Localized hyperhidrosis may occur on the face during eating, especially spicy foods—gustatory reflex sweating. Boswell says of Johnson: 'While in the act of eating the veins of his forehead swelled and generally a strong perspiration was visible.' Such gustatory sweating, which may affect only one half of the face, can occur as a congenital abnormality or may sometimes develop for no apparent cause during adult life; it can often be relieved by the use of propantheline. The 'syndrome of crocodile tears', in which lacrimation occurs during eating may follow facial paralysis and is presumed to be due to the fact that during nerve fibre regeneration, parasympathetic fibres intended for the salivary glands are misdirected to the lacrimal gland. Flushing and hyperhidrosis in the temple may occur after injury in the region of the parotid gland—the auriculotemporal syndrome. Hyperhidrosis is also seen in the distribution of a cutaneous nerve which is the site of a partial lesion, as in causalgia. Cerebral lesions causing hemiplegia may lead to excessive sweating on the paralysed half of the body.

When necessary, hyperhidrosis can be treated by sympathectomy.

DISTURBANCES OF THE FUNCTIONS OF THE AUTONOMIC NERVOUS SYSTEM AFTER LESIONS OF THE SPINAL CORD

The difference in the distribution of the sympathetic and somatic nervous outflow from the spinal cord accounts for the occurrence in many cases of a difference in the distribution of the sympathetic and somatic (motor and sensory) disturbances after lesions of the spinal cord. Since the sympathetic outflow to the whole body leaves the cord below the eighth cervical spinal segment, lesions at and above this level may cause a disturbance of sympathetic function over the whole body, though the motor and sensory innervation of the head and neck and of a part of the upper limbs remains undisturbed. At the mid-thoracic level of the cord the upper levels of the sympathetic and somatic disturbances approximately coincide. When the lesion of the cord is situated below the first lumbar spinal segment the somatic innervation is alone affected, the sympathetic outflow leaving the cord entirely above the lesion. The following disturbances of sympathetic function are found in cases of complete transection of the cord and in cases of less severe lesions which interrupt the intraspinal paths of the sympathetic. The pilomotor reflex elicited by a massive stimulus applied to the skin above the level of the lesion does not extend to areas innervated by parts of the cord below the lesion, but the reflex is excitable from these regions after the disappearance of spinal shock. The cutaneous temperature over the paralysed parts is higher than over normal parts of the body and vasoconstriction in response to exposure of the whole body to cold is diminished below the level of the lesion. Dermographism is diminished at the level of the lesion but usually somewhat increased below. (See also section on Compression of the Spinal Cord, p. 639.)

SWEATING

Excessive sweating after complete division of the spinal cord usually appears over parts of the body which are thus separated from the control of higher autonomic centres. Such sweating develops *pari passu* with the recovery of other reflex functions in the divided cord. It varies in intensity from time to time and may be reflexly excited by cutaneous stimuli, flexor spasms of the lower limbs, distension of the bladder, and exposure to heat.

Disturbances of sweating are rarely observed after partial lesions of the spinal cord, except in syringomyelia. In this disease loss of sweating may occur when the sympathetic ganglion cells in the lateral horns of grey matter are destroyed, and is most often seen over the face and upper limb. Excessive sweating with a similar distribution may, however, occur, sometimes spontaneously and sometimes being excited reflexly when the patient takes hot or highly seasoned food.

THE AUTONOMIC NERVOUS SYSTEM AND PAIN

REFERRED PAIN

Since most viscera are innervated only by the autonomic nervous system, it follows that the sensation of visceral pain must be mediated by afferent autonomic fibres. The most potent cause of visceral pain is an increase in the tension of the viscus. Visceral pain is a diffuse and poorly localized sensation, and is frequently associated with pain referred to, and tenderness of, the superficial tissues of the body over an area which is innervated by the same segments of the nervous system as the painful viscus. The physiological explanation of referred pain is uncertain. It has been attributed to a heightened excitability of the fibres and synapses concerned in pain conduction in the spinal cord, which receive impulses from the segments innervating the viscus, and also to a branching of axons, so that the same fibre supplies both somatic and visceral structures (Sinclair, Weddell, and Feindel, 1948). Referred pain may or may not be accompanied by cutaneous hyperalgesia.

Since most viscera receive a double nerve supply, both sympathetic and parasympathetic, both of which may conduct painful impulses, a visceral lesion, as Head (1893, 1894, 1896) showed, may be associated with two areas of referred pain. The area of reference corresponding to innervation through the sympathetic nervous system involves one or more spinal segments. When the viscus is also innervated by the vagus, the area of referred pain is found within the distribution of the trigeminal or upper cervical areas which constitute the somatic sensory distribution corresponding to the vagus. Individuals differ greatly in their susceptibility to referred pain, and the extent of the area of reference varies from time to time in the same individual in correspondence with the state of the viscus. One of the commonest examples of referred pain is that associated with disease of the coronary arteries, such as occurs in angina pectoris. In angina, pain is usually referred into the third, fourth, and fifth cervical and first, second, and third thoracic segments on the left side and often into the same or a somewhat similar area on the right side. The corresponding area in the trigeminal distribution extends on to the forehead and cheek around the eyes.

The autonomic nervous system sometimes provides an alternative path for painful sensations from areas deprived of their somatic sensory nerves. When pain can be evoked in such circumstances the painful impulse is probably conducted to the central nervous system by the autonomic nerves supplying the blood vessels. Autonomic painful impulses have been held responsible for some forms of neuralgia, especially in the face, but the interruption of the cervical sympathetic in such conditions has yielded uncertain results. Sympathectomy is also performed for causalgia.

FAMILIAL DYSAUTONOMIA

Familial dysautonomia (The Riley–Day syndrome) is a rare disorder occurring mainly in Jewish children and inherited by an autosomal recessive mechanism. Clinically it is characterized by defective lacrimation, hyperhidrosis, episodic hypertension, hyperpyrexia and vomiting, and attacks of epilepsy. Most patients also show dysphagia, ageusia, areflexia and a relative insensitivity to pain sensation and they die as a rule from respiratory infection or uraemia in infancy or childhood. The condition appears to be due to an inborn error of catecholamine metabolism which results in the excretion of homovanillic acid in the urine (Smith, Taylor, and Wortis, 1963). The presence of parasympathetic denervation is confirmed by the instillation of 2·5 per cent. methacholine into the eye; this produces miosis (Dancis and Smith, 1966).

REFERENCES

DANCIS, J., and SMITH, A. A. (1966) Familial dysautonomia, *New Engl. J. Med.*, **274**, 207.

RILEY, C. M., DAY, R. L., GREELY, D. M., and LANGFORD, N. S. (1949) Central autonomic dysfunction with defective lacrimation. Report of five cases, *Pediatrics*, **3**, 468.

SMITH, A. A., TAYLOR, T., and WORTIS, S. B. (1963) Abnormal catechol amine metabolism in familial dysautonomia, *New Engl. J. Med.*, **268**, 705.

AUTONOMIC AND METABOLIC CENTRES

Recent increase in knowledge has made this subject a vast and complex one. For details readers are referred to reviews by Ingram (1960), Harris (1960), Ortmann (1960), Brobeck (1960), Sawyer (1960), Glees (1961), and Walsh (1964). Here it is possible to give only a brief summary, and to deal more particularly with points of special clinical importance.

ANATOMY

The autonomic nervous system and many metabolic functions are under the control of nerve centres, many of which are situated in the hypothalamus. This is the region of the brain lying ventrally to the thalamus and constituting the floor of the third ventricle. The most important part of the hypothalamus is the tuber cinereum, which forms part of the floor of the third ventricle and extends from the optic chiasma anteriorly to the corpora mamillaria behind. In the centre of the tuber is the infundibulum, from which rises the stalk of the hypophysis. The hypothalamus contains a large number of scattered ganglion cells, which have been differentiated into a number of nuclei. The nuclei themselves are arranged in three groups and there is some evidence that a functional differentiation corresponds to this anatomical arrangement. The following are the principal nuclei of the preoptic area and the hypothalamus (Le Gros Clark, 1948):

Preoptic Area   .   .   .   Medial Preoptic nucleus.
                                     Lateral Preoptic nucleus.

Hypothalamus—
  Pars Supraoptica
    Hypothalami.   ,   .   Nucleus Supraopticus.
                                       Nucleus Paraventricularis.
                                       Nucleus Suprachiasmaticus.

                         Nucleus Hypothalamicus Anterior.
  Pars Tuberalis
    Hypothalami.   .   .   Nucleus Hypothalamicus Dorsomedialis.
                                       Nucleus Hypothalamicus Ventromedialis.
                                       Nucleus Arcuatus.
                                       Nucleus Hypothalamicus Lateralis.

                         Nucleus Hypothalamicus Posterior.
  Pars Mamillaris
    Hypothalami.   .   .   Nucleus Mamillaris Medialis.
                                       Nucleus Mamillaris Lateralis.
                                       Nucleus Intercalatus.
                                       Nucleus Premamillaris.
                                       Nucleus Supramamillaris.

The projections of the hypothalamus are not yet completely known. The following tracts, however, are probably of special importance. From the supraoptic nucleus arises a tract which terminates in the pars intermedia and the posterior lobe of the hypophysis. The fornix system runs from the hippocampus to the mamillary region and the mamillothalamic tract (bundle of Vicq d'Azyr) runs from the mamillary body to the anterior nucleus of the thalamus. There are also both efferent and afferent tracts running between the mamillary body and the midbrain.

The hypothalamus is richly supplied with blood from the vessels of the circle of Willis.

The importance of the frontal lobe for autonomic function has recently been established. Its anatomical relations with the hypothalamus are described by Le Gros Clark (1948): their functional relationships are discussed by Fulton (1949). Respiratory and vasomotor changes can be evoked from area 13, incision of the posterior part of area 14 on both sides causes 'sham rage' in monkeys [see p. 960], and removal of area 24, the anterior cingulate gyrus, renders monkeys unusually tame and alters their social adjustments [see FIG. 121 and p. 960].

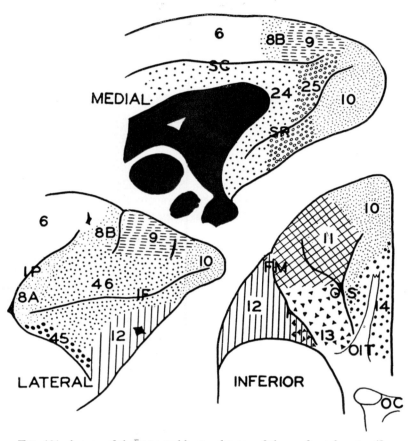

FIG. 121. A map of the cyto-architectural areas of the prefrontal cortex (from Walker, 1940)

THE FUNCTIONS OF THE HYPOTHALAMUS

The functions of the hypothalamus have been investigated by means of stimulation and experimental lesions. The posterior and lateral hypothalamus is an important centre for the activity of the sympathetic nervous system—the dynamogenic or ergotropic zone of Hess (1954). Stimulation of the posterior hypothalamus causes an increase of the heart rate, rise of blood pressure, dilatation of the pupil, erection of the hair, and inhibition of movements of the gut and of the tone of the bladder. The nuclei of the posterior hypothalamus are also responsible for the massive reaction known as 'sham rage' which occurs in animals when this region has been released from higher control. Destruction of this area, on the other hand, causes lethargy and parasomnia.

The nuclei of the tuber, on the other hand, appear to be concerned with the functions of the parasympathetic—the endophylactic or trophotropic zone of Hess. Stimulation of this region causes slowing of the heart rate and increase in the atrioventricular conduction time. There is also an increase in the peristaltic movements of the stomach and of the tone of the bladder. Lesions of this region may cause haemorrhagic erosions of the mucosa of the body of the stomach. The hypothalamus influences the release of gonadotrophic hormones from the hypophysis, and adiposogenital dystrophy, characterized by great obesity and genital atrophy, may be produced by experimental lesions of the tuber.

The hypothalamus is also concerned with the regulation of the temperature of the body, in which shivering, sweating, vasoconstriction, and vasodilatation as well as other factors play a part. The role of the hypothalamus in carbohydrate metabolism is not completely understood, but glycosuria, which is usually transitory, may follow lesions of this region. The hypothalamus is also concerned in water and sleep regulation.

The Relationship between the Hypothalamus and the Hypophysis

An important part of the influence of the hypothalamus upon bodily functions is exerted through the hypophysis. The anterior lobe of the hypophysis is under nervous control though it has no blood supply. This paradox is explained by the hypophysial portal system, through which humoral substances secreted by nerve cells in the hypothalamus are conveyed to, and excite, the hypophysis. Thus electrical stimulation of the hypothalamus excites gonadotrophic, adrenocorticotrophic, and thyrotrophic hypophysial secretion while direct electrical stimulation of the hypophysis has no such effect.

SYNDROMES OF THE HYPOTHALAMUS

ADIPOSITY

Adiposity, which is generally associated with genital hypoplasia or atrophy, may occur as a symptom of a variety of pathological states involving either the hypothalamus or the hypophysis, or both of these structures.

1. *Chromophobe adenoma of the hypophysis* may produce it [see p. 248].
2. *Tumours above the hypophysis*, especially craniopharyngiomas [see p. 251].
3. *Internal hydrocephalus* from any cause may lead to obesity and genital hypoplasia as a result of distension of the floor of the third ventricle which compresses the sella turcica and the hypophysis. In this way the syndrome may result from a tumour remote from the sella turcica, for example, a tumour of the cerebellum. More often, however, it is secondary to aqueduct stenosis or communicating hydrocephalus.
4. The syndrome may be produced by *infective conditions of the nervous system*, especially by encephalitis lethargica and, rarely, basal syphilitic meningitis. Granulomatous meningitis, say in sarcoidosis, may have a similar effect.
5. *Idiopathic adiposogenital dystrophy*. In the majority of cases of this syndrome,

including those in which the disturbance of function is most marked, none of the above cases can be held responsible. The disorder appears to be present from birth, and it is usually noticed at an early age that the child is exceptionally fat [FIG. 122]. Both sexes are affected, though boys appear to suffer more often than girls. The cheeks are rosy, and the skin is soft and hairless, except on the scalp. In these cases obesity is often associated with skeletal overgrowth, the child being exceptionally tall as well as exceptionally fat. There is often a marked genital hypoplasia, though exceptionally genital function may be normal. This is the case more often in females than in males. Sugar tolerance is usually increased. Polyuria, lethargy, and narcolepsy are exceptional associated symptoms. There is no evidence of a lesion involving the visual paths and the sella turcica is radiographically normal. These negative findings, together with the early onset, render it possible to distinguish the idiopathic variety of adiposogenital dystrophy (Fröhlich's syndrome) from other conditions of which similar disturbances are symptomatic.

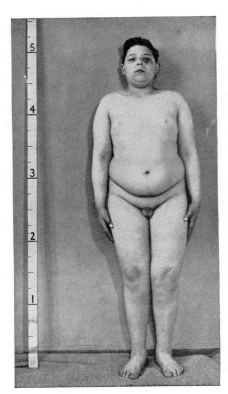

FIG. 122. Adiposogenital dystrophy in a boy aged 11; weight, 12 st. 4lb.

CACHEXIA

Cachexia is much less frequently encountered as a symptom of a lesion of the hypothalamus than obesity. It is occasionally produced, however, by suprasellar tumours and is common in the advanced stages of Parkinsonism due to encephalitis lethargica. A hypothalamic syndrome causing severe wasting in infancy and childhood has also been described (White and Ross, 1963).

SEXUAL FUNCTIONS

Failure of the sexual functions to develop at the normal age, or retrogression after normal development, may be the result of lesions either of the hypothalamus or of the hypophysis. Sexual infantilism, or, in the adult, impotence or amenorrhoea, according to sex, is then usually associated with obesity as described in the last section.

Sexual precocity is much rarer. It may be a symptom either of endocrine or of nervous disorder. In the endocrine sphere it may be produced by tumours of the ovary, testis, or suprarenal. Pineal tumours cause sexual precocity in a proportion of cases, almost exclusively in males [see p. 247], but sexual precocity may also be produced by other tumours of the midbrain and by hydrocephalus from any cause. It has also been reported after encephalitis lethargica and in association with tuberous sclerosis and suprasellar tumours as well as in rare cases of glioma of the hypothalamus.

So far we have been considering bodily changes in the reproductive organs resulting from disease of the nervous system. Loss of sexual desire without concurrent bodily change may be encountered in patients with a tumour involving the base of the brain and sometimes occurs after head injury, and in association with extensive destructive cerebral lesions of any kind. Excessive libido, on the other hand, may be experienced by patients in whom a tumour or a more diffuse lesion, such as general paresis in an early stage, diminishes inhibition.

Impotence implies a condition in the male in which sexual desire is normal but the patient cannot achieve an erection of the penis adequate for sexual intercourse. Erection of the penis and ejaculation of semen depend in the first instance upon the integrity of reflex arcs at the sacral level of the spinal cord. Injury to these reflex arcs, such as may occur in tabes, spina bifida, or a tumour or injury of the cauda equina, may cause impotence. Since, however, higher centres also play a part in the sexual act, impotence may be produced by lesions of the spinal cord at a higher level, as, for example, in multiple sclerosis. If the nervous system is normal and there is no debilitating general disease, impotence is neurotic in origin. Simple anxiety may cause impotence, which may be associated with ejaculatio praecox, which is explained by the fact that the sympathetic nervous system, which is over-active during anxiety, is inhibitory to erection of the penis but motor to the vesiculae seminales. Often, however, the cause of neurotic impotence lies deeply in the personality and can only be exposed by psychological analysis.

DIABETES INSIPIDUS

Mode of Production. It has been shown experimentally that diabetes insipidus follows bilateral destruction of the supra-optic nuclei, or removal of the posterior lobe of the hypophysis and its stalk. The subject has been reviewed by Kuhlenbeck (1954), who discussed the complex relations between the hypothalamus, the hypophysis, and the hypophysioportal circulation, and by Campbell and Dickinson (1960). The antidiuretic hormone (ADH) is probably produced by the nerve cells of the supra-optic and paraventricular nuclei, and reaches the neuro-hypophysis by their descending tracts. The hormone is necessary for the resorption of water by the renal tubules. The presence of the anterior lobe of the hypophysis and the thyroid appears to be necessary for the full effects of absence of the antidiuretic hormone to occur.

The secretion of ADH is excited by an increase in plasma osmolarity, and by a reduction in the circulating blood volume, and emotional stimuli: it is inhibited by decrease in plasma osmolarity and a rise in circulating blood volume.

Aetiology. Diabetes insipidus usually occurs as a result of lesions involving either the tuber cinereum or the hypophysis, though in the latter case the polyuria is usually less severe than in the former. Tuberal lesions responsible for diabetes insipidus include trauma, ranging from gun-shot wounds of the suprahypophysial region to closed head injury with concussion, basal meningitis, which is usually syphilitic but may be due to sarcoidosis, torula or a variety of other causes, epidemic encephalitis, cerebral malaria, internal hydrocephalus, and tumours of the third ventricle; and the syndrome may be produced by primary and secondary neoplasms and tuberculoma of the hypophysis. It may also occur in essential xanthomatosis.

Symptoms. Diabetes insipidus causes extreme thirst and the passage of large volumes of urine of low specific gravity, amounting in severe cases to several gallons a day. Sleep is disturbed by thirst and the necessity for frequent micturition. Excessive hunger is a rare accompaniment. There are several tests for diabetes insipidus (see Campbell and Dickinson, 1960), of which the simplest is that water deprivation does not lead to release of ADH and hence the specific gravity of the urine does not rise above 1,014.

Diagnosis. The polyuria of diabetes insipidus must be distinguished from that which occurs in other conditions, especially renal failure, hereditary nephrogenic diabetes insipidus, and psychogenic compulsive water-drinking (de Wardener and Barlow, 1958). The last is prone to occur in middle-aged women, who show a low plasma osmolarity in contrast to the high one of diabetes insipidus, and fail to respond to vasopressin.

Prognosis. The prognosis of diabetes insipidus is considerably influenced by the nature of the causative lesion. Polyuria following encephalitis lethargica is rarely severe. There are often marked fluctuations in the urinary output from day to day, and spontaneous recovery may occur. In syphilitic cases benefit may follow antisyphilitic treatment. When the cause is tumour or hydrocephalus, relief may follow if the primary disorder can be treated surgically.

Prognosis in traumatic cases is uncertain. Some patients improve or recover after a few months: in others the disorder is permanent.

Treatment. In severe cases, extract of the posterior lobe of the hypophysis affords the only palliative treatment. Nasal insufflation of posterior lobe extract may be tried but is sometimes ineffective. Often it is necessary to inject vasopressin subcutaneously to obtain a few hours' relief from the polyuria and thirst. It may be necessary to give more than one dose during the day. If one dose only is given, it should be administered at bedtime, in order to ensure several hours' sleep. Vasopressin tannate in oil is more slowly acting.

DISTURBANCES OF SLEEP

The role of the hypothalamus in the normal regulation of sleep is still uncertain, but clinical experience shows that lesions in the region of the tuber cinereum may lead either to persistent somnolence or to paroxysmal attacks of sleep similar to those occurring in idiopathic narcolepsy [see p. 966].

It has been suggested that a syndrome of periodic hypersomnolence and megaphagia which usually occurs in adolescent males (the Kleine-Levin syndrome, see p. 969) is of hypothalamic origin but the aetiology is not yet known.

OTHER HYPOTHALAMIC DISTURBANCES

Sugar Metabolism. The disturbances of sugar metabolism which have been produced by experimental lesions of the hypothalamus find a clinical counterpart in the occurrence of glycosuria as a result of lesions of this part of the brain. Glycosuria is most often seen in patients with a tumour in the region of the hypothalamus or the fourth ventricle. It is more often due to a lowered renal threshold than to hyperglycaemia. 'Cerebral glycosuria' may also occur after head injury and spontaneous subarachnoid haemorrhage, and in meningitis and encephalitis.

Temperature Regulation. Irregular pyrexia may occur in patients with a lesion in the region of the tuber cinereum, and the hyperpyrexia which not uncommonly follows operations in this region is probably the result of injury to a hypothalamic temperature-regulating mechanism.

Ulceration of the Alimentary Canal. Many years ago Schiff demonstrated that lesions in the neighbourhood of the hypothalamus were followed by acute ulceration of the upper part of the alimentary canal, and this has since been confirmed. Perforating ulcers may thus be produced in the oesophagus, stomach, and duodenum of experimental animals. Cushing has drawn attention to the occurrence of similar ulceration in man, as a rare sequel of head injury and cerebral operations, and it may also follow operation on the spinal cord.

Respiratory Disturbances. There is evidence that abnormalities in the rate and amplitude of respiration may be produced by lesions of the hypothalamus, and it is probable that this is the explanation of the respiratory disturbances which have sometimes been seen as sequels of encephalitis lethargica.

REFERENCES

ANDRÉ-THOMAS, (1926) Les moyens d'exploration du système sympathique et leur valeur, *Rev. neurol.*, **33**, (i), 767.

BANNISTER, R., ARDILL, L., and FENTEM, P. (1967) Defective autonomic control of blood vessels in idiopathic orthostatic hypotension, *Brain*, **90**, 725.

BARD, P. (1929) The central representation of the sympathetic system, *Arch. Neurol. Psychiat.(Chicago)*, **22**, 230.

BEATTIE, J., BROW, G. R., and LONG, C. N. H. (1930) Physiological and anatomical evidence for the existence of nerve tracts connecting the hypothalamus with spinal sympathetic centres, *Proc. roy. Soc. B*, **106**, 253.

BROBECK, J. R. (1960) Regulation of feeding and drinking, in *Handbook of Physiology*, Vol. 2, ed. FIELD, J., Washington, D.C.

CAMPBELL, E. J. M., and DICKINSON, G. (1960) *Clinical Physiology*, Oxford.

CLARK, W. E. LE G. (1948) The connexions of the frontal lobes of the brain, *Lancet*, i, 353.

CLARK, W. E. LE G., BEATTIE, J., RIDDOCH, G., and DOTT, N. M. (1938) *The Hypothalamus*, London.

DE WARDENER, H. E., and BARLOW, E. D. (1958) Compulsive water-drinking, *Quart. J. Med.*, **27**, 567.

FULTON, J. F. (1943) *Physiology of the Nervous System*, 2nd ed., Chapters 12 and 13, New York.

FULTON, J. F. (1949) *Functional Localization in the Frontal Lobes and Cerebellum*, Oxford.

FULTON, J. F., and INGRAHAM, F. D. (1929) Emotional disturbances following experimental lesions of the base of the brain (pre-chiasmal), *J. Physiol. (Lond.)*, **67**, 27.

GLEES, P. (1961) *Experimental Neurology*, Chap. xii, Oxford.

GUTTMANN, L. (1940) Topographic studies of disturbances of sweat secretion after complete lesions of peripheral nerves, *J. Neurol. Psychiat.*, N.S. **3**, 197.

HARRIS, G. W. (1960) Central control of pituitary secretion, in *Handbook of Physiology*, Vol. 2, ed. FIELD, J., Washington, D.C.

HEAD, H. On disturbances of sensation with especial reference to the pain of visceral disease. Part I, *Brain*, 1893, **16**, 1; Part II, *Brain*, 1894, **17**, 339; Part III, *Brain*, 1896, **19**, 153.

HESS, W. R. (1954) *Diencephalon*, New York.

INGRAM, W. R. (1960) Central autonomic mechanisms, in *Handbook of Physiology*, Vol. 2, ed. FIELD, J., Washington, D.C.

KUHLENBECK, H. (1954) *The Human Diencephalon*, Basel.

LE MARQUAND, H. S., and RUSSELL, D. S. (1934–5) A case of pubertas praecox (macrogenitosomia praecox) in a boy associated with a tumour in the floor of the third ventricle, *Roy. Berks. Hosp. Rep.*, p. 31.

LEWIS, T. (1937) The nocifensor system of nerves and its reactions, *Brit. med. J.*, **1**, 431.

LEWIS, T. (1938) Suggestions relating to the study of somatic pain, *Brit. med. J.*, **1**, 321.

LIST, C. F., and PEET, M. M. (1938) Sweat secretion in man. IV. Sweat secretion of the face and its disturbances, *Arch. Neurol. Psychiat. (Chicago)*, **40**, 442.

MUNCH-PETERSON, C. J. (1931) Glycosurias of cerebral origin, *Brain*, **54**, 72.

ORTMANN, R. (1960) Neurosecretion, in *Handbook of Physiology*, Vol. 2, ed. FIELD, J., Washington, D.C.

RANSON, S. W. (1926) Anatomy of the sympathetic nervous system with reference to sympathectomy and ramisection, *J. Amer. med. Ass.*, **86**, 1886.

RICHTER, C. P. (1930) Experimental diabetes insipidus, *Brain*, **53**, 76.

SACHS, E., and MACDONALD, M. E. (1925) Blood sugar studies in experimental pituitary and hypothalamic lesions, with a review of literature, *Arch. Neurol. Psychiat. (Chicago)*, **13**, 335.

SAWYER, C. H. (1960) Reproductive behaviour, in *Handbook of Physiology*, Vol. 2., ed. FIELD, J., Washington, D.C.

SINCLAIR, D. C., WEDDELL, G., and FEINDEL, W. H. (1948) Referred pain and associated phenomena, *Brain*, **71**, 184.

SÖDERBERGH, G. (1926) Les moyens actuels d'exploration du système sympathique en clinique et leur valeur, *Rev. neurol.*, **33**, 721.

WALKER, A. E. (1940) A cyto-architectural study of the prefrontal area of the macaque monkey, *J. comp. Neurol.*, **73**, 59.

WALSH, E. G. (1964) *Physiology of the Nervous System*, 2nd ed., Chap. 12, London.

WECHSLER, I. S. (1956) Hypothalamic syndromes, *Brit. med. J.*, **2**, 375.

WHITE, J. C., and SMITHWICK, R. H. (1942) *The Autonomic Nervous System: Anatomy, Physiology and Surgical Application*, 2nd ed., London.

WHITE, P. T., and ROSS, A. T. (1963) Inanition syndrome in infants with anterior hypothalamic neoplasms, *Neurology (Minneap.)*, **13**, 974.

21

DISEASES OF THE BONES OF THE SKULL

OSTEITIS DEFORMANS

Synonym. Paget's disease.

Definition. A chronic disease of the bones characterized by absorption and new bone formation and leading to enlargement of the skull, deformity of the vertebral column, and bowing of the clavicles and long bones of the extremities, and in some cases to nervous symptoms secondary to the bone changes.

AETIOLOGY AND PATHOLOGY

Osteitis deformans is a rare disease of unknown aetiology developing in middle life and affecting both sexes.

Histologically, the changes in the bones are those of a rarefying osteitis, with secondary new bone formation both beneath the periosteum and on the inner side of the corticalis. The deformities are the result of the softening of the bones. The skull becomes thickened, and the distinction between the inner and the outer tables and the diploë is obliterated. The cranial cavity is increased in breadth and to a less extent in length, but its vertical diameter becomes diminished. The base tends to sink relatively to the region of the foramen magnum, which is supported by the vertebral column, and platybasia or basilar impression may result [see p. 917]. Thickening of the skull also leads to a reduction of the size of the vascular and neural foramina and is thus responsible for symptoms of compression of cerebral hemispheres, cerebellum, and cranial nerves. Similar changes in the bones of the vertebral column lead to kyphosis and reduction in the height of the patient, and sometimes to compression of the spinal cord. The clavicles and the long bones of the limbs may also become softened, thickened, and bowed. Generalized atheroma of the arteries is frequently present.

OSSEOUS SYMPTOMS

The onset of the disease is insidious, the patient usually complaining first of pains in the head and limbs. The gradual enlargement of the skull necessitates an increase in the size of the hat worn, and the deformities of the spine and long bones are noticed, together with the resulting diminution in height, which in extreme cases may amount to as much as a foot. The enlarged skull bulges in the frontal and parietal regions. Affected bones often feel unusually warm to the touch. Radiograms show a characteristic appearance, the thickened bone being mottled and 'woolly': rarely there are large islands of osteoporosis in the skull [FIG. 123].

NERVOUS SYMPTOMS

Mental deterioration and epileptiform attacks may occur as a result of compression of the cerebral hemispheres, and symptoms of cerebellar deficiency have also been observed.

Any of the cranial nerves may be compressed owing to reduction in the calibre of their foramina, the olfactory, optic, and vestibulocochlear nerves being most

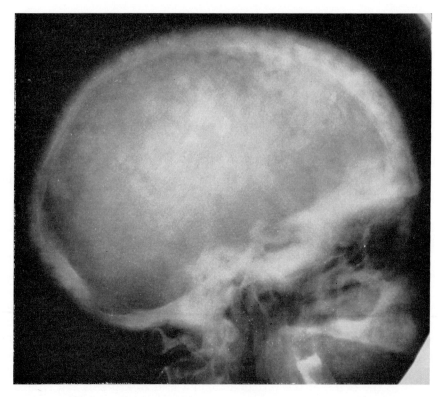

Fig. 123. Paget's disease of the skull. Lateral radiograph demonstrating thickening and the typical 'woolly' appearance of the skull vault with some platybasia. (Kindly provided by Dr. G. L. Gryspeerdt)

often affected. I have seen unilateral optic atrophy, paralysis of one lateral rectus, and also trigeminal neuralgia occurring as isolated nervous symptoms of osteitis deformans. In spite of deformity of the spine associated with vertebral collapse, symptoms of compression of the spinal roots are rare, but compression of the cord itself has been reported in a number of cases and may be associated with cranial nerve lesions, such as optic atrophy. Symptoms of spinal compression are described on page 639. Retinitis pigmentosa may be present.

DIAGNOSIS

The diagnosis is readily made by X-ray examination of the bones, and this should always be carried out in middle-aged patients who complain of obscure pains in the head or limbs or exhibit unexplained cranial nerve palsies or paraplegia. A systolic bruit, due to increased blood flow through the affected bone, may be heard over the skull or spine. The serum alkaline phosphatase is usually raised.

PROGNOSIS

Osteitis deformans is an extremely chronic and slowly progressive disease. Local sarcoma of bone sometimes occurs as a complication. The associated arterial atheroma may prove fatal, for example by causing coronary thrombosis.

Rarely, in severe cases, owing to multiple arteriovenous communications in the affected bones, 'high-output' cardiac failure occurs.

TREATMENT

Treatment is unsatisfactory. Analgesics are often required and radiotherapy has been said to relieve bone pain in some cases. Calcium and vitamin D should probably be given. Laminectomy is necessary when the spinal cord is compressed; and when platybasia causes compression of the lower medulla or upper spinal cord, decompression at the foramen magnum may be indicated but operation is invariably difficult as the affected bone is excessively vascular.

REFERENCES

BOGAERT, L. VAN (1933) Über eine hereditäre und familiäre Form der Pagetschen Ostitis deformans mit Chorioretinitis pigmentosa, Z. ges. Neurol. Psychiat., 147, 327.

BOLL, J. (1946–7) Paget's disease of the skull with platybasia, Proc. roy. Soc. Med., 40, 85.

GREGG, D. (1926) Neurologic symptoms in osteitis deformans (Paget's disease), Arch. Neurol. Psychiat. (Chicago), 15, 613.

GRÜNTHAL, E. (1931) Über den Hirnbefund bei Pagetscher Krankheit des Schädels, Z. ges. Neurol. Psychiat., 136, 656.

GURDJIAN, E. S., WEBSTER, J. E., and LATIMER, F. R. (1952) Paget's disease of the spine with compression of the spinal cord, Trans. Amer. neurol. Ass., 77, 243.

KAUFMAN, M. R. (1929) Psychosis in Paget's disease, Arch. Neurol. Psychiat. (Chicago), 21, 828.

PAGET, J., FRICKER, G., and VER BRUGGHEN, A. (1950) Osteitis fibrosa cystica localisata of the skull, J. Neurosurg., 7, 447.

WYLLIE, W. G. (1923) The occurrence in osteitis deformans of lesions of the central nervous system, with a report of four cases, Brain, 46, 336.

LEONTIASIS OSSEA AND POLYOSTOTIC FIBROUS DYSPLASIA

Leontiasis ossea is characterized by hyperostoses of the bones of the face and skull; sometimes all of the bones of the skull and face are involved and the condition is then similar clinically and pathologically to Paget's disease, but in other cases the overgrowth is limited to one or both cranial bones or to one or both jaws. The name of the condition derives from the leonine facial appearance of many cases. Unlike typical Paget's disease, the condition, which may give rise to convulsions due to compression of the brain, or to cranial nerve palsies, usually begins in childhood and is slowly progressive.

Polyostotic fibrous dysplasia (Albright's syndrome) is limited as a rule to young girls; changes in the long bones, cutaneous pigmentation, and precocious puberty may be accompanied by cranial nerve palsies and/or optic atrophy due to involvement of the bones of the skull base.

REFERENCES

ALBRIGHT, F. (1947) Polyostotic fibrous dysplasia, *J. clin. Endocr.*, **7**, 307.
SMITH, A. G., and ZAVALETA, A. (1952) Osteoma, ossifying fibroma and fibrous dysplasia of the facial and cranial bones, *Arch. Path.*, **54**, 507.

CRANIOSTENOSIS

Synonyms. Oxycephaly; acrocephaly; turricephaly; tower skull.

Definition. A congenital abnormality of the skull due to premature synostosis of the sutures and characterized by an abnormal shape of the head, exophthalmos, optic atrophy, and symptoms of increased intracranial pressure.

AETIOLOGY AND PATHOLOGY

It is generally agreed that craniostenosis is due to premature synostosis of the skull bones. This usually begins in the coronal, sagittal, and lambdoidal sutures, but variations are encountered, and the synostosis may be asymmetrical. It has been attributed to displacement of the centres of ossification towards the sutures. Mann (1937) considers that it is due to a localized arrest of development of the post-optic visceral mesoderm (maxillary process) possibly of atavistic significance. The condition is congenital and sometimes hereditary. Though the sutures are closed, the brain continues to grow at the usual rate. Compensatory enlargement of the skull occurs by means of expansion where the sutures are not united and by thinning of the bone—convolutional atrophy—from pressure of the growing brain. The ultimate break-down of this compensatory process leads to the development of symptoms of increased intracranial pressure. The optic atrophy has been attributed to various causes, including compression of the optic nerves by narrowing of their canals, stretching of the nerves by elongation, pressure upon them by the brain, and papilloedema due to increased intracranial pressure. It is probable that different factors operate in different cases, and that the optic nerves may be damaged in more than one of these ways simultaneously. The exophthalmos appears to be due to abnormal shallowness of the orbits.

Craniostenosis is a feature of the acrocephalosyndactyly of Apert, in which oxycephaly is associated with syndactyly, and of the craniofacial dysostosis of Crouzon.

SYMPTOMS

Since oxycephaly is due to a congenital abnormality, the deformity of the skull may be present at birth, but the patient may not come under observation until other symptoms, such as headache and failing vision, develop, which usually occur in childhood.

The skull is brachycephalic and dome-shaped, with a high forehead, and there may be flattening of the maxillae or asymmetrical facial deformity. The short upper lip is highly characteristic. Owing to the shallowness of the orbits the eyes are prominent, and may even become spontaneously dislocated, and a divergent

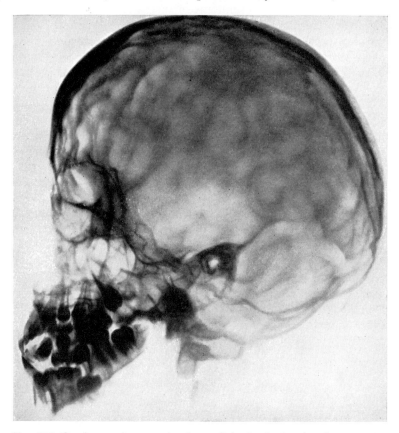

FIG. 124. Craniostenosis: note the shape of the head, the closed sutures, the convolutional thinning, and the prognathism

squint and nystagmus are common. Papilloedema may be present or optic atrophy, either primary or secondary, with impairment of vision, which may reach complete blindness. Other symptoms due either directly to the bone changes or indirectly to increased intracranial pressure include anosmia and deafness. The mental state is usually normal. Radiograms of the skull show the premature synostosis of the sutures and compensatory enlargement, with marked and sometimes extreme convolutional thinning of the calvarium, especially in the frontal region [FIG. 124].

Craniofacial Dysostosis. This disorder, described by Crouzon, is closely related to oxycephaly, and is usually hereditary. The forehead recedes to the high, rather pointed vertex—trigonocephaly. There are also hyperplasia of the maxillae and relative prognathism, together with exophthalmos, divergent squint, and in some cases optic atrophy.

DIAGNOSIS

The condition can usually be recognized at a glance from the shape of the skull. In microcephaly the abnormally small size of the skull is secondary to hypoplasia of the brain, and symptoms of increased intracranial pressure are absent. In hydrocephalus the skull is enlarged in all its diameters and its total volume, which in oxycephaly tends to be subnormal, is increased. Oxycephaly is not likely to be confused with intracranial causes of increased intracranial pressure, such as tumour, if attention is paid to the shape of the skull.

PROGNOSIS

In mild cases compensatory enlargement of the skull may be adequate to prevent the development of symptoms. When, however, headache is present or vision is threatened, no improvement can be anticipated, and the patient's condition is likely to become worse.

TREATMENT

Only surgical treatment is effective. Attempts have been made to deal radically with the cause by opening the sutures and paring their edges. Since in some cases it is possible that the optic nerves are directly compressed in their canals, radiograms of the optic canals should be taken, and if they appear to be unusually small their surgical enlargement should be considered. King (1938) reviewed the surgical treatment and described a new technique, and reviews of modern surgical methods of treatment have been given by Pemberton and Freeman (1962) and Anderson and Geiger (1965).

REFERENCES

ANDERSON, F. M., and GEIGER, L. (1965) Craniosynostosis. A survey of 204 cases, *J. Neurosurg.*, **22**, 229.
CROUZON, O. (1929) *Études sur les maladies familiales nerveuses et dystrophiques*, Paris.
DAVIS, F. A. (1925) Tower skull, oxycephalus, *Amer. J. Ophthal.*, **8**, 513.
KING, J. E. J. (1938) Oxycephaly: a new operation and its results, *Arch. Neurol. Psychiat. (Chicago)*, **40**, 1205.
MANN, I. C. (1937) *Developmental Abnormalities of the Eye*, London.
PEMBERTON, J. W., and FREEMAN, J. M. (1962) Craniosynostosis. A review of experience with forty patients with particular reference to ocular aspects and comments on operative indications, *Amer. J. Ophthal.*, **54**, 641.
SAETHRE, H. (1931) Ueber den Turmschädel, seine Erblichkeit, Pathogenese und neuro-psychiatrischen Symptome, *Acta psychiat. (Kbh.)*, **6**, 405.
WORMS, G., and CARILLON, R. (1930) Oxycephaly, *Rev. Oto-neuro-ophtal.*, **8**, 736.

CLEIDOCRANIAL DYSOSTOSIS

In this rare developmental disorder absence of part or the whole of both clavicles is accompanied by an increase in the width of the forehead. Sometimes there is an associated absence of one or more shoulder-girdle muscles but there are no associated neurological manifestations except in occasional cases in which there are also congenital malformations of the brain and/or other parts of the nervous system.

HYPERTELORISM

In this developmental disorder the distance between the eyes is increased; there is a vertical ridge on the forehead and the bridge of the nose is excessively broad. Usually there is no neurological defect but in occasional rare and severe cases associated maldevelopment of the forebrain gives rise to mental deficiency.

REFERENCES

CURRARINO, G., and SILVERMAN, F. N. (1960) Orbital hypertelorism, arhinencephaly and trigonocephaly, *Radiology*, **74**, 206.
KLEMMER, R. N., SNOKE, P. O., and COOPER, H. K. (1931) Cleidocranial dysostosis, *Amer. J. Roentgenol.*, **25**, 710.

BASILAR IMPRESSION

Basilar impression is an abnormality of the base of the skull in which the angle between the basisphenoid and the basilar portion of the occipital bone—normally between 110 and 140 degrees—is widened. In the congenital form the foramen magnum is deformed, the atlas is occipitalized, and the medulla is unusually low, so that it and the upper part of the cervical spinal cord may be compressed by the dens. In a lateral radiograph the line drawn from the posterior end of the hard palate to the posterior lip of the foramen magnum normally lies above the cervical spine, but in basilar impression it cuts the cervical spine at some point (Chamberlain, 1939), but Bull, Nixon, and Pratt (1955) point out that the plane of the axis relative to that of the hard palate is a more reliable guide. Normally these are roughly parallel: in basilar impression they form an acute angle. The condition is often identified, particularly in the American literature, by the term 'platybasia', but the latter term, which simply means a flat base of skull, can equally be applied to the changes in the skull base which occur, for instance, in Paget's disease. Basilar impression is a name best reserved for the congenital disorder in which, perhaps because of a congenital abnormality of the occipital bone, the posterior part of the atlas vertebra is partially invaginated into the cranial cavity.

Basilar impression is therefore congenital and may be associated with fusion of the bodies of some cervical vertebrae—the Klippel-Feil syndrome—or it may be due to osteogenesis imperfecta (Hurwitz and McSwiney, 1960).

It may lead to hydrocephalus, and, Gustafson and Oldberg (1940) suggested, may be responsible for the Arnold-Chiari syndrome, but they are more probably associated congenital abnormalities. The spinal cord may exhibit hydromyelia. In adults the clinical picture may resemble multiple sclerosis, syringomyelia, or high cervical tumour. The head is sometimes mushroom-shaped and the neck abnormally short, but the diagnosis can only be made by X-ray examination. If symptoms occur the treatment is surgical decompression.

REFERENCES

BULL, J., NIXON, W. L. B., and PRATT, R. T. C. (1955) The radiological criteria and familial occurrence of primary basilar impression, *Brain*, **78,** 229.

CHAMBERLAIN, W. E. (1939) Basilar impression (platybasia), *Yale J. Biol. Med.*, **11,** 487.

GUSTAFSON, W. A., and OLDBERG, E. (1940) Neurologic significance of platybasia, *Arch. Neurol. Psychiat. (Chicago)*, **44,** 84.

HURWITZ, L. J., and MCSWINEY, R. R. (1960) Basilar impression and osteogenesis imperfecta in a family, *Brain*, **83,** 138.

22

PAROXYSMAL AND CONVULSIVE DISORDERS

EPILEPSY

Definition. Epilepsy is a paroxysmal and transitory disturbance of the functions of the brain which develops suddenly, ceases spontaneously, and exhibits a conspicuous tendency to recurrence. Though in its most typical forms it is characterized by the sudden onset of loss of consciousness, which may or may not be associated with tonic spasm and clonic contractions of the muscles, many varieties of epileptic attack occur, their distinctive features depending upon differences in the site of origin, extent of spread, and nature of the disturbance of function. Epilepsy is thus a symptom. In some cases a local lesion of the brain plays the chief part in causation; in others hereditary predisposition seems the important factor: in others again the cause is quite unknown. A generalized attack has long been known as 'grand mal', an attack characterized by loss of consciousness only without falling and without, as a rule, motor accompaniments, as 'petit mal'.

THE PHYSIOLOGICAL NATURE OF EPILEPSY

The invention of electroencephalography [see p. 138], though it has posed many problems which are still unsolved, has thrown much new light upon the nature of epilepsy. The electroencephalograms obtained in epilepsy are described in more detail later. For our present purpose it is sufficient to say that epileptic attacks are usually accompanied by abnormal changes in the electrical potentials of the brain; hence epilepsy has been described as 'paroxysmal cerebral dysrhythmia' (Gibbs, Gibbs, and Lennox, 1937). In spite of this advance many problems remain unsolved, for cortical dysrhythmias similar to those found in epilepsy may be present in patients suffering from disorders other than epilepsy, and also in non-epileptic relatives of epileptics. Furthermore, in certain unquestionable attacks of epilepsy, EEG recordings taken through the intact skull may show no abnormality.

Nevertheless, this work supports the view that the physiological basis of a convulsion is a discharge of neurones rather than a primary impairment or loss of cortical function. Experimentally it can be shown in animals that convulsant drugs induce fits, the pattern of which can be modified by the successful removal of different levels of the nervous system from the cortex downwards. Moreover, electrical stimulation of the cortex in man, as shown especially by Foerster, results in convulsions which can only be satisfactorily interpreted as the expression of a regional cortical discharge. Transitory post-epileptic symptoms, whether loss or disorder of consciousness, paralysis or sensory loss, have been interpreted as being due to temporary exhaustion of neurones which have been the site of discharge. However, Efron (1961) has given cogent reasons for suggesting that an active process of inhibition rather than 'exhaustion', resulting from persistent subclinical epileptic discharge, is a more probable explanation for post-epileptic paralysis (Todd's paralysis).

Excitation, however, is not the most likely explanation of loss of consciousness occurring as the sole, or almost the sole, manifestation of epilepsy, as in petit mal. The bilaterally synchronous wave-and-spike cortical discharge which characterizes petit mal appears to originate at a subcortical centre, perhaps the interthalamic adhesion (Jasper and Droogleever-Fortuyn, 1947) and the resulting impairment of consciousness has been interpreted by Grey Walter (1947) as the result of an abnormal synchronization of cortical rhythms, and by Williams (1950) as indicating a blockage of afferent impulses to the cortex. In the light of experimental work and the behaviour of the EEG in man, Gastaut and Fischer-Williams (1960) put forward the hypothesis that 'a grand mal seizure seems to depend on a thalamic discharge which involves the non-specific reticular structures and is projected to the cortex in what may be considered a generalized recruiting response transmitted along the diffuse cortical projection pathways'. They compare 'the hypersynchronous discharge of generalized epilepsy' with a sort of 'paroxysmal sleep' localized to the thalamocortical system and provoking a functional exclusion of this system; if it be supposed that the same factor also precipitates hypersynchrony of the reticular formation, it is possible to explain all the features of a grand mal attack, the thalamic discharge being responsible for the loss of consciousness and the discharge of the brain stem reticular formation for the tonic and clonic element in the convulsions. According to the same authors petit mal may be explained as the result of a thalamic discharge occurring in a subject with a very effective inhibitory mechanism. The lack of convulsions may depend on the fact that the reticular formation is rhythmically inhibited. The site of origin of the myoclonic jerks which occur in some forms of epilepsy has been studied also by Gastaut and Fischer-Williams. Such jerks may be evoked by sensory stimuli, especially after the administration of convulsant drugs, and appear to originate in the mesencephalon and thalamus. The disturbances of consciousness, mood, and behaviour which occur as a result of discharges originating in the temporal lobe have been interpreted as disorders of a specific integrating role in respect of consciousness played by this part of the brain (Penfield and Jasper, 1954).

Epilepsy, then, is to be regarded as an uncontrolled neural discharge, that is, as an abnormal conversion of the potential energy of the neurones into kinetic energy. Fundamentally, therefore, it is a physico-chemical disturbance, and it is to be expected that the causative abnormal physico-chemical state of the neurones should be produced by a wide variety of agencies. How they operate is most likely to be elucidated by study of the physiological disorder underlying the onset and cessation of a focal attack. Symonds (1959) considered possible regulatory biochemical factors. He suggested that γ-aminobutyric acid (GABA) may be 'a natural anticonvulsant' formed in the brain. Local lesions may cause seizures either by allowing the accumulation of an excitatory substance or by depressing the tonic inhibitory control of afferent impulses. Recent experimental work has shown that the application of acetylcholine to the cerebral cortex may provoke focal convulsions, while generalized fits may follow the intravenous injection of this substance; thus fits may be due to exogenous or endogenous factors which influence its local or generalized release in excess of the normal quantities required for synaptic transmission. GABA and acetylcholine have opposite effects upon brain excitability so that an imbalance between these two substances within the brain could be one factor predisposing to seizure production (Jurgelsky and Thomas, 1966).

AETIOLOGY

The following classification of the principal causes of epilepsy is for convenience arranged schematically, but it must be remembered that the precise way in which a cause operates is often obscure and in some instances a single pathological condition might be placed in more than one category.

1. *Local Causes*

   (*a*) Conditions associated with increased intracranial pressure:
   Intracranial tumour; cerebral abscess; subdural haematoma; subarachnoid haemorrhage.

   (*b*) Inflammatory conditions:
   Meningitis; all forms of acute and subacute encephalitis; toxoplasmosis; neurosyphilis; multiple sclerosis; cerebral cysticercosis.

   (*c*) Trauma:
   Perinatal brain injury and/or haemorrhage; head injuries of later life.

   (*d*) Congenital abnormalities:
   Congenital diplegia; tuberous sclerosis; porencephaly.

   (*e*) Degenerations:
   The cerebral lipidoses; diffuse sclerosis; encephalopathies of infancy and childhood, including 'infantile spasms'; Pick's disease; Alzheimer's disease; progressive myoclonic epilepsy; subacute spongiform encephalopathy; Jakob-Creutzfeldt disease.

   (*f*) Circulatory disturbances:
   Cerebral atheroma, haemorrhage, thrombosis, embolism; eclampsia; hypertensive encephalopathy; cerebral complications of 'connective tissue' or 'collagen diseases'; polycythaemia; acute cerebral ischaemia from any cause.

2. *General Causes*

   (*a*) Exogenous poisons:
   Alcohol; absinthe; thujone; cocaine; strychnine; lead; chloroform; ether; insulin; amphetamines; camphor; *Metrazol*, organophosphorus and organochlorine compounds used as insecticides, and fluoracetic acid derivatives; amine-oxidase inhibitors, imipramine and its derivatives; and *withdrawal* of alcohol, barbiturates, and other drugs.

   (*b*) Anoxia:
   Asphyxia; carbon monoxide poisoning; nitrous oxide anaesthesia; profound anaemia.

(c) Disordered metabolism:

Uraemia; hepatic failure; hypo–adrenalism; water intoxication; porphyria; hypoglycaemia; hyperpyrexia; alkalosis; pyridoxine deficiency.

(d) Endocrine disorders:

Parathyroid tetany; idiopathic hypoparathyroidism and pseudohypoparathyroidism.

(e) Allergy:

Epilepsy associated with asthma or other allergic states.

(f) Conditions associated particularly with childhood:

Rickets; acute infections ('febrile convulsions').

3. *Psychological Factors*

These are relatively unimportant. It is doubtful if psychological factors alone are sufficient to cause epileptiform convulsions. In individuals otherwise predisposed, however, fright or anxiety may precipitate attacks.

4. *Constitutional Epilepsy*

When all the above factors have been excluded there remains a large group of patients who suffer from convulsions for which no local or general cause can be found. We seem, therefore, compelled to regard these individuals as suffering from a predisposition to convulsions, the nature of which is not yet understood, but it must be borne in mind that the distinction between constitutional and symptomatic epilepsy is not clear-cut. There is an intermediate group of patients in whom predisposition determines the development of epilepsy after a focal cerebral lesion such as a head injury. (See Lennox's (1947) study of twin pairs with seizures.) Thus while a division of cases of epilepsy into symptomatic and idiopathic ('constitutional' or 'cryptogenic' or 'centrencephalic') groups is of some clinical value it should be recognized that, in a sense, to make a diagnosis of idiopathic epilepsy is a confession of failure as it simply implies that even with modern methods of investigation the cause of the epilepsy cannot be demonstrated.

The History of Patients Suffering from Epilepsy

The following inquiries should be made of a patient suffering from convulsions.

When did the first attack occur? Was it precipitated by an accident or associated with an acute illness? How soon was it followed by the second? What is the usual interval between the attacks? Are they increasing in frequency? Do the attacks occur in bouts? Has the patient had a series of attacks without recovering consciousness? Do the attacks occur at any special time of the day? Do they occur only by day or only by night? In the case of a woman, are they related to the menstrual periods? Is any factor known to precipitate the attacks? Does the patient have any warning? If so, what, and by how long does it precede the attack? How does an attack begin? Is its onset local or general, gradual or sudden? Is consciousness lost? Do convulsive movements occur in the attack? If so, are they symmetrical or asymmetrical? Has the patient injured himself in an attack? Does he bite his tongue and pass urine? How long do the attacks last? What is his condition afterwards? Are the attacks followed by headache, sleepiness, paralysis, or mental disturbance, such as automatism? What treatment has he had and how has he responded to it? Has he at any time suffered from head injury? If the attacks did not begin in infancy, did he suffer from infantile convulsions? Is there a family history of epilepsy or of fainting fits or of mental disorder?

Heredity

Inherited predisposition plays a considerable part in the aetiology of epilepsy. In a series of 200 epileptics there was a family history of the disease in 28 per cent. We must distinguish, however, between the inheritance of a predisposition and the inheritance of epilepsy. What seems to be inherited is the physical or neurophysiological basis of a cortical dysrhythmia, but only a small proportion of those with cortical dysrhythmia become epileptic. Lennox, Gibbs, and Gibbs (1940) studied the EEG in the parents of epileptics; only in 5 per cent. were both normal; in 35 per cent. both were abnormal. The same authors state that an abnormal EEG is six times as common among the relatives of epileptics as in controls, and this is true both of 'symptomatic' and 'idiopathic' epileptics. However, clinical evidence indicates that a history of epilepsy in other members of the family is obtained twice as commonly in patients with idiopathic epilepsy as in those whose seizures are symptomatic. Lennox (1947) believes that the dysrhythmia is inherited as a Mendelian dominant. For the reasons given above, it is difficult to estimate the liability of an epileptic parent to transmit the disorder to his or her offspring, since it often remains latent and the condition reappears in a collateral line. Not more than one in thirty-six of the children of a mixed group of epileptics develops epilepsy, but in some families the incidence is higher. The risk is greater if there are several cases in the family and if the non-epileptic conjugal partner has a cortical dysrhythmia.

Trauma

The role of trauma in causing epilepsy is difficult to estimate. It is well known that severe head injuries may be followed by epilepsy [p. 348]. In adults, post-traumatic epilepsy rarely follows closed head injury unless the latter was severe enough to cause twenty-four hours of post-traumatic amnesia or unless 'early fits' occurred within the first forty-eight hours after the injury, in which case the development of post-traumatic epilepsy subsequently is much more common (Jennett, 1961). The incidence is much greater after penetrating wounds of the brain and in young children in whom less severe closed head injuries may be followed by fits, which usually begin within the first year after the injury. Epilepsy is relatively commoner among firstborn children than among later members of the family, and this is probably explained by the increased liability of the firstborn to head injury during birth.

Other Local Cerebral Lesions

There is evidence also that other lesions of the nervous system predispose to epileptic attacks, for example, infantile hemiplegia. That minor cerebral lesions are also of some aetiological importance is indicated by the frequency with which slight abnormalities are found in the nervous system in epileptics.

For example, Hodskins and Yakovlev (1930) found a completely normal nervous system in only 17 per cent. of three hundred epileptics in an institution. In addition to a wide range of congenital abnormalities, cerebral birth lesions, and lesions caused by encephalitis in childhood, certain other disorders predispose towards epilepsy which may, however, be delayed for many years. These are eclampsia and hypertension complicating pregnancy, acute otitis media and mastoiditis, probably only when complicated by cortical venous thrombosis. Epilepsy is associated with rheumatic heart disease more frequently than can be explained by chance. In mitral stenosis a small cerebral embolus may cause epilepsy, as may a small asymptomatic infarct in patients with intracranial atheroma (Dodge, Richardson, and Victor, 1954).

Metabolic and Endocrine Factors

Prolonged search has not revealed any constant metabolic abnormality in epileptic patients, though hints are not wanting that some metabolic disturbance may play a part in the production of the fits. Generalized convulsions may occur in tetany due either to alkalosis, to destruction of the parathyroids, or to idiopathic hypoparathyroidism, and in epileptics, as Rosett has shown, a fit can often be precipitated if alkalosis is induced by over-breathing. There is no evidence, however, that normally alkalosis is responsible for the attacks. Attacks may be induced in some epileptics by water retention or by excessive alcohol consumption. A small proportion of patients are of the obese type associated with hypopituitarism. In fact some epileptics fall into the group which Kretschmer describes as dysplastic. The role of menstruation in precipitating the attacks in women is unexplained, but supports the view which attributes importance to metabolic factors. Pregnancy may also influence the attacks. It is not uncommon for an epileptic woman to be free from attacks during pregnancy or even to be free when she is pregnant with children of one sex and not with the other. Others, again, are worse when pregnant. The truth probably is that epileptics are usually made worse by any change in their internal environment.

Febrile Convulsions

Convulsions accompanying febrile illnesses in infancy and early childhood have been regarded by some authorities as carrying a good prognosis. Certainly some infants may have one or two such attacks and no more but many go on to develop spontaneous fits later and a proportion have definite epileptic discharges in the EEG. The condition should be considered to be one form (possibly a benign form) of idiopathic infantile epilepsy.

Allergy

Allergy may be a causal factor in a few cases, especially in patients who also suffer from asthma or other allergic states.

Migraine

While loss of consciousness during an attack of migraine or at the height of the headache is usually syncopal, there is a slightly increased incidence of epilepsy in migraine sufferers, even in those who have no evidence of a cerebral lesion (such as an angioma) of which both the migraine and the epilepsy could be symptomatic.

Sex and Age Incidence

Females have been said to suffer from epilepsy slightly more frequently than males. In Gowers' series of 3,000 cases the ratio of females to males was 13:12. However, the sex incidence may be changing as Lennox and Lennox (1960) found that whereas under the age of 5 years there were 105 females for every 100 affected males, over the age of 20 years the male:female incidence was 100:59. In three-quarters of all cases the disorder first manifests itself under the age of 20, almost half the cases beginning during the second decade of life. Only in 10 per cent. does it develop after the age of 30 (Gowers). During the first twenty years of life the onset of convulsions occurs more frequently at certain ages than at others. The liability is high during the first three years; there is a peak at 7, corresponding to the second dentition; and a further peak at 14, 15, and 16. Apart from cases in which the attacks begin during infancy and continue without remission, epileptics exhibit a special liability to infantile convulsions, with a subsequent period of freedom from fits, which may last for years. Infantile convulsions have been noted to occur up to ten times as often in patients subsequently developing epilepsy as in the non-epileptic adult population.

Estimates of the incidence of epilepsy in the population of Switzerland, Holland, and America are all about 5 per 1,000 and a similar figure was recently obtained for England and Wales (Report by Research Committee of General Practitioners, 1960).

PATHOLOGY

There is no constant pathological change to be found in the brains of epileptics, though abnormalities are common. The difficulty is to determine which pathological changes may be the cause of epilepsy and which may result from the seizures that, if severe and frequent, may undoubtedly cause cerebral anoxia. In patients with symptomatic epilepsy secondary to identifiable organic disease of the brain little difficulty will usually arise but the interpretation of minor abnormalities in cases of presumed idiopathic epilepsy is much more difficult (Meyer, 1963). Probably in most such cases loss of nerve cells in the cortex and cerebellum, a finding described by many authors, is the result, rather than the cause of the epilepsy. Microscopically much attention has been directed to focal lesions in Ammon's horn. When recent these consist of foci of tissue destruction which are later followed by gliosis. Spielmeyer considered that these changes were the results of vascular spasm, but recent work suggests that they may be the cause and not the result of epileptic attacks (Falconer, 1953). Such changes appear to be responsible for temporal lobe epilepsy in a high proportion of cases and Earle, Baldwin, and Penfield (1953) suggest that hippocampal herniation at birth is the aetiological factor of greatest importance. However, similar pathological changes in Ammon's horn and in the region of the amygdala may be a sequel of anoxia. Cavanagh (1958) has reported eight cases of temporal lobe epilepsy of many years' standing associated with small tumours, considered most likely to be hamartomas, but a few showing early evidence of neoplastic transformation.

SYMPTOMS

Major Epilepsy (Grand Mal)

Pre-convulsive Symptoms. Epileptic patients frequently exhibit symptoms which precede an attack for hours, or even for a day or two, and which enable those about them to recognize that a fit is likely to occur. These pre-convulsive symptoms include mental changes such as irritability and depression, abnormal feelings referred to the head, giddiness, and sudden myoclonic twitches.

Precipitating Factors. Usually these are absent. Rarely the kind of stimulus which more often causes syncope may precipitate an epileptic attack [see p. 285]. Severe coughing may do so (so-called laryngeal epilepsy). Eating or drinking alcohol sometimes brings on an attack. Lastly there are the varieties of evoked or reflex epilepsy [see p. 930].

The Aura. The aura, or warning of the attack, occurs according to Gowers in three-fifths of all cases. It is a symptom produced by the beginning of the epileptic discharge and perceived by the patient before consciousness is lost. In the remaining cases the patient experiences no warning, but becomes unconscious at the onset of the fit. Since the focus of origin of the fit may be situated in a variety of localities within the brain there is a corresponding variety of auras. The aura may take the form of a complex mental state, such as a feeling of unreality (*jamais vu*) or, on the other hand, of familiarity (*déjà vu*), as though events being experienced have happened before. The patient may feel that he is disembodied, or he may experience an intense but inexplicable fear. This last aura is sometimes associated with running, the patient running several yards before falling unconscious—'cursive epilepsy'. The aura may be referred to one of the special senses: olfactory and gustatory hallucinations may occur; visual auras may consist of complex scenes (formed visual hallucinations) or simple flashes of light or balls of fire (crude visual hallucinations); auditory auras may take the form of hallucinations of hearing words or phrases uttered, or may consist merely of crude sounds. Vertigo is a common aura, and Foerster has shown that a convulsion beginning with an aura of vertigo can be excited by electrical stimulation of the intraparietal sulcus. Sensory auras may consist of sensations of numbness, tingling or electric shocks referred to part of the body, or there may be a sensation as though a limb were shrivelling up. Painful sensory auras occur, but are rare. Abnormal visceral sensations frequently constitute the aura, the patient experiencing a peculiar sensation ('butterflies' in the stomach) or sometimes even pain in the epigastrium. There are many forms of motor aura. There may be a strong impulse to speak associated with a feeling of inability to do so or else chewing or 'smacking' of the lips may occur. The fit may begin with spasm or clonic movement of part of the body, for example turning of the head to one side or flexion of the upper limb, and the patient may be aware of the movement before he loses consciousness. Sometimes the whole body is rotated to one side.

Frequently the aura is so brief and takes the form of no more than a transient indefinable sensation that the patient is unable to describe it though he knows that he has a warning of insufficient duration for him to be able to reach a place of safety.

The Convulsion. The convulsion may begin with the epileptic cry, a harsh scream due to forcible expiration of air through the partly closed vocal cords, but this is more often absent than present. Consciousness is lost either immediately after the aura or at the very beginning of the attack, and the patient falls to the ground. He usually has no recollection of falling. In the fall he may injure himself, and permanent scars on the face, limbs or trunk from this cause are common in epileptics. The first motor manifestation of the convulsion proper is usually a phase of tonic spasm of the muscles. This is for the most part symmetrical on the two sides of the body, though it is common for the head and eyes to be rotated to one side and for the mouth to be drawn to one side by asymmetry in the degree of facial spasm. The upper limbs are usually adducted at the shoulders and flexed at the elbows and wrists. The fingers are flexed at the metacarpophalangeal and extended at the interphalangeal joints, the thumb being adducted. The lower limbs are usually extended, with the feet inverted. The respiratory and trunk muscles partake in the spasm, and respiration is arrested. The tonic phase may last only a few seconds and rarely endures more than half a minute.

It is followed by the clonic phase, in which sustained tonic contraction of the muscles gives place to sharp, short, interrupted jerks. As Gowers pointed out, the clonic phase is probably a series of interruptions of the tonic contraction, rather than an essentially different phenomenon, and Cobb (1932) has shown electromyographically that both are tetanic. The tonic phase may be so intense that occasionally compression fracture of the body of one or more thoracic vertebrae may occur in a fit and this should be borne in mind if the patient complains of pain in the back after recovery.

In the clonic phase the tongue may be bitten if it is caught between the teeth when the jaw is closed. Foaming at the mouth may occur, and the saliva may be blood-stained if the tongue has been bitten. Incontinence of urine often occurs: incontinence of faeces is less common.

At the onset of an epileptic fit the patient may be either pale or flushed. He becomes progressively cyanosed during the arrest of respiratory movements which occurs in the tonic stage, the cyanosis passing off when respiration is re-established in the clonic stage. Subconjunctival or cutaneous petechial haemorrhages may occur. There is often profuse sweating. The pupils become dilated at the beginning of the attack and the reaction to light is usually lost. The corneal reflexes are also lost in a severe attack; the tendon reflexes may be abolished and the plantar reflexes may be extensor for a short time after the attack.

The Post-convulsive Phase. Towards the end of the clonic phase the intervals between the muscular contractions become longer and the jerks finally cease. The patient remains unconscious for a variable time, usually from a few minutes to half an hour and on recovering consciousness often sleeps for several hours.

Headache is common after an attack. Usually after recovering consciousness the patient is mentally normal. Exceptionally, however, a convulsion is followed by an abnormal mental state which may last a few minutes or even for several hours. In post-epileptic automatism the patient, though apparently conscious, may carry out a series of complex actions which are often inappropriate to the circumstances and of which he subsequently has no recollection. Sometimes the epileptic attack passes into an hysterical attack. Rarely the epileptic patient may become maniacal after a convulsion. Post-epileptic mental aberration follows temporal lobe epilepsy more frequently than it does major epilepsy.

Minor Epilepsy

Minor epilepsy is a term applied to slight epileptic attacks in which impairment or loss of consciousness is the most prominent symptom.

Petit Mal

Whereas in the past the term petit mal was often used to identify all forms of minor epilepsy unaccompanied by convulsions, the term is now reserved for transient minor 'absences' or 'blank spells' which invariably begin in childhood and never in adult life though in occasional cases, having begun in a child, they may continue for many years. In the present state of knowledge, true petit mal is invariably idiopathic, never symptomatic. The child, without warning, stares blankly into space, the eyes may roll up beneath the upper lids, and for a second or two he will stop talking or whatever he is doing and then will continue with his activity, often unaware that an attack has taken place. Occasionally a single myoclonic twitch of the head and upper limbs may accompany such episodes. Falling does not occur and the attacks often occur many times in the day. Some patients with attacks of petit mal also have major seizures or develop these as they grow older.

Other Forms of Minor Epilepsy

These may occur at any age and may be idiopathic or symptomatic, the pattern depending upon the origin and spread of the epileptic discharge. Some such attacks, occurring either in childhood or in adult life, may be clinically indistinguishable from true petit mal.

The slightest form of minor epilepsy, often described by the patient as a 'sensation', consists of a disturbance of consciousness often similar to the aura of a major attack, and sometimes associated with giddiness. In a 'sensation' consciousness may not be completely lost. Next in severity comes complete loss of consciousness, preceded or not by an aura, but the motor and postural functions of the brain are so little affected that the patient remains standing and does not fall. He looks somewhat dazed and stares as in an attack of petit mal. After a few seconds he recovers and may continue what he was doing before the attack. In more severe attacks the motor and postural functions are affected, and the patient, besides losing consciousness, may fall to the ground or may exhibit slight muscular rigidity or carry out a brief stereotyped movement. Attacks in which falling occurs but in which there are no convulsive movements are often called akinetic epilepsy. Transitory pallor may occur in minor epilepsy. Incontinence of urine may occur, though it is less frequent than in major attacks. There is no post-ictal coma.

Temporal Lobe Epilepsy. The clinical picture of temporal lobe epilepsy depends upon whether the epileptic discharge remains localized to the temporal lobe (in which case focal features related to temporal lobe dysfunction are consistently noted) or whether it spreads rapidly throughout the remainder of the brain, in which case there may be a major fit with a 'temporal lobe aura' or even a major fit without an aura which is then indistinguishable from an attack of idiopathic grand mal. The EEG is of considerable value in the diagnosis. In these attacks the patient may become confused, often anxious and negativistic, and carries out movements of a highly organized but semi-automatic character (automatism).

Automatism may take various forms; sometimes it is purposeless, occasionally purposive (e.g. undressing in public) and, rarely, aggressive or violent behaviour can occur. Attacks may last for only a few seconds or for minutes or longer, whether or not a major convulsion follows the aura. Varied disturbances of the content of consciousness may occur: these include hallucinations of smell and taste (uncinate epilepsy), vision and hearing, perceptual illusions, disordered sense of reality or of the body, disturbances of memory, and paroxysms of fear. Visual phenomena may include formed hallucinations, macropsia and micropsia, while depersonalization (*jamais vu* or unreality) suggests to the patient a dream or 'trance-like' state and *déjà vu*, an intense feeling of familiarity, may be accompanied by vivid visual or auditory memory patterns which the patient is subsequently unable to recall though remembering that they were familiar and a constantly-recurring pattern of his attack. Depression is also an occasional feature. Uncinate attacks are characterized by hallucinations of smell or taste. They are often accompanied by movements of the lips, tongue, and jaw, for example, those of tasting or chewing, and are associated with a disturbance of memory. Uncinate attacks are usually the result of organic disease in the region of the uncus [see p. 243].

Jacksonian Epilepsy. Jacksonian epilepsy usually begins in one of three foci, the thumb and index finger, the angle of the mouth, or the great toe. A convulsion with such a focal onset and the type of spread described on page 24 is almost always a symptom of organic disease of the brain in the region of the precentral gyrus. A similar focal onset is not unknown in presumed idiopathic epilepsy, particularly in children, but in such cases the spread of the convulsion is more rapid than in a typical Jacksonian attack and consciousness is lost early.

Sensory Epilepsy. This is the sensory equivalent of motor Jacksonian epilepsy and consists of paraesthesiae, such as tingling or 'electric shocks', less frequently of painful sensation, involving usually a part or the whole of one side of the body. The attacks may occur without loss of consciousness and are usually the result of a lesion in the opposite parietal lobe.

Epilepsia Partialis Continua. This is a rare form of focal convulsion in which Jacksonian epilepsy, confined to a limited part of the body, continues for hours, days, weeks, or rarely months, without stopping. It is invariably due to a focal lesion of the brain though the nature of the lesion may not be immediately apparent.

Adversive Attacks. These begin with turning of the head and eyes and some-times of the body to the opposite side: they originate in front of the precentral gyrus in the region of the so-called frontal eye field (Brodmann's area 8).

Inhibitory Epilepsy. This is a very rare form of attack in which transitory loss of power occurs in a limb or in one-half of the body without precedent tonic spasm or clonic movements. It may or may not be associated with impairment or loss of consciousness.

'Drop' Attacks. In these the patient falls to the ground without warning. The only evidence for loss of consciousness is unawareness of the fall itself. The patient can get up at once. There are two varieties of these: (1) a form of akinetic epilepsy (see above); and (2) sudden falls occurring chiefly in elderly women. It is unlikely that the latter attacks are epileptic; they seem most often to be a symptom of atheromatous ischaemia of the brain stem (vertebro-basilar insufficiency).

'Tonic Epilepsy.' A convulsion may consist of an attack of muscular rigidity associated with loss of consciousness, but not followed by clonic movements. In the usual form of tonic convulsion the posture of the body differs from that of the tonic phase of a major epileptic attack. The head is extended, the upper limbs are thrown out in front of the patient, extended at the elbows, internally rotated and hyperpronated, with the fingers somewhat flexed. The lower limbs are extended. This type of fit is usually the result of organic disease of the brain [see p. 921] but occurs occasionally in idiopathic epilepsy. Focal 'tonic fits' in which similar attacks may involve one or two limbs without loss of consciousness have been described in multiple sclerosis and have been attributed to the presence of a brain stem lesion (Matthews, 1954).

Vestibular and Vestibulogenic Attacks. Behrman and Wyke (1958) dis-tinguish these two varieties of attack both of which have an aura of vertigo. They suggest that vestibular attacks originate in the cortical vestibular centre in the mid-temporal region and that vestibulogenic attacks are excited by labyrinthine discharge, often from an abnormal labyrinth, which excites discharge from neurones in the brain stem reticular system.

Evoked or Reflex Epilepsy. It occasionally happens that a convulsion may be excited by some form of external stimulation. This may be a sudden loud noise—*acoustico-motor epilepsy*—or music—*musicogenic epilepsy*—or a visual—*photic*—or cutaneous stimulus. So-called 'television epilepsy' has been in-creasingly recognized in recent years. Both childhood petit mal but more par-ticularly grand mal in children and less commonly in adults may be precipitated by watching television, particularly when the set is flickering or poorly adjusted so that flickering lines appear. Sometimes a voluntary movement will precipitate an attack. In such cases sudden movement is particularly likely to induce a type of 'tonic fit' in the limb which is moved (Lishman *et al.*, 1962). Numerous activities which may act in this way are described by Symonds (1959). An attack may be self-induced; this particularly occurs in children with petit mal who may rapidly move their fingers between their eyes and the sun to induce an attack (Whitty, 1960).

There may be visceral concomitants; not only may gastric distension precipitate an attack, but in some patients the onset is always associated with diarrhoea.

Reflex inhibition of a fit is an allied phenomenon. When a convulsion has a focal onset and begins with movement, for example, of one limb, a strong stimulus, such as a firm grip, rubbing, or passive movement applied to the limb, will often abort an attack, if it is begun immediately after the onset. Efron (1957) has shown that uncinate attacks may sometimes be arrested by smelling a powerful odour.

Pyknolepsy. Pyknolepsy is a term which has been applied to a form of epilepsy characterized by very frequent attacks of petit mal. It occurs in children, and the patient may have over a hundred attacks in a day. As the condition is in no way different from petit mal the term has now been discarded.

Infantile Spasms

This name has been given to brief attacks, beginning almost invariably in infants within the first few months of life in which there is a sudden shock-like flexion of the arms and often flexion of the head, neck, and trunk with drawing up of the knees (so-called salaam attacks). These momentary attacks may occur many times in the day; their development sometimes in infants who appear to be of normal intellect is followed by progressive mental deterioration so that when they eventually cease the child is often left spastic and severely retarded. The EEG usually shows a pattern of almost continuous irregular slow spike-and-wave activity which has been called hypsarrhythmia (Gibbs and Gibbs, 1952; Bower and Jeavons, 1959; Kiloh and Osselton, 1967). In most cases coming to autopsy the degenerative changes seen in the cortex and white matter of the cerebrum are non-specific but the syndrome has been observed in children with hypoglycaemia, phenylketonuria, and tuberous sclerosis (della Rovere, Hoare, and Pampiglione, 1964). The cause is unknown; while anticonvulsants are relatively ineffective, ACTH or steroid drugs, if given early enough, may arrest the process.

Myoclonus Epilepsy. See page 956.

The Time-relationship of Attacks

Individuals differ greatly in respect of the frequency of their attacks. At one extreme are those who have only one, or perhaps two, in a lifetime; at the other, those who convulse several times a day.

As Gowers pointed out, there are three common modes of onset of the convulsions. A patient may have petit mal for a long period before beginning to have major fits. Alternatively, the first attack may be a severe one and thereafter major fits may occur at short intervals, with or without attacks of petit mal in addition; or there may be major attacks separated by long intervals of months or even years. In 76 per cent. of Gowers' cases the intervals between attacks were less than one month. Some patients always have attacks in groups of two or more within a few hours.

Time of day is an important factor in determining the occurrence of fits. In 42 per cent. of a series of cases attacks occurred by day only, in 24 per cent. by night only, and in the remainder both by day and by night. When the attacks were confined to the day they occurred only half as frequently as in the other two groups. Nocturnal fits are most likely to occur shortly after going to sleep and between 4 and 5 a.m., while the commonest time for diurnal attacks is during the first hour after awakening. Menstruation markedly influences the occurrence of fits in women. Many women have attacks only at the menstrual period, usually just before the period begins, less frequently during or immediately after Laidlaw (1956). 'Long-distance rhythms', i.e. the regular recurrence of attacks at intervals of many months, have been studied by Griffiths and Fox (1938).

Status Epilepticus. An epileptic patient may have a succession of convulsions with recovery of consciousness between the attacks—serial epilepsy. In some cases, however, one attack follows another without any intervening period of consciousness—status epilepticus. Unless the convulsions can be arrested, coma deepens, and pyrexia, or even hyperpyrexia, develops, and death occurs. Some patients exhibit a special tendency to develop status epilepticus, and do so on many occasions.

Mental and Physical Abnormalities

No mental or physical abnormalities are constantly associated with epilepsy, and many epileptic patients exhibit neither. As already indicated, however, there are a number of organic or metabolic disorders of the brain which may produce both dementia and epilepsy. Epilepsy is sometimes associated with mental deficiency, and one easily recognizable type of mentally defective, epileptic child is excitable, noisy, destructive, and difficult to control ('the hyperkinetic syndrome'). The commonest mental abnormality in adult epileptics is a tendency to a certain morose egotism. The cause of the progressive mental deterioration which sometimes accompanies epilepsy is obscure. It is probably not always a direct result of the fits, since it may be absent in patients having frequent severe attacks, but recurrent anoxia occurring in major fits and giving rise to progressive brain damage is certainly the cause in some cases.

Behaviour disorders, with aggressive outbursts and paranoid traits, are particularly common in some adults and children with severe temporal lobe epilepsy. Furthermore, epilepsy is known to occur occasionally in patients suffering from psychotic illnesses, particularly paranoid schizophrenia, while spontaneous fits may develop following electroconvulsive therapy.

Thus is may be concluded that epilepsy itself does not *produce* mental changes unless the fits are severe or frequent enough to produce anoxic damage to the brain, in which case progressive dementia may develop. Mental dullness and lack of concentration with a deteriorating performance in school or at work is sometimes due to the drugs being given to treat the epilepsy rather than to the condition itself and folic-acid deficiency as a result of anticonvulsant therapy should be considered as a possible aetiological factor in causing mental deterioration.

Petit mal status should also be considered as a possible cause of such a syndrome in children (Brett, 1966).

Physical signs which have been described in some cases of epilepsy in previous reports, including nystagmus, dysarthria, and ataxia are in some instances due to the treatment rather than to the disease. Other features such as evidence of pyramidal tract disease, when present, should invariably suggest that the epilepsy is symptomatic of some underlying organic lesion of the brain.

No constant endocrine abnormality has been found to be associated with epilepsy, though minor disorders of skeletal growth and genital development are common. Many adolescent epileptics are exceptionally tall for their age. Obesity of the hypopituitary and eunuchoid type is sometimes seen, together with a heterosexual distribution of pubic hair. Scattered spots of *café-au-lait* pigmentation of the skin are occasionally present. Facial naevus should suggest an intracranial angioma on the same side, which may cause an audible bruit on auscultation of the skull. In spite of numerous investigations no constant metabolic abnormality has been generally recognized in cases of 'idiopathic' epilepsy. Frequent major fits, mental backwardness and tetany, associated sometimes with intracranial calcification, may occur in cases of idiopathic hypoparathyroidism and in pseudohypoparathyroidism (Simpson, 1952; Glaser and Levy, 1960); the fits may be improved by treatment with dihydrotachysterol (*A.T. 10*) given in an initial dosage of 1·25 mg. three times daily until the serum calcium is normal, and then a smaller maintenance dose is required.

In 'idiopathic' epilepsy the cerebrospinal fluid is normal except that during or after frequent fits or an attack of status epilepticus there may be a rise in pressure to above 200 mm. of fluid and a modest rise in protein content of the fluid. A consistently raised C.S.F. protein and a pleocytosis should suggest that the epilepsy is symptomatic. Air encephalography and/or ventriculography usually give normal findings but in some cases of long-standing epilepsy and epilepsy of late onset signs of ventricular dilatation and cortical atrophy are apparent (Hunter *et al.*, 1962). It is not certain as to whether these findings indicate that the cortical atrophy is the result of frequent fits or whether an unspecified degenerative process causing the cortical atrophy is also the cause of the fits.

Electroencephalography

The diagnostic importance of the EEG in epilepsy lies in the fact that an abnormal record obtained in the interval between the attacks may establish the diagnosis when this is otherwise in doubt. Further, the effect of different drugs upon the abnormal rhythm, and in general the response to treatment can be studied. It is important to stress the present limitations of electroencephalography in the diagnosis of epilepsy. From 10 to 20 per cent. of epileptics have a normal EEG, and the percentage is higher in those having grand mal only and after the age of 40. A normal EEG, therefore, does not exclude epilepsy. Patients with petit mal usually exhibit the wave-and-spike pattern [see FIG. 125] or a three-per-second wave, but the abnormal rhythm may be present only after over-ventilation. These rhythms, however, are not pathognomonic of petit mal, but may occur in other forms of epilepsy. Grand mal is not associated with any single characteristic form of EEG, but paroxysmal diffuse multiple spikes in rapid rhythm or isolated generalized paroxysmal outbursts of spike or sharp-wave activity are usually associated with grand mal. Temporal lobe epilepsy is often identified by means of focal spike or sharp wave discharges arising in one

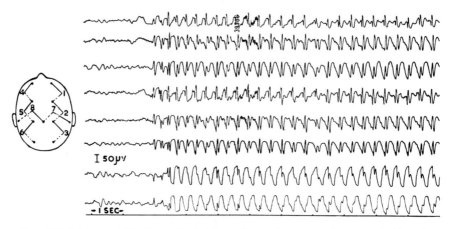

FIG. 125. Male, aged 18. Generalized, bilaterally synchronous and symmetrical 3 cycles per second wave-and-spike discharges during a petit mal attack

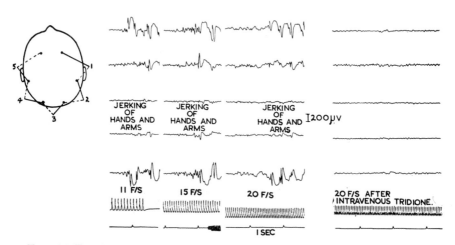

FIG. 126. Female, aged 19. Epilepsy, myoclonic. Photo-myoclonic response at various flash frequencies and subsequent effect of intravenous tridione

or other temporal region or by paroxysmal outbursts of rhythmical slow theta activity which are similarly located. These discharges may only become apparent during early sleep so that sleep recordings induced by sedative drugs may be helpful. Recording with sphenoidal or pharyngeal electrodes before, during, and after thiopentone-induced sleep is a valuable technique and the unilateral absence of barbiturate-induced fast activity over one temporal lobe is a valuable guide to the presence of a focal epileptogenic lesion. Focal epileptogenic cortical lesions in other areas are often similarly associated with corresponding focal, abnormal EEG discharges. With the possible exception of the wave-and-spike pattern and its fast and slow variants there is no abnormal EEG which is pathognomonic of epilepsy, and non-specific abnormalities may be found in epilepsy, psychoneurosis, psychopathy, or psychosis. It follows that an abnormal EEG can be interpreted only in relation to the clinical history of the patient (Gibbs,

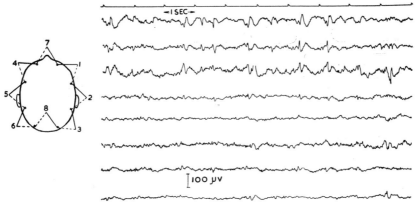

FIG. 127. Male, aged 30. Temporal lobe epilepsy. Focal sharp and slow waves in the right temporal region

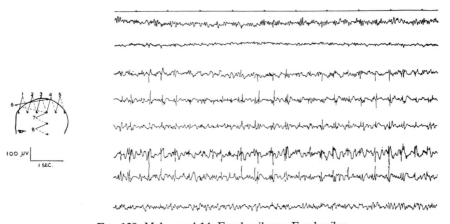

FIG. 128. Male, aged 14. Focal epilepsy. Focal spikes

Gibbs, and Lennox, 1937, 1938, 1943; Jasper and Kershman, 1941; Williams, 1941; Kiloh and Osselton, 1967). An epileptic dysrhythmia is much more likely to be detected during sleep than during waking life (Gibbs and Gibbs, 1947) and may be evoked by an injection of leptazol (*Metrazol*) or bemegride (*Megimide*) (Ziskind and Bercel, 1947; Hill and Parr, 1963). Electrocorticography is used for the precise localization of an epileptic focus at operation.

DIAGNOSIS

The diagnosis of epilepsy falls into two parts. It is first necessary to distinguish epileptic attacks from other paroxysmal disturbances, and secondly, to decide whether the attacks are symptomatic of organic disease or metabolic disorder, or whether the patient is suffering from constitutional or idiopathic epilepsy.

Both minor and major attacks must be distinguished from *syncope*. Syncope usually occurs in individuals with vasomotor instability or as the result of exhaustion, haemorrhage, an emotional shock, sudden change of posture, or standing for long periods [see p. 286]. Both the onset and the cessation of syncopal attacks are more gradual than is usually the case in epilepsy, and the former is usually preceded by a feeling of faintness. In syncope also the patient is limp, whereas the occurrence of slight rigidity is in favour of epilepsy; on the other hand, transient rigidity and twitching and even incontinence may occur in severe syncope. Perspiration and severe pallor favour a diagnosis of fainting. Nevertheless, in some individuals pressure upon the carotid sinus or circumstances which usually induce syncope may cause an epileptic attack. For a discussion of the relationship between syncope and epilepsy, see page 285.

In *narcolepsy* consciousness is lost, but convulsive movements are absent and the patient, unlike the epileptic, shows all the features of natural sleep and can be immediately roused. In *cataplexy* voluntary power is lost but consciousness is retained.

Aural vertigo may be confused with minor and major epilepsy, in which vertigo may also occur, often as a transient aura. In vertigo of aural origin, however, consciousness is retained and other symptoms of aural disease, such as tinnitus and deafness, are usually present. Though an attack of aural vertigo may be brief, it usually lasts longer than a minor attack or an aura, and passes away more gradually. But the relationship between the labyrinth and epilepsy is complex [see p. 183].

Hysterical convulsions are usually easily distinguished from epileptic attacks if the patient is seen when convulsed. Their onset is usually gradual, and they occur only in the presence of an audience. Consciousness is not completely lost, for the patient can usually be roused by forcible measures, and an attempt to elicit the corneal reflex usually evokes a vigorous contraction of the orbicularis oculi. If the patient cries out during the attack he usually articulates words or phrases, and laughing and crying may occur. The movements which constitute an hysterical convulsion are not clonic jerks as in epilepsy, but such as can be carried out voluntarily, for example, clutching at objects in the neighbourhood. The tongue is not bitten, nor does incontinence of urine usually occur in an hysterical attack. However, there is a particular type of hysterical attack which occurs usually in young females, less often in males, in which sudden falling without convulsive movements occurs and the picture may be indistinguishable from that of akinetic epilepsy. After being asked frequently by one or more doctors the patient may oblige by passing urine in an attack. These attacks are often very frequent, occur particularly at times of stress, appear to cause the patient little concern and show virtually no response to anticonvulsant drugs. The difficulty of differential diagnosis is increased by the fact that epileptic and hysterical attacks may coexist in the same individuals. A similar type of attack occasionally occurs in a medicolegal context in adults after trivial head injury and frequently ceases abruptly after settlement of a compensation claim.

Anxiety attacks are occasionally confused with epilepsy. In these consciousness is not lost, but the predominant symptom is an intense sense of anxiety, which is often associated with a feeling of giddiness, palpitation, and sweating.

The panic attacks of the phobic anxiety-depersonalization syndrome (Harper and Roth, 1962) may be readily confused with temporal lobe epilepsy as in these episodes mounting panic and angor animi (fear of 'impending doom') are often associated with a sense of intense depersonalization or unreality and if there is associated hyperventilation, syncope sometimes occurs or even tetany. Usually, however, consciousness remains unimpaired and there are associated phobias about going out of the house alone, crossing roads or entering crowded places which are not a feature of epilepsy. Similar symptoms sometimes occur in depressive illness.

Under the term *vasovagal attacks*, Gowers described 'prolonged seizures, the symptoms of which consist chiefly in disturbance of some of the functions of the pneumo-gastric'. The patient complains of gastric, respiratory, or cardiac discomfort, and these symptoms are often associated with vasoconstriction and coldness of the extremities. Women are more subject to these paroxysms than men. They are distinguished from epilepsy by their gradual onset and longer duration, and by the usual absence of loss of consciousness. It is doubtful if they represent a nosological entity [see p. 948].

Migraine is a paroxysmal disturbance which may simulate epilepsy. The onset of an attack of migraine, however, is gradual. Consciousness is not lost, and headache usually occurs. It must be remembered, however, that the same individual may suffer from both migraine and epilepsy, and that very exceptionally a severe attack of migraine may terminate in an epileptic fit.

When it has been established that a patient suffers from epileptiform attacks, it remains to exclude the various focal and metabolic causes of convulsions enumerated on page 921.

Gross organic lesions such as *hydrocephalus* and *infantile hemiplegia* give rise to no difficulty.

Tuberous sclerosis can be diagnosed as a cause of epilepsy associated with mental defect only when adenoma sebaceum is present, when there are phakomata to be seen in the retina or by the characteristic X-ray changes.

Renal disease and *hypertensive encephalopathy* may be excluded by examination of the cardiovascular system, including the blood pressure, and of the urine and the blood urea.

The diagnosis of *syphilis* can be established by means of the history, the presence of signs of the infection of the nervous system, and a positive V.D.R.L. reaction in the blood or cerebrospinal fluid.

When alcohol or *amphetamines* or *drug intoxication* or *withdrawal* is the cause of the convulsions a history of alcoholism or of drug-taking can usually be obtained.

Heart block offers little difficulty in diagnosis if the possibility of its occurrence is borne in mind. If an attack is witnessed it is found to coincide with cardiac asystole and flushing usually accompanies the return of consciousness. When complete atrioventricular block is established the pulse rate is usually about 30. Even if the pulse rate is normal between the attacks, impaired conduction in the atrioventricular bundle can be demonstrated by an electrocardiogram.

Spontaneous hypoglycaemia may cause syncopal or epileptic attacks, or in milder cases, fatigability, anxiety, sweating, giddiness, diplopia, or mental confusion. The subject is well reviewed by Conn (1947). Apart from gross disease of the liver, hypophysis, or adrenals, the two chief causes are: (1) adenoma, carcinoma, or hyperplasia of the islet cells of Langerhans of the pancreas; and (2) reactive hyperinsulinism. The former is the more likely to give rise to epilepsy. The diagnosis is based upon the low fasting blood sugar in the former, and abnormal sugar tolerance tests and the correlation between the attacks and the low blood sugar in both (Wauchope, 1933; Prunty, 1944; Conn, 1947).

Special consideration must be given to two common causes of convulsions developing after the age of 30, namely intracranial tumour and cerebral arteriosclerosis. In *intracranial tumour* convulsions may precede other symptoms by months or years, and when this is the case the cause can often only be suspected. Though convulsions due to cerebral tumour may be generalized, a focal origin for the attacks should suggest tumour, especially when they are followed by temporary aphasia or paresis. Sooner or later headache and other symptoms of increased intracranial pressure make their appearance, together with signs of a progressive cerebral lesion. The EEG may suggest the presence of a focal lesion, radiographs of the skull or echo-encephalography may indicate a 'shift' of midline structures and gamma-encephalography, air encephalography, ventriculography, or angiography may be required. Epileptiform attacks due to *cerebral arteriosclerosis* occur in late middle life and old age. They may follow upon clinically-evident episodes of cerebral infarction (post-hemiplegic epilepsy), but sometimes the cause of the attacks is a previous asymptomatic minor cortical infarct. Vascular thickening is usually demonstrable in the arteries of the retina and of the limbs, and the blood pressure may be raised.

Cysticercosis should be considered when epilepsy begins in adult life in men who have lived abroad, especially in India, and search should be made for subcutaneous cysts. Calcified cysts may be demonstrated radiographically in the muscles and less often in the brain.

PROGNOSIS

The risk that death will occur during an epileptic attack is slight, except in status epilepticus, in which condition the patient's life is always threatened until consciousness returns, and death may occur even after recovery of consciousness.

When death occurs as the result of an attack it is not usually due to the fit itself but is an accidental result of the loss of consciousness. Thus a patient who convulses in bed may turn over and become asphyxiated through his face being buried in the pillow, and drowning may follow a convulsion which occurs when a patient is in the bath.

Minor accidents occurring from the attacks include injuries induced by the fall, though these are rarely serious, and dislocation of the shoulder, which is produced by muscular action, and which, having once occurred, is liable to recur in subsequent attacks. The violence of the convulsions may cause compression fracture of vertebral bodies, usually in the thoracic region, a possibility which should always be considered when the patient complains of pain in the back after a fit. Fractures of limb bones occur less frequently. The prognosis as to recovery from the attacks depends upon a number of factors. To achieve recovery it is necessary to abolish the attacks by means of treatment for a sufficient length of time for the patient to lose the epileptic habit. Persevering and thorough treatment is therefore essential, and must be continued for at least three years after the attacks have ceased and in many cases indefinitely. Treatment should always be withdrawn gradually but even so, fits recur, even after three or more years of freedom in over 30 per cent. of cases. The sooner the treatment can be begun after the first fit, the better the outlook, and the prognosis is best in those in whom the attacks begin after the age of 20. A family history of the disease is not necessarily an adverse factor in prognosis, and patients with an epileptic heredity often do better than those without. Individuals suffering from frequent severe attacks are least likely to be completely cured. According to Gowers the outlook is best when the attacks occur only during sleep, and treatment is most likely to be successful when they take place at a regular time of the day or of the month, so that intensive treatment can be timed so as to avert them. Marked mental deterioration makes the outlook worse. Thus few patients in institutions become free from attacks, and the death rate among institutional epileptics is four times that of the general population. Probably about 30 per cent. of non-institutional epileptics are cured, in the sense of remaining free from attacks indefinitely but in over 60 per cent. the attacks can be completely controlled with treatment. (See also Bridge, Kajdi, and Livingston, 1947.)

There has been some controversy concerning the prognosis of childhood petit mal. Lees and Liversedge (1962) suggested that in many children with this form of minor epilepsy attacks continued into adult life. However, Livingston *et al.* (1965) found that the attacks eventually ceased in adolescence in over three-quarters of their cases, but grand mal eventually developed in 54 per cent. of those who started with 'pure' petit mal seizures.

TREATMENT
General Management

Symptomatic epilepsy, resulting, say, from an intracranial tumour, is best treated by curing the condition of which the epilepsy is but a symptom, but this is only rarely possible and thus, in many symptomatic cases, the same treatment as that given for idiopathic epilepsy must be employed.

It is desirable that an epileptic patient should as far as possible live a normal life. Children should attend school and should be subjected to ordinary discipline. Adults should carry on an occupation, though certain trades will necessarily be ruled out. Occupations involving working at heights, or near machinery, or driving vehicles are obviously unsuitable, and sufferers from epilepsy have been precluded by law from obtaining a motor-driver's licence in Great Britain. After a single fit, however, for which investigation demonstrates no obvious cause, many neurologists are prepared to recommend that driving should be banned for one year only and that anticonvulsant drugs should only be taken for the first six months of this period. After a second or subsequent fits it is now usual to recommend that the restoration of a driving licence cannot be considered until the patient has had at least three years of freedom from attacks.

A change in the law to allow an epileptic to drive, while continuing to take treatment, after such a period of freedom, or when his attacks are nocturnal only, is now pending.

Children should be allowed to take part in sports; an individual decision must be made in every case depending upon the frequency and severity of the attacks but the riding of horses or of bicycles can often be allowed if the attacks are well controlled. A regular occupation is a considerable prophylactic against attacks. Certain risks of everyday life must be explained to the patient and his friends, but it is difficult, if not impossible, to guard him against them all. The water in his bath should be shallow, and he should not bathe in deep water unaccompanied. Institutional treatment may be necessary for mentally defective patients, and those having severe and frequent fits, if adequate home care is not available. Those in whom the disorder renders an ordinary occupation impossible often do well at an epileptic colony.

No general rule can be laid down concerning the marriage of epileptics. There is no evidence that marriage affects the tendency to fits either beneficially or adversely, though pregnancy may prove either beneficial or the reverse. The risk of transmitting the disorder to the children must be individually assessed in each case. This risk is clearly greatest when there is a family history of epilepsy or when an EEG shows that the non-epileptic parent has an abnormal record, and least when a focal lesion of the brain can be held partly responsible for the attacks. Even when the epileptic tendency is hereditary it is exceptional for a patient to transmit the disorder in the direct line, and the chances are thirty-five to one against any individual child of an epileptic parent developing epilepsy.

Careful attention must be paid to general hygiene in epilepsy. Moderate exercise is desirable, but violent exertion sometimes precipitates attacks. Any factor adversely affecting the general health, especially enlarged tonsils, adenoids, and intestinal worms in children, should receive attention. If there is evidence of an allergic reaction to certain foods these should be avoided, or desensitization may be tried. Alcohol should be avoided, as over-indulgence, or even a modest intake, may precipitate attacks.

The Investigation of Epilepsy of Late Onset

In many centres there has been a vogue which has demanded the full investigation with contrast radiological studies of all patients over the age of 30 years who develop epilepsy. However, under 10 per cent. of such individuals eventually prove to have intracranial tumours and in the early stages such tumours, most of which are gliomas, are not often revealed by angiography or air encephalography. Indications for full investigation include symptoms of raised intracranial pressure and clinical or electroencephalographic indications of a focal cerebral lesion. Otherwise patients with late-onset epilepsy should be treated in the same way as any case of presumed idiopathic epilepsy arising in childhood or early adult life until or unless such manifestations develop.

Treatment of the Epileptic Attack

Treatment of a patient in an epileptic attack consists merely in preventing him from injuring himself. A gag should be placed between the teeth and an airway maintained. The attack is self-limited, and no immediate treatment will shorten its course.

Surgical Treatment

From the most ancient times trephining the skull has played a part in the treatment of epilepsy. Apart from intracranial tumours, however, this operation is probably of benefit only in a very narrowly restricted group of cases. When there is clear evidence of an organic lesion of the brain, especially one of traumatic origin, and the attacks have a focal onset which can be related to the lesion, and the site of which can be demonstrated by electrocorticography, excision of the affected area may abolish the attacks (Penfield and Jasper, 1954). Surgical treatment is, however, indicated only, as a rule, when the attacks are intractable and inadequately controlled by drugs (because the surgeon in removing one scar must leave another) and when the lesion is situated in an area of the brain which, when excised, is unlikely to result in permanent and severe neurological deficit. Even in temporal lobe epilepsy, in which good results have followed anterior temporal lobectomy in appropriate cases (Falconer and Serefitinides, 1963), probably less than one per cent. of cases require, and are suitable for, surgical treatment.

Treatment with Drugs

Certain drugs have been found to diminish the severity and frequency of epileptic attacks and in favourable cases to abolish them completely. The object of drug treatment is to secure an abolition of the attacks for a sufficient length of time to enable the patient to lose the epileptic habit. When the attacks occur regularly at the same hour of the day or period of the month, the doses are timed correspondingly so as to produce their maximal effect when the attack is expected. Thus when the attacks are nocturnal or occur in the early morning, a single dose at bedtime may be sufficient. When they occur only at the monthly periods, medication can sometimes be increased in the previous and subsequent weeks. When the fits are irregular a dose must be taken two or three times a day. Perseverance in treatment is essential, and the patient must continue to take the effective drug for at least three years after the attacks cease, if a relapse is to be avoided. Electroencephalography may prove helpful in assessing the results of treatment, but even if the EEG remains abnormal and the patient is free from attacks after three years, withdrawal of treatment should be attempted.

Bromides. For many years the bromides were the most effective drugs in the treatment of epilepsy, but they are now outmoded.

DRUG TREATMENT

General Principles

These have been well stated in a recent article in the *British Medical Journal* in the section on Today's Drugs (1968). It is first important to recognize that one group of drugs, including the barbiturates, hydantoinates, and acetylureas, together with a number of modern synthetic remedies, are effective in major epilepsy (whether idiopathic or symptomatic) and also in focal epilepsy (including the temporal lobe variety) as well as in some cases of myoclonic epilepsy (see below) but not in petit mal. A second group, including the diones and suximides, may control petit mal but on occasion may even seem to make associated major epilepsy worse or may appear to precipitate major attacks in patients with petit mal who have never suffered such episodes before. There is also some recent evidence to indicate that the prognosis of petit mal in the long-term is better if the child is treated with at least one drug effective in the control of major epilepsy (usually a hydantoin derivative) as well as with one or more of those which are effective in petit mal.

In all cases patients or their parents must be warned not to discontinue treatment without medical advice as this may precipitate dangerous episodes of status epilepticus. Difficulties which arise in the management of epilepsy are one of the major justifications for the existence of neurological follow-up clinics, as regular and careful supervision of such patients, and patient regulation and alteration in anticonvulsant medication and dosage, may pay considerable dividends. In general, combined tablets, containing more than one drug, are to be condemned, as when using these remedies it is not possible to adjust the dosage of the individual constituents of the tablet independently.

Major and Focal Epilepsy

The principle must be to give the minimum dose of drugs sufficient to control the attacks for as long as may be necessary. Occasionally a single drug suffices but more often it is necessary to give a combination of at least two, and occasionally of three or more drugs in combination, in order to achieve maximum control, bearing in mind the fact that often one drug may potentiate the effect of another, but always remembering that not only are the therapeutic effects of these remedies additive but also that the same may apply to their side-effects. Sometimes, therefore, the addition of a new drug to the patient's existing medication may result in psychomotor retardation and a paradoxical increase in the number of fits. All of the drugs in common use tend to produce some slowing of mental processes to a greater or lesser extent but this is particularly true of the barbiturates and occasionally satisfactory control of the attacks is only achieved at the expense of a disabling degree of drowsiness. It must, however, be remembered that as patients become accustomed to their medication such side-effects may noticeably diminish with the passage of time so that such symptoms are not invariably an indication for a reduction in treatment if attacks are under control. Small doses of amphetamine derivatives may help to control drowsiness.

However, all of the drugs to be considered below, apart from toxic effects common to the individual remedy, which will be mentioned, have a tendency at times to produce an unacceptable degree of drowsiness, dysarthria and ataxia, often with nystagmus, blurred vision, and even diplopia. These manifestations often develop relatively suddenly in a patient who has been receiving a stable regimen of treatment for some time; the patient has a 'drugged' and almost drunken appearance which is virtually diagnostic but may be misconstrued by the unwary as being due to organic intracranial disease. Such toxic effects are particularly common in those taking primidone and hydantoinates; complete withdrawal of these remedies is not as a rule necessary as the level of dosage at which they appear is finely balanced in the individual and a reduction in dosage of a single tablet or capsule per day sometimes results in rapid amelioration of these symptoms, though more often a more substantial reduction in daily dosage is required. Macrocytic anaemia due to folic acid deficiency has long been recognized to be an occasional complication of anticonvulsant therapy but recent evidence (Reynolds, 1968) suggests that such a deficiency may also account for some other side-effects of these drugs and that improvement may follow the regular administration of folic acid, 5 mg. daily. Paradoxically, however, this remedy sometimes results in an increase in the number of seizures. Drug rashes also occur not infrequently in patients receiving phenobarbitone and hydantoinates; they can sometimes be controlled with antihistamine drugs but more often necessitate withdrawal of the offender and the substitution of another remedy.

The Treatment Routine

It is usual to begin in an adult with phenobarbitone, 30 mg. twice daily, increasing if need be to three times a day, or to give 15 mg. daily in a tablet or elixir to a young child. The drug is contra-indicated in mentally-defective and hyperkinetic children in whom the hyperkinesis may be accentuated. A few adults may tolerate up to 60 mg. three times a day but even smaller doses may produce intolerable drowsiness. Less soporific in its effects and useful as an alternative anticonvulsant is methylphenobarbitone (*Prominal, Phemitone*) which is given in a dosage of 100–200 mg. two or three times daily.

If modest doses of phenobarbitone are insufficient to control the attacks it is usual to add sodium hydantoinate (*Epanutin, Dilantin*) in a dosage of 100 mg. two or three times a day (the dose suitable for a child is 50 mg. twice or three times daily); few patients can take more than four such daily doses without developing the side-effects mentioned above. In a high proportion of patients phenobarbitone and *Epanutin* in combination will produce an acceptable degree of attack control but when seizures continue it is then reasonable gradually to substitute primidone (*Mysoline*) for the phenobarbitone, while continuing the hydantoin. This powerful drug is given in a dosage of 250 mg. three or four times daily (125 mg. twice daily for a young child). Even on low dosage some patients develop nausea and vomiting and others drowsiness and ataxia; more patients fail to tolerate this drug than any other but, by contrast, some individuals find that they can take up to six tablets a day without ill-effect. Usually the combined use of primidone and phenobarbitone is contra-indicated because of their combined sedative effects.

In patients whose seizures continue to resist treatment with the standard and established remedies mentioned above, there are a number of newer drugs which may usefully be given in addition. One of the most useful is sulthiame (*Ospolot*) which is given in a dosage of 200 mg., two, three, or four times daily (50 mg. tablets are available for children). In some cases of major and temporal lobe epilepsy it is a remarkably effective adjuvant to the more traditional remedies and it often improves behaviour in epileptic children. It has few side-effects (apart from occasional irritating paraesthesiae in the extremities) and can be given in maximum dosage along with other remedies. Also valuable in some cases are other hydantoinates including methoin (*Mesontoin*) (which has unfortunately been known to produce marrow aplasia) and the rather less toxic ethotoin (*Peganone*); the dose of the former is 100 mg. two or three times a day and of the latter 250–500 mg. two or three times daily for an adult, with correspondingly lower doses for children. While these drugs can be added in modest dosage to primidone and sodium hydantoin, they may produce additive side-effects. Commonly used in the past was phenylacetylurea (*Phenurone*), particularly in temporal lobe and myoclonic epilepsy, but this drug is particularly toxic, producing nausea and vomiting in many patients, liver and renal damage in some, and carrying the risk of marrow aplasia. More recently introduced and much less toxic is phenylethylacetylurea (*Benuride*) of which the adult dose is 200 mg. three times a day. When sulthiame is ineffective it can usefully be tried as an adjuvant remedy along with phenobarbitone, hydantoinates and/or primidone. An alternative powerful new anticonvulsant, which may well prove to be an alternative adjuvant remedy, but which has not yet been fully evaluated, is carbamazepine (*Tegretol*) of which the adult dose is also 200 mg. three times a day.

Drugs with weaker anticonvulsant effects but worthy of a trial along with established remedies in resistant cases include chlordiazepoxide (*Librium*), 5–10 mg. three times daily, diazepam (*Valium*), 2–5 mg. three times daily, and beclamide (*Nydrane*), 500 mg. three or four times daily. The latter drug is remarkably non-toxic, and like sulthiame, has proved to be of particular value in some children with behaviour disorders.

Petit Mal

As already mentioned it is now regarded as essential in children with petit mal to give, in addition to the specific remedies for this form of epilepsy, another remedy (usually sodium hydantoin, 50 mg. two or three times a day) in order to guard against the immediate or subsequent development of major seizures.

The drug of choice is now ethosuximide (*Zarontin*) which can be given, even to young children, in a dosage of 250 mg. two, three, or four times daily. Often the attacks cease abruptly but sometimes petit mal is remarkably resistant and it may be necessary to add one or two other remedies, also in full dosage, in order to achieve control of the attacks. These include the older remedies trimethadione (*Tridione*) and paramethadione (*Paradione*) each of which is given in a dosage of 300 mg. three times a day. Sometimes these two drugs produce an unpleasant visual glare phenomenon, and agranulocytosis, aplastic anaemia, nephrosis, and liver damage have been described but are all rare. Routine regular white blood cell counts were once advised in patients receiving these drugs but are of little value; it is wiser to advise the parents to seek medical advice if the child under treatment develops a sore throat or high temperature.

Other suximide drugs which may be tried in petit mal in place of ethosuximide and possibly with one or both of the dione drugs, but which are usually less effective are phensuximide (*Milontin*), 250–500 mg. three or four times daily, and methsuximide (*Celontin*), 300 mg. up to three or four times a day. In occasional cases, for reasons which are not clearly understood, chlortetracycline

(*Aureomycin*), 250 mg. three times a day, is effective in petit mal and so, too, are diuretics including frusemide (*Lasix*), (but regular measurement of serum potassium is necessary with this drug and is inconvenient), and acetazolamide (*Diamox*), 250–500 mg. once or twice daily.

Amphetamine sulphate and dextroamphetamine sulphate in a dosage of 5–10 mg. at 8 a.m. and 12 noon have been found to be of occasional value in patients with petit mal and are also of some benefit in patients with major or temporal lobe epilepsy when drowsiness due to medication is a problem. Paradoxically, a small dose of amphetamine, tried with caution, may improve and sedate some hyperkinetic children and those with aggressive behaviour disorders.

In the treatment of petit mal, toxic side-effects of medication are in general less of a problem, because of the character of the drugs being used, than in the management of major and temporal lobe epilepsy. In all forms of epilepsy, however, the aim must be to achieve a balance between the control of the attacks on the one hand and the preservation of mental capacity, concentration, and alertness on the other.

Treatment of Status Epilepticus

Paraldehyde is the most effective drug, being given in doses of 10 ml. intramuscularly to an adult and repeated as necessary. In an emergency it can be given by intravenous drip in a dosage of 0·05 to 0·1 ml. per kg. of body weight in normal saline. Unfortunately the intramuscular injections are painful and occasionally give abscess formation while phlebitis usually follows intravenous administration. In mild cases the patient may respond to 120–250 mg. of phenobarbitone sodium intramuscularly followed by 120 mg. every hour for several hours. General anaesthetics have long been used; recently thiopentone has been used by intravenous drip (Mortimer, 1961) and in severe cases muscle relaxants and positive pressure respiration have been employed. Another useful drug introduced recently is diazepam (*Valium*) (Gastaut *et al.*, 1965), which is given intravenously in a drip in successive 10 mg. doses every 15 minutes until control is achieved or until 50–60 mg. has been given over one or two hours. EEG monitoring is valuable to show when the cerebral epileptic discharge has been controlled (James and Whitty, 1961; Mortimer, 1961).

The lower bowel should be well washed out with enemata, and nasal feeding should be used if unconsciousness is prolonged. The patient should be nursed flat and preferably in the semiprone position.

Petit mal status, which may give prolonged disorientation, accompanied by almost continuous spike-and-wave activity in the child's EEG, is best treated by ethosuximide (*Zarontin*), in a dosage of 250 mg. four-hourly but hydantoin sodium (*Epanutin*) should be given as well (at least 50 mg. two or three times daily) to guard against the development of major seizures. ACTH has also been recommended in such cases (80 Units daily intramuscularly for a week).

Dietetic Treatment

Geyelin, in 1921, observed that complete starvation caused a marked reduction in the number of fits in epileptics. Other workers, acting on the hypothesis that the benefit derived from starvation was due to the associated ketosis, tried the effects of inducing ketosis by administering a diet rich in fats and poor in carbohydrates. A ketogenic diet has been found to be of some value in the treatment of epilepsy in children, but adults are less responsive. On such a diet about 30 per cent. of children have been said to become free from attacks, and in a further 20 per cent. the frequency of the attacks is reduced. However, the diet is rather unpleasant and though still used in some parts of the world, it has few advocates.

Psychotherapy

There is no reason to regard epilepsy as primarily a psychological disorder. In a few cases, however, mental stress and emotional difficulties appear to precipitate attacks. Depression, anxiety, and hysterical manifestations may also occur in epileptic individuals. When such subordinate causes can be found, benefit may result from a course of psychological treatment. More often help is obtained by the addition of antidepressive and/or tranquillizing remedies to the patient's anticonvulsant medication, always remembering that certain antidepressive drugs (particularly imipramine—*Tofranil*) may potentiate epileptic discharges whereas some tranquillizers (e.g. chlordiazepoxide—*Librium*) have an anticonvulsant effect.

REFERENCES

BALDWIN, M., and BAILEY, P. (1958) *Temporal Lobe Epilepsy*, Springfield, Ill.

BEHRMAN, S., and WYKE, B. D. (1958) Vestibulogenic seizures, *Brain*, **81**, 529.

BIRD, C. A. K., GRIFFIN, B. P., MIKLASZEWSKA, J. M., and GALBRAITH, A. W. (1966) Tegretol (carbamazepine): a controlled trial of a new anticonvulsant, *Brit. J. Psychiat.*, **112**, 737.

BOWER, B. D., and JEAVONS, P. M. (1959) Infantile spasms and hypsarrhythmia, *Lancet*, i, 605.

BRAIN, W. R. (1925–6) The inheritance of epilepsy, *Quart. J. Med.*, **19**, 299.

BRETT, E. M. (1966) Minor epileptic status, *J. neurol. Sci.*, **3**, 52.

BRIDGE, E. M., KAJDI, L., and LIVINGSTON, S. (1947) A fifteen year study of epilepsy in children, *Res. Publ. Ass. nerv. ment. Dis.*, **26**, 451.

CAVANAGH, J. B. (1958) On certain small tumours—encountered in the temporal lobe, *Brain*, **81**, 389.

COBB, S. (1932) Causes of epilepsy, *Arch. Neurol. Psychiat. (Chicago)*, **27**, 1245.

CONN, J. W. (1947) The diagnosis and management of spontaneous hypoglycaemia, *J. Amer. med. Ass.*, **134**, 130.

COX, P. J. N., and MARTIN, E. (1959) Infantile spasms and hypsarrhythmia, *Lancet*, i, 1099.

DAVIS, J. P., and LENNOX, W. G. (1947) The effect of trimethyloxazolidine dione and dimethylethyloxazolidine dione on seizures and the blood, *Res. Publ. Ass. nerv. ment. Dis.*, **26**, 423.

DODGE, P. R., RICHARDSON, E. P., JNR., and VICTOR, M. (1954) Recurrent convulsive seizures as a sequel to cerebral infarction, *Brain*, **77**, 610.

EARLE, K. M., BALDWIN, M., and PENFIELD, W. (1953) Incisural sclerosis and temporal lobe seizures produced by hippocampal herniation at birth, *Arch. Neurol. Psychiat. (Chicago)*, **69**, 27.

EFRON, R. (1957) The conditioned inhibition of uncinate fits, *Brain*, **80**, 251.

EFRON, R. (1961) Post-epileptic paralysis. Theoretical critique and report of a case, *Brain*, **84**, 381.

FALCONER, M. A. (1953) Discussion of the surgery of temporal lobe epilepsy, *Proc. roy. Soc. Med.*, **46**, 971.

FALCONER, M. A., and SEREFITINIDES, F. A. (1963) A follow-up study in temporal lobe epilepsy, *J. Neurol, Neurosurg. Psychiat.*, **26**, 154.

GARLAND, H., and SUMMER, D. (1964) Sulthiame in treatment of epilepsy, *Brit. med. J.*, **1**, 454.

GASTAUT, H., and FISCHER-WILLIAMS, M. (1960) The physiopathology of epileptic seizures, in *Handbook of Physiology*, ed. FIELD, J., Sect. 1, Vol. 1, p. 329, Washington, D.C.

GASTAUT, H., NAQUET, R., POIRE, R., and TASSINARI, C. A. (1965) Treatment of status epilepticus with diazepam (*Valium*), *Epilepsia (Amst.)* **6**, 167.

GIBBS, E. L., and GIBBS, F. A. (1947) Sleep records in epilepsy, *Res. Publ. Ass. nerv. ment. Dis.*, **26**, 366.

GIBBS, F. A., and GIBBS, E. L. (1952) *Atlas of Electroencephalography*, Vol. 2, p. 24, Cambridge, Mass.

GIBBS, F. A., GIBBS, E. L., and LENNOX, W. G. (1937) Epilepsy: a paroxysmal cerebral dysrhythmia, *Brain*, **60**, 377.

GIBBS, F. A., GIBBS, E. L., and LENNOX, W. G. (1938) Cerebral dysrhythmias of epilepsy. Measures for their control, *Arch. Neurol. Psychiat. (Chicago)*, **34**, 298.

GIBBS, F. A., GIBBS, E. L., and LENNOX, W. G. (1943) Electro-encephalographic classification of epileptic patients and control subjects, *Arch. Neurol. Psychiat. (Chicago)*, **1**, 111.

GIBBS, F. A., LENNOX, W. G., and GIBBS, E. L. (1936) The electro-encephalogram in diagnosis and in localization of epileptic seizures, *Arch. Neurol. Psychiat. (Chicago)*, **36**, 1225.

GIRDWOOD, R. H. (1959) The role of folic acid in blood disorders, *Brit. med. Bull.*, **15**, 17.

GLASER, G. H., and LEVY, L. L. (1960) Seizures and idiopathic hypoparathyroidism, *Epilepsia*, **1**, 454.

GOWERS, W. R. (1901) *Epilepsy and Other Chronic Convulsive Diseases*, London.

GRIFFITHS, G. M., and FOX, J. T. (1938) Rhythm in epilepsy, *Lancet*, ii, 409.

HARPER, M., and ROTH, M. (1962) Temporal lobe epilepsy and the phobic-anxiety-depersonalisation syndrome, *Comprehens. Psychiat.*, **3**, 129.

HAWKINS, C. F., and MEYNELL, M. J. (1958) Macrocytosis and macrocytic anaemia caused by anti-convulsant drugs, *Quart. J. Med.*, **27**, 45.

HILL, J. D. N., and PARR, G. (1963) *Electroencephalography*, 2nd ed., London.

HODSKINS, M. B., and YAKOVLEV, P. I. (1930) Neurosomatic deterioration in epilepsy, *Arch. Neurol. Psychiat. (Chicago)*, **23**, 986.

HUNTER, R., HURWITZ, L. J., FULLERTON, P. M., NIEMAN, E. A., and DAVIES, H. (1962) Unilateral ventricular enlargement. A report of 75 cases, *Brain*, **85**, 295.

INTERNATIONAL BUREAU FOR EPILEPSY (1966) *Epilepsy and Driving Licences*, Social studies in epilepsy, No. 4 Supplement to *British Epilepsy Association Journal*, London.

JACKSON, J. H. (1931) Epilepsy and epileptiform convulsions, *Selected Writings*, Vol. 1, London.

JAMES, J. L., and WHITTY, C. W. M. (1961) The electroencephalogram as a monitor of status epilepticus suppressed peripherally by curarisation, *Lancet*, ii. 239.

JASPER, H. H., and DROOGLEEVER-FORTUYN, J. (1947) Experimental studies on the functional anatomy of petit mal epilepsy, *Res. Publ. Ass. nerv. ment. Dis.*, **26**, 272.

JASPER, H. H., and KERSHMAN, J. (1941) Electro-encephalographic classification of the epileptics, *Arch. Neurol. Psychiat. (Chicago)*, **45**, 903.

JELLIFFE, S. E., and NOTKIN, J. (1934–5) The pyknolepsies, *Amer. J. Psychiat.*, **91**, 679.

JENNETT, W. B. (1961) *Late Epilepsy after Blunt Head Injury*, Hunterian Lecture to Royal College of Surgeons, London.

JURGELSKY, W., JNR., and THOMAS, J. A. (1966) The *in vivo* protection of gamma-amino-butyric acid against organic phosphate inhibition of ACHE, *Life Sci.*, **5**, 1525.

KILOH, L. G., and OSSELTON, J. W. (1967) *Clinical Electroencephalography*, 2nd ed., London.

LAIDLAW, J. (1956) Catamenial epilepsy, *Lancet*, ii, 1235.

LEES, F., and LIVERSEDGE, L. A. (1962) The prognosis of petit mal and minor epilepsy, *Lancet*, ii, 797.

LENNOX, W. G. (1945) The petit mal epilepsies, *J. Amer. med. Ass.*, **129**, 1069.

LENNOX, W. G. (1947) Sixty-six twin pairs affected by seizures, *Res. Publ. Ass. nerv. ment. Dis.*, **26**, 11.

LENNOX, W. G., GIBBS, E. L., and GIBBS, F. A. (1940) The inheritance of epilepsy as revealed by the electro-encephalograph, *Arch. Neurol. Psychiat. (Chicago)*, **44**, 1155.

LENNOX, W. G., and LENNOX, M. A. (1960) *Epilepsy and Related Disorders*, Boston, Mass.

LISHMAN, W. A., SYMONDS, C. P., WHITTY, C. W. M., and WILLISON, R. G. (1962) Seizures induced by movement, *Brain*, **85**, 93.

LIVINGSTON, S., TORRES, I., PAULI, L. L., and RIDER, R. V. (1965) Petit mal epilepsy. Results of a prolonged follow-up study of 117 patients, *J. Amer. med. Ass.*, **194**, 227.

MATTHEWS, W. B. (1954) Tonic seizures in multiple sclerosis, *Brain*, **81**, 193.

MEYER, A. (1963) Epilepsy, in *Greenfield's Neuropathology*, 2nd ed., ed. BLACKWOOD, W., McMENEMEY, W. H., MEYER, A., NORMAN, R. M., and RUSSELL, D. S., London.

MORTIMER, P. L. F. (1961) The encephalogram as a monitor of status epilepticus, *Lancet*, ii, 776.

PENFIELD, W., and JASPER, H. (1954) *Epilepsy and the Functional Anatomy of the Human Brain*, Boston.

PRUNTY, F. T. G. (1944) Reactive hyperinsulinism, *Brit. med. J.*, **2**, 398.

REYNOLDS, E. H. (1968) Mental effects of anticonvulsants and folic acid metabolism, *Brain*, **91**, 197.

DELLA ROVERE, M., HOARE, R. D., and PAMPIGLIONE, G. (1964) Tuberose sclerosis in children, an E.E.G. study, *Develop. med. Child. Neurol.*, **6**, 149.

SIMPSON, J. A. (1952) Neurological manifestations of hypoparathyroidism, *Brain*, **75**, 76.

SLATER, E., and BEARD, A. W. (1963) The schizophrenia-like psychoses of epilepsy, *Brit. J. Psychiat.*, **109**, 95.

SYMONDS, C. (1959) Excitation and inhibition in epilepsy, *Brain*, **82**, 133.

TODAY'S DRUGS (1968) Drug treatment of epilepsy, *Brit. med. J.*, **1**, 350.

WALTER, W. G. (1947) Analytical means of discovering the origin and nature of epileptic disturbances, *Res. Publ. Ass. nerv. ment. Dis.*, **26**, 237.

WAUCHOPE, G. M. (1933) Hypoglycaemia, *Quart. J. Med.*, N.S. **2**, 117.

WHITTY, C. W. M. (1960) Photic and self-induced epilepsy, *Lancet*, i, 1207.

WILLIAMS, D. (1941) The significance of an abnormal electro-encephalogram, *J. Neurol. Psychiat.*, N.S. **4**, 257.

WILLIAMS, D. (1950) New orientations in epilepsy, *Brit. med. J.*, **1**, 685.

WILSON, J., WALTON, J. N., and NEWELL, D. J. (1959) Beclamide in intractable epilepsy: a controlled trial, *Brit. med. J.*, **1**, 1275.

ZISKIND, E., and BERCEL, N. A. (1947) Preconvulsive paroxysmal electro-encephalographic changes after metrazol injection, *Res. Publ. Ass. nerv. ment. Dis.*, **26**, 487.

VASOVAGAL ATTACKS

The terms 'vagal' and 'vasovagal' attacks were first used by Gowers to describe 'prolonged seizures, the symptoms of which consist chiefly in disturbance of some of the functions of the pneumogastric'. Vasovagal attacks are uncommon and occur more frequently in women than in men. As a rule no precipitating cause can be discovered. Gowers was careful to state that he used the term 'vagal' for purposes of description 'without implying causation' and vasovagal attacks are not a nosological entity. Though the attacks are characterized by some symptoms which may reasonably be attributed to a disturbance both of the sensory and of the motor functions of the vagus, other symptoms may be regarded as indicating overaction of the sympathetic. Their cause is unknown but some may be a manifestation of an epileptic dysrhythmia, and Gowers included them in 'the borderland of epilepsy'. Others seem more allied to syncope; and others again may be psychogenic.

REFERENCE

GOWERS, W. R. (1907) *The Borderland of Epilepsy*, London.

TETANY

Definition. Tetany, or carpopedal spasm, is a form of muscular spasm beginning in, and sometimes remaining limited to, the peripheral muscles of the limbs. It is associated with an increased excitability of the neuromuscular apparatus to all forms of stimuli. It is a symptom of a variety of disorders which either reduce the calcium content of the blood or increase its alkalinity.

AETIOLOGY

Modern investigations of the metabolism of calcium and of the biochemistry of the blood have rendered it possible to reduce the immediate causes of tetany to two. It is probable that in all cases the patient is suffering from either a subnormal calcium content of the blood, or from an alkalosis, though a few conditions remain which have not yet been sufficiently investigated to enable them to be placed in either class. An attempt has been made to attribute all forms of tetany to calcium deficiency, on the hypothesis that alkalosis diminishes the amount of ionized calcium in the blood, even though its total calcium content remains normal. This at present, however, remains unproved, and there are indications that tissue anoxaemia may be of some importance.

Conditions characterized by a Subnormal Blood Calcium

Parathyroid Deficiency. The important role of the parathyroids in the metabolism of calcium and their influence upon the calcium content of the blood are comparatively recent discoveries. Hyperparathyroidism due to a parathyroid tumour causes the blood calcium content to rise above its normal figure of between 9 and 11 mg. per 100 ml. Hypoparathyroidism leads to a subnormal blood-calcium content which may be as low as 4 or 5 mg. per 100 ml., and in such cases tetany may occur—tetania parathyreopriva. Hypoparathyroidism, which is rare, is usually the result of accidental removal of the parathyroid glands during thyroidectomy but may occur spontaneously, the cause then being unknown. Pseudohypoparathyroidism is a rare cause.

Defective Intestinal Calcium Absorption. Fatty diarrhoea, when severe and of long duration, may lead to a fall in the blood calcium content sufficient to cause tetany. Thus tetany may occur in sprue, in cases of idiopathic steatorrhoea, and, exceptionally, in tuberculous enteritis. The low blood calcium in such cases has been attributed to loss of calcium from the intestine in combination with fatty acids in the form of soaps. It appears, however, that the chief cause of the calcium defect is a failure to absorb vitamin D (Hunter, 1930). No hard and fast line can be drawn between defective absorption and excessive loss.

Rickets and Osteomalacia. In the past, dietary deficiency of vitamin D or lack of exposure to sunlight was the commonest cause of rickets which often gave rise to infantile tetany (spasmophilia). About 10 per cent. of such cases also suffered epileptic seizures. The widespread use of vitamin supplements in infancy has virtually abolished rickets due to dietary deficiency but a number of forms of vitamin-D resistant rickets have been described; in one of these, hypophosphatasia, a single enzyme defect has been identified (Fraser, 1957). Some cases of adult osteomalacia are due to an inadequate dietary intake of calcium and vitamin D.

Increased Demand for Calcium. Pregnancy and lactation may cause tetany, owing to the increased demand which they make upon the calcium resources of the mother. The likelihood of tetany's occurring is much increased when the intake of vitamin D and calcium is subnormal, as in osteomalacia.

High Urinary Calcium Loss. Renal failure in chronic nephritis and in certain other forms of renal disease may lead to tetany as a result of hypocalcaemia and raised serum phosphate, which is present also in hypoparathyroidism. A raised blood potassium is sometimes a contributory factor.

Conditions characterized by Alkalosis

Alkalosis occurs when the ratio of acid to base in the blood is diminished, with the result that the pH, normally between 7·3 and 7·5, rises as does the serum bicarbonate. This may occur in the following conditions:

Excessive Ingestion of Alkali. Overdosage with sodium bicarbonate and other alkalis used in the treatment of dyspepsia may cause alkalosis and hence tetany, especially if the power of the kidney to excrete alkali is diminished by nephritis.

Hyperpnoea. Overbreathing, by washing out CO_2 from the blood, may lead to alkalosis and hence to tetany. Tetany may thus be induced by voluntary forced breathing, by hysterical hyperpnoea, or by hyperpnoea occurring as a result of disturbance of function of the respiratory centre, for example in encephalitis.

High Intestinal Obstruction. It has long been known that tetany may complicate disorders associated with repeated vomiting—gastric tetany—and McCallum suggested that in such cases alkalosis was produced by a loss of acid from the body in the vomit. Since, however, alkalosis may occur in cases of pyloric obstruction due to carcinoma of the stomach, in which the vomit may be free from acid, this hypothesis cannot be the whole explanation. It has been shown experimentally that high intestinal obstruction in itself leads to a fall in the chloride content and a rise in the bicarbonate content of the blood.

Other Causes of Tetany

So-called idiopathic tetany occurs in epidemic form in some of the countries of central Europe, usually in the spring months. Tetany also occurs in association with a low blood potassium, e.g. in hyperaldosteronism.

PATHOPHYSIOLOGY

The pathophysiology of tetany has been reviewed by Alajouanine, Contamin, and Cathala (1958). They believe that it is essentially a functional disorder of the peripheral sensorimotor fibres resulting from various metabolic disturbances. Electrically the nerves show hyperexcitability, diminished capacity for accommodation, and a tendency to show repetitive responses to single stimuli. These authors discount a cerebral origin for tetany, a point discussed by Matthews (1958).

SYMPTOMS

An attack of tetany is usually preceded by tingling sensations in the periphery of the limbs, especially in the hands and there are often similar paraesthesiae with a sense of stiffness in the lips and tongue. The attack itself consists of muscular spasm which develops spontaneously, but its intensity may be increased by external stimuli, such as manipulation of the limbs. In mild cases the spasm is confined to the hands and feet, or even to the hands. The tonic contraction of the interossei of the hands leads to a typical attitude—*la main d'accoucheur*. The fingers are slightly flexed at the metacarpophalangeal joints and extended at the interphalangeal joints. They are strongly adducted, and the thumb is similarly adducted and usually extended. The cause of the limitation of the muscular spasm in mild cases to the small muscles of the hands is unknown. Exceptionally the fingers become flexed at all joints, and Rosett, in investigating the tetany produced by voluntary hyperpnoea, has shown that the limbs will become rigid in any posture in which they are previously fixed. The characteristic attitude of the feet is one of plantar-flexion at the ankle and adduction of the toes.

In severe attacks the muscular spasm spreads to the proximal muscles of the limbs. In the upper limbs it predominates as a rule in the flexors of the elbow and in the adductors of the shoulder. In the lower limbs the knees are usually extended and the hips adducted. In such cases the muscles of the head may also go into spasm, the masseters closing the jaw and the angles of the mouth being retracted in a *risus sardonicus*. The eyes may be partly closed and the bulbar muscles may also be affected, especially those of the larynx. Laryngospasm with resultant stridor has been described, particularly in children with rickets. Dysarthria and dyspnoea may thus be produced. Spasm of the trunk muscles may also occur, leading to slight opisthotonos. Generalized convulsions may occur, especially in childhood.

Though slight attacks of tetany are painless, considerable cramp-like pain attends the more violent spasms. Sweating and tachycardia and even rise of temperature may occur in severe attacks.

The increased excitability of the neuromuscular apparatus is demonstrable in the response to certain tests, even in the absence of actual attacks of tetany.

Chvostek's sign consists of a brisk contraction of the facial muscles in response to a light tap over the facial nerve in front of the ear. Pressure upon the main artery supplying a limb or upon the peripheral nerves may precipitate an attack of tetany—*Trousseau's sign*. This test is simply applied by means of the cuff of a sphygmomanometer. The response to electrical stimulation of the nerves is also abnormal, as Erb first demonstrated. There is increased excitability of the motor nerves, and when the galvanic current is employed a response is most readily evoked by the anodal closing current (*Erb's electrical reaction*). The ulnar nerve is the most convenient for this test. Bourguignon and Haldane have shown that during tetany induced by voluntary hyperpnoea there is an increase in chronaxie as determined by stimulation both of the nerve trunk and of the motor point. Electromyographic changes are discussed by Alajouanine *et al*.

In hypoparathyroidism generalized epileptiform convulsions associated with loss of consciousness may occur, but are rare except in children with idiopathic hypoparathyroidism in whom mental backwardness is usual. Confusion and intellectual blunting may occur in acquired hypoparathyroidism. Papilloedema may be present, with or without lenticular cataract. The EEG may show spikes and slow waves in the frontal areas. X-rays of the skull may demonstrate calcification in the basal ganglia and dentate nuclei. For a discussion of this see Roberts (1959) and Glaser and Levy (1960).

DIAGNOSIS

The symptoms of tetany are so striking that they are not likely to be confused with other conditions. The onset of the muscular spasm in the hands and feet and the associated signs of increased neuromuscular excitability are pathognomonic of tetany. Tetanus is distinguished by the fact that in this disease muscular spasm, though subject to exacerbations, is constant and not, as in tetany, intermittent. Moreover, in tetanus the *main d'accoucheur* attitude does not occur and spasm of the masseters as a rule develops early, whereas in tetany this is a late symptom occurring only in severe attacks. Hysteria may be associated with tetany when the latter is produced by hysterical hyperpnoea. In addition hysterical muscular rigidity may simulate tetany. In hysteria, however, the typical attitude of tetany is as a rule absent, though I have seen one hysterical patient who had suffered from tetany as a child and who in later life reproduced the attitude of tetany as an hysterical symptom with remarkable accuracy. Other hysterical symptoms, such as anaesthesia, are usually to be found in such cases, and the patient's emotional reaction to his symptoms is characteristic.

In every case of tetany the underlying cause must be ascertained. This is usually easy if the common causes are borne in mind and appropriate inquiries are made. It is, however, always desirable that the pH and bicarbonate content of the blood plasma and the calcium and phosphate content of the serum should be ascertained in order to determine whether the condition is due to a low blood calcium or alkalosis.

PROGNOSIS

Recovery from an attack of tetany is almost invariable, though death may occur in a severe attack, owing to laryngeal or bronchial spasm. The prognosis as to cessation of the attacks depends upon the nature of their cause and the efficiency of treatment.

TREATMENT

In hypocalcaemic tetany the blood calcium may be raised by administering calcium lactate as a powder taken fasting in repeated doses up to a total of 10 to 30 G. daily (Hunter) together with calciferol in the dose appropriate to the individual. Effervescent calcium tablets (e.g. *Calcium-Sandoz*) may be more palatable and convenient than calcium lactate. Dihydrotachysterol (*A.T. 10*), has a more rapid effect and is given in a dosage of 1·25 mg. three times daily until the serum calcium is normal after which a single daily maintenance dose may suffice. A severe attack may be cut short by slowly injecting 20 ml. of 5 per cent. solution of calcium gluconate intravenously.

In tetany due to steatorrhoea the intake of fat in the diet should be restricted to a minimum and the patient should be given calciferol. This vitamin, with or without irradiation with ultraviolet light, is all that is required in the treatment of tetany associated with rickets, and the same treatment should be given in osteomalacia and when tetany occurs in pregnancy, together with calcium by the mouth and a diet rich in calcium. Parathyroid extract should not be given in these conditions, since it raises the blood calcium by withdrawing calcium from the bones.

When tetany is due to vitamin-resistant rickets or some other inborn error of metabolism the appropriate treatment will depend upon the identification of the underlying biochemical disorder.

REFERENCES

ALAJOUANINE, T., CONTAMIN, F., and CATHALA, H. P. (1958) *Le Syndrome Tétanie*, Paris.
BICKNELL, F., and PRESCOTT, F. (1953) *The Vitamins in Medicine*, 3rd ed., London.
FOLEY, J. (1951) Calcification in a family, *J. Neurol. Neurosurg. Psychiat.*, N.S. **14**, 253.
FRASER, D. (1957) Hypophosphatasia, *Amer. J. Med.*, **22**, 730.
GLASER, G. H., and LEVY, L. L. (1960) Seizures and idiopathic hypoparathyroidism, *Epilepsia*, **1**, 454.
GRANT, D. K. (1953) Papilloedema and fits in hypoparathyroidism, *Quart. J. Med.*, N.S. **22**, 243.
HUNTER, D. (1930) Goulstonian Lectures. The significance to clinical medicine of studies in calcium and phosphorus metabolism, *Lancet*, i, 897, 947, 999.
MATTHEWS, W. (1958) Tonic seizures in disseminated sclerosis, *Brain*, **81**, 193.
ROBERTS, P. D. (1959) Familial calcification of the basal ganglia and its relation to hypoparathyroidism, *Brain*, **82**, 599.
SALVESEN, H. A. (1930, 1931) Observations on human tetany. I. Spontaneous tetany in adults, *Acta med. scand.*, **73**, 511; II. Postoperative tetany, ibid., **74**, 13.
WEST, R. (1935) Studies in the neurological mechanism of parathyroid tetany, *Brain*, **58**, 1.

MYOCLONUS

The term 'myoclonus' is applied to a brief, shock-like muscular contraction which may involve a whole muscle or may rarely be limited to a small number of muscle fibres. Myoclonus may be confined to a single muscle or may involve many muscles, either successively or simultaneously. Frequently contractions occur symmetrically in muscles on the opposite sides of the body. The contraction may be too slight to cause movement of a segment of the limb, or may cause such violent movements as to throw the patient to the ground. The contraction never involves groups of muscles which are normally synergically associated, nor does it as a rule affect mutually antagonistic muscles.

The situation of the disorder of function responsible for myoclonus has been much discussed. When myoclonus is associated with epilepsy the disturbance appears to arise at a situation deeply placed which is able to activate both cerebral hemispheres and it seems likely that it originates in the reticular substance of the brain stem. There is also evidence that myoclonus without epilepsy may be caused by disorders of the olivo-dentate system. Myoclonus may occur without any demonstrable pathological lesion—essential myoclonus. Bradshaw (1954) and Aigner and Mulder (1960) have reviewed this topic and it has been shown that no fewer than 30 different entities have been described in which myoclonus may occur.

The Causes of Myoclonus

While the sharp, transient muscular contractions or 'jerks' which constitute the myoclonic phenomena are in most cases to be regarded as representing a type of transient epileptic discharge arising in cerebral or brain stem neurones, other forms of epileptic attack are not invariably associated with myoclonus. Myoclonic jerks which occur on falling asleep in the 'drifting' stage are physiological and probably depend upon a transient reactivation of reticular system neurones. When, however, nocturnal myoclonus continues during deep sleep, it is often found that major fits, possibly nocturnal, eventually occur in such cases and this syndrome is undoubtedly to be regarded as a form of epilepsy. Recurrent myoclonic jerks in the early morning after waking, causing the patient to spill the breakfast tea or coffee or even to 'throw' cutlery across the room, is not infrequently seen in some children with idiopathic epilepsy, and a single myoclonic jerk in the upper limbs occasionally occurs in an attack of petit mal. 'Jerking' or 'jumping' of the limbs and trunk in response to a sudden noise may sometimes be so intense as to be undoubtedly pathological. It has been called hyperekplexia or the 'essential startle disease' (Gastaut and Villeneuve, 1967), is occasionally familial and may be indistinguishable from myoclonus, except that it is always precipitated by noise. Physiological evidence which suggests that evoked potentials may easily be recorded in scalp EEG recordings as a result of peripheral sensory stimuli suggests that perhaps in patients with the benign forms of myoclonus, inhibitory mechanisms in the brain stem reticular substance are defective.

In Unverricht's progressive myoclonic epilepsy degenerative changes have been described in cortical ganglion cells and in cerebellar dentate nuclei. Myoclonus may occur also in encephalitis lethargica, inclusion encephalitis, and the cerebral lipidoses. Jones and Nevin (1954) describe it as a symptom of subacute spongiform encephalopathy [see p. 608]. The olivo-dentate form may be the result of an abiotrophic degeneration, as in Hunt's dyssynergia cerebellaris myoclonica, vascular lesions, tumours, and multiple sclerosis. Myoclonus in the legs has been described as a result of pathological changes in the spinal cord (Campbell and Garland, 1956).

Myoclonus is thus a symptom which may be produced by a variety of different lesions, and in some cases the nature of the underlying disorder of function is still obscure. The classification of varieties of myoclonus is, therefore, necessarily somewhat arbitrary.

VARIETIES OF MYOCLONUS

FACIAL MYOCLONUS

This name has been given, erroneously, by some authors to hemifacial spasm [see p. 171].

MYOCLONUS IN ENCEPHALOMYELITIS

Myoclonus is a somewhat uncommon symptom of encephalitis lethargica. It occurred with special frequency in some epidemics [see p. 441]. It may also occur in subacute encephalitis and in cervical herpes zoster, especially in those cases in which there is evidence that the infection has spread in the spinal cord beyond the first sensory neurone. Campbell and Garland (1956) described a condition which they called progressive myoclonic spinal neuronitis in which myoclonic jerking in the lower limbs was followed by the development of a progressive paraplegia.

PALATO-PHARYNGO-LARYNGO-OCULO-DIAPHRAGMATIC MYOCLONUS

This syndrome, as its name implies, is characterized by the synchronous occurrence of a rhythmical myoclonus of the soft palate, pharynx, larynx, eyes, and diaphragm, and sometimes of other muscles. The distribution of the myoclonus may be unilateral or bilateral. The palatal movement has been described as 'nystagmus of the soft palate'. The rate of the movements varies from 80 to 180 to the minute, and is usually about 120 to 130 contractions to the minute. It is uninfluenced by drugs, and apparently by sleep, but may be inhibited at first by voluntary effort, and disappears if paralysis supervenes in the myoclonic muscles. It appears to be due to a degenerative process of unknown cause in most cases, but has been observed in multiple sclerosis and as a sequel to brain stem infarction. The disorder appears to be one of the olivo-cerebellar modulatory projection on to the rostral brain stem (Hermann and Brown, 1967).

PARAMYOCLONUS MULTIPLEX

The term 'paramyoclonus multiplex' and its synonyms, myoclonus simplex and essential myoclonus, should be reserved for the syndrome first described by Friedreich in 1881 and characterized by the onset during adult life of frequent myoclonic muscular contractions. These are most frequently observed in the facial muscles and in the biceps, triceps, and brachioradialis in the upper limbs and in the quadriceps, and to a less extent in the adductors of the hip, biceps, and semitendinosus in the lower limbs. The muscular contraction involves the whole muscle or groups of muscles and occurs regularly with a frequency varying from ten to fifty times a minute. The jerking movements are increased by tension and anxiety and may be inhibited by volitional contraction; though they may affect symmetrically muscles on the two sides of the body, these do not contract synchronously. The myoclonic movements disappear during sleep. The electrical reactions of the muscles are normal, sensation is unimpaired, and the only associated abnormality is an exaggeration of the tendon reflexes. The disorder is a benign and chronic one which does not threaten life, and in some cases recovery occurs. These patients do not as a rule develop epileptic seizures, dementia, or ataxia; no consistent pathological changes have been discovered in the brain in this condition, which Mahloudji and Pikielny (1967) suggest should be called 'hereditary essential myoclonus'. Treatment with sedative drugs should be carried out on the same lines as for epilepsy.

PROGRESSIVE FAMILIAL MYOCLONIC EPILEPSY

Myoclonic contractions are common in patients suffering from idiopathic epilepsy, occurring between the epileptic attacks and usually becoming intensified before the attack occurs. In addition epileptic attacks have been described rarely in patients regarded as suffering from paramyoclonus multiplex, though it is difficult to say on what grounds such cases are distinguished from idiopathic epilepsy with myoclonus. The term 'progressive familial myoclonus epilepsy' is best reserved for the rare but well-defined syndrome first described by Unverricht in 1891, and later carefully studied by Lundborg (1903). Recent reports are by Harriman and Millar (1955) and Noad and Lance (1960). Myoclonus epilepsy thus defined is usually familial, and occurs in several sibs, being inherited as an autosomal recessive disorder.

The distinctive pathological feature is the presence of inclusion bodies in the cytoplasm of the nerve cells. Harriman and Millar describe two types: (1) the Lafora bodies staining like amyloid; and (2) lipid inclusions resembling those of amaurotic family idiocy. The most striking pathological changes are observed in cerebral cortical neurones and in the dentate nuclei of the cerebellum. Millar and Neill (1959) have found that in such cases an abnormal mucoprotein may be detected in the serum. Yokoi et al. (1968) have shown that isolated Lafora bodies contain insoluble aggregates of an unusual polyglucosan and suggest that progressive myoclonic epilepsy should be regarded as one of the 'glycogen deposition diseases'.

The onset of symptoms occurs as a rule between the ages of 6 and 16, usually when the patient is about 10, development up to that point having been normal. Generalized epileptiform attacks with loss of consciousness appear first, and, to begin with, frequently occur only at night. After several years the characteristic myoclonic contractions develop. These are shock-like muscular contractions simultaneously involving symmetrical muscles on both sides of the body, sufficiently strong to produce movements of the limb segments. They involve the muscles of the face, trunk, and of both upper and lower limbs. They disappear during sleep and are intensified by emotional excitement. They often increase in severity before a generalized epileptic attack but are not attended by loss of consciousness. Myoclonus may occur in the ocular muscles, the lips, and the tongue, interfering with speech and with swallowing. In the limbs the flexors are more often attacked than the extensors. Writing may become impossible, and sudden contractions of the flexors of the lower limbs when the patient is standing or walking may throw him violently to the ground. After some years, during which myoclonic and epileptic attacks are associated, a progressive dementia develops, and the patient passes into the third stage of the disease, in which the epileptic attacks tend to disappear, though myoclonus continues. Dysarthria and dysphagia increase, and death follows progressive cachexia. Noad and Lance (1960) report a family with signs of cerebellar disorder. The EEG shows bilaterally synchronous sharp waves associated with the myoclonus, which Harriman and Millar think indicates that the discharge originates in the brain stem. Noad and Lance found that the EEG discharge resembled that seen in the lipidoses.

The relationship of this condition to Hunt's dyssynergia cerebellaris myoclonica is uncertain but in the latter disorder myoclonus and cerebellar ataxia, rather than major fits and dementia, predominate. The two disorders also differ pathologically (de Barsy et al., 1969).

Treatment is merely palliative. The usual treatment of epilepsy may control the generalized epileptic attacks, but has less influence upon the myoclonus.

REFERENCES

AIGNER, B. R., and MULDER, D. W. (1960) Myoclonus, Arch. Neurol. (Chic.), 2, 600.

DE BARSY, T., MYLE, G., TROCH, C., MATTHYS, R., and MARTIN, J. J. (1969) La dyssynergie cérébelleuse myoclonique (R. Hunt): affection autonome ou variante du type dégénératif de l'épilepsie myoclonique progressive (Unverricht-Lundborg) (approche anatomo-chimique), J. neurol. Sci., in press.

BRADSHAW, J. P. P. (1954) A study of myoclonus, Brain, 77, 138.

CAMPBELL, A. M. G., and GARLAND, H. G. (1956) Progressive myoclonic spinal neuronitis, J. Neurol. Neurosurg. Psychiat., 19, 268.

GASTAUT, H., and VILLENEUVE, A. (1967) The startle disease or hyperekplexia, J. neurol. Sci., 5, 523.

GUILLAIN, G. (1937–8) The syndrome of synchronous and rhythmic palato-pharyngolaryngo-oculo-diaphragmatic myoclonus, Proc. roy. Soc. Med., 31, 1031.

HARRIMAN, D. G. F., and MILLAR, J. H. D. (1955) Progressive familial myoclonic epilepsy in three families; its clinical features and pathological basis, Brain, 78, 325.

HERRMANN, C., JR., and BROWN, J. W. (1967) Palatal myoclonus: a reappraisal, J. neurol. Sci., 5, 473.

JACQUIN, G., and MARCHAND, L. (1913) Myoclonie épileptique progressive, Encéphale, 8, (1), 205.

JONES, D. P., and NEVIN, S. (1954) Rapidly progressive cerebral degeneration (Subacute vascular encephalopathy with mental disorder, focal disturbances, and myoclonic epilepsy), J. Neurol. Neurosurg. Psychiat., N.S. 17, 148.

LUNDBORG, H. (1903) Die progressive Myoklonus-Epilepsie, Uppsala.

MAHLOUDJI, M., and PIKIELNY, R. T. (1967) Hereditary essential myoclonus, Brain, 90, 669.

MILLAR, J. H. D., and NEILL, D. W. (1959) Serum mucoproteins in progressive familiar myoclonic epilepsy, Epilepsia, 1, 115.

NOAD, K. B., and LANCE, J. W. (1960) Familial myoclonic epilepsy and its association with cerebellar disturbance, Brain, 83, 618.

PÉLISSIER, F. (1911) Des Myoclonies épileptiques, Thèse de Montpellier.

REIMOLD, W. (1925) Über die myoklonische Form der Encephalitis, Z. ges. Neurol. Psychiat., 95, 21.

UNVERRICHT, H. (1891) Die Myoclonie, Leipzig.

YOKOI, S., AUSTIN, J., WITMER, F., and SAKAI, M. (1968) Studies in myoclonus epilepsy (Lafora body form), Arch. Neurol. (Chic.), 19, 15.

23

PSYCHOLOGICAL ASPECTS OF NEUROLOGY

THE growth of medical psychology has rendered it necessary to restrict the scope of the psychological section of a textbook of neurology. Much of psychiatry and psychotherapy falls outside the province of neurology. Nevertheless, since the brain is the organ of the mind the neurologist has unique opportunities of observing the effects of nervous disease upon mental functions, and in particular of studying disorders of perception, memory, and emotion. He is also concerned with the psychoses and psychoneuroses in the differential diagnosis of organic nervous disease. This section, therefore, deals with psychological medicine primarily from the standpoint of the neurologist. But since the neurologist is a doctor it falls to his lot to treat large numbers of patients suffering from psychological disorders. He cannot avoid, therefore, being at times a psychotherapist; hence some consideration of the relationships between neurology and psychiatry is called for in this chapter.

ANATOMY AND PHYSIOLOGY

GENERAL CONSIDERATIONS

The principal difference between the human and the subhuman brain consists in the great development of the cerebral cortex in man. The cortex is, in the first instance, an end-station at which are received nervous impulses derived from the eyes, the ears, and other sensory organs. The corresponding regions of the cortex are linked by association paths by means of which the sensations which form the raw material of perception evoke memories and become enriched with meanings, which can be communicated to others by means of speech, writing, and gesture. The function of the cerebral cortex, therefore, as Head pointed out in relation to sensation, is primarily discriminative, and the massive development of the cortex in man compared with that in the lower animals is paralleled by the great enhancement of the range of his discriminative faculties, which has occurred in spite of there having been little improvement, and in some cases an actual retrogression, of his sensory acuity.

By contrast there is far less difference between man and the lower animals in respect of the development of subcortical centres, and in particular of the thalamus and hypothalamus. It is these regions of the brain, basal alike in situation and in function, which are intimately concerned with the affective element in feeling, with the emotional and instinctive life, and the regulation of the autonomic nervous system and to some extent of metabolic and endocrine function. The brain, however, works as a whole and there is a constant interplay between cortical and subcortical functions. Perception evokes emotion and, conversely, emotion provides the interest which activates perception.

There is another aspect, however, of the relationship between the cerebral cortex and subcortical function. Discrimination, the function of the cortex, implies inhibition, for, if an organism is to react appropriately to a stimulus, inappropriate modes of reaction must be simultaneously inhibited. This is true even at the level of a simple reflex arc; it is far more essential when the range both of potential stimuli and of potential reactions has been so greatly enlarged by the development of the cerebral cortex. The cortex, therefore, acquires inhibitory functions as the complement of its discriminative functions.

Anatomy and Physiology of the Diencephalon

As Pribham (1958) has shown, it is convenient to begin with the thalamus which seems in many ways both physiologically and anatomically basic to the organization of animal behaviour. The dorsal thalamus is divided into an external portion and an internal core. Each of these has nuclei which receive impulses from outside the thalamus and other nuclei which, as far as is known, do not. These are distinguished as extrinsic and intrinsic nuclei. The extrinsic nuclei of the external division receive the somatic sensory tracts, and the optic and auditory pathways: the intrinsic nucleus is the posterior nucleus. The extrinsic nuclei of the internal core receive impulses from the posterior hypothalamus and the central reticular formation: the intrinsic nucleus is the medial. Turning now to the projections from these nuclei we find that the extrinsic nuclei of the external portion project to the primary sensory cortical areas concerned with somatic sensibility, hearing, and vision in the parietal, temporal, and occipital lobes, while the intrinsic, posterior, nucleus projects to the rest of the parieto-temporo-occipital cortex. The extrinsic nuclei of the internal core project to the limbic areas of the medial aspect of the frontal and parietal lobes and to the anterior rhinencephalon and the basal ganglia, and the medial, the intrinsic, nucleus projects to the antero-frontal cortex. There is an important corticifugal pathway running from the mediobasal part of the frontal lobe to the thalamus and the hypothalamic nuclei, including the corpora mamillaria.

Experimental stimulation and destruction of these regions in animals leads to the following conclusions. The projections from the extrinsic nuclei of the external part of the dorsal thalamus are the familiar sensory afferent pathways, and interference with them causes sensory loss in the corresponding modalities. Damage to the parts of the cerebral cortex supplied by the projections from the intrinsic nuclei of the external part lead to a failure to differentiate and respond to patterns of sensory stimuli—a condition resembling that known in man as agnosia. These nuclei, their projections and the corresponding cortical areas must therefore be regarded as constituting a higher-level perceptual discriminative mechanism.

On the other hand, ablations and stimulations of the anatomical systems represented by the nuclei of the internal core of the thalamus, and their projections through the medial and basal telencephalon, affect feeding (eating and drinking), fighting and aggression, fleeing and avoidance, mating, and maternal behaviour: they are therefore concerned with what may in the broadest sense be termed instinctive behaviour. All such activities, when they occur in man, are linked with emotion to a greater or a lesser extent, and it seems a reasonable inference that the same is true of animals.

The Neurological Basis of Emotion

Psychophysiologically, emotion implies a number of factors: there is (1) some external object which excites it. (2) There are specific feelings characteristic of particular emotions, and (3) the emotion tends to find expression in some characteristic action. Accompanying the feelings and the motor activities there are (4) certain other physiological states in which the autonomic nervous system and the endocrines play an important part. And, finally, there is often (5) a pre-existing physiological state which is necessary if the appetite, or emotional need, is to be experienced. This is most obvious in the case of hunger, thirst, and the sexual impulse.

Many years ago Head's work drew attention to the possible role of the optic thalamus in emotion, but Head was specifically concerned with abnormal reactions to sensory stimuli, and Lashley (1960), reviewing the subject, concluded that there was no evidence that the thalamus is in any way related to emotional feelings, but that it might be concerned with the patterns of the motor manifestations or expressions of emotion. It has been found in monkeys that whereas bilateral lesions of the anterior nuclei of the thalamus produce no change in behaviour, similar lesions of the dorsomedial nuclei lead to restlessness, loss of fear and distractability, symptoms resembling those of frontal lobectomy in the same animals (Brierley and Beck, 1958).

Bard (1928) observed that lesions cephalad to the hypothalamus in cats led to the manifestation of what he called 'sham rage', whereas lesions caudal to the hypothalamus were followed by states of abnormal tranquillity. The possible role of the hypothalamus in emotion has been reviewed by Masserman (1943), who concluded that there is little or no evidence that the hypothalamus governs, or mediates, the emotional experiences themselves, but that it is well established that it reinforces and co-ordinates the neural and hormonal mechanisms of emotional expression and activity.

Dell (1958) draws a distinction between two factors in instinctive or appetitive behaviour: there is a specific perceptual one, which is concerned with the recognition of the object which will satisfy the instinctive need, and there is a non-specific one common to all forms of instinctive behaviour, which consists of 'a heightened level of sensory and motor excitation', and which in his view depends upon activation of the brain stem reticular formation. This is aroused by the appropriate perceptual experience and provides the 'drive' which leads to the activity necessary to satisfy the need. Consummation of the instinctive act produces changes which have a depressing effect on the reticular activity and vigilance.

The relationship between the hypothalamus and the endocrine system is considered elsewhere [see p. 905].

Certain experimental and clinical facts appear to link the temporal lobe with at any rate certain emotions or instinctive activities. Ablation experiments first carried out by Klüver (1958), and confirmed by Denny-Brown and Chambers (1958), have shown that the bilateral removal of the temporal lobe produces profound effects upon the behaviour of monkeys. Those which particularly concern the emotions are loss of normal fear, and hypersexuality. Denny-Brown and Chambers have also shown that parietal lobectomy in monkeys produces the reverse effect, leading to excessive avoidance reactions. The temporal lobe is a unity only in the sense that it is so to the naked eye: the more research is done upon it, the greater the complexity and variety of its functions appears. The experimental evidence that some part of it is concerned with the

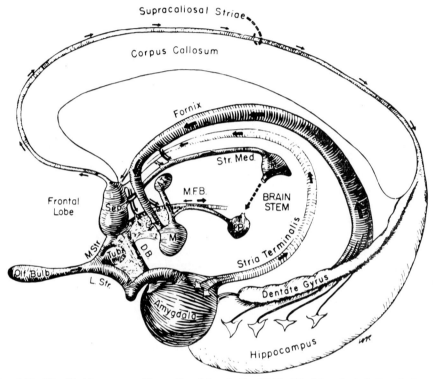

FIG. 129. The limbic system. (From Smythies, J. R. (1966) *The Neurological Foundations of Psychiatry*, by kind permission of the author and Blackwell's Scientific Publications.)

emotion of fear is supported by the clinical observation that fear may be experienced as a subjective element in an epileptic attack originating in the temporal lobe (Williams, 1956). Experimental work suggests that the hypersexuality which follows temporal-lobe ablation may be induced by small lesions restricted to an area in the posterolateral part of the piriform cortex (Green, 1958).

Papez (1937) suggested that the central emotional process of cortical origin is built up in the hippocampus and then transferred via the fornix to the mamillary body, whence it reaches the anterior thalamic nucleus and irradiates to the cortex of the gyrus cinguli [see FIG. 129]. As will be seen later, a very similar pathway has been held to be involved in memory. In the light of subsequent work it now seems probable that while any or all the structures mentioned by Papez may play some part in emotion, its neurological basis, viewed as a whole, must be much more diffuse than this. That does not exclude the existence of localized

afferent and efferent (motor and autonomic) pathways concerned in the evocation of emotions which are localizable. Between them, however, lies a diffuse
process concerned with the heightening of the specific activities concerned with
each individual emotion.

Smythies (1966) regards the 'Papez circuit' as being of fundamental importance, but draws attention, in a detailed review, to the role of the entire
integrated 'limbic system' (which includes the amygdala, hippocampus, mamillary bodies, fornix, thalamus, cingulate gyrus, and possibly the brain stem
reticular system) as being involved in emotional control. The same pathways
appear to be involved in memory function (see below).

Memory

Disturbances of memory, resulting from lesions of the temporal lobe, have
been known for many years, particularly in relation to what is now often described as temporal lobe epilepsy. Penfield (1958) and Penfield and Jasper (1954),
in a series of communications, have stressed the temporal lobe as the region
from which the revival of past memories can be excited by electrical stimulation,
or by epileptic attacks. Recent work has thrown further light on this. Bickford
et al. (1958) have produced a syndrome of loss of memory for recent events up
to several days (with a normal recall for events preceding the amnesia) by
electrical stimulation in the general region of the posterior part of the middle
temporal gyrus. Scoville and Milner (1957) have observed persistent, profound,
and generalized loss of recent memory in ten cases of bilateral hippocampal
excision, the amnesia being unrelated to any deterioration of the intellect or
personality of the subject. Milner (1958, 1966) and Walker (1957) both report
cases of recent memory impairment after *unilateral* temporal lobe lesions. It is
suggested in explanation either that in such cases the corresponding area on the
opposite side must previously have been damaged, or that individual differences,
perhaps variations in the use of imagery, in some way influence the lateralization
of memory function in the brain. However this may be, there is no doubt that
bilateral hippocampal lesions are likely to cause permanent and continuing loss
of memory for recent events, and this disability has also been observed by Rose
and Symonds (1960) and by Brierley et al. (1960) in patients who have suffered
from encephalitis, which the latter authors were able to show selectively damaged
the limbic brain, including the hippocampus. The important area seems to lie
from 5·5 cm. to 8 cm. behind the tip of the temporal lobe.

Sweet, Talland, and Erwin (1959) have reported a case in which severe and
persistent loss of recent memory followed surgical division of the anterior pillars
of the fornix [see Fig. 129] in the course of removal of a colloid cyst of the third
ventricle, but it is possible that other structures were also damaged. In reviewing the literature of anatomical lesions causing the amnesic syndrome, they
found that in addition to the sites mentioned above it had followed lesions of
the mamillary bodies and of the mamillothalamic tracts. The neuropathology
of amnesic states has recently been reviewed by Brierley (1966). The similarity
between the pathways, damage to which causes loss of recent memory, and those
postulated by Papez [see p. 961] as the anatomical basis of emotion is striking.
Indeed, Sweet et al. suggest that the amnesic defect may be due in part to the

loss of an emotional factor necessary for the 'embedding' of experience. A patient of mine suffering from the amnesic syndrome after encephalitis, and usually unable to recall any recent event, told me that to his surprise he found he could recall all the events connected with his wife's death which happened after his own illness. He said: 'It seems that it is only if I feel something strongly that I can remember it.'

The fact that the structures mentioned seem to be essential to the storage and evocation of memories must not be taken to imply that they are also the site of storage. Practically nothing is understood about this, but it seems much more probable that the storage of memories is a complex function involving extensive areas of the brain.

The Functions of the Frontal Lobe

Pribram points out that in animals experimental damage to the frontal cortex which derives its thalamic input from the medial nuclear group affects the ability of the animal to solve problems which depend upon the use of past experience. It has long been believed that the frontal lobes play a particularly important part in the mental life. Penfield and Evans (1935) found that the maximum amputation of the right or left frontal lobe produced little change in the mental life except for some impairment of those processes necessary for planned initiative, and Jefferson (1937) concluded from 8 cases of unilateral frontal lobectomy that the role of the fontal lobes in the mental life is quantitative rather than qualitative. Rylander (1939) reported 32 cases of operation on the frontal lobe. Emotional changes consisted of diminished inhibition of affective responses and a tendency to euphoria, less often to depression. Changes in psychomotor activity took the form either of restlessness or lack of initiative and interest. In the intellectual life the more automatic forms of intelligence were relatively well preserved, together with attention and memory, but the higher forms of reasoning, thinking in symbols, and judgement had deteriorated. All of these features were exhibited by Brickner's (1936, 1939) patient who was observed for eight years after bilateral frontal lobectomy.

The operation of prefrontal leucotomy or lobotomy has thrown new light upon the functions of the frontal lobes which may be summarized as follows: 'According to Freeman and Watts, the prefrontal regions in man are concerned with foresight, imagination and the apperception of the self. These psychological functions are invested with emotion by way of the association fibres that link the hippocampus and cingulate gyrus with the thalamus and the hypothalamus. It would seem, then, that the functions of the prefrontal lobes are concerned with the adjustment of the personality as a whole to future contingencies. The imagination, therefore, in the pure sense of the term, may be said to reside in the prefrontal areas. Pure intellection in the sense of analysis, synthesis, and selectivity does not appear to require the integrity of the frontal and prefrontal areas to the extent that was previously thought necessary' (Brain and Strauss, 1945). This view receives support from the observations of Hebb and Penfield (1940) and Hebb (1941) that extensive resection of one or both frontal lobes is not necessarily followed by intellectual deterioration, though Penfield (1948) in a later study found a slight drop in general intelligence after frontal gyrectomy and lobotomy, which he attributed to the patients' greater distractibility. But, as Smythies (1966) points out, despite much speculation and the virtual certainty that the frontal lobe is concerned with storage of certain social behaviour patterns, its exact functions are still poorly understood.

Destruction of the dorsomedial nuclei of the thalamus has been shown to produce similar effects to frontal leucotomy. Since the efferent frontothalamic pathways are comparatively scanty it has been suggested that leucotomy works by interrupting the afferent pathways from the dorsomedial nuclei to the granular frontal cortex and from the anteromedial nuclei to the cingulate gyri. Modern selective operations aim at the relief of emotional tension with minimal effects upon other parts of the mental life (Knight, 1964).

REFERENCES

BARD, P. (1928) A diencephalic mechanism for the expression of rage with special reference to the sympathetic nervous system, *Amer. J. Physiol.*, 84, 490.

BICKFORD, R. C., MULDER, D. W., DODGE, H. W., JNR., SVIEN, H. J., and ROME, H. P. (1958) Changes in memory function induced by electrical stimulation of the temporal lobe in man, *Res. Publ. Ass. nerv. ment. Dis.*, 36, 227.

BRAIN, W. R., and STRAUSS, E. B. (1945) *Recent Advances in Neurology and Neuropsychiatry*, London.

BRICKNER, R. M. (1936) *The Intellectual Functions of the Frontal Lobes*, New York.

BRICKNER, R. M. (1939) Bilateral frontal lobectomy. Follow-up report of case, *Arch. Neurol. Psychiat. (Chicago)*, 41, 580.

BRIERLEY, J. B. (1966) The neuropathology of amnesic states, in *Amnesia*, ed. WHITTY, C. W. M., and ZANGWILL, O. L., London.

BRIERLEY, J. B., and BECK, E. (1958) The effects upon behaviour of lesions in the dorsomedial and anterior thalamic nuclei of cat and monkey, *Ciba Foundation Symposium on the Neurological Basis of Behaviour*, p. 90, London.

BRIERLEY, J. B., CORSELLIS, J. A. N., HIERONS, R., and NEVIN, S. (1960) Subacute encephalitis of later adult life, *Brain*, 83, 357.

DELL, P. (1958) Some basic mechanisms of the translation of bodily needs into behaviour, *Ciba Foundation Symposium on the Neurological Basis of Behaviour*, p. 187, London.

DENNY-BROWN, D., and CHAMBERS, R. A. (1958) The parietal lobe and behavior, *Res. Publ. Ass. nerv. ment. Dis.*, 36, 35.

GREEN, J. D. (1958) The rhinencephalon and behaviour, *Ciba Foundation Symposium on the Neurological Basis of Behaviour*, p. 222, London.

HEBB, D. O. (1941) Human intelligence after removal of cerebral tissue from the right frontal lobe, *J. genet. Psychol.*, 25, 257.

HEBB, D. O., and PENFIELD, W. (1940) Human behavior after extensive bilateral removal from the frontal lobes, *Arch. Neurol. Psychiat. (Chicago)*, 44, 421.

JEFFERSON, G. (1937) Removal of right and left frontal lobes in man, *Brit. med. J.*, 2, 199.

KLÜVER, H. (1958) 'The temporal lobe syndrome' produced by bilateral ablations, *Ciba Foundation Symposium on the Neurological Basis of Behaviour*, p. 175, London.

KNIGHT, G. (1964) The orbital cortex as an objective in the surgical treatment of mental illness, *Brit. J. Surg.*, 51, 114.

LASHLEY, K. (1960) The thalamus and emotion, in *The Neuropsychology of Lashley*, ed. BEACH, F. A., HEBB, D. O., MORGAN, C. T., and NISSEN, H. W., New York.

MASSERMAN, J. H. (1943) *Behavior and Neurosis*, Chicago.

MILNER, B. (1958) Psychological defects produced by temporal lobe excision, *Res. Publ. Ass. nerv. ment. Dis.*, 36, 244.

MILNER, B. (1966) Amnesia following operations on the temporal lobe, in *Amnesia*, ed. WHITTY, C. W. M., and ZANGWILL, O. L., London.

PAPEZ, J. W. (1937) A proposed mechanism of emotion, *Arch. Neurol. Psychiat. (Chicago)*, **38**, 725.

PENFIELD, W. (1948) Bilateral frontal gyrectomy and postoperative intelligence, *Res. Publ. Ass. nerv. ment. Dis.*, **27**, 519.

PENFIELD, W. (1958) The role of the temporal cortex in the recall of past experiences and interpretation of the present, *Ciba Foundation Symposium on the Neurological Basis of Behaviour*, p. 149, London.

PENFIELD, W., and EVANS, J. (1935) The frontal lobes in man. A clinical study of maximum removals, *Brain*, **58**, 115.

PENFIELD, W., and JASPER, H. (1954) *Epilepsy and the Functional Anatomy of the Human Brain*, Boston.

PRIBRAM, K. (1958) Comparative neurology and the evolution of behavior, in *Behavior and Evolution*, ed. ROE, A., and SIMPSON, G. G., New Haven.

ROSE, F. C., and SYMONDS, C. P. (1960) Persistent memory defect following encephalitis, *Brain*, **83**, 195.

RYLANDER, G. (1939) *Personality Changes after Operations on the Frontal Lobes*, Copenhagen.

SCOVILLE, W. B., and MILNER, B. (1957) Loss of recent memory after bilateral hippocampal lesions, *J. Neurol. Neurosurg. Psychiat.*, **20**, 11.

SMYTHIES J. R., (1966) *The Neurological Foundations of Psychiatry*, Oxford.

SWEET, W. H., TALLAND, G. A., and ERWIN, F. R. (1959) Loss of recent memory following section of the fornix, *Trans. Amer. neurol. Ass.*, p. 76.

TALLAND, G. A. (1958) Psychological studies of Korsakow's psychosis. II. Perceptual functions, *J. nerv. ment. Dis.*, **127**, 197.

TALLAND, G. A. (1959) The interference theory of forgetting and the amnesic syndrome, *J. abnorm. soc. Psychol.*, **59**, 10.

TALLAND, G. A., and EKDAHL, M. (1959) Psychological studies of Korsakow's psychosis. IV. The rate and mode of forgetting narrative material, *J. nerv. ment. Dis.*, **129**, 391.

WALKER, A. E. (1957) Recent memory impairment in unilateral temporal lobe lesions, *Arch. Neurol. Psychiat. (Chicago)*, **78**, 543.

WILLIAMS, D. (1956) The structure of emotions reflected in epileptic experiences, *Brain*, **79**, 29.

WILSON, S. A. K. (1928) The psychical components of temporal (uncinate) epilepsy, in *Modern Problems of Neurology*, p. 51, London.

CONSCIOUSNESS AND UNCONSCIOUSNESS

The Neural Basis of Consciousness

Consciousness is a primary element in experience and cannot be defined in terms of anything else. Neurology lends support to the distinction between the content of consciousness and the state of consciousness itself. The content of consciousness consists of sensations, emotions, images, memories, ideas, and similar experiences, and these depend upon the activities of the cerebral cortex and the thalamus and the relations between them, in the sense that lesions of these structures alter the content of consciousness without as a rule changing the state of consciousness as such. On the other hand, recent work has shown that other structures, particularly that part of the central reticular formation of the brain stem, which is known as the ascending reticular activating system and which extends at least from the lower border of the pons to the ventromedial thalamus, profoundly influence the state of consciousness. Magoun and his collaborators (Magoun, 1952), and Gellhorn (1954) have shown that, in Gellhorn's words, 'the cortex receives at least two kinds of afferent impulses, those which alter the activity of the greater part or the whole of the cortex and those which activate specific cortical projection areas (visual, auditory, &c.)', and, again quoting Gellhorn, 'destruction of the reticulo-hypothalamic system does not interfere with the action of the sensory impulses on a specific projection area, but it eliminates the tonic impulses from the hypothalamic-reticular system on the cortex as a whole. Under these conditions no conscious processes are elicited.' There is evidence that drugs which tend to produce unconsciousness, such as anaesthetics and hypnotics, selectively depress the ascending reticular alerting system, while those which cause wakefulness have the opposite, facilitatory effect upon it.

SLEEP

Sleep is to be regarded as a periodical physiological depression of function of those parts of the brain concerned with consciousness, induced by the appropriate state of the reticulo-hypothalamic system. Electroencephalography shows that as sleep deepens there is a transition from normal alpha waves to a phase of bursts of more rapid waves to the development of slow random waves. Dreams have been shown to be associated with a burst of alpha waves in the second stage of sleep. As Plum and Posner (1966) point out, sleep is an active physiological process during which some neurones show decreased activity while in others activity is increased. Normal sleep has been shown to have several stages, one of which is the so-called 'rapid eye-movement' (R.E.M.) phase during which most dreams occur. This phase, also called 'paradoxical sleep', occurs shortly after falling asleep and again shortly before waking and seems to be the most important stage of sleep in relieving fatigue. Recent work has shown that a disordered relationship between the R.E.M. and non-R.E.M. phases of sleep may occur in various disorders of brain function (Jouvet, 1962). Bremer has shown that barbiturate anaesthetics produce electroencephalographic changes similar to those accompanying normal sleep. Though sleep-like states can be induced by electrical stimulation of an area in the diencephalon it is an oversimplification to regard this as a 'sleep centre'. Sleep is the result of complex processes whereby, facilitated by fatigue, the withdrawal of afferent impulses leads to a reversible depression of the alerting system, which inactivates the cerebral cortex (see Wolstenholme and O'Connor, 1961).

During sleep not only is consciousness lost, but certain bodily changes occur. The pulse rate, blood pressure, and the respiratory rate fall; the eyes usually deviate upwards, the pupils are contracted, but usually react to light, but slowly; the tendon reflexes are abolished and the plantar reflexes may become extensor.

NARCOLEPSY AND OTHER SLEEP DISTURBANCES

Narcolepsy is sleep which is abnormal by reason of its onset's being irresistible, though the circumstances may be inappropriate and excessive fatigue is absent. The patient can be roused from the narcoleptic attack as from normal sleep.

It is necessary to consider with narcolepsy four other forms of sleep disturbance which, since they may be associated with narcolepsy or with each other in the same patient, are closely related to one another. These are cataplexy, sleep paralysis, hallucinatory states associated with sleep, and somnambulism.

The first case of narcolepsy was described by Westphal in 1877, but the term 'narcolepsy' was first used by Gélineau (1880).

Narcolepsy

The irresistible attacks of sleep characteristic of narcolepsy may be very numerous, occurring many times a day. In the attacks the patient suddenly becomes unconscious and the condition resembles normal sleep in that he can be aroused immediately by appropriate stimuli. The attacks are most likely to occur in circumstances normally conducive to drowsiness, such as after a heavy meal, during a lecture, in the cinema, in church, or during a monotonous occupation, especially when driving a car. They are usually worse in the afternoon. They are occasionally precipitated by strong emotion. The sleep is usually brief, lasting only for seconds or minutes, but if the patient remains undisturbed he may sleep for hours.

Cataplexy

By cataplexy is understood an attack to which sufferers from narcolepsy are liable, but which differs from sleep in that, though the patient suddenly loses all power of movement and of maintaining posture, consciousness is preserved. Sometimes tremor of the head or muscular twitching occurs at the onset, but these may be absent. The patient sinks limply to the ground with the eyes closed. The muscles are hypotonic, the pupils may fail to react to light, the tendon reflexes may be diminished or lost, and during the attacks the plantar reflexes may be extensor. Though completely unable to move or to utter a sound, the patient is fully aware of all that is happening. Cataplectic attacks usually last less than a minute and recovery is rapid. They are commonly precipitated by strong emotion, pleasurable or otherwise, especially by laughter or excitement, and the patient may be unable to move until he has controlled his emotion.

Sleep Paralysis

Sleep paralysis resembles cataplexy except that instead of being precipitated during the day by emotion, it usually occurs during the period of falling asleep or of awakening. The patient, though fully conscious, is unable to move hand or foot and often experiences intense anxiety. A touch will rapidly disperse the paralysis. So-called 'night-nurse's paralysis' is undoubtedly a similar phenomenon.

Hallucinatory States associated with Sleep

Sufferers from narcolepsy sometimes experience vivid hallucinations. These, which are more often visual than auditory, may occur as the patient is falling asleep, when they are termed hypnagogic hallucinations. Sometimes, however, they occur during the night, when the patient is apparently awake. These hallucinations are often elaborate and terrifying, and though they seem real at the time their true character is readily recognized during normal waking life. The night-terrors of childhood appear to be of a similar nature.

Somnambulism

Somnambulism may be regarded as the reciprocal of cataplexy in that the patient, though partly asleep, is able to stand and walk in an automatic fashion. It is occasionally associated with narcolepsy, but usually occurs in adolescents who are of a neurotic disposition but otherwise normal. It may occur as an isolated incident following exposure to unusual stress (e.g. during examinations).

The Nature of Narcolepsy and Allied Disorders

Some authors—for example, Wilson (1928)—have thought that narcolepsy is allied to epilepsy. Adie, however, and others have put forward the view that it is a disturbance of sleep and thus no more than an exaggeration of physiological processes. This is supported by the fact that narcoleptic subjects, as has already been shown, are liable to various disturbances of their nocturnal sleep. Narcolepsy, on this hypothesis, is to be regarded as sleep of sudden and irresistible onset, and cataplexy as a localized sleep affecting the centres concerned in movement and posture only. Sleep paralysis is the outcome of a failure of the uniform spread of sleep over the nervous system, the levels concerned with consciousness remaining awake when the motor and postural levels have fallen asleep, or, conversely, awakening before them. The hallucinatory states appear to be the product of a dissociation of consciousness, akin to dreaming, when the subject is partially awake; and somnambulism, the converse of cataplexy, is a condition in which the highest levels are asleep, but lower levels are awake. Thus an imbalance of activity in the various parts of the reticular activating mechanism may be postulated. Nevertheless, in a minority of cases there seems to be a relationship between narcolepsy and epilepsy, and occasionally the latter follows the former.

The Causes of Narcolepsy

Narcolepsy may be symptomatic or idiopathic. Symptomatic narcolepsy may follow head injury or may be due to cerebral arteriosclerosis, neurosyphilis, encephalitis lethargica, or intracranial tumour involving the posterior part of the hypothalamus. In such cases it is probably due to disturbance of function of the sleep centre. Much more often no cause can be found, and the disorder is then designated idiopathic narcolepsy. Males are more subject to this than females and the onset usually occurs during adolescence or, at any rate, under the age of thirty. Idiopathic narcolepsy is probably in many instances in the true sense a functional disorder, that is, a disturbance of function consisting of an exaggeration of a normal tendency to drowsiness. Physical abnormalities indicative of disorder of other functions of the hypothalamus may be present, especially obesity, with or without genital atrophy.

DIAGNOSIS

Both narcolepsy and cataplexy are so distinctive that diagnosis usually presents no difficulty. Narcolepsy is distinguished from both epilepsy and syncope in the circumstances in which the attacks occur and in that when consciousness is lost the patient can be immediately aroused. Cataplexy is distinguished from these disorders by the preservation of consciousness. Careful investigation should be made for evidence of organic disease involving the hypothalamus. The skull should be X-rayed as a routine to make certain that there is no enlargement of the sella or parasellar calcification. Recording of the EEG and of eye movements shows that in narcoleptic attacks the sleep is usually immediately of the R.E.M. (rapid eye-movement) type but nocturnal recordings from such patients may show an abnormal relationship between the R.E.M. and non-R.E.M. phases (Dement, Rechtshaffen, and Gulevich, 1966).

PROGNOSIS

The disorder does not threaten life unless the patient should be unfortunate enough to have an attack in a dangerous situation. The response to treatment is sometimes disappointing and the attacks usually continue indefinitely, though occasionally they cease spontaneously. I have known one patient who, after suffering from narcolepsy for twenty years, developed typical epileptic attacks, but this is rare.

TREATMENT

The sufferer from narcolepsy will necessarily be debarred from occupations in which an attack of sleep may endanger him, and should not usually be allowed to drive a car if his attacks are severe. Ephedrine and amphetamine have a specific action upon both narcolepsy and cataplexy. Amphetamine is usually the more effective and the treatment should begin with 10 mg. two or three times a day. A slower and more prolonged action is produced by giving it in 'Spansule' form. To avoid disturbing nocturnal sleep the last dose should not be given later than late afternoon. When narcolepsy or cataplexy by day are associated with disturbances of nocturnal sleep it is wise to give a nightly dose of a barbiturate. Recent work suggests that imipramine (*Tofranil*) in a dosage of 25–50 mg. three times a day, is effective in some cases, but desmethylimipramine (*Pertofran*) in similar dosage is even more effective in controlling cataplexy but may have to be given along with amphetamine for full control of narcolepsy (Hishikawa *et al.*, 1966).

PERIODIC SOMNOLENCE AND MORBID HUNGER

Kleine (1925) and Levin (1936) described a rare disorder characterized by periodic attacks of excessive appetite followed by profound sleepiness which may last for days. During this phase the patient's personality may be profoundly altered, but in the intervals between the attacks he is usually normal. In the attacks of prolonged somnolence the patient awakens only as a rule to eat ravenously (often of a wide variety of unusual foods) and abnormal sexual behaviour with frequent masturbation and hypersexuality may be seen (Critchley 1962; Garland, Sumner, and Fourman, 1965). The condition is almost invariably seen in adolescent males but a case in a young female has been described (Duffy and Davison, 1968). Depression, delusions and amnesia may be noted temporarily after an attack. The cause is unknown and in my experience no abnormality, clinical, biochemical, or electroencephalographic can be discovered during the attack. Amphetamine has been used with some success (Gallinek, 1954) in the treatment of the condition and Duffy and Davison (1968) found that intravenous methedrine cut short the attacks.

STUPOR AND COMA

In the past the term hypersomnia has been used to describe a state in which the patient has been thought to be pathologically sleepy, the resemblance to sleep lying in the fact that he can be to some extent aroused by the kind of stimuli which arouse a healthy person from sleep. Since, however, the mental state of such patients when aroused is often far from normal Jefferson proposed the term parasomnia for this condition. Between full consciousness and pathological complete unconsciousness or coma there exist states which differ not only in degree but also in quality, but much work remains to be done before they can be completely differentiated. At present it is convenient to distinguish broadly two different states of unconsciousness, namely, coma and stupor. In coma the patient cannot be aroused by any stimulus however vigorous and painful. Semi-coma can be defined as complete loss of consciousness with a response only at the reflex level, while less severe degrees of impairment of consciousness have been entitled severe, moderate, and mild confusion. Lethargy is a state of drowsiness and indifference in which increased stimulation may be needed to obtain a response, while stupor is a term used to define a state 'from which the subject can only be aroused by vigorous and continuous external stimulation' (Plum and Posner, 1966). Parasomnia may be regarded as one variety of stupor. Akinetic mutism, another state of stupor described by Cairns, resembles sleep in being associated with general muscular relaxation, but differs from sleep in that, although the patient's eyes remain alert to moving objects, strong afferent stimuli are incapable of arousing him. So-called 'coma vigil' is similar. Skultety (1968), on the basis of experimental work in animals and clinicopathological observations in man, points out that whereas lesions of the periaqueductal grey matter of the brain stem have been found to be associated with akinetic mutism in some cases, lesions in this area alone are insufficient as a rule to produce the syndrome which may result from disease involving the afferent input to the reticular activating system, of this system itself, or even of its efferent pathways. This clinical picture represents only part of a spectrum of altered states of responsiveness.

Lesions Responsible for Stupor and Coma

The experimental work described above and the clinico-pathological studies of Cairns (1952) and French (1952) have established that stupor or coma may occur as the result of lesions involving the central portion of the brain stem between the anterior end of the third ventricle and the medulla. A wide range of pathological processes may therefore be responsible, the chief of which are head injury, tumour, vascular and inflammatory lesions, and it may well be that toxic states lead to unconsciousness primarily through their effect upon this part of the brain. The chief importance of recent work in this field lies in its implication that the effect of cerebral lesions in general upon consciousness must now be considered mainly in terms of their effect upon the reticular substance in the brain stem [see Plum and Posner (1966)].

THE CAUSES OF UNCONSCIOUSNESS

In this section we shall discuss the principal causes of unconsciousness as a necessary preliminary to considering how the cause is to be discovered in any particular case. It will be noted that even though the cause of unconsciousness may be described in general terms, it is often impossible to say in detail how that cause operates, or it may act in so complex a way that one cannot say which of a number of factors is the more important.

CEREBRAL VASCULAR LESIONS

A cerebral vascular lesion is one of the commonest causes of coma. It is probable that in most cases the unconsciousness is due to the fact that the cerebral vascular lesion directly or indirectly interferes with the functions of the ascending reticular alerting formation. Ischaemia of this structure may be the result either of a rise in intracranial pressure or of local pressure upon the diencephalon or brain stem, or impairment of blood supply secondary to pathological narrowing of the relevant arteries. The conditions most likely to produce these results are: (1) a massive subarachnoid haemorrhage; (2) a subarachnoid haemorrhage invading one cerebral hemisphere; (3) a massive intracerebral haemorrhage, or one rupturing into one cerebral ventricle; (4) an area of infarction of one cerebral hemisphere large enough to cause considerable oedema of the hemisphere; and (5) atheroma of the cerebral arteries, particularly those of the vertebro-basilar system, of which the superior cerebellar artery is one of the most important. The symptomatology of these lesions is described elsewhere, but in general it may be said that a vascular cause for unconsciousness is suggested by the presence of atheroma or hypertension, a sudden or relatively sudden onset of the symptoms, focal signs corresponding to those produced by a vascular lesion, or signs of meningeal irritation of sudden onset. The presence of red blood cells or xanthochromia and a raised protein in the cerebrospinal fluid would support the diagnosis. [See also p. 299.]

SPACE-OCCUPYING LESIONS

Unconsciousness due to intracranial tumour or abscess usually comes on much more slowly than that due to a cerebral vascular lesion, though occasionally haemorrhage into a tumour or the sudden development of oedema around it may cause a rapid loss of consciousness. A history of symptoms of increased intracranial pressure, especially headache increasing in severity, is therefore usually obtainable, and papilloedema is likely to be present, and is often severe. Signs of vascular disease are usually absent, but the diagnosis may be difficult when a tumour develops late in life in a patient who suffers from hypertension or atheroma. Subdural haematoma is most commonly encountered in the middle-aged or elderly, in whom it may develop without discoverable cause or insidiously after a head injury. Headache is usually a prominent symptom, and unconsciousness, when it develops, often fluctuates strikingly in depth.

Papilloedema and signs of focal cerebral compression are often present, but may be absent.

HEAD INJURY

When unconsciousness is due to head injury, there is usually a history of the injury, and there may be bruising of the scalp or signs of fracture of the vault or of the base of the skull. It must be remembered, however, that a patient who becomes unconscious from some other cause may injure his head in falling, and that a head injury may indirectly affect the brain, for example, by leading to thrombosis of one internal carotid artery. Traumatic intracranial arterial haemorrhage leads to progressively deepening coma, with signs of a focal lesion of one hemisphere, often beginning with convulsions and producing hemiplegia. Herniation of the medial portion of the temporal lobe through the tentorial hiatus will often cause compression of the third nerve as it crosses the free border of the tentorium and as a result the pupil on the same side becomes fixed and dilated and other signs of a third nerve palsy on the same side may develop later. By contrast, cerebellar tonsillar herniation due to a space-occupying lesion (whether haemorrhage, tumour, or abscess) in the posterior fossa usually gives occipital headache and neck stiffness, possibly with bradycardia and depression of respiration due to brain stem compression. However, it may be impossible clinically to distinguish between traumatic intracranial arterial haemorrhage and a rapidly progressive subdural haematoma or haemorrhage from a cerebral laceration.

MENINGITIS AND ENCEPHALITIS

When meningitis is the cause of coma, the onset of symptoms is usually subacute, and before losing consciousness the patient complains of intense headache, which is associated with fever, cervical rigidity, and Kernig's sign. The diagnosis is confirmed by the discovery of the characteristic changes in the cerebrospinal fluid, from which it may be possible to isolate the causal organism. The onset of encephalitis is also usually subacute, and associated with fever, though the development of herpes simplex encephalitis [p. 449] may be explosive. The physical signs are those of more or less diffuse damage to the brain, and in many cases also the spinal cord, the precise distribution and character of which varies in relation to the aetiology. Signs of meningeal irritation are usually absent but may be present, and there is often, but not invariably, a pleocytosis in the cerebrospinal fluid.

METABOLIC DISORDERS

Uraemic Coma. Uraemic coma may occur in chronic nephritis and other conditions causing renal destruction. The metabolic changes produced by renal failure are complex, and it is probable that a raised blood urea, though in general an important index of their severity, is not in itself the main cause of unconsciousness. There is usually metabolic acidosis, accompanied by complex disturbances of the body sodium and potassium. The blood calcium may be subnormal and the administration of alkalis to correct the acidosis may precipitate tetany. There is usually a raised blood pyruvic acid, and the cerebral consumption of oxygen is reduced. Headache, vomiting, dyspnoea, mental confusion, drowsiness or rest-lessness, and insomnia are early symptoms, and later muscular twitchings or generalized convulsions are likely to precede the coma. The raised blood urea establishes the diagnosis.

Diabetic Coma. When diabetes leads to ketosis and acidosis, deep coma is unlikely to develop until the blood carbon dioxide falls below 25 volumes per 100 ml. Here again the mode of production of the coma is complex. The oxygen con-sumption of the brain is diminished, and the blood pyruvic acid is raised. The patient is usually wasted, pale, and dehydrated. Both the rate and amplitude of the respirations are increased, and the ocular tension is very low. The pulse is rapid and feeble, and the blood pressure tends to fall. The tendon reflexes are sometimes depressed due to the presence of an associated diabetic neuropathy but may be normal, and the plantar responses are usually flexor until the patient is actually comatose. The breath has the characteristic odour of acetone. Large quantities of sugar are demonstrable, together with diacetic acid and acetone, in the urine, and the blood sugar is much raised.

Hypoglycaemic Coma. Hypoglycaemic coma is not difficult to recognize if it is due to an overdose of insulin which the patient is known to be taking. The presence of sugar in the urine does not exclude this, since the urine may have been excreted before the patient became hypoglycaemic. Spontaneous hypo-glycaemia sufficient to cause coma is usually the result in an adult of the excessive production of insulin by a tumour composed of cells of the islets of Langerhans in the pancreas. In such cases fainting fits or convulsions or periods of mental disorder may precede the onset of coma by weeks or months. On the other hand, the coma may occur without warning in a patient apparently previously healthy, and the patient may then live on in an unconscious state for weeks or months. Hypoglycaemia may also occur spontaneously in early infancy and may then be responsible for severe brain damage if not recognized and treated early, and in adult life it has been observed to arise spontaneously in patients with liver disease, hypopituitarism, and Addison's disease. At the time of the onset the hypoglycaemic patient sweats profusely, the pupils are dilated, the tendon reflexes increased, and the plantar reflexes may be extensor. The diagnosis can be made by examination of the blood sugar, which is found to be extremely low, in the region of 40 or 50 mg. per 100 ml. or even much lower.

Unless treated promptly and effectively, hypoglycaemia can result in irre-versible brain damage and the pathological changes, affecting the Purkinje cells of the cerebellum, the cerebral cortex, basal ganglia, and hippocampus, are similar to those of severe anoxia. Dementia and cerebellar ataxia are the main clinical features of this syndrome.

Heat Stroke. After prolonged exertion in hot surroundings (as in racing cyclists) the normal rise in body temperature with profuse sweating can be followed by an ominous clinical picture of hyperpyrexia, an abrupt cessation of sweating, the rapid onset of coma, convulsions, and death. The condition may be pre-cipitated by the use of amphetamine drugs. Hyperpyrexia may also be seen in tetanus and a result of lesions involving the floor of the third ventricle (such as intraventricular haemorrhage) or pons (e.g. pontine haemorrhage).

Hypothermia. An abnormally low body temperature may give rise to deepening coma. While hypothermia has been described in cases of myxoedema and hypopituitarism (see below) accidental hypothermia can result from a failure of the normal temperature-regulating mechanism of the body, the reverse of that which occurs in heat stroke. It can result from prolonged exposure in cold conditions (as in mountaineers or fell-walkers) and has also been described in elderly patients, often suffering from disorders such as arthritis or Parkinsonism which reduce mobility, who live in unheated rooms in winter conditions. Drugs such as chlorpromazine may also precipitate hypothermic coma which can be fatal.

Hepatic Coma. The cause of hepatic coma is still incompletely understood [see p. 719]. The diagnosis is not usually difficult when the patient is known to be suffering from liver failure. Jaundice, however, may be absent. In patients with liver disease coma tends to be precipitated by gastro-intestinal haemorrhage, hypotension, infection, the rapid removal of large quantities of ascitic fluid, the use of certain diuretics, the administration of some sedatives, particularly morphine, and the ingestion of high protein foods or ammonium compounds. Except when it is of sudden onset, hepatic coma is usually preceded by the neurological symptoms of hepatic insufficiency, especially tremor [see p. 720]. Otherwise the diagnosis rests upon the presence of physical signs of liver disease, including hepatic foetor, and biochemical evidence of disturbed liver function.

Porphyria. Porphyria is an occasional cause of coma.

COMA OF ENDOCRINE ORIGIN

This may present a difficult diagnostic problem when it occurs in patients in whom the pre-existing endocrine disease has not been recognized.

Hypopituitary Coma. In hypopituitary coma again the unconsciousness appears to be the result of a complexity of interacting factors, of which the most important would appear to be hypoglycaemia, hypotension, and diminished suprarenal cortical function. The onset may be sudden, for example, if it is precipitated by an infection. The patient is usually a woman who exhibits the endocrine changes of hypopituitarism. The blood pressure and blood sugar are likely to be low, and the body temperature may be subnormal or above normal. The thyroid gland is likely to be impalpable, while the urinary excretion of 17-ketosteroids and the serum cortisol are very low.

Coma in Myxoedema. A myxoedematous patient may gradually become comatose, more usually in the winter months. The characteristic feature is profound hypothermia, temperatures between 70° and 80°F. being by no means uncommon. A low-reading thermometer must be used to record these and on suspicion the temperature should be taken rectally. The patient presents the usual clinical features of myxoedema, and the blood cholesterol is often but not invariably raised.

Suprarenal Cortical Failure. Coma from this cause may be difficult to recognize if it occurs suddenly as the result of stress, for example, in a patient not known to be suffering from Addison's disease. The low blood pressure, and electrolyte disturbances, however, are characteristic.

Abnormalities of Blood Calcium. Hypercalcaemia as a cause of mental confusion or coma may be missed if the blood calcium is not routinely examined. Hypercalcaemia may be due to parathyroid tumour, carcinoma, with or without bone secondaries, myelomatosis, or sarcoidosis (Lemann and Donatelli, 1964; Watson, 1963; Dent and Watson, 1964). Hypocalcaemia, due to spontaneous hypoparathyroidism, may also cause coma.

CARBON DIOXIDE INTOXICATION

Carbon dioxide retention may be the result of acute or chronic pulmonary disease, or respiratory failure of neuromuscular origin in, for example, motor neurone disease, poliomyelitis, polyneuritis, myopathy, and myasthenia. It causes a fall in the pH and a rise in the pCO_2 in the blood. Though the patient is hypoxic, the state of consciousness is related to the level of CO_2 in the blood. In chronic CO_2 retention the respiratory centre fails to react to the raised level of CO_2 and respiration is then maintained by the receptors which respond to oxygen lack. Consequently, administering oxygen to such patients may remove the stimulus to respiration, raise the blood CO_2 still further, and precipitate coma. The same result may be produced by sedatives, particularly morphine, or even by barbiturates. Milder degrees of CO_2 intoxication cause drowsiness and confusion. In some cases there is papilloedema due to cerebral oedema. Estimation of the pCO_2 in arterial blood will usually confirm the diagnosis.

CARBON MONOXIDE INTOXICATION

In carbon monoxide intoxication there is almost always a history of exposure to coal-gas or the exhaust fumes of a motor-car, or some other source of carbon monoxide. In doubtful cases the diagnosis can be made by the spectroscopic examination of the blood.

NARCOTIC AND SEDATIVE DRUGS

When a narcotic drug is the cause of coma, there is usually evidence of this, sometimes in the patient's own statement before becoming unconscious, sometimes in the fact that he or she is known to have had a supply of such a drug. In practice the drugs most commonly taken for suicidal purposes are aspirin and barbiturates, less frequently pethidine, methadone, morphine, or heroin. Drugs which may produce coma as the result of a therapeutic overdosage include the barbiturates, any of the drugs generally used in the treatment of epilepsy, the tranquillizers, and bromides.

When alcohol is the cause of coma, this can usually be established from the history; the face is flushed, the conjunctivae congested, the pulse rapid, and the blood pressure low. The size of the pupils varies according to the toxic agent: they tend to be dilated in alcoholic coma, contracted in coma due to morphine, but in the case of other drugs are intermediate in size. The reaction to light is usually sluggish, and may be lost. The tendon reflexes tend to be diminished or lost, and the plantar reflexes extensor. Respiration is shallow, and the pulse rapid and of low tension. The drug responsible should be sought in the stomach washings, and its level estimated in the blood.

EPILEPSY

In the case of post-epileptic coma there is usually a history of epilepsy, or at least of the attack which preceded the coma. In the absence of this information, scars on the face or a bitten tongue may provide a clue. Focal signs of a cerebral lesion are usually absent, but the plantar reflexes may be extensor. After a single epileptic attack the period of unconsciousness is usually short, not more than from half an hour to an hour, but status epilepticus may be followed by prolonged coma.

HYSTERIA

In hysterical trance the patient, though apparently unconscious, usually shows some response to external stimuli. For example, an attempt to elicit the corneal reflex may cause a vigorous contraction of the orbicularis oculi. Rigidity of the hysterical type may be present, and signs of organic disease are absent.

THE INVESTIGATION OF THE UNCONSCIOUS PATIENT

The patient who presents with coma will require a most detailed and systematic examination, since any part of the body may provide a clue to the cause of the unconsciousness.

THE HEAD

The head should be examined for evidence of injury indicated by cuts or abrasions. The skull should be palpated for a depressed fracture, and the ears and nose examined for haemorrhage and leakage of cerebrospinal fluid. The ears should also be investigated for infection of the middle ear. Scars on the face may point to injuries received in previous epileptic attacks, and the tongue should be examined to see if it has been recently bitten or is the site of similar scars.

THE BREATH

The smell of the breath may provide a clue, for example, in alcoholic intoxication the characteristic odour of alcohol can be detected, and that of acetone in diabetic coma. In hepatic coma there is the characteristic foetor, but the smell of the breath in uraemia may be simulated by that present in many unconscious patients with oral infection.

THE NECK

An attempt should be made gently to flex the cervical spine. Cervical rigidity may indicate meningitis or subarachnoid haemorrhage. Gross inequality in the pulsation of the internal carotid arteries or a systolic bruit would suggest atheroma or thrombosis of the one on the side of the diminished pulsation or murmur as a possible cause of cerebral infarction.

THE SKIN

Cyanosis will be present when coma is due to CO_2 intoxication, while carbon monoxide poisoning causes a cherry-red colour. Patients with Addison's disease will show the characteristic brown pigmentation. Multiple telangiectases are found in hereditary telangiectasia, in which condition a cerebral telangiectasis may give rise to cerebral haemorrhage, and spider naevi over the upper part of the body are characteristic of hepatic disease. Purpura may be associated with an intracranial haemorrhage in thrombocytopenic purpura or scurvy, with a cerebral embolus in subacute infective endocarditis, and also with meningococcal meningitis. The characteristic skin changes of myxoedema and hypopituitarism (with loss of body hair) will be present in patients suffering from coma due to those conditions. The scars of injections may be found in diabetics and drug addicts.

RESPIRATION

After voluntary hyperventilation patients with diffuse metabolic or structural brain disease may demonstrate post-hyperventilation apnoea (Plum and Posner, 1966) but the performance of this test demands that the patient should be sufficiently conscious to be able to perform it. Periodic (Cheyne-Stokes) respiration in which hyperpnoea alternates with apnoea usually occurs in patients with central cerebral or high brain stem lesions. Central neurogenic hyperventilation (Plum and Swanson, 1959) has been described in patients with dysfunction of the brain stem tegmentum while brain stem lesions may also give apneustic breathing (a pause at full inspiration—Plum and Alvord, 1964) or ataxic, irregular respiration with random deep and shallow breaths; the latter pattern occurs particularly with medullary lesions (Plum and Swanson, 1958).

THE PUPILS

Plum and Posner (1966) have summarized the pupillary changes which may occur in comatose patients. Midbrain tectal lesions give round, regular, medium-sized pupils which do not react to light but may show hippus; nuclear midbrain lesions also as a rule give medium-sized pupils, fixed to all stimuli, which are often irregular and unequal. A third nerve lesion distal to the nucleus gives a fixed, dilated pupil on the side of the lesion. Tegmental lesions in the pons give bilaterally small pupils which in pontine haemorrhage may be pinpoint. A lateral medullary lesion may give an ipsilateral Horner's syndrome, while the pupil on the side of an occluded carotid artery giving cerebral infarction is often small. Bilateral pupillary dilatation during neck flexion can be a sign of uncal herniation (Norris and Fawcett, 1965). Drugs such as atropine, and cerebral anoxia dilate the pupils, morphine constricts, and many metabolic encephalopathies give small pupils with a normal light reflex.

OCULAR MOVEMENTS

In unconscious patients with bilateral or diffuse disorders of the cerebrum the eyes look straight ahead, oculocephalic movements (on head rotation) are brisk, and caloric stimulation gives sustained deviation of the eyes. A frontal lobe lesion may cause deviation of the eyes towards the side of the lesion, while a lateral pontine lesion may cause conjugate deviation to the opposite side with absence of oculocephalic and caloric responses. Skew deviation results from a dorsolateral pontine lesion. Conjugate deviation downwards means a midbrain lesion, while dysconjugate ocular deviation means a structural brain stem lesion if strabismus can be excluded. Oculocephalic and caloric responses are normal in metabolic disorders unless severe (Plum and Posner, 1966).

OTHER SYSTEMS

The examination of other parts of the nervous system is obviously of special importance in view of the large number of nervous disorders which give rise to coma. Special attention should be paid to the fundi where papilloedema will indicate increased intracranial pressure, or may be associated with hypertensive retinopathy. The cardiovascular system may yield evidence of hypertension, atheroma, or mitral stenosis and atrial fibrillation, a common cause of cerebral embolism. The lungs may yield evidence of the cause of CO_2 retention. X-rays of the lungs will be necessary to exclude a primary carcinoma. The abdomen may show the venous congestion and hepatomegaly of chronic liver disease, or the renal enlargement of polycystic kidneys, or one of the abdominal or pelvic organs may be the site of a neoplasm.

LABORATORY INVESTIGATIONS

Routine investigations of the urine and blood should be carried out. In addition, the blood sugar and blood urea should always be examined, and the blood electrolytes will also need to be investigated if it is thought that the coma is the result of their derangement, and to make sure that they are maintained at a normal level in the management of the unconscious patient. Provided there is no special contra-indication such as the signs of uncal or cerebellar herniation as described, examination of the cerebrospinal fluid should be carried out. This is essential to establish the diagnosis of meningitis or subarachnoid haemorrhage.

OTHER INVESTIGATIONS

Other investigations which may be necessary include X-rays of the skull, cerebral angiography, electroencephalography, and electrocardiography.

The EEG in Coma

The EEG may be of value in the diagnosis of coma in several ways: (1) it may indicate the presence of a focal lesion as opposed to a diffuse inflammatory or metabolic cause for the coma; (2) it may provide some evidence as to the probable nature of the focal lesion, as described elsewhere in the relevant sections of this book; (3) if there is a diffuse disturbance, the EEG may throw some light on its nature, distinguishing, for example, between encephalitis, epilepsy, and a metabolic disorder; and (4) changes in the degree of abnormality, and particularly in a metabolic disorder, may provide evidence of improvement or deterioration in the patient's condition.

THE MANAGEMENT OF THE UNCONSCIOUS PATIENT

During recent years improvements in the technique of dealing with the unconscious patient have been so great that it is now possible to maintain unconscious patients in a condition of otherwise good health indefinitely.

Nursing. The unconscious patient should be nursed in the semiprone position with the head on a thin pillow, and turned at least every two hours, the usual attention being paid to the care of the skin, especially the pressure areas.

The Respiratory Tract. The mouth and pharynx should be cleansed regularly by means of a swab held in forceps, and mucus and saliva prevented from accumulating in the pharynx by sucking the mouth periodically with a soft rubber catheter attached to a mechanical sucker. Regular turning of the patient will improve the ventilation of the lungs, and a physiotherapist should carry out regular percussion over the chest, especially over the bases of the lungs. If there are signs of pulmonary collapse the patient will require bronchoscopy in order that an obstructed bronchus may be cleared by suction. An oral airway will be required by a deeply unconscious patient, and if there is severe respiratory depression artificial respiration will also be necessary. This is usually best carried out by a positive pressure mechanical respirator combined with tracheal intubation, or tracheostomy. The latter measure is preferable if unconsciousness is likely to be prolonged, and a cuffed tracheostomy tube has the advantage of preventing the aspiration of food or saliva. Penicillin should be given regularly as a prophylactic against pneumonia, but if chest infection occurs a broad-spectrum antibiotic should be substituted.

Feeding. A patient who is unconscious for more than a few hours will require both food and drink, and since he cannot swallow this must be given by an oesophageal tube. This, however, is not a complete safeguard against the aspiration of food, since a feed may be regurgitated and vomiting may occur. Unless a special diet is indicated the following will prove satisfactory. A fortified milk mixture is made consisting of four pints of milk, 8 oz. of skimmed milk powder, 4 oz. of dextrose, and 1 teaspoonful of Marmite. This provides 160 g. of protein as well as carbohydrate, mineral salts, and vitamins, and has a calorie value of 2,880: $2\frac{1}{2}$ pints will provide the daily requirement of fluid and calories for an adult of average weight. Alternatively *Complan* may be used. Additional vitamins and a liquid preparation of iron should be added if liquid feeding has to be continued for long periods, or the necessary vitamins can be given by intramuscular injection.

The Blood Electrolytes. There are several ways in which the blood electrolytes may become disordered in the unconscious patient. When the unconsciousness is itself the result of a metabolic disturbance the biochemical changes which that produces will be present. The blood biochemistry may also be disordered as the result of an excessive or inadequate intake of water, or an excessive amount of protein in the diet. A cerebral lesion may itself lead to hypernatraemia as the result of disorder of the thirst mechanisms, or hyponatraemia unresponsive to corticosteroids which may sometimes be due to inappropriate secretion of antidiuretic hormone (A.D.H.). The fluid intake and output of the unconscious patient should therefore be carefully recorded, and from time to time also the blood urea, sodium, potassium, chloride, and glucose. It may also be necessary to estimate the urinary sugar, sodium, potassium, chloride, and nitrogen.

The Sphincters. The unconscious patient will have retention or incontinence of urine, and this is best dealt with by the use of a self-retaining catheter which should be changed every three days. The urine should be examined for infection. Constipation is best dealt with by enemas.

HALLUCINATIONS AND ALLIED DISORDERS OF PERCEPTION

Hallucinations may be defined as mental impressions of sensory vividness occurring without external stimulus, but appearing to be located, or to possess a cause located, outside the subject. An illusion is defined as a misinterpretation of an external stimulus, but illusions in some cases are closely related to hallucinations and may occur as symptoms of hallucinatory states. Psychophysiologically, though hallucinations manifest themselves as changes in the content of consciousness, there is considerable evidence that they are often the result of disordered function of the reticulo-hypothalamic and associated pathways concerned with the state of consciousness as a whole.

The principal circumstances in which hallucinations may occur are: (1) in dreaming and the hypnagogic state; (2) in the pathological disturbances of sleep; (3) as a result of organic disease of the sense organs or of the central nervous system (including focal epilepsy); (4) in states of intoxication, particularly after the administration of certain drugs such as mescaline and lysergic acid or after withdrawal of alcohol, amphetamines, or barbiturates; and (5) in certain psychoses.

Lhermitte (1951) has reviewed the subject of hallucinations with particular reference to those resulting from nervous disease. Visual hallucinations may occur in patients suffering from severe visual loss as a result of disease of the eyes, or with lesions in any part of the visual pathways as well as elsewhere in the nervous system. When a hemianopia is present the hallucinations may be seen in the normal half fields or in the blind half fields. Lhermitte himself has described what he terms the peduncular hallucinosis, which is the occurrence of hallucinations, especially visual hallucinations, as a result of lesions of the upper part of the brain stem. Lhermitte interprets these hallucinations as an expression of a dissociation of the state of sleep in which, although bodily activity remains awake, the mind is plunged into a special condition which permits the appearance of images analogous to those which normally occur only in dreams. Clearly any explanation of hallucinations occurring in association with organic lesions of the sense organs or the central nervous system must also take into account the mental state of the patient as a whole.

Hallucinations involving various sensory modalities, together with perceptual illusions and other disorders of consciousness, are particularly liable to occur as a result of lesions of the temporal lobes. The perceptual illusions include disordered visual perception, for example macropsia or micropsia and a similar alteration in auditory perception, feelings of unreality of the self or the surroundings, and disturbances of awareness of the body. Visual hallucinations may occur on occasion as a result of epileptic discharge arising in the posterior part of the temporal lobe or in the parieto-occipital lesion and, when 'formed', invariably indicate the presence of a focal cortical lesion when toxic causes can be excluded.

DISORDERS OF MEMORY

Memory may be defined as the power to retain and recall past experiences. A little reflection, however, will show that memory thus defined includes functions of differing complexity. Perhaps the simplest form of memory is that involved in remembering a series of digits or a passage of meaningless jargon. In such an act of recollection of mechanical memory there is little emphasis upon the 'pastness' of what is recollected. The emphasis is rather upon the persistence into the present of a series of acts which have become habitual, perhaps through repetition. In such an act of remembering there is nothing more than the three fundamental elements of memory—registration, retention, and recall. Compare this, however, with the recollection, evoked by a place or a scent, of a single past experience fraught with strong emotion. Such an act is initiated by an associative process and there is considerable emphasis upon the 'pastness' of the experience by contrast with a present in which it is no longer occurring. Moreover, one of two such episodes in the past is remembered as having been experienced prior to the other, so that arising out of the function of memory is the experience of a personal past time as an extended dimension in which past experiences bear a constant and linear relation to each other. Furthermore, these past experiences are all felt as being the experiences of the same person, hence it follows that memory is essential to the experience of personal identity.

There is also a function of memory which seems to be intermediate between the reproduction of a passage of jargon and the recollection of an isolated incident. This is the recall of an image built up as a result of repeated experiences as, for example, that of a house or a person with whom one is familiar. A similar function of remembering enters not only into the act of representing to oneself the familiar house or face in its absence, but also into the act of recognizing it when it is presented to one again.

Loss of memory is known as amnesia.

The Anatomical Basis of Memory

This is discussed on page 962.

Tests of Memory

It will be clear from what has been said that the function of remembering cannot be adequately tested by means of the ordinary simple tests which usually investigate the patient's power to retain and recall a series of digits or similar data. Inquiry must also be made into the patient's power to recall the events of his past life, both remote and recent, as well as his capacity for mechanical memory as illustrated by the recollection of digits or passages learnt by heart [see p. 988]. Other tests designed to investigate other functions of memory described above will suggest themselves in particular cases.

Some Organic Causes of Amnesia

The importance of the temporal lobe in memory mechanisms has already been stressed [p. 962] and it is well recognized that bilateral temporal lobe disease or resection (Kluver and Bucy, 1939) may seriously impair memory. Among the conditions which may cause severe memory loss, characterized particularly by an inability to record, retain, and recall recent impressions with, as a rule, comparative sparing of the memory for remote events, are inflammatory and degenerative diseases of the brain which cause dementia (including general paresis, the presenile and senile dementias and diffuse cerebral atherosclerosis), temporal lobe tumours, severe head injury with diffuse brain damage, chronic alcoholism and, in some cases, bilateral rostral leucotomy (Whitty and Lishman, 1966). Transient amnesia may occur as a result of various toxic confusional states, anoxic episodes, acute alcoholic or drug intoxication, encephalitis and meningitis, epilepsy (particularly of the temporal lobe type), migraine and other forms of cerebral ischaemia, and a variety of deficiency disorders (particularly of thiamine, giving the Korsakow syndrome—*vide infra*).

Transient Global Amnesia

This syndrome, believed to be due to transient ischaemia in one or both temporal lobes, as it usually occurs in middle-aged or elderly individuals with evidence of cerebral atherosclerosis, is a disorder of sudden onset (Fisher and Adams, 1958). Memory loss for recent events develops rapidly and in the attacks, despite their inability to register new impressions the patients retain their personal identity, show no abnormality of behaviour apart from anxiety and no evidence of impaired perception. Recovery is usually complete within a few hours, and retrograde amnesia shrinks rapidly, leaving the patient with no disability other than amnesia for the events occurring in the attack itself.

Hysterical Amnesia

This is considered on page 997.

KORSAKOW'S SYNDROME

The characteristic feature of Korsakow's syndrome is a certain type of amnesia. The patient has a gross defect of memory for recent events so that he has no recollection of what has happened even half an hour previously. He is disorientated in space and time and he fills the gaps in his memory by confabulating, that is, by giving imaginary accounts of his activities. Thus a bedridden patient will describe a walk which he asserts he has just taken. The subject was reviewed by Lewis (1961).

The amnesia of Korsakow's syndrome appears to be due to a lesion in the same situation as that which causes amnesia for current events. Other psychological disorders include a reduced capacity for retention and a disturbance of perception except for the immediate apprehension of spatially and temporally unitary patterns (Talland, 1958, 1959; Talland and Ekdahl, 1959). Lidz (1942) states that in this 'amnestic syndrome' the patient can neither evoke the past nor relate the current experience to it. The defect of appreciation of time is secondary to the amnesia.

Korsakow's psychosis is seen typically in chronic alcoholism, and Victor (1964) identifies it with Wernicke's encephalopathy, speaking of the Korsakow–Wernicke syndrome. The lesions involve the medial parts of the medial, dorsal pulvinar and antero-ventral thalamic nuclei, the mamillary bodies, and the terminal portions of the fornices, and consist of loss of medullated fibres and nerve cells, large numbers of adventitial histiocytes and microglia, increased cellularity of capillaries, and in a few cases haemorrhages.

Korsakow's syndrome may result from other kinds of lesion involving the same structures, e.g. head injury, anoxia, carbon monoxide poisoning, epilepsy, electroconvulsive therapy, acute encephalitis, dementia paralytica, other forms of dementia, intracranial tumour, cerebral arteriosclerosis, and the operation of cingulectomy.

REFERENCES

ADIE, W. J. (1926) Idiopathic narcolepsy: a disease *sui generis*; with remarks on the mechanism of sleep, *Brain*, **49**, 257.

BRAIN, W. R. (1939) Sleep normal and pathological, *Brit. med. J.*, **2**, 51.

BRAIN, W. R. (1947) Some observations on visual hallucinations and cerebral metamorphopsia, *Acta psychiat. scand.*, Suppl. 46.

BRAIN, W. R. (1958) The physiological basis of consciousness, *Brain*, **81**, 426.

CAIRNS, H. (1952) Disturbances of consciousness with lesions of the brain-stem and diencephalon, *Brain*, **75**, 109.

CRITCHLEY, M. (1939) Neurological aspects of visual and auditory hallucinations, *Brit. med. J.*, **2**, 634.

CRITCHLEY, M. (1962) Periodic hypersomnia and megaphagia in adolescent males, *Brain*, **85**, 627.

DANIELS, L. E. (1934) Narcolepsy, *Medicine (Baltimore)*, **13**, 1 (contains 268 references).

DEMENT, W., RECHTSHAFFEN, A., and GULEVICH, G. (1966) The nature of the narcoleptic sleep attack, *Neurology (Minneap.)*, **16**, 18.

DENT, C. E., and WATSON, L. C. A. (1964) Hyperparathyroidism and cancer, *Brit. med. J.*, **2**, 218.

DUFFY, J. P., and DAVISON, K. (1968) A female case of the Kleine–Levin syndrome, *Brit. J. Psychiat.*, **114**, 77.

FISHER, M., and ADAMS, R. D. (1958) Transient-global amnesia, *Trans. Amer. neurol. Ass.*, **83**, 143.

FRENCH, J. B. (1952) Brain lesions associated with prolonged unconsciousness, *Arch. Neurol. Psychiat. (Chicago)*, **68**, 727.

GALLINEK, A. (1954) The syndrome of episodes of hypersomnia, bulimia and abnormal mental states, *J. Amer. med. Ass.*, **154**, 1081.

GARLAND, H., SUMNER, D., and FOURMAN, P. (1965) The Kleine–Levin syndrome. Some further observations, *Neurology (Minneap.)*, **15**, 1161.

GÉLINEAU, (1880) De la narcolepsie, *Gaz. Hôp. (Paris)*, **53**, 626 and 635.

GELLHORN, E. (1954) Physiological processes related to consciousness and perception, *Brain*, **67**, 401.

HISHIKAWA, Y., IDA, H., NAKAI, K., and KANEKO, Z. (1966) Treatment of narcolepsy with imipramine (Tofranil) and desmethylimipramine (Pertofran), *J. neurol. Sci.*, **3**, 453.

JOUVET, M. (1962) Recherches sur les structures nerveuses et les méchanismes responsables des différentes phases du sommeil physiologique, *Arch. ital. Biol.*, **100**, 125.

KLEINE, W. (1925) Periodische Schlafsucht, *Mschr. Psychiat. Neurol.*, **57**, 285.

KLEITMAN, N. (1929) Sleep, *Physiol. Rev.*, **9**, 624.

KLUVER, H., and BUCY, P. C. (1939) Preliminary analysis of functions of the temporal lobes in monkeys, *Arch. Neurol. Psychiat. (Chicago)*, **42**, 979.

LEMANN, J., and DONATELLI, A. A. (1964) Calcium intoxication due to primary hyper-parathyroidism; a medical and surgical emergency, *Ann. intern Med.*, **60**, 447.

LEVIN, M. (1932) Cataplexy, *Brain*, **55**, 397.

LEVIN, M. (1936) Periodic somnolence and morbid hunger: a new syndrome, *Brain*, **59**, 494.

LEWIS, A. (1961) Amnesic syndromes: the pyschopathological aspect, *Proc. roy. Soc. Med.*, **54**, 955.

LHERMITTE, J. (1951) *Les Hallucinations*, Paris.

LHERMITTE, J., and TOURNAY, A. (1927) Le sommeil normal et pathologique, *Rev. neurol.*, **34**, (i), 751.

LIDZ, T. (1942) The amnestic syndrome, *Arch. Neurol. Psychiat.* (*Chicago*), **47**, 588.

MAGOUN, H. W. (1952) The ascending reticular activating system, *Res. Publ. Ass. nerv. ment. Dis.*, **30**, 480.

NORRIS, F. H., and FAWCETT, J. (1965) A sign of intracranial mass with impending uncal herniation, *Arch. Neurol.* (*Chic.*), **12**, 381.

PAVLOV, I. P. (1928) *Lectures on Conditioned Reflexes*, p. 305, New York.

PLUM, F., and ALVORD, E. C., JR. (1964) Apneustic breathing in man, *Arch. Neurol.* (*Chic.*), **10**, 101.

PLUM, F., and POSNER, J. B. (1966) *The Diagnosis of Stupor and Coma*, Oxford.

PLUM, F., and SWANSON, A. G. (1958) Abnormalities in the central regulation of respira-tion in acute and convalescent poliomyelitis, *Arch. Neurol. Psychiat.* (*Chicago*), **80**, 267.

PLUM, F., and SWANSON, A. G. (1959) Central neurogenic hyperventilation in man, *Arch. Neurol. Psychiat.* (*Chicago*), **81**, 535.

RANSON, S. W. (1939) Somnolence caused by hypothalamic lesions in the monkey, *Arch. Neurol. Psychiat.* (*Chicago*), **41**, 1.

ROSENBAUM, M., and MERRITT, H. H. (1939) Korsakoff's syndrome. Clinical study of the alcoholic form, with special regard to prognosis, *Arch. Neurol. Psychiat.* (*Chicago*), **51**, 978.

SKULTETY, F. M. (1968) Clinical and experimental aspects of akinetic mutism, *Arch. Neurol.* (*Chic.*), **19**, 1.

TALLAND, G. A. (1958) Psychological studies of Korsakow's psychosis. II. Perceptual functions, *J. nerv. ment. Dis.*, **127**, 197.

TALLAND, G. A. (1959) The interference theory of forgetting and the amnesic syndrome, *J. abnorm. soc. Psychol.*, **59**, 10.

TALLAND, G. A., and EKDAHL, M. (1959) Psychological studies of Korsakow's psychosis. IV. The note and mode of forgetting narrative material, *J. nerv. ment. Dis.*, **129**, 391.

VICTOR, M. (1964) RNA and brain function, memory and learning, in *Brain Function*, Vol. ii, ed. BRAZIER, M. A. B., Berkeley, Calif.

WALTER, W. G., GRIFFITHS, G. M., and NEVIN, S. (1939) The electro-encephalogram in a case of pathological sleep due to hypothalamic tumour, *Brit. med. J.*, **1**, 107.

WATSON, L. C. A. (1963) Hypercalcaemia and cancer, *Postgrad. med. J.*, **39**, 646.

WHITTY, C. W. M., and LISHMAN, W. A. (1966) Amnesia in cerebral disease, in *Amnesia*, ed. WHITTY, C. W. M., and ZANGWILL, O. L., London.

WILSON, S. A. K. (1928) The narcolepsies, *Brain*, **51**, 63.

WOLSTENHOLME, G., and O'CONNOR, M. (1961) *Ciba Foundation Symposium on the Nature of Sleep*, London.

DISORDERS OF MOOD

The neural basis of the registration of emotion and the integration of the accompanying bodily changes have been discussed on page 960 It is to dis-orders of this mechanism and of its relationship with higher levels of the nervous system that we must look for the explanation of disorders of mood occurring as a result of organic nervous disease.

Emotional Instability

Emotional instability or lability is a very common symptom of nervous diseases, especially of those in which the lesions are diffuse. The patient is easily moved by almost any form of emotion. He is quickly irritated or angered, easily becomes apprehensive, is readily depressed or reduced to tears. Less often, he experiences pleasurable emotion with abnormal facility and is readily moved to laughter. Emotional instability of this kind is commonly encountered after head injury, after massive cerebral infarction, and in elderly patients with cerebral arteriosclerosis. It is frequently present in the early stages of dementia, however produced, and is highly characteristic of the later stages of multiple sclerosis. The animal experiments already quoted suggest that this exaggerated emotional activity common to so many disorders is the result of an impairment of the control which higher levels normally exercise over the thalamus and hypothalamus.

Impulsive Disorders of Conduct

The emotional instability described in the previous paragraph does not usually lead to disorder of conduct, perhaps because conduct is normally more strongly inhibited than feeling. Exceptionally, however, impairment of higher control releases emotions which pass into action. This most often happens in children or adolescents in whom the control of impulsive action, which it is the object of education to impose, is as yet incomplete. The misdemeanours and acts of violence sometimes committed by children and adolescents who have had encephalitis lethargica are examples of this, and similar acts may be committed by aggressive psychopaths, and epileptics, either before an epileptic attack or in the phase of post-epileptic automatism or in the intervals between attacks. Such acts of aggression seem most likely to occur in patients with temporal lobe lesions.

Emotional Apathy

A general loss of emotional responsiveness without a proportionate intellectual deterioration is most characteristically seen in association with Parkinsonism due to encephalitis lethargica. In view of the known predilection of the virus of this disease for the diencephalic grey matter, it is reasonable to attribute the apathy to injury to the posterior hypothalamus. A similar picture is seen associated with mental deterioration in the later stages of dementia from any cause. Here it is probable that the apathy is in part, at least, secondary to the deterioration of thought and perception. The apathetic patient loses all his former interests and affections and, lacking the drive of the instinctive life, becomes incapable of effort, and sinks into a vegetative existence.

Euphoria

Euphoria is the term used to indicate a mood characterized by feelings of cheerfulness and happiness, a sense of mental well-being. Transitory euphoria is induced in many people by the consumption of alcohol. As a prevailing mood, it is seen most characteristically in multiple sclerosis. Many sufferers from this disease remain persistently serene and happy in spite of their increasing physical disabilities. Euphoria is also encountered occasionally in patients with intra-cranial tumours, especially when the tumour is situated in the temporal lobe or, less frequently, in the frontal lobe or corpus callosum. Euphoria is common also in general paralysis and is the predominating emotional state in the milder degrees of maniacal excitement. The psychophysiological basis of euphoria is little understood.

Excitement

Excitement is a term somewhat loosely applied to several forms of mental over-activity, which may predominantly involve the intellectual, emotional, or psychomotor spheres. All three may be affected together, as in acute mania, characterized by flight of ideas, elation, and psychomotor restlessness. Disordered ideas may be linked with excitement in some delirious and confusional states, and in catatonic schizophrenia. Delirium has been defined as confusion with an overlay of excitement. It may occur as a result of head injury, diffuse inflamma-tion of the brain or in a variety of toxic and metabolic confusional states including those resulting from drug withdrawal. Psychomotor restlessness is associated with anxiety in agitated depression; and the prevailing mood is rage in the out-bursts of aggressive psychopaths. Meyer (1944) discusses the evidence for the view that states of excitement may be caused by lesions of the anterior hypo-thalamus.

Depression

Depression may be regarded as the opposite of euphoria. It is a mood of dejection and gloom for which frequently the patient can offer no explanation. It is encountered in a variety of states. It is sometimes produced by infections, especially influenza, and certain drugs, especially the sulphonamides. It may be a reaction to an adequate external cause, such as failure or bereavement, or a neurotic reaction to internal difficulties. In sufferers from cyclothymia, depression is liable to occur as a recurrent disorder of mood, sometimes alternating with phases of excitement, though often these are no more than a mild general sense of elation. In cyclothymic individuals the depression is likely to be associated with some mental retardation, manifesting itself in a difficulty in concentrating, and with insomnia and loss of appetite. Such patients typically wake early and feel at their worst in the early part of the day. Depression also occurs as the predominant feature of involutional melancholia, in which it may be associated with agitation. Patients suffering from psychotic depression in a severe form often have delusions of guilt or of a hypochondriacal nature. Individuals with such a so-called endogenous depression frequently have physical symptoms including headache, fatigue, and facial and/or limb or low back pain; often they show a typical pattern of early-morning waking. Depression is also a mood which is common in patients suffering from organic disease of the brain. This may be in part a natural reaction to their disabilities and it is most likely to occur in individuals of a cyclothymic temperament in whom the nervous disease may be regarded as having released a pre-existing tendency to depression. Thus we sometimes encounter depression after head injury, in a minority of patients suffering from multiple sclerosis, and sometimes in patients with intracranial tumour or general paresis.

Anxiety

Fear is the emotional reaction to an imminent danger; anxiety is the reaction to a possible future danger—fear linked with anticipation. Anxiety may be produced in a variety of ways. It may, of course, be a normal emotional reaction. It may be the effect of certain toxins which appear to stimulate directly the nervous centres concerned. These are all toxins which have a stimulating effect upon the sympathetic nervous system, namely adrenaline, ephedrine, amphetamine, nicotine, and thyroxine. Anxiety may be the prevailing mood in patients suffering from organic disease of the brain, for example, following head injury, and it is then probably in part the outcome of diminished control of emotional reactions by higher centres, and in part a reaction to the disability produced by the injury or disease. Fear may be very evident in delirious states, when it appears as the reaction to terrifying hallucinations, and may be linked with depression in involutional melancholia. In very many cases, however, anxiety is neurotic—that is, it is the product of unconscious mental processes.

REFERENCES

COTTRELL, S. S., and WILSON, S. A. K. (1926) The affective symptomatology of disseminated sclerosis, *J. Neurol. Psychopath.*, **7**, 1.

FULTON, J. F., and INGRAHAM, F. D. (1929) Emotional disturbances following experimental lesions of the base of the brain (pre-chiasmal), *J. Physiol. (Lond.)*, **67**, 27.

MEYER, A. (1944) The Wernicke syndrome, *J. Neurol. Neurosurg. Psychiat.*, **7**, 66.

SMYTHIES, J. R. (1966) *The Neurological Foundations of Psychiatry*, Oxford.

THE INVESTIGATION OF MENTAL CHANGES AFTER CEREBRAL LESIONS

It is only during recent years that much attention has been devoted to the psychological investigation of patients with lesions of the brain, and the Second World War gave a great impetus to this study. The complexity of mental function makes progress slow, but certain facts of theoretical and practical importance have emerged already. Numerous tests and several batteries of tests have been employed (Babcock, 1930; Wechsler, 1941; Reynell, 1944). Though there is much of theoretical interest to be learned from patients in states of confusion, the chief practical importance of psychometric investigation is in the diagnosis of dementia, and the assessment of the nature of the residual psychological change after head injury in relation to prognosis and rehabilitation.

Specific Defects of Speech and Perception

It is first necessary to recognize defects of a specific kind, such as aphasia, acalculia, and the various forms of apraxia and agnosia. Two types of defect are of special importance, as emphasized by Zangwill (1945). Minor degrees of aphasia, which are a substantial handicap to a patient in formulating and expressing his thoughts with fluency, may be shown only by special tests of high-grade comprehension and reasoning. And disorders of spatial judgement and manipulative skill—minor degrees of spatial agnosia or constructive apraxia—may interfere with the performance of skilled and semi-skilled manual occupations. These disorders are discussed elsewhere in this book [see pp. 113 and 566]. The Wechsler intelligence scale for children (W.I.S.C.) is particularly useful in childhood, when a discrepancy between the results obtained on the verbal and performance scales may indicate a specific inability to carry out certain performance tasks (motor skills) thus indicating some degree of apraxia. The assessment of Schonell's 'reading age' is also valuable in the assessment of suspected dyslexia. Similar tests are available for adults. The topic is reviewed in detail by Klein and Mayer-Gross (1957).

Intellectual Defects

The study of intellectual defects by appropriate tests has brought to light the fact that after damage to the brain 'certain abilities or attainments, such as vocabulary, general information, and powers of comprehension suffer less in deterioration than do such capacities as reasoning ability, attention, recent memory, and "relational thinking" ' (Reynell, 1944). Babcock's and Reynell's batteries are designed to detect this difference. It is clear that the functions which suffer are themselves complex. Trist and Trist (1942–3) find Weigl's 'form-colour sorting test' of special value as a test of conceptual thought: failure is interpreted as meaning that the patient cannot abstract from the perceptual fields. (See Rapaport, 1945.) Piercy (1964) has given a valuable review of current methods, and Allison (1962) describes techniques of particular value in the elderly.

Defects of Memory

Memory defects are common after cerebral lesions and play an important part in causing intellectual defect. Inquiry should first be made about everyday events in the patient's immediate past. His memory for remote events is also tested. Specific tests are also useful. Some form of digit test is simple to carry out. Zangwill (1942–3) first ascertains the normal span, i.e. the number of digits which the patient can repeat correctly after one hearing, and then the number of hearings necessary for correct repetition when one more digit is added. The deteriorated patient will be able to repeat fewer than normal (7) and may exhibit a sharp threshold, i.e. he may fail completely to remember one more. Reynell scores the total number of digits repeated forwards correctly added to the number repeated backwards, the average being $7+5$. It is also customary to use the name, address, and flower test, in which the patient is given a name, an address, and the name of a flower to recall several minutes later after other tests have been interposed. Zangwill also uses the Rey Davis performance test and one of the Babcock Sentences, No. 23, which runs as follows: 'One thing a nation must have to become rich and great is a large, secure supply of wood.' The observer ascertains the number of hearings necessary before the patient can repeat it correctly. More than four is abnormal.

Emotional Factors and Personality Changes

Psychometric tests have proved of value in distinguishing between failures of performance due to intellectual defects and those resulting from emotional disturbances. Thus Zangwill (1942–3) finds the 'organic' reaction-type characterized by impairment of learning capacity and the 'neurotic' reaction-type by exaggerated variability of response and a tendency to fail on easy tasks. The importance of personality change needs no emphasis. It can be interpreted only in the light of the patient's previous personality, of which the new personality is often a 'caricature' as Patterson (1942) points out; i.e. the previous trends are exaggerated. In other cases the change is rather an inversion (Reynell), and the previously cheerful, sociable, alert person may become depressed, unsocial, and lacking in initiative. After brain damage, which to an uncertain and variable extent may involve cortex and subcortical 'affective' centres, the distinction made by Zangwill between 'organic' and 'neurotic' would perhaps be better described as between intellectual and emotional; for it is artificial to distinguish between organic and psychogenic symptoms in such patients: once again we are dealing with a brain-mind unity.

REFERENCES

ALLISON, R. S. (1962) *The Senile Brain*, London.
BABCOCK, H. (1930) An experiment in the measurement of mental deterioration, *Arch. Psych.*, **117**, 5, New York.
KLEIN, R., and MAYER-GROSS, W. (1957) *The Clinical Examination of Patients with Organic Cerebral Disease*, London.
PATTERSON, A. (1942) Emotional and cognitive changes in the post-traumatic confusional state, *Lancet*, ii, 717.
PIERCY, M. (1964) The effects of cerebral lesions on intellectual function: a review of current research trends, *Brit. J. Psychiat.*, **110**, 310.
RAPAPORT, D. (1945) *Diagnostic Psychological Testing*, Chicago.
REYNELL, W. R. (1944) A psychometric method of determining intellectual loss following head injury, *J. ment. Sci.*, **90**, 710.
TRIST, E. L., and TRIST, V. (1942–3) Discussion on the quality of mental test performance in intellectual deterioration, *Proc. roy. Soc. Med.*, **36**, 243.
WECHSLER, D. (1941) *Measurement of Adult Intelligence*, Baltimore.
ZANGWILL, O. L. (1942–3) Clinical tests of memory impairment, *Proc. roy. Soc. Med.*, **36**, 576.
ZANGWILL, O. L. (1945) A review of psychological work at the brain injuries unit, Edinburgh, 1941–5, *Brit. med. J.*, **2**, 248.

DEMENTIA

Dementia is the term applied to a diffuse deterioration in the mental functions manifesting itself primarily in thought and memory and secondarily in feeling and conduct. It may be produced by a large number of pathological agencies and the clinical picture varies somewhat according to the previous temperament of the patient, the age of onset, the localization, rate of progress, and nature of the causal disorder.

SYMPTOMS
Judgement and Reasoning

The earliest disability is often an impairment of judgement and reasoning manifesting itself in a failure to grasp the meaning of a situation as a whole and hence to react to it appropriately. At this stage a man's business judgement begins to fail, though in the semi-automatic activities of life no defect may be noticed.

Memory

Memory becomes impaired, the recollection of recent events suffering more than that of early periods of life [see p. 962]. Even when both are grossly defective, mechanical memory may remain for a time. In more severe stages of dementia, defect of memory linked with defective perception leads to disorientation in space and time.

The Emotional Life

Although in some patients the emotional life is little disturbed, in others impairment of higher control leads to emotional instability which finds expression in irritability and impulsive conduct. Acts of violence, alcoholic excess, and sexual aberrations are thus explained. The prevailing mood may be one of euphoria, with hilariousness and hyperactivity, depression, anxiety, or maniacal excitement, and will be influenced by the pre-existing psychological constitution. In the late stages the patient is apathetic.

Delusions

Delusions are the outcome of emotional disorder, associated with impairment of judgement and defective appreciation of reality. Delusions centred on the self are likely to be grandiose in a state of euphoria and self-condemnatory or hypochondriacal in a state of depression. Delusions regarding others are often hostile and express fear, suspicion, or jealousy.

Care of the Person

In the later stages of dementia the patient becomes careless in dress and in personal cleanliness, and finally incontinent. This may be attributed at first to a decay of the self-regarding sentiment and later also to the lack of perception.

Speech

In the later stages also, speech undergoes a progressive disintegration. Though the forms of aphasia caused by focal lesions of the brain may be present in dementia, there is also a destruction of the speech function as a whole, so that speech becomes increasingly meaningless and ends in jargon or isolated words or phrases, 'logoclonia'. Agnosia and apraxia may also develop.

Physical Concomitants

The condition of the somatic nervous functions will depend upon the causal disorder, but, whatever the cause, there is usually a general physical deterioration with loss of weight, and depression of endocrine function.

AETIOLOGY

The causes of dementia, many of which have already been considered in detail, are:

1. Syphilis—general paresis, cerebral meningovascular syphilis, &c.
2. Cerebral arteriosclerosis.
3. The presenile dementias—a mixed group of degenerative diseases of unknown origin—Pick's disease, Alzheimer's disease (presbyophrenia), Creutzfeld-Jakob disease, subacute spongiform encephalopathy, Huntington's chorea.
4. Intracranial tumour, 'low-pressure' or communicating hydrocephalus.
5. Non-syphilitic inflammatory diseases—encephalitis (various forms), intracranial abscess, meningitis.
6. Intoxications and deficiency diseases—alcoholism, drug addiction, carbon monoxide poisoning, uraemia, vitamin B_{12} neuropathy, pellagra, Wernicke's encephalopathy, myxoedema, liver failure.
7. Dementia supervening in chronic psychotic states.
8. Miscellaneous demyelinating and metabolic disorders, including multiple sclerosis, the diffuse cerebral scleroses, the lipidoses, and tuberous sclerosis, many of which may cause dementia in childhood.
9. Injury to the brain.
10. Severe and diffuse brain damage due to anoxia (as in some cases of intractable epilepsy).
11. Dementia in the hereditary ataxias (some forms).

Since in most of these disorders the dementia is an inconstant and sometimes a rare symptom, an account of them must be sought in the appropriate sections of this book. The presenile dementias, however, which, with the exception of Huntington's chorea, are predominantly mental disorders, are most conveniently considered at this point, and will also provide an opportunity of considering the diagnosis of dementia.

THE PRESENILE DEMENTIAS

Alzheimer's Disease

Alzheimer's disease is a progressive cerebral degeneration with the pathological picture of senility occurring in middle life. The essential lesion is a diffuse degeneration of the cerebral cortex involving all its layers and most marked in the frontal lobes. The basal ganglia and the cerebellum escape. The brain is atrophic. Histologically, besides degeneration of the ganglion cells of the cortex there is a profusion of senile plaques in the cortex. These are silver-staining masses, often ring- or star-shaped, and probably of neuroglial origin. In addition, there are intraneural fibrillary tangles. These changes are regarded as characteristic of senile degeneration of the cortex. Their occurrence in middle age is unexplained, but there seems no doubt that Alzheimer's disease is essentially a premature senile change. Woodard (1962) has shown that granulovacuolar degeneration in the nerve cells of the hippocampal pyramidal layer can be even more closely correlated with dementia than senile plaques in the cortex. Tomlinson, Blessed, and Roth (1968) have shown that all of the changes described, with the possible exception of granulo-vacuolar degeneration, can be found in the brains of non-demented elderly people, but there is a quantitative relationship between the severity of dementia and the severity and ubiquity of the pathological changes described (Roth, Tomlinson, and Blessed, 1966).

Alzheimer's disease usually develops between the ages of 40 and 60. The symptoms are those of a progressive dementia with apraxia and speech disturbances. The onset is insidious. In the early stages the patient suffers from loss of memory and becomes careless in dress and conduct. Epileptiform attacks may occur. Speech becomes slurred, and there is difficulty in recalling words. As the disease progresses there is complete disorientation. The patient recognizes none of his friends, becomes restless, and may wander about. A progressive deterioration takes place in the faculty of speech, which, from paraphasic talkativeness, becomes reduced to isolated words and phrases, so-called 'logoclonia'. Movements become stereotyped and the sucking reflex is often elicitable in the late stages. Spastic contractures usually develop. The duration of the disease is from one and a half to thirteen years. Treatment does not influence its course.

Pick's Disease

Synonym. Circumscribed cortical atrophy.

This condition is characterized by circumscribed atrophy of the cerebral cortex, usually confined to the frontal and temporal regions. The upper three cortical layers are principally affected, exhibiting chromatolysis and disappearance of ganglion cells. There is some glial increase in the atrophic areas, but senile plaques and intraneural fibrils are absent and arteriosclerosis plays no part in causation. The cause of the disease is unknown. It may be toxic in origin or a form of primary degeneration developing in middle life. Multiple cases have been described in one sibship. The age of onset is usually between 50 and 60, and the disease has a duration of from three to twelve years, always terminating fatally. Females are said to be affected more often than males. It is characterized by a progressive dementia and aphasia. Restlessness and loss of normal inhibitions are prominent in the early stages. The patient is often voluble and tends to make jokes and puns. At first the more abstract intellectual functions suffer, but the more concrete type of behaviour is well-preserved and the patient emotionally accessible. Later, mental dullness becomes pronounced and epileptic attacks may occur. Speech is reduced to a few stereotyped phrases. In the terminal stages there is much loss of weight, and the patient becomes bed-ridden, and tends to develop contractures.

SENILE DEMENTIA

Many of the causes of dementia listed on page 991 may operate in old age. Is there a distinctive senile dementia apart from them, and especially from cerebral atheromatosis? This has been much debated (see McMenemey, 1958), but on the whole the evidence suggests that 'idiopathic' senile dementia is usually due to Alzheimer's disease of late onset and that it simply represents an ageing process which is observed in lesser degree in elderly non-demented subjects. Pathological evidence indicates that except in the presence of a history of recurrent cerebral infarction, atherosclerotic dementia is rare, even in old age and cerebral softening must be severe and widespread for dementia to occur (Tomlinson, Blessed, and Roth, 1968).

THE DIAGNOSIS OF THE CAUSE OF DEMENTIA

The cause of dementia is sometimes obvious, as when the condition follows head injury, acute encephalitis, epilepsy, or chronic alcoholism. Dementia of syphilitic origin, whether due to general paralysis or meningovascular syphilis, is associated with characteristic serological reactions and usually with abnormal physical signs in the nervous system. In cases of intracranial tumour the history is usually short, and the course of the dementia steadily progressive. The diagnosis is easy if symptoms and signs of increased intracranial pressure are present. In their absence an encephalogram is often necessary. Air encephalography is usually diagnostic in cases of low-pressure or communicating hydrocephalus which may present with fluctuating confusion, dementia, and ataxia. Air will outline dilated ventricles but in this condition none passes over the cortex and deterioration often follows the procedure. Isotope encephalography may confirm the diagnosis. Arteriosclerotic dementia is usually encountered after the age of 60. The onset is usually insidious, and there is almost always a history of focal cerebral vascular lesions, slight 'strokes'. Evidence of arteriosclerosis is to be found as a rule in the retinal and peripheral circulation, with or without high blood pressure. The differentiation of the presenile dementias may be difficult. These usually begin between 45 and 60. The commoner causes of dementia can readily be excluded. Encephalograms demonstrate some general dilatation of the cerebral ventricles with an excess of air over the anterior part of the hemispheres in Pick's disease, but more diffuse in Alzheimer's disease. Early psychomotor restlessness and jocularity and a family history of presenile dementia would favour Pick's disease as against Alzheimer's disease.

The possibility of a metabolic or endocrine cause for dementia must always be borne in mind. In vitamin B_{12} deficiency, dementia may antedate symptoms and signs of anaemia and spinal cord involvement and estimation of the serum B_{12} or a Schilling test may be necessary for diagnosis. Myxoedema will usually be apparent clinically, if considered. The fluctuating confusion of subdural haematoma is sometimes mistaken for dementia, but there is usually associated drowsiness and headache and an angiogram will give diagnostic findings.

It must also be remembered that the retardation of severe endogenous depression may be misconstrued as being due to dementia, while many patients with receptive aphasia due to focal cerebral lesions are wrongly regarded as suffering from dementia in view of their failure to communicate. Hysteria in young patients and hysterical 'pseudodementia' in adults, sometimes arising as a result of a desire for financial compensation after relatively minor head injury may also give rise to occasional difficulty.

REFERENCES

ALEXANDER, L., and LOONEY, J. M. (1938) Histologic changes in senile dementia and related conditions, *Arch. Neurol. Psychiat.* (*Chicago*), **40**, 1075.

ALLISON, R. S. (1962) *The Senile Brain*, London.

BENEDEK, L., and LEHOCZKY, T. (1939) The clinical recognition of Pick's disease. Report of three cases, *Brain*, **62**, 104.

DELAY, J., BRION, S., and BADARACIO, J. G. (1955) Le diagnostic différentiel des maladies de Pick et de Alzheimer, *Encéphale*, **44**, 454.

GRÜNTHAL, E. (1926) Ueber die Alzheimersche Krankheit, *Z. ges. Neurol. Psychiat.*, **101**, 128.

GRÜNTHAL, E. (1930) Über ein Brüderpaar mit Pickscher Krankheit, *Z. ges. Neurol. Psychiat.*, **129**, 350.

HENDERSON, D. K., and MACLACHAN, S. H. (1930) Alzheimer's disease, *J. ment. Sci.*, **76**, 646.

HERZ, E., and FUNFGELD, E. (1928) Zur Klinik und Pathologie der Alzheimerschen Krankheit, *Arch. Psychiat. (Berlin)*, **84**, 633.

HORN, L., and STENGEL, E. (1930) Zur Klinik und Pathologie der Pickschen Atrophie, *Z. ges. Neurol. Psychiat.*, **128**, 673.

LARSSON, T., SJÖGREN, T., and JACOBSON, G. (1963) Senile dementia, *Acta psychiat. (Kbh.)*, **39**, Suppl. 167.

MALAMUD, W., and LOWENBERG, K. (1929) Alzheimer's disease, *Arch. Neurol. Psychiat. (Chicago)*, **21**, 805.

MANSVELT, J. VAN (1954) *Pick's Disease*, Enschede.

MAYER-GROSS, W., and others (1937–8) Discussion on the presenile dementias: symptomatology, pathology and differential diagnosis, *Proc. roy. Soc. Med.*, **31**, 1443.

McMENEMEY, W. H. (1958) in *Neuropathology*, ed. GREENFIELD, J. G., BLACKWOOD, W., McMENEMEY, W. H., MEYER, A., and NORMAN, R. M., p. 475, London.

NICHOLS, I. C., and WEIGNER, W. C. (1938) Pick's disease—a specific type of dementia, *Brain*, **61**, 237.

ONARI, K., and SPATZ, H. (1926) Anatomische Beiträge zur Lehre von der Pickschen umschriebenen Großhirnrinden-Atrophie ('Picksche Krankheit'), *Z. ges. Neurol. Psychiat.*, **101**, 470.

ROTH, M., TOMLINSON, B. E., and BLESSED, G. (1966) Correlation between scores for dementia and counts of 'senile plaques' in cerebral grey matter of elderly subjects, *Nature (Lond.)*, **209**, 109.

SJÖGREN, T., SJÖGREN, H., and LINDGREN, A. G. H. (1952) Morbus Alzheimer and Morbus Pick, *Acta psychiat. scand.*, Suppl. 82.

THORPE, F. T. (1932) Pick's disease (circumscribed senile atrophy) and Alzheimer's disease, *J. ment. Sci.*, **78**, 303.

TOMLINSON, B. E., BLESSED, G., and ROTH, M. (1968) Observations on the brains of non-demented old people, *J. neurol. Sci.*, **7**, 331.

URECHIA, C. I., and MIHALESCU, S. (1928) La maladie de Pick (atrophie sénile circonscrite), *Encéphale*, **23**, 803.

WOODARD, J. S. (1962) Clinico-pathological significance of granulo-vacuolar degeneration in Alzheimer's disease, *J. Neuropath. exp. Neurol.*, **21**, 85.

HYSTERIA

Definition. A disorder characterized by mental dissociation leading in severe cases to multiple personality and amnesia, but more often to somatic symptoms such as 'fits', paralysis, and sensory disturbances in the absence of organic disease of the nervous system.

AETIOLOGY

In hysteria the type of abnormal reaction exhibited by the patient is determined by the peculiar tendency of the hysterical personality to mental dissociation.

In response to mental stress of a kind to be described later, the personality becomes split, certain psychophysiological elements becoming separated from the conscious life. In general, all hysterical syndromes may be regarded as representing the subconscious results of an attempt to escape from some stressful situation. In the most severe cases the dissociated part of the mental life is so extensive that the patient may be regarded as suffering from multiple personality, since his body is at different times under the control of different personalities, which exhibit differences in temperament and which may or may not have access to each other's memories. A similar profound mental dissociation is responsible for the state known as hysterical fugue, in which the patient disappears from home and wanders about, having lost his sense of identity. During the period of fugue he has no access to the memories of his normal personality, and on recovery he may have no recollection of the events of his fugue. Such profound degrees of dissociation are, however, uncommon, and usually the splitting of the personality finds expression at the physiological level, part of the body being functionally cut off from the rest of the mental life, so that the patient is unable to move it or to feel with it, hysterical paralysis or anaesthesia resulting.

The nature of the hysterical tendency to dissociation is little understood. It appears to be associated with a peculiarity of the emotional life of the hysterical patient. The poverty of the affective reactions of such individuals is well known—la belle indifférence of Janet—and Golla has shown that in spite of the violence of their somatic reactions the psycho-galvanic response to nocuous stimuli is greatly depressed in hysterical patients. The underlying abnormality which finds expression in hysteria may well in many cases be inborn or at least may develop at an early age. But certain organic nervous diseases seem to predispose to hysteria, especially multiple sclerosis, and typically hysterical symptoms may occur in patients with a focal abnormality in the temporal lobe, which suggests that mental dissociation may sometimes have an organic basis. Women suffer from hysteria more frequently than men.

It is also important to recognize that hysterical manifestations occurring for the first time in adult life, unless there is some obvious motive (such as, for instance, escape from stress, or the desire for material gain such as compensation after injury) may be the result of either an underlying organic disorder (such as early dementia) or else of a more serious psychiatric illness (such as endogenous depression). Slater (1965) has drawn attention to the frequency with which symptoms regarded by experienced clinicians as being due to hysteria may conceal evidence of underlying organic disease of the nervous system. He suggests that all too often this diagnosis is 'a disguise for ignorance and a fertile source of clinical error'. His warning that such a diagnosis does not necessarily imply the absence of, as yet, unrecognized organic disease, is timely.

The Mode of Production of Hysterical Symptoms

The hysterical symptom is at the same time (1) a product of suggestion, (2) the expression of an idea in the patient's mind, and (3) a means to achieve a purpose.

1. The precise nature of a hysterical symptom in a given case is usually, probably always, determined by suggestion. The suggestion frequently emanates from an organic disorder from which the patient actually suffers. Thus laryngitis

may lead to aphonia, which is perpetuated as a hysterical symptom. Accidents of all kinds, for reasons which are discussed elsewhere, are apt to cause hysterical symptoms which perpetuate or exaggerate the disabilities produced by an injury. A doctor, nurse, or friend of the patient may unwittingly evoke a hysterical symptom by seeming to imply that a disability is to be expected. There are fashions in hysterical symptoms which seem partly to be determined by the expectations of doctors interested in the subject at the time. Finally, the symptom may be an imitation of an organic disorder in a person whom the patient has seen and with whom for some reason he identifies himself.

2. Suggestion operates through the patient's acceptance on irrational grounds of the idea that he is suffering from a certain symptom. It follows that the hysterical symptom is always the expression of an idea in the patient's mind. Thus hysterical aphonia expresses the idea 'I have lost my voice', hysterical paralysis the idea 'I cannot move my limb', and so on. This fact is of great diagnostic importance, for it is impossible that the patient's idea of a symptom should correspond with a similar symptom produced by organic disease, and the resulting discrepancy renders possible the diagnosis of the one from the other.

3. The purposive character of the hysterical symptom is important in connexion with treatment. The purpose served by the symptom can usually be expressed as the unconscious solution, however unsatisfactory, of a mental conflict. The patient finds himself in a situation in which a course of action which he desires to follow conflicts with his sense of duty or self-respect. The development of the hysterical symptom unconsciously solves this conflict, though at the price of a neurotic disability. For example, a girl was compelled to give up her work to look after her invalid mother. She developed a hysterical paralysis of her right hand which prevented her from doing housework, and assistance had to be obtained to look after both her mother and herself. Her hysterical illness saved her from her unpleasant duty and also preserved her self-respect, since she felt that no one could blame her for being ill. At the same time she ceased to do any work at all, unconsciously revenged herself on her exacting parent, and became an object of sympathy to those with whom she came in contact. It is important to recognize that hysteria may fulfil other purposes than the solution of such a conflict, and that one symptom may achieve more than one object. The symptom frequently expresses a demand for sympathy, especially when the patient feels that he is neglected or insufficiently appreciated. Tyrannical parents and unfaithful spouses excite such a demand directly, while invalid parents and delicate brothers and sisters evoke it competitively. The hysterical symptom frequently possesses the further significance of being a symbol which expresses the patient's feelings. An example is the adoption of a crucifixion attitude in a hysterical fit.

The patient suffering from hysteria is thus often an individual confronted with a mental difficulty, often a conflict between two opposing wishes. While in this situation he receives a suggestion of ill health emanating either from an actual organic disease or from some outside source. He accepts this suggestion and manifests hysterical symptoms which provide a solution, albeit a pathological and unsatisfactory one, of his difficulty, and may also express in symbolic form his emotional reaction to his problem.

SYMPTOMS

Amnesia and Multiple Personality

Loss of memory and multiple personality are among the most striking symptoms of hysteria, and in outspoken forms are rare. The commonest example is the hysterical fugue, in which the patient disappears from home and wanders about, having lost his sense of identity. This state may last for hours, days, or even months, and on recovery the patient usually has no recollection of the events of his period of fugue. During the fugue he may be dazed and confused or he may be apparently normal and live as a normal individual, carrying on an occupation and exhibiting a mode of life different from his usual one. Hysterical amnesias and fugues are usually reactions to difficulties which render normal life intolerable. A wife has been known to react in this way to the infidelity of her husband and to adopt during her fugue the name of his mistress. A patient already in financial difficulties had a quantity of uninsured stock stolen from his car. He drove for miles in a state of fugue, subsequently returning home exhausted and without any recollection of the events of the day, including the theft. In such a case the fugue and the amnesia constituted an escape from an unbearable situation which composed so large a part of the patient's life that he could only escape from it by suppression of a large field of consciousness. Amnesia may also occur in association with hysterical fits, the events of the attack being subsequently forgotten. Patients suffering from hysterical fugue may justly be regarded as examples of multiple or dissociated personality, since they exhibit alternating phases of consciousness with mutually isolated memories. More complicated cases of multiple personality have been described in which more than two sub-personalities alternated or coexisted, some having access to the memories of the others. It is interesting to note that it has sometimes been possible to produce these dissociations of personality by hypnotic suggestion, and that the subject-matter of a hysterical amnesia can often be restored to consciousness under hypnosis.

By no means all cases of 'loss of memory' are hysterical in origin. Many other mental disorders lead to mental confusion or impairment of memory such that the patient may become lost and be unable to give an account of himself.

Pseudodementia

Hysterical pseudodementia, or the Ganser syndrome, is characterized by failure of memory, and the acting out of the patient's idea of a psychosis, i.e. bizarre behaviour, excitement, or stupor.

Hysterical 'Fits'

It is sometimes difficult to decide from the history whether attacks are hysterical or epileptic, but the question is usually easily settled if the doctor is fortunate enough to witness a fit himself. The hysterical fit is often a dramatic performance appropriately staged, hence it does not occur when the patient is alone or at least out of reach of an audience. Often the attack is directly precipitated by the emotional situation responsible for the neurosis. The onset is usually gradual and never of the fulminating suddenness of an epileptic fit. Whereas the epileptic falls to the ground with alarming violence and may injure himself, the hysteric subsides with some care, leaning, for example, against a wall or slipping slowly from a chair on to the ground. The epileptic fit follows a more or less stereotyped course, beginning sometimes with a cry and passing through a tonic phase, a phase of clonic, purposeless, jerking movements, and ending in post-convulsive coma of variable length, sometimes followed by automatism. In hysterical fits these phases do not occur. Crying-out often occurs during the attack, but unlike the convulsive cry of the epileptic, which is merely an inarticulate phonation, consists of emotional reactions, e.g. laughing and crying, or the articulate utterance of words or sentences. The movements of the hysterical fit are not of a low order like the clonic movements of epilepsy, but are co-ordinated and purposive. The hysteric clutches at surrounding objects, struggles, and may attempt to fall out of bed or to tear off his clothes. Opisthotonos is common, and bizarre attitudes may be adopted. The tongue is not bitten in a hysterical convulsion, and incontinence of urine does not usually occur, but if the patient becomes aware that micturition is a characteristic of epileptic attacks, this symptom may be reproduced. Some hysterical 'fits', particularly in adolescent girls are not accompanied by movement, but the patient simply slumps to the floor and gets up again a few minutes later. These attacks may be difficult to distinguish from akinetic epilepsy but they usually occur at work or at school, do not cause injury and usually fail to respond to anticonvulsant drugs. In the convulsions of epilepsy consciousness is lost at the onset, so that the patient during and immediately after the fit makes no response to external simuli. The hysteric when in a 'fit', though in an abnormal state of consciousness, is not completely unconscious and can usually be roused by sufficiently firm handling, whence the time-honoured practice of administering a douche of cold water. The corneal reflex accordingly is absent in an epileptic during a fit and during the phase of post-convulsive coma. The corneal reflex is sometimes absent in hysteria, but an attempt to elicit it during a hysterical fit often evokes a violent contraction of the orbicularis oculi. The hysterical 'fit', unlike the epileptic, has no well-defined termination but tails away in sighs and groans and motor restlessness. After the attack the hysterical patient, though shaken and exhausted, does not usually exhibit the tendency to sleep which follows most epileptic fits. The plantar reflexes are for a time extensor after a proportion of epileptic fits. Flexor plantar responses after a fit do not exclude epilepsy, but extensor responses in similar circumstances exclude hysteria as the cause of the fit, provided there is no coexisting corticospinal tract lesion to which they are attributable.

Paralysis

Hysterical paralysis may affect any part of the body over which there is normally voluntary control. Most commonly it involves one limb or part of a limb, the movements at one joint being alone affected. Less frequently more than one limb is affected, as in hysterical hemiplegia, paraplegia, and diplegia. The paralysis may be associated with flaccidity or rigidity, or there may be no gross disturbance of muscle tone. Hysterical paralysis of the face and tongue is rare and is usually associated with spasm of the corresponding muscles on the opposite side. The diagnosis of hysterical paralysis rests upon the following points:

found in polyneuritis and in subacute combined degeneration, but in these disorders the transition from impaired to normal sensibility is always gradual. Hysterical patients often exhibit striking discrepancies in their sensory symptoms which are incompatible with an organic origin. Thus co-ordination may be perfect in spite of complete loss of postural sensibility and appreciation of passive movement in a limb. Or a patient with hysterical hemianaesthesia may state that he is unable to feel a vibrating tuning-fork placed over the affected half of the sternum or skull, although the bone conducts the stimulus perfectly to the opposite side. In hysterical persons sensory loss can readily be, and perhaps always is, produced by suggestion.

Deafness. There is little difficulty in detecting hysterical deafness when examination reveals that the ears and vestibular reactions are normal, but the diagnosis is more difficult when hysterical deafness is superimposed upon a reduction of hearing due to organic disease of the ears. Hysterical deafness may disappear during sleep, so that the patient can be aroused by sounds, and the blinking reflex on auditory stimulation may be retained by the hysterically deaf. When Bárány's noise-box is used, a patient suffering from hysterical deafness will raise his voice, but this does not occur when deafness is due to disease of the ear. Hysterical vertigo is rare.

Pain. There has been some discussion as to whether hysterical pain is qualitatively the same as the pain produced by organic disease, and this has been denied on the ground that the hysterical patient, though complaining of severe pain, usually exhibits none of the physical reactions which are associated with pain of organic origin and presents an appearance which belies his allegations of intense suffering. Nevertheless, since pain is essentially a psychical state, there seems no reason why it should not sometimes be psychogenic, and it does not follow that pain thus induced would necessarily be associated with the physiological concomitants of pain excited at lower levels of the nervous system. Hysterical pain is especially common in the head. The recognition of its nature depends upon the absence of symptoms of organic disease sufficient to explain it, its failure to respond to analgesic drugs, often including morphine, and to local anaesthetic block of the nerves innervating the affected region, and upon the mental state of the patient, who is usually distressed and agitated by the pain to an abnormal degree.

Ocular Symptoms

Hysterical blindness may be unilateral or bilateral and may be complete or consist merely of a reduction of visual acuity. Bilateral blindness may be a perpetuation of the transitory visual impairment associated with syncope or with head injury. Unilateral blindness may be associated with hysterical hemianaesthesia on the same side. In hysterical blindness the optic discs and the pupillary reactions to light are normal, and it may be possible to evoke blinking by a sudden feint with the hand towards the eyes. Moreover, the blind hysteric may avoid obstacles in his path, but so, too, may the patient with visual agnosia due to organic brain disease. There are a number of tests for the detection of unilateral hysterical blindness. Diplopia may be produced by covering one eye with an appropriate prism, or one eye may be covered with a red, and the other with a green glass, the patient being then asked to read a word-test of alternate red and green letters. Since one colour is invisible to each eye, if all the letters are read the patient must be using both eyes. Visual field defects are common in hysteria and are usually the result of suggestion at the time of examination. The commonest type is a concentric defect of the field which takes the form of a spiral with the field progressively diminishing with each circuit of the test object but 'tubular vision' may also occur.

Disturbances of the ocular movements include spasm of convergence, which is almost always hysterical, and may be associated with spasm of accommodation. Defects and dissociation of conjugate ocular movements in the lateral and vertical planes may be produced by spasm of the ocular muscles, and a coarse nystagmus may occur. Hysterical ptosis is the result of spasm of the palpebral fibres of the orbicularis oculi, and when the lid is passively raised this spasm can be felt to increase. Blepharospasm is similarly produced.

Symptoms referred to the Alimentary Canal

Hysterical dysphagia may occur, but is rare. Air-swallowing is common and is usually begun by straining to bring up wind. It may lead to extreme gastric distension. Globus hystericus, described as a sensation of constriction or a lump in the throat, is probably also usually the result of air-swallowing and is a referred sensation produced by the presence of air in the lower part of the oesophagus. It must be distinguished from the similar sensation which can occur in some patients with hiatus hernia.

Hysterical vomiting when mild may lead to no loss of weight, when severe may cause marked acidosis and emaciation. It is usually symbolic of an intense aversion from some task or situation, of which the patient is literally, as well as metaphorically, sick.

Hysterical anorexia—'anorexia nervosa'—may arise as a primary hysterical reaction to the patient's difficulties, or may be secondary to other hysterical symptoms referred to the alimentary canal, and which the patient believes are exacerbated by taking food. It occurs in adolescent girls and young women, and may lead to extreme emaciation, and to amenorrhoea.

Hysterical diarrhoea and constipation may occur, and it is probable that many of the abdominal and pelvic symptoms which used to be attributed to visceroptosis are in part or entirely hysterical.

Cardiac Symptoms

Tachycardia and palpitation play a prominent part in the symptoms of neurotic anxiety. In hysteria, however, such symptoms may occur in a patient who is outwardly placid. The recognition of their nature is of great importance, lest sufferers from these symptoms should be confined to bed for long periods with a mistaken diagnosis of organic heart disease or thyrotoxicosis.

Respiratory Symptoms

Respiratory tics have already been described. Hysterical hyperpnoea is sometimes seen and usually follows a fright. It also occurs in some panic attacks of the phobic anxiety-depersonalization syndrome. I have known it produced by suggestion in a patient with congenital dextrocardia. The excessive ventilation of the lungs may lead to tetany and even to syncope. The hysterical nature of the symptom can usually be detected by the fact that the hyperpnoea disappears or is much diminished when the patient is engaged in conversation, whereas talking increases the dyspnoea due to organic disease.

Urinary Symptoms

Nocturnal enuresis in childhood is the perpetuation of, or a reversion to, the infantile lack of control over the bladder. Its motive is frequently a desire to attract attention, and the symptom tends to be maintained by punishment and by suggestions emanating from a household in which the lapse comes to be expected. Pathological polyuria and organic causes of enuresis, especially spina bifida occulta, must be excluded. Hysterical retention of urine usually occurs in young girls.

The Skin

'Dermatitis artefacta' is the term applied to cutaneous lesions voluntarily produced by a hysterical patient, either by scratching or rubbing, or by the use of external agents, including corrosives. These are usually easily recognized by their appearance and by the fact that they quickly heal when covered by an occlusive dressing. Pruritus is frequently a hysterical symptom. Cyanosis and oedema may occur in a limb which is the site of hysterical paralysis and has been described as a result of the purposive use of tight elastic bands applied to the limb by the hysterical patient.

The Spine

The spine may be the site of hysterical pain and tenderness, and occasionally remarkable deformities occur in hysteria, sometimes leading to an apparent shortening of several inches in the vertebral column.

Pyrexia

Probably in most cases of apparent pyrexia occurring in hysteria, the thermometer is manipulated by the patient. This source of error can readily be detected by adequate supervision when the temperature is taken. In certain cases, however, it appears that an actual rise of body temperature may occur as a hysterical symptom.

The 'von Munchausen Syndrome'

The 'desire to be ill' is classified by some authorities as a condition which shows some affinities with hysteria though it would appear that many of the affected individuals have psychopathic personalities. Not only may the patients feign illness by manipulation of clinical thermometers but some may actually produce illness in themselves by injecting themselves with insulin or with their own bath water. *E. coli* arthritis is invariably due to this cause. This type of phenomenon is almost always seen in nurses or doctors.

The 'von Munchausen syndrome' is a name given to a group of patients who move from hospital to hospital, cleverly feigning physical illness, including cardiac infarction, renal colic, perforated peptic ulcer or even cerebral vascular accidents. While some such individuals are addicted to morphine or pethidine and simply seek injections of the appropriate drugs and others seek nothing more than a bed for the night, others undertake these activities for complex psychological reasons related to the 'desire to be ill' (Mayer-Gross, Slater, and Roth, 1960).

Speech

Hysterical speech disturbances—mutism and aphonia—are described elsewhere.

DIAGNOSIS

The diagnosis of individual hysterical symptoms has already been considered. In general it may be said that the diagnosis of hysteria depends upon the presence of positive signs of hysteria already described in connexion with individual symptoms, and the absence of signs of organic disease. It is also essential, when possible, to identify a motive. It is essential in every case, therefore, that a thorough examination should be made both of the nervous system and of other systems to which symptoms may be referred. The organic nervous disease most likely to be confused with hysteria is multiple sclerosis, on account of the transitory occurrence in the early stages of this disorder of weakness and sensory disturbances. Careful examination of a patient with multiple sclerosis, however, will almost always reveal signs of organic disease of the nervous system, the commonest of which are pallor of the optic discs, nystagmus, diminution or absence of the abdominal reflexes, and extensor plantar responses.

The distinction between hysteria (subconscious motivation) and malingering (conscious motivation) may be a matter of considerable difficulty in individuals who are seeking compensation after injury or in others accused of criminal offences (who may feign amnesia) as the clinical manifestations of the two conditions are similar. Unfortunately we possess no definitive objective tests by means of which this distinction can be made (Miller, 1966).

PROGNOSIS

The prognosis as to recovery from an individual symptom of hysteria is good in most cases, though relapses are frequent unless the patient can be induced to carry out a considerable psychological readjustment. Chronic cases are common in which a single symptom persists for years, often because it is the patient's reaction to a domestic situation which also persists unchanged. Victims of chronic hysteria are often persons in whom the expectation of compensation for an injury or the receipt of a pension puts a premium upon the persistence of their disability.

TREATMENT

General Considerations

When a hysterical symptom is a neurotic solution of a mental conflict, symptomatic treatment alone is inadequate. It is essential that the cause of the conflict should be discovered and that the patient should be induced to deal with it in a manner which does not involve resort to a neurosis. Analytical psychological methods, however, are often rendered difficult by lack of intelligence or by resistance in the patient, and in severely dissociated individuals with amnesia, hypnosis or narco-analysis may be necessary to recover forgotten episodes. When the cause of the symptom has been discovered and dealt with, treatment may also be directed towards the relief of the symptom itself. A careful physical examination must be made in order that the patient may be assured that no organic cause for the disability exists, but that it is due to a faulty mental habit. The patient must be convinced that he can overcome the disability, but care should be taken to avoid the suggestion that this requires a great effort of will, since this attitude implies that the achievement is difficult. In some cases recovery is best effected by a gradual process of persuasion and re-education extending over a considerable time. Some, however, prefer to attempt to remove the symptom at one sitting. This method requires great tact and patience on the part of the physician and is not without risk, since the failure of a protracted attempt to cure will only reinforce the patient's belief in the intractable nature of his disorder. The removal of a symptom by hypnotic suggestion is usually undesirable in adult patients, since it tends to strengthen the abnormal suggestibility which is an undesirable characteristic of the hysteric. This method, however, is admissible in dealing with children, in whose education suggestion plays a legitimate part.

Treatment of Individual Symptoms

Hysterical 'Fits'. A hysterical attack can usually be quickly terminated by firm handling, especially if the patient is isolated from a sympathetic audience.

Paralysis and Rigidity. These symptoms are commonly associated, and, since they depend in part upon involuntary muscular contraction, this should be explained to the patient, who should first be directed to relax the muscles of the affected region and should be told that when the muscles are relaxed movement will be easy. Electrical stimulation may be employed to demonstrate that the muscles are still capable of contraction, the patient then being made to imitate the movements excited electrically.

Abasia. Abasia is a symptom which lends itself to cure at a single treatment. The patient is first encouraged to walk with adequate support, the doctor walking on one side. The support is gradually diminished until the patient can be told that he is now walking alone, and finally he should be induced to run.

Enuresis. Before regarding enuresis in childhood as a neurosis it is necessary to exclude irritative lesions of the urinary tract, polyuria, and organic lesions which impair sphincter control, especially spinal dysraphic syndromes associated with spina bifida occulta. An attempt should be made to ascertain the cause of the symptom, which may be the symbol of a wish to remain infantile or express a desire to attract attention. Both the parents and the patient should be encouraged to expect a cure, and neither blame nor punishment for lapses should be permitted. Propantheline or ephedrine in full doses given before retiring may be used to depress reflex evacuation of the bladder until the habit of continence is established. Hypnotic suggestion or various deconditioning techniques will often bring about a cure in hitherto intractable cases.

Vomiting. The psychological cause of the vomiting must first be ascertained and discussed with the patient, who must be reassured that no organic cause for it exists. Special diets, alkalies, and nutrient enemas may often have been employed in treatment. These and the apparatus connected with them should all be removed from the room. An ordinary light meal should then be obtained and the patient persuaded to consume it with the assurance that no vomiting will follow. An attempt should always be made to cure hysterical vomiting at one sitting, a cure once effected usually being permanent.

Anorexia Nervosa. The patient should be isolated from relatives and friends and the cause of the anorexia ascertained. It is often necessary to explain that the symptoms which the patient attributes to taking food are really the result of taking too little. A beginning should be made with frequent small feeds, and no effort should be spared to make the diet attractive. An acid mixture will often relieve flatulence and improve appetite, and it is usually necessary to treat constipation. In severe cases treatment with insulin, tube-feeding, or even leucotomy may be called for. Chlorpromazine in increasing doses has been found to be helpful in some cases but for details the reader is referred to textbooks of psychiatry.

OCCUPATIONAL NEUROSIS

Synonyms. Craft palsy; occupational cramp.

Definition. A functional nervous disorder prone to afflict those whose occupation entails the persistent use of finely co-ordinated movements, especially of the hand, and characterized by a progressive occupational disability, due to spasm of the muscles employed, which are often the site of pain and sometimes of tremor.

AETIOLOGY

Occupational neurosis has been attributed to fatigue of cortical ganglion cells and has also been regarded as a disorder of the basal ganglia. It seems more probable, however, that it is primarily psychogenic, but irreversible abnormal cortical motor dispositions may in time become established. We know of no organic disorder in which the movements are impaired when they take part in one co-ordinated act but remain unaffected in others. The muscular spasm evoked by an attempt to carry out the act involves both prime movers and their antagonists, and thus resembles the disorder of function which occurs in hysterical paralysis. The disability in occupational neurosis may be influenced by external factors in a manner which seems inexplicable if it is due to an organic disorder. For example, a solicitor who suffered from severe writers' cramp was almost totally unable to write when sitting, but could write quite well when standing. Occupational neurosis, moreover, may be associated with typical hysterical symptoms, and investigation may elicit an adequate psychological cause. Thus a woman who developed writers' cramp after an unhappy marriage suffered also from vaginismus. Finally, in some cases, occupational neurosis is curable by psychotherapy. It thus presents many points of resemblance to stammering, another functional disorder of finely co-ordinated movements; indeed, occupational neurosis may be described as a manual stammer. It must be admitted, however, that sufferers from occupational neurosis may possess a physiological predisposition which determines the character of their neurosis, as, for example, left-handedness appears to predispose to stammering.

Fatigue and the effort to carry out accurate work against time are important precipitating factors, and since in most cases the sufferer's livelihood depends upon his speed and accuracy, an impairment of his efficiency evokes anxiety, which probably plays a part in the psychogenesis of the disorder. Numerous occupational neuroses have been described, writers', telegraphists', gold-beaters', violinists', and piano-players' cramps being the most familiar, but there is probably no occupation involving the repetition of fine movements which is immune. Both sexes are affected, but males more often than females.

SYMPTOMS

The symptoms of writers' cramp will alone be described, since the disorder is essentially the same in other occupations. The onset of symptoms is gradual, and the disorder shows itself at first only when the patient is fatigued, when a difficulty in controlling the pen leads to inaccurate writing. When the condition is well developed the attempt to write evokes a spasm of the muscles concerned in holding and moving the pen, and this may spread to the whole of the upper limb. The whole limb may thus become rigid, so that the act is brought to an abrupt stop. More usually the attempt to write leads to jerky and inco-ordinate movements of the fingers, so that the writing is completely illegible. The pen may be driven into the paper. In some cases a tremor of the hand develops. No two patients present precisely the same disorder of function. An attempt is often made to circumvent the disability by various tricks and unusual methods of holding the pen. Extension of the muscular spasm beyond the upper limb is rare. Sensory symptoms are common and are the result of the muscular spasm, the patient complaining of a sense of fatigue or an aching pain in the muscles, not only of the upper limb but sometimes also of the neck. Muscular wasting, sensory loss, and reflex changes are absent. In the early stages the disability is limited to the single act in which it originates. Later it may extend to other acts which are carried out by the same hand. Thus the woman already mentioned, after developing writers' cramp, learned to use a typewriter. Her disability then extended to typing and finally to the use of a paint-brush in water-colour sketching. The sufferer from writers' cramp who learns to write with the left hand may develop the same disorder in this.

DIAGNOSIS

Occupational neurosis must be distinguished from organic disorders of the nervous system which may lead to a difficulty in carrying out fine movements. A careful history and physical examination usually render the diagnosis easy, since in such cases signs of organic disease are always present and the disability usually involves all finely co-ordinated acts, and not writing alone, to an equal extent from the beginning.

PROGNOSIS

The prognosis of occupational neurosis is usually bad, since in many cases the disability is progressive, though recovery may occur and some patients may be able to continue their occupation in spite of their disorder.

TREATMENT

Prolonged rest from the occupation is essential if practicable, and the period of rest should be occupied by psychological investigation and appropriate psychological treatment. The way in which muscular spasm interferes with the act should be explained to the patient, and he should be taught muscular relaxation under skilled supervision. This should later be combined with re-educational exercises for the affected limb, and return to work should be gradual, fatigue being avoided. Learning to write with the other hand, or using a typewriter may be helpful, but not infrequently the second hand, and even the movements involved in typewriting, may later be affected. Liversedge and Sylvester (1955) have devised a method of 'deconditioning' the patient. Some patients obtain benefit from the use of drugs such as chlordiazepoxide (*Librium*), 10 mg. three or four times a day, or diazepam (*Valium*), 2–5 mg. three or four times daily, but while these may partially relieve muscular spasms they are in no sense curative.

REFERENCES

EYSENCK, H. J. (1960) *Handbook of Abnormal Psychology*, London.
KRETSCHMER, E. (1952) *A Textbook of Medical Psychology*, trans. STRAUSS, E. B., 2nd ed., London.
LIVERSEDGE, L. R., and SYLVESTER, J. D., (1955) Conditioning techniques in the treatment of writer's cramp. *Lancet*, i, 1147.
MAYER-GROSS, W., SLATER, E., and ROTH, M. (1960) *Clinical Psychiatry*, 2nd ed., London.
MILLER, H. (1966) Mental sequelae of head injury, *Proc. roy. Soc. Med.*, **59**, 257.
SIM, M. (1968) *Guide to Psychiatry*, 2nd ed., Edinburgh.
SLATER, E. (1965) Diagnosis of 'hysteria', *Brit. med. J.*, **1**, 1395.

INDEX

PRINTED IN GREAT BRITAIN
AT THE UNIVERSITY PRESS, OXFORD
BY VIVIAN RIDLER
PRINTER TO THE UNIVERSITY